# Myeloma

## BIOLOGY AND MANAGEMENT

# *Myeloma*

## BIOLOGY AND MANAGEMENT

## THIRD EDITION

### James S. Malpas, MD, DPhil, FRCP, FRCPCH
Professor of Medicine, Emeritus
London University
ICRF Department of Medical Oncology
St. Bartholomew's Hospital
London, United Kingdom

### Daniel E. Bergsagel, CM, MD, DPhil
Professor of Medicine, Emeritus
University of Toronto
Ontario Cancer Institute
Toronto, Ontario, Canada

### Robert A. Kyle, MD
Professor of Medicine,
Laboratory Medicine, and Pathology
Mayo Clinic College of Medicine
Mayo Clinic
Rochester, Minnesota

### Kenneth C. Anderson, MD
Kraft Family Professor of Medicine
Harvard Medical School
Chief, Division of Hematologic Neoplasia
Director, Jerome Lipper Multiple Myeloma Center
Dana-Farber Cancer Institute
Boston, Massachusetts

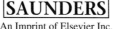

An Imprint of Elsevier Inc.

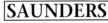

An Imprint of Elsevier Inc.

The Curtis Center
Independence Square West
Philadelphia, Pennsylvania 19106

Second edition © Oxford University Press 1998, First edition © Oxford University Press 1995

**Library of Congress Cataloging-in-Publication Data**

Myeloma : biology and management / [edited by] James S. Malpas ... [et al.] — 3rd ed.
   p. ; cm
   Includes bibliographical references and index.
   ISBN 0-7216-0006-9
   1. Multiple myeloma. I. Malpas, J. S.
   [DNLM: 1. Multiple Myeloma—complications. 2. Multiple Myeloma—diagnosis.
    3. Multiple Myeloma—therapy. WH 540 M9965 2004]
   RC280.B6M94 2004
   616.99'471—dc21                                      2003054299

*Acquisitions Editor:*   Dolores Meloni
*Publishing Services Manager:*   Joan Sinclair
*Project Manager:*   Mary Stermel

Printed in the United States

Last digit is the print number:   9   8   7   6   5   4   3   2   1

To our wives:
Joyce, Joyce, Charlene, and Cynthia

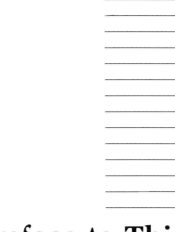

# Preface to Third Edition

Interest in multiple myeloma has shown such an increase and knowledge of its pathology has grown so rapidly that we feel no apology is required for a third edition of this book. It has also been most encouraging to see the introduction of many new drugs, but this has increased the complexities of management. We are fortunate to have a number of new contributors who we hope will help guide the reader through these advances.

We appreciate the efforts of the staff of our new publisher who have helped bring about the publication of this book.

*London*                                                                       J.S.M.
*Toronto*                                                                      D.E.B.
*Rochester*                                                                  R.A.K.
*Boston*                                                                       K.C.A.
November 2003

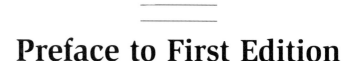

# Preface to First Edition

In a conversation with Professor Tim McElwain in the late 1980s, we came to the conclusion that the time had arrived for a new book on myeloma. Sadly, Tim did not live to take part in the project. It is evident that there is now a renewed interest in the biology of the disease, new concepts with regard to its clinical evolution (which in some senses makes it a "role model" for cancer), and options for therapy that have not been available before. Myeloma has always involved many systems and caused many problems for the clinician. Recent discoveries in the field of renal disease, disorders of calcium metabolism and amyloid, for example, impinge on the management of the disease and are ripe for review.

Myeloma has become a focus of attention for the scientist and clinician. In the past co-operation produced a major advance in our knowledge of proteins and immunity. It is possible that similar co-operation will now help to shed light on the complexities of cytokines, among many other topics. We hope this book will help to promote this interest, and are grateful to the authors from Europe, the UK, Australia, Canada, and the United States who agreed to contribute.

*London*                                                                                 J.S.M.
*Toronto*                                                                                D.E.B.
*Rochester*                                                                            R.A.K.
July 1994

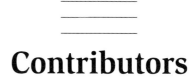

# Contributors

**Kenneth C. Anderson, MD**
Kraft Family Professor of Medicine
Harvard Medical School
Chief, Division of Hematologic
    Neoplasia
Director, Jerome Lipper Multiple
    Myeloma Center
Dana-Farber Cancer Institute
Boston, Mass.

**Dalsu Baris, MD, PhD**
Staff Scientist, Epidemiologist
National Cancer Institute
Bethesda, Md.

**James R. Berenson, MD**
Chief Executive Officer
Institute for Myeloma & Bone Cancer
    Research
Los Angeles, Calif.

**Daniel E. Bergsagel, CM, MD, DPhil**
Professor of Medicine, Emeritus
University of Toronto
Ontario Cancer Institute
Toronto, ON, Canada

**Karin Isgur Bergsagel, RN, BA**
Williamsburg, Va.

**P. Leif Bergsagel, MD**
Associate Professor of Medicine
Weill Medical College of Cornell
    University
Associate Attending Physician
New York Presbyterian Hospital
New York, N.Y.

**Joan Bladé, MD**
Hematology and Oncology
    Institute
Department of Hematology
Postgraduate School of
    Hematology
"Farreras Valentí"
Institut d' Investigacions
    Biomediques August Pi i Sunyer
    (IDIBAPS)
Hospital Clínic
Barcelona, Spain

**Jamie D. Cavenagh, MD**
Senior Lecturer in
    Haematology
Honorary Consultant, Department of
    Haematology
St. Bartholomew's and The Royal
    London School of Medicine and
    Dentistry
London, United Kingdom

**Dharminder Chauhan, PhD**
Principal Associate in
    Medicine
Department of Medicine
Harvard Medical School
Dana-Farber Cancer Institute
Boston, Mass.

**Selina Chen-Kiang, PhD**
Professor of Pathology, Microbiology,
    and Immunology
Weill Medical College of Cornell
    University
New York, N.Y.

**J. Anthony Child, MD**
Professor
Consultant: Clinical
  Haematologist
The General Infirmary at Leeds
Leeds, United Kingdom

**Faith E. Davies, MBBCh, MRCP, MD**
Department of Health Clinician
  Scientist
Academic Department of Haematology
  and Oncology
University of Leeds
Department of Haematology
Leeds General Infirmary
Leeds, United Kingdom

**Anneclaire J. De Roos, MPH, PhD**
Assistant Professor
University of Washington
Seattle, Wash.

**Meletios A. Dimopoulos, MD**
Professor
University of Athens School of
  Medicine
Alexandra Hospital
Department of Clinical
  Therapeutics
Athens, Greece

**Rafael Fonseca, MD**
Associate Professor of Medicine
  Consultant
Mayo Clinic College of
  Medicine
Rochester, Minn.

**Jeffrey Gawler, MD**
Neurology Department
Royal London Hospital
London, United Kingdom

**Philip R. Greipp, MD**
Professor of Laboratory Medicine
  and Medicine
Mayo Clinic College of
  Medicine
Consultant
Division of Hematology
Mayo Clinic
Rochester, Minn.

**Philip N. Hawkins, PhD, FRCP**
Professor of Medicine
Clinical Director, National
  Amyloidosis Centre
Centre for Amyloidosis and Acute
  Phase Proteins
Royal Free and University College
  Medical School
University College London
London, United Kingdom

**Lisa Herrinton, PhD**
Epidemiologist/Research Scientist
Kaiser Permanente Medical Care
  Program
Oakland, Calif.

**Teru Hideshima, MD, PhD**
Principal Associate in Medicine
Medical Oncology
Dana-Farber Cancer Institute
Harvard Medical School
Boston, Mass.

**D. E. Joshua, BSc., MB, BS, DPhil,
FRACP, FRCPA**
Clinical Professor in Medicine
University of Sydney
Head, Institute of
  Haematology
Royal Prince Alfred Hospital
Sydney, Australia

**Michael S. Katz, BS, MBA**
Vice President
International Myeloma
  Foundation
Los Angeles, Calif.

**W. Michael Kuehl, MD**
Senior Investigator and Chief
Molecular Pathogenesis of Myeloma
  Section
National Cancer Institute
Bethesda, Md.

**Robert A. Kyle, MD**
Professor of Medicine, Laboratory
  Medicine, and Pathology
Mayo Clinic College of Medicine
Mayo Clinic
Rochester, Minn.

**James S. Malpas, MD, DPhil, FRCP, FRCPCH**
Professor of Medicine, Emeritus
London University
ICRF Department of Medical Oncology
St. Bartholomew's Hospital
London, United Kingdom

**Lia A. Moulopoulos, MD**
Assistant Professor
University of Athens School of
    Medicine
Aretaieio Hospital
Department of Radiology
Athens, Greece

**S. Vincent Rajkumar, MD**
Associate Professor of Medicine
Mayo Clinic College of Medicine
Consultant
Division of Hematology
Mayo Clinic
Rochester, Minn.

**Paul G. Richardson, MD**
Assistant Professor of Medicine
Harvard Medical School
Attending Physician
Clinical Director
Jerome Lipper Myeloma Center
Division of Hematologic Oncology
Dana-Farber Cancer Institute
Boston, Mass.

**Jesus F. San Miguel, MD**
Professor of Hematology
University of Salamanca
Head of Hematology
Hospital Universitario de Salamanca
Salamanca, Spain

**John D. Shaughnessy, Jr., PhD**
Associate Professor of Medicine
Director, Donna D. and
    Donald M. Lamberty Laboratory of
    Myeloma Genetics
Chief, Division of Basic Sciences
Myeloma Institute for Research and
    Therapy
University of Arkansas for Medical
    Sciences
Little Rock, Ark.

**David P. Steensma**
Assistant Professor of Medicine and
    Oncology
Mayo Clinic College of
    Medicine
Senior Associate Consultant
Division of Hematology
Department of Medicine
Mayo Clinic
Rochester, Minn.

**A. Keith Stewart, MB, CHB, FRCT(C)**
Associate Professor
University of Toronto
Toronto General Research
    Institute
Toronto, ON, Canada

**Dietlind L. Wahner-Roedler, MD**
Assistant Professor of Medicine
Mayo Clinic College of
    Medicine
Rochester, Minn.

**Noel S. Weiss, MD, DrPH**
Professor
University of Washington
Seattle, Wash.

# Contents

PART IV
*Other Disorders Associated with*
*Paraproteinemia* . . . . . . . . . . . . . . . . . . . . . . . . . . . . . . . . . . **313**

# PART I

*Pathophysiology*

# CHAPTER 1

# Immunoglobulins

## D. E. JOSHUA

## Introduction

In 1937, Tiselius separated serum globulins by electrophoresis into three components, which he termed alpha, beta, and gamma globulins. The gamma globulins of normal human serum are composed of five different globulins, which were termed "immunoglobulin" by Heremans (1959). The five immunoglobulins are designated IgG, IgA, IgM, IgD, and IgE. Immunoglobulins are present in all higher vertebrates and constitute the humoral arm of a sophisticated adaptive immune system. They consist of a heterogeneous group of molecules whose structural features enable them to bind firmly to a spectrum of foreign antigens. Despite the fact that the term "immunoglobulin" was only introduced in 1959, their property of antigen recognition was in fact recognized by Tiselius who demonstrated the association between antigen binding activity and the gamma globulin fraction of serum.

### Structure

The immunoglobulin molecule consists of two heavy chains and two light chains, each divided into classes designated by Greek lower case letters. There are five heavy chains designated $\mu$, $\delta$, $\gamma$, $\alpha$, and $\varepsilon$ and two light chains, $\kappa$ and $\lambda$. Only one heavy chain and only one light chain are present in any given immunoglobulin molecule, and the name is taken from the combination of the heavy and light chain designations. The five immunoglobulin molecules and their properties are listed in Table 1-1 and their structure in Figure 1-1.

## TABLE 1-1

### Properties of the Five Major Immunoglobulin Molecules

| Properties | IgG | IgA | IgM | IgD | IgE |
|---|---|---|---|---|---|
| Molecular weight ($H_2I_2$) | 150,000 | 170,000 | 900,000 | 180,000 | 196,000 |
| Subclass | 4(IgG 1-4) | 2(IgA 1-2) | None | None | None |
| Light chain isotype | κ & λ | κ & λ | κ & λ | κ & λ | κ & λ |
| Sedimentation coefficient | 6.7S | 7-15S | 19S | 7.0S | 8.05 |
| Half-life | 21 days* | 5.8 days | 5.1 days | 2.8 days | 2.3 days |
| Daily synthetic rate (mg/kg) | 33 | 24 | 6.7 | 0.4 | 0.02 |
| Complement fixation | IgG, IgG3 | Alternate pathway | Yes | Yes | Yes |
| Placental transfer | Yes | No | No | No | No |

* Subclass IgG3 has a half-life of 7 days.

The heavy chain has approximately 440 to 450 amino acid residues and the light chains have 210 to 220. Amino acid sequencing of a large number of immunoglobulin chains has shown that approximately 110 residues at the amino terminal ends of each light and heavy chain constitute a region where the amino acid sequences differ considerably. This is the variable or "V" region and is the site that determines the "idiotype" or unique antigen binding ability of the antibody. However, not every variable residue is equally involved in the process of antigen binding, and three subregions stand out as being "hypervariable." The hypervariable regions of light and heavy chains are the regions specifically responsible for the binding of the antigen for that individual immunoglobulin molecule. The remainder of the molecule, which is not involved in antigen recognition, is termed the "constant region" and is identical to other immunoglobulin molecules of the same class, subclass, and allotype (Stewart and Schwartz, 1994; Virella and Wang, 1993).

The region between the antigen binding part of the immunoglobulin and the constant part is the hinge region. The length of the hinge region varies between the immunoglobulin classes and subclasses. The heavy chains are linked by interchain disulphide bridges varying between 2 ($IgG_1$) and 5 ($IgG_3$). The light chain is joined to the heavy chain by one disulphide bridge. The number of interchain heavy chain disulphide bridges in each subclass is listed in Table 1-2.

Two intrachain disulphide bridges are found in light chains and four such bridges are found in heavy chains. Each bridge encloses a peptide loop of 60 to 70 amino acids residues, and there is a high degree of sequence homology between sections of peptide chains contained within the disulphide-bridged loops.

These regions are indicated by a specific name, the so-called "homology" regions. For example, there are three "homology regions" in the constant part of the γ chain designated $C\gamma^1$, $C\gamma^2$, $C\gamma^3$. Each homology region is folded in a compact globular structure or domain.

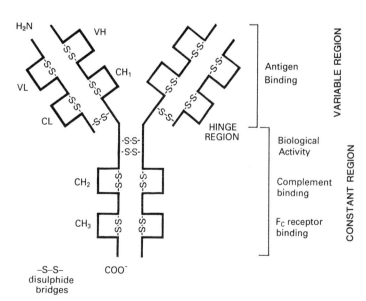

**Figure 1-1** *Structure of the normal immunoglobulin molecule. Heavy and light chains are bonded together by interchain disulphide bridges. The intrachain disulphide bridges enclose the four domains (VH, CH1, CH2, CH3) of the heavy chains and the two domains of the light chains. The antigen-binding region is at the amino terminal portion of the heavy and light chains and the hypervariable region consists of three portions of the terminal part of that region. The constant-region is responsible for biologic activity, complement binding, and Fc receptive binding.*

=== **TABLE 1-2** ===

### Immunoglobulins and Number of Disulphide Bridges

| Immunoglobulin Subclass | Disulphide Bridges |
|---|---|
| $IgG_1$ | 2 |
| $IgG_2$ | 4 |
| $IgG_3$ | 5 |
| $IgG_4$ | 2 |
| $IgA_1$ | 1 |
| $IgA_2$ $A_2m'$ | 0 |
| IgM | 1 |
| IgD | 1 |
| IgE | 2 |

Each domain is believed to play a particular biologic role. Macrophage binding is a function of the $C\gamma_3$ region and complement binding a function of the $C\gamma_2$ region. In the $\gamma$ heavy chain the amino terminal homology region is called the $V_H$ region.

There are four subclasses of IgG heavy chains and two of IgA. The half-life of one of the IgG subclasses, $IgG_3$, is shorter than the other three subclasses (7 vs. 21 days), whereas the half-life of the two IgA subclasses is identical.

IgM and IgA have the propensity to form polymers; indeed, IgM normally exists as a pentameric structure of molecular weight 900,000 daltons (d). IgA polymers have sedimentation coefficients of 7S to 15S. Dimers often form and the concentration of IgA polymers has been found to correlate with serum viscosity (Chandy et al., 1981).

## Normal Immunoglobulin Levels

The normal adult serum concentration of IgG is 6.5 to 15.0 g/L, IgA is 0.6 to 4.0 g/L, and IgM 0.5 to 3.2 g/L. The production of all immunoglobulin classes does not reach adult levels until after the first decade.

Because maternal IgG crosses the placenta, neonatal levels of IgG are within the normal adult range but rapidly fall to reach their nadir at 4 to 6 months according to the half-life of IgG and the onset of endogenous synthesis. The normal and age-related range of immunoglobulin levels is shown in Table 1-3.

### Light Chains

The two distinct light chain varieties ($\kappa$ and $\lambda$) were described in 1956 by Korngold and Lipari. Two-thirds of serum light chains are $\kappa$ and one-third $\lambda$. Light chains have a molecular weight of 22,000 d and contain 210 to 220 amino acids. Like heavy chains, they contain a constant and variable region. The variable region extends from the amino terminal for approximately 110 amino acids and is responsible for the unique thermal solubility and antigen binding properties.

Measurement of free $\kappa$ and $\lambda$ light chains in serum by enzyme-linked immunoassay (Nelson et al., 1992) has demonstrated the normal range for free $\kappa$ to be 1.6 to 15.2 mg/L and free $\lambda$ to be 0.4 to 4.2 mg/L. Recent measurements using a highly specific immunoassay for free light chains suggested a mean free $\kappa$ concentration pf 13.7 mg/L (95% confidence interval [CI], 7.0–22.6 mg/L) and a mean free $\lambda$ of 18.6 mg/L (95% CI, 9.9–34.4 mg/L), producing a mean $\kappa/\lambda$ ratio of 0.77 (Drayson et al., 2001; Bradwell et al., 2001).

There are three known human allotypes for $\kappa$ chains: termed Km(1), Km(2), and Km(3). There are no known allotypic markers for $\lambda$ chains.

The *de novo* synthesis of $\kappa$ and $\lambda$ chains is by plasma cells and is in slight excess. These chains can play a role in immunoregulation of the immune response (Joshua, 1991). Light chains are catabolized by the kidney (Wochner et al., 1967). The nephrotoxic properties of light chains are not clearly understood. Clyne et al. postulated that nephrotoxicity is related to the isoelectric point (Clyne et al., 1979) with cationic light chains being more nephrotoxic than anionic chains

=== **TABLE 1-3** ===

### Age-Related Ranges of Immunoglobulin Levels

| Age | IgG (g/L) | IgA (g/L) | IgM (g/L) | IgE* (mg/L) |
|---|---|---|---|---|
| Neonates | 6.5–150 | <0.06 | 0.11–0.35 | — |
| 6 mo | 1.98–8.6 | 0.1–0.96 | 0.25–1.20 | 0–0.02 |
| 1–2 y | 3.5–11.8 | 0.36–1.65 | 0.72–1.60 | 0–0.025 |
| 2–3 y | 5.0–13.6 | 0.45–1.35 | 0.46–1.90 | 0–0.035 |
| 3–4 y | 5.4–14.4 | 0.52–2.10 | 0.52–2.00 | 0–0.035 |
| 4–7 y | 5.7–13.2 | 0.65–2.40 | 0.60–1.75 | 0–0.07 |
| 7–10 y | 7.3–13.5 | 0.7–2.22 | 0.80–1.50 | 0–0.18 |
| Adults | 6.5–15.0 | 0.6–4.0 | 0.5–3.2 | 0–0.2 |

*IgE values from the Department of Immunology, Royal Prince Alfred Hospital.

(Melcion et al., 1984; McIntyre et al., 1988). To investigate the nephrotoxic potential of Bence Jones proteins, Solomon et al. (1991) injected mice intraperitoneally with purified Bence Jones protein from 40 patients with myeloma, and studied the renal pathology both in the mice and, in some cases, the corresponding human kidney biopsy material. This investigation found the nephrotoxic properties of the Bence Jones protein unrelated to isoelectric point, molecular weight, and light chain isotype. Similar studies by Johns et al. (1986) came to the same conclusions. Light chains, however, appear to be inhibitors of phosphate and glucose transport in proximal tubular cells (Batuman et al., 1994), but the specific features responsible for the nephrotoxicity remain unknown.

High-resolution two-dimensional electrophoresis has demonstrated patient-specific microheterogeneity in monoclonal light chains. In patients with myeloma, up to six isoforms of light chains can be seen. Most patients have at least two isoforms. Light chain isoforms are the result of both charge and mass differences and have been attributed to post-translation glycosylation and/or deamination. Other investigators have suggested abnormal truncated proteins could be the cause of the two-dimensional microheterogeneity (Goldfarb, 1992). There is no correlation between the heavy and light chain microheterogeneity patterns (Harrison, 1992).

## Proteolytic Cleavage of Immunoglobulins

Treatment of immunoglobulins with proteolytic enzymes produces well-defined fragments. Papain splits IgG into three fragments. Two are identical and are known as the fragments (Fab); they are composed of the variable region of the heavy chain and the complete light chains, and thus possess the antigen-binding site. Fab fragments have a molecular weight of 52,000 d. The other fragment (Fc) cannot combine with antigen but possesses other important biologically active sites such as complement fixation, binding of receptors for macrophages, and catabolic regulation.

In contrast, pepsin hydrolysis releases an F(ab′)$_2$ fragment that possesses both the antigen binding sites of the parent molecule and is incapable of complement fixation. The lack of Fc antibody binding and immunologic determinants has led to the use of F(ab′)$_2$ fragments for diagnostic clinical testing. The fragments produced by proteolytic cleavage are illustrated in Figure 1-2.

## Immunoglobulin Allotypes

GM factors are allotypic markers present on IgG heavy chains. Rheumatoid factors (RF) are a diverse group of antibodies with specificity for determinants

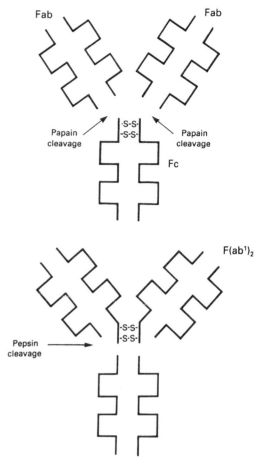

**Figure 1-2** *The result of proteolytic cleavage of the immunoglobulin molecule. Papain splits the molecule providing two identical Fab fragments and one Fc fragment. Pepsin on the other hand splits off an F(ab¹)$_2$ fragment, which contains both antigen-combining sites of the molecule.*

on the Fc region of IgG. GM factors often behave as antigens in RF reactions and were initially described using anti-GM antibodies from patients with rheumatoid arthritis. The first GM marker described as G1m(a) is localized exclusively on IgG$_1$ molecules and has been studied in Caucasians (it is present in 100% of non-Caucasian populations). It is inherited in an autosomal codominant fashion (Gaarder and Natvig, 1970; Grubb, 1956) and is thus expressed in heterozygotes. In total, four allotypes have been recognized: G1m(z), (a), (x), and (f). G1m(z) and (f) are mutually exclusive and cannot be coexpressed on the same chain. G1m(f) is predominantly Caucasian and G1m(fa) is typically Asian. G2m(n) is the only known allotype of IgG$_2$ chains. It is absent in African-Americans but common in Europeans and Asians and is also present in Australian aborigines (De Lange, 1991).

At present two allotypes of the IgA$_2$ subclass have been described, and it appears to be a two-allelic system. The frequency of the allele A$_2$m$^1$ and A$_2$m$^2$

varies considerably in different races, the $A_2m^2$ allele being very rare in Caucasians.

Only one IgE allotype has been discovered, Em(1) (Van Loghem et al., 1984). It is very common in all races and difficult to type.

Kappa allotypes are termed Km and occur in all classes of immunoglobulin. The genes involved are inherited as autosomal-dominant genes and are independent of the GM locus (Ropartz et al., 1961; Vyas and Fudenberg, 1969). The presence of Km allotypes is dependent on the amino acids 153 and 191 of the κ chain with variations of valine or alanine at position 153 and leucine or valine at 191 giving rise to the three known alleles (De Lange, 1991).

## Nomenclature

1. **Idiotype.** This refers to the unique antigen-binding site comprising the variable region of the heavy and light chain. Different antibodies may share idiotypic determinants (known as cross reactivity). Both heavy and light chains are involved in antigen binding. The interaction between antigen and antibody is due to noncovalent bonding.

2. **Isotype.** Antigenic determinants present on all molecules of a certain class or subclass, e.g., IgG, IgA, κ and λ. Isotypes are monomorphic determinants, they are present in all normal individuals. They are located on the constant part of the immunoglobulin molecule.

3. **Allotypes.** Genetically determined antigenic markers on human immunoglobulins, e.g., GM antigens. These are found on the constant part of the molecule and are autosomally dominantly inherited. Most allotypes have originated by mutations of only one or a few nucleotides resulting in differences of one or two amino acids.

4. **Subclass.** This refers to diversity of immunoglobulin molecules within a major group, for example (IgG$_{1-4}$). All subclass proteins share structural features common to the class.

## Properties of Individual Immunoglobulins

### IgG

Normal human IgG contains a mixture of all four IgG subclasses. IgG$_1$ and IgG$_3$ fix complement by the classic pathway, whereas IgG$_2$ and IgG$_4$ do not. Other varying properties of the IgG subclasses include the presence of the receptor for macrophages (IgG$_1$ and IgG$_3$) and the failure to react with staphylococcal A protein (IgG$_3$). IgG$_1$ antibodies are directed against isoagglutinins and viruses, whereas IgG$_2$ antibodies are directed against polysaccharides. IgG$_4$ antibodies are involved in the circulating anticoagulants against coagulation factors VIII and IX. All classes of IgG cross the placenta and are responsible for passive immunity in the newborn. IgG interacts with the Fc receptors on neutrophils, monocytes, and macrophages. With the exception of the IgG$_3$ subclass, IgG has a half-life of 21 days and is the only immunoglobulin exhibiting a concentration catabolic relationship. This is of relevance in patients with IgG myeloma in whom the high IgG levels result in more rapid catabolism. In contrast, the catabolism of IgA and IgM is independent of serum concentration (Waldmann and Strober, 1969). Owing to an extended hinge region, IgG$_3$ has the highest molecular weight of the four IgG subclasses (Michaelson et al., 1977). The distribution of IgG subclasses among the paraproteins in patients with myeloma or monoclonal gammopathies of undetermined significance (MGUS) does not differ from the normal serum distribution (Kyle and Gleich, 1982).

### IgM

The IgM molecule is a pentamer composed of five $H_2L_2$ subunits (Fig. 1-3). It is found in all vertebrate orders and fulfills several important biologic functions. IgM antibodies are the first to appear in the immune response and are very effective in the activation of complement by the classic pathway. Low molecular weight IgM occurs in normal serum at low concentrations. Its role is unknown but it appears to be synthesized *de novo* and is not a result of catabolism of the pentamer (Solomon and McLaughlin, 1970). IgM is the major protein found on the surface of B lymphocytes.

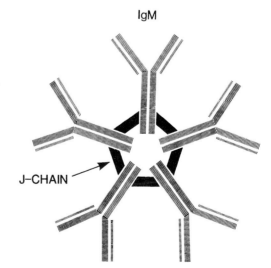

**IgM**

**J–CHAIN**

*Figure 1-3* IgM exist as a pentamer with five IgM immunoglobulin molecules joined by J chain.

Such membrane IgM is a monomer and has a carboxyl terminal hydrophobic segment that allows it to be anchored through the plasma membrane with a small cytoplasmic tail. IgM antibodies occurring naturally include cold agglutinins and ABO isoagglutinins.

### IgA

IgA accounts for approximately 20% of normal serum immunoglobulins. It is produced in areas adjacent to secretory surfaces. Most IgA is monomeric, although approximately 15% of serum IgA circulates as a dimer linked by a joining or J chain (Fig. 1-4). The J chain combines covalently with the H chain of IgA (and IgM) and is structurally unrelated to heavy and light immunoglobulin chains. It has a molecular weight of 15,000 d (Koshland, 1975). Secretory IgA differs from serum IgA in its association with a peptide chain called the secretory component (molecular weight 70,000 d). The role of secretory component is to increase the resistance of the IgA molecule to proteolytic digestion in secretions such as those in the digestive system.

Secretory IgA has a molecular weight of 380,000 d, and the complete molecule is a dimer of IgA together with a J chain and secretory component. Secretory IgA has antibacterial and antiviral activity and prevents microorganisms from penetrating mucosal surfaces (Decoteau, 1974). Aggregated IgA can fix complement by the alternate pathway. There are two subclasses of IgA: IgA$_1$ and IgA$_2$. Approximately 90% of serum IgA is IgA$_1$, but external secretions contain equal proportions of both subclasses. The incidence of IgA subclasses in myeloma reflects the serum distribution of IgA$_1$ and IgA$_2$, and the major source of serum IgA production is the bone marrow. Naturally occurring IgA is associated with Henoch-Schönlein purpura.

In a recent study, the isotypic and allotypic distribution of monoclonal IgA from patients with myeloma in France and Japan has been defined (Aucouturier et al., 1992). No significant difference could be found between French and Japanese patients with the exception of a higher evidence of A$_2$M(z) allotype in Japan. The IgA subclass IgA$_1$ accounted for over 90% of all monoclonal proteins in both groups.

### IgD

IgD was first described in a patient with myeloma (Rowe and Fahey, 1965). Its role in normal immune regulation is unclear. Although present in normal serum in very small amounts (less than 1% of total serum Ig), it is found on the surface of most B lymphocytes. The molecular weight of IgD is 180,000 d, and it is rapidly catabolized, having a half-life of 2.8 days. Ninety percent of normal serum IgD and IgD myeloma paraproteins are of λ light chain isotype. Surface IgD is usually found in association with IgM and, in this situation, both molecules have the same VH and VL regions (Tu et al., 1974; Vitella and Uhr, 1975).

### IgE

IgE is the reaginic antibody of man. Such antibodies mediate the wheal and flare reactions and are often present in highly allergic individuals. IgE is present on the surface of mast cells and basophils, and a variety of immune mediators, including histamine, are released on antibody-antigen interaction.

IgE has a molecular weight of 180,000 d, approximately 12% of which is carbohydrate. The serum level of IgE is low because of a very low synthetic rate and short intravascular half-life.

## Monoclonal Proteins

Monoclonal proteins result from the overproduction of immunoglobulin molecules by plasma cells and are the hallmark of multiple myeloma and related conditions. However, the presence of a monoclonal protein *per se* is not a marker of malignancy, and a number of benign conditions, such as collagen vascular disease, can be associated with monoclonal immunoglobulin production. In addition, monoclonal proteins can occur in the elderly, apparently without malignant potential (for example, MGUS or benign paraproteins). Several benign and other malignant lymphoproliferative neoplasms can be associated with monoclonal gammopathies.

Restricted immunoglobulin components, even to the extent of a single heavy and light chain, can be produced experimentally by immunization, especially with carbohydrate moieties (Krause, 1970). Balb/c mice, in particular, show a propensity to form large and uniform clones in response to immunization (Cerny et al., 1971), and this could be related to their propensity to form plasmacytomas after pristane injection. With the current availability of genetic markers (Alexander

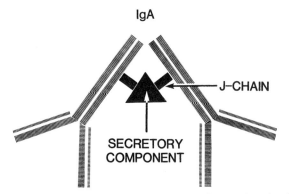

**IgA**

J–CHAIN

SECRETORY
COMPONENT

*Figure 1-4* IgA exists as a dimer consisting of two IgA molecules joined by a J chain and secretory component.

et al., 1985), it is clear that myeloma proteins are composed solely of an individual antibody and are the product of a single clone of plasma cells. This was suggested in the late 1960s by Kunkel (1968) and is supported by light chain restriction of all myeloma proteins. In most patients with myeloma, production of heavy chains is associated with excess secretion of light chains; these are excreted in the urine and are a significant cause of renal toxicity in myeloma. In approximately 20% of patients with myeloma no heavy chain is secreted, and only light chains are found in the serum. This is termed light chain myeloma.

The mechanism for the lack of production of heavy chains is not known. A few myeloma clones do not secrete heavy or light chains at all and are termed "nonsecretory myeloma." Recent studies involving both immunofluorescent and immunoperoxidase techniques demonstrate the presence of immunoglobulin in the plasma cells of most cases of "nonsecretory myeloma." The current availability of *in situ* hydridization with RNA probe for κ and λ mRNA demonstrates that the block in secretion is mostly posttranscriptional (Akhtar et al., 1989). Finally, the entity of heavy chain disease is characterized by cells that secrete an abnormal (usually truncated) heavy chain and usually fail to produce light chain (Frangione and Franklin, 1977).

# Immunoglobulin Gene Structure

Immunoglobulin genes consist of three groups (heavy chain, κ, and λ) encoded on three separate chromosomes (14, 2, and 22, respectively). Each group consists of a number of variable and constant-region gene segments, which are noncontiguous in the germline DNA. This section summarizes the principles of gene structure, gene rearrangements, the generation of antibody diversity, and affinity maturation of Ig molecules. Detailed reviews are available elsewhere (Alexander et al., 1985; Alt et al., 1992; Liebler et al., 1994; Tonegawa, 1983).

## κ Gene

In humans the κ gene is localized to chromosome 2 (Malcolm et al., 1982) and comprises three segments termed V, J, and C. The variable gene segments (Vκ) number approximately 70 in four Vκ families whose members are interspersed. They are located at the 5′ end of the gene complex, and the most proximal Vκ gene is 23 kb from the Jκ-Cκ complex.

The Vκ gene segments encode a promoter, a leader segment, and the first 95 amino acids of the V region of the light chain protein. The constant-region gene segment encodes the constant region amino acids, the termination codon, and a polyadenylation signal. Between the Vκ and Cκ regions are four Jκ segments,

which immediately precede the DNA of the constant region (Proudfoot and Brownlee, 1976). Up to 25 orphan Vκ genes have been located on other chromosomes (Zimmer et al., 1990).

## λ Gene

The λ gene locus is on chromosome 22 (Erickson et al., 1981). At least 40 human germline Vλ regions belonging to four families have been defined. The number of Cλ genes varies in different human racial groups, and three polymorphic forms of the λ locus have been described (Vasicek and Leder, 1990).

## Heavy Chain Genes

The genes coding for the human immunoglobulin heavy chains are located on chromosome 14 (Shander et al., 1980). The gene consists of variable genes (VH), diversity genes (DH), and joining (JH) genes followed by the constant (CH) gene of the appropriate heavy chain subclass. A number of pseudogenes have also been mapped using linkage disequilibrium studies (Bech-Hansen et al., 1983). Analysis of the structural repertoire of the human VH segments reveals approximately 100 to 150 groups of VH segments with different hypervariable loops of which 60 to 70 are functional and available for recombination. This is believed to account for the structural diversity of the germline repertoire for antigen binding (Stewart and Schwartz, 1994; Tomlinson et al., 1992).

The major difference between heavy and light chain immunoglobulin genes is the presence of diversity genes (D) 3′ to the V regions of the heavy chain genes (Siebenlist et al., 1981). Each D segment contains approximately 30 nucleotides and there are at least 30 D segments. The D locus comprises two clusters, major and minor, which are linked to the VH locus.

There is little restriction-site polymorphism in the D locus (Chastagner et al., 1992), and it is postulated that the conserved DH locus is related to its critical role in determining the function of the third complementarity-determining region. Close to the JH region is the switch region, a 3-kb stretch of DNA, which is involved in class switching and allows different heavy chain classes to be combined with the same V region.

Detailed studies involving the physical organization of the immunoglobulin heavy chain gene using two-dimensional DNA electrophoresis have been reported but are beyond the scope of this chapter (Walter et al., 1990).

## VH Families

The VH gene segments, coding for the first 95 amino acids of the heavy chain, have been subdivided into six families, VH 1–6, on the basis of regions of DNA homology.

Unlike the situation in the mouse, the individual human immunoglobulin VH genes are apparently interspersed. There are approximately 25 VH1, 5 VH2, 28 VH3, 14 VH4, 3 VH5, and 1 VH6 gene segments (Walter et al., 1990). It has been found that nonstochastic use of certain VH families occurs in a variety of conditions. For example, preferential use of the VH5 family has been reported in chronic lymphocytic leukemia (CLL) and acute lymphoblastic leukemia (ALL) (Humphries et al., 1988). Such non-stochastic use of VH families could account for the restricted immunoglobulin repertoire seen in CLL and could reflect an increase in "malignant potential" in certain heavy and light chain recombinations.

VH gene families have been shown to have a developmentally regulated pattern of use in B cells. Rearranged VH3 genes are rarely found in the germinal centre but are abundant in blood. Studies on individuals with HIV have shown failure of VH3 use suggesting a block of B-cell maturation at germinal center stage (Berberian et al., 1991). Low-affinity IgM antibody in the preimmune state is predominantly of the $VH_3$ subfamily, whereas high-affinity antibodies produced after immunization contain all families (Veki et al., 1990).

In myeloma there is conflicting evidence, with reports of nonpreferential use of VH5 (Clofent et al., 1989) and preferential non-stochastic use of the later VH families VH4 to VH6 (Rettig et al., 1996).

## Gene Rearrangements

The rearrangement of immunoglobulin genes during B cell development is sequential and ordered. Heavy chain genes undergo rearrangement before light chain genes, and κ gene rearrangement precedes λ (Blackwell and Alt, 1989; Ravetch et al., 1981).

In the initial steps of heavy chain gene rearrangement, D and J segments are joined, followed by V and DJ joining (Fig. 1-5). Complete VDJ rearrangements appear to only occur in B cells, but T cells appear to be able to carry out the preliminary steps of joining DJH.

The product of successful VDJ joining activates rearrangement of the κ locus. The mechanism of how B lineage cells sense that a rearranged locus is productive has recently been clarified with the discovery of two new genes in the mouse, the V preB and λ5. These genes encode proteins that associate with each other to form a light chain-like structure, the "surrogate" L chain. This can be bound covalently to the $D_H J_H C\mu$ protein and μ heavy chains, and is expressed on the surface of B lineage precursors only. The surrogate light chains disappear when mature B cells develop. This expression allows the variable regions of the heavy chain and the surrogate light chain to be exposed to the stroma cells, which are known to be required for the production of cytokines involved in B cell development. These cytokine signals can trigger the next round of immunoglobulin gene rearrangements (Melchers et al., 1993).

Light chain rearrangement commences with VJ joining. If this is successful, the rearrangement stops. However, if both κ alleles fail to produce a functional protein, then the λ genes rearrange. This is the principle of allelic exclusion or, in the case of κ and λ light chains, isotypic exclusion. The control mechanisms involved appear to differ in different species. A key feature involves recognition by the cell of productive rearrangements. Each of the immunoglobulin genes contains segments related to the regulation of expression. The heavy chain and κ genes carry segments that have the capacity to increase their rate of transcription (Queen and Baltimore, 1983; Rajewsky, 1996). VDJ recombinations are catalyzed by a series of enzymes coded for by the RAG genes on chromosome 11 (Oettinger et al., 1990). This common recombinase is used for T cell receptor variable region gene combination (Yancopoulos et al., 1986).

The Cμ heavy chain is first expressed during B cell differentiation followed by the δ chain. Class switching

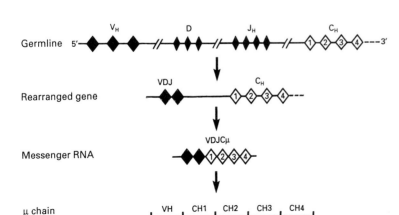

*Figure 1-5* DNA gene arrangements resulting in production of a heavy chain. The first DNA rearrangement results in a unique VD and J segment, which is joined to the CH segments in the second DNA rearrangement. This is transcribed into messenger RNA, followed by translation into the protein.

to an alternate heavy chain as the immune response proceeds is the result of the deletion of the unwanted heavy chain constant-region genes between the VH and the Cκ region. This is the result of a deletional recombination mechanism involving distinct switch-region segments in the JH-Cμ intron (Mountz et al., 1990).

T cells play an important role in regulating isotype switch. Cytokines secreted by T cells (e.g., interleukin-4 and γ-interferon) play crucial roles in regulating class switching, probably by selectively inducing transcription activation of the heavy chain class that is eventually used (Snapper and Mond, 1993). This process of VDJ rearrangement and class switching allows a single B cell clone to produce antibodies of the different heavy chain classes to the same antigenic epitope.

### Antibody Diversity

The generation of antibody diversity over and above that seen in the germline results from a specialized process called somatic hypermutation (Tonegawa, 1983). After interaction with antigen, somatic mutation of the immunoglobulin variable chain region is introduced by site-directed mutation processes and occurs in the germinal center phase of the immune response (MacLennan, 1991).

This mechanism leads to sequence heterogeneity in the third complementarity-determining region (CDRIII) of the assembled heavy chain variable region. This region encompasses the D region and the VHD and DJ junctions, and the resulting variation in the CDR III region is the basis of a precise PCR-based test of monoclonality of B cell tumours (Billadeau et al., 1991; Brisco et al., 1990; Yamada et al., 1989).

In myeloma, the immunoglobulin heavy chain genes contain somatic mutations characteristic of an antigen-driven process (Bakkus et al., 1992; Ralph et al., 1993).

Analysis of the immunoglobulin gene sequence of patients in varying stages of their disease has demonstrated that ongoing somatic mutation does not occur in myeloma. This is unlike the situation in B cell acute leukemia, which undergoes clonal evolution, or indolent follicular lymphoma, which undergoes continual somatic mutation (Bird et al., 1988; Meeker et al., 1985; Ralph et al., 1993). It has been suggested that the ongoing somatic mutation in follicular lymphoma is related to positive selection for altered antigen binding (Zelenetz et al., 1992).

It has recently been demonstrated that preclass switch immunoglobulin gene sequences can be detected in some patients with myeloma (Corradini et al., 1993) and although there is some controversy about the significance of the findings (Berenson et al., 1995), it raises the possibility of the clonogenic cell in myeloma being a preswitch B cell.

## Immunoglobulins: Members of a Family of Proteins

The number of proteins homologous to immunoglobulins is large; the term "immunoglobulin supergene family" is used for these proteins. This presumes a common genetic ancestry. Members of the immunoglobulin family include the α and β chains of the T cell receptor, the α chain of the MHC class I tissue antigens, β2 microglobulin, and N-CAM, which mediates adhesion of several cell types.

# Immunoglobulins: Laboratory Recognition and Measurement

Electrophoresis has made it possible to separate the proteins of serum into albumin, α, β, and γ globulins. The speed of different proteins during electrophoresis depends on their size and electrical charge at the pH of the buffer. Electrophoresis on cellulose acetate is useful for detecting the presence of a monoclonal protein; however, ultimate identification of the protein requires immunoelectrophoresis or immunofixation to distinguish the immunoglobulin heavy chain class and the light chain isotype. Serum and urine electrophoresis is most commonly performed at pH 8.6 with cellulose acetate or agarose gels (Jeppson et al., 1979).

High-resolution, two-dimensional polyacrylamide gel electrophoresis has been used to evaluate specimens in which standard immunofixation did not provide definitive analysis (Harrison et al., 1993; Tissot et al., 1993). These techniques are limited in their use and are largely replaced by molecular sequencing of immunoglobulin genes.

Quantitation of immunoglobulins is performed by radial immunodiffusion or automated-rate nephelometry, although the former is currently rarely used in routine laboratories.

### Electrophoresis

The indications for performing electrophoresis are multiple and include myeloma, macroglobulinemia, or amyloidosis, and numerous causes of benign paraproteinemia (MGUS). In addition, paraproteins are found in association with other diseases such as lichen myxoedematosis and peripheral neuropathies. Because paraproteins represent a homogeneous population of immunoglobulin molecules, they are identified as a characteristic narrow band or peak in the γ, β, and α$_2$ region of the electrophoresis tracing. An excess of polyclonal immunoglobulins shows as a broad-based band, which is usually restricted to the γ region. Serum is preferred to plasma as a source sample because fibrinogen forms a band in the β-γ region. Other factors

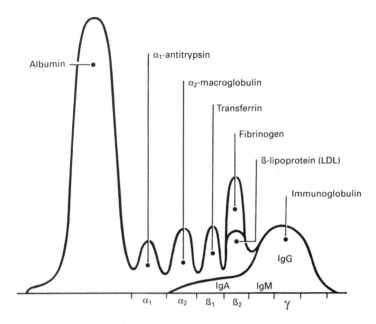

**Figure 1-6** *Schematic representation of the quantitatively dominating proteins of plasma separated by electrophoresis. Fibrinogen comprises the major portion of the γ region, and this is removed when serum is used. Immunoglobulins are present in the gamma region.*

might give restricted "bands." These include the hemoglobin-haptoglobin complex of hemolyzed serum, which forms a band between the $\alpha_2$ and $\beta$ region, whereas free hemoglobin forms a band in the $\beta$ region. Large quantities of transferrin in patients with iron deficiency can produce a band in the $\beta$ region.

The technical considerations for good-quality electrophoresis have been reviewed by Kohn (1976).

Isolated heavy chains can be missed on simple electrophoresis. In γ heavy chain disease, for example, a broad band in the β-γ regions might be all that is seen. Alternatively, hypogammaglobulinemia could be the only abnormality. Light chain disease, as well as IgD and IgE myeloma, either might not display a monoclonal peak or the peak produced might be so small as not to be evident visually. Distinct electrophoresis patterns are characteristic of several conditions: chronic liver disease, chronic infections, and HIV infection, for example, are associated with a large broad-based polyclonal hypergammaglobulinemia (Vega et al., 1990). In the nephrotic syndrome hypoalbuminemia is associated with relatively increased α and β globulins and often decreased γ globulins.

A diagrammatic representation of the dominant proteins of fresh human plasma is given in Figure 1-6;

Tables 1-4 and 1-5 outline the major components of the serum electrophoretic pattern and possible causes of pseudomonoclonal proteins, respectively.

## Immunoelectrophoresis

Immunoelectrophoresis is a suitable technique for the identification of a monoclonal protein but is not as sensitive as immunofixation, which has largely replaced it (Guinan et al., 1989). Monospecific antisera to IgG, IgA, IgM, IgD, IgE, κ, and λ light chains produce localized bowing when they react with the appropriate antigen of heavy and light chains (Graber and Williams, 1955). Polyclonal hypergammaglobulinemia can often produce an apparent localized bowing of the IgG heavy chain arc, but this is not associated with corresponding bowing of the κ or λ light chain arc.

Caution is necessary when interpreting immunoelectrophoresis data because soluble immune complexes do not precipitate and can lead to erroneous results. Neat serum and also a 1:5 (1:3–1:10) dilution should be used to avoid antigen excess and soluble complex formation. The detection of a light chain arc without a correspondingly heavy chain is representative of free light chain.

| | | TABLE 1-4 | | |
|---|---|---|---|---|
| | | Major Components of the Serum Electrophoretic Pattern | | |
| (+) Albumin | $\alpha^1$ Globulin | $\alpha^2$ Globulin | β Globulin | Globulin (−) α |
| Albumin | $\alpha^1$ Lipoprotein | $\alpha^2$ Macroglobulin | Haemopexin | Immunoglobulins |
| Pre-albumin | $\alpha^1$ Antitrypsin | Ceruloplasmin | Transferrin | |
| | Orosomucoid | Haptoglobin | β Lipoprotein | |

═══════ **TABLE 1-5** ═══════

Pseudomonoclonal Proteins

| Mobility of Pseudomonoclonal Spike | Possible Cause of Pseudomonoclonal Spike |
| --- | --- |
| Albumin | Bisalbuminaemia |
| $\alpha^2$ Globulin | $\alpha^2$ Macroglobulin |
| $\beta$ Globulin | Transferrin |
| $\beta$–$\gamma$ Globulin | Haemoglobin |
| | Fibrinogen (in plasma) |
| $\gamma$ Globulin | C reactive protein |
| | Muramidase |

This technique has largely been replaced by immunofixation, but immunoelectrophoresis still has a place in smaller routine laboratories, especially when assessing paraproteins of over 7g/L, which are rarely missed by the latter technique.

## Immunofixation

Immunofixation is the recommended method when investigating abnormal bands detected by electrophoresis or in patients with suspected B cell malignancies. The technique was originally described by Wilson (1964) and refined by Calper and Johnson (1969). It is easier to interpret than immunoelectrophoresis and more sensitive and useful when the results of immunoelectrophoresis are equivocal (Ritchie and Smith, 1976).

Immunofixation relies on a combination of protein electrophoresis on agarose and subsequent reaction of the separated proteins with monospecific antibodies, resulting in the deposition of insoluble immune complexes.

The washing step that follows fixation with the specific antiserum removes all protein with the exception of the insoluble immune complexes. These are then visualized with a protein stain and the presence of a monoclonal protein is demonstrated by a localized well-defined band.

A similar reaction to a single light chain ($\kappa$ or $\lambda$) with the same electrophoretic mobility will identify a monoclonal protein. A polyclonal protein population will give a diffuse band with anti-heavy chain immunoglobulin, but with no discrete bands and similar diffuse staining with both $\kappa$ and $\lambda$ chains.

Bence Jones protein is identified when there is reaction with light chain antiserum but no corresponding heavy chain reaction. Light chain bands might occasionally be seen in the serum, especially in cases of renal impairment (Solomon and Fahey, 1964) and will have the same mobility as the urinary Bence Jones protein.

The presence of Bence Jones protein only in the serum might indicate polymerization of Bence Jones

protein. $\lambda$ chains are especially prone to dimerization because of the availability of a penultimate cystine residue. Heavy chain disease proteins are identified by a reaction with heavy chain antisera, but no corresponding light chain reaction. Nevertheless, some heavy chain proteins have been reported with unreactive light chains and caution in interpretation is required. Biclonal gammopathies are best visualized by immunofixation.

The limitations of immunofixation require mention. The technique will be impaired if excess antigen (immunoglobulin) is applied to the gel. This often leads to fixing of the perimeter of the antigen band, while, in the central region, where the concentration of the antigen is highest, soluble antigen-antibody complexes form, which can then be washed away. Like in immunoelectrophoresis, dilution of the patient sample (1:3–1:10) should be performed to avoid this phenomenon.

In addition, some monoclonal proteins bind to the agarose gel mixture, which results in identical precipitin bands with all five antisera. The true reaction is often more intense, however, and can usually be identified.

Typing of immunoglobulins using abnormalities in $\kappa/\lambda$ ratios has been used to identify immunoglobulins. This method is not as sensitive as immunofixation and is rarely used in routine clinical testing (Guinan et al., 1989; Whicher et al., 1987).

Despite the fact that immunofixation is the most sensitive technique for detecting immunoglobulins, the clinical significance of small paraproteins might be doubtful in the general patient population. Multiple paraproteins of low concentration can be documented in "intensive care" hospitalized patients (Keshgegian, 1982); they are usually transient and the result of a restricted antibody response. Nevertheless, in patients with myeloma, especially those who receive high-dose therapies with or without stem-cell rescue, the importance of documenting the total disappearance of paraprotein to determine complete response requires the use of immunofixation as the most sensitive routine technique. Examples of immunofixation and electrophoresis patterns are illustrated in Figures 1-7, 1-8, and 1-9.

### Immunoisoelectric Focusing

Immunoisoelectric focusing (Sheehan et al., 1985; Sinclair et al., 1984, 1986) is one of the most sensitive means of detecting monoclonal immunoglobulins, but is not in general clinical use with the exception of testing for oligoclonal bands in cerebrospinal fluid for multiple sclerosis. It is 10 times more sensitive than immunoelectrophoresis, therefore enabling the detection of protein bands in cases of apparent nonsecretory myeloma and the confirmation of complete remission status after transplantation. However, molecular

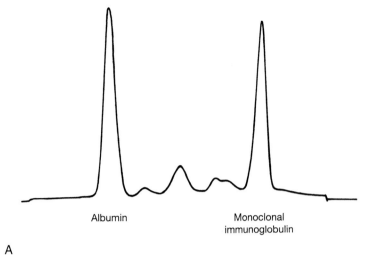

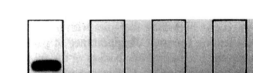

A

B

*Figure 1-7* A monoclonal spike identified by electrophoresis (*A*) identified as IgGκ by immunofixation. (*B*) Albumin migrates the fastest (most anodic) and immunoglobulin the slowest (most cathodic).

polymerase chain reaction (PCR)-based tests for minimal residual disease are more sensitive and have superseded the latter application.

## Quantitation of Immunoglobulins

There are a number of satisfactory methods for the quantitation of serum immunoglobulins; these are based on radial immunodiffusion and immunonephelometry and immunoturbidimetry.

## Nephelometry

Nephelometry is the method of choice for the quantitation of paraproteins (Markowitz and Tschida, 1972). Turbidity produced by the antigen-antibody interaction in liquid media is less affected by the inherent problems of diffusion. Rate nephelometry is superior to end-point nephelometry.

Under conditions of antibody excess, the reduction in light transmission is proportional to the original concentration of antigen (Ig) present in the solution.

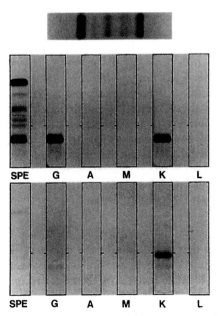

*Figure 1-8* Electrophoresis, serum, and urinary immunofixation of a patient with myeloma. The heavy band identified in electrophoresis is shown to be IgGκ and urinary-free κ (Bence Jones protein) is identified.

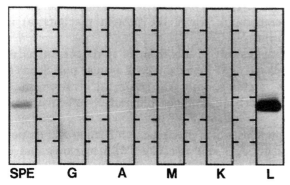

**SPE    G    A    M    K    L**

*Figure 1-9  Urinary immunofixation: demonstration of free λ light chains identified by immunofixation.*

Direct nephelometric assays are meant to function with the antibody present in excess. When quantitating monoclonal proteins, samples with large amounts of antigen must be diluted until the concentration of the protein being assayed falls within the range of the system. These conditions apply to all antigen-antibody assay systems. Nevertheless, with adequate precautions it is the most accurate method for the quantitation of monoclonal proteins (Bouzek and Mancol, 1989).

Radial immunodiffusion has been a widely used method for measuring immunoglobulins. Although suitable for normal immunoglobulins, it has significant inaccuracies when used to measure monoclonal proteins and this technique is not recommended.

## ELISA Techniques

A recently described technique uses magnetic beads as a solid phase in an ELISA method. This method has the advantage of brevity with short incubation reaction times. Similar assays for immunoglobulin subclasses have been described (Jimeno-Hagales et al., 1990; Ronning and Christophersen, 1991). In addition, a rapid protein A-based affinity chromatography technique has been described for analysis of IgG concentrations in solutions in which IgG is present in small amounts. This technique has a detection limit of 100 ng of IgG (Compton et al., 1989).

### Cryoglobulins

Cryoglobulins are proteins that precipitate in the cold and redissolve when heated. Most cryoglobulins are immunoglobulins and are usually classified as type I, II, or III depending on the immunofixation analysis of the cold-precipitated proteins (Brouet et al., 1974).

Type I cryoglobulins are monoclonal proteins (usually IgM or IgG). Type II cryoglobulins are the so-called "mixed cryoglobulins," which consist of two or more proteins with at least one being monoclonal.

In type III cryoglobulins, no monoclonal protein is found and the cold-sensitive proteins represent a polyclonal proliferation of immunoglobulins. Patients with monoclonal cryoglobulinemia might present with pain, Raynaud's phenomenon, and ulceration on cold exposure, but there is not a clear-cut relationship between the level of cryoglobulins and symptoms. The thermal amplitude (i.e., the range of temperature in which the protein precipitates) is probably more important than the quantity.

Mixed cryoglobulemia usually results from an IgM-IgG antibody-antigen immune complex with monoclonal IgM being directed against polyclonal IgG. The clinical presentation includes vasculitis with skin and renal involvement. The cryoproteins might result from an underlying lymphoproliferative, infective, or collagen vascular disease process.

Pyroglobulins are proteins that precipitate on heating and do not redissolve when cooled. They are usually IgG and associated with myeloma and other monoclonal proliferation. They are of limited clinical significance (Ivernizzi et al., 1973).

### Analysis of Immunoglobulins in Urine

The analysis of immunoglobulins in dilute body fluids such as cerebrospinal fluid and urine is of considerable importance in a number of clinical conditions.

The detection and quantitation of urinary light chains is an essential component in the diagnosis and monitoring of patients with myeloma. "Screening" tests for Bence Jones protein, while of historic interest, have little place in the modern laboratory where electrophoresis is required as an essential diagnostic evaluation procedure. Screening tests rely on the unusual thermal properties of Bence Jones protein. Most light chains in urine precipitate at 40 to 60°C, dissolve at 100°C, and reprecipitate on cooling. False-positive heat tests can be seen in renal and malignant disease and also in collagen vascular diseases.

Normal urine contains small amounts of protein and requires concentration (50 × or more) for electrophoresis. The normal nephron will exclude proteins of molecular weight greater than 100,000 d, but κ and λ light chains (22,000 d) are freely filtered. However, they are subsequently reabsorbed and metabolized by the renal tubular cells. Urinary excretion is therefore increased in either glomerular or tubular abnormalities as well as in conditions in which a high concentration of protein (e.g., myeloma) overwhelms the capacity of the renal tubule to metabolize the light chain.

A urinary monoclonal protein is most often seen as a dense, localized band on electrophoresis and is usually found in the γ region. A polyclonal increase is seen as a broad band within the γ region. In glomerular disease, nonspecific leakage of albumin, α-1-antitrypsin, and transferrin can occur. $\beta_2$ microglobulin, which runs in the mid-$\beta$ region, is present.

Immunofixation is more sensitive than immuno-electrophoresis of urine and is particularly of value for small paraproteins in the presence of glomerular damage or polyclonal increases in light chains. In heavy chain disease, heavy chain fragments in the urine can easily be detected. No evaluation of urine immuno-chemistry in myeloma is complete without a 24-hour collection and quantification. Quantification of urinary light chains is very important in the management of a patient with light chain myeloma; in patients with myeloma with an M protein, the appearance of new light chain fragments of different electrophoretic mobility can occur with progressive disease. Occasionally heavy chain secretion can be disassociated from light chain secretion in progressive disease states; this is known as light chain escape.

## Analysis of Immunoglobulin Heavy Chain Variants

Heavy chain disease is a lymphoproliferative disorder in which malignant cells secrete a monoclonal protein consisting of an abnormal heavy chain in the serum or urine but fail to secrete light chains.

### $\gamma$ Heavy Chain Variants

In $\gamma$ heavy chain disorders the $\gamma$ chain is a truncated protein, with deletions mainly in the Fc portion. Molecular weights range from 27,000 to 49,000 d.

The electrophoretic pattern in $\gamma$ heavy chain disease is variable, often just showing a broad-based increase in the $\gamma$ region or hypogammaglobulinemia. If a sharp band is seen it might occur in the $\beta$ and not the $\gamma$ region. The IgG subclass in $\gamma$ heavy chain disease reflects the proportion of those subclasses in normal sera, with the exception of IgG$_2$, which seems under-represented (Schur, 1972).

### $\mu$ Heavy Chain Proteins

The $\mu$ heavy chain disease proteins have molecular weights of up to 520,000 d. The proteins so far studied have shown deletion of the VH domain and occasionally the CH1 and CH2 domain (Bakhshi et al., 1986). The diagnosis depends on finding $\mu$ chain by immunofixation without a reaction with either $\kappa$ or $\lambda$ antisera (O'Reilly et al., 1981).

### $\alpha$ Heavy Chain Proteins

The molecular weights of $\alpha$ chain proteins are usually approximately 30,000 d. Internal deletions mostly involve the VH regions.

All the reported molecules are of the $\alpha_1$ subclass, and thus not representative of the normal distribution of the $\alpha_1$ and $\alpha_2$ classes (Mihaesco et al., 1971). Serum protein electrophoresis might not reveal any evidence of the abnormal protein or an abnormal broad band in the $\alpha_2$ or $\beta$ region related to polymer formation. No light chain synthesis has been identified. Caution, however, must be used in the interpretation of immunofixation patterns because occasionally the light chain of the intact IgA molecule might not react with light chain antisera, and a spurious diagnosis of $\alpha$ heavy chain disease can be made.

## REFERENCES

Akhtar, N., Ruprai, A., Pringle, J. H., Lauder, I., and Durrant, S. T. (1989). In situ hybridization detection of light chain MRNA in routine bone marrow trephines from patients with suspected myeloma. *British Journal of Haematology, 73,* 296–301.

Alexander, A., Rosen, S., and Buxbaum, J. (1985). Immunoglobulin genes in health and disease. *Clinical Immunology, 4,* 31.

Alt, F. W., Rosenberg, N., Casanova, R. J., Thomas, E., and Baltimore, D. (1982). Immunoglobulin heavy-chain expression and class switching in a murine leukaemia cell line. *Nature, 296,* 325–331.

Aucouturier, P., Musset, L., Itoh, Y., Ko, Y. C., Silvan, C., and Preud'homme, L. (1992). Isotypic and allotypic analysis with monoclonal antibodies and jacalin of serum monoclonal IgA from French and Japanese myeloma patients. *Immunology Letters, 32,* 31.

Bakhshi, A., Guglielmi, P., Coligan, J. E., Gamza, F., Waldmann, T. A., Korsmeyer, S. J. (1986). A pre-translational defect in a case of human mu heavy chain disease. *Molecular Immunology, 23,* 725–732.

Bakkus, M. H. C., Heirman, C., Van Reit, I. V., Van Camp, B., and Thielmans, K. (1992). Evidence that multiple myeloma Ig heavy chain VDJ genes contain somatic mutations but show no intraclonal variation. *Blood, 80,* 2326.

Batuman, V., Guan, S., O'Donovan, R., Puschett, J. B. (1994). Effect of myeloma light chains on phosphate and glucose transport in renal proximal tubule cells. *Renal Physiology & Biochemistry, 17,* 294–300.

Bech-Hansen, N. T., Linsley, P. S., and Cox, D. W. (1983). Restriction fragment length polymorphisms associated with immunoglobulin C genes reveal linkage disequilibrium and genomic organisation. *Proceedings of the National Academy of Science, USA, 80,* 6952.

Berberian, L., Valles Ayoub, Y., Sun, N., Martiez-Maza, O., and Braun, J. (1991). A VH clonal deficit in human immunodeficiency virus-positive individuals reflects a B cell maturational arrest. *Blood, 78,* 175.

Berenson, J. R., Vescio, R. A., Hong, C. H., Cao, J., Kim, A., Lee, C. C., Schiller, G., Berenson, R. J., and Lichtenstein, A. K. (1995). Multiple myeloma clones are derived from a cell late in B lymphoid development. *Current Topics in Immunology and Microbiology, 194,* 25.

Billadeau, D., Blackstadt, M., Greipp, P., Kyle, R. A., Oken, M. M., Kay, N., and Van-Ness, B. (1991). Analysis of 13 lymphoid malignancies using allele-specific polymerase chain reaction. A technique for sequential quantitation of residual disease. *Blood, 78,* 3021.

Bird, J., Galili, N., Link, M., Stites, D., and Sklar, J. (1988). Continuing rearrangement but absence of somatic hypermutation in immunoglobulin genes of human B cell precursor leukaemia. *Journal of Experimental Medicine,168,* 229.

Blackwell, T. K., and Alt, F. W. (1989). Immunoglobulin genes. In B. D. Hames, and D. M. Glover (Eds.), *Molecular Immunology* (p. 60). Oxford: IRL Press.

Bouzek, J., and Mancol, P. (1989). Comparability of serum protein determination by radial immunodiffusion laser nephelometric, and

Tubidometric assays employing Q antisera SEVAC. *Journal Hygiene of Epidemiology, Microbiology and Immunology, 33,* 105.

Bradwell, A. R., Carr-Smith, H. D., Mead, G. P., Tang, T. X., Showell, P. J., Drayson, M. T., Drew, R. (2001). Highly sensitive, automated immunoassay for immunoglobulin free light chains in serum and urine. *Clinical Chemistry, 47,* 673–680.

Brisco, M. J., Tan, L. W., Osborn, A. M., and Morley, A. A. (1990). Development of a highly sensitive assay based on the polymerase chain reaction for rare B lymphocyte clones in a polyclonal population. *British Journal of Haematology, 75,* 163.

Brouet, J. C., Clauvel, J. P., Danon, F., et al. (1974). Biological and clinical significance of cryoglobulins. A report of 86 cases. *American Journal of Medicine, 57,* 775.

Calper, C. A., and Johnson, A. M. (1969). Immunofixation electrophoresis: A technique for the study of protein polymorphism. *Vox. Sanguinis, 17,* 445.

Cerny, J., McAlack, R. E., Sajid, M. A., and Friedman, H. (1971). Genetic differences in the immunocyte response of mice to separate determinants on one bacterial antigen. *Nature New Biology, 230,* 247.

Chandy, K. G., Stockley, R. A., Leonard, R. C. F., et al. (1981). Relationship between serum viscosity and intravascular IgA polymer concentration in IgA myeloma. *Clinical and Experimental Immunology, 46,* 653.

Chastagner, P., Theze, J., and Zomali, M. (1992). Monomorphic organization of human diversity (DH) heavy chain variable region. *European Journal of Immunogenetics, 19,* 303.

Clofent, G., Brockly, F., Commes, T., Lefrac, M., Bataille, R., and Klein, B. (1989). No preferential use of VH5 family in human multiple myeloma. *British Journal of Haematology, 73,* 486.

Clyne, D. H., Amadeo, J. P., and Thompson, R. E. (1979). Nephrotoxicity of Bence Jones proteins in the rat: Importance of protein isoelectric point. *Kidney International, 16,* 345.

Compton, B. J., Lewis, M. A., Whigham, F., Gerald, J. S., and Countrymen, G. E. (1989). Analytical potential of protein A for affinity chromatography of polyclonal and monoclonal antibodies. *Analytical Chemistry, 61,* 1314.

Corradini, P., Boccadoro, M., Voena, C., and Pileri, A. (1993). Evidence for a bone marrow B cell transcribing malignant plasma cell VDJ joined to C mu sequence in immunoglobulin IgG- and IgA-secreting multiple myelomas. *Journal of Experimental Medicine, 178,* 1091.

Decoteau, W. E. (1974). The role of secretory IgA in defense of the distal lung. *Annals of the New York Academy of Science, 221,* 214.

De Lange, G. (1991). Allotypes and other epitopes of immunoglobulins. *Clinical Haematology, 4,* 903.

Drayson, M., Tang, L. X., Drew, R., Mead, G. P., Carr-Smith, H., Bradwell, A. R. (2001). Serum free light-chain measurements for identifying and monitoring patients with nonsecretory multiple myeloma. *Blood, 97,* 2900–2902.

Erickson, J., Martinis, J., and Croce, C. (1981). Assignment of the genes for human λ immunoglobulin genes to chromosome 22. *Nature, 294,* 173.

Frangione, B., and Franklin, E. (1977). Structural variants of human and murine immunoglobulins. *Contemporary Topics in Molecular Immunology, 4,* 89.

Gaarder, P. I., and Natvig, J. B. (1970). Hidden rheumatoid factors reacting with a "non a" and other antigens of native autologous IgG. *Journal of Immunology, 105,* 928.

Goldfarb, M. F. (1992). Two dimensional electrophoretic analysis of immunoglobulin patterns in monoclonal gammopathies. *Electrophoresis, 13,* 440.

Graber, P., and Williams, C. (1955). Methode immuno-electrophoretic d'analyse de milanges de substance anteniques. *Biochimica Biophysica Acta, 17,* 67.

Grubb, R. (1956). Agglutination of erythrocytes coated with incomplete anti Rh by certain rheumatoid arthritic sera and some other sera—the existence of human serum groups. *Acta Pathology Microbiology Scandinavia, 39,* 195.

Guinan, J., Kenny, D., and Gatenby, P. (1989). Detection and typing of paraproteins: Comparison of different methods in a routine laboratory. *Pathology, 21,* 35.

Harrison, H. (1992). Patient-specific microheterogeneity patterns of monoclonal immunoglobulin light chain as revealed by high resolution two dimensional electrophoresis. *Clinical Biochemistry, 25,* 235.

Harrison, H. H., Miller, K. L., Abu-Alfa, A., and Podlasek, S. J. (1993). Immunoglobulin clonality analysis. Resolution of ambiguities in immunofixation electrophoresis results by high-resolution, two-dimensional electrophoretic analysis of paraprotein bands eluted from agarose gels. *American Journal of Clinical Pathology, 100,* 550.

Heremans, J. F. (1959). Immunochemical studies on protein pathology. The immunoglobulin concept. *Clinica Chemica Acta, 4,* 639.

Humphries, C. G., Shen, A., Kuzel, A., Capra, J. D., Blattner, F. R., and Tucker, P. W. (1988). A new human immunoglobulin VH family preferentially rearranged in immature B cell tumours. *Nature, 331,* 446.

Ivernizzi, F., Cattaneo, R., Rosso di San Secondo, V., et al. (1973). Pryoglobulins: a report of eight patients with associated paraproteinaemia. *Acta Haematologica (Basel), 50,* 65.

Jeppson, J. E., Laurell, C. B., and Franzen, B. (1979). Agarose gel electrophoresis. *Clinical Chemistry, 25,* 629.

Jimeno-Hagales, L., Carreira, J., and Lombardero, M. (1990). Obtention of monoclonal antibodies against IgG4 using two different immunization strategies: Development of biotin-based ELISA for IgG4. *International Archives of Allergy and Applied Immunology, 92,* 175.

Johns, E. A., Turner, R., Cooper, E. H., and MacLennan, I. C. M. (1986). Isoelectric points of urinary light chains in myelomatosis: Analysis in relation to nephrotoxicity. *Journal Clinical Pathology, 39,* 833.

Joshua, D. E. (1991). Multiple myeloma: Host-tumor and tumor host interactions. Cambridge Medical Reviews. *Haematology Oncology, 1,* 225.

Keshgegian, A. (1982). Prevalence of small monoclonal proteins in the serum of hospitalized patients. *American Journal of Clinical Pathology, 77,* 436.

Kohn, J. (1976). Cellulose acetate electrophoresis and immunoelectrophoresis. In I. Smith (Ed.), *Chromatographic and Electrophoretic Techniques, 2,* 90.

Korngold, L., and Lipari, R. (1956). Multiple-myeloma proteins III. The antigenic relationship of Bence Jones proteins to normal gamma globulin and multiple myeloma serum proteins. *Cancer, 9,* 262.

Koshland, M. E. (1975). Structure and function of the J chain. *Advances in Immunology, 20,* 41.

Krause, R. M. (1970). The search for antibodies with molecular uniformity. *Advances in Immunology, 12,* 1.

Kunkel, H. G. (1968). The abnormality of myeloma proteins. *Cancer Research, 28,* 1351.

Kyle, R. A., and Gleich, G. J. (1982). IgG subclasses in monoclonal gammopathy of undermined significance. *Journal of Laboratory and Clinical Medicine, 100,* 806.

Liebler, M. R., Chang, C. P., Gallo M., et al. (1994). The mechanism of V(D)J recombination. Site-specificity reaction fidelity and immunologic diversity. *Seminars in Immunology, 6,* 143–153.

McIntyre, O. R., Kochwa, S., and Propert, K. J. (1988). Prognostic value of light chain isoelectric point (IEP) in multiple myeloma. *Proceedings of the American Society of Clinical Oncology, 7,* 8844.

MacLennan, I. C. M. (1991). The centre of hypermutation. *Nature, 354,* 352.

Malcolm, S., Barton, P., Murphy, Y., et al. (1982). Localization of κ light chain variable genes to the short arm of chromosome 2. *Proceedings of the National Academy of Science, USA, 79,* 4957.

Markowitz, H., and Tschida, A. R. (1972). Automated quantitative immunochemical analysis of human immunoglobulins. *Clinical Chemistry, 18,* 1364.

Mecker, T., Lowder, J., Cleary, M. L., Stewart, S., Wainke, R., Sklar, J., and Levy, R. (1985). Emergence of idiotype variants during treatment of B cell lymphoma with anti-idiotype antibody. *New England Journal of Medicine, 312,* 1685.

Melchers, F., Karasuyama, H., Haasner, D., Bauer, S., Kudo, A., Sakaguchi, N., Jameson, B., and Rolink, A. (1993). The surrogate light chains in B cell development. *Immunology Today, 14,* 60.

Melcion, C., Mougenot, B., Baudouin, B., et al. (1984). Renal failure in myeloma; Relationship with isoelectric point of immunoglobulin light chains. *Clinical Nephrology, 22,* 138.

Michaelson, T. E., Fragione, B., and Franklin, E. C. (1977). Primary structure of the "hinge" region of human IgG₃. *Journal of Biological Chemistry, 253,* 883.

Mihaesco, E., Seligmann, M., and Frangione, B. (1971). Studies of alpha chain disease. *Annals of the New York Academy of Science, 190,* 487–500.

Mountz, J. D., Mushinski, J. F., Owens, J. D., and Finkelman, F. D. (1990). The in vivo generation of murine IgD secreting cells is accompanied by deletion of the Cμ gene and occasional deletion of the gene for the CSI domain. *Journal of Immunology, 145,* 1583.

Nelson, M., Brown, R. D., Gibson, J., and Joshua, D. E. (1992). Measurement of free κλ chains in serum and the significance of their ratio in patients with multiple myeloma. *British Journal of Haematology, 81,* 223.

Oettinger, M. A., Schatz, D. G., Gorka, C., Baltimore, D. (1990). RAG-1 and RAG-2, adjacent genes that synergistically activate V(D)J recombination. *Science, 248,* 1517–1523.

O'Reilly, D., Adjukiewicz, A., and Whicher, J. T. (1981). Biochemical findings in a case of μ-chains disease. *Clinical Chemistry, 27,* 331.

Proudfoot, N., and Brownlee, G. (1976). 3′ Non-coding regions sequences in eukaryotic messenger RNA. *Nature, 263,* 211.

Queen, C., and Baltimore, D. (1983). Immunoglobulin gene transcription is activated by downstream enhancer elements. *Cell, 33,* 741.

Rajewsky, K. (1996). Clonal selection and learning in the antibody systems. *Nature, 381,* 751.

Ralph, Q., Brisco, M., Joshua, D. E., Brown, R. D., Gibson, J., and Morley, A. A. (1993). Advancement of multiple myeloma from diagnosis through plateau phase to progressive does not involve a new B cell clone: evidence from the immunoglobulin heavy chain gene. *Blood, 82,* 202.

Ravetch, J., Siekenlist, V., Korsmeyer, S., et al. (1981). Structure of the human immunoglobulins mu locus. Characteristics of embryonic and rearranged D and J genes. *Cell, 27,* 583.

Rettig, M. B., Vescio, R. A., Cas, J., et al. (1996). VH gene usage in multiple myeloma complete absence of the VH4.21 (VH4.34) gene. *Blood, 87,* 2846.

Ritchie, R. F., and Smith, R. (1976). Immunofixation III. Applications to the study of monoclonal proteins. *Clinical Chemistry, 22,* 1982.

Ronning, O. W., and Christophersen, A. C. (1991). An ELISA method using magnetic beads as solid phase for rapid quantitation of mouse and human immunoglobulins. *Hybridoma, 10,* 641.

Ropartz, C., Lenoir, J., and Rivat, L. (1961). A new inheritable property of human sera: The Inv factor. *Nature, 189,* 586.

Rowe, D. S., and Fahey, J. L. (1965). A new class of human immunoglobulins. A unique myeloma protein. *Journal of Experimental Medicine, 121,* 171

Schur, P. H. (1972). Human gamma-G subclasses. *Progress in Clinical Immunology, 1,* 71.

Shander, M., Martinis, J., and Croce, C. M. (1980). Genetics of human immunoglobulins: Assignment of the genes for μ and δ immunoglobulin chains to human chromosome 14. *Transplantation Proceedings, 12,* 417.

Sheehan, T., Sinclair, D., Tansey, P., and O'Donnell, J. R. (1985). The potential value of immuno-isoelectric focusing in the diagnosis and management of solitary plasmacytoma. *Clinical Laboratory Haematology, 7,* 375–377.

Siebenlist, V., Ravetch, J., Korsemyer, S., et al. (1981). Human immunoglobulin D segments encoded in tandem multigenic families. *Nature, 294,* 631.

Sinclair, D., Kumararatne, D. S., and Stott, D. (1984). Detection and identification of serum monoclonal immunoglobulin by immuno-isoelectric focusing. Limits of sensitivity and use during relapse of multiple myeloma. *Journal of Clinical Pathology, 37,* 255.

Sinclair, D., Parrott, D. M., and Stott, D. I. (1986). Quantitation of monoclonal immunoglobulins by immuno-isoelectric focusing and its application for monitoring secretory B cell neoplasia. *Journal of Immunology Methods, 90,* 247.

Snapper, C., and Mond, J. (1993). Towards a comprehensive view of immunoglobulin class switching. *Immunology Today, 14,* 15.

Solomon, A., and Fahey, J. (1964). Bence Jones proteinaemia. *American Journal of Medicine, 37,* 206.

Solomon, A., and McLaughlin, C. L. (1970). Biosynthesis of low molecular weight (7S) and high molecular weight (19S) immunoglobulin. *Journal of Clinical Investigation, 49,* 150.

Solomon, A., Weiss, D., and Kaltine, A. (1991). Nephrotoxic potential of Bence Jones proteins. *New England Journal of Medicine, 324,* 1845.

Stewart, A. K., and Schwartz, R. S. (1994). Immunoglobulin V regions and the B cell. *Blood, 83,* 1717.

Tiselius, A. (1937). Electrophoresis of serum globin II. Electrophoretic and analysis of normal and immune sera. *Biochemical Journal, 31,* 1464.

Tissot, J. D., Hochstrasser, D. F., Spertini, F., Schifferli, J. A., and Schneider, P. (1993). Pattern variations of polyclonal and monoclonal immunoglobulins of different isotypes analyzed by high-resolution two-dimensional electrophoresis. *Electrophoresis, 41,* 227.

Tomlinson, I. M., Water, G., Marks, J. D., Llevelyn, M. B., and Winter, G. (1992). The repertoire for human germline VH sequences reveals about fifty groups of VH segments with different hypervariable loops. *Journal of Molecular Biology, 5,* 776.

Tonegawa, S. (1983). Somatic generation of antibody diversity. *Nature, 302,* 575.

Tu, S. M., Winchester, R. J., and Kunkel, H. G. (1974). Occurrence of surface IgM, IgD and free light chains in human lymphocytes. *Journal of Experimental Medicine, 139,* 451.

Van Loghem, E., Aalbersc, R. C., and Matsumato, H. (1984). A genetic marker of human IgE heavy chains Em(1). *Vox Sanguinis, 46,* 195.

Vasicek, T. J., and Leder, P. (1990). Structure and expression of the human immunoglobulin λ gene. *Journal of Experimental Medicine, 170,* 609.

Vega, M. A., Guigo, R., and Smith, T. F. (1990). Autoimmune response in AIDS. *Nature, 345,* 26.

Veki, Y., Goldfarb, I.S., Harindranath, N., Gore, M., Koprowski, H., Notkins, A., and Casali, P. (1990). Clonal analysis of a human antibody response. Quantitation of precursors of antibody producing cells and generation and characterization of monoclonal IgM, IgG, and IgA to rabies virus. *Journal of Experimental Medicine, 19,* 34.

Virella, G., and Wang A. C. (1993). Immunoglobulin structure. *Immunology Series, 58,* 75–90.

Vitella, E. A., and Uhr, J. W. (1975). Immunoglobulin receptors revisited. A model for the differentiation of bone marrow derived lymphocytes is described. *Science, 189,* 964.

Vyas, G. N., and Fudenberg, H. H. (1969). Immunogenetic study of Am(1), the first allotype of human IgA. *Clinical Research, 17,* 469.

Waldmann, T. A., and Strober, W. (1969). Metabolism of immunoglobulins. *Progress in Allergy, 13,* 1.

Walter, M., Surti, V., Hofker, M., and Cox, D. (1990). The physical organisation of the human immunoglobulin heavy chain gene complex. *EMBO Journal, 9,* 3303.

Whicher, J. T., Wallage, M., and Fifield, K. (1987). Use of immunoglobulin heavy and light chain measurements compared with existing techniques as a means of typing monoclonal immunoglobulins. *Clinical Chemistry, 33,* 1771.

Wilson, A. T. (1964). Direct immunoelectrophoresis. *Journal of Immunology, 92,* 431.

Wochner, R. D., Strober, W., and Waldman, T. A. (1967). The role of the kidney in the catabolism of Bence Jones proteins and immunoglobulin fragments. *Journal of Experimental Medicine, 126,* 207.

Yamada, M., Hudson, S., Fournay, D., Bitenbander, S., Shane, S. S., Lange, B., Tsujimotoy Carton, A. J., and Rovera, G. (1989). Detection of minimal disease in hemopoietic malignancies of the B cell lineage by using their complimentarity determining (CDR III) specific probes. *Proceedings of the National Academy of Science, USA, 86,* 5123.

Yancopoulos, G. D., Brackwell, T. K., Suh, H., et al. (1986). Introduced T cell receptor variable gene segments recombine in pre B cells: evidence that B and T cells use a common recombinase. *Cell, 44,* 251.

Zelenetz, A. D., Chen, T. T., and Levy, R. (1992). Clonal expansion in follicular lymphoma occurs subsequent to antigen selection. *Journal of Experimental Medicine, 176,* 1137.

Zimmer, F. J., Hameister, H., Schek, H., and Zachua, H. (1990). Transposition of human immunoglobulin VK genes within the same chromosome and mechanism of the amplification. *EMBO Journal, 9,* 1535.

# CHAPTER 2

# Multiple Myeloma and Plasma Cells: Cell-Cycle and Apoptotic Controls

## SELINA CHEN-KIANG

## Introduction

Multiple myeloma (MM) is a cancer of plasmacytoid cells. It represents a collection of plasma cell dyscrasias sharing 2 prominent features: elevated production of monoclonal antibodies and bone destruction. Although it is widely accepted that MM cells are malignant counterparts of normal plasmacytoid cells arrested at progressive stages of B cell terminal differentiation, there is no unified genetic basis or mechanism of pathogenesis. Most MM cells do not cycle; therefore, they accumulate in the bone marrow microenvironment principally as a result of loss of apoptotic controls. Although the initiation event for MM pathogenesis remains unknown, dysregulation of the cell cycle must have occurred earlier to account for the expansion of monoclonal MM cells. Thus, MM is a cancer that has lost both cell-cycle and apoptotic controls at disparate stages of oncogenesis. Until now, progress in understanding the mechanism of MM pathogenesis has been hindered in part due to the lack of understanding of normal plasma cell differentiation at the cellular and molecular levels.

Plasma cells are essential for humoral immunity because they alone synthesize and secrete large amounts of antigen-specific antibodies. Until recently, virtually nothing was known about the molecular mechanism of B cell terminal differentiation. This complex process requires timely orchestration of cell-cycle control, cellular differentiation, and apoptosis, yet each of these parameters had not been defined in primary plasma cells. Exciting new findings have now begun to shed light on these 3 subjects. By integrating the recent advances in cell-cycle control of normal plasma cell differentiation, the mechanism of plasma cell apoptosis and the transcriptional control of plasma cell differentiation, we may significantly advance our understanding of MM pathogenesis and therapeutic design.

This chapter focuses on our current thinking about coordinated cell-cycle and apoptotic controls of normal plasma cell differentiation and MM pathogenesis.

# B Cell Terminal Differentiation

## Plasma Cell Differentiation Is a Multistep Process

Plasma cells are generated by terminal differentiation of antigen-stimulated B cells. Most antibody responses to protein antigens require the participation of T cells, the so-called T cell-dependent antibody response, whereas those responding to carbohydrate antigens can proceed without the help of T cells, the so-called T-independent antibody response. In both cases, the primary antibody response begins with antigen activation of resting mature B cells and expansion of the activated B cell population by cell division. In the T cell-independent response, terminal differentiation rapidly ensues to generate mostly IgM-secreting plasma cells in the extrafollicular foci. In the T cell-dependent response, the activated B cells also form germinal centers where isotype switching and hypermutation of the Ig variable region occur (Jacob et al.,

1993; Liu et al., 1991; Smith et al., 1997). During terminal differentiation, antigen-activated B cells are either eliminated by apoptosis due to low affinity or self-reactivity, or differentiated to affinity-matured memory B cells or antibody-secreting plasma cells (Liu and Banchereau, 1997). In successive immunizations, the antibody response is accelerated and amplified by the activation of long-lived, antigen-specific memory B cells (Ahmed and Gray, 1996) (Fig. 2-1).

Homeostasis in each of these steps is tightly regulated by the cell-cycle, apoptosis, and cell migration. Plasma cells are permanently withdrawn from the cell cycle and memory cell cycle infrequently, if at all. Both arrest in the G1 phase of the cell cycle, raising an important question of how the cell cycle controls plasma cell and memory cell fate, decision, and differentiation. However, the mechanism of cell-cycle control in B cell terminal differentiation is not known (Fig. 2-1).

## Hallmarks of Primary Plasma Cells

Primary plasma cells have been only partially characterized at the cellular level. We know, for example, that coinciding with a prominent increase in Ig synthesis and secretion, primary plasma cells cease to express MHC class II and have markedly reduced surface expression of Ig, B220, and CD19. CD38 is expressed on human but not mouse plasma cells. The only cell surface protein known to be highly expressed on normal human and mouse plasma cells is CD138 (syndecan-1). This proteoglycan also appears on cells of other lineages during early development and on malignant plasma cells (Sanderson et al., 1989; Sneed et al., 1994), but not mature B cells before terminal differentiation. Although its function in plasma cells remains obscure, syndecan-1 has served as a useful cell surface marker for identification of plasmacytoid cells.

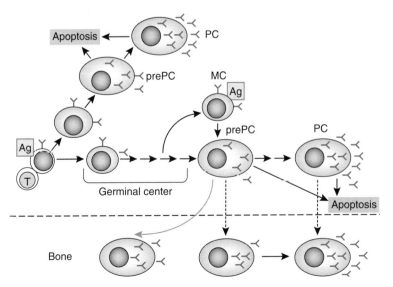

**Figure 2-1** *B cell terminal differentiation. Cell-cycle control in plasma cell. The schematic depicts a T cell-dependent antibody response. Differentiation of preplasma cells (prePC) and plasma cells (PC) occurs in the extrafollicular foci directly following germinal center reactions. The cell cycle is activated on stimulation with antigen and interacting with T cells. PrePC cycles, memory B cells (MC), and PC are arrested in the G1 phase of the cell cycle.*

# Mechanism of Normal Plasma Cell Death

Most plasma cells are rapidly eliminated by cell death following Ig secretion. The only exceptions are certain long-lived populations found in the bone marrow and the lamina propria of the gut (Ho et al., 1986; Manz et al., 1997; Slifka et al., 1998). Thus, apoptosis represents a major determinant of plasma cell homeostasis *in vivo*. Virtually nothing was known, however, of the mechanism that underlies primary plasma cell death.

## Fas Mediates Apoptosis of Activated B Cells

Extensive investigation of B cell death has established that homeostasis of antigen-activated B cells at the germinal center is principally controlled by apoptosis mediated by Fas expressed on the cell surface (Krammer et al., 1994; Nagata, 1997; Rathmell et al., 1995). Fas-signaled apoptosis is in turn attenuated by CD40 signaling in response to CD40 ligand (CD40L) expressed on activated T cells (Banchereau et al., 1994), by B cell receptor signaling (Rathmell et al., 1996), and by the expression of appropriate Bcl-2 family proteins (Cory, 1995; Grillot et al., 1996; McDonnell et al., 1989). Although CD40 signaling promotes cell-cycle progression and cell survival, it also enhances the expression of Fas (Garrone et al., 1995; Rothstein et al., 1995; Schattner et al., 1995). In this manner, CD40 signaling is subject to feedback regulation by enhancing Fas-mediated apoptosis. Apoptosis of activated B cells is thus determined, at least in part, by the balance between the dual functions of CD40 signaling.

## TRAIL Induces Apoptosis of Primary Plasma Cells

By contrast, the extrinsic and intrinsic factors that determine the longevity of plasma cell survival are not known. A recent study (Ursini-Siegel et al., 2002) suggests that differential susceptibility to TRAIL/Apo2L (tumor necrosis factor-related apoptosis-inducing ligand) (Pitti et al., 1996; Wiley et al., 1995) may play a role. The expression of both TRAIL/Apo2L and the death receptors DR4 (TRAIL-1R1) and DR5 (TRAIL-R1) (Ashkenazi and Dixit, 1998; Bodmer et al., 2000; Kischkel et al., 2000; Sprick et al., 2000) is sustained in primary mouse plasma cells as well as in IL-6-differentiated Ig-secreting human plasma cells (Ursini-Siegel et al., 2002). Plasma cell apoptosis is induced by both endogenous and exogenous TRAIL *ex vivo*, suggesting that TRAIL-mediated killing may, in part, be an autonomous property of plasma cells. By contrast, resting and activated B cells resist TRAIL killing despite comparable expression of TRAIL and

DRs (Ursini-Siegel et al., 2002). Collectively, these results provide the first evidence that primary plasma cells synthesize TRAIL and are direct targets of TRAIL-mediated apoptosis.

The preferential killing of plasma cells by TRAIL is novel, given that TRAIL was initially thought to predominantly kill tumor cells (Ashkenazi et al., 1999; Walczak et al., 1999). Further studies of primary plasma cell apoptosis reveal that the sensitivity to TRAIL correlates with decreased expression of Fas and CD40 and inactivation of NF-κB (nuclear factor kappa B), a key signal transducer and transcription factor. Moreover, apoptosis of primary plasma cells can only be partially inhibited by caspase inhibitors, unlike that of activated B cells (Ursini-Siegel et al., 2002). These results underscore the complexity of plasma cell death and suggest that plasma cells differ from activated B cells in the intrinsic determinants for cell survival. CD40, Fas, and TRAIL all belong to the tumor necrosis factor (TNF) family. Thus, the intrinsic determinants for plasma cell death are in part governed by a dynamic shift in the balance between TNF receptors that mediate signals for positive and negative control of the cell cycle and apoptosis during plasma cell differentiation (Fig. 2-2).

## Attenuation of IL-6 Signaling in Plasma Cells

IL-6 is a cytokine specifically required for the generation of IgG and IgA antibody responses in mice (Kopf et al., 1994; Ramsay et al., 1994). It has an essential role in plasma cell tumorigenesis, given the requirement for

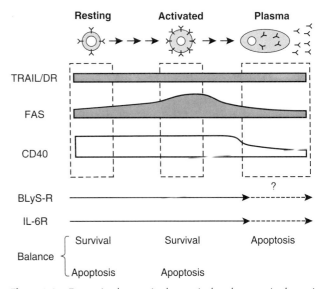

**Figure 2-2** *Dynamic changes in the survival and apoptotic determinants during plasma cell differentiation. The schematic depicts the dynamic changes of the expression of survival and apoptotic receptors during B cell terminal differentiation. The balance between survival and apoptotic signals mediated by these receptors determines survival and apoptosis of resting and activated B cells and plasma cells.*

IL-6 in plasmacytoma development (Hilbert et al., 1995) and its ability to promote the survival of plasmacytoma cells (Nordan and Potter, 1986) and MM cells *in vitro*. IL-6 has been proposed to enhance both cell proliferation and survival of MM cells and nonmalignant human plasmablasts (Jego et al., 2001). Emerging evidence favors the view that IL-6 functions predominantly as a survival factor for B cells and plasmacytoid cells, and through attenuation of apoptosis, IL-6 permissively augments the expansion of cycling B cells (Zhang and Chen-Kiang, unpublished data). Based on studies of plasma cell differentiation in response to IL-6 in a IgG-bearing human lymphoblastoid cell line, increasing the level of Mcl-1, but not other antiapoptotic proteins of the Bcl-2 family, represents one means by which IL-6 protects human plasma cells from apoptosis (Altmeyer et al., 1997).

The IL-6 receptor is a tetramer comprised of 2 glycoproteins, the ligand-binding subunit, gp80 (CD126), and the signaling subunit, gp130. Recent work suggests that IL-6-induced B cell terminal differentiation is associated with a drastic reduction of both subunits of the IL-6 receptor (Zhang and Chen-Kiang, unpublished data). Importantly, this observation has been confirmed in primary plasma cells generated in a T cell-dependent antibody response *in vivo* (Ursini-Siegel and Chen-Kiang, unpublished data). A reduced capacity to mediate the IL-6 survival signals that would result from repression of IL-6 receptor expression represents another potent mechanism by which the survival and death of primary plasma cells is modulated (Fig. 2-2).

### A Potential Role for BLyS in Plasma Cell Survival

BLyS (B Lymphocyte Stimulator [BAFF]) is a recently identified member of the TNF family (Moore et al., 1999; Schneider et al., 1999) that plays a key role in antibody response, possibly including plasma cell differentiation (reviewed in Do and Chen-Kiang, 2002; Rolink and Melchers, 2002). BLyS is produced in activated monocytes and is required for peripheral B cell development (Gross et al., 2001; Harless et al., 2001; Schiemann et al., 2001; Yan et al., 2001). It is unique among TNF family proteins in that it acts on just cells of the B lineage (Gross et al., 2000; Yan et al., 2001) and a subset of T cells (Huard et al., 2001). In addition to mature B cells, the BLyS targets now include the immature transitional type 2 B cells on their migration to the spleen from the bone marrow (Batten et al., 2000). Plasmablasts, the cycling preplasma cells present in the extrafollicular foci in a T cell-independent antibody response, also appear to be responsive to BLyS (Balazs et al., 2002).

The primary mechanism of BLyS action is attenuation of apoptosis that is independent of the cell-cycle status. This was first shown in quiescent and activated splenic mature B cells *in vivo* and *ex vivo* (Do et al., 2000). Further studies in primary B cells *in vitro* point to an extraordinary collaboration between BLyS and CD40 signaling (Do et al., 2000) and BLyS and the cell-cycle control (Huang and Chen-Kiang, unpublished data) in maintaining B cell homeostasis. BLyS signaling leads to activation of both the classic NF-κB pathway (Do et al., 2000) and the newly uncovered, alternative NF-κB pathway (Claudio et al., 2002; Hatada et al., 2003; Kayagaki et al., 2002). Thus, by activating the NF-κB pathways, BLyS signaling converges with CD40 signaling to ensure temporally restricted cell survival during plasma cell differentiation. Whether BLyS signals in the terminally differentiated, Ig-secreting plasma cells or MM cells is currently unknown. This is a subject under intense investigation because of its potential importance in modulating the longevity of plasma cells and MM cells.

## Dysregulation of MM Apoptosis

Dysregulation of MM apoptosis has been amply documented, initially in studies of MM cell lines established from extramedullary MM cells that have lost bone marrow dependence, and more recently in the investigation of primary MM cells freshly isolated from patient marrow aspirates. The data point to a loss of apoptotic control in MM cells as a consequence of dysregulation of multiple survival pathways stemming from oncogenic transformation and interaction with the bone microenvironments. Therefore, to understand the basis for dysregulation of MM apoptosis, we need to answer several questions: What is the origin of MM cells in relationship to long-lived plasma cells generated in B cell terminal differentiation? What are the key differences in migration of MM and plasma cells to the bone? Finally, in what ways do the MM and long-lived plasma cells interact differently with the bone marrow microenvironments? Above all is the need to understand the mechanism of normal plasma cell death. Although our current understanding of primary plasma cell death is incomplete, it nonetheless serves as a normal reference and a basis for dissecting the myriad of events associated with dysregulation of MM apoptosis and accumulation.

### Induction of MM Apoptosis by Fas and TRAIL

Induction of MM apoptosis by Fas and TRAIL has been described. Fas is expressed at varying levels on MM cells and subject to killing by Fas (Shain et al.,

2000), marking them as the malignant counterparts of early preplasma cells before losing Fas expression or, alternatively, preplasma cells which have reduced ability to inhibit Fas expression (Fig. 2-3). The killing of MM cells by TRAIL (Lincz et al., 2001; Liu et al., 2001; Mitsiades et al., 2001) indicates that these cells continue to express the TRAIL death receptor (Fig. 2-3). These findings are consistent with the ability of TRAIL to preferentially kill tumor cells (Ashkenazi et al., 1999; Walczak et al., 1999). The ability of TRAIL signaling to activate caspases in MM cells (Mitsiades et al., 2002), however, differs significantly from the lack of caspase activation in primary plasma cell apoptosis mediated by TRAIL (Ursini-Siegel et al., 2002). Resolving the basis of this distinction between normal and malignant plasma cells in TRAIL-mediated apoptosis, as well as the contribution of a caspase-independent mechanism to normal plasma cell apoptosis, should help to advance our understanding of the specificity of TRAIL killing (Fig. 2-3).

TRAIL is expressed in normal plasma cells (Ursini-Siegel et al., 2002). Currently there is no information on the status of TRAIL expression in MM cells. The survival of MM cells is known to be prolonged by paracrine survival factors provided by the bone marrow, and MM cells expand at the expense of skeletal integrity. A recent report suggests that TRAIL might play a role in this process. OPG (Simonet et al., 1997) (osteoprotegerin), the decoy receptor of OPGL (osteoprotegerin ligand) necessary for osteoclast differentiation (Lacey et al., 1998), can bind to and inhibit the

TRAIL apoptotic function in MM cells (Shipman and Croucher, 2003). This implies that the TRAIL–OPG interaction might cause the release of OPGL and augment osteoclast differentiation. In this way, TRAIL would play a key role in modulating the MM–bone marrow interaction in addition to apoptosis of MM cells. This, and the source of TRAIL in the bone marrow microenvironment, are important questions to address in terms of MM cell survival and MM-associated bone destruction.

## Dysregulation of the IL-6 Signaling Pathway in MM Cells

The IL-6 signaling pathway appears to be dysregulated at multiple levels in MM cells. In some MM cells, the identified mechanistic defect is sustained expression of IL-6 receptor gp80 (CD126) (Rawstron et al., 2000). In others, activation of Stat3 by tyrosine phosphorylation appears to be constitutive instead of being transiently activated by cytokines (Catlett-Falcone et al., 1999). In still others, the expression of Mcl-1 is significantly heightened (Zhang et al., 2003), which appears to be essential for MM cell survival (Derenne et al., 2002). Given that the reduction of IL-6 signaling pathway permits apoptosis in primary plasma cells (Ursini-Siegel and Chen-Kiang, unpublished data), the maintenance of this pathway in MM cells must contribute significantly to MM cell survival. Having a functional IL-6 signaling pathway in MM cells may do more than potentiate cell survival, because IL-6 signaling leads to cell-cycle arrest through activation of a cyclin-dependent kinase inhibitor p18$^{INK4C}$ (discussed in later sections) (Morse et al., 1997). Whether this aspect of IL-6 signaling occurs in MM cells needs to be determined because it might account for cell-cycle arrest in concert with cell survival in most MM cells (Fig. 2-3).

## Dysregulation of CD40 Signaling in MM Cells

In contrast to the drastic reduction of CD40 in primary plasma cells, this protein is expressed at varying levels on primary MM cells (Hatada and Chen-Kiang, unpublished data). However, the functional consequence of CD40 expression in primary MM cells remains to be defined, because it has been suggested to mediate cell migration (Tai et al., 2003), enhance the secretion of IL-6 (Urashima et al., 1995) or the vascular endothelial growth factor (Tai et al., 2002), among others. Whether stimulation of CD40 leads to augmented proliferation, survival, or even death (Tong et al., 2000) is presently unclear. Whether BLyS functions in MM cells also

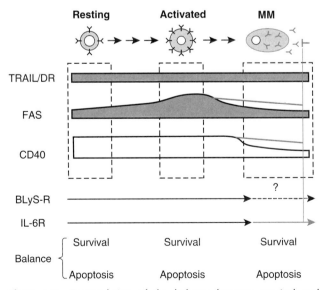

**Figure 2-3** *Dysregulation of the balance between survival and apoptotic receptors in MM cells. The schema depicts the failure of MM cells to fully differentiate into plasma cells, and the inappropriate retention of IL-6 receptor, CD40, and possibly Fas expression.*

remains to be determined. Given that activation of the NF-κB pathways by CD40 and BlyS (Do et al., 2000; Hatada et al., 2003) will undoubtedly contribute to the attenuation of apoptosis, elucidation of these 2 pathways in primary MM cells should provide new insights into dysregulation of MM apoptosis (Fig. 2-3).

## Cell-Cycle Dysregulation in Multiple Myeloma Pathogenesis

Although the accumulation of noncycling MM cells in the bone marrow stems mainly from dysregulation of apoptosis, the expansion of monoclonal MM cells cannot be achieved without dysregulation of the cell cycle earlier during MM pathogenesis. The findings of cyclin D overexpression (Chesi et al., 1996; Shaughnessy et al., 2001) and the inactivation of cyclin-dependent kinase (CDK) inhibitor p16$^{INK4a}$ (Ng et al., 1997; Tasaka et al., 1998) in MM cells support this notion, because both of these changes would potentiate cell-cycle progression. Beyond these descriptions, however, there is no information regarding the mechanism for cell-cycle dysregulation in MM pathogenesis. The basic biochemical mechanism of mammalian cell-cycle control has been established, and a specific CDK inhibitor, p18$^{INK4C}$, has been determined to be required for the generation of functional plasma cells. These are discussed in the context of normal plasma cell differentiation and cell-cycle dysregulation in MM pathogenesis.

## The Mammalian Cell Cycle

The mammalian somatic cell cycle is regulated primarily at the G1 to S transition by a family of serine/threonine protein kinases consisting of the regulatory cyclin subunits and the catalytic cyclin-dependent kinases (CDK) (Hunter and Pines, 1994). Two CDK enzymes, CDK4 and CDK6, in combination with 3 D-type cyclins (D1, D2, and D3), usher cell-cycle progression to mid G1, then CDK2-cyclin E catalyzes late G1 cell-cycle progression (Weinberg, 1995). Phosphorylation of the retinoblastoma protein pRb (p105) and the related p107 and p130 by CDKs leads to the release of E2F/DP-1 transcription factors from pRB and S phase entry (Fig. 2-4).

The CDK catalytic activity is in turn negatively regulated by 7 inhibitory proteins of the INK4 and Cip/Kip families (Sherr and Roberts, 1999). The INK4 family proteins (p16$^{INK4a}$, p15$^{INK4b}$, p18$^{INK4c}$, and p19$^{INK4d}$) function solely as negative cell-cycle regulators by forming stable binary complexes with CDK4 and CDK6.

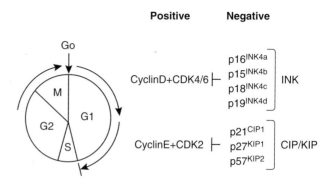

**Figure 2-4** *Positive and negative control of G1-S cell cycle progression. The schematic depicts the control of G1-S transition by the balance between positive and negative cell cycle regulators.*

The Cip/Kip proteins (p21$^{Cip1}$, p27$^{Kip1}$, and p57$^{Kip2}$) have broader substrate specificity and range of functions. Their principal role is to inhibit CDK2-cyclin E by forming inactive ternary complexes. However, they may also facilitate the formation of stable CDK4-cyclin D complexes, thereby acting as positive cell-cycle regulators (Cheng et al., 1999). Thus, G1 to S cell-cycle progression is determined not by the absolute level of any given cell-cycle regulator, but by the aggregate balance between positive and negative cell-cycle regulators and the interplay among them.

## CDK Inhibitor 18$^{INK4c}$ Is Required for the Generation of Functional Plasma Cells

### Cell-Cycle Control in B Cells

Gene targeting studies show that specific CDK inhibitors are needed for some aspects of development (Sherr and Roberts, 1999). Beyond that, the physiological functions of CDK inhibitors, in particular cell-cycle control of immunity, remain largely uncharacterized. Several CDK inhibitors (p19$^{INK4d}$, p21$^{Cip1}$, and p27$^{Kip1}$), CDKs, and D-type cyclins were shown to be regulated *in vitro* in primary mouse splenic B cells in response to IL-4 and anti-IgM (Lam et al., 2000; Mullins et al., 1998; Solvason et al., 1996; Tanguay and Chiles, 1996). Activation of Rb phosphorylation by antigen–receptor crosslinking appeared to be inhibited by cocrosslinking of Fcγ receptors (Tanguay et al., 1999). These results brought to light the regulation of individual positive and negative cell-cycle regulators by major B cell signaling pathways, but did not address the functional consequence in cell-cycle control or the relevance to the humoral response.

## p18[INK4c] Mediates IL-6 Signals for Cell-Cycle Arrest in Human Plasma Cell Differentiation

A role for p18[INK4c] (p18) (Guan et al., 1994; Hirai et al., 1995) in plasma cell differentiation was first indicated in studies of a human IgG lymphoblastoid cell line in which IL-6 simultaneously induces reverse EBV immortalization (Altmeyer et al., 1997) and B cell terminal differentiation (Morse et al., 1997; Natkunam et al., 1994). p18, but not any other CDK inhibitor, was increased at the protein level in response to IL-6, leading to inhibition of CDK6, the preferred substrate for p18 (Guan et al., 1994; Hirai et al., 1995), and cell-cycle arrest in G1 (Morse et al., 1997). In addition, forced expression of p18 was sufficient to cause G1 arrest of IgM lymphoblastoid cells by sequestration of CDK6 (Morse et al., 1997). Therefore, p18 is regulated by IL-6 and mediates IL-6 signals for cell-cycle arrest during human plasma cell differentiation.

## Enhanced B Cell Expansion in the Absence of p18

p18 is expressed in many tissues (Guan et al., 1994), but it is dispensable for mouse development (Franklin et al., 1998). The absence of p18, however, leads to increased numbers of peripheral B and T cells *in vivo* and enhanced expansion of B cells in response to CD40L *in vitro* as a result of elevated CDK activity (Franklin et al., 1998). Hyperproliferation of lymphocytes in the absence of p18 was subsequently confirmed by the induction of lymphocyte proliferation with the mitogens phorbol myristic acid (PMA) and concanavalin A *in vitro* (Latres et al., 2000). Thus, a gain of p18 function in IL-6 signaling is sufficient to cause cell-cycle arrest in B cell terminal differentiation, whereas the loss of p18 function leads to enhanced B cell activation in response to mitogens.

## p18 Is Required Within B Cells for the Generation of Ig-Secreting Plasma Cells

Characterization of the p18 function in antibody response to a well-characterized T cell-dependent antigen NP-CGG (4-hydroxy-3-nitropheny acetyl linked to chicken γ-globulin) further demonstrates that p18 is required for the generation of functional plasma cells (Tourigny et al., 2002). In the absence of p18, antibody secretion is notably reduced during, and even before, primary immunization and is virtually absent in the secondary response. The requirement for p18 is differentiation stage-specific, because p18 deficiency does not impair germinal center formation, Ig switch recombination, V-region hypermutation, or memory cell generation. In the absence of p18, antigen-specific,

antibody-containing extrafollicular plasmacytoid cells form, but they fail to terminate the cell cycle or to differentiate into antibody-secreting plasma cells. Instead, the plasmacytoid cells undergo accelerated apoptosis *in vivo*. These findings provide the first direct evidence for cell-cycle control of plasma cell differentiation in the humoral immune response, and they suggest an extraordinary specificity with which cell-cycle CDK inhibitors control B cell terminal differentiation *in vivo* (Tourigny et al., 2002) (Fig. 2-5).

For simplicity, "plasma cell" refers to a functional, Ig-secreting plasma cell, whereas "preplasma cell (prePC)" refers to nonsecreting plasmacytoid cells that are morphologically indistinguishable from functional plasma cells.

p18 is dispensable for homing of prePCs to the bone and for their survival in the bone marrow microenvironment (Tourigny et al., 2002). However, both lymphoid and bone marrow p18-deficient prePCs are defective in Ig secretion, suggesting that p18 is required within B cells for the generation of plasma cells. This is confirmed by reconstituting primary plasma cell differentiation *in vitro* in which both the p18 cell cycle and Ig secretion defects are recapitulated (Tourigny et al., 2002). The requirement for p18 within B cells for the final step of plasma cell differentiation raises 3 important questions: What biochemical mechanism underlies the specificity of p18 action in plasma cell differentiation? How does p18-mediated cell-cycle control relate to transcriptional regulation of plasma cell differentiation and plasma cell survival? Also, do p18-deficient prePCs resemble the recently identified self-renewing prePC present in the bone marrow (O'Connor et al., 2002)?

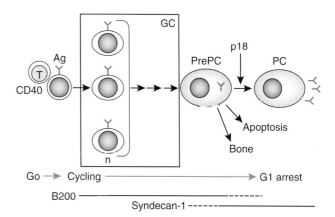

**Figure 2-5**  *p18 is required for the generation of Ig-secreting plasma cells. B cells enter the cell cycle and expand by cell division to a predetermined number (N) in the germinal center (GC). In the absence of p18, the cycling preplasma cells (prePC) do not efficiently differentiate into Ig-secreting plasma cells (PC). They undergo accelerated apoptosis but are not defective in homing to the bone.*

# Specificity of Negative Cell-Cycle Control by p18: Cooperation Between CD40 and IL-6

The specificity for the control of G1 to S transition is primarily determined by the molar ratios and the relative affinity between positive and negative cell-cycle regulators. It follows that modulation of the molar ratios in response to extracellular stimuli will profoundly regulate cell-cycle progression. With respect to the role of p18 in cell-cycle control in a T-dependent antibody response, CDK inhibitors and CDKs are differentially regulated in primary B cells during terminal differentiation mediated by CD40 (Tourigny et al., 2002). The expression of p18 and the structurally similar protein, p19[INK4d] (Chan et al., 1995; Guan et al., 1996; Hirai et al., 1995) are sustained throughout cell-cycle activation and G1 arrest. Both p21[Cip1] (Harper et al., 1993; Xiong et al., 1993) and p27[Kip1] (Fero et al., 1996; Kiyokawa et al., 1996; Nakayama et al., 1996) of the CIP/Kip family are expressed in resting B cells and declined on cell-cycle activation. Although p21 levels continue to decline, the p27 levels are partially restored in G1-arrested cells. Whether 19 and p27 have a functional role in plasma cell differentiation has not yet been defined, but they clearly cannot compensate for the loss of p18 in B cells *in vivo* and *in vitro*.

The CDK6 levels rise and fall with cell-cycle activation and arrest, whereas CDK4 levels change only modestly. Most importantly, the loss of p18 markedly enhances CDK6 activity. p18 is upregulated in response to IL-6 in a model cellular system (Morse et al., 1997) and in plasma cells *in vivo* in T cell-dependent antibody responses (Tourigny et al., 2002). Together, these results suggest a model in which CD40 and IL-6 regulate G1 to S by balancing the ratio between p18 and CDK6.

# Cell-Cycle Control of Cellular Differentiation and Apoptosis

The p18-deficient prePCs turn over more rapidly than their wild-type counterparts in the extrafollicular foci of the spleen (Tourigny et al., 2002). If terminal differentiation occurs within a restricted period of time, apoptosis might preclude the p18-deficient prePCs from final differentiation into functional plasma cells. However, the preservation of the prePC Ig secretion defect in the absence of accelerated turnover in the bone marrow and *in vitro* argues that impaired cellular differentiation in the absence of p18 is not secondary to apoptosis. A better understanding of the mechanism

for plasma cell death is needed to resolve the role of apoptosis in defective cellular differentiation in the absence of p18.

In any case, cell-cycle control is upstream of cellular differentiation. The role of p18 in coordinating cell-cycle control and cellular differentiation of plasma cells necessitates that it acts in concert with transcription factors. One candidate is Blimp-1 (B cell maturation protein-1) (Turner et al., 1994), which appears to control a regulatory cascade leading to activation of genes expressed and repression of genes extinguished in plasma cells (Calame et al., 2003; Piskurich et al., 2000). Given that the loss of p18 does not affect the expression of Blimp-1 in prePCs (Tourigny et al., 2002), p18 might function downstream of Blimp-1 or in a complementary pathway to coordinately regulate the final differentiation of plasma cells. A second potential collaborator for p18 is XBP-1 (X-box-binding protein 1). Chimera studies have shown that the loss of XBP-1 leads to defective Ig secretion without impairment in germinal center formation during plasma cell differentiation (Reimold et al., 2001). This is strikingly similar to the Ig-secretion defect observed in p18-/- mice in an antibody response. Although XBP-1 is unlikely to be directly involved in Ig secretion, it regulates the unfolded protein response in cell line systems *in vitro* (Calfon et al., 2002; Yoshida et al., 2001). In addition, XBP-1 is regulated by IL-4 and in turn regulates IL-6 in primary B cells, suggesting that XBP-1 might link the unfolded protein response to a cytokine circuitry necessary for Ig secretion (Iwakoshi et al., 2003). The functional relationship between cell-cycle control and XBP-1 is a fascinating question to follow.

# Overexpression of D-Type Cyclins in MM Cells

Studies of cell-cycle dysregulation in MM cells have been limited to the characterization of individual cell-cycle regulators at the level of RNA or protein expression. Overexpression of cyclin D1 and D3 frequently associates with multiple myeloma. Dysregulation of the cyclin D genes might be caused by translocation into the IgH switch region (Chesi et al., 1996; Shaughnessy et al., 2001) or might occur independently of chromosomal translocation. In either case, it is reasonable to postulate that overexpression of cyclin D contributes to myeloma pathogenesis by dysregulating cell-cycle progression.

However, cyclin D overexpression has not been associated with an overt increase in the proliferation of myeloma cells. This presents a paradox. The D-type cyclins appear to be highly redundant functionally, as evidenced by the ability of cyclin D3 to compensate for the loss of cyclin D2 in B lymphocyte activation (Lam et al., 2000). It is possible that overexpression of cyclin D without a corresponding increase of CDK4 or CDK6 is insufficient to promote cell-cycle progression. Alternatively, cyclin D overexpression might promote the proliferation of myeloma precursor cells, thereby contributing to the precursor cell expansion without directly promoting an accumulation of noncycling myeloma cells.

## Inactivation of CDK Inhibitors in MM Cells

By contrast, a loss of a CDK inhibitor in the absence of functional compensation may have a severe consequence in cell-cycle control by lowering the threshold of kinase inhibition. Increasing evidence supports a role for inactivation of CDK inhibitors of the INK4 family in myeloma pathogenesis (Drexler, 1998). Formally, the INK4 genes are tumor-suppressor genes. For example, the loss of the INK4 family member p18 in mice leads to the development of pituitary adenoma (Franklin et al., 1998) and sensitizes the animals to carcinogen-induced tumorigenesis (Bai et al., 2003). Homozygous deletion of $p18^{INK4c}$ has been reported in myeloma cell lines (Kulkarni et al., 2002), but is infrequently detected in primary myeloma cells (Tasaka et al., 1997). Whether this is the result of the elimination of p18-deficient malignant cells by death, likely would be predicted by the phenotype of p18-deficient prePCs, is not known.

A more frequent occurrence in primary myeloma cells is inactivation of $p16^{INK4a}$ and $p15^{INK4b}$ genes by methylation (Ng et al., 1997; Tasaka et al., 1998). This is interesting given that $p16^{INK4a}$ is a putative genetic modifier involved in plasmacytoma susceptibility in the BALB/c strain mouse (Zhang et al., 1998, 2001). The loss of p18 does not affect homing of plasma cell precursors to the bone, but it inhibits them from further differentiation (Tourigny et al., 2002). The inactivation of p16 or p15 might contribute to myeloma pathogenesis by similarly promoting the expansion of bone marrow myeloma precursors without affecting their ability to differentiate to noncycling myeloma cells. Although p18 might or might not be the precise CDK inhibitor that is pivotal in controlling cell-cycle progression in MM cells, understanding the mechanism of p18 action provides a much needed framework for investigating cell-cycle control of MM pathogenesis.

Taken together, cell-cycle dysregulation by either gain of cyclin D function or loss of INK4 CDK inhibitor function may contribute to myeloma pathogenesis by enhancing the expansion of proliferating myeloma precursor cells in conjunction with losing apoptotic control of noncycling myeloma cells (Fig. 2-6).

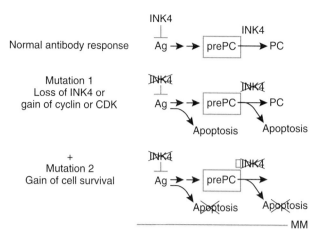

**Figure 2-6** *Dysregulation of cell-cycle control and apoptosis in MM pathogenesis. The model depicts the cooperation between dysregulation of cell cycle and apoptosis in the pathogenesis of multiple myeloma. The p18 is used as an example. p18 is required for negative control of B cell expansion in response to antigen challenge (Huang et al., unpublished data) and for plasma cell differentiation (Tourigny et al., 2002). Loss of p18 or another INK4 family gene, or gain of cyclin or CDK function resulting from mutation 1 would lead to apoptosis. This prevents the accumulation of cell-cycle mutants. If the mutant cells also lack apoptotic control as a result of a second mutation, they expand and then accumulate as a result of the cooperation between the 2 mutations.*

## Concluding Remarks

Cell-cycle control and apoptosis are 2 major determinants for homeostasis in both normal plasma cell generation and MM pathogenesis. Cell-cycle progression is controlled by the aggregate balance between positive and negative cell-cycle regulators. One such negative cell-cycle regulator, the CDK inhibitor $p18^{INK4c}$, is specifically required for final differentiation of pre-plasma cells to Ig-secreting plasma cells. Dysregulated expression of a related CDK inhibitor, $p16^{INK4a}$, and the D-type cyclins has been described in MM cells. The understanding of p18-mediated cell-cycle control of plasma cell differentiation in response to IL-6 and CD40L provides a framework for investigating the mechanism of cell-cycle dysregulation in MM pathogenesis. Apoptosis of normal plasma cells is determined, at least in part, by the dynamic regulation of IL-6, CD40, Fas, and TRAIL signaling pathways during B cell terminal differentiation. This coordination is disrupted in MM cells. Induction of primary plasma cell apoptosis by TRAIL/Apo-2L gives the first glimpse of the molecular mechanism that underlies normal plasma cell death. Much more needs to be learned, but this finding suggests new avenues for modulating MM cell survival in the bone marrow. Collectively, the recent advances in cell-cycle control and apoptosis in primary plasma cells suggest that a thorough investigation of these processes in primary MM cells in the bone microenvironment, at the molecular level and in the context of clinical outcome, will give new insights into myeloma pathogenesis and therapeutic design.

# Acknowledgments

The author thanks Drs. Josie Ursini-Siegel, Eunice Hatada, Maurizio DiLiberto, Xiangao Huang, and Lin Kang for helpful discussions and Dr. Beth Schachter for critical reading of the manuscript. The work was supported by grants from NIH (CA80204, AR49436) and a SCOR grant from the Leukemia and Lymphoma Society of America.

## REFERENCES

Ahmed, R., and Gray, D. (1996). Immunological memory and protective immunity: understanding their relation. *Science, 272,* 54–60.

Altmeyer, A., Simmons, R. C., Krajewski, S., Reed, J. C., Bornkamm, G. W., and Chen-Kiang, S. (1997). Reversal of EBV immortalization precedes apoptosis in IL-6-induced human B cell terminal differentiation. *Immunity, 7,* 667–677.

Ashkenazi, A., and Dixit, V. M. (1998). Death receptors: signaling and modulation. *Science, 281,* 1305–1308.

Ashkenazi, A., Pai, R. C., Fong, S., Leung, S., Lawrence, D. A., Marsters, S. A., Blackie, C., Chang, L., McMurtrey, A. E., Hebert, A., et al. (1999). Safety and antitumor activity of recombinant soluble Apo2 ligand. *Journal of Clinical Investigation, 104,* 155–162.

Bai, F., Pei, X. H., Godfrey, V. L., and Xiong, Y. (2003). Haploinsufficiency of p18(INK4c) sensitizes mice to carcinogen-induced tumorigenesis. *Molecular Cell Biology, 23,* 1269–1277.

Balazs, M., Martin, F., Zhou, T., and Kearney, J. (2002). Blood dendritic cells interact with splenic marginal zone B cells to initiate T-independent immune responses. *Immunity, 17,* 341–352.

Banchereau, J., Bazan, F., Blanchard, D., Briere, F., Galizzi, J. P., van Kooten, C., Liu, Y. J., and Saeland, R. S. (1994). The CD40 antigen and its ligand. *Annual Review of Immunology, 12,* 881–922.

Batten, M., Groom, J., Cachero, T. G., Qian, F., Schneider, P., Tschopp, J., Browning, J. L., and Mackay, F. (2000). BAFF mediates survival of peripheral immature B lymphocytes. *Journal of Experimental Medicine, 192,* 1453–1466.

Bodmer, J. L., Holler, N., Reynard, S., Vinciguerra, P., Schneider, P., Juo, P., Blenis, J., and Tschopp, J. (2000). TRAIL receptor-2 signals apoptosis through FADD and caspase-8. *Nature Cell Biology, 2,* 241–243.

Calame, K. L., Lin, K. I., and Tunyaplin, C. (2003). Regulatory mechanisms that determine the development and function of plasma cells. *Annual Review of Immunology, 21,* 205–230.

Calfon, M., Zeng, H., Urano, F., Till, J. H., Hubbard, S. R., Harding, H. P., Clark, S. G., and Ron, D. (2002). IRE1 couples endoplasmic reticulum load to secretory capacity by processing the XBP-1 mRNA. *Nature, 415,* 92–96.

Catlett-Falcone, R., Landowski, T. H., Oshiro, M. M., Turkson, J., Levitzki, A., Savino, R., Ciliberto, G., Moscinski, L., Fernandez-Luna, J. L., Nunez, G., et al. (1999). Constitutive activation of Stat3 signaling confers resistance to apoptosis in human U266 myeloma cells. *Immunity, 10,* 105–115.

Chan, F. K., Zhang, J., Cheng, L., Shapiro, D. N., and Winoto, A. (1995). Identification of human and mouse p19, a novel CDK4 and CDK6 inhibitor with homology to p16ink4. *Molecular Cell Biology, 15,* 2682–2688.

Cheng, M., Olivier, P., Diehl, J. A., Fero, M., Roussel, M. F., Roberts, J. M., and Sherr, C. J. (1999). The p21(Cip1) and p27(Kip1) CDK 'inhibitors' are essential activators of cyclin D-dependent kinases in murine fibroblasts. *Embo Journal, 18,* 1571–1583.

Chesi, M., Bergsagel, P. L., Brents, L. A., Smith, C. M., Gerhard, D. S., and Kuehl, W. M. (1996). Dysregulation of cyclin D1 by translocation into an IgH gamma switch region in two multiple myeloma cell lines. *Blood, 88,* 674–681.

Claudio, E., Brown, K., Park, S., Wang, H., and Siebenlist, U. (2002). BAFF-induced NEMO-independent processing of NF-kappaB2 in maturing B cells. *Nature Immunology, 3,* 958–965.

Cory, S. (1995). Regulation of lymphocyte survival by the Bcl-2 gene family. *Annual Review of Immunology, 13,* 513–543.

Derenne, S., Monica, B., Dean, N. M., Taylor, J. K., Rapp, M. J., Harousseau, J. L., Bataille, R., and Amiot, M. (2002). Antisense strategy shows that Mcl-1 rather than Bcl-2 or Bcl-x(L) is an essential survival protein of human myeloma cells. *Blood, 100,* 194–199.

Do, R. K., and Chen-Kiang, S. (2002). Mechanism of BLyS action in B cell immunity. *Cytokine Growth Factor Review, 13,* 19–25.

Do, R. K., Hatada, E., Lee, H., Tourigny, M. R., Hilbert, D., and Chen-Kiang, S. (2000). Attenuation of apoptosis underlies B lymphocyte stimulator enhancement of humoral immune response. *Journal of Experimental Medicine, 192,* 953–964.

Drexler, H. G. (1998). Review of alterations of the cyclin-dependent kinase inhibitor INK4 family genes p15, p16, p18 and p19 in human leukemia-lymphoma cells. *Leukemia, 12,* 845–859.

Fero, M. L., Rivkin, M., Tasch, M., Porter, P., Carow, C. E., Firpo, E., Polyak, K., Tsai, L. H., Broudy, V., Perlmutter, R. M., et al. (1996). A syndrome of multiorgan hyperplasia with features of gigantism, tumorigenesis, and female sterility in p27(Kip1)-deficient mice. *Cell, 85,* 733–744.

Franklin, D. S., Godfrey, V. L., Lee, H., Kovalev, G. I., Schoonhoven, R., Chen-Kiang, S., Su, L., and Xiong, Y. (1998). CDK inhibitors p18(INK4c) and p27(Kip1) mediate two separate pathways to collaboratively suppress pituitary tumorigenesis. *Genes and Development, 12,* 2899–2911.

Garrone, P., Neidhardt, E.-M., Garcia, E., Galibert, L., van Kooten, C., and Banchereau, J. (1995). Fas ligation induces apoptosis of CD40-activated human B lymphocytes. *Journal of Experimental Medicine, 182,* 1265–1273.

Grillot, D. A., Merino, R., Pena, J. C., Fanslow, W. C., Finkelman, F. D., Thompson, C. B., and Nunez, G. (1996). Bcl-x exhibits regulated expression during B cell development and activation and modulates lymphocyte survival in transgenic mice. *Journal of Experimental Medicine, 183,* 381–391.

Gross, J. A., Dillon, S. R., Mudri, S., Johnston, J., Littau, A., Roque, R., Rixon, M., Schou, O., Foley, K. P., Haugen, H., et al. (2001). Taci-ig neutralizes molecules critical for b cell development and autoimmune disease. Impaired B cell maturation in mice lacking blys. *Immunity, 15,* 289–302.

Gross, J. A., Johnston, J., Mudri, S., Enselman, R., Dillon, S. R., Madden, K., Xu, W., Parrish-Novak, J., Foster, D., Lofton-Day, C., et al. (2000). TACI and BCMA are receptors for a TNF homologue implicated in B-cell autoimmune disease. *Nature, 404,* 995–999.

Guan, K.-L., Jenkins, C. W., Li, Y., Nichols, M. A., Wu, X., O'Keefe, C. L., Matera, A. G., and Xiong, Y. (1994). Growth suppression by p18$^{INK4C}$, a p16$^{INK4A/MTS1}$ and p14$^{INK4B/MTS2}$-related CDK inhibitor, correlates with wild-type pRb function. *Gene and Development, 8,* 2939–2952.

Guan, K. L., Jenkins, C. W., Li, Y., O'Keefe, C. L., Noh, S., Wu, X., Zariwal, A. G., and Xiong, Y. (1996). Isolation and characterization of p19INK4d, a p16-related inhibitor specific to CDK6 and CDK4. *Molecular Biology of the Cell, 7,* 57–70.

Harless, S. M., Lentz, V. M., Sah, A. P., Hsu, B. L., Clise-Dwyer, K., Hilbert, D. M., Hayes, C. E., and Cancro, M. P. (2001). Competition for BLyS-mediated signaling through Bcmd/BR3 regulates peripheral B lymphocyte numbers. *Current Biology, 11,* 1986–1989.

Harper, J. W., Adami, G. R., Wei, N., Keyomarsi, K., and Elledge, S. J. (1993). The p21 Cdk-interacting protein Cip1 is a potent inhibitor of G1 cyclin-dependent kinases. *Cell, 75,* 850–866.

Hatada, E., Do, R. K., Orlofsky, A., Liou, H.-C., Prystowsky, M., MacLennan, I. C. M., Caamano, J., and Chen-Kiang, S. (2003). NF-κB1 p50 is required for BLyS attenuation of apoptosis but dispensable for processing of NF-κB2 p100 to p52 in quiescent mature B cells. *Journal of Immunology.*

Hilbert, D. M., Kopf, M., Mock, B. A., Kohler, G., and Rudikoff, S. (1995). Interleukin 6 is essential for in vivo development of B lineage neoplasms. *Journal of Experimental Medicine, 182,* 243–248.

Hirai, H., Roussel, M. F., Kato, J. Y., Ashmun, R. A., and Sherr, C. J. (1995). Novel INK4 proteins, p19 and p18, are specific inhibitors of the cyclin D-dependent kinases CDK4 and CDK6. *Molecular and Cellular Biology, 15,* 2672–2681.

Ho, F., Lortan, J. E., MacLennan, I. C. M., and Khan, M. (1986). Distinct short-lived and long-lived antibody-producing cell populations. *European Journal of Immunology, 16,* 1297–1301.

Huard, B., Schneider, P., Mauri, D., Tschopp, J., and French, L. E. (2001). T cell costimulation by the TNF ligand BAFF. *Journal of Immunology, 167,* 6225–6231.

Hunter, T., and Pines, J. (1994). Cyclins and cancer II: cyclin D and Cdk inhibitors come of age. *Cell, 79,* 573–582.

Iwakoshi, N. N., Lee, A. H., Vallabhajosyula, P., Otipoby, K. L., Rajewsky, K., and Glimcher, L. H. (2003). Plasma cell differentiation and the unfolded protein response intersect at the transcription factor XBP-1. *Nature Immunology, 4,* 321–329.

Jacob, J., Przylepa, J., Miller, C., and Kelsoe, G. (1993). In situ studies of the primary immune response to (4-hydroxy-3-nitrophenyl) acetyl. III. The kinetics of V region mutation and selection in germinal center B cells. *Journal of Experimental Medicine, 178,* 1293–1307.

Jego, G., Bataille, R., and Pellat-Deceunynck, C. (2001). Interleukin-6 is a growth factor for nonmalignant human plasmablasts. *Blood, 97,* 1817–1822.

Kayagaki, N., Yan, M., Seshasayee, D., Wang, H., Lee, W., French, D. M., Grewal, I. S., Cochran, A. G., Gordon, N. C., Yin, J., et al. (2002). BAFF/BLyS receptor 3 binds the B cell survival factor BAFF ligand through a discrete surface loop and promotes processing of NF-kappaB2. *Immunity, 17,* 515–524.

Kischkel, F. C., Lawrence, D. A., Chuntharapai, A., Schow, P., Kim, K. J., and Ashkenazi, A. (2000). Apo2L/TRAIL-dependent recruitment of endogenous FADD and caspase-8 to death receptors 4 and 5. *Immunity, 12,* 611–620.

Kiyokawa, H., Kineman, R. D., Manova-Todorova, K. O., Soares, V. C., Hoffman, E. S., Ono, M., Khanam, D., Hayday, A. C., Frohman, L. A., and Koff, A. (1996). Enhanced growth of mice lacking the cyclin-dependent kinase inhibitor function of p27^Kip1. *Cell, 85,* 721–732.

Kopf, M., Baumann, H., Freer, G., Freudenberg, M., Lamers, M., Kishimoto, T., Zinkernagel, R., Bluethmann, H., and Kohler, G. (1994). Impaired immune and acute-phase responses in interleukin-6-deficient mice. *Nature, 368,* 339–342.

Krammer, P. H., Dhein, J., Walczak, H., Behrmann, I., Mariani, S., Matiba, B., Fath, M., Daniel, P. T., Knipping, E., Westendorf, M. O., et al. (1994). The role of APO 1-mediated apoptosis in the immune system. *Immunological Reviews, 142,* 175–191.

Kulkarni, M. S., Daggett, J. L., Bender, T. P., Kuehl, W. M., Bergsagel, P. L., and Williams, M. E. (2002). Frequent inactivation of the cyclin-dependent kinase inhibitor p18 by homozygous deletion in multiple myeloma cell lines: ectopic p18 expression inhibits growth and induces apoptosis. *Leukemia, 16,* 127–134.

Lacey, D. L. T. E., Tan, H.-L., Kelley, M. J., Dunstan, C. R., Burgess, T., Elliott, R., Colombero, A., Elliott, G., Scully, S., Hsu, H., Sullivan, J., Hawkins, N., Davy, E., Capparelli, C., Eli, A., Qian, Y.-X., Kaufman, S., Sarosi, I., Shalhoub, V., Senaldi, G., Guo, J., Delaney, J., and Boyle, W. J. (1998). Osteoprotegerin ligand is a cytokine that regulates osteoclast differentiation and activation. *Cell, 93,* 165–176.

Lam, E. W., Glassford, J., Banerji, L., Thomas, N. S., Sicinski, P., and Klaus, G. G. (2000). Cyclin D3 compensates for loss of cyclin D2 in mouse B-lymphocytes activated via the antigen receptor and CD40. *Journal of Biological Chemistry, 275,* 3479–3484.

Latres, E., Malumbres, M., Sotillo, R., Martin, J., Ortega, S., Martin-Caballero, J., Flores, J. M., Cordon-Cardo, C., and Barbacid, M. (2000). Limited overlapping roles of P15(INK4b) and P18(INK4c) cell cycle inhibitors in proliferation and tumorigenesis. *Embo Journal, 19,* 3496–3506.

Lincz, L. F., Yeh, T. X., and Spencer, A. (2001). TRAIL-induced eradication of primary tumour cells from multiple myeloma patient bone marrows is not related to TRAIL receptor expression or prior chemotherapy. *Leukemia, 15,* 1650–1657.

Liu, Q., El-Deiry, W. S., and Gazitt, Y. (2001). Additive effect of Apo2L/TRAIL and Adeno-p53 in the induction of apoptosis in myeloma cell lines. *Experimental Hematology, 29,* 962–970.

Liu, Y. J., and Banchereau, J. (1997). Regulation of B-cell commitment to plasma cells or to memory B cells. *Seminars in Immunology, 9,* 235–240.

Liu, Y. J., Zhang, J., Lane, P. J., Chan, E. Y., and MacLennan, I. C. (1991). Sites of specific B cell activation in primary and secondary responses to T cell-dependent and T cell-independent antigens. *European Journal of Immunology, 21,* 2951–2962.

Manz, R. A., Thiel, A., and Radbruch, A. (1997). Lifetime of plasma cells in the bone marrow [Letter]. *Nature, 388,* 133–134.

McDonnell, T. J., Deane, N., Platt, F. M., Nunez, G., Jaeger, U., McKearn, J. P., and Korsmeyer, S. J. (1989). Bcl-2-immunoglobulin transgenic mice demonstrate extended B cell survival and follicular lymphoproliferation. *Cell, 57,* 79–88.

Mitsiades, C. S., Treon, S. P., Mitsiades, N., Shima, Y., Richardson, P., Schlossman, R., Hideshima, T., and Anderson, K. C. (2001). TRAIL/Apo2L ligand selectively induces apoptosis and overcomes drug resistance in multiple myeloma: therapeutic applications. *Blood, 98,* 795–804.

Mitsiades, N., Mitsiades, C. S., Poulaki, V., Chauhan, D., Richardson, P. G., Hideshima, T., Munshi, N., Treon, S. P., and Anderson, K. C. (2002). Biologic sequelae of nuclear factor-kappaB blockade in multiple myeloma: therapeutic applications. *Blood, 99,* 4079–4086.

Moore, P. A., Belvedere, O., Orr, A., Pieri, K., LaFleur, D. W., Feng, P., Soppet, D., Charters, M., Gentz, R., Parmelee, D., et al. (1999). BLyS: member of the tumor necrosis factor family and B lymphocyte stimulator. *Science, 285,* 260–263.

Morse, L., Chen, D., Franklin, D., Xiong, Y., and Chen-Kiang, S. (1997). Induction of cell cycle arrest and B cell terminal differentiation by CDK inhibitor p18(INK4c) and IL-6. *Immunity, 6,* 47–56.

Mullins, M. W., Pittner, B. T., and Snow, E. C. (1998). CD40-mediated induction of p21 accumulation in resting and cycling B cells. *Molecular Immunology, 35,* 567–580.

Nagata, S. (1997). Apoptosis by death factor. *Cell, 88,* 355–365.

Nakayama, K., Ishida, N., Shirane, M., Inomata, A., Inoue, T., Shishido, N., Horii, I., and Loh, D. Y. (1996). Mice lacking p27(Kip1) display increased body size, multiple organ hyperplasia, retinal dysplasia, and pituitary tumors. *Cell, 85,* 707–720.

Natkunam, Y., Zhang, X., Liu, Z., and Chen-Kiang, S. (1994). Simultaneous activation of Ig and Oct-2 synthesis and reduction of surface MHC class II expression by IL-6. *Journal of Immunology, 153,* 3476–3484.

Ng, M. H., Chung, Y. F., Lo, K. W., Wickham, N. W., Lee, J. C., and Huang, D. P. (1997). Frequent hypermethylation of p16 and p15 genes in multiple myeloma. *Blood, 89,* 2500–2506.

Nordan, R. P., and Potter, M. (1986). A macrophage-derived factor required by plasmacytomas for survival and proliferation in vitro. *Science, 233,* 566–569.

O'Connor, B. P., Cascalho, M., and Noelle, R. J. (2002). Short-lived and long-lived bone marrow plasma cells are derived from a novel precursor population. *Journal of Experimental Medicine, 195,* 737–745.

Piskurich, J. F., Lin, K. I., Lin, Y., Wang, Y., Ting, J. P., and Calame, K. (2000). BLIMP-I mediates extinction of major histocompatibility class II transactivator expression in plasma cells. *Nature Immunology, 1,* 526–532.

Pitti, R. M., Marsters, S. A., Ruppert, S., Donahue, C. J., Moore, A., and Ashkenazi, A. (1996). Induction of apoptosis by Apo-2 ligand, a new member of the tumor necrosis factor cytokine family. *Journal of Biological Chemistry, 271,* 12687–12690.

Ramsay, A. J., Husband, A. J., Ramshaw, I. A., Bao, S., Matthaei, K. I., Koehler, G., and Kopf, M. (1994). The role of interleukin-6 in mucosal IgA antibody responses in vivo. *Science, 264,* 561–563.

Rathmell, J. C., Cooke, M. P., Ho, W. Y., Grein, J., Townsend, S. E., Davis, M. M., and Goodnow, C. C. (1995). CD95 (Fas)-dependent elimination of self-reactive B cells upon interaction with CD4 + T cells. *Nature, 376,* 181–184.

Rathmell, J. C., Townsend, S. E., Xu, J. C., Flavell, R. A., and Goodnow, C. C. (1996). Expansion or elimination of B cells in vivo: dual roles for CD40– and Fas (CD95)-ligands modulated by the B cell antigen receptor. *Cell, 87,* 319–329.

Rawstron, A. C., Fenton, J. A., Ashcroft, J., English, A., Jones, R. A., Richards, S. J., Pratt, G., Owen, R., Davies, F. E., Child, J. A., et al. (2000). The interleukin-6 receptor alpha-chain (CD126) is expressed by neoplastic but not normal plasma cells. *Blood, 96,* 3880–3886.

Reimold, A. M., Iwakoshi, N. N., Manis, J., Vallabhajosyula, P., Szomolanyi-Tsuda, E., Gravallese, E. M., Friend, D., Grusby, M. J., Alt, F., and Glimcher, L. H. (2001). Plasma cell differentiation requires the transcription factor XBP-1. *Nature, 412,* 300–307.

Rolink, A. G., and Melchers, F. (2002). BAFFled B cells survive and thrive: roles of BAFF in B-cell development. *Current Opinions in Immunology, 14,* 266–275.

Rothstein, T. L., Wang, J. K. M., Panka, D. J., Foote, L. C., Wang, Z., Stanger, B., Cui, H., Ju, S.-T., and Marshak-Rothstein, A. (1995). Protection against Fas-dependent Th1-mediated apoptosis by antigen receptor engagement in B cells. *Nature, 374,* 163–165.

Sanderson, R. D., Lalor, P., and Bernfield, M. (1989). B lymphocytes express and lose syndecan at specific stages of differentiation. *Cell Regulation, 1,* 27–35.

Schattner, E. J., Elkon, K. B., Yoo, D.-H., Tumang, J., Krammer, P. H., Crow, M. K., and Friedman, S. M. (1995). CD40 ligation induces Apo-1/Fas expression on human B lymphocytes and facilitates apoptosis through the Apo-1/Fas pathway. *Journal of Experimental Medicine, 182,* 1557–1565.

Schiemann, B., Gommerman, J. L., Vora, K., Cachero, T. G., Shulga-Morskaya, S., Dobles, M., Frew, E., and Scott, M. L. (2001). An essential role for BAFF in the normal development of B cells through a BCMA-independent pathway. *Science, 293,* 2111–2114.

Schneider, P., MacKay, F., Steiner, V., Hofmann, K., Bodmer, J. L., Holler, N., Ambrose, C., Lawton, P., Bixler, S., Acha-Orbea, H., et al. (1999). BAFF, a novel ligand of the tumor necrosis factor family, stimulates B cell growth. *Journal of Experimental Medicine, 189,* 1747–1756.

Shain, K. H., Landowski, T. H., Buyuksai, I., Cantor, A. B., and Dalton, W. S. (2000). Clona variability in CD95 expression is a major determinant in Fas-mediated, but not chemotherapy-mediated apoptosis in the RPMI 8226 multiple myeloma cell line. *Leukemia, 14,* 830–840.

Shaughnessy, J., Jr., Gabrea, A., Qi, Y., Brents, L., Zhan, F., Tian, E., Sawyer, J., Barlogie, B., Bergsagel, P. L., and Kuehl, M. (2001). Cyclin D3 at 6p21 is dysregulated by recurrent chromosomal translocations to immunoglobulin loci in multiple myeloma. *Blood, 98,* 217–223.

Sherr, C. J., and Roberts, J. M. (1999). CDK inhibitors: positive and negative regulators of G1-phase progression. *Genes and Development, 13,* 1501–1512.

Shipman, C. M., and Croucher, P. I. (2003). Osteoprotegerin is a soluble decoy receptor for tumor necrosis factor-related apoptosis-inducing ligand/Apo2 ligand and can function as a paracrine survival factor for human myeloma cells. *Cancer Research, 63,* 912–916.

Simonet, W. S., Lacey, D.L., Dunstan, C. R., Kelley, M. J., Chang, M. S., Luthy, R., Nguyen, H. Q., Wooden, S., Bennett, L., Boone, T., Shimamoto, G., DeRose, M., Elliott, R., Colombero, A., Tan, H.-L., Trail, G., Sullivan, J., Davy, E., Bucay, N., Renshaw-Gegg, L., Hughes, T. M., Hill, D., Pattison, W., Campbell, P., Sander, S., Van, G., Tarpley, J., Derby, P., Lee, R., Amgen EST Program, and Boyle, W. J. (1997). Osteoprotegerin: a novel secreted protein involved in the regulation of bone density. *Cell, 89,* 309–319.

Slifka, M. K., Antia, R., Whitmire, J. K., and Ahmed, R. (1998). Humoral immunity due to long-lived plasma cells. *Immunity, 8,* 363–372.

Smith, K. G., Light, A., Nossal, G. J., and Tarlinton, D. M. (1997). The extent of affinity maturation differs between the memory and antibody-forming cell compartments in the primary immune response. *Embo Journal, 16,* 2996–3006.

Sneed, T. B., Stanley, D. J., Young, L. A., and Sanderson, R. D. (1994). Interleukin-6 regulates expression of the syndecan-1 proteoglycan on B lymphoid cells. *Cellular Immunology, 153,* 456–467.

Solvason, N., Wu, W. W., Kabra, N., Wu, X., Lees, E., and Howard, M. C. (1996). Induction of cell cycle regulatory proteins in anti-immunoglobulin-stimulated mature B lymphocytes. *Journal of Experimental Medicine, 184,* 407–417.

Sprick, M. R., Weigand, M. A., Rieser, E., Rauch, C. T., Juo, P., Blenis, J., Krammer, P. H., and Walczak, H. (2000). FADD/MORT1 and caspase-8 are recruited to TRAIL receptors 1 and 2 and are essential for apoptosis mediated by TRAIL receptor 2. *Immunity, 12,* 599–609.

Tai, Y. T., Podar, K., Gupta, D., Lin, B., Young, G., Akiyama, M., and Anderson, K. C. (2002). CD40 activation induces p53-dependent vascular endothelial growth factor secretion in human multiple myeloma cells. *Blood, 99,* 1419–1427.

Tai, Y. T., Podar, K., Mitsiades, N., Lin, B., Mitsiades, C., Gupta, D., Akiyama, M., Catley, L., Hideshima, T., Munshi, N. C., et al. (2003). CD40 induces human multiple myeloma cell migration via phosphatidylinositol 3-kinase/AKT/NF-kappa B signaling. *Blood, 101,* 2762–2769.

Tanguay, D., Pavlovic, S., Piatelli, M. J., Bartek, J., and Chiles, T. C. (1999). B cell antigen receptor-mediated activation of cyclin-dependent retinoblastoma protein kinases and inhibition by co-cross-linking with Fc gamma receptors. *Journal of Immunology, 163,* 3160–3168.

Tanguay, D. A., and Chiles, T. C. (1996). Regulation of the catalytic subunit (p34PSK-J3Cdk4) for the major D-type cyclin in mature B cells. *Journal of Immunology, 156,* 539–548.

Tasaka, T., Asou, H., Munker, R., Said, J. W., Berenson, J., Vescio, R. A., Nagai, M., Takahara, J., and Koeffler, H. P. (1998). Methylation of the p16INK4A gene in multiple myeloma. *British Journal of Haematology, 101,* 558–564.

Tasaka, T., Berenson, J., Vescio, R., Hirama, T., Miller, C. W., Nagai, M., Takahara, J., and Koeffler, H. P. (1997). Analysis of the p16INK4A, p15INK4B and p18INK4C genes in multiple myeloma. *British Journal of Haematology, 96,* 98–102.

Tong, A. W., Seamour, B., Chen, J., Su, D., Ordonez, G., Frase, L., Netto, G., and Stone, M. J. (2000). CD40 ligand-induced apoptosis is Fas-independent in human multiple myeloma cells. *Leukemia Lymphoma, 36,* 543–558.

Tourigny, M. R., Ursini-Siegel, J., Lee, H., Toellner, K. M., Cunningham, A. F., Franklin, D. S., Ely, S., Chen, M., Qin, X. F., Xiong, Y., et al. (2002). CDK inhibitor p18(INK4c) is required for the generation of functional plasma cells. *Immunity, 17,* 179–189.

Turner, C. A., Jr., Mack, D. H., and Davis, M. M. (1994). Blimp-1, a novel zinc finger-containing protein that can drive the maturation of B lymphocytes into immunoglobulin-secreting cells. *Cell, 77,* 297–306.

Urashima, M., Chauhan, D., Uchiyama, H., Freeman, G. J., and Anderson, K. C. (1995). CD40 Ligand triggered interleukin-6 secretion in multiple myeloma. *Blood, 85,* 1903–1912.

Ursini-Siegel, J., Zhang, W., Altmeyer, A., Hatada, E. N., Do, R. K., Yagita, H., and Chen-Kiang, S. (2002). TRAIL/Apo-2 ligand induces primary plasma cell apoptosis. *Journal of Immunology, 169,* 5505–5513.

Walczak, H., Miller, R. E., Ariail, K., Gliniak, B., Griffith, T. S., Kubin, M., Chin, W., Jones, J., Woodward, A., Le, T., et al. (1999). Tumoricidal activity of tumor necrosis factor-related apoptosis-inducing ligand in vivo. *Nature Medicine, 5,* 157–163.

Weinberg, R. A. (1995). The retinoblastoma protein and cell cycle control. *Cell, 81,* 323–330.

Wiley, S. R., Schooley, K., Smolak, P. J., Din, W. S., Huang, C. P., Nicholl, J. K., Sutherland, G. R., Smith, T. D., Rauch, C., and Smith, C. A. (1995). Identification and characterization of a new member of the TNF family that induces apoptosis. *Immunity, 3,* 673–682.

Xiong, Y., Hannon, G. J., Zhang, H., Casso, D., Kobayashi, R., and Beach, D. (1993). p21 is a universal inhibitor of cyclin kinases. *Nature, 366,* 701–704.

Yan, M., Brady, J. R., Chan, B., Lee, W. P., Hsu, B., Harless, S., Cancro, M., Grewal, I. S., and Dixit, V. M. (2001). Identification of a novel receptor for B lymphocyte stimulator that is mutated in a mouse strain with severe B cell deficiency. *Current Biology, 11,* 1547–1552.

Yoshida, H., Matsui, T., Yamamoto, A., Okada, T., and Mori, K. (2001). XBP1 mRNA is induced by ATF6 and spliced by IRE1 in response to ER stress to produce a highly active transcription factor. *Cell, 107,* 881–891.

Zhang, B., Potyagaylo, V., and Fenton, R. G. (2003). IL-6-independent expression of Mcl-1 in human multiple myeloma. *Oncogene, 22,* 1848–1859.

Zhang, S., Ramsay, E. S., and Mock, B. A. (1998). Cdkn2a, the cyclin-dependent kinase inhibitor encoding p16INK4a and p19ARF, is a candidate for the plasmacytoma susceptibility locus, Pctr1. *Proceeding of the National Academy of Science of the United States of America, 95,* 2429–2434.

Zhang, S. L., DuBois, W., Ramsay, E. S., Bliskovski, V., Morse, H. C. III, Taddesse-Heath, L., Vass, W. C., DePinho, R. A., and Mock, B. A. (2001). Efficiency alleles of the Pctr1 modifier locus for plasmacytoma susceptibility. *Molecular and Cellular Biology, 21,* 310–318.

# CHAPTER 3

# The Molecular Biology of Multiple Myeloma

P. LEIF BERGSAGEL

W. MICHAEL KUEHL

## Introduction

Multiple myeloma is an incurable plasma cell (PC) malignancy with a yearly incidence of 5.6 per 100,000 individuals (or approximately 1% of all malignancies). The rate increases dramatically with age: it is 2 (per 100,000) in the population under 65 and 30 in those 65 and older. In the United States in 1999 it is estimated that there were 13,700 new patients diagnosed and 10,565 deaths from multiple myeloma (MM). The incidence is twofold higher in African-American than Caucasians, with a significantly higher incidence in males for each population (Ries et al., 2002). The roles of genetic background and environment are poorly defined, although there is suggestive evidence of some clustering within families (Lynch et al., 2001). The hallmarks of MM are a monoclonal Ig (M-protein) by serum electrophoresis or a urinary Ig L chain (Bence Jones protein), a content of >10% PC distributed at multiple foci in the bone marrow (BM), and bone resorption ranging from mild osteoporosis to multiple lytic lesions. The malignant PC secretes IgG (60%), IgA (20%), IgD (2%), free light chain (17%), or no Ig (1%), but rarely IgE or IgM (Chapter 9).

# Multiple Myeloma Is a Low Proliferative Tumor of Postgerminal Center Plasma Cells (Fig. 3-1)

Three B cell-specific DNA remodeling mechanisms that modify Ig genes are involved at different stages of B cell development (Kuppers et al., 1999): VDJ recombination, somatic hypermutation, and IgH switch recombination. Following sequential and regulated VDJ recombination, immature B cells that express functional surface IgM exit the bone marrow and home to secondary lymphoid tissues as mature B cells. Productive interaction of mature B cells with antigen results in proliferation and differentiation. The primary immune response generates pregerminal center plasma cells that typically are short-lived, and usually secrete IgM but can secrete other Ig isotypes as a result of IgH switch recombination (Calame, 2001; MacLennan, 1998; Sze et al., 2000). *Germinal centers* are generated during the primary immune response. Antigen-activated lymphoblasts that enter a germinal center are subjected to multiple rounds of somatic hypermutation of IgH and IgL V(D)J sequences and antigen selection. Cells expressing high-affinity antigen receptors are selected for survival, with subsequent differentiation to memory B cells or postgerminal center plasma cells. Postgerminal center plasmablasts/plasma cells, including those generated from memory B cells, that undergo IgH switch recombination, typically home to the bone marrow where they reside as terminally differentiated, nonproliferating long-lived plasma cells for >30 days but sometimes years.

Nearly 80% of B cell tumors arise from germinal-center or postgerminal center B cells, indicating that the intrinsic genetic instability of B cells that is unleashed in the germinal center is important for their development. Although somatic hypermutation can cause mutations in some non-Ig genes (Kuppers and Dalla-Favera, 2001; Pasqualucci et al., 2001), it is unclear if the germinal center environment is responsible for any oncogenetic changes other than primary Ig translocations. Multiple myeloma cells are the transformed counterparts of postgerminal center bone marrow plasmablast/plasma cells (Bergsagel and Kuehl, 1998; Klein et al., 1995).

## Stages of Multiple Myeloma

Plasma cell neoplasms are distinguished by an idiotypic rearrangement of immunoglobulin genes. The clone that develops must increase to approximately $5 \times 10^8$ cells before it produces enough of the idiotypic immunoglobulin to be recognized as a monoclonal "spike" (M-protein) in a serum electrophoresis pattern. Most subjects with a serum M-protein are asymptomatic; if other causes of an M-protein can be ruled out, they are labeled as *monoclonal gammopathies of undetermined significance* (MGUS). By definition the clone in MGUS is stable and the serum M-protein concentration remains level for many years. However, prolonged followup of a large group of MGUS subjects at the Mayo Clinic has shown that approximately 1% of patients with non-IgM MGUS progress per year to develop symptomatic multiple myeloma (MM). In fact, this rate of progression varies from 0.6% to 3% per year as the level of the M-spike increases, a result that suggests the probability of progression is directly related to the number of MGUS tumor cells (Kyle et al., 2002). MGUS is considered to be a premalignant lesion

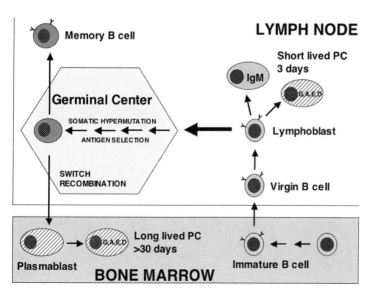

**Figure 3-1** *Normal PC development. Functional V(D)J rearrangements of IgH and IgL genes in pre-B cells in the BM generate an immature B cell that expresses a functional immunoglobulin on the cell surface, which then exits the BM as a virgin (mature) B cell and homes to the secondary lymphoid tissues. Early in the immune response productive interaction with antigen stimulates formation of a lymphoblast, which differentiates into a short-lived nonswitched (IgM) or switched (IgG, IgA, IgE, or IgD) PC. Later in the primary response or in a secondary response, the lymphoblast generated by productive interaction with antigen enters a germinal center, where it undergoes somatic hypermutation of its IgH and IgL genes, and antigen selection of cells with high-affinity Ig receptor. A germinal center plasmablast that undergoes productive IgH switch recombination typically homes to the BM where it differentiates into a long-lived PC (cf. MM cell).*

*Figure 3-2* Stages of multiple myeloma. This diagram depicts the linear progression of multiple myeloma, starting from a normal germinal center B cell. It appears that at least 30% to 50% of malignant multiple myeloma arises from the benign plasma cell neoplasm MGUS (Kyle, 1994). It does not always pass through a period of smoldering myeloma. Initially, multiple myeloma is confined to the bone marrow (intramedullary), but with time the tumor might acquire the ability to grow in extramedullary locations (blood, pleural fluid, skin, and so on). Some of these extramedullary multiple myelomas can establish immortalized cell lines in vitro. The transition of MGUS to intramedullary multiple myeloma is manifested by increased tumor mass at multiple foci, but also associated angiogenesis and osteolytic bone destruction.

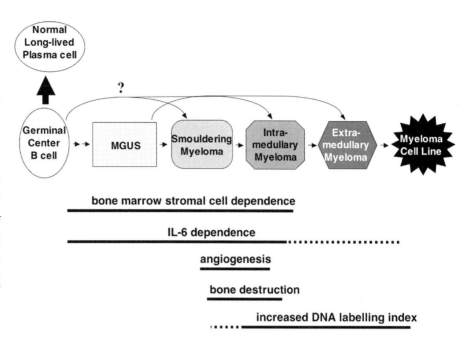

because the clone does not grow progressively, but is stable and asymptomatic. Almost all of the genetic aberrations identified in MM (aneuploidy, monosomy 13, 14q32 chromosome translocations) are also present in MGUS (Avet-Loiseau et al., 1999b). Additional neoplastic changes are required to convert this large, stable clone into MM, a progressively expanding tumor with malignant characteristics.

*Amyloidosis*, which accounts for approximately 4000 deaths per year in the United States, usually has the same pathology as MGUS except that the monoclonal Ig (generally the intact or fragmented Ig light chain) forms pathologic deposits in various tissues (Hayman et al., 2001). Multiple myeloma is distinguished from MGUS by having a greater intramedullary (i.e., within the bone marrow) tumor cell content (>10%), osteolytic bone lesions, and/or an increasing tumor mass. *Smoldering myeloma* has a stable intramedullary tumor cell content of >10% but no osteolytic lesions or other complications of malignant MM. At least 30% to 50% of patients with MM progress from a preceding MGUS, and there is not always a recognizable smoldering stage (Kyle, 1994). Although it has been proposed that MM can arise *de novo* without passing through the MGUS stage, there is no convincing evidence that this occurs at a significant frequency (Avet-Loiseau et al., 1999d, 2002). In fact, Figure 3-2 attempts to illustrate that a linear progression connecting the major stages might be bypassed in a variety of ways, as indicated by a question mark and alternative arrows. Progression of *intramedullary myeloma* is associated with increasingly severe secondary features

(lytic bone lesions, anemia, immunodeficiency, renal impairment) and in a fraction of patients the occurrence of tumor in extramedullary locations. *Extramedullary myeloma* is a more aggressive tumor that often is called secondary or primary plasma cell leukemia, depending on whether preceding intramedullary myeloma has been recognized. Human multiple myeloma cell lines (HMCL) can sometimes be generated, but usually only from extramedullary tumors. Although HMCL might not precisely reflect the incidence of genetic abnormalities found in *in vivo* tumors, they might still be viewed as the ultimate stage of tumor progression. Multiple myeloma is a low proliferative tumor. The *plasma cell labeling index*, typically detecting less than 1% of tumor cells actively synthesizing DNA until late in the disease, is a better prognostic indicator than the tumor cell content in the bone marrow (Rajkumar et al., 1999).

## Overview of Oncogenic Changes Found in Tumors

Cancer is an acquired genetic disease that rarely might involve only a single genetic change (e.g., the t[9;22] translocation that creates a bcr-abl fusion protein, which inhibits the normal differentiation process in chronic myelogenous leukemia) (Druker, 2002). More often, tumors are generated by the stepwise accumulation of half a dozen or more genetic and epigenetic changes in somatic cells that sometimes might start with an intrinsic germline mutation that represents one step in oncogenesis (Kinzler and Vogelstein, 1996). The acquisition of each genetic change is thought to alter the phenotype of the cell and confer an increased survival and/or proliferation advantage, so that tumor development might be considered to be a process similar to evolution. At one time it was thought that the accumulation of genetic changes led to autonomous changes in the phenotype of the tumor cell. However, it has become increasingly apparent that there are intimate mutual heterotypic interactions between the tumor cell and other cells in its environment, with the phenotypes of both the tumor cells and the "normal" cells being altered as a result of this interaction (Olumi et al., 1999; Tlsty, 2001).

Genetic changes in tumors can include, for example, point mutations that alter the level of expression or function of a gene; small deletions or insertions that can have a similar effect or even generate chimeric genes; amplification; balanced or unbalanced chromosome translocations that can alter the structure or regulation of genes, or differentially effect gene dosage; or differential changes in the number of copies of different chromosomes. Although we understand the molecular consequences of some of these genetic abnormalities (e.g., activating mutations in RAS; amplification of c-MYC; increased expression of translocated BCL-2 by juxtaposition to an Ig enhancer), in many instances we do not understand the molecular consequences (e.g., most trisomies and unbalanced translocations). It is also suspected that there might be many genetic changes (e.g., point mutations, small deletions) that are not apparent. In any case, the large number of genetic alterations that have been identified in many kinds of tumors suggest that one or more of the steps in oncogenesis promotes genomic instability (Marx, 2002).

Genetic changes that occur in the tumors often are classified as dominant activation of proto-oncogenes or recessive inactivation of tumor-suppressor genes. However, our increasing knowledge of the interlocking metabolic processes and genes involved in oncogenesis is rapidly reaching a state of sophistication for which it seems inadequate to label an affected gene only as an oncogene or a tumor-suppressor gene. There are a limited number of tumors, with colorectal carcinoma representing by far the best but still incompletely understood example, for which we can catalog the stages of tumorigenesis and correlate those stages with the acquisition of specific genetic and epigenetic abnormalities (Kinzler and Vogelstein, 1996, 1998; Zhou et al., 1999). However, certain specific pathways are altered in many human tumors (activation of RAS in approximately 25% of tumors; alteration of one of the components of the RB pathway in most tumors). Hanahan and Weinberg have suggested that the vast array of human cancer cell genotypes is manifested by six

essential alterations in cell physiology, which together are responsible for the malignant growth of most tumors (Hanahan and Weinberg, 2000). Their list includes self-sufficiency in growth signals (e.g., activating RAS mutations), insensitivity to growth-inhibitory signals (e.g., disruption of RB pathway), evasion of programmed cell death (e.g., disruption of p53 pathway), unlimited replicative potential (activation of telomerase), sustained angiogenesis, and tissue invasion and metastasis. For any given tumor, each of these six alterations might be accomplished by one or more genetic or epigenetic changes that remain to be fully identified. Although there has been remarkable progress in our understanding of oncogenesis in the past 20 years, it is clear that much remains to be learned.

# Murine Models to Study the Pathogenesis, Prevention, and Treatment of MM

Although the ideal animal model would fully mimic all aspects of human MM, there presently is no model that accomplishes this goal. Instead there are several imperfect models. Some involve only murine cells. Others use a mouse host plus human MM tumor cells, HMCL, or a combination of human MM tumor cells and human stromal cells.

## Pristane-Induced Plasmacytoma in Balb/c Mice

Three critical features of this model include formation of peritoneal oil granulomas that produce IL-6 and other cytokines that support the survival, proliferation, and differentiation of plasmablasts; a critical role for three recessive susceptibility loci (one of which appears to be a partially defective p16INK4a gene) on Balb/c chromosome 4; and the early and essentially universal occurrence of Ig translocations that dysregulate the c-MYC oncogene. Similar kinds of plasmacytoma, sometimes without pristane induction or in mouse strains other than Balb/c, can occur in transgenic mice with B cell-specific expression of BCL-2, v-ABL, or IL-6, or in mice infected by retroviruses that contain v-ABL, or v-MYC together with v-ABL, v-RAF, or H-RAS. In each of these cases, the plasmacytoma almost always has a translocation that dysregulates endogenous c-MYC (or an exogenous dysregulated c- or v-MYC gene). Unlike human MM, the plasmacytoma does not localize to the bone marrow but has a phenotype that is rather similar to advanced extramedullary human MM, a stage of MM in which c-MYC is often dysregulated by a secondary translocation (see previously) (Gado et al., 2001; Potter, 1997; Zhang et al., 2001).

## Spontaneous MGUS and MM Tumors in C57 BL/KaLwRij Mouse Strain

At the age of 1 year, approximately 25% of these mice develop a premalignant tumor similar to MGUS, and by 2 years of age, MM tumors occur in approximately 0.5% of these mice. Unlike the murine plasmacytoma (discussed previously), but similar to early human MM, the C57 BL MM tumors do not have Ig translocations that involve c-MYC. The MGUS tumors can be serially transplanted no more than three or four times, whereas the MM tumors usually can be transplanted indefinitely. Both MGUS and MM tumors are localized predominantly in the bone marrow, but unlike their human counterparts, they often localize to the spleen or lymph nodes as well. In contrast to murine plasmacytoma but similar to human MM, C57 BL MM tumors cause osteolytic bone disease. In several cases, these MM tumors have generated cell lines that retain the *in vivo* growth properties of the original MM tumor. Despite the obvious similarities to human MGUS and MM, the C57 BL model has the disadvantages of a relatively low incidence plus its propensity to grow in lymphoid tissues other than bone marrow (Dallas et al., 1999; Garrett et al., 1997; Radl, 1999; Radl et al., 1990; van den Akker et al., 1996; Vanderkerken et al., 1997; Zhu et al., 1998).

## Growth of Human MM Tumors or HMCL in SCID or NOD SCID Murine Hosts

Often it has been possible to grow HMCL in these immunodeficient murine hosts, but with one notable exception there has been little success growing primary MM tumor cells in these hosts. Part of the problem might be that murine IL-6 cannot appropriately stimulate human IL-6 receptors, although it is likely that other critical properties of human bone marrow stromal cells cannot be replaced by murine bone marrow stromal cells. Another problem with this model is that the human HMCL or tumor cells grow in the spleen, lymph nodes, and sometimes other tissues in addition to bone marrow, so that interaction of human tumor and normal mouse cells is distinctly different than the interaction of tumor and normal cells in the human (Alsina et al., 1996; Gado et al., 2001; Pilarski et al., 2000; Rebouissou et al., 1998; Tsunenari et al., 1997).

## Growth of Human MM Tumors in SC ID-hu Host

Implantation of human fetal bone subcutaneously into a SCID mouse provides a human microenvironment of bone marrow stromal cells. Injection of intramedullary human MM tumor cells into the fetal bone resulted in growth of the MM tumor cells, osteolytic lesions, and associated angiogenesis that involved human cells. The tumor grew only in the human bone and not in mouse tissues, but could spread to a second human bone placed elsewhere in the mouse. The tumor could be serially passaged into the fetal bone of other SCID-hu hosts without apparent changes in the properties of the tumor cells. Selection of CD38+CD45– tumor cells from bone marrow or blood of an MM patient grew in this assay, whereas tumor cells depleted of CD38+ did not grow, suggesting that the tumor stem cell has a plasma cell and not a B cell phenotype. Extramedullary MM tumor cells grew on as well as within the bone, suggesting a dependence on the human microenvironment but not the bone marrow microenvironment. Inhibition of osteoclast activity inhibited osteolysis and growth of intramedullary MM tumor cells, indicating a critical role of osteoclasts in tumor growth. However, inhibition of osteoclast activity did not affect growth of extramedullary MM tumor cells. Recombinant endostatin inhibited angiogenesis and MM tumor growth, providing evidence that angiogenesis is required for MM growth. Although this is a cumbersome model, it presently appears to provide the best model to assess tumor-host interactions and novel therapies (Pearse et al., 2001; Urashima et al., 1997a; Yaccoby and Epstein, 1999; Yaccoby et al., 2002a, 2002b).

# Karyotypic Abnormalities and Karyotypic Instability

The karyotypes of multiple myeloma are more similar to epithelial tumors and the blast phase of chronic myelogenous leukemia than are other hematopoietic tumors. However, the ratio of balanced translocations versus unbalanced translocations might be somewhat higher in multiple myeloma than in epithelial tumors (Mitelman et al., 2001; Sawyer et al., 1998a, 2000). Numeric chromosomal abnormalities are present in virtually all multiple myeloma tumors, and most, if not all, MGUS tumors (Avet-Loiseau et al., 1999b; Drach et al., 1995; Flactif et al., 1995; Fonseca et al., 1998a; Zandecki et al., 1997). There is nonrandom involvement of different chromosomes in different myeloma tumors and often heterogeneity among cells within a tumor. Comparative genomic hybridization (CGH) studies show that unbalanced chromosome structural changes are present in all plasma cell leukemias and most, if not all, multiple myeloma tumors (Aalto et al., 1999; Avet-Loiseau et al., 1997; Cigudosa et al., 1998; Gutierrez et al., 2001). Chromosomal gains that recur in more than 30% of multiple myeloma tumors include 1q, 3q, 9q, 11q, and 15q, the consequences of which remain to be determined. The most frequent chromosome loss is 13q (below). Because CGH does not detect balanced translocations, a more comprehensive view is provided by spectral karyotype (SKY) analyses, although these studies are complicated by the fact that metaphase spreads can only be obtained in approximately 30% of cases (Sawyer et al., 1998a, 2000). Karyotypic complexity increases during tumor progression (Sawyer et al., 1998b). Understanding how karyotype correlates with disease severity is important because the detection of an abnormal karyotype correlates with a poor prognosis (Rajkumar et al., 1999). In addition, hypodiploidy is associated with a poorer prognosis than hyperdiploidy (Smadja et al., 2001).

## Primary Versus Secondary (Ig) Translocations

Primary translocations provide a very early and possibly initiating event in the pathogenesis of many plasma cell tumors. By contrast, secondary translocations are later events that contribute to tumor progression. Most primary translocations appear to be simple reciprocal translocations that juxtapose an oncogene and one of the Ig enhancers, resulting in increased and dysregulated expression of the oncogene. These primary translocations are mediated mainly by errors in IgH switch recombination, but sometimes by errors in somatic hypermutation during the generation of plasma cells in germinal centers. Although errors in the third B cell-specific DNA modification process, VDJ recombination, often mediate translocations in B lymphomas, there is no evidence to date that this mechanism is involved in translocations in plasma cell tumors. Because all three B-cell DNA modification mechanisms seem to be inactive in normal and tumor plasma cells, it seems apparent that secondary translocations must be mediated by other mechanisms that are active in tumor cells. The only definitive way to

distinguish primary from secondary translocations would be to document the time(s) at which translocations occur during the pathogenesis of individual tumors. In the absence of this definitive test, we propose other criteria that help to distinguish primary from secondary translocations in multiple myeloma (Table 3-1) (Bergsagel and Kuehl, 2001; Kuehl and Bergsagel, 2002).

## Anatomy of Primary IgH Translocations in MM

Whereas chromosome translocations in myeloid cells typically result in the formation of a fusion protein with a novel or dysregulated function, most Ig translocations in B cell tumors, including MM, result in the dysregulated expression of oncogenes by juxtaposition to Ig regulatory elements (Dalla-Favera and Gaidano, 2001). There are at least three important enhancer elements that regulate IgH expression in B cells: the intronic enhancer (Eμ) located in the intron between the JH and switch mu sequences, and two powerful 3′ IgH enhancers downstream of the alpha genes (Eα1 and Eα2) (Max, 1999). In a translocation with a breakpoint in the JH region, all three enhancers remain on the der14 chromosome so that the dysregulated oncogene is on der14. In contrast, as a result of a reciprocal translocation into a switch region, these enhancers become dissociated so that each derivative chromosome has the potential to dysregulate juxtaposed oncogenes (Fig. 3-3). The t(4;14) translocation that we identified in MM is the first example of a translocation that simultaneously dysregulates two apparent oncogenes: FGFR3 by juxtaposition to Eα1 or Eα2 on der14 and MMSET by juxtaposition to Eμ on der4 (Chesi et al., 1997, 1998b).

---

**TABLE 3-1**

### Primary Versus Secondary Translocations in Plasma Cell Tumors

| Characteristics | Primary | Secondary |
|---|---|---|
| Timing | Early (initiation) | Late (progression) |
| B-cell specific double strand cleavage* | Usually | No |
| Breakpoint in/near J or switch regions | Usually | Rarely |
| Juxtaposition of Ig enhance† | Usually | Sometimes |
| Present in MGUS | Yes | Rarely |
| Heterogeneity in tumor population | No | Sometimes |
| Type of karyotypic abnormalities‡ | Mostly simple | Often complex |

*Somatic hypermutation and IgH switch recombination are active in germinal center B cells but not in normal plasma cells or plasma cell tumors.
†The B cell-specific DNA modification process specifically targets an immunoglobulin (Ig) locus in most primary translocations.
‡Simple usually is a balanced reciprocal translocation involving two chromosomes; complex often is a nonreciprocal translocation or insertion that can involve more than two chromosomes and sometimes is associated with inversion, deletion, duplication, or amplification.
*Abbreviations:* J, JH, or JL joining segments; MGUS, monoclonal gammopathy of undetermined significance.

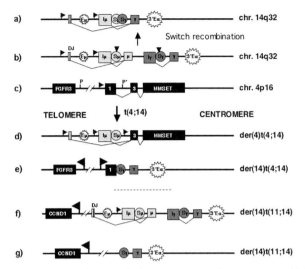

*Figure 3-3* IgH locus and chromosome translocations in multiple myeloma. The relative location of the promoters (triangles), exons (rectangles), enhancers (stars), and switch regions (circles) involved in the t(4;14) and t(11;14) are diagrammed. Deletional switch recombination (**A**) occurs at the same time on both the productive and nonproductive alleles; errors in this process can contribute to chromosome translocations in MM. Following the t(4;14) translocation, the intronic enhancer (Eμ) on der4 (**d**) is juxtaposed to MMSET resulting in mRNA transcripts that initiate in the Jh and Iμ exons, and downstream of the breakpoint on 4p16. The 3′ enhancer (3′Eα) on der14 (**E**) dysregulates the expression of FGFR3 and occasionally also results in reciprocal hybrid mRNA transcripts between the noncoding exons of MMSET and a constant region (γ). Whereas the t(4;14) breakpoints always occur in the switch regions, the t(11;14) breakpoints can also occur in the JH region (**F** and **G**).

In contrast to t(4;14), which has all breakpoints into or near switch regions, t(11;14) translocation breakpoints in at least two of seven cases analyzed involved the JH region, consistent with these translocations being mediated by an error in somatic hypermutation (Bergsagel and Kuehl, 2001). Preliminary analyses of the t(11;14) translocation in four additional HMCL indicates that for three HMCL there is no evidence for an illegitimate switch recombination event so that an error in IgH switch recombination is unlikely to be responsible for the translocation (Bergsagel and Kuehl, unpublished data). Translocation breakpoints were near or within IgH switch regions in five of seven cases analyzed, consistent with an error in IgH switch recombination; it is of interest that in this case, cyclin D1 is dysregulated by juxtaposition to Eα1 and/or Eα2 on der14, whereas MYEOV (a possible oncogene, see later in this chapter) is dysregulated by juxtaposition to Eμ on der11 (Bergsagel and Kuehl, 2001; Janssen et al., 2000). We have cloned only one reciprocal pair of breakpoints, but this unique example provides convincing evidence that translocations into IgH switch regions occur at the time of normal IgH switch recombination (Gabrea et al., 1999).

# Dysregulation of c-MYC as a Paradigm for Secondary Translocations in MM

Chromosomal translocations that dysregulate c-MYC by juxtaposing it with one of the three Ig loci appear to represent a virtually invariant primary event in human Burkitt's lymphoma and murine plasmacytoma tumors (Dalla-Favera and Gaidano, 2001; Potter, 1997). These translocations, which are thought to be mediated by errors in one of the three B cell-specific DNA modification processes described previously, usually are simple reciprocal translocations (e.g., the classic t[8;14] as depicted in Fig. 3-4A). The nontranslocated c-MYC allele is not expressed, corresponding to the absence of c-MYC expression in resting germinal center B cells and terminally differentiated plasma cells (Kakkis et al., 1989). Recently, it was determined that L-MYC (one HMCL) or one c-MYC allele is expressed selectively in all 13 informative HMCL, consistent with cis-dysregulation of L-MYC or one c-MYC allele in all HMCL (Peterson T, unpublished data; Shou et al., 2000). In addition, by RNA microarray analysis, N-MYC, which is not expressed in normal PB or PC, is expressed in two of 82 primary MM tumors (Tarte et al., 2002; Zhan et al., 2002). Three-color FISH analyses of metaphase chromosomes show that 28 of 32 (88%) HMCL and 18 of 38 (47%) advanced primary MM tumors have similar, complex karyotypic abnormalities involving c-MYC, L-MYC (one HMCL), or N-MYC (one tumor) (Shou et al., 2000; Martelli M, Gabrea A, unpublished data). Strikingly, classic t(8;14) and t(8;22) reciprocal translocations comprise only 10% and 5%, respectively, of the c-MYC karyotypic abnormalities that were detected. Most karyotypic abnormalities are complex translocations and insertions that often are nonreciprocal and frequently involve three different chromosomes (Figs. 3-4A–C). In addition, associated deletions, inversions, duplications, and amplification sometimes are seen. Most of these c-MYC karyotypic abnormalities would not be detected by conventional cytogenetics, but many would be detected by SKY analyses (Sawyer et al., 1998a, 2000). The karyotypic abnormalities often, but not always, juxtapose c-MYC and an Ig enhancer, with 11 of 28 (39%) MM cell lines and 8 of 17 (47%) primary tumors having a karyotypic abnormality of c-, L-, or N-MYC that does not involve an apparent association with an Ig enhancer (Fig. 3-4). This suggests the possibility that secondary translocations can dysregulate c-MYC by juxtaposition to non-Ig enhancers. By interphase FISH analyses, it is reported that the c-MYC locus is rearranged in 3% of MGUS/SMM tumors, 10% of MM tumors with a low tumor mass, and 19% of MM tumors with a high tumor mass (beta-2 microglobulin >3), and frequently is

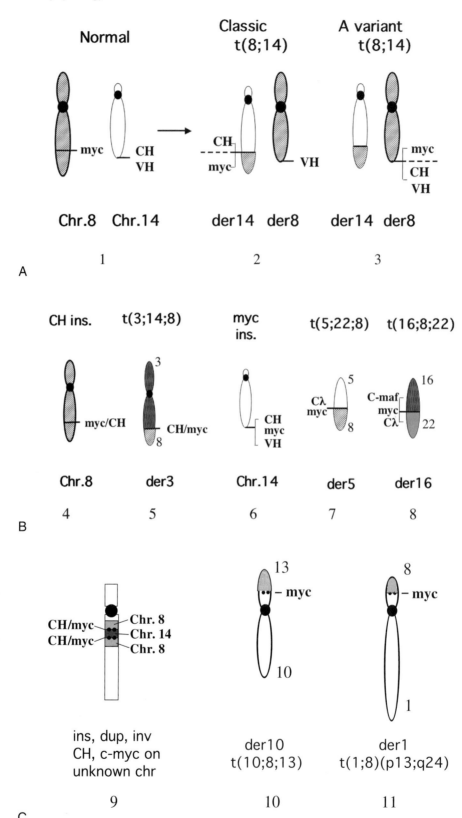

**Figure 3-4** *Examples of simple and complex translocations in multiple myeloma. Translocations involving c-MYC are shown as examples of the kinds of translocations seen in MM. (**A**) Normal chr 8 with c-MYC at 8q24 and chr 14 with the IgH locus bracketed by the centromeric 3′ IgH enhancer (CH) and the telomeric V region (VH) with a simple reciprocal classic t(8;14) translocation and one kind of variant t(8;14 translocation) that occurs in MM. (**B**) Examples of complex translocations in which c-MYC is juxtaposed to an Ig enhancer. (**C**) Other examples of c-MYC translocations that juxtapose c-MYC at a translocation breakpoint, but sometimes without juxtaposition to an Ig enhancer.*

heterogeneous within a tumor (Avet-Loiseau et al., 2001). Cloned t(8;14) translocation/insertion breakpoints often do not occur at the IgH sites targeted by the three B cell-specific DNA modifications (Bergsagel and Kuehl, 2001). Together, these results support a model for MM in which dysregulation of c-, L-, or N-MYC occurs as a late, progressive event that is mediated by secondary translocations that do not involve the three B cell-specific DNA modification mechanisms.

## Identification of Ig Translocations in MM

Karyotypic analyses of MM tumors using conventional cytogenetic methods greatly underestimated the incidence of IgH translocations, and rarely identified the partner chromosome except for t(11;14) (Calasanz et al., 1997; Dewald et al., 1985; Lai et al., 1995; Sawyer et al., 1995). At least three problems are responsible for the inability of conventional cytogenetic analyses of metaphase chromosomes to detect IgH translocations in MM. First, MM tumors have a very low mitotic index even when tumors are cultured *in vitro* with a variety of cytokines, including IL-6. Metaphase chromosomes can be obtained from approximately 30% of MM tumors, with this success rate being directly correlated with the extent of karyotypic abnormality and the stage of the tumor. Second, all MM tumors have abnormal karyotypes, and many tumors have numerous and complex chromosome rearrangements, including nonreciprocal rearrangements, that complicate the identification of specific chromosomes. Third, the IgH locus (14q32) has a telomeric location, and many of the partner loci have telomeric (4p16; 6p25) or subtelomeric (16q23) locations. Interphase FISH analyses using probes that flank an Ig locus to detect split signals or a probe from one end of an Ig locus together with a probe from a specific chromosomal region to detect fusion signals permit a comprehensive assessment of Ig translocations in all tumor cells, including MGUS. To minimize the significant background problems with interphase FISH assays, tumor cells have been enriched by pre-selection (e.g., CD-138 magnetic bead selection) or by restricting analysis to cells that express cytoplasmic kappa or lambda IgL (Ahmann et al., 1998; Avet-Loiseau et al., 1999a).

## Incidence of Ig Translocations in MM, MGUS, PCL, and HMCL

Recent studies have shown that a majority of MM tumors have an IgH translocation that nonrandomly involves one of many potential chromosomal partners (Anderson et al., 2002; Avet-Loiseau et al., 2002; Bergsagel and Kuehl, 2001; Fonseca et al., 2002a). The incidence of IgH translocations varies with the stage of disease: 46–48% in MGUS or SMM, 55–73% in intramedullary MM, 85% in primary plasma cell leukemia, and >90% in HMCL that are generated from extramedullary MM. Limited studies indicate a much lower incidence of Igκ translocations: 11% in MGUS, 17% in advanced intramedullary tumors that generate abnormal metaphase chromosomes, and 23% in HMCL. The incidence of Igκ translocations is even lower, and appears to be no more than 2% to 3% based on studies of advanced intramedullary MM tumors and HMCL (Martelli M, unpublished data; Sawyer et al., 1998a, 2000). Importantly, although all 34 HMCL fully analyzed have either an IgH or Igλ translocation, nearly 50% of MGUS tumors and 26% of advanced intramedullary MM tumors do not have an IgH or IgL translocation (Martelli M, Gabrea A, unpublished data).

## Four Chromosomal Partners Account for Most Primary Ig Translocations

### 11q13-Cyclin D1

By conventional cytogenetics and interphase FISH analyses the t(11;14)(q13;q32) is present in 15% to 26% of MGUS/SMM, 15% to 18% of MM, and 29% of HMCL (Avet-Loiseau et al., 1998, 2002; Fonseca et al., 1998b, 2002a). The cloned breakpoints on 14q32 fall near or within either the JH region, or the switch regions, and are compatible with being mediated by either somatic hypermutation or switch recombination, respectively (Fig. 3-3). On 11q13, the breakpoints are dispersed over 330 kb centromeric to cyclin D1, with no evidence of clustering in the Major Translocation Cluster (MTC) described for mantle cell lymphoma (MCL) (Janssen et al., 2000). This difference could reflect the different mechanisms responsible for the translocations, because those in MCL are ascribed to errors in V(D)J recombination, which might more specifically target the MTC. Alternatively, it might reflect differences in accessibility of the bcl-1 locus at different stages of B cell development.

Normally B cells express cyclin D2 and cyclin D3, but not cyclin D1. As a result of the translocation, cyclin D1 is juxtaposed to the powerful IgH 3′ enhancer (s) on der (14) and its expression is dysregulated. The exact nature of this dysregulation has not been well characterized, and it is not known if it results in an amplification of cyclic levels of cyclin D1 mRNA expression or in a loss of cell cycle control of mRNA levels and high-level tonic expression of cyclin D1 mRNA. When the translocation breakpoint falls within a switch region, the intronic enhancer (and Eα1 if the breakpoint occurs downstream of this enhancer) end up on der (11) where they might be associated with the ectopic expression of a gene, *myeov* (myeloma over-expressed gene), located 360 kb centromeric to cyclin D1. This gene, which was identified using DNA from a gastric carcinoma in a transformation assay, has no significant sequence homology to other proteins and was found upregulated in 3 of 7 MM cell lines with 11q13 translocations (Janssen et al., 2000).

## 6p21-Cyclin D3

Recently we identified a translocation of 6p21 into switch gamma sequence in an MM cell line (Shaughnessy et al., 2001). The breakpoint is located 65 kb centromeric to the 5′ end of cyclin D3 and is associated with a sixfold increase level of cyclin D3 expression. We identified the t(6;14) in 1 of 30 MM cell lines and in 6 of 150 patients with abnormal metaphase karyotypes. By microarray analysis we found 3 of 53 patients with high levels of cyclin D3 expression, and determined that these patients had a juxtaposition of the IgH locus and cyclin D3 by interphase FISH analysis. Another MM tumor had a t(6;22)(p21;q11), so that cyclin D3 is bracketed by the centromeric IgH and telomeric IgL breakpoints. The finding of dysregulation of cyclin D1 in approximately 15% to 18% and of cyclin D3 in 4% of patients highlights the importance of the D-type cyclins in MM. There is one report of a t(12;22)(p13;q11) in a lymphoma with a breakpoint in the negative regulatory element of the cyclin D2 promoter (Qian et al., 1999). Although no expression data was shown, it was postulated to dysregulate cyclin D2. There is also a report of an MM tumor and an MM cell line in which there is a t(12;14) translocation that could reflect dysregulation of cyclin D2 (Avet-Loiseau et al., 1999a).

## 4p16.3-FGFR3 and MMSET

The t(4;14) is identified in approximately 2% to 9% of MGUS/SMM, 10% to 18% of MM tumors, and 26% of HMCL (Avet-Loiseau et al., 1998; Chesi et al., 1998b, 2001; Malgeri et al., 2000). The t(4;14) translocation appears to dysregulate two potential oncogenes, FGFR3 on der (14) and MMSET on der (4), but FGFR3 on der (14) is lost or not expressed in 20% to 25% of MM tumors that have a t(4;14) translocation (Chesi et al., 2002; Keats et al., 2003; Santra et al., 2003). As a result, studies that have focused only on FGFR3 have underestimated the incidence of the t(4;14) translocation. The breakpoints occur in the telomeric region of chromosome 4 and result in a karyotypically silent translocation; it cannot be identified by either G-banding or spectral karyotype analysis. In the IgH locus the breakpoints all occur in the switch region and dissociate the intronic enhancer from the 3′ enhancer. The 4p16 breakpoints fall 50 to 100 kb centromeric to FGFR3 that becomes associated with the 3′ enhancer (s) on der14 (Fig. 3-3). This region includes the 5′ noncoding (largely) exons of MMSET/WHSC1 that becomes dysregulated by juxtaposition to the IgH intronic enhancer, resulting in formation of hybrid mRNA transcripts with the JH and I-mu exons. The hybrid transcripts provide a very specific and sensitive means of detecting this translocation. We have not identified any variant translocations, nor any translocations into the JH region, suggesting that dysregulation of *both* MMSET and FGFR3 might be important in the pathogenesis of MM.

MMSET encodes a nuclear protein with two predicted dominant forms: a short form that includes an HMG domain and a long form that additionally includes four PHD-type zinc fingers and a SET domain. It thus shares homology to other PHD and SET domain proteins such as ASH1 and trithorax in drosophila. It also shares these features with MLL1/HRX/ALL1, the gene on 11q23 involved in translocations in acute leukemia, suggesting that it could play a role in the oncogenic transformation of MM cells. This gene falls with the minimally deleted region identified for Wolf-Hirschorn syndrome, a multiple malformation syndrome characterized by mental retardation and developmental defects resulting from partial deletion of the short arm of one chromosome 4 (Stec et al., 1998). Although it is thought to be a contiguous gene syndrome, it could be predicted that patients with this syndrome have only one copy of MMSET and it is a likely candidate to contribute to this phenotype.

FGFR3 is one of four high-affinity tyrosine kinase receptors for the FGF family of ligands. It is not normally expressed in plasma cells and is ectopically expressed as a result of the translocation. Activating mutations of the t(4;14) translocated FGFR3 allele are present in one-third of the MM cell lines and in some patients, substantiating an oncogenic role for FGFR3 in MM. Interestingly, some of the lines with t(4;14) translocation without FGFR3 mutations contained activating mutations of N or K-RAS, but no lines contained mutations of both FGFR3 and RAS (Chesi et al., 2001). This suggests that during tumor progression, activation of FGFR3 or RAS could provide an equivalent stimulus to the cells. Activated FGFR3 has been shown to be an oncogene that can induce transformation in fibroblasts that is inhibited by dominant negative inhibitors of the ras/MAPK pathway. Signaling from FGFR3 in MM has been shown to result in phosphorylation of STAT3 and MAPK, and to synergize with IL-6 signals in an IL-6-dependent plasmacytoma cell line. FGFR3 signaling can substitute for IL-6 for the growth and survival of this line, and inhibition of these signals results in apoptosis (Plowright et al., 2000). These experiments validate

FGFR3 as an important target for experimental therapeutics in t(4;14) MM.

## 16q23-c-maf

Translocation t(14;16)(q32;q23) is identified in 1% to 5% of MGUS/SMM, 2% to 9% of MM, and 21% of MM cell lines (Avet-Loiseau et al., 2002; Chesi et al., 1998b; Fonseca et al., 2002a; Sawyer et al., 1998a, 2000). The five cloned breakpoints on 16q23 occur over a region 550 to 1350 kb centromeric to c-*maf*, all but one of them within the 800 kb intron of an oxidoreductase gene, WWOX/FOR (Bednarek et al., 2000; Ried et al., 2000). This region is a common fragile site, FRA16D, which has been found to undergo frequent homozygous deletion in adenocarcinomas of the stomach, lung, colon, and ovary. Allelic deletions of this region have not been associated with inactivation of the remaining allele so that a possible role as a tumor-suppressor gene is unclear. Presumably, the DNA double strand breaks that occur frequently in this fragile site contribute to the pathogenesis of the t(14;16) translocation. Perhaps only in MM cells is the 3' enhancer sufficiently active to dysregulate c-*maf* located at such a distance from the breakpoints, providing a possible reason for the apparent lack of 16q23 translocations in other B cell tumors.

The identification of t(16;22)(q23;q11) translocations with breakpoints telomeric to c-*maf* (not involving WWOX) serves to delineate the targeted region of dysregulation, and indicates that inactivation of one allele of WWOX by translocation is not required for MM cell transformation by 16q23 translocation. C-*maf* is the cellular homolog of v-*maf*, the transforming gene in the avian maf retrovirus. It is a basic zipper transcription factor that can heterodimerize with jun and fos and small maf proteins. In lymphoid cells it has been characterized as a T cell transcription factor expressed specifically in TH2 lymphocytes that controls the expression of IL-4 (Ho et al., 1996). It is expressed at a high level in MM cells with a 16q23 translocation and at a low to undetectable level in the other MM cell lines. How c-*maf* contributes to the pathogenesis of MM tumors with t(14;16) remains to be determined.

# Other Recurrent Chromosomal Partners for Ig Translocations

## 8q24 (c-MYC)

Translocations of 8q24 in MM are complex and appear to be late events involved in the progression of the disease (Shou et al., 2000). This is in surprising contrast to their role as a primary event in Burkitt's lymphoma and mouse plasmacytoma. It serves to highlight the importance of c-MYC in MM, and suggests that in early stages of MM there could be transfactors present only in the bone marrow microenvironment that serve to upregulate c-MYC. With disease progression, c-MYC dysregulation by chromosome translocation might abrogate the requirement for these transfactors and allow for increased and/or extramedullary growth of the MM cells.

## 6p25-MUM1/IRF-4

A t(6;14)(p25;q32) translocation breakpoint was cloned from an MM cell line and found to occur immediately downstream of the IRF-4 gene, a member of the interferon regulatory factor family active in the control of B cell proliferation and differentiation (Iida et al., 1997). This translocation was identified by metaphase FISH analyses in three of 17 (18%) MM cell lines that were screened (Yoshida et al., 1999). Although IRF-4 is normally expressed in most MM cell lines, the three lines with the translocation expressed much higher levels. IRF-4 was shown to be transforming in fibroblasts, suggesting that it might contribute to the oncogenesis of the MM tumors. The incidence of the t(6;14)(p25;q32) translocation in various stages of primary PC tumors, and role in tumor initiation and/or progression are not clearly established at this time.

## 1q21-24-IRTA1 and IRTA2

Unbalanced nonrandom translocations of 1q and trisomy 1q21-31 were identified in 20% to 31% of MM (Hatzivassiliou et al., 2001). A breakpoint from this region was cloned from the FR4 MM cell line and resulted in the identification of two novel cell surface receptors homologous to the Fc and inhibitory families. IRTA2 is upregulated in most Burkitt lymphoma cell lines with 1q21 abnormalities. It was also upregulated in one of three MM cell lines with 1q21 translocations. How this contributes to the pathogenesis of MM remains to be determined. The location of the t(1;14)(q21;q32) breakpoint far downstream of the Sα region suggests that this likely represents a secondary translocation, at least in this tumor cell line. From SKY analyses of 150 tumors, the incidence of the t(1;14)(q21;q32) translocation is approximately 1% to 2% of advanced intramedullary MM tumors (Sawyer et al., 1998a, 2000).

## 20q12-mafB

Balanced t(14;20) translocations have been identified in 5% to 10% of HMCL (Avet-Loiseau et al., 2002; Hanamura et al., 2001; Cultraro C, unpublished data) and approximately 1% of advanced tumors analyzed by spectral karyotyping (SKY) (Sawyer et al., 1998a, 2000). The apparent dysregulated oncogene is mafB, a basic zipper transcription factor that is closely related to c-maf. Similar to translocations that dysregulate c-myc, translocations that dysregulate mafB sometimes are complex, and can have breakpoints that are not near or within J or switch sequences (Cultraro C, unpublished data). Thus, it appears that at least some of the translocations that dysregulate mafB are secondary translocations.

## Chromosomal Partners for Ig Translocations: Promiscuous Partners

The recurrent translocation partners described previously do not account for many of the IgH translocations that have been identified. For example, a French group reports that 30% of MGUS/SMM and 43% of intramedullary MM have IgH translocations that do not involve c-MYC or three (11q13, 4p16, 16q23) of the four (6p21 was not assessed) recurrent chromosomal partners described previously (Avet-Loiseau et al., 2002). A second group at the Mayo Clinic reports that 10% of MGUS/SMM and 21% of intramedullary myeloma have IgH translocations that do not involve three (11q13, 4p16, 16q23) of the four (6p21 and c-MYC were not assessed) recurrent chromosomal partners described previously (Fonseca et al., 2002a, Fonseca R, personal communication, 3/19/2003). The reason for the differences between the MGUS/SMM and MM, and the differences for the two groups is not clear. However, SKY analyses of metaphase chromosomes from 150 advanced intramedullary MM tumors show that approximately 17% of tumors have IgH translocations that do not involve c-MYC or one of the four recurrent partners described previously; but none of these other chromosomal loci is an IgH translocation partner in more than 1% of MM tumors (Sawyer et al., 1998a, 2000).

## Primary and Secondary Translocations Usually Involve Different Oncogenes

As indicated previously, there are four chromosomal loci (oncogenes) that are recurrently involved in primary translocations: 11q13 (cyclin D1), 6p21 (cyclin D3), 4p16 (FGFR3 and MMSET), and 16q23 (c-maf). However, the occurrence of a t(11;14) translocation in a subset of MGUS tumor cells that all contain a t(4;14) translocation suggests the possibility that 11q13 sometimes can be involved in secondary translocations during tumor progression (Fonseca et al., 2002a). The

apparent involvement of many other loci in MGUS/SMM suggests that at least some of these might represent primary translocations, although this remains to be confirmed. Compared with MGUS/SMM, we suspect that the increased incidence of IgH translocations in MM and at later stages of disease is partially explained by the accumulation of secondary translocations, although this explanation needs to be validated in longitudinal studies. Using the criteria in Table 3-1, we have tentatively identified several recurrent loci involved in secondary translocations: 8q24 (c-myc), 2p23 (N-myc), 20q12 (mafB), 6p25 (MUM-1/IRF-4), and 1q21 (IRTA 1 and 2). The apparent differential involvement of specific oncogenes in primary versus secondary translocations might reflect specific functional properties of oncogenes, but might also reflect susceptibility to translocation at different stages of tumorigenesis.

## Dysregulation of Cyclin D1, 2, or 3 in MM: A Potential Unifying Event

A critical feature shared by premalignant MGUS and malignant MM tumors is the presence of a substantial intramedullary tumor burden despite an extremely low rate of tumor cell proliferation. The PC labeling index (PCLI) measures the fraction of cells that incorporate thymidine, or BUDR as a thymidine analog, during a 2-hour labeling period in vitro. Typically, the PCLI is <0.2% for MGUS and <1.0% (often much lower) for MM tumor cells until terminal stages of the disease (Rajkumar et al., 1999). There is a somewhat higher but still low fraction of MGUS or MM cells that express the Ki67 antigen that is a marker for cells that are cycling. In terms of proliferation, both tumors seem closer to normal, nonproliferating PC than to normal, but highly proliferating plasmablasts (PB), for which 30% or more of the cells can be in S phase (Tarte et al., 2002). Strikingly, however, our analysis of combined RNA expression microarray data from two laboratories (Olumi et al., 1999; Tlsty, 2001; Zhan et al., 2002) shows that expression levels of cyclin D1, cyclin D2, or cyclin D3 mRNA in myeloma tumors is extremely high, apparently comparable to the levels of cyclin D2 mRNA expressed in normal proliferating PB and distinctly different from normal PC (Fig. 3-5).

Normal hematopoietic cells, including normal B lymphocytes and PB, predominantly express cyclin D2, usually together with lower levels of cyclin D3, but do not express cyclin D1 (Shaughnessy et al., 2001). Lymphocytes in a cyclin D2 null mouse upregulate expression of cyclin D3 but still do not express cyclin D1 (Lam et al., 2000). Given the lack of cyclin D1 expression in normal lymphocytes and the occurrence of Ig translocations that dysregulate cyclin D1 or cyclin

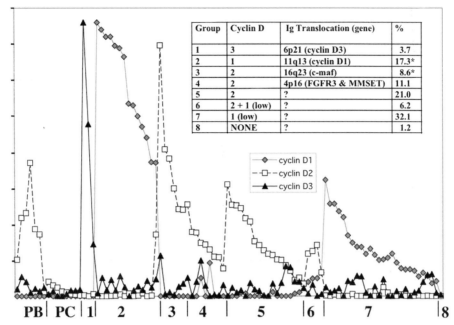

| Group | Cyclin D | Ig Translocation (gene) | % |
|---|---|---|---|
| 1 | 3 | 6p21 (cyclin D3) | 3.7 |
| 2 | 1 | 11q13 (cyclin D1) | 17.3* |
| 3 | 2 | 16q23 (c-maf) | 8.6* |
| 4 | 2 | 4p16 (FGFR3 & MMSET) | 11.1 |
| 5 | 2 | ? | 21.0 |
| 6 | 2 + 1 (low) | ? | 6.2 |
| 7 | 1 (low) | ? | 32.1 |
| 8 | NONE | ? | 1.2 |

***Figure 3-5*** *Cyclin D RNA expression in normal PB, normal PC, and MM tumors. Microarray expression data (Affymetrix FL6800 chips) published by Tarte et al. (Tarte et al., 2002) and Zhan et al. (Zhan et al., 2002) was pooled and analyzed. Relative expression values for cyclins D1, 2, and 3 are shown for normal PB and PC, and for 82 MM tumors. The MM tumors are divided into eight groups as described in the text, and the level of the predominantly expressed cyclin D is arranged by level of expression within each group. Because c-maf is not on the FL6800 chip, the t(14;16) group is predicated on surrogate markers (β7 integrin and CX3CR1) that are associated with the t(14;16) translocation in HMCL. The t(4;14) group is based only on FGFR3 expression because MMSET is not on the FL6800 chip; therefore, three or four tumors in group 5 are likely to have t(4;14) translocations and express MMSET but not FGFR3. The inserted table provides additional information for each group. The asterisks in the table indicate that one tumor appears to have both t(11;14) and t(14;16) translocations with this tumor depicted at the border of groups 2 and 3.*

D3 in a subset of MM tumors, the cyclin D expression results shown in Figure 3-5 suggest the possibility that all myeloma tumors dysregulate at least one of the cyclin D genes. In many tumors, there is prominent expression of only one of the cyclin D genes. The presence of one of the four recurrent primary Ig translocations, together with the cyclin D expression profile shown in Figure 3-5, allows us to separate the myeloma tumors into eight groups. Groups 1 and 2 have Ig translocations that dysregulate, respectively, cyclin D3 (6p21) and cyclin D1 (11q13). Groups 3 and 4, both of which predominantly express cyclin D2, have Ig translocations that appear to involve 16q23 (c-maf) and 4p16 (MMSET, FGFR3), respectively. It seems possible that cyclin D2 expression is dysregulated as a consequence of these translocations, an hypothesis that is supported by the fact that the only tumor with a t(11;14) translocation that expresses high levels of cyclin D2 in addition to cyclin D1 also appears to have a translocation that dysregulates c-maf. Group 5 tumors, several of which must have t(4;14) translocations and express MMSET but not FGFR3, predominantly express cyclin D2. Curiously, although cyclin D3 is expressed at low and variable levels in many tumors, the level of cyclin D3 expression in group 5 tumors

seems to correlate inversely with the level of cyclin D2 expression. Group 6 tumors show expression of cyclin D2 together with ectopic expression of low levels of cyclin D1. Group 7 tumors, representing the largest group and accounting for nearly one-third of all tumors, show ectopic expression of cyclin D1 despite the likely absence of a t(11;14) translocation. Finally, there is a single tumor in group 8 that seems to express virtually no cyclin D. This final group might represent an experimental error, or could represent a tumor, for example, that expresses no functional retinoblastoma gene product (Rb1) and thus needs no cyclin D expression to facilitate G1 progression. Results for five MGUS tumors suggest that there is similar overexpression of a cyclin D gene in MGUS tumors, despite their even lower proliferative index (Zhan et al., 2002).

From cyclin D1 transgenic mice and cyclin D transfection experiments, it is known that overexpression of cyclin D is insufficient by itself to cause cell cycle progression (Bodrug et al., 1994; Lovec et al., 1994; Sherr and McCormick, 2002). Instead, it has been suggested that the overexpression of cyclin D renders a cell more sensitive to growth-activating signals and/or less sensitive to growth inhibitory signals. The apparent universal enhanced expression/dysregulation of one of the cyclin D genes in low proliferative myeloma tumors seems consistent with what is known about the effect of dysregulated cyclin D expression in these model systems. Clearly, there are many questions that need to be answered to test the hypothesis that dysregulation of a cyclin D gene is a seminal event in the pathogenesis of MM.

## Additional Thoughts about Ig Translocations and Cyclin D Dysregulation

As indicated previously, the incidence of Ig translocations is correlated with the stage of disease. Moreover, the occurrence of multiple independent IgH translocations in the same tumor also is correlated with the stage of disease. Two independent IgH translocations are infrequent in SMM/MGUS or MM, but occur in approximately 10% of advanced MM tumors and primary PCL and in nearly 50% of HMCL. Moreover, we identified three or more independent IgH translocations in 13% of HMCL (unpublished data). In addition, the incidences of specific primary and secondary translocations is lower in intramedullary tumors than in HMCL that are derived from extramedullary tumors representing both primary PC leukemia and terminal progression of intramedullary MM. The increased incidence of secondary translocations is consistent with accumulation of these translocations during disease progression. However, the increased incidence of primary translocations in HMCL compared with intramedullary tumors most likely occurs as a result of selective progression of intramedullary tumors with Ig translocations to an extramedullary phase from which virtually all HMCL are generated. Consistent with this latter hypothesis, the third of MM tumors that ectopically express cyclin D1 without a t(11;14) translocation (Fig. 3-5) are not represented among the 34 HMCL that we have analyzed. On the basis of these results, we suggest the hypothesis that progression from stromal-dependent, intramedullary MM to stromal-independent, extramedullary MM requires a minimum of two genetic events, one of which can be an Ig translocation that dysregulates expression of one of the cyclin D genes. As a corollary to this hypothesis, we suggest that the ectopic expression of cyclin D1 in the absence of a t(11;14) translocation requires the interaction of the MM tumor cells with bone marrow stromal cells.

## Chromosome 13 Monosomy

Monoallelic loss of 13q sequences is one of the most frequent abnormalities in multiple myeloma (approximately 50% of untreated cases by interphase FISH analyses) and is an independent predictor of a poor prognosis (Avet-Loiseau et al., 1999d, 2000; Desikan et al., 2000; Dewald et al., 1985; Facon et al., 2001; Fonseca et al., 2001; Konigsberg et al., 2000; Perez-Simon et al., 1998; Seong et al., 1998; Shaughnessy et al., 2000; Worel et al., 2001; Zojer et al., 2000). Most often there is 13 monosomy, with selective loss of 13q sequences by interstitial deletion or translocation occurring much less frequently. The minimum region of deletion appears to be at 13q14, but bi-allelic deletion is rare. Notably, trisomy of chromosome 13 is also rare. The frequency of chromosome 13q loss increases with disease stage, from 20% in MGUS (but 50% of MGUS patients in one study (Fonseca et al., 2002a) to nearly 70% in plasma cell leukemia or HMCL. With the exception of one study (Fonseca et al., 2002a), only a subset of MGUS tumour cells has the 13q abnormality, whereas for MM patients with an abnormality of 13q, virtually all tumour cells have this abnormality. These results indicate that chromosome 13 losses begin in MGUS and increase in myeloma, but the nearly uniform presence of this abnormality in MGUS and myeloma tumors with t(4;14) or t(14;16) raises the possibility that this abnormality might occur as a very early event in tumors with these translocations (Avet-Loiseau et al., 2001; Fonseca et al., 2001; Sawyer et al., 1998a, 1998b). Studies on other kinds of tumors show that both copies of the retinoblastoma (RB) gene at 13q14 must be inactivated to eliminate its tumor-suppressor function. However, bi-allelic deletion, inactivating mutations, and lack of RB expression appear to occur only infrequently (i.e., perhaps a few percent), even in advanced myeloma tumors and cell lines (Juge-Morineau et al., 1997; Kramer et al., 2002; Zandecki et al., 1995). Notably, loss of 13q14 sequences is frequent in chronic lymphocytic leukemia, but is not associated with a poor prognosis (Dohner et al., 1999; Kipps, 2000). Therefore, there might be a tumor-suppressor gene on 13q that is unique to multiple myeloma.

## Tumor-Suppressor Genes: p16, p18, PTEN, p53, Rb, WWOX

### TP53

Inactivating mutations of TP53 (which encodes the p53 tumor suppressor), which has a major role in regulating genomic stability, represents the most frequent genetic abnormality in human tumors. Mutations and/or deletion of p53 occur in only a few percent of intramedullary multiple myelomas, but are present in up to 40% of advanced multiple myelomas and in greater than 60% of HMCL (Avet-Loiseau et al., 1999c; Corradini et al., 1994; Mazars et al., 1992; Neri et al., 1993; Ollikainen et al., 1997; unpublished data).

## CDKN2A

This tumor-suppressor gene encodes the cyclin-dependent kinase (CDK) inhibitor INK4A (also known as p16), which associates with CDK4 and CDK6, inhibiting phosphorylation of RB and subsequent progression from the G1 to the S phase of the cell cycle. In many kinds of tumors it is inactivated, mainly by deletion or promoter methylation and rarely by mutations. It has been reported to be expressed in multiple myeloma but not in plasma cell leukemia or HMCL (Taniguchi et al., 1999; Urashima et al., 1997b). There are no reports of deletion or mutation of CDKN2A in multiple myeloma, but promoter methylation is present in 15% of purified MGUS or multiple myeloma cells, and in most plasma cell leukemia and HMCL (Urashima et al., 1997c; Guillerm et al., 2001; Uchida et al., 2001). Retroviral transfection of *CDKN2A* or treatment with the demethylating agent 5-deoxyazacytidine restored *CDKN2A* expression and induced G1 growth arrest in plasma cell leukemia cells and HMCL (Urashima et al., 1997c).

## CDKN2C

Also known as p18INK4C, this gene encodes a cyclin-dependent kinase inhibitor that associates primarily with CDK6 and to a lesser extent with CDK4. It has not been found mutated in tumors; however, it has been reported to have an important role in terminal PC differentiation (Tourigny et al., 2002). It has been found to be homozygously deleted in 32% of HMCL and in approximately 3% to 5% of intramedullary MM tumors (Kulkarni et al., 2002; Dib A, unpublished data).

## PTEN

Inactivation of this tumor-suppressor gene, the product of which negatively regulates the phosphatidylinositol 3-kinase (PI 3K)-mediated phosphorylation of AKT and BAD, inhibits apoptosis. Recently, inactivating mutations of PTEN were identified in two of eight HMCL, and transfection of normal PTEN into one HMCL inhibited *in vivo* tumor development (Ge and Rudikoff, 2000; Hyun et al., 2000).

## *WWOX*

Recently, *WWOX* has been shown to behave as a tumor-suppressor gene *in vitro*. As noted previously, translocations that inactivate a WWOX allele (16q23 translocations) do occur in multiple myeloma, but the other allele seems to be expressed normally and does not contain mutations (Bednarek et al., 2001; unpublished data). In addition, variant 16q23 translocations that do not disrupt *WWOX* are seen, indicating that it does not play an important role in multiple myeloma (Chesi et al., 1998a).

## RB

As noted previously, bi-allelic inactivation of RB is involved only infrequently in multiple myeloma.

## Activating Mutations of K- or N-*RAS*, or FGFR3

Activating mutations of N- or K-*RAS* oncogenes distinguish multiple myeloma from MGUS. In one large study, activating mutations of *RAS* at codons 12, 13, or 61 were identified in approximately 40% of multiple myeloma tumors at the time of diagnosis, with a limited analysis indicating mutations in 49% of tumors at the time of relapse; 60% of the mutations were in N-*RAS* and 40% in K-*RAS* (Liu et al., 1996). A second large study reports a slightly higher incidence of *RAS* mutations, with K-*RAS* affected more often than N-*RAS* (Bezieau et al., 2001). The frequency of activating *RAS* mutations is relatively independent of the plasma cell labeling index and stage of myeloma. The same mutations are found in 17 of 38 (45%) of HMCL (Chesi et al., 2001 and unpublished data). Strikingly, less than 5% of MGUS tumors have *RAS* mutations (Bezieau et al., 2001; Corradini et al., 1993; Rasmussen T, personal communication, 11/15/2002). Although H-*RAS* is expressed at high levels in some multiple myeloma tumors, most studies have focused on K- and N-*RAS*. Recently, an unusual activating H-RAS mutation was described in one MM cell line (Crowder et al., 2003). Tumors that overexpress *FGFR3* as a result of a t(4;14) translocation can have activating mutations of *RAS* or *FGFR3* but not both, consistent with constitutive activation of the mitogen-activated protein kinase (MAPK) pathway in each case (Chesi et al., 2001). Transfection studies of an interleukin 6 (IL-6)-dependent HMCL show that activating mutations of either N- or K-*RAS*, or *FGFR3*, enhance growth and decrease the amount of IL-6 that is required for survival and growth (Billadeau et al., 1995, 1997; Plowright et al., 2000). K-*RAS* mutation is associated with a shortened survival, whereas patients whose myeloma tumors have N-*RAS* mutations have a similar prognosis to those who do not have *RAS* mutations (Liu et al., 1996).

## Other Genetic Changes

The complex genetic changes identified on MM karyotypes are reminiscent of the changes seen in solid tumors, some of which have been linked to emergence from senescence and telomere crisis. In the majority of cases the telomere length in the MM cells is significantly shorter than in the patient's normal granulocytes and lymphocytes. In addition, telomerase activity is elevated in 70% of patients (Wu et al., 2001). Further study is required to determine the role of telomere shortening and telomerase activity in the development of genetic changes and progression of MM.

# A Current Model for the Molecular Pathogenesis of Multiple Myeloma (MM)

The apparent normal counterpart of an MM tumor cell is a long-lived bone marrow PC. It is derived from a germinal center B cell that has undergone repeated rounds of Ig somatic hypermutation and antigen selection followed by productive IgH switch recombination to express an isotype other than IgM. These genetically modified cells, which differentiate into proliferating plasmablasts and then to terminally differentiated PC, ultimately home to the bone marrow where they can remain for many months, perhaps years, in intimate contact with bone marrow stromal cells. Typically, approximately 0.5% to 2% of bone marrow mononuclear cells are normal long-lived, polyclonal PC, although the fraction of polyclonal PC can be somewhat higher in some instances. By definition, premalignant MGUS tumors have a stable tumor mass that comprises less than 10% to often only 1% or 2% of bone marrow mononuclear cells. This suggests the possibility that for many MGUS tumors there could be a competition with normal PC for a unique niche within the bone marrow. Consistent with this possibility, in some MGUS patients the polyclonal immunoglobulin levels are below normal. By contrast, SMM, which has a stable tumor mass greater than 10% of bone marrow mononuclear cells, and most frankly malignant MM tumors, appear to have expanded beyond the bone marrow niche that supports normal PC and MGUS tumor cells. Therefore, competition with normal PC must occur in SMM and MM, perhaps accounting for the reduced polyclonal immunoglobulin levels that usually are observed. Overall, this scenario seems similar to premalignant versus malignant epithelial tumors, for which the former usually remain within the same tissue boundaries as their normal counterpart, whereas the latter extends beyond these tissue boundaries.

The pathways that generate the various bone marrow PC tumors are indicated in Figure 3-6. It is well documented that premalignant non-IgM MGUS tumors convert to SMM or frankly malignant MM at an average rate of approximately 1% per year. The rate of progression is directly related to the level of monoclonal serum immunoglobulin, consistent with the rate of progression being determined by the number of MGUS tumor cells. Not surprisingly, it is thought that SMM progresses to frankly malignant MM at an even higher rate (Kyle R, personal communication, 12/5/2002). As indicated previously, it has been reported that at least 30% of MM tumors are preceded by MGUS, and it has been proposed that although some MM tumors represent progression of MGUS, other MM tumors occur *de novo* without passing through an MGUS phase. Unfortunately, however, there are no longitudinal studies that provide a definitive answer regarding the fraction of MM tumors that were preceded by MGUS.

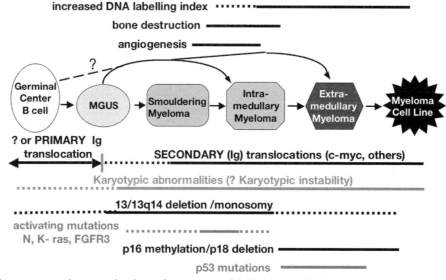

**Figure 3-6** *Multistep molecular pathogenesis model for MM. Defined stages of pathogenesis are depicted, with arrows indicating potential pathways. The approximate timing of several clinical features and oncogenic changes are depicted as thick horizontal lines, with dashed regions reflecting some uncertainty as to the precise time that these changes occur. The vertical line that separates primary and secondary translocations is meant to depict the cessation of IgH switch recombination and somatic hypermutation during B cell maturation.*

As noted previously, each of these bone marrow PC tumors has a very low incidence of proliferating cells, with the PCLI typically less than 0.1% for MGUS and less than 1% for MM until terminal stages of disease. Unfortunately, we know very little about the phenotype of the cell that is proliferating versus the phenotype of the nonproliferating cell, the relationship between the proliferating and nonproliferating compartments, the lifetime of the cells, the basis for the expansion of tumor cells beyond the normal boundaries that delimit normal PC, and so on. It has been proposed that together with the predominant malignant and clonal PC population in the bone marrow, a minor population of clonal cells with a B cell phenotype is present in the bone marrow, peripheral blood, or other sites (Pilarski et al., 2000). There is some evidence that the clonal B cells and malignant PC share the same chromosomal abnormalities, but it remains to be determined if the malignant PC and clonal B cells are in an ongoing asymmetric but reversible equilibrium, or one of these kinds of cells is a precursor for the other (Pilarski et al., 2002; Zojer et al., 2002).

Although not adequately investigated at this time, there is minimal evidence for germline mutations that contribute to the pathogenesis of MM. In addition, there is no convincing evidence for or against the hypothesis that some genetic changes begin to accumulate before the generation of germinal center B cells. Given the intrinsic genomic instability of germinal center B cells, as manifested by somatic hypermutation and IgH switch recombination, it is attractive to speculate that errors in these processes can spill over and cause genetic mishaps in nonimmunoglobulin loci. Thus far, the only consistent abnormality in MGUS and MM tumors is numeric chromosomal changes. As noted previously, unbalanced chromosomal structural changes occur in all plasma cell leukemia tumors and in most, if not all, MM tumors, but unfortunately this issue has not been addressed in MGUS tumors. Although the numeric or structural chromosome abnormalities are nonrandom, there is substantial heterogeneity in the reported abnormalities. Thus, the significance of these changes remains uncertain. Curiously, the number of chromosomes in an MM tumor seems to suggest two pathways of pathogenesis: hyperdiploid tumors with 47–74 chromosomes and non-hyperdiploid tumors that can be hypodiploid (45 or less chromosomes), pseudo-diploid (46 chromosomes), or subtetraploid (75 or more chromosomes). Importantly, the non-hyperdiploid tumors have a much poorer prognosis than hyperdiploid tumors. The basis for this difference is unclear, but it is noteworthy that non-hyperdiploid tumors have a substantially higher incidence of chromosome 13 deletions and IgH translocations than hyperdiploid tumors (Smadja et al., 2001; Fonseca R, personal communication, 3/19/2003).

Primary IgH translocations appear to be mediated mainly by errors in IgH switch recombination, and less often by errors in somatic hypermutation, in germinal center B cells en route to terminal PC differentiation. As summarized previously, at least 50% of MGUS and MM tumors seem to have primary IgH translocations that might represent an initial immortalizing event that occurs in germinal center B cells, but at least 25% of MM tumors have no IgH or IgL translocation. In light of the apparent relationship of primary Ig translocations and cyclin D dysregulation as summarized previously, we propose the following model for the molecular pathogenesis of MM. In 50% of MGUS/SMM tumors and possibly two-thirds of MM tumors, a primary chromosome translocation, mediated mostly by aberrant switch recombination and less frequently by aberrant somatic mutation, results in the ectopic expression of an oncogene. This could lead directly (11q13-cyclin D1 and 6p21-cyclin D3) or indirectly (4p16, 16q23, other–cyclin D2) to cyclin D dysregulation. Alternatively, in approximately one-third of MM tumors there is no Ig translocation, and cyclin D1 is dysregulated by an as-yet undefined mechanism that might involve aberrant interaction with bone marrow stromal cells. The dysregulation of one of three cyclin D genes, which provides a unifying model for the pathogenesis of MM, could render these clonal cells more susceptible to proliferative stimuli, resulting in selective expansion of this clone. Numeric (and possibly structural) karyotypic abnormalities, including monosomy of chromosome 13 or deletion of 13q14, often are present in premalignant MGUS, the earliest identified stage of tumorigenesis. It remains to be determined if karyotypic abnormalities occur before or after primary IgH translocations. However, it is notable that monosomy of chromosome 13 (or 13q14 deletion), which is present in approximately 50% of MM tumors, is present in most MM tumors that have a t(4;14) or t(14;16) translocation, perhaps consistent with the occurrence of this karyotypic abnormality preceding these translocations.

Although we do not understand the molecular basis for the progression from premalignant MGUS to frankly malignant MM, we do have one clue. Mutually exclusive activating mutations of K- or N-*RAS* (or FGFR3 when there is a t[4;14] translocation) are rare or absent in MGUS, whereas RAS mutations are present in 40% of early MM but perhaps 50% of advanced MM, and FGFR3 mutations are more frequent in the advanced stages of MM. Although it seems possible that acquisition of RAS or FGFR3 mutations causes progression from premalignant MGUS to frankly malignant MM, some other as-yet unidentified event must be responsible in the majority of cases. In any case, this progression appears to turn on a molecular switch that results in osteolytic bone lesions mediated by osteoclastogenesis, neo-angiogenesis, and enhanced growth of the myeloma clone. Although poorly understood, this process seems likely to be mediated by the intimate reciprocal interaction of the tumor cells and bone marrow stromal cells (Kuehl and Bergsagel, 2002).

It is not well established whether there is a high rate of ongoing karyotypic instability in MM, but tumor progression is associated with secondary chromosome translocations, of which c-MYC provides a paradigm. The secondary translocations of c-MYC, which are associated with mono-allelic expression of c-MYC, are present at a low frequency in intramedullary MM tumors, but occur in nearly 50% of advanced tumors that generate metaphase chromosomes and are almost universally present in HMCL. The dysregulation of c-MYC would appear to be associated with progression to a more aggressive, proliferative phenotype. Mutations and/or mono-allelic deletion of p53 are seen late in the course of the disease. Interestingly, although dysregulation of cyclin D appears to be a universal event in the pathogenesis of MM, inactivation of RB or the INK4 cyclin-dependent kinase inhibitors still occurs, but apparently late in the more aggressive phase of the disease: p16INK4a by methylation, and Rb or p18INK4a by bi-allelic deletions.

# Concluding Thoughts

A better understanding of the molecular pathogenesis of MM will result in improved diagnosis and management of patients with MM, and eventually should result in more effective, rational, targeted therapy of this uniformly fatal disease. Therefore, it is encouraging that research from many laboratories during the past 5 years has led to steady progress regarding our understanding of the stages and molecular events involved in the pathogenesis of MM, as summarized previously and in Figure 3-6. Nonetheless, in contrast to the paradigm of the pathogenesis of colorectal carcinoma that has been pioneered by Vogelstein, Kinzler, and their colleagues (Kinzler and Vogelstein, 1996, 1998), the extent of our knowledge still seems rather limited. Hopefully, however, building on what we have learned thus far, the application of new genomic technologies, such as RNA microarray profiling, array CGH, and SNP analysis, will lead to identification of additional genetic and epigenetic changes that occur during the pathogenesis of MM.

## What Is the Significance of the Genetic Changes That Have Been Identified Thus Far?

First, we are particularly intrigued by the possibility that the dysregulation of one of the cyclin D genes, as proposed previously, might represent a unifying early event that could provide a potential therapeutic target in a premalignant stage. As indicated, each of the four major primary Ig translocations seems to directly or indirectly dysregulate one of the cyclin D genes, but it will be of particular importance to determine the mechanism responsible for ectopic expression of cyclin D1 that occurs in approximately one-third of MM tumors lacking a t(11;14) translocation. As suggested previously, this ectopic expression of cyclin D1 might be abrogated by inhibiting interactions between the tumor cells and stromal cells.

Second, despite significant heterogeneity, immunoglobulin translocations that target specific oncogenes appear to represent critical events that can affect the phenotype of the tumor cell and also impact prognosis. Patients with IgH translocations that target 4p16 (FGFR3; MMSET) or 16q23 (c-maf) have an extremely poor prognosis compared with patients lacking these translocations. By contrast, patients with IgH translocations that target 11q13 (cyclin D1) have somewhat different clinical features and a slightly better prognosis than patients lacking this translocation (Avet-Loiseau et al., 2002; Fonseca et al., 2002b). In one recent study examining patients treated with single or tandem autologous stem cell transplants, there was a remarkable difference in outcome depending on the IgH translocation present: 23% versus 88% survival at 80 months for patients with t(4;14) and t(11;14), respectively. These results suggest that the oncogenes dysregulated by the early translocation event are likely to represent potential therapeutic targets even in the frankly malignant MM tumor. Although this possibility has not yet been firmly established, there are encouraging studies, which show that pharmacologic inhibitors of FGFR3 can efficiently cause differentiation and death of some HMCL that express FGFR3 as a result of a t(4;14) translocation (Trudel et al., 2002).

Third, activating mutations of K- or N-RAS are present in 40% to 50% of MM tumors, but are rarely present in premalignant MGUS. It seems possible that RAS pathway inhibitors (such as lovastatin or the farnesyltransferase inhibitor R115777) might be effective in patients with RAS mutations. This might also provide an opportunity for chemoprevention, for which nontoxic RAS pathway inhibitors (such as lovastatin) might be used to prevent the emergence of RAS mutations that are associated with the progression from MGUS to MM. Finally, monosomy of chromosome 13 or 13q14 deletion occurs in a substantial fraction of MGUS tumors, but in nearly 50% of MM tumors, and is an independent indicator of a poor prognosis. Clearly, it is critical to determine the molecular target of this abnormality. Apart from identifying additional specific oncogenic events, it seems apparent that an improved understanding of the pathogenesis of myeloma must focus on some of the following areas.

## Biology of Normal Plasmablasts and Plasma Cells

It seems well established that MGUS and MM are tumors of postgerminal center, long-lived bone marrow plasmablasts (PB), and/or PC. Yet we know little about the biology of these normal cells. Are there molecular markers that distinguish different types of PB and PC? What determines homing and maintenance of these cells in the bone marrow and other sites (e.g., mucosa)? Most importantly, what regulates their growth and determines their turnover?

## MGUS and SMM

These premalignant tumors can be diagnosed by a simple noninvasive blood test long before conversion to frankly malignant MM. What limits the growth of these tumors? Can we identify molecular markers that will predict the progression of these tumors to MM so that we can develop preventive pharmacologic or immune therapies?

## Biology of Bone Marrow Cells and Their Interactions with Normal and Tumor PC

Normal PC, and MGUS, SMM, or intramedullary MM tumor cells are dependent on intimate mutual interactions with a variety of bone marrow stromal cells and extracellular matrix factors to achieve differentiation, growth, and survival. A better understanding of these interactions not only will improve our understanding of the pathogenesis of PC tumors, but is almost certain to impact on the development of effective therapies.

## Development of Improved Animal and *Ex Vivo* Models

As summarized briefly in this chapter, each of the various animal models has significant limitations that prevent us from testing hypotheses about the pathogenesis and treatment of PC tumors. Much work is needed to improve existing animal models. However, an even more critical need is the development of an *ex vivo* model that will allow more rapid and precise manipulation and analysis of cells in tumorigenesis or treatment assays.

## REFERENCES

Aalto, Y., Nordling, S., Kivioja, A. H., Karaharju, E., Elomaa, I., and Knuutila, S. (1999). Among numerous DNA copy number changes, losses of chromosome 13 are highly recurrent in plasmacytoma. *Genes Chromosomes Cancer, 25*, 104–107.

Ahmann, G. J., Jalal, S. M., Juneau, A. L., Christensen, E. R., Hanson, C. A., Dewald, G. W., and Greipp, P. R. (1998). A novel three-color, clone-specific fluorescence in situ hybridization procedure for monoclonal gammopathies. *Cancer Genetics Cytogenetics, 101*, 7–11.

Alsina, M., Boyce, B., Devlin, R. D., Anderson, J. L., Craig, F., Mundy, G. R., and Roodman, G. D. (1996). Development of an in vivo model of human multiple myeloma bone disease. *Blood, 87*, 1495–1501.

Anderson, K. C., Shaughnessy, J. D., Jr., Barlogie, B., Harousseau, J. L., and Roodman, G. D. (2002). Multiple myeloma. *Hematology (Am Soc Hematol Educ Program)*, 214–240.

Avet-Loiseau, H., Andree-Ashley, L. E., Moore, D. II, Mellerin, M. P., Feusner, J., Bataille, R., and Pallavicini, M. G. (1997). Molecular cytogenetic abnormalities in multiple myeloma and plasma cell leukemia measured using comparative genomic hybridization. *Genes Chromosomes Cancer, 19*, 124–133.

Avet-Loiseau, H., Brigaudeau, C., Morineau, N., Talmant, P., Lai, J. Y., Daviet, A., Li, J. Y., Praloran, V., Rapp, M. J., Harousseau, J. L., Facon, T., and Bataille, R. (1999a). High incidence of cryptic translocations involving the Ig heavy chain gene in multiple myeloma as shown by fluorescence in situ hybridization. *Genes Chromosomes Cancer, 24*, 9–15.

Avet-Loiseau, H., Daviet, A., Sauner, S., and Bataille, R. (2000). Chromosome 13 abnormalities in multiple myeloma are mostly monosomy 13. *British Journal of Haematology, 111*, 1116–1117.

Avet-Loiseau, H., Facon, T., Daviet, A., Godon, C., Rapp, M. J., Harousseau, J. L., Grosbois, B., and Bataille, R. (1999b). 14q32 translocations and monosomy 13 observed in monoclonal gammopathy of undetermined significance delineate a multistep process for the oncogenesis of multiple myeloma. Intergroupe Francophone du Myelome. *Cancer Research, 59*, 4546–4550.

Avet-Loiseau, H., Li, J. Y., Facon, T., Brigaudeau, C., Morineau, N., Maloisel, F., Rapp, M. J., Talmant, P., Trimoreau, F., Jaccard, A., Harousseau, J. L., and Bataille, R. (1998). High incidence of translocations t(11;14)(q13;q32) and t(4;14)(p16;q32) in patients with plasma cell malignancies. *Cancer Research, 58*, 5640–5645.

Avet-Loiseau, H., Facon, T., Grosbois, B., Magrangeas, F., Rapp, M. J., Harousseau, J. L., Minvielle, S., and Bataille, R. (2002). Oncogenesis of multiple myeloma: 14q32 and 13q chromosomal abnormalities are not randomly distributed, but correlate with natural history, immunological features, and clinical presentation. *Blood, 99*, 2185–2191.

Avet-Loiseau, H., Gerson, F., Margrangeas, F., Minvielle, S., Harousseau, J. L., and Bataille, R. (2001). Rearrangements of the c-myc oncogene are present in 15% of primary human multiple myeloma tumors. *Blood, 98*, 3082–3086.

Avet-Loiseau, H., Li, J. Y., Godon, C., Morineau, N., Daviet, A., Harousseau, J. L., Facon, T., and Bataille, R. (1999c). P53 deletion is not a frequent event in multiple myeloma. *British Journal of Haematology, 106*, 717–719.

Avet-Loiseau, H., Li, J. Y., Morineau, N., Facon, T., Brigaudeau, C., Harousseau, J. L., Grosbois, B., and Bataille, R. (1999d). Monosomy 13 is associated with the transition of monoclonal gammopathy of undetermined significance to multiple myeloma. Intergroupe Francophone du Myelome. *Blood, 94*, 2583–2589.

Bednarek, A. K., Keck-Waggoner, C. L., Daniel, R. L., Laflin, K. J., Bergsagel, P. L., Kiguchi, K., Brenner, A. J., and Aldaz, C. M. (2001). WWOX, the FRA16D gene, behaves as a suppressor of tumor growth. *Cancer Research, 61*, 8068–8073.

Bednarek, A. K., Laflin, K. J., Daniel, R. L., Liao, Q., Hawkins, K. A., and Aldaz, C. M. (2000). WWOX, a novel WW domain-containing protein mapping to human chromosome 16q23.3-24.1, a region frequently affected in breast cancer. *Cancer Research, 60*, 2140–2145.

Bergsagel, P. L., and Kuehl, W. M. (1998). Molecular biology of multiple myeloma. In J. S. Malpas, D. E. Bergsagel, R. Kyle, and K. C. Anderson (Eds.). *Myeloma: Biology and Management*. Oxford: Oxford University Press.

Bergsagel, P. L., and Kuehl, W. M. (2001). Chromosomal translocations in multiple myeloma. *Oncogene, 20*, 5611–5622.

Bezieau, S., Devilder, M. C., Avet-Loiseau, H., Mellerin, M. P., Puthier, D., Pennarun, E., Rapp, M. J., Harousseau, J. L., Moisan, J. P., and Bataille, R. (2001). High incidence of N and K-Ras activating mutations in multiple myeloma and primary plasma cell leukemia at diagnosis. *Human Mutation*, 18, 212–224.

Billadeau, D., Jelinek, D. F., Shah, N., LeBien, T. W., and Van Ness, B. (1995). Introduction of an activated N-ras oncogene alters the growth characteristics of the interleukin 6-dependent myeloma cell line ANBL6. *Cancer Research*, 55, 3640–3646.

Billadeau, D., Liu, P., Jelinek, D., Shah, N., LeBien, T. W., and Van Ness, B. (1997). Activating mutations in the N- and K-ras oncogenes differentially affect the growth properties of the IL-6-dependent myeloma cell line ANBL6. *Cancer Research*, 57, 2268–2275.

Bodrug, S. E., Warner, B. J., Bath, M. L., Lindeman, G. J., Harris, A. W., and Adams, J. M. (1994). Cyclin D1 transgene impedes lymphocyte maturation and collaborates in lymphomagenesis with the myc gene. *Embo Journal*, 13, 2124–2130.

Calame, K. L. (2001). Plasma cells: finding new light at the end of B cell development. *Nature Immunology*, 2, 1103–1108.

Calasanz, M. J., Cigudosa, J. C., Odero, M. D., Ferreira, C., Ardanaz, M. T., Fraile, A., Carrasco, J. L., Sole, F., Cuesta, B., and Gullon, A. (1997). Cytogenetic analysis of 280 patients with multiple myeloma and related disorders: Primary breakpoints and clinical correlations. *Genes Chromosomes Cancer*, 18, 84–93.

Chesi, M., Bergsagel, P. L., and Kuehl, W. M. (2002). The enigma of ectopic expression of FGFR3 in multiple myeloma: A critical initiating event or just a target for mutational activation during tumor progression. *Current Opinion in Hematology*, 9, 288–293.

Chesi, M., Bergsagel, P. L., Shonukan, O. O., Martelli, M. L., Brents, L. A., Chen, T., Schrock, E., Ried, T., and Kuehl, W. M. (1998a). Frequent dysregulation of the c-maf proto-oncogene at 16q23 by translocation to an Ig locus in multiple myeloma. *Blood*, 91, 4457–4463.

Chesi, M., Nardini, E., Brents, L. A., Schrock, E., Ried, T., Kuehl, W. M., and Bergsagel, P. L. (1997). Frequent translocation t(4;14)(p16.3;q32.3) in multiple myeloma is associated with increased expression and activating mutations of fibroblast growth factor receptor 3. *Nature Genetics*, 16, 260–264.

Chesi, M., Nardini, E., Lim, R. S. C., Smith, K. D., Kuehl, W. M., and Bergsagel, P. L. (1998b). The t(4;14) translocation in myeloma dysregulates both FGFR3 and a novel gene, MMSET, resulting in IgH/MMSET hybrid transcripts. *Blood*, 92, 3025–3034.

Chesi, M., Brents, L. A., Ely, S. A., Bais, C., Robbiani, D. F., Mesri, E. A., Kuehl, W. M., and Bergsagel, P. L. (2001). Activated fibroblast growth factor receptor 3 is an oncogene that contributes to tumor progression in multiple myeloma. *Blood*, 97, 729–736.

Cigudosa, J. C., Rao, P. H., Calasanz, M. J., Odero, M. D., Michaeli, J., Jhanwar, S. C., and Chaganti, R. S. (1998). Characterization of nonrandom chromosomal gains and losses in multiple myeloma by comparative genomic hybridization. *Blood*, 91, 3007–3010.

Corradini, P., Inghirami, G., Astolfi, M., Ladetto, M., Voena, C., Ballerini, P., Gu, W., Nilsson, K., Knowles, D. M., Boccadoro, M., et al. (1994). Inactivation of tumor suppressor genes, p53 and Rb1, in plasma cell dyscrasias. *Leukemia*, 8, 758–767.

Corradini, P., Ladetto, M., Voena, C., Palumbo, A., Inghirami, G., Knowles, D. M., Boccadoro, M., and Pileri, A. (1993). Mutational activation of N- and K-ras oncogenes in plasma cell dyscrasias. *Blood*, 81, 2708–2713.

Crowder, C., Kopantzev, E., Williams, K., Lengel, C., Miki, T., and Rudikoff, S. (2003). An unusual H-*Ras* mutant isolated from a human multiple myeloma line leads to transformation and factor-independent cell growth. *Oncogene*, 22, 649–659.

Dalla-Favera, R., and Gaidano, G. (2001). Molecular biology of lymphoma. In V. T. DeVita, S. Hellman, and S. A. Rosenberg (Eds.), *Cancer: Principles and Practice of Oncology* (pp. 2215–2235). Philadelphia: Lippincott Williams and Wilkins.

Dallas, S. L., Garrett, I. R., Oyajobi, B. O., Dallas, M. R., Boyce, B. F., Bauss, F., Radl, J., and Mundy, G. R. (1999). Ibandronate reduces osteolytic lesions but not tumor burden in a murine model of myeloma bone disease. *Blood*, 93, 1697–1706.

Desikan, R., Barlogie, B., Sawyer, J., Ayers, D., Tricot, G., Badros, A., Zangari, M., Munshi, N. C., Anaissie, E., Spoon, D., Siegel, D., Jagannath, S., Vesole, D., Epstein, J., Shaughessy, J., Fassas, A., Lim, S., Roberson, P., and Crowley, J. (2000). Results of high-dose therapy for 1000 patients with multiple myeloma: Durable complete remissions and superior survival in the absence of chromosome 13 abnormalities. *Blood*, 95, 4008–4010.

Dewald, G. W., Kyle, R. A., Hicks, G. A., and Greipp, P. R. (1985). The clinical significance of cytogenetic studies in 100 patients with multiple myeloma, plasma cell leukemia, or amyloidosis. *Blood*, 66, 380–390.

Dohner, H., Stilgenbauer, S., Dohner, K., Bentz, M., and Lichter, P. (1999). Chromosome aberrations in B-cell chronic lymphocytic leukemia: Reassessment based on molecular cytogenetic analysis. *Journal of Molecular Medicine*, 77, 266–281.

Drach, J., Schuster, J., Nowotny, H., Angerler, J., Rosenthal, F., Fiegl, M., Rothermundt, C., Gsur, A., Jager, U., Heinz, R. (1995). Multiple myeloma: High incidence of chromosomal aneuploidy as detected by interphase fluorescence in situ hybridization. *Cancer Research*, 55, 3854–3859.

Druker, B. J. (2002). Inhibition of the Bcr-Abl tyrosine kinase as a therapeutic strategy for CML. *Oncogene*, 21, 8541–8546.

Facon, T., Avet-Loiseau, H., Guillerm, G., Moreau, P., Genevieve, F., Zandecki, M., Lai, J. L., Leleu, X., Jouet, J. P., Bauters, F., Harousseau, J. L., Bataille, R., and Mary, J. Y. (2001). Chromosome 13 abnormalities identified by FISH analysis and serum beta2-microglobulin produce a powerful myeloma staging system for patients receiving high-dose therapy. *Blood*, 97, 1566–1571.

Flactif, M., Zandecki, M., Lai, J. L., Bernardi, F., Obein, V., Bauters, F., and Facon, T. (1995). Interphase fluorescence in situ hybridization (FISH) as a powerful tool for the detection of aneuploidy in multiple myeloma. *Leukemia*, 9, 2109–2114.

Fonseca, R., Ahmann, G. J., Jalal, S. M., Dewald, G. W., Larson, D. R., Therneau, T. M., Gertz, M. A., Kyle, R. A., and Greipp, P. R. (1998a). Chromosomal abnormalities in systemic amyloidosis. *British Journal of Haematology*, 103, 704–710.

Fonseca, R., Bailey, R. J., Ahmann, G. J., Rajkumar, S. V., Hoyer, J. D., Lust, J. A., Kyle, R. A., Gertz, M. A., Greipp, P. R., and Dewald, G. W. (2002a). Genomic abnormalities in monoclonal gammopathy of undetermined significance. *Blood*, 100, 1417–1424.

Fonseca, R., Blood, E. A., Oken, M. M., Kyle, R. A., Dewald, G. W., Bailey, R. J., Van Wier, S. A., Henderson, K. J., Hoyer, J. D., Harrington, D., Kay, N. E., Van Ness, B., and Greipp, P. R. (2002b). Myeloma and the t(11;14)(q13;q32); evidence for a biologically defined unique subset of patients. *Blood*, 99, 3735–3741.

Fonseca, R., Oken, M. M., Harrington, D., Bailey, R. J., Van Wier, S. A., Henderson, K. J., Kay, N. E., Van Ness, B., Greipp, P. R., and Dewald, G. W. (2001). Deletions of chromosome 13 in multiple myeloma identified by interphase FISH usually denote large deletions of the q arm or monosomy. *Leukemia*, 15, 981–986.

Fonseca, R., Witzig, T. E., Gertz, M. A., Kyle, R. A., Hoyer, J. D., Jalal, S. M., and Greipp, P. R. (1998b). Multiple myeloma and the translocation t(11;14)(q13;q32): A report on 13 cases. *British Journal of Haematology*, 101, 296–301.

Gabrea, A., Bergsagel, P. L., Chesi, M., Shou, Y., and Kuehl, W. M. (1999). Insertion of excised IgH switch sequences causes overexpression of cyclin D1 in a myeloma tumor cell. *Molecular Cell*, 3, 119–123.

Gado, K., Silva, S., Paloczi, K., Domjan, G., and Falus, A. (2001). Mouse plasmacytoma: An experimental model of human multiple myeloma. *Haematologica*, 86, 227–236.

Garrett, I. R., Dallas, S., Radl, J., and Mundy, G. R. (1997). A murine model of human myeloma bone disease. *Bone*, 20, 515–520.

Ge, N. L., and Rudikoff, S. (2000). Expression of PTEN in PTEN-deficient multiple myeloma cells abolishes tumor growth in vivo. *Oncogene, 19,* 4091–4095.

Guillerm, G., Gyan, E., Wolowiec, D., Facon, T., Avet-Loiseau, H., Kuliczkowski, K., Bauters, F., Fenaux, P., and Quesnel, B. (2001). p16(INK4a) and p15(INK4b) gene methylations in plasma cells from monoclonal gammopathy of undetermined significance. *Blood, 98,* 244–246.

Gutierrez, N. C., Hernandez, J. M., Garcia, J. L., Canizo, M. C., Gonzalez, M., Hernandez, J., Gonzalez, M. B., Garcia-Marcos, M. A., and San Miguel, J. F. (2001). Differences in genetic changes between multiple myeloma and plasma cell leukemia demonstrated by comparative genomic hybridization. *Leukemia, 15,* 840–845.

Hanahan, D., and Weinberg, R. A. (2000). The hallmarks of cancer. *Cell, 100,* 57–70.

Hanamura, I., Iida, S., Akano, Y., Hayami, Y., Kato, M., Miura, K., Harada, S., Banno, S., Wakita, A., Kiyoi, H., Nowe, T., Shirugu, S., Sonta, S. I., Nifta, M., Taniwaki, M., and Veda, R. (2001). Ectopic expression of MAFB gene in human myeloma cells carrying (14;20)(q32;q11) chromosomal translocations. *Japanese Journal of Cancer Research, 92,* 638–644.

Hatzivassiliou, G., Miller, I., Takizawa, J., Palanisamy, N., Rao, P. H., Iida, S., Tagawa, S., Taniwaki, M., Russo, J., Neri, A., Cattoretti, G., Clynes, R., Mendelsohn, C., Chaganti, R. S., and Dalla-Favera, R. (2001). Irta1 and irta2, novel immunoglobulin superfamily receptors expressed in B cells and involved in chromosome 1q21 abnormalities in B cell malignancy. *Immunity, 14,* 277–289.

Hayman, S. R., Bailey, R. J., Jalal, S. M., Ahmann, G. J., Dispenzieri, A., Gertz, M. A., Greipp, P. R., Kyle, R. A., Lacy, M. Q., Rajkumar, S. V., Witzig, T. E., Lust, J. A., and Fonseca, R. (2001). Translocations involving the immunoglobulin heavy-chain locus are possible early genetic events in patients with primary systemic amyloidosis. *Blood, 98,* 2266–2268.

Ho, I. C., Hodge, M. R., Rooney, J. W., and Glimcher, L. H. (1996). The proto-oncogene c-maf is responsible for tissue-specific expression of interleukin-4. *Cell, 85,* 973–983.

Hyun, T., Yam, A., Pece, S., Xie, X., Zhang, J., Miki, T., Gutkind, J. S., and Li, W. (2000). Loss of PTEN expression leading to high Akt activation in human multiple myelomas. *Blood, 96,* 3560–3568.

Iida, S., Rao, P. H., Butler, M., Corradini, P., Boccadoro, M., Klein, B., Chaganti, R. S., and Dalla-Favera, R. (1997). Deregulation of MUM1/IRF4 by chromosomal translocation in multiple myeloma. *Nature Genetics, 17,* 226–230.

Janssen, J. W., Vaandrager, J. W., Heuser, T., Jauch, A., Kluin, P. M., Geelen, E., Bergsagel, P. L., Kuehl, W. M., Drexler, H. G., Otsuki, T., Bartram, C. R., and Schuuring, E. (2000). Concurrent activation of a novel putative transforming gene, myeov, and cyclin D1 in a subset of multiple myeloma cell lines with t(11;14)(q13;q32). *Blood, 95,* 2691–2698.

Juge-Morineau, N., Harousseau, J. L., Amiot, M., and Bataille, R. (1997). The retinoblastoma susceptibility gene RB-1 in multiple myeloma. *Leukemia Lymphome, 24,* 229–237.

Kakkis, E., Riggs, K. J., Gillespie, W., and Calame, K. (1989). A transcriptional repressor of c-myc. *Nature, 339,* 718–721.

Keats, J. J., Reiman, T., Maxwell, C. A., Taylor, B. J., Larratt, L. M., Mant, M. J., Belch, A. R., and Pilarski, L. M. (2003). In multiple myeloma, t(4;14)(p16;q32) is an adverse prognostic factor irrespective of FGFR3 expression. *Blood, 101,* 1520–1529.

Kinzler, K. W., and Vogelstein, B. (1996). Lessons from hereditary colorectal cancer. *Cell, 87,* 159–170.

Kinzler, K. W., and Vogelstein, B. (1998). Landscaping the cancer terrain. *Science, 280,* 1036–1037.

Kipps, T. J. (2000). Genetics of chronic lymphocytic leukaemia. *Hematology Cell Therapy, 42,* 5–14.

Klein, B., Zhang, X. G., Lu, Z. Y., and Bataille, R. (1995). Interleukin-6 in human multiple myeloma. *Blood, 85,* 863–872.

Konigsberg, R., Ackermann, J., Kaufmann, H., Zojer, N., Urbauer, E., Kromer, E., Jager, U., Gisslinger, H., Schreiber, S., Heinz, R., Ludwig, H., Huber, H., and Drach, J. (2000). Deletions of chromosome 13q in monoclonal gammopathy of undetermined significance. *Leukemia, 14,* 1975–1979.

Kramer, A., Schultheis, B., Bergmann, J., Willer, A., Hegenbart, U., Ho, A. D., Goldschmidt, H., and Hehlmann, R. (2002). Alterations of the cyclin D1/pRb/p16(INK4A) pathway in multiple myeloma. *Leukemia, 16,* 1844–1851.

Kuehl, W. M., and Bergsagel, P. L. (2002). Multiple myeloma: Evolving genetic events and host interactions. *National Review of Cancer, 2,* 175–187.

Kulkarni, M. S., Daggett, J. L., Bender, T. P., Kuehl, W. M., Bergsagel, P. L., and Williams, M. E. (2002). Frequent inactivation of the cyclin-dependent kinase inhibitor p18 by homozygous deletion in multiple myeloma cell lines: Ectopic p18 expression inhibits growth and induces apoptosis. *Leukemia, 16,* 127–134.

Kuppers, R., and Dalla-Favera, R. (2001). Mechanisms of chromosomal translocations in B cell lymphomas. *Oncogene, 20,* 5580–5594.

Kuppers, R., Klein, U., Hansmann, M. L., and Rajewsky, K. (1999). Cellular origin of human B-cell lymphomas. *New England Journal of Medicine, 341,* 1520–1529.

Kyle, R. A. (1994) Monotonal gammopathy of undetermined significance. *Blood Review. 8,* 135–141.

Kyle, R. A., Therneau, T. M., Rajkumar, S. V., Offord, J. R., Larson, D. R., Plevak, M. F., and Melton, L. J. III. (2002). A long-term study of prognosis in monoclonal gammopathy of undetermined significance. *New England Journal of Medicine, 346,* 564–569.

Lai, J. L., Zandecki, M., Mary, J. Y., Bernardi, F., Izydorczyk, V., Flactif, M., Morel, P., Jouet, J. P., Bauters, F., and Facon, T. (1995). Improved cytogenetics in multiple myeloma: A study of 151 patients including 117 patients at diagnosis. *Blood, 85,* 2490–2497.

Lam, E. W., Glassford, J., Banerji, L., Thomas, N. S., Sicinski, P., and Klaus, G. G. (2000). Cyclin D3 compensates for loss of cyclin D2 in mouse B-lymphocytes activated via the antigen receptor and CD40. *Journal of Biologic Chemistry, 275,* 3479–3484.

Liu, P., Leong, T., Quam, L., Billadeau, D., Kay, N. E., Greipp, P., Kyle, R. A., Oken, M. M., and Van Ness, B. (1996). Activating mutations of N- and K-ras in multiple myeloma show different clinical associations: Analysis of the Eastern Cooperative Oncology Group Phase III Trial. *Blood, 88,* 2699–2706.

Lovec, H., Grzeschiczek, A., Kowalski, M. B., and Moroy, T. (1994). Cyclin D1/bcl-1 cooperates with myc genes in the generation of B-cell lymphoma in transgenic mice. *Embo Journal, 13,* 3487–3495.

Lynch, H. T., Sanger, W. G., Pirruccello, S., Quinn-Laquer, B., and Weisenburger, D. D. (2001). Familial multiple myeloma: A family study and review of the literature. *Journal of the National Cancer Institute, 93,* 1479–1483.

MacLennan, I. C. M. (1998). Antibody-secreting cells and their origins. In J. S. Malpas, D. E. Bergsagel, R. A. Kyle, and K. C. Anderson (Eds.), *Myeloma: Biology and Management* (pp. 29–47). Oxford: Oxford University Press.

Malgeri, U., Baldini, L., Perfetti, V., Fabris, S., Vignarelli, M. C., Colombo, G., Lotti, V., Compasso, S., Bogni, S., Lombardi, L., et al. (2000). Detection of t(4;14)(p16.3;q32) chromosomal translocation in multiple myeloma by reverse transcription-polymerase chain reaction analysis of IGH-MMSET fusion transcripts. *Cancer Research, 60,* 4058–4061.

Marx, J. (2002). Debate surges over the origins of genomic defects in cancer. *Science, 297,* 544–546.

Max, E. E. (1999). Immunoglobulins: Molecular genetics. In W. E. Paul (Eds.), *Fundamental Immunology* (pp. 113–184). Philadelphia: Lippincott-Raven.

Mazars, G. R., Portier, M., Zhang, X. G., Jourdan, M., Bataille, R., Theillet, C., and Klein, B. (1992). Mutations of the p53 gene in human myeloma cell lines. *Oncogene, 7,* 1015–1018.

Mitelman, F., Johansson, B., and Mertens, F. (2001). Mitelman Database of Chromosome Aberrations in Cancer http://egap.nci.nih.gov/chromosomes.Mitelman

Neri, A., Baldini, L., Trecca, D., Cro, L., Polli, E., and Maiolo, A. T. (1993). p53 gene mutations in multiple myeloma are associated with advanced forms of malignancy. *Blood*, 81, 128–135.

Ollikainen, H., Syrjanen, S., Koskela, K., Pelliniemi, T. T., and Pulkki, K. (1997). p53 gene mutations are rare in patients but common in patient-originating cell lines in multiple myeloma. *Scandinavian Journal of Clinical Laboratory Investigation*, 57, 281–289.

Olumi, A. F., Grossfeld, G. D., Hayward, S. W., Carroll, P. R., Tlsty, T. D., and Cunha, G. R. (1999). Carcinoma-associated fibroblasts direct tumor progression of initiated human prostatic epithelium. *Cancer Research*, 59, 5002–5011.

Pasqualucci, L., Neumeister, P., Goossens, T., Nanjangud, G., Chaganti, R. S., Kuppers, R., and Dalla-Favera, R. (2001). Hypermutation of multiple proto-oncogenes in B-cell diffuse large-cell lymphomas. *Nature*, 412, 341–346.

Pearse, R. N., Sordillo, E. M., Yaccoby, S., Wong, B. R., Liau, D. F., Colman, N., Michaeli, J., Epstein, J., and Choi, Y. (2001). Multiple myeloma disrupts the TRANCE/osteoprotegerin cytokine axis to trigger bone destruction and promote tumor progression. *Proceeding of the National Academy of Sciences of the United States of America*, 98, 11581–11586.

Perez-Simon, J. A., Garcia-Sanz, R., Tabernero, M. D., Almeida, J., Gonzalez, M., Fernandez-Calvo, J., Moro, M. J., Hernandez, J. M., San Miguel, J. F., and Orfao, A. (1998). Prognostic value of numerical chromosome aberrations in multiple myeloma: A FISH analysis of 15 different chromosomes. *Blood*, 91, 3366–3371.

Pilarski, L. M., Hipperson, G., Seeberger, K., Pruski, E., Coupland, R. W., and Belch, A. R. (2000). Myeloma progenitors in the blood of patients with aggressive or minimal disease: Engraftment and self-renewal of primary human myeloma in the bone marrow of NOD SCID mice. *Blood*, 95, 1056–1065.

Pilarski, L. M., Seeberger, K., Coupland, R. W., Eshpeter, A., Keats, J. J., Taylor, B. J., and Belch, A. R. (2002). Leukemic B cells clonally identical to myeloma plasma cells are myelomagenic in NOD/SCID mice. *Experimental Hematology*, 30, 221–228.

Plowright, E. E., Li, Z., Bergsagel, P. L., Chesi, M., Barber, D., Branch, D. R., Hawley, R. G., and Stewart, A. K. (2000). Ectopic expression of fibroblast growth factor receptor 3 promotes myeloma cell proliferation and prevents apoptosis. *Blood*, 95, 992–998.

Potter, M. (1997). Experimental plasmacytomagenesis in mice. *Hematology/Oncology Clinics of North America*, 11, 323–347.

Qian, L., Gong, J., Liu, J., Broome, J. D., and Koduru, P. R. (1999). Cyclin D2 promoter disrupted by t(12;22)(p13;q11.2) during transformation of chronic lymphocytic leukaemia to non-Hodgkin's lymphoma. *British Journal of Haematology*, 106, 477–485.

Radl, J. (1999). Multiple myeloma and related disorders. Lessons from an animal model. *Pathol Biol (Paris)*, 47, 109–114.

Radl, J., Punt, Y. A., van den Enden-Vieveen, M. H., Bentvelzen, P. A., Bakkus, M. H., van den Akker, T. W., and Benner, R. (1990). The 5T mouse multiple myeloma model: absence of c-myc oncogene rearrangement in early transplant generations. *British Journal of Cancer*, 61, 276–278.

Rajkumar, S. V., Fonseca, R., Dewald, G. W., Therneau, T. M., Lacy, M. Q., Kyle, R. A., Greipp, P. R., and Gertz, M. A. (1999). Cytogenetic abnormalities correlate with the plasma cell labeling index and extent of bone marrow involvement in myeloma. *Cancer Genetics Cytogenetics*, 113, 73–77.

Rebouissou, C., Wijdenes, J., Autissier, P., Tarte, K., Costes, V., Liautard, J., Rossi, J. F., Brochier, J., and Klein, B. (1998). A gp130 interleukin-6 transducer-dependent SCID model of human multiple myeloma. *Blood*, 91, 4727–4737.

Ried, K., Finnis, M., Hobson, L., Mangelsdorf, M., Dayan, S., Nancarrow, J. K., Woollatt, E., Kremmidiotis, G., Gardner, A.,

Venter, D., et al. (2000). Common chromosomal fragile site FRA16D sequence: Identification of the FOR gene spanning FRA16D and homozygous deletions and translocation breakpoints in cancer cells. *Human Molecular Genetics*, 9, 1651–1663.

Ries, L. A. G., Eisner, M. P., Kosary, C. L., Hankey, B. F., Miller, B. A., Clegg, L., and Edwards, B. K. (2002). *SEER Cancer Statistics Review, 1973–1999*. Bethesda: National Cancer Institute.

Santra, M., Zhan, F., Tian, E., Barlogie, B., and Shaughnessy, J. (2003). A subset of multiple myeloma harboring the t(4;14)(p16;q32) translocation lack FGFR3 expression but maintain an IGH/MMSET fusion transcript. *Blood*. 15, 2374–2376.

Sawyer, J. R., Lukacs, J. L., Munshi, N., Desikan, K. R., Singhal, S., Mehta, J., Siegel, D., Shaughnessy, J., and Barlogie, B. (1998a). Identification of new nonrandom translocations in multiple myeloma with multicolor spectral karyotyping. *Blood*, 92, 4269–4278.

Sawyer, J. R., Lukacs, J. L., Thomas, E. L., Swanson, C. M., Goosen, L. S., Sammartino, G., Gilliland, J. C., Munshi, N. C., Tricot, G., Shaughnessy, J. D., et al. (2000). Multicolour spectral karyotyping identifies new translocations and a recurring pathway for chromosome loss in multiple myeloma. *British Journal of Haematology*, 112, 1–9.

Sawyer, J. R., Tricot, G., Mattox, S., Jagannath, S., and Barlogie, B. (1998b). Jumping translocations of chromosome 1q in multiple myeloma: Evidence for a mechanism involving decondensation of pericentromeric heterochromatin. *Blood*, 91, 1732–1741.

Sawyer, J. R., Waldron, J. A., Jagannath, S., and Barlogie, B. (1995). Cytogenetic findings in 200 patients with multiple myeloma. *Cancer Genetics Cytogenetics*, 82, 41–49.

Seong, C., Delasalle, K., Hayes, K., Weber, D., Dimopoulos, M., Swantkowski, J., Huh, Y., Glassman, A., Champlin, R., and Alexanian, R. (1998). Prognostic value of cytogenetics in multiple myeloma. *British Journal of Haematology*, 101, 189–194.

Shaughnessy, J., Gabrea, A., Qi, Y., Brents, L. A., Zhan, F., Tian, E., Sawyer, J., Barlogie, B., Bergsagel, P. L., and Kuehl, W. M. (2001). Cyclin D3 at 6p21 is dysregulated by recurrent Ig translocations in multiple myeloma. *Blood*, 98, 217–223.

Shaughnessy, J., Tian, E., Sawyer, J., Bumm, K., Landes, R., Badros, A., Morris, C., Tricot, G., Epstein, J., and Barlogie, B. (2000). High incidence of chromosome 13 deletion in multiple myeloma detected by multiprobe interphase FISH. *Blood*, 96, 1505–1511.

Sherr, C. J., and McCormick, F. (2002). The RB and p53 pathways in cancer. *Cancer Cell*, 2, 103–112.

Shou, Y., Martelli, M. L., Gabrea, A., Qi, Y., Brents, L. A., Roschke, A., Dewald, G., Kirsch, I. R., Bergsagel, P. L., and Kuehl, W. M. (2000). Diverse karyotypic abnormalities of the c-myc locus associated with c-myc dysregulation and tumor progression in multiple myeloma. *Proceedings of the National Academy of Sciences of the United States of America*, 97, 228–233.

Smadja, N. V., Bastard, C., Brigaudeau, C., Leroux, D., and Fruchart, C. (2001). Hypodiploidy is a major prognostic factor in multiple myeloma. *Blood*, 98, 2229–2238.

Stec, I., Wright, T. J., van Ommen, G. J., de Boer, P. A., van Haeringen, A., Moorman, A. F., Altherr, M. R., and den Dunnen, J. T. (1998). WHSC1, a 90 kb SET domain-containing gene, expressed in early development and homologous to a Drosophila dysmorphy gene maps in the Wolf-Hirschhorn syndrome critical region and is fused to IgH in t(4;14) multiple myeloma. *Human Molecular Genetics*, 7, 1071–1082.

Sze, D. M., Toellner, K. M., Garcia de Vinuesa, C., Taylor, D. R., and MacLennan, I. C. (2000). Intrinsic constraint on plasmablast growth and extrinsic limits of plasma cell survival. *Journal of Experimental Medicine*, 192, 813–821.

Taniguchi, T., Chikatsu, N., Takahashi, S., Fujita, A., Uchimaru, K., Asano, S., Fujita, T., and Motokura, T. (1999). Expression of p16INK4A and p14ARF in hematological malignancies. *Leukemia*, 13, 1760–1769.

Tarte, K., De Vos, J., Thykjaer, T., Zhan, F., Fiol, G., Costes, V., Reme, T., Legouffe, E., Rossi, J. F., Shaughnessy, J., Jr., Orntoft, T. F., and Klein, B. (2002). Generation of polyclonal plasmablasts from peripheral blood B cells: A normal counterpart of malignant plasmablasts. *Blood*, *100*, 1113–1122.

Tlsty, T. D. (2001). Stromal cells can contribute oncogenic signals. *Seminars in Cancer Biology*, *11*, 97–104.

Tourigny, M. R., Ursini-Siegel, J., Lee, H., Toellner, K. M., Cunningham, A. F., Franklin, D. S., Ely, S., Chen, M., Qin, X. F., Xiong, Y., MacLennan, I. C., and Chen-Kiang, S. (2002). CDK inhibitor p18(INK4c) is required for the generation of functional plasma cells. *Immunity*, *17*, 179–189.

Trudel, S., Ely, S., Farooqui, Y., Robbiani, D. F., Affer, M., Chesi, M., and Bergsagel, P. L. (2002). Rational therapy targeting the initial genetic event in multiple myeloma: FGFR3 as a drug target in t(4;14) MM. *Blood*, *100*, 396a.

Tsunenari, T., Koishihara, Y., Nakamura, A., Moriya, M., Ohkawa, H., Goto, H., Shimazaki, C., Nakagawa, M., Ohsugi, Y., Kishimoto, T., et al. (1997). New xenograft model of multiple myeloma and efficacy of a humanized antibody against human interleukin-6 receptor. *Blood*, *90*, 2437–2444.

Uchida, T., Kinoshita, T., Ohno, T., Ohashi, H., Nagai, H., and Saito, H. (2001). Hypermethylation of p16INK4A gene promoter during the progression of plasma cell dyscrasia. *Leukemia*, *15*, 157–165.

Urashima, M., Chen, B. P., Chen, S., Pinkus, G. S., Bronson, R. T., Dedera, D. A., Hoshi, Y., Teoh, G., Ogata, A., Treon, S. P., et al. (1997a). The development of a model for the homing of multiple myeloma cells to human bone marrow. *Blood*, *90*, 754–765.

Urashima, M., Teoh, G., Ogata, A., Chauhan, D., Treon, S. P., Hoshi, Y., DeCaprio, J. A., and Anderson, K. C. (1997b). Role of CDK4 and p16INK4A in interleukin-6-mediated growth of multiple myeloma. *Leukemia*, *11*, 1957–1963.

Urashima, M., Teoh, G., Ogata, A., et al. (1997c). Characterization of p16(INK4A) expression in multiple myeloma and plasma cell leukemia. *Clinical Cancer Research*, *3*, 2173–2179.

van den Akker, T. W., Radl, J., Franken-Postma, E., Hagemeijer, A. (1996). Cytogenetic findings in mouse multiple myeloma and Waldenström's macroglobulinemia. *Cancer, Genetics, and Cytogenetics*, *86*, 156–161.

Vanderkerken, K., De Raeve, H., Goes, E., Van Meirvenne, S., Radl, J., Van Riet, I., Thielemans, K., and Van Camp, B. (1997). Organ involvement and phenotypic adhesion profile of 5T2 and 5T33 myeloma cells in the C57BL/KaLwRij mouse. *British Journal of Cancer*, *76*, 451–460.

Worel, N., Greinix, H., Ackermann, J., Kaufmann, H., Urbauer, E., Hocker, P., Gisslinger, H., Lechner, K., Kalhs, P., and Drach, J. (2001). Deletion of chromosome 13q14 detected by fluorescence in situ hybridization has prognostic impact on survival after high-dose therapy in patients with multiple myeloma. *Annals of Hematology*, *80*, 345–348.

Wu, K., Orme, L., Shaughnessy, J., Bumm, K., Barlogie, B., and Moore, M. A. S. (2001). Telomerase expression and telomere length in purified myeloma cells: A study of 158 cases. *Blood*, *11*, 374a.

Yaccoby, S., and Epstein, J. (1999). The proliferative potential of myeloma plasma cells manifest in the SCID-hu host. *Blood*, *94*, 3576–3582.

Yaccoby, S., Johnson, C. L., Mahaffey, S. C., Wezeman, M. J., Barlogie, B., and Epstein, J. (2002a). Antimyeloma efficacy of thalidomide in the SCID-hu model. *Blood*, *100*, 4162–4168.

Yaccoby, S., Pearse, R. N., Johnson, C. L., Barlogie, B., Choi, Y., and Epstein, J. (2002b). Myeloma interacts with the bone marrow microenvironment to induce osteoclastogenesis and is dependent on osteoclast activity. *British Journal of Haematology*, *116*, 278–290.

Yoshida, S., Nakazawa, N., Iida, S., Hayami, Y., Sato, S., Wakita, A., Shimizu, S., Taniwaki, M., and Ueda, R. (1999). Detection of MUM1/IRF4-IgH fusion in multiple myeloma. *Leukemia*, *13*, 1812–1816.

Zandecki, M., Facon, T., Preudhomme, C., Vanrumbeke, M., Vachee, A., Quesnel, B., Lai, J. L., Cosson, A., and Fenaux, P. (1995). The retinoblastoma gene (RB-1) status in multiple myeloma: A report on 35 cases. *Leukemia and Lymphoma*, *18*, 497–503.

Zandecki, M., Lai, J. L., Genevieve, F., Bernardi, F., Volle-Remy, H., Blanchet, O., Francois, M., Cosson, A., Bauters, F., and Facon, T. (1997). Several cytogenetic subclones may be identified within plasma cells from patients with monoclonal gammopathy of undetermined significance, both at diagnosis and during the indolent course of this condition. *Blood*, *90*, 3682–3690.

Zhan, F., Hardin, J., Kordsmeier, B., Bumm, K., Zheng, M., Tian, E., Sanderson, R., Yang, Y., Wilson, C., Zangari, M., et al. (2002). Global gene expression profiling of multiple myeloma, monoclonal gammopathy of undetermined significance, and normal bone marrow plasma cells. *Blood*, *99*, 1745–1757.

Zhang, S. L., DuBois, W., Ramsay, E. S., Bliskovski, V., Morse, H. C. III, Taddesse-Heath, L., Vass, W. C., DePinho, R. A., and Mock, B. A. (2001). Efficiency alleles of the Pctr1 modifier locus for plasmacytoma susceptibility. *Molecular and Cell Biology*, *21*, 310–318.

Zhou, S., Kinzler, K. W., and Vogelstein, B. (1999). Going mad with Smads. *New England Journal of Medicine*, *341*, 1144–1146.

Zhu, D., van Arkel, C., King, C. A., Meirvenne, S. V., de Greef, C., Thielemans, K., Radl, J., and Stevenson, F. K. (1998). Immunoglobulin VH gene sequence analysis of spontaneous murine immunoglobulin-secreting B-cell tumours with clinical features of human disease. *Immunology*, *93*, 162–170.

Zojer, N., Konigsberg, R., Ackermann, J., Fritz, E., Dallinger, S., Kromer, E., Kaufmann, H., Riedl, L., Gisslinger, H., Schreiber, S., et al. (2000). Deletion of 13q14 remains an independent adverse prognostic variable in multiple myeloma despite its frequent detection by interphase fluorescence in situ hybridization. *Blood*, *95*, 1925–1930.

Zojer, N., Schuster-Kolbe, J., Assmann, I., Ackermann, J., Strasser, K., Hubl, W., Drach, J., and Ludwig, H. (2002). Chromosomal aberrations are shared by malignant plasma cells and a small fraction of circulating CD19 + cells in patients with myeloma and monoclonal gammopathy of undetermined significance. *British Journal of Haematology*, *117*, 852–859.

# CHAPTER 4

# Cytokines, Cytokine Receptors, and Signal Transduction in Human Multiple Myeloma

TERU HIDESHIMA
DHARMINDER CHAUHAN
KENNETH C. ANDERSON

## Introduction

We have characterized the role of growth factors in multiple myeloma (MM) pathogenesis and derived novel therapies to improve patient outcome based on targeting cytokines and their signaling cascades both in the MM cell as well as its bone marrow (BM) microenvironment. To achieve this goal, we have developed systems for studying the growth, survival, and drug resistance mechanisms intrinsic to MM cells. Importantly, we have also developed both *in vitro* systems and *in vivo* animal models to characterize mechanisms of MM cell homing to BM, as well as cytokines promoting MM cell growth and drug resistance in the BM milieu. These model systems have allowed for the development of several promising biologically based therapies, including thalidomide (Thal) and its immunomodulatory analogs (IMiDs), proteasome inhibitor PS-341, and arsenic trioxide (As$_2$O$_3$) (see Chapter 14). Once preclinical promise had been demonstrated, we rapidly translated these laboratory studies to phase I and II clinical trials to evaluate their clinical use and toxicity. Importantly, ongoing gene array studies of samples obtained from patients treated using these protocols is directed to identify *in vivo* targets and mechanisms of drug action on the one hand versus mechanisms of drug resistance on the other. These studies have suggested the critical role of cytokines in growth, survival, drug resistance, and migration of MM cells, providing the framework for validating their role in MM pathogenesis and as targets for novel therapies.

## Role of Cytokines in MM Pathogenesis

Multiple myeloma cells home to the BM and adhere to extracellular matrix proteins and BM stromal cells (BMSCs), which not only localizes tumor cells in the BM milieu, but also has important functional sequelae (Teoh and Anderson, 1997). Specifically, binding of MM cells to the extracellular matrix protein fibronectin triggers upregulation of p27 and cell adhesion-mediated drug resistance (CAM-DR) (Damiano et al., 1999; Hazlehurst et al., 2000), related directly to cell contact and mediated independent of cytokines. In addition, however, our studies have identified adhesion molecules mediating MM cell binding to BMSCs, as well as growth, survival, and drug resistance conferred by this binding (Teoh and Anderson, 1997; Uchiyama et al., 1992). Importantly, adhesion of MM cells to BMSCs not only similarly mediates resistance to drug-induced

apoptosis, but also triggers the paracrine nuclear factor (NF)-κB dependent transcription and secretion of interleukin (IL)-6, the major cytokine-mediating MM cell growth and survival in BMSCs (Chauhan et al., 1996; Hideshima et al., 2002c; Uchiyama et al., 1993). Second, we have shown that MM cells localized in the BM milieu secrete cytokines (tumor necrosis factor α [TNFα], transforming growth factor [TGF]-β, vascular endothelial growth factor [VEGF]), which further upregulate IL-6 secretion in BMSCs (Gupta et al., 2001; Hideshima et al., 2001a; Urashima et al., 1996). Within the BM microenvironment, we have demonstrated that these cytokines mediate growth (IL-6, insulin-like growth factor [IGF]-1, VEGF), survival (IL-6, IGF-1), drug resistance (IL-6, IGF-1), and migration (VEGF, stromal cell-derived factor [SDF]-1α) of MM cells; and also trigger angiogenesis (VEGF) (Chauhan et al., 1997b, 1999; Hideshima et al., 2001b, 2002b, 2002c; Mitsiades et al., 2002c; Ogata et al., 1997; Podar et al., 2001, 2002) (Fig. 4-1). After establishing the biologic significance of these cytokines in MM pathogenesis, we then delineated the signaling cascades mediating their effects to target these cascades with novel therapies.

## Interleukin-6

This cytokine has been implicated in autocrine and paracrine growth of MM cells within the BM milieu. Some MM cells spontaneously secrete IL-6, and IL-6 secretion can be induced by CD 40 activation of tumor cells (Urashima et al., 1995) or by cytokines (TNF-α, VEGF, IL-1) within the BM microenvironment (Costes et al., 1998; Lust and Donovan, 1999). Most IL-6 in the BM milieu is secreted by BMSCs; transcription and

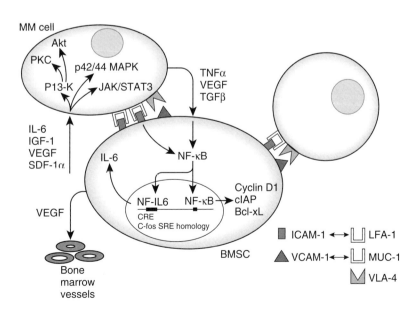

**Figure 4-1** Cytokines induce signaling cascades, mediating growth, survival, adhesion molecules, expression, drug resistance, and angiogenesis in the MM BM milieu.

secretion of IL-6 in BMSCs is further enhanced both by binding of tumor cells to BMSCs (Chauhan et al., 1996; Gupta et al., 2001; Uchiyama et al., 1993) and by secretion of cytokines (VEGF, TGF-β, TNFα) from MM cells (Dankbar et al., 2000; Gupta et al., 2001; Hideshima et al., 2001a, 2002c, 2003; Urashima et al., 1996). Our studies have shown that IL-6-induced proliferation is associated with activation of Ras/Raf/mitogen-activated protein kinase (MEK)/p42/44 MAPK signaling cascade (Ogata et al., 1997), which is abrogated by MAPK antisense oligonucleotide or by the ERK inhibitor PD98059 (Hideshima et al., 2001b). Survival of MM cells triggered by IL-6 is conferred through Janus kinase2 (JAK2)/signal transducers and activators of transcription (STAT) 3 signaling and can be blocked by dominant/negative STAT3 (Catlett-Falcone et al., 1999; Oshiro et al., 2001). Activation of STAT3 induces Bcl-xL (Catlett-Falcone et al., 1999) and Mcl-1 expression (Epling-Burnette et al., 2001; Puthier et al., 1999; Wei et al., 2001), which can contribute to MM cell survival. Drug (dexamethasone [Dex]) resistance is mediated through phosphatidylinositol-3 kinase (PI3-K)/Akt signaling cascade, which can be neutralized by wartmannin or LY294002 (Hideshima et al., 2001b; Tu et al., 2000) (Fig. 4-2). Importantly, we have shown that gamma irradiation (IR), Fas, and Dex-induced MM cell apoptosis is mediated by distinct signaling cascades (Chauhan et al., 1997a, 1997b, 1997c). For example, Dex- (but not IR or Fas) triggered apoptosis is mediated through activation of related adhesion focal tyrosine kinase (RAFTK) (Chauhan et al., 1999). Moreover, Dex-mediated MM apoptosis is not associated with mitochondrial cytochrome c release (Chauhan et al., 1997b), but is mediated by Second mitochondria activator of caspase (Smac) release from mitochondria (Chauhan et al., 2001b); cytosolic Smac disrupts the inhibitor of apoptosis XIAP/caspase 9 complex, thereby allowing activation of caspase 9, caspase 3 cleavage,

and apoptosis. Importantly, IL-6 inhibits apoptosis triggered by Dex (but not IR) through PI3-K/Akt signaling (Hideshima et al., 2001b) and specific activation of SHP2 phosphatase, thereby blocking activation of RAFTK (Chauhan and Anderson, 2001a). We have most recently used gene microarray both to further delineate this cytokine-induced growth and anti-apoptotic pathways (Chauhan et al., 2002a) and to derive targeted therapeutic strategies to overcome drug resistance based on interrupting growth or triggering apoptotic signaling cascades (Chauhan and Anderson, 2001a). For example, these studies have demonstrated that IL-6 induces the XBP-1 transcription factor (Chauhan et al., 2003), which is implicated in differentiation of normal B cells to plasma cells (Claudio et al., 2002; Reimold et al., 2001) and is markedly upregulated in freshly isolated MM patient samples (Chauhan et al., 2003). Finally, we have also developed animal models for the evaluation of cytokine-induced cellular and molecular events regulating the growth, survival, and migration of human MM cells *in vivo*. Specifically, we pioneered the SCID-hu model of human MM in which human fetal bone grafts are implanted bilaterally in the flanks of SCID mice (Urashima et al., 1997). Human MM cells implanted into these grafts proliferate, trigger human IL-6 secretion in BMSCs, secrete MM idiotypic protein detectable in mouse serum, and migrate to the contralateral human BM graft, but not to murine BM. This *in vivo* model of human MM therefore provides a means for identifying adhesion molecules mediating specific homing of human MM cells to the human, as opposed to murine, BM microenvironment; as well as for studying the role of microenvironmental factors (cytokines, angiogenesis) in MM pathogenesis.

Most importantly, serum IL-6 and IL-6 receptors are prognostic factors in MM and reflect the proliferative fraction of MM cells within patients (Kyrtsonis et al., 1996; Pulkki et al., 1996; Stasi et al., 1998). C reactive protein (CRP), an acute phase reactant synthesized in the liver in response to IL-6, can serve as a surrogate prognostic factor (Pelliniemi et al., 1995). IL-6 or CRP, either alone or coupled with β2 microglobulin (β2m) as a measure of MM cell mass (Calasanz et al., 1997; Tricot et al., 2002), provides the framework for a biologically based staging system in MM. Attempts to target IL-6 in treatment strategies to date have included antibodies to IL-6 and IL-6 receptor (Ogata et al., 1996), as well as IL-6 superantagonists which bind to IL-6R but do not trigger downstream signaling. Although anti-MM activities *in vivo* have been observed, responses have only been transient. Of interest, novel agents, including proteasome inhibitor PS-341 and $As_2O_3$, can overcome the growth survival, and drug resistance induced by IL-6 and thereby overcome classic drug resistance.

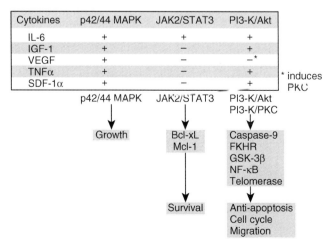

**Figure 4-2** *Cytokines induce p42/44 MAPK, JAK2/STAT3, and/or PI3-K/Akt and downstream signaling cascades.*

# Tumor Necrosis Factor α

TNFα secreted by MM cells does not induce significant growth, survival, or drug resistance in tumor cells. However, TNFα secreted by MM cells is a more potent stimulus of IL-6 secretion in BMSCs than is VEGF or TGF-β (Hideshima et al., 2001a); it binds directly to a TNFα response element in the IL-6 promotor and thereby augments IL-6 mediated sequelae, including growth, survival, and drug resistance. Importantly, TNFα secreted by MM cells can induce NF-κB-dependent upregulation of adhesion molecules in MM cells and BMSCs (CD49d, CD54) (Hideshima et al., 2001a), thereby increasing binding of MM cells, and associated further induction of IL-6 transcription and secretion in BMSCs (Hideshima et al., 2001a, 2002c) (Fig. 4-2), as well as CAM-DR. Therefore, novel agents targeting TNFα, including Thal and the IMiDs (Corral et al., 1999; Hideshima and Anderson, 2002), might act, at least in part, by inhibiting IL-6 mediated sequelae.

# Vascular Endothelial Growth Factor

VEGF is produced both by MM cells and by BMSCs and can account, at least in part, for the increased angiogenesis observed in MM patient BM. Our most recent studies further show that CD40 activation induces p53-dependent VEGF secretion in human MM cells (Tai et al., 2002). Of interest, our studies have shown that some MM cell lines and patient cells express VEGF receptor Flt-1, and that VEGF triggers its phosphorylation (Podar et al., 2001, 2002). Exogenous VEGF triggers modest ERK activation and proliferation in MM cell lines and patient cells, which can be neutralized by antibody to VEGF, the VEGF receptor tyrosine kinase inhibitor PTK787 (Lin et al., 2002), or by PD98059 (Podar et al., 2001). Most importantly, VEGF induces MM cell migration, assayed in a Transwell migration assay, to a greater extent in patient plasma cell leukemia cells than in patient MM cells. This VEGF-induced migration of MM cells is associated with β1 integrin- and PI3-K-dependent PKCα activation, but not with ERK activation (Podar et al., 2002) (Fig. 4-2). This migration is abrogated by bisindolylmaleimide or antibody to VEGF, but not by PD98059 (Podar et al., 2001). These direct effects of VEGF on tumor cells, coupled with its induction of cytokines (i.e., IL-6) and angiogenesis in the BM milieu, provide the framework for targeting VEGF in treatment strategies. The VEGF receptor tyrosine kinase inhibitor PTK787 is active preclinically and will soon undergo clinical protocol testing in MM (Lin et al., 2002).

# Insulin-Like Growth Factor-1

IGF-1 activates MAPK and PI3K/Akt signaling cascades in MM cells (Ge and Rudikoff, 2000; Qiang et al., 2002), which promotes proliferation and drug resistance. We have recently delineated the molecular mechanism whereby IGF-1 promotes MM cell survival and drug resistance (Mitsiades et al., 2002c) (Fig. 4-2). Specifically, IGF-1 stimulates sustained activation of NF-κB and PI3-K/Akt; induces phosphorylation of FKHR/forkhead transcription factor; upregulates a series of intracellular antiapoptotic proteins, including FLIP, survivin, cIAP-2, A1/Bfl-1, and XIAP; and decreases drug sensitivity of MM cells. It is more potent than IL-6 in mediating these effects, setting the stage for novel MM treatments targeting IGF-1. Most recently, we have shown that both IL-6 and IGF-1 increase telomerase activity through PI3-K/Akt activation (Akiyama et al., 2002). Therapies targeting IGF-1, inhibitors of IGF-1 receptor, already have shown preclinical anti-MM activity and will soon undergo clinical evaluation (Mitsiades et al., 2002a).

# Stromal Cell-Derived Factor-1α

SDF-1α mediates migration of normal hematopoietic stem cells. We have recently detected SDF-1α in BM plasma from patients with MM and in supernatants from MM patient BMSCs (Hideshima et al., 2002b). Moreover, CXCR4, a receptor for SDF-1α, is expressed on some MM cells. SDF-1α promotes proliferation, induces migration, and protects against Dex-induced apoptosis in MM cells. SDF-1α activates MAPK, PI3-K/Akt, and NF-κB in MM cells (Fig. 4-2). Within the BM microenvironment, SDF-1α upregulates secretion of IL-6 and VEGF in BMSCs, thereby promoting tumor cell growth survival, drug resistance, and migration. However, these effects of SDF-1α are only modest compared with other cytokines, and SDF-1α therefore does not represent a promising target for novel therapeutics for MM.

# Other Cytokines

A variety of other cytokines have been reported to play a role in MM pathogenesis. Recombinant IL-1β stimulates MM cells to produce IL-6, which consequently augments proliferation of MM cells (Costes et al., 1998). TGF-β is secreted by MM cells and triggers IL-6 secretion in BMSCs (Urashima et al., 1996), augmenting paracrine IL-6-mediated tumor cell growth. TGF-β secreted by MM cells likely also contributes to the immunodeficiency characteristic of MM by downregulating B cells, T cells, and natural killer cells without similarly inhibiting the growth of MM cells. IL-10 is a proliferation factor, but not a differentiation factor, for human MM cells (Gu et al., 1996; Lu et al., 1995). Macrophage inflammatory protein-1α (MIP-1α) is a potential osteoclast stimulatory factor in MM (Abe et al., 2002; Choi et al., 2000). Autocrine growth mediated by IL-15 (Hjorth-Hansen et al., 1999; Tinhofer et al., 2000), and most recently by IL-21 (Brenne et al., 2002), has been demonstrated in both MM cell lines and patient cells. Cytokines other that IL-6 that use gp130 signaling have also been implicated in MM pathogenesis including oncostatin M (Chauhan et al., 1995), IL-11, and leukemia inhibitory factor 1 (Nishimoto et al., 1994).

# Therapeutic Implications and Future Directions

Many conventional therapies downregulate cytokine production or bioactivity. For example, Dex downregulates IL-6 transcription in BMSCs through binding to the glucocorticoid response element in the IL-6 promoter. As mentioned previously, novel agents, including PS-341 and $As_2O_3$, inhibit transcription of IL-6 by blocking activation of NF-κB. Our recent studies shed new insights into an additional mechanism whereby MM therapies might target cytokine signaling. gp130/ CD130, the β-subunit of IL-6 family member receptors, plays an essential role in IL-6 mediating signaling. After IL-6 binds to gp80 (IL-6 receptor α-subunit), gp130 dimerizes and is phosphorylated, thereby triggering multiple downstream signaling pathways, such as Ras/Raf/MEK/p42/44 MAPK, JAK2/STAT3, and PI3-K/Akt. These signaling cascades promote MM cell growth, drug resistance, and antiapoptosis in the BM microenvironment. Our previous studies demonstrated that proteasome inhibitor PS-341 and $As_2O_3$ overcome the protective effect of IL-6 against Dex-induced apoptosis in MM by inducing caspase-8 and/or -9 cleavage, followed by caspase-3 cleavage (Hayashi et al., 2002; Hideshima et al., 2000c, 2001; Mitsiades et al., 2002b). Most recently, we have shown that PS-341 and $As_2O_3$ induce gp130 cleavage *in vitro*, before MM cell death (Hideshima et al., submitted for publication). Importantly, gp130 cleavage triggered by these agents is completely abrogated by the pan-caspase inhibitor Z-VAD-FMK, but not by caspase-8 inhibitor Z-IETD-FMK or caspase-9 inhibitor Z-LEHD-FMK. Moreover, phosphorylation of p42/44 MAPK, STAT3, and PI3-K/Akt induced in MM.1S cells by exogenous IL-6 and in the BM microenvironment is abrogated by PS-341. Our results therefore suggest that cleavage of gp130 is one mechanism accounting for the inability of IL-6 to protect MM cells against cytotoxicity of these agents *in vivo*. Future cytokine-targeted therapies will similarly be directed to inhibit cytokine production and/or signaling, to overcome drug resistance and improve patient outcome.

# REFERENCES

Abe, M., Hiura, K., Wilde, J., Moriyama, K., Hashimoto, T., Ozaki, S., Wakatsuki, S., Kosaka, M., Kido, S., Inoue, D., and Matsumoto, T. (2002). Role for macrophage inflammatory protein (MIP)-1alpha and MIP-1beta in the development of osteolytic lesions in multiple myeloma. *Blood, 100,* 2195–2202.

Akiyama, M., Hideshima, T., Hayashi, T., Tai, Y. T., Mitsiades, C. S., Mitsiades, N., Chauhan, D., Richardson, P., Munshi, N. C., and Anderson, K. C. (2002). Cytokines modulate telomerase activity in a human multiple myeloma cell line. *Cancer Research, 62,* 3876–3882.

Brenne, A. T., Baade Ro, T., Waage A., Sundan, A., Borset, M., and Hjorth-Hansen, H. (2002). Interleukin-21 is a growth and survival factor for human myeloma cells. *Blood, 99,* 3756–3762.

Calasanz, M. J., Cigudosa, J. C., Odero, M. D., Ferreira, C., Ardanaz, M. T., Fraile, A., Carrasco, J. L., Sole, F., Cuesta, B., and Gullon, A. (1997). Cytogenetic analysis of 280 patients with multiple myeloma and related disorders: Primary breakpoints and clinical correlations. *Genes Chromosomes Cancer, 18,* 84–93.

Catlett-Falcone, R., Landowski, T. H., Oshiro, M. M., Turkson, J., Levitzki, A., Savino, R., Ciliberto, G., Moscinski, L., Fernandez-Luna, J. L., Nunez, G., Dalton, W. S., and Jove, R. (1999). Constitutive activation of Stat3 signaling confers resistance to apoptosis in human U266 myeloma cells. *Immunity, 10,* 105–115.

Chauhan, D., and Anderson, K. C. (2001a). Apoptosis in multiple myeloma: therapeutic implications. *Apoptosis, 6,* 47–55.

Chauhan, D., Auclair, D., Robinson, E. K., Hideshima, T., Li, G., Podar, K., Gupta, D., Richardson, P., Schlossman, R. L., Krett, N., Chen, L. B., Munshi, N. C., and Anderson, K. C. (2002a). Identification of genes regulated by dexamethasone in multiple myeloma cells using oligonucleotide arrays. *Oncogene, 21,* 1346–1358.

Chauhan, D., Hideshima, T., Pandey, P., Treon, S., Teoh, G., Raje, N., Rosen, S., Krett, N., Husson, H., Avraham, S., Kharbanda, S., and Anderson, K. C. (1999). RAFTK/PYK2-dependent and -independent apoptosis in multiple myeloma cells. *Oncogene, 18,* 6733–6740.

Chauhan, D., Hideshima, T., Rosen, S., Reed, J. C., Kharbanda, S., and Anderson, K. C. (2001b). Apaf-1/cytochrome c-independent and Smac-dependent induction of apoptosis in multiple myeloma (MM) cells. *Journal of Biological Chemistry, 276,* 24453–24456.

Chauhan, D., Kharbanda, S. M., Ogata, A., Urashima, M., Frank, D., Malik, N., Kufe, D. W., and Anderson, K. C. (1995). Oncostatin M induces association of Grb2 with Janus kinase JAK2 in multiple myeloma cells. *Journal of Experimental Medicine, 182,* 1801–1806.

Chauhan, D., Kharbanda, S., Ogata, A., Urashima, M., Teoh, G., Robertson, M., Kufe, D. W., and Anderson, K. C. (1997a). Interleukin 6 inhibits Fas-induced apoptosis and stress-activated protein kinase activation in multiple myeloma cells. *Blood, 89,* 227–234.

Chauhan, D., Li, G., Hideshima, T., Auclair, D., Richardson, P., Schlossman, R. L., Podar, K., Li, C., Kim, R. S., Li, W. W., and Anderson, K. C. (2003). Identification of genes regulated by 2-methoxyestradiol (2ME2) in multiple myeloma (MM) cels using oligonucleotide array. *Blood, 101,* 3606–3614.

Chauhan, D., Pandey, P., Hideshima, T., Treon, S., Raje, N., Davies, F. E., Shima, Y., Tai, Y. T., Rosen, S., Avraham, S., Kharbanda, S., and Anderson, K. C. (2000). SHP2 mediates the protective effect of interleukin-6 against dexamethasone-induced apoptosis in multiple myeloma cells. *Journal of Biological Chemistry, 275,* 27845–27850.

Chauhan, D., Pandey, P., Ogata, A., Teoh, G., Krett, N., Halgren, R., Rosen, S., Kufe, D., Kharbanda, S., and Anderson, K. (1997b). Cytochrome c-dependent and -independent induction of apoptosis in multiple myeloma cells. *Journal of Biological Chemistry, 272*, 29995–29997.

Chauhan, D., Pandey, P., Ogata, A., Teoh, G., Treon, S., Urashima, M., Kharbanda, S., and Anderson, K. C. (1997c). Dexamethasone induces apoptosis of multiple myeloma cells in a JNK/SAP kinase independent mechanism. *Oncogene, 15*, 837–843.

Chauhan, D., Uchiyama, H., Akbarali, Y., Urashima, M., Yamamoto, K., Libermann, T. A., and Anderson, K. C. (1996). Multiple myeloma cell adhesion-induced interleukin-6 expression in bone marrow stromal cells involves activation of NF-κB. *Blood, 87*, 1104–1112.

Choi, S. J., Cruz, J. C., Craig, F., Chung, H., Devlin, R. D., Roodman, G. D., and Alsina, M. (2000). Macrophage inflammatory protein 1-alpha is a potential osteoclast stimulatory factor in multiple myeloma. *Blood, 96*, 671–675.

Claudio, J. O., Masih-Khan, E., Tang, H., Goncalves, J., Voralia, M., Li, Z. H., Nadeem, V., Cukerman, E., Francisco-Pabalan, O., Liew, C. C., Woodgett, J. R., and Stewart, A. K. (2002). A molecular compendium of genes expressed in multiple myeloma. *Blood, 100*, 2175–2186.

Corral, L. G., Haslett, P. A., Muller, G. W., Chen, R., Wong, L. M., Ocampo, C. J., Patterson, R. T., Stirling, D. I., and Kaplan, G. (1999). Differential cytokine modulation and T cell activation by two distinct classes of thalidomide analogues that are potent inhibitors of TNF-alpha. *Journal of Immunology, 163*, 380–386.

Costes, V., Portier, M., Lu, Z. Y., Rossi, J. F., Bataille, R., and Klein, B. (1998). Interleukin-1 in multiple myeloma: Producer cells and their role in the control of IL-6 production. *British Journal of Haematology, 103*, 1152–1160.

Damiano, J. S., Cress, A. E., Hazlehurst, L. A., Shtil, A. A., and Dalton, W. S. (1999). Cell adhesion-mediated drug resistance (CAM-DR): Role of integrins and resistance to apoptosis in human myeloma cell lines. *Blood, 93*, 1658–1667.

Dankbar, B., Padro, T., Leo, R., Feldmann, B., Kropff, M., Mesters, R. M., Serve, H., Berdel, W. E., and Kienast, J. (2000). Vascular endothelial growth factor and interleukin-6 in paracrine tumor—stromal cell interactions in multiple myeloma. *Blood, 95*, 2630–2636.

Epling-Burnette, P. K., Liu, J. H., Catlett-Falcone, R., Turkson, J., Oshiro, M., Kothapalli, R., Li, Y., Wang, J. M., Yang-Yen, H. F., Karras, J., Jove, R., and Loughran, T. P., Jr. (2001). Inhibition of STAT3 signaling leads to apoptosis of leukemic large granular lymphocytes and decreased Mcl-1 expression. *Journal of Clinical Investigations, 107*, 351–362.

Ge, N. L., and Rudikoff, S. (2000). Insulin-like growth factor I is a dual effector of multiple myeloma cell growth. *Blood, 96*, 2856–2861.

Gu, Z. J., Costes, V., Lu, Z. Y., Zhang, X. G., Pitard, V., Moreau, J. F., Bataille, R., Wijdenes, J., Rossi, J. F., and Klein, B. (1996). Interleukin-10 is a growth factor for human myeloma cells by induction of an oncostatin M autocrine loop. *Blood, 88*, 3972–3986.

Gupta, D., Treon, S. P., Shima, Y., Hideshima, T., Podar, K., Tai, Y. T., Lin, B., Lentzsch, S., Davies, F. E., Chauhan, D., Schlossman, R. L., Richardson, P., Ralph, P., Wu, L., Payvandi, F., Muller, G., Stirling, D. I., and Anderson, K. C. (2001). Adherence of multiple myeloma cells to bone marrow stromal cells upregulates vascular endothelial growth factor secretion: Therapeutic applications. *Leukemia, 15*, 1950–1961.

Hayashi, T., Hideshima, T., Akiyama, M., Richardson, P., Schlossman, R. L., Chauhan, D., Munshi, N. C., Waxman, S., and Anderson, K. C. (2002). Arsenic trioxide inhibits growth of human multiple myeloma cells in the bone marrow microenvironment. *Molecular Cancer Therapy, 1*, 851–860.

Hazlehurst, L. A., Damiano, J. S., Buyuksal, I., Pledger, W. J., and Dalton, W. S. (2000). Adhesion to fibronectin via β1 integrins regulates p27kip1 levels and contributes to cell adhesion-mediated drug resistance (CAM-DR). *Oncogene, 19*, 4319–4327.

Hideshima, T., Akiyama, M., Hayashi, T., Richardson, P., Schlossman, R., Chauhan, D., and Anderson, K. C. (2003a). Targeting p38 MAPK inhibits multiple myeloma cell growth in the bone marrow milieu. *Blood, 101*, 703–705.

Hideshima, T., and Anderson, K. C. (2002). Molecular mechanisms of novel therapeutic approaches for multiple myeloma. *National Review of Cancer, 2*, 927–937.

Hideshima, T., Chauhan, D., Hayashi, T., Akiyama, M., Mitsiades, N., Mitsiades, C., Podar, K., Munshi, N. C., Richardson, P. G., and Anderson, K. C. (2001). Caspase-dependent cleavage of gp130/interleukin-6 receptor β-subunit in multiple myeloma: Therapeutic implications. *Cancer Research, 61*, 3071–3076.

Hideshima, T., Chauhan, D., Hayashi, T., Podar, K., Masaharu, A., Gupta, D., Richardson, P., Munshi, N., and Anderson, K. C. (2002b). The biologic sequelae of stromal cell-derived factor-1α in multiple myeloma. *Molecular Cancer Therapy, 1*, 539–544.

Hideshima, T., Chauhan, D., Richardson, P., Mitsiades, C., Mitsiades, N., Hayashi, T., Munshi, N., Dang, L., Castro, A., Palombella, V., Adams, J., and Anderson, K. C. (2002c). NF-κB as a therapeutic target in multiple myeloma. *Journal of Biological Chemistry, 277*, 16639–16647.

Hideshima, T., Chauhan, D., Schlossman, R., Richardson, P., and Anderson, K. C. (2001a). The role of tumor necrosis factor α in the pathogenesis of human multiple myeloma: Therapeutic applications. *Oncogene, 20*, 4519–4527.

Hideshima, T., Mitsiades, C., Akiyama, M., Hayashi, T., Chauhan, D., Richardson, P., Schlossman, R., Munshi, N., Mitsiades, N., and Anderson, K. C. (2003). Molecular mechanisms mediating antimyeloma activity of proteasome inhibitor PS-341. *Blood, 101*, 1530–1534.

Hideshima, T., Nakamura, N., Chauhan, D., and Anderson, K. C. (2001b). Biologic sequelae of interleukin-6 induced PI3-K/Akt signaling in multiple myeloma. *Oncogene, 20*, 5991–6000.

Hideshima, T., Richardson, P., Chauhan, D., Palombella, V. J., Elliot, P. J., Adams, J., and Anderson, K. C. (2000c). The proteasome inhibitor PS-341 inhibits growth, induces apoptosis, and overcomes drug resistance in human multiple myeloma. *Cancer Research, 61*, 3071–3076.

Hjorth-Hansen, H., Waage, A., and Borset, M. (1999). Interleukin-15 blocks apoptosis and induces proliferation of the human myeloma cell line OH-2 and freshly isolated myeloma cells. *British Journal of Haematology, 106*, 28–34.

Kyrtsonis, M. C., Dedoussis, G., Zervas, C., Perifanis, V., Baxevanis, C., Stamatelou, M., and Maniatis, A. (1996). Soluble interleukin-6 receptor (sIL-6R), a new prognostic factor in multiple myeloma. *British Journal of Haematology, 93*, 398–400.

Lin, B., Podar, K., Gupta, D., Tai, Y. T., Hideshima, T., Lentzsch, S., Davies, F., Weisberg, E., Schlossman, R. L., Richardson, P. G., Griffin, J. D., Wood, J., and Anderson, K. C. (2002). The vascular endothelial growth factor receptor kinase inhibitor PTK787/ZK222584 inhibits growth and migration of multiple myeloma cells in the bone marrow microenvironment. *Cancer Research, 62*, 5019–5026.

Lu, Z. Y., Zhang, X. G., Rodriguez, C., Wijdenes, J., Gu, Z. J., Morel-Fournier, B., Harousseau, J. L., Bataille, R., Rossi, J. F., and Klein, B. (1995). Interleukin-10 is a proliferation factor but not a differentiation factor for human myeloma cells. *Blood, 85*, 2521–2527.

Lust, J. A., and Donovan, K. A. (1999). The role of interleukin-1 beta in the pathogenesis of multiple myeloma. *Hematology Oncology Clinic of North America, 13*, 1117–1125.

Mitsiades, C. S., Mitsiades, N., Kung, A. L., Shringapurne, R., Poulaki, V., Richardson, P. G., Libermann, T. A., Munshi, N. C., Loukopoulos, D., and Anderson, K. C. (2002a). The IGF/IGF-1R system is a major therapeutic target for multiple myeloma, other hematologic malignancies and solid tumors. *Blood, 100,* 170a.

Mitsiades, N., Mitsiades, C. S., Poulaki, V., Chauhan, D., Gu, X., Bailey, C., Joseph, M., Libermann, T. A., Treon, S. P., Munshi, N. C., Richardson, P. G., Hideshima, T., and Anderson, K. C. (2002b). Molecular sequelae of proteasome inhibition in human multiple myeloma cells. *Proceedings of the National Academy of Sciences of the United States of America, 99,* 14374–14379.

Mitsiades, C. S., Mitsiades, N., Poulaki, V., Schlossman, R., Akiyama, M., Chauhan, D., Hideshima, T., Treon, S. P., Munshi, N. C., Richardson, P. G., and Anderson, K. C. (2002c). Activation of NF-kappaB and upregulation of intracellular anti-apoptotic proteins via the IGF-1/Akt signaling in human multiple myeloma cells: Therapeutic implications. *Oncogene, 21,* 5673–5683.

Nishimoto, N., Ogata, A., Shima, Y., Tani, Y., Ogawa, H., Nakagawa, M., Sugiyama, H., Yoshizaki, K., and Kishimoto, T. (1994). Oncostatin M, leukemia inhibitory factor, and interleukin 6 induce the proliferation of human plasmacytoma cells via the common signal transducer, gp 130. *Journal of Experimental Medicine, 179,* 1343–1347.

Ogata, A., and Anderson, K. C. (1996). Therapeutic strategies for inhibition of interleukin-6 mediated multiple myeloma cell growth. *Leukemia Research, 20,* 303–307.

Ogata, A., Chauhan, D., Teoh, G., Treon, S. P., Urashima, M., Schlossman, R. L., and Anderson, K. C. (1997). Interleukin-6 triggers cell growth via the *ras*-dependent mitogen-activated protein kinase cascade. *Journal of Immunology, 159,* 2212–2221.

Oshiro, M. M., Landowski, T. H., Catlett-Falcone, R., Hazlehurst, L. A., Huang, M., Jove, R., and Dalton, W. S. (2001). Inhibition of JAK kinase activity enhances Fas-mediated apoptosis but reduces cytotoxic activity of topoisomerase II inhibitors in U266 myeloma cells. *Clinical Cancer Research, 7,* 4262–4271.

Pelliniemi, T. T., Irjala, K., Mattila, K., Pulkki, K., Rajamaki, A., Tienhaara, A., Laakso, M., and Lahtinen, R. (1995). Immunoreactive interleukin-6 and acute phase proteins as prognostic factors in multiple myeloma. Finnish Leukemia Group. *Blood, 85,* 765–771.

Podar, K., Tai, Y. T., Davies, F. E., Lentzsch, S., Sattler, M., Hideshima, T., Lin, B. K., Gupta, D., Shima, Y., Chauhan, D., Mitsiades, C., Raje, N., Richardson, P., and Anderson, K. C. (2001). Vascular endothelial growth factor triggers signaling cascades mediating multiple myeloma cell growth and migration. *Blood, 98,* 428–435.

Podar, K., Tai, Y. T., Lin, B. K., Narsimhan, R. P., Sattler, M., Kijima, T., Salgia, R., Gupta, D., Chauhan, D., and Anderson, K. C. (2002). Vascular endothelial growth factor-induced migration of multiple myeloma cells is associated with $\beta$1 integrin- and phosphatidylinositol 3-kinase-dependent PKC$\alpha$ activation. *Journal of Biological Chemistry, 277,* 7875–7881.

Pulkki, K., Pelliniemi, T. T., Rajamaki, A., Tienhaara, A., Laakso, M., and Lahtinen, R. (1996). Soluble interleukin-6 receptor as a prognostic factor in multiple myeloma. Finnish Leukaemia Group. *British Journal of Haematology, 92,* 370–374.

Puthier, D., Bataille, R., and Amiot, M. (1999). IL-6 up-regulates Mcl-1 in human myeloma cells through JAK/STAT rather than ras/MAP kinase pathway. *European Journal of Immunology, 29,* 3945–3950.

Qiang, Y. W., Kopantzev, E., and Rudikoff, S. (2002). Insulinlike growth factor-I signaling in multiple myeloma: Downstream elements, functional correlates, and pathway cross-talk. *Blood, 99,* 4138–4146.

Reimold, A. M., Iwakoshi, N. N., Manis, J., Vallabhajosyula, P., Szomolanyi-Tsuda, E., Gravallese, E. M., Friend, D., Grusby, M. J., Alt, F., and Glimcher, L. H. (2001). Plasma cell differentiation requires the transcription factor XBP-1. *Nature, 412,* 300–307.

Stasi, R., Brunetti, M., Parma, A., Di Giulio, C., Terzoli, E., and Pagano, A. (1998). The prognostic value of soluble interleukin-6 receptor in patients with multiple myeloma. *Cancer, 82,* 1860–1866.

Tai, Y. T., Podar, K., Gupta, D., Lin, B., Young, G., Akiyama, M., and Anderson, K. C. (2002). CD40 activation induces p53-dependent vascular endothelial growth factor secretion in human multiple myeloma cells. *Blood, 99,* 1419–1427.

Teoh, G., and Anderson, K. C. (1997). Interaction of tumor and host cells with adhesion and extracellular matrix molecules in the development of multiple myeloma. *Hematology Oncology Clinic of North America, 11,* 27–42.

Tinhofer, I., Marschitz, I., Henn, T., Egle, A., and Greil, R. (2000). Expression of functional interleukin-15 receptor and autocrine production of interleukin-15 as mechanisms of tumor propagation in multiple myeloma. *Blood, 95,* 610–618.

Tricot, G., Spencer, T., Sawyer, J., Spoon, D., Desikan, R., Fassas, A., Badros, A., Zangari, M., Munshi, N., Anaissie, E., Toor, A., and Barlogie, B. (2002). Predicting long-term (> or = 5 years) event-free survival in multiple myeloma patients following planned tandem autotransplants. *British Journal of Haematology, 116,* 211–217.

Tu, Y., Gardner, A., and Lichtenstein, A. (2000). The phosphatidylinositol 3-kinase/AKT kinase pathway in multiple myeloma plasma cells: Roles in cytokine-dependent survival and proliferative responses. *Cancer Research, 60,* 6763–6770.

Uchiyama, H., Barut, B. A., Chauhan, D., Cannistra, S. A., and Anderson, K. C. (1992). Characterization of adhesion molecules on human myeloma cell lines. *Blood, 80,* 2306–2314.

Uchiyama, H., Barut, B. A., Mohrbacher, A. F., Chauhan, D., and Anderson, K. C. (1993). Adhesion of human myeloma-derived cell lines to bone marrow stromal cells stimulates interleukin-6 secretion. *Blood, 82,* 3712–3720.

Urashima, M., Chauhan, D., Uchiyama, H., Freeman, G. J., and Anderson, K. C. (1995). CD40 ligand triggered interleukin-6 secretion in multiple myeloma. *Blood, 85,* 1903–1912.

Urashima, M., Chen, B. P., Chen, S., Pinkus, G. S., Bronson, R. T., Dedera, D. A., Hoshi, Y., Teoh, G., Ogata, A., Treon, S. P., Chauhan, D., and Anderson, K. C. (1997). The development of a model for the homing of multiple myeloma cells to human bone marrow. *Blood, 90,* 754–765.

Urashima, M., Ogata, A., Chauhan, D., Hatziyanni, M., Vidriales, M. B., Dedera, D. A., Schlossman, R. L., and Anderson, K. C. (1996). Transforming growth factor-beta1: Differential effects on multiple myeloma versus normal B cells. *Blood, 87,* 1928–1938.

Wei, L, H., Kuo, M. L., Chen, C. A., Chou, C. H., Cheng, W. F., Chang, M. C., Su, J. L., and Hsieh, C. Y. (2001). The anti-apoptotic role of interleukin-6 in human cervical cancer is mediated by up-regulation of Mcl-1 through a PI 3-K/Akt pathway. *Oncogene, 20,* 5799–5809.

# CHAPTER 5

# Cytogenetics of Multiple Myeloma

RAFAEL FONSECA

## Introduction

Multiple and complex chromosomal abnormalities are present in plasma cells (PCs) of multiple myeloma (MM) (Dewald et al., 1985; Tabernero et al., 1996; Zandecki et al., 1996). Through the use of interphase FISH, we know chromosomal abnormalities are early events because they are present in monoclonal gammopathy of undetermined significance (MGUS) and smoldering multiple myeloma (SMM) (Avet-Loiseau et al., 2002; Drach et al., 1995c; Fonseca et al., 1997, 2002a; Tabernero et al., 1996; Zandecki et al., 1996). The recurrent nature and biologic plausibility make the abnormalities highly suspect for disease pathogenesis (Kuehl and Bergsagel, 2002). We have just begun to understand the clinical and biologic importance of specific abnormalities (Bergsagel and Kuehl, 2001; Kuehl and Bergsagel, 2002). We review current information with special emphasis on the clinical implications of these aberrations.

The karyotype analysis in MM by conventional cytogenetics (CC) has long been hampered by the low proliferative index of the clone. In most cases (50–70%) the karyotype reveals normal metaphases that originate from the myeloid elements, with the consequent limitations for the clinical applicability of results (Debes-Marun et al., 2002; Dewald et al., 1985; Gould et al., 1988; Lai et al., 1995; Sawyer et al., 1995; Smadja et al., 1998, 2001; Zandecki, 1996). In an effort to improve on the yield of abnormal metaphases, the use of cytokines has been attempted without much success (Lai et al., 1995). In addition, because of their cryptic nature, some of the important abnormalities in MM are not detectable in CC analysis (e.g., t(4;14)(p16.3;q32)) (Chesi et al., 1997, 1998a; Sawyer et al., 1998). The detection of an abnormal karyotype in MM is highly correlated with an elevated PC labeling index (PCLI), reflective of a higher mitotic rate, and also with a higher bone marrow plasmacytosis (Rajkumar et al., 1999). However, the interest into the role of specific genetic aberrations in the outcome of MM was sparked by reports showing clinical implications for aberrations (Dewald et al., 1985; Seong et al., 1998; Smadja et al., 1998, 2001; Tricot et al., 1995). A seminal observation made by Tricot was that monosomy of chromosome 13 ($\Delta$13) was associated with a significantly shorter survival (Desikan et al., 2000; Tricot et al., 1995, 1997).

To improve on the accuracy of conventional karyotype analysis, other methods of investigation have been attempted. For instance, multicolor metaphase FISH has been used to provide greater details of complex karyotypes (Sawyer et al., 1998, 2001). This technique is still limited by the need of cells to undergo mitosis. Another technique that does not require metaphases is comparative genomic hybridization (CGH). However, CGH allows only for the detection of net DNA gain or loss and cannot detect balanced structural abnormalities. CGH has been used for the study of MM, and several areas of recurrence have been identified (Avet-Loiseau and Bataille, 1998; Cigudosa et al., 1998; Gutierrez et al., 2001) (Table 5-1).

MM has also been successfully studied by interphase FISH, because this is an assay that can be done in nondividing cells (Avet-Loiseau et al., 2002; Drach et al., 1995c; Fonseca et al., 1997, 2001b, 2001c, 2002b, 2002c; Hayman et al., 2001; Tabernero et al., 1996; Zandecki et al., 1996). To better estimate for the prevalence of chromosomal abnormalities, interphase FISH is best done in purified cells (e.g., CD138 micro-bead selection) or by using simultaneous immunofluorescence (Ahmann et al., 1998; Avet-Loiseau et al., 1998, 1999a, 2000, 2002; Fonseca et al., 2001b, 2001c, 2002a, 2002c, 2003; Konigsberg et al., 2000a). Both techniques can be used for the study of PC conditions with a low-percentage plasmacytosis (Avet-Loiseau et al., 1999b; Fonseca et al., 1998a, 2002a; Hayman et al., 2001). The availability of large-scale gene expression profiling has revolutionized the field of human genetics. The details of this technique are discussed elsewhere in this book.

## Translocations Involving the Immunoglobulin (Ig) Locus

Translocations that involve both the Ig heavy (IgH) and light chain (IgL) genes have been implicated as seminal events in the pathogenesis of MM (Bergsagel et al., 1995, 1996). In most cases these translocations involve IgH locus, but in a minority they involve the IgL. Of interest those translocations that involve the IgL genes predominantly involve IgL-$\lambda$ translocations. IgH translocations are observed in 50% to 70% of all MM cases and in a similar proportion of patients with

---

**TABLE 5-1**

### Prevalence of Chromosomal Gains and Losses as Determined by Metaphase CGH

| Chromosome | Cigudosa (Cigudosa et al., 1998) | Avet-Loiseau (Avet-Loiseau et al., 1997) 8 patients and 13 cell lines | Gutierrez (Gutierrez et al., 2001) MM cases n = 25, PCL 5 |
|---|---|---|---|
| 1 | | +1q12–qter (40–80%) | +1q11–q41 (36%) in PCL (100%) |
| 3 | | +3q22q29 (>10%) +3p25–pter (>10%) | +3q25–q27 (40%) |
| 6 | –6q21 (13%) | –6q22.1–q23 (>10%) | |
| 7 | | +7 (45%) | |
| 8 | | +8q21–qter (30–40%) | |
| 9 | +9q (10%) | | +9q (40%) |
| 11 | +11q (20%) | +11q13.1 (50–60%) | +11q (44%) |
| 12 | +12q24 (10%) | | |
| 13 | –13q14–21 (30%) | –13 (40–60%) (13q12.1–q21) (13q32–34) | |
| 14 | | –14 (40–60%) (14q11.2–q13) (14q23–q31–) | |
| 15 | +15q32–qter (10%) | | +15q (48%) |
| 16 | –16q (17%) | | |
| 17 | +17q22–24 (13%) | –17p11.2–p13 (>10%) | |
| 22 | +22q (10%) | | |

**TABLE 5-2**

### Prevalence and Clinical Importance of IgH Translocations

| Abnormality | MGUS/SMM (%) | MM (%) | Upregulated Oncogenes | Effect on Prognosis |
|---|---|---|---|---|
| IgL translocations | 30 | 30 | *c-myc* and others | Unknown |
| IgH translocations | 50 | 75 | See below | Mixed |
| t(4;14)(p16.3;q32) | 10 | 15 | *FGFR3* and *MMSET* | Adverse |
| t(11;14)(q13;q32) | 30 | 16 | *Cyclin D1* and *myeov* | Favorable |
| t(14;16)(q32;q23) | 5 | 5 | *C-maf WWOX?* | Adverse |
| *Other IgH* | 5 | ~35 | *Cyclin D3, MUM1* Others | Unknown |

MGUS (Avet-Loiseau et al., 1999b; Fonseca et al., 2002a; Nishida et al., 1997) (Table 5-2).

IgH translocations in MM include an array of nonrandom recurrent chromosomal partners, including 4p13, 6p21, 6p2511q13, and 16q23 (Kuehl and Bergsagel, 2002). Some of the IgH translocations (i.e., t(4;14)(p16.3;q32) and t(14;16)(q32;q23)) are associated with aggressive variants of MM and are overrepresented in human MM cell lines. IgH translocations are also likely associated with a higher predisposition of independence of the bone marrow microenvironment like they are more commonly seen in PC leukemia (Avet-Loiseau et al., 2001a; Bergsagel et al., 1996). Some translocations might represent secondary or progression events because they are mostly seen in the advanced stages of the disease. One such example is translocations that involve *c-myc* (both at Ig sites and other) (Avet-Loiseau et al., 2001b; Shou et al., 2000).

The importance of IgH translocations in the pathogenesis of MM is based on several pieces of evidence. First, IgH translocations form plausible pathogenetic founder lesions in a multitude of other B-cell neoplasms (Hallek et al., 1998; Willis and Dyer, 2000). IgH translocations are highly favored with clonal expansion because they are seen in the majority of clonotypic cells in MM (Avet-Loiseau et al., 1999a, 2002; Fonseca et al., 2001b, 2002c). IgH translocations are recurrent and at similar prevalence as reported by multiple investigators (Avet-Loiseau et al., 1999a, 2002; Fonseca et al., 2001b, 2002c). IgH translocations in MM result in transcriptional activation of putative oncogenes (Kuehl and Bergsagel, 2002). In serially tested samples translocations are conserved and not lost (Fonseca R, unpublished observations). These cytogenetic aberrations are seen since the early stages of the plasma cell neoplasms (MGUS) (Avet-Loiseau et al., 1999b; Fonseca et al., 2002a). However, the specific partner chromosomes dictate biologic variability in patients with MM (Fonseca et al., 2002b; Moreau et al., 2002). Based on this information, it is currently believed that translocations are early and important events for the immortalization of the clone in at least 60% of patients. While translocations are insufficient to elicit progression to MM form MGUS, they still dictate biologic variability when present in the MM stages of the disease (Fonseca et al., 2002b; Moreau et al., 2002).

The powerful transcriptional influence of IgH enhancers is best exemplified by the upregulation of oncogenes located hundreds of kilobases away from the breakpoints (Chesi et al., 1998a). Unlike other B-cell neoplasms, IgH translocations in MM are thought to occur because of deranged isotype class switching (Bergsagel and Kuehl, 2001). The breakpoints at 14q32 result in IgH enhancers (intronic or Eμ and Eα enhancers) being present in both derivative chromosomes, with two or more oncogenes being upregulated (Kuehl and Bergsagel, 2002). Selected cases of the t(11;14)(q13;q32) might be produced as a consequence of nonswitch-mediated IgH recombination (Bergsagel and Kuehl, 2001). The recurrent nature of the chromosomal partners to IgH translocations is not currently understood (Bergsagel and Kuehl, 2001; Kuehl and Bergsagel, 2002). In some instances such as the t(14;16)(q32;q23), the breakpoints at 16q23 appeared to be occurring in chromosomal fragile sites (FRA16D) (Krummel et al., 2000; Ried et al., 2000).

## t(11;14)(q13;q32)

The t(11;14)(q13;q32) was the first described translocation in MM because of its conspicuous karyotypic appearance (Dewald et al., 1985). Like seen in mantle cell lymphoma, this translocation results in increased gene expression of *cyclin D1* upregulation (Chesi et al., 1996). The use of interphase FISH has now conclusively established the prevalence of the abnormality at 16% (Fonseca et al., 2002c). The translocation is readily detectable by karyotype analysis (in patients with informative karyotypes), interphase FISH, and gene expression profiles (Zhan et al., 2002) (Fig. 5-1). We have described a higher prevalence of the t(11;14)(q13;q32) in the early-stage PC neoplasms, because it seems to be more prevalent in MGUS (30%) and in light chain-associated amyloidosis (AL) (50%) (in AL the BM plasma cell percent is usually <10%) (Avet-Loiseau et al., 1999b; Fonseca et al.,

# t(11;14)(q13;q32)

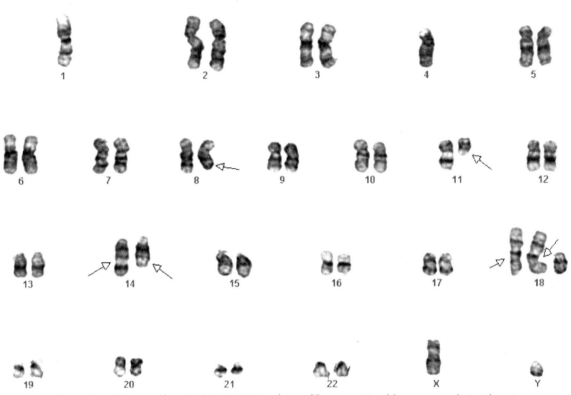

**Figure 5-1** *Patients with a t(11;14)(q13;q32) as detected by conventional karyotype analysis. Also −1, −4, and other structural abnormalities are depicted. (Picture courtesy of Dr. Gordon Dewald, Mayo Clinic, Rochester, MN.)*

2002a; Harrison et al., 2001; Hayman et al., 2001). These observations suggest that the chromosome abnormality is associated with a lower likelihood of progression to MM (Fonseca et al., 2002a; Hayman et al., 2001). However, others have found a similar incidence of the t(11;14)(q13;q32) in MGUS and MM indicating no particular effect on the progression of the disease (Avet-Loiseau et al., 1999b). The breakpoints at 11q13 are scattered over at least 700 kb (Janssen et al., 2000; Meeus et al., 1995; Raynaud et al., 1993; Ronchetti et al., 1999; Vaandrager et al., 1997).

In human MM cell lines, high levels of expression of *cyclin D1* are tightly linked to the presence of the t(11;14)(q13;q32). In primary MM samples, *cyclin D1* positivity is noted in 15% to 30% of MM patients (as detected by immunohistochemistry) (Hoyer et al., 2000; Ronchetti et al., 1999; Vasef et al., 1997). We have recently noted that there are some cases of MM and MGUS with the t(11;14)(q13;q32) but no evidence of *cyclin D1* nuclear positivity (Hoyer et al., 2000). This is likely the result of the presence of unbalanced IgH translocations, like is apparent as well for other partner chromosomes. Upregulation of the cyclin/CDK pathway is seen in human cancers (Sherr, 1996), but is specifically implicated in mantle cell lymphoma

(Vandenberghe et al., 1991) and parathyroid adenomas (Tahara et al., 1996).

It was previously suspected the t(11;14)(q13;q32) was associated with an adverse outcome and shortened survival (Fonseca et al., 1998b; Konigsberg et al., 2000b; Tricot et al., 1995). This was likely the result of the notorious nature of the abnormality in patients with abnormal karyotypes. It is now clear the ability to obtain abnormal metaphases is highly correlated with bone marrow plasmacytosis and proliferative index of the clone. It has become clear in recent years that the abnormality is associated with an improved survival, especially apparent in patients treated with high-dose chemotherapy and stem cell support (Fonseca et al., 2002c; Moreau et al., 2002) (Fig. 5-2). There is an association of the t(11;14)(q13;q32) with oligosecretory variant MM and lymphoplasmacytic morphology (Fonseca et al., 2002c; Hoyer et al., 2000; Moreau et al., 2002).

## t(4;14)(p16.3;q32)

The t(4;14)(p16.3;q32) is karyotypically silent and was first detected by cloning experiments in the human MM cell lines (Chesi et al., 1997, 1998b). The translocation is seen in 15% to 20% of primary MM samples

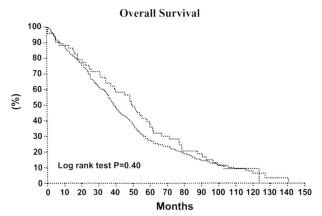

**Overall Survival**

*Figure 5-2* Overall survival curves for patients stratified according to the presence or absence of t(11;14)(q13;q32). In general, patients with t(11;14)(q13;q32) tend to have a more favorable outcome and be more responsive to therapy. (Reprinted with permission from Fonseca, R., Blood, E. A., Oken, N. M., Kyle, R. A., Dewald, G. W., Bailey, R. J., Van Wier, S. A., Henderson, K. J., Hoyer, J. D., Harrington, D., Kay, N. E., Van Ness, B., and Greipp, P. R. (2002). Myeloma and the t(11;14) (q13;q32): Evidence for a biologically defined unique subset of patients. Blood, 99, 3735–3741.)

and in 25% of human MM cell lines (Chesi et al., 1997, 1998b; Fonseca et al., 2001b; Moreau et al., 2002; Richelda et al., 1997). This translocation can be detected by interphase FISH or by an RT-PCR strategy to detect IgH-MMSET transcripts (*or MMSET-IgH transcripts*) (Chesi et al., 1997, 1998b) (Fig. 5-3). The t(4;14)(p16.3;q32) has been detected in 10% of MGUS cases by some investigators (Fonseca et al., 2002a; Malgeri et al., 2000), whereas others have failed to observe the abnormality in MGUS (Avet-Loiseau et al., 2002). Other investigators have noted the abnormality in patients (15%) with AL (Perfetti et al., 2001). When described in MGUS, the abnormality has been found as insufficient for further progression to MM, because patients might stay in the stable MGUS phase for years (Fonseca et al., 2002a; Malgeri et al., 2000).

The breakpoints at 4p16.3 are centromeric to the FGFR3 and dispersed over 200 kb, usually within the 5' intron of MMSET (Chesi et al., 1997, 1998b). The t(4;14)(p16.3;q32) was the first human translocation to be associated with upregulation of two oncogenes, FGFR3 (fibroblast growth factor receptor 3) and MMSET (MM SET domain). In a small minority of patients, and in human MM cell lines, activating mutations of FGFR3, akin to those of thanatophoric dwarfism, are detected (Chesi et al., 2001; Intini et al., 2001; Ronchetti et al., 2001). In MM, the t(4;14) (p16.3;q32) might be unbalanced but the loss appears to be that of the der14 invariably. The perceived need of persistence of MMSET suggests this might be the responsible oncogene in MM with the t(4;14) (p16.3;q32). The work of several groups has now

shown that in almost all cases of the t(4;14)(p16.3;q32) there is coexistence of Δ13 in both MM and MGUS (Avet-Loiseau et al., 2002; Fonseca et al., 2001b). We have postulated that because of this strong association, at least in some cases, Δ13 precedes the translocation.

The t(4;14)(p16.3;q32) is an unfavorable prognostic factor for MM patients treated with either conventional or high-dose chemotherapy (Fonseca et al., 2002b; Moreau et al., 2002). The focus of future research should be on how to best treat patients with this specific aberration.

## t(14;16)(q32;q23) and Other *maf* Translocations

The t(14;16)(q32;q23) is the third most common translocation in MM and is seen in about 5% to 10% of patients and in about 25% of human MM cell lines (Avet-Loiseau et al., 2002; Chesi et al., 1998a; Fonseca et al., 2002b). C-*maf* is transcriptionally upregulated as a result of this translocation (Chesi et al., 1998a). The translocation is difficult to detect by conventional cytogenetic analysis but has been described in 7% of MM patients with abnormal metaphases and that were multicolor metaphase FISH (Sawyer et al., 1998). In a large study of 350 patients with MM, a prevalence of 5% was reported (Fonseca et al., 2002b). In addition to c-*maf*, a small fraction of patients and two human MM cell lines harbor translocations that involve b-*maf* (Hanamura et al., 2001; Fonseca R, Kuehl M, unpublished data). Like the case with the t(4;14)(p16.3;q32), the t(14;16)(q32;q23) has also been described in MGUS, although some investigators have failed to observe it (Avet-Loiseau et al., 1999b; Fonseca et al., 2002a). Likewise, the t(14;16)(q32;q23) is also associated with shorter survival among patients treated with conventional chemotherapy (Fonseca et al., 2002b). Variant c-*maf* translocations also include the IgL-λ locus in the human MM cell lines 8226 and XG-6.

## Other IgH Translocations

An array of other chromosomal partners has been detected in human MM cases. One of these other partners is *cyclin D3* (t(6;14)(p21;q32)) (Shaughnessy et al., 2001). This translocation is also detectable by interphase FISH, conventional cytogenetics, and multicolor metaphase FISH (Sawyer et al., 2001). There is no known clinical or prognostic information for this translocation and whether it is also seen in MGUS. Another IgH translocation that involves chromosome 6 is the t(6;14)(p25;q32). It has been described in human MM cell lines (Iida et al., 1997) and results in transcriptional upregulation of the MUM1/IRF4 (Yoshida et al., 1999). The role and biology of this translocation is less clear because it might be seen only in a fraction of clonotypic cells and has not known clinical implications.

# IgH-MMSET Hybrid Transcripts

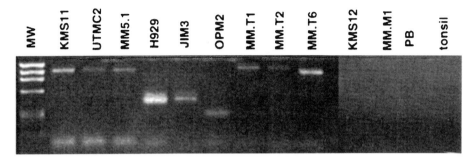

**Iμ-MMSET on der(4)**

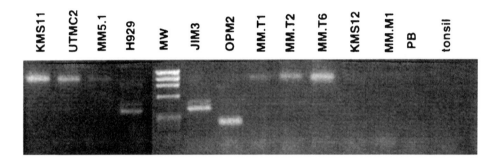

**Jh-MMSET on der(4)**

*Figure 5-3* *Detection of the t(4;14)(p16.3;q32) is also possible through the use of RT-PCR to amplify the IgH-MMSET hybrid transcript. Alternatively, the MMSET-IgH transcript is also detectable. Two sets of sense primers (Iμ and $J_H$ respectively) are used with a common MMSET antisense primer. The technique can be applied with samples with heterogeneous cell populations (i.e., unsorted plasma cells) and in samples with low percent of plasma cells (e.g., MGUS). (Reprinted with permission from Chesi, M., Nardini, E., Lim, R. S., Smith, K. D., Kuehl, W. M., and Bergsagel, P. L. (1998). The t(4;14) translocation in myeloma dysregulates both FGFR3 and a novel gene, MMSET, resulting in IgH/MMSET hybrid transcripts. Blood, 92, 3025–3034.)*

## Translocations That Involve *c-myc* and Other IgL-λ Translocations

Because of the invariable presence of c-*myc* translocations in the mouse plasmacytoma model, *myc* involving translocations were initially thought to be likely in human MM (Adams et al., 1985; Crews et al., 1982; Erikson et al., 1985; Keath et al., 1984; Piccoli et al., 1984; Stanton et al., 1983). However, careful analysis of abnormal karyotypes revealed the abnormality only in a minority of patients (Sawyer et al., 2001). It is now known that *myc* aberrations correlate with advanced stages of the disease because they are common in human MM cell lines but seldom seen in MM patients (Avet-Loiseau et al., 2001b; Shou et al., 2000). The clinical and prognostic implications for *myc* abnormalities are unknown but will likely be negative for overall survival, given that *myc* aberrations are

suspected to represent progression events. Some of these c-*myc* translocations involve the IgH and IgL-λ loci, but in some occasions might involve nonimmunoglobulin sites. Of interest we note that translocations involving the Ig light chain genes are less common in MM and almost always involve IgL-γ (Sawyer et al., 2001).

# Chromosome 13 Abnormalities

## Prevalence and Biology

Chromosome 13 (Δ13) abnormalities are highly prevalent in MM (40–50%) (Avet-Loiseau et al., 1999b; Drach et al., 2000; Fonseca et al., 2001a). They are observed in all stages of the disease, including MGUS (Avet-Loiseau et al., 1999b; Facon et al., 2001; Fonseca et al., 2002a; Zojer et al., 2000). The prevalence of Δ13 in MM reported by the different investigators is by necessity linked to its method of detection. When MM patient samples are tested by standard metaphase analysis, the abnormality is seen in 9% to 18% of cases (depending on the rate of abnormal metaphases, usually 18–30%) (Dewald et al., 1985; Sawyer et al., 1995). However, among cases with abnormal karyotypes, the prevalence is quite constant at 50%, which is the same prevalence reported by interphase FISH (Avet-Loiseau et al., 2002; Fonseca et al., 2001c; Sawyer et al., 2001; Zojer et al., 2000) (Table 5-3). In 85% of cases with Δ13, the abnormality is a monosomy, whereas in the remaining 15% it represents an interstitial deletion (Avet-Loiseau et al., 2000; Fonseca et al., 2001c) (Fig. 5-4). Δ13 are clonally selected because the abnormality, when present, is detectable in the majority of clonotypic PCs (Avet-Loiseau et al., 1999c, 2000; Fonseca et al., 2001a, 2001c) (Fig. 5-5). Chromosome 13 trisomy is exceedingly rare (Avet-Loiseau et al., 2000; Dewald et al., 1985; Fonseca et al., 2001c; Sawyer et al., 2001; Tabernero et al., 1996). Δ13 is likely not the critical event in the progression form MGUS to MM because it is seen in similar proportions of patients at both stages (Avet-Loiseau et al., 1999c; Fonseca et al., 2002a; Konigsberg et al., 2000a).

## Clinical and Pathologic Implications, Including Prognosis

We and others have shown Δ13 are associated with a higher frequency of λ-type light chain, female gender, higher PCLI and MM with lower serum M-spike concentrations (Fonseca et al., 2002c; Moreau et al., 2002).

Independent of the mode of treatment (standard vs. high-dose chemotherapy) and the mode of detection (karyotype vs. FISH), Δ13 are associated with shorter survival and lower response rate to treatment (Desikan et al., 2000; Facon et al., 2001; Fonseca et al., 2002b; Zojer et al., 2000) (Fig. 5-6). Because of its robust prognostic ability, Δ13 has been combined with an elevated β₂-microglobulin (>2.5 mg/dL) to categorize patients into the following three prognostic groups: good, average, and poor prognosis according to the number of unfavorable variables (0, 1, and 2) (Facon et al., 2001; Fonseca et al., 2002b). The median survival for each one of the groups was >111, 47.3 and 25.3 months, respectively (for patients treated with high-dose chemotherapy) (Facon et al., 2001). Among patients treated with conventional chemotherapy, similar observations are pertinent with survivals of 61, 45, and 33.2 months, respectively ($p < .0001$) (Fonseca et al., 2002b). This information strongly suggests that high-dose chemotherapy is of much greater benefit for patients without Δ13 (Fonseca et al., 2002b). Of interest we have found that the administration of interferon-α to patients with Δ13 results in shorter survival (Fonseca et al., 2002b).

# Aneuploidy, Including Hypodiploid MM

## Prevalence

MM is characterized by the frequent occurrence of aneuploidy as detected by karyotype and DNA flow cytometry (Dewald et al., 1985; Drach et al., 1995c; Fonseca et al., 1997, 2000; Gould et al., 1988; Lai et al.,

## TABLE 5-3
### Prevalence and Effect on Survival of Δ13

| Author | Total Number of Patients | Percent with Abnormality | Median Overall Survival | | Median Progression-Free Survival | | Independent Significance |
|---|---|---|---|---|---|---|---|
| | | | Months | P Value | Months | P Value | |
| Fonseca | 325 | 54 | 34.9 | .021 | 24.7 | .03 | Yes |
| | | | 51.0 | | 33.0 | | |
| Zojer | 97 | 46 | 24.2 | <.005 | NA | NA | Yes |
| | | | >60.0 | | | | |
| Perez-Simon | 48 | 33 | 14.0 | .0012 | NA | NA | Yes |
| | | | 60.0 | | | | |
| Facon | 110 | 38 | 27.9 | <.0001 | 17.0 | .0005 | Yes |
| | | | 65.0 | | 33.0 | | |
| *Conventional Cytogenetics* | | | | | | | |
| Tricot | 155 | 14 | 29.0 | .001 | 22.0 | .001 | Yes |
| | | | >50.0 | | 43.0 | | |
| Desikan | 1000 | 16 | 16.0 | <.001 | NA | NA | Yes |
| | | | 44.0 | | | | |

NA, not available.

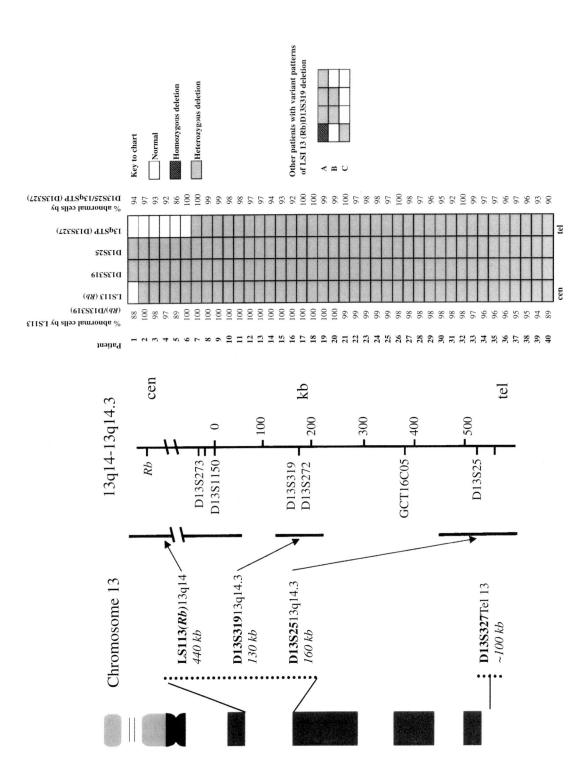

**Figure 5-4** A mapping study of deletions at 13q14 in MM. This figure shows a normal human chromosome 13 and the location of the Δ13 marker probes and their relative size. The map of 13q14 is only at an approximate scale and has been drawn and modified from the map of Kalachikov and the manufacturer map of the probes (http://www.vysis.com/). The cartoon on the right shows that in most cases with 13q14 deletions, there was simultaneous loss of the telomeric probes in the 40 cases with deletions of LSI 13 (Rb)/D13S319 studied. There is loss of LSI 13 (Rb), D13S319, and D13S25 in all cases studied except one, and in only six cases is there a remaining signal from the 13qSTP probe. The percentages of abnormal cells for each one of the pairs of probes for a patient are shown in the second (LSI 13 (Rb)/D13S319) and seventh (D13S25/13qSTP) columns. In the right side of the figure the results for three patients with variant patterns of 13q14 deletion are depicted. (Adapted with permission Fonseca, R., Oken, M. M., Harrington, D., Bailey, R. J., Van Wier, S. A., Henderson, K. J., Kay, N. E., Van Ness, B., Greipp, P. R., and Dewald, G. W. (2001). Deletions of chromosome 13 in multiple myeloma identified by interphase FISH usually denote large deletions of the q arm or monosomy. Leukemia, 62, 981–986.)

74

**Percent of Abnormal cells with Δ13**

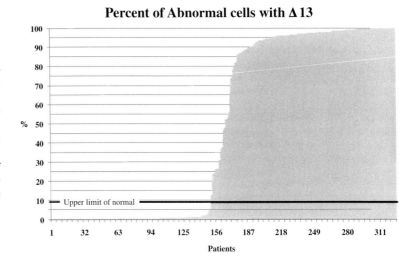

*Figure 5-5* Graph depicting the percentage of cells with loss of LSI 13 (Rb)/D13S319 signals indicative of deletion. The dark line marks the upper limit of normal value used for this study. The values for percentage of abnormal cells were arranged in incremental order from left to right, and all patients tested are shown. (Reprinted with permission from Fonseca, R., Oken, M. M., Harrington, D., Bailey, R. J., Van Wier, S. A., Henderson, K. J., Kay, N. E., Van Ness, B., Greipp, P. R, and Dewald, G. W. (2001). Deletions of chromosome 13 in multiple myeloma identified by interphase FISH usually denote large deletions of the q arm or monosomy. Leukemia, 15, 981–986.)

1995; Latreille et al., 1982; Sawyer et al., 1995; Tabernero et al., 1996; Zandecki et al., 1996). The most common trisomies are of chromosomes 3, 5, 7, 9, 11, 15, and 19 and the most common monosomies are of chromosomes 13, 14, 22, and X in women (Fig. 5-7). However, no specific numeric chromosomal abnormality is constant or predictive of disease progression. In some studies the presence of certain trisomies (6, 9, and 17) was associated with an improved survival (Perez-Simon et al., 1998). The prevalence of aneuploidy seems to be independent of stage (i.e., MGUS vs. MM) (Drach et al., 1995a, 1995b, 1995c; Fonseca et al., 1998a; Zandecki, 1996; Zandecki et al., 1994, 1995, 1997).

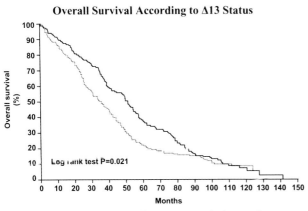

*Figure 5-6* Overall survival of patients stratified according to D13 status. (Reprinted with permission from Fonseca, R., Harrington, D., Oken, M. M., Dewald, G. W., Bailey, R. J., Van Weir, S. A., Henderson, K. J., Blood, E. A., Rajkumar, S. V., Kay, N. R., Van Ness, B., and Greipp, P. R. (2002). Biological and prognostic significance of interphase fluorescence in situ hybridization detection of chromosome 13 abnormalities (delta13) in multiple myeloma: An Eastern cooperative oncology group study. Cancer Research, 62, 715–720.)

## Hyperdiploid Versus Non-Hyperdiploid MM

A detailed and careful analysis of abnormal karyotypes in MM reveals certain order among aneuploid tumors (Debes-Marun et al., 2002; Smadja et al., 1998, 2001). Specifically, it is evident that there are two major types of MM: hyperdiploid MM and non-hyperdiploid MM (Fig. 5-8) (Debes-Marun et al., 2002; Smadja et al., 2001). The non-hyperdiploid MM is composed of cases with pseudo-diploid, hypodiploid, and near-tetraploid karyotypes (Debes-Marun et al., 2002; Smadja et al., 1998, 2001). The near-tetraploid cases have been found to represent duplications of the pseudo-diploid or hypodiploid karyotypes (Debes-Marun et al., 2002). This last group is best characterized by a high prevalence of IgH translocations ( > 85%), whereas IgH translocations are sharply less common in the hyperdiploid MM ( <30%) (Fonseca R et al., 2003). The hypo-diploid variant MM is generally associated with a shorter survival (Calasanz et al., 1997; Fassas et al., 2002; Greipp et al., 1999; Smadja et al., 2001; Smith et al., 1986). Hypodiploidy has been found to supersede the prognostic ability of Δ13 in some studies but not by others (Debes-Marun ct al., 2002; Fassas et al., 2002; Smadja et al., 2001).

## Other Abnormalities

### Abnormalities of *ras* and *p53*

*Ras* mutations have been noted in 30% to 50% of MM patients. The prevalence of the mutations seems to increase with advancing stages of the disease (Matozaki et al., 1991; Neri et al., 1989). Mutations of K-*ras*, but not N-*ras*, have been associated with shorter

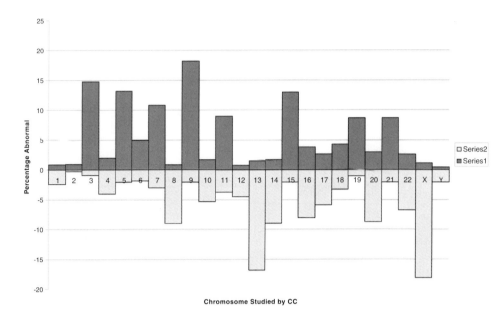

**Figure 5-7** *Prevalence of numerical chromosomal abnormalities in MM. The data is a composite of karyotypes reported in the literature. (Reprinted with permission from Fonseca, R., Coignet, L. J., and Dewald, G. W. (1999). Cytogenetic abnormalities in multiple myeloma.* Hematology Oncology Clinics of North America, 13, *1169–1180.)*

survival (Liu et al., 1996). *Ras* mutations appear to be rare in the early stages of the plasma cell neoplasms as reported in one study (Bezieau et al., 2001).

Inactivation of *p53* by either deletion or mutation seems to be a rare event in human MM (Drach et al., 1998; Schultheis et al., 1999). Deletions of the tumor-suppressor gene *p53* locus, 17p13, have been detected

in approxiamtely 10% and are associated with a shorter survival (Drach et al., 1998; Fonseca et al., 2002b). Much like for *ras*, deletions of 17p13 appear to be rare in MGUS (Ackermann et al., 1998). Inactivating mutations of *p53* have also been observed in MM, but more often in the advanced stages of the disease: 5% at diagnosis versus 20% to 40% of PC leukemia

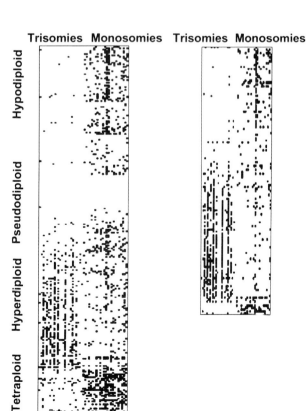

**Figure 5-8** *Chromosome clustering analysis done in 254 patients with abnormal karyotypes. The graph depicts the distinction of the four major types of MM according to total chromosome number: hypodiploid, pseudodiploid, hyperdiploid, and near-tetraploid. The diagram was used to provide a graphic representation of the distribution of chromosomal abnormalities in MM and their relation to ploidy status. Each one of the rows represents a patient (n = 254) and each one of the columns represents the different chromosome abnormalities. These are ordered (from left to right) as structural chromosomal abnormalities, trisomies (left to right chromosome 1 to Y), and monosomies (left to right chromosome 1 to Y). A square is blank if no abnormality was reported, white if a specific trisomy or monosomy was present. The cartoon on the left is the same analysis performed in the series of patients published by Smadja and colleagues (Blood 98:2229), which shows the same results. (Reprinted with permission from Debes-Marun, C. S., Dewald, G. W., Bryant, S., Picken, E., Santana-Davila, R., Gonzalez-Paz, N., Winkler, J. M., Kyle, R. A., Gertz, M. A., Witzig, T. E., Dispenzieri, A., Lacy, M. Q., Rajkumar, S. V., Lust, J. A., Greipp, P. R., and Fonseca, R. (2003). Chromosome abnormalities clustering and its implication for pathogenesis and prognosis in myeloma.* Leukemia, 17, *427–436.*

(Corradini et al., 1994; Mazars et al., 1992; Neri et al., 1993; Preudhomme et al., 1992).

### Methylation of *p16*

Inactivation of *p16* by the methylation of its promoter has been associated with advancement through the different stages of the PC neoplasms (Arora and Jelinek, 1998; Gonzalez et al., 2000; Lo et al., 1999; McClure et al.; Ng et al., 1999; Uchida et al., 2001). Methylation of the *p16* promoter appears to be rare in MGUS, but is seen in up to 40% of MM cases at diagnosis (Arora and Jelinek, 1998; Gonzalez et al., 2000; Lo et al., 1999; McClure et al.; Ng et al., 1999; Uchida et al., 2001). Furthermore, methylation of *p16* is common in cases of MM with a significant extramedullary compartment (Uchida et al., 2001).

# Conclusion

It is clear that while we have learned much about the biology of MM, many questions remain. It is of interest that all available data suggest that IgH translocations are seminal events for many patients, yet are not sufficient to exert the full malignant potential of the clone. It is also uncertain what the genetic events required are for the transformation from MGUS to MM. It seems that the genetic heterogeneity of the disease suggests that MM is composed of several variants identified best by these chromosomal abnormalities.

## REFERENCES

Ackermann, J., Meidlinger, P., Zojer, N., Gisslinger, H., Ludwig, H., Huber, H., and Drach, J. (1998). Absence of p53 deletions in bone marrow plasma cells of patients with monoclonal gammopathy of undetermined significance. *British Journal of Haematology*, 103, 1161–1163.

Adams, J. M., Harris, A. W., Pinkert, C. A., Corcoran, L. M., Alexander, W. S., Cory, S., Palmiter, R. D., and Brinster, R. L. (1985). The c-myc oncogene driven by immunoglobulin enhancers induces lymphoid malignancy in transgenic mice. *Nature*, 318, 533–538.

Ahmann, G. J., Jalal, S. M., Juneau, A. L., Christensen, E. R., Hanson, C. A., Dewald, G. W., and Greipp, P. R. (1998). A novel three-color, clone-specific fluorescence in situ hybridization procedure for monoclonal gammopathies. *Cancer Genetics Cytogenetics*, 101, 7–11.

Arora, T., and Jelinek, D. F. (1998). Differential myeloma cell responsiveness to interferon-alpha correlates with differential induction of p19(INK4d) and cyclin D2 expression. *Journal of Biological Chemistry*, 273, 11799–11805.

Avet-Loiseau, H., Andree-Ashley, L. E., Moore, D. II, Mellerin, M. P., Feusner, J., Bataille, R., and Pallavicini, M. G. (1997). Molecular cytogenetic abnormalities in multiple myeloma and plasma cell leukemia measured using comparative genomic hybridization. *Genes, Chromosomes and Cancer*, 19, 124–133.

Avet-Loiseau, H., and Bataille, R. (1998). Detection of nonrandom chromosomal changes in multiple myeloma by comparative genomic hybridization. *Blood*, 92, 2997–2998.

Avet-Loiseau, H., Brigaudeau, C., Morineau, N., Talmant, P., Lai, J. L., Daviet, A., Li, J. Y., Praloran, V., Rapp, M. J., Harousseau, J. L., Facon, T., and Bataille, R. (1999a). High incidence of cryptic translocations involving the Ig heavy chain gene in multiple myeloma, as shown by fluorescence in situ hybridization. *Genes, Chromosomes, Cancer*, 24, 9–15.

Avet-Loiseau, H., Daviet, A., Brigaudeau, C., Callet-Bauchu, E., Terre, C., Lafage-Pochitaloff, M., Desangles, F., Ramond, S., Talmant, P., and Bataille, R. (2001a). Cytogenetic, interphase, and multicolor fluorescence in situ hybridization analyses in primary plasma cell leukemia: A study of 40 patients at diagnosis, on behalf of the Intergroupe Francophone du Myelome and the Groupe Francais de Cytogenetique Hematologique. *Blood*, 97, 822–825.

Avet-Loiseau, H., Daviet, A., Saunier, S., and Bataille, R. (2000). Chromosome 13 abnormalities in multiple myeloma are mostly monosomy 13. *British Journal of Haematology*, 111, 1116–1117.

Avet-Loiseau, H., Facon, T., Daviet, A., Godon, C., Rapp, M. J., Harousseau, J. L., Grosbois, B., and Bataille, R. (1999b). 14q32 translocations and monosomy 13 observed in monoclonal gammopathy of undetermined significance delineate a multistep process for the oncogenesis of multiple myeloma. Intergroupe Francophone du Myelome. *Cancer Research*, 59, 4546–4550.

Avet-Loiseau, H., Facon, T., Grosbois, B., Magrangeas, F., Rapp, M. J., Harousseau, J. L., Minvielle, S., and Bataille, R. (2002). Oncogenesis of multiple myeloma: 14q32 and 13q chromosomal abnormalities are not randomly distributed, but correlate with natural history, immunological features, and clinical presentation. *Blood*, 99, 2185–2191.

Avet-Loiseau, H., Gerson, F., Magrangeas, F., Minvielle, S., Harousseau, J. L., and Bataille, R. (2001b). Rearrangements of the c-myc oncogene are present in 15% of primary human multiple myeloma tumors. *Blood*, 98, 3082–3086.

Avet-Loiseau, H., Li, J. Y., Morineau, N., Facon, T., Brigaudeau, C., Harousseau, J. L., Grosbois, B., and Bataille, R. (1999c). Monosomy 13 is associated with the transition of monoclonal gammopathy of undetermined significance to multiple myeloma. Intergroupe Francophone du Myelome. *Blood*, 94, 2583–2589.

Bergsagel, P. L., Chesi, M., Brents, L. A., and Kuehl, W. M. (1995). Translocations into IgH Switch Regions—The Genetic Hallmark of Multiple Myeloma. *Blood*, 86, 223.

Bergsagel, P. L., Chesi, M., Nardini, E., Brents, L. A., Kirby, S. L., and Kuehl, W. M. (1996). Promiscuous translocations into immunoglobulin heavy chain switch regions in multiple myeloma. *Proceedings of the National Academy of Science USA*, 93, 13931–13936.

Bergsagel, P. L., and Kuehl, W. M. (2001). Chromosome translocations in multiple myeloma. *Oncogene*, 20, 5611–5622.

Bezieau, S., Devilder, M. C., Avet-Loiseau, H., Mellerin, M. P., Puthier, D., Pennarun, E., Rapp, M. J., Harousseau, J. L., Moisan, J. P., and Bataille, R. (2001). High incidence of N and K-Ras activating mutations in multiple myeloma and primary plasma cell leukemia at diagnosis. *Human Mutation*, 18, 212–224.

Calasanz, M. J., Cigudosa, J. C., Odero, M. D., Garcia-Foncillas, J., Marin, J., Ardanaz, M. T., Rocha, E., and Gullon, A. (1997). Hypodiploidy and 22q11 rearrangements at diagnosis are associated with poor prognosis in patients with multiple myeloma. *British Journal of Haematology*, 98, 418–425.

Chesi, M., Bergsagel, P. L., Brents, L. A., Smith, C. M., Gerhard, D. S., and Kuehl, W. M. (1996). Dysregulation of cyclin D1 by translocation into an IgH gamma switch region in two multiple myeloma cell lines. *Blood*, 88, 674–681.

Chesi, M., Bergsagel, P. L., Shonukan, O. O., Martelli, M. L., Brents, L. A., Chen, T., Schrock, E., Ried, T., and Kuehl, W. M. (1998a). Frequent dysregulation of the c-maf proto-oncogene at 16q23 by translocation to an Ig locus in multiple myeloma. *Blood*, 91, 4457–4463.

Chesi, M., Brents, L. A., Ely, S. A., Bais, C., Robbiani, D. F., Mesri, E. A., Kuehl, W. M., and Bergsagel, P. L. (2001). Activated fibroblast growth factor receptor 3 is an oncogene that contributes to tumor progression in multiple myeloma. *Blood, 97*, 729–736.

Chesi, M., Nardini, E., Brents, L. A., Schrock, E., Ried, T., Kuehl, W. M., and Bergsagel, P. L. (1997). Frequent translocation t(4;14)(p16.3;q32.3) in multiple myeloma is associated with increased expression and activating mutations of fibroblast growth factor receptor 3. *Nature Genetics, 16*, 260–264.

Chesi, M., Nardini, E., Lim, R., Smith, K., Kuehl, W., and Bergsagel, P. (1998b). The t(4;14) translocation in myeloma dysregulates both FGFR3 and a novel gene, MMSET, resulting in IgH/MMSET hybrid transcripts. *Blood, 92*, 3025–3034.

Cigudosa, J. C., Rao, P. H., Calasanz, M. J., Odero, M. D., Michaeli, J., Jhanwar, S. C., and Chaganti, R. S. (1998). Characterization of nonrandom chromosomal gains and losses in multiple myeloma by comparative genomic hybridization. *Blood, 91*, 3007–3010.

Corradini, P., Inghirami, G., Astolfi, M., Ladetto, M., Voena, C., Ballerini, P., Gu, W., Nilsson, K., Knowles, D. M., Boccadoro, M., Pileri, A., and Dalla-Favera, R. (1994). Inactivation of tumor suppressor genes, p53 and Rb1, in plasma cell dyscrasias. *Leukemia, 8*, 758–767.

Crews, S., Barth, R., Hood, L., Prehn, J., and Calame, K. (1982). Mouse c-myc oncogene is located on chromosome 15 and translocated to chromosome 12 in plasmacytomas. *Science, 218*, 1319–1321.

Debes-Marun, C., Dewald, G., Bryant, S., Picken, E., Santana-Dávila, S., González-Paz, N., Kyle, R., Gertz, M., Witzig, T., Dispenzieri, A., Lacy, M., Rajkumar, S., Lust, J., Greipp, P., and Fonseca, R. (2002). Chromosome abnormalities clustering and its implications for pathogenesis and prognosis in myeloma. *Leukemia, 17*, 427–436.

Desikan, R., Barlogie, B., Sawyer, J., Ayers, D., Tricot, G., Badros, A., Zangari, M., Munshi, N. C., Anaissie, E., Spoon, D., Siegel, D., Jagannath, S., Vesole, D., Epstein, J., Shaughnessy, J., Fassas, A., Lim, S., Roberson, P., and Crowley, J. (2000). Results of high-dose therapy for 1000 patients with multiple myeloma: Durable complete remissions and superior survival in the absence of chromosome 13 abnormalities. *Blood, 95*, 4008–4010.

Dewald, G. W., Kyle, R. A., Hicks, G. A., and Greipp, P. R. (1985). The clinical significance of cytogenetic studies in 100 patients with multiple myeloma, plasma cell leukemia, or amyloidosis. *Blood, 66*, 380–390.

Drach, J., Ackermann, J., Fritz, E., Kromer, E., Schuster, R., Gisslinger, H., DeSantis, M., Zojer, N., Fiegl, M., Roka, S., Schuster, J., Heinz, R., Ludwig, H., and Huber, H. (1998). Presence of a p53 gene deletion in patients with multiple myeloma predicts for short survival after conventional-dose chemotherapy. *Blood, 92*, 802–809.

Drach, J., Angerler, J., Schuster, J., Rothermundt, C., Thalhammer, R., Haas, O. A., Jager, U., Fiegl, M., Geissler, K., and Ludwig, H. (1995a). Interphase fluorescence in situ hybridization identifies chromosomal abnormalities in plasma cells from patients with monoclonal gammopathy of undetermined significance. *Blood, 86*, 3915–3921.

Drach, J., Angerler, J., Schuster, J., Thalhammer, R., Jager, U., Geissler, K., Lechner, K., Ludwig, H., and Huber, H. (1995b). Clonal chromosomal aberrations in plasma cells from patients with monoclonal gammopathy of undetermined significance (MGUS) (Meeting abstract). *Proceedings of the Annual Meeting of the American Association for Cancer Research, 36*, 144.

Drach, J., Kaufmann, H., Urbauer, E., Schreiber, S., Ackermann, J., and Huber, H. (2000). The biology of multiple myeloma. *Journal of Cancer Research and Clinical Oncology, 126*, 441–447.

Drach, J., Schuster, J., Nowotny, H., Angerler, J., Rosenthal, F., Fiegl, M., Rothermundt, C., Gsur, A., Jager, U., Heinz, R., Lechner, K., Ludwig, H., and Huber, H. (1995c). Multiple myeloma: high incidence of chromosomal aneuploidy as detected by interphase fluorescence in situ hybridization. *Cancer Research, 55*, 3854–3859.

Erikson, J., Miller, D. A., Miller, O. J., Abcarian, P. W., Skurla, R. M., Mushinski, J. F., and Croce, C. M. (1985). The c-myc oncogene is

translocated to the involved chromosome 12 in mouse plasmacytoma. *Proceedings of the National Academy of Sciences of the United States of America, 82*, 4212–4216.

Facon, T., Avet-Loiseau, H., Guillerm, G., Moreau, P., Geneviève, F., Zandecki, M., Laï, J., Leleu, X., Jouet, J., Bauters, F., Harousseau, J., Bataille, R., Mary, J., and On the behalf of the Inter Groupe Francais du Myelome (IFM). (2001). Chromosome 13 abnormalities identified by FISH analysis and serum beta-2-microglobulin produce a powerful myeloma staging system for patients receiving high-dose therapy. *Blood, 97*, 1566–1571.

Fassas, A. B., Spencer, T., Sawyer, J., Zangari, M., Lee, C. K., Anaissie, E., Muwalla, F., Morris, C., Barlogie, B., and Tricot, G. (2002). Both hypodiploidy and deletion of chromosome 13 independently confer poor prognosis in multiple myeloma. *British Journal of Haematology, 118*, 1041–1047.

Fonseca, R., Ahmann, G. J., Jalal, S. M., Dewald, G. W., Larson, D. R., Therneau, T. M., Gertz, M. A., Kyle, R. A., and Greipp, P. R. (1998a). Chromosomal abnormalities in systemic amyloidosis. *British Journal of Haematology, 103*, 704–710.

Fonseca, R., Ahmann, G. J., Juneau, A. L., Jalal, S. M., Dewald, G. W., Larson, D. M., Therneau, T. M., Gertz, M. A., and Greipp, P. R. (1997). Cytogenetic abnormalities in multiple myeloma and related plasma cell disorders; a comparison of conventional cytogenetic analysis to fluorescent in-situ hybridization with simultaneous cytoplasmic immunoglobulin staining [Meeting abstract]. *Blood, 90*:1558a, 349.

Fonseca, R., Bailey, R., Ahmann, G., Aguayo, P., Jalal, S., Rajkumar, S., Kyle, R., Gertz, M., Dispenzieri, A., Lust, J., Lacy, M., Witzig, T., Greipp, P., and Dewald, G. (2001a). Translocations involving 14q32 are common in patients with the monoclonal gammopathy of undetermined significance. *Blood.*

Fonseca, R., Bailey, R. J., Ahmann, G. J., Rajkumar, S. V., Hoyer, J. D., Lust, J. A., Kyle, R. A., Gertz, M. A., Greipp, P. R., and Dewald, G. W. (2002a). Genomic abnormalities in monoclonal gammopathy of undetermined significance. *Blood, 100*, 1417–1424.

Fonseca, R., Dewald, G. W., Ahmann, G. J., Bailey, R. J., Larson, D. M., Therneau, T. M., Børset, M., Seidel, C., Hoyer, J. D., Rajkumar, S. V., Dispenzieri, A., Lacy, M. Q., Lust, J. A., Witzig, T. E., Gertz, M. A., Kyle, R. A., Greipp, P. R., and Jalal, S. M. (2000). Aneuploidy is universal and clonally restricted in plasma cell dyscrasias. *Submitted.*

Fonseca, R., Blood, E., Rue, M., Harrington, D., Oken, M., Dewald, G., Kyle, R., Van Wier, S., Henderson, K., Bailey, R., and Greipp, P. (2003). Clinical and biologic implications of recurrent genomic aberrations in myeloma. *Blood, 101*, 4569–4575.

Fonseca, R., Harrington, D., Oken, M., Dewald, G., Bailey, R., Van Wier, S., Henderson, K., Blood, E., Rajkumar, S., Kay, N., Van Ness, B., and Greipp, P. (2002b). Biologic and prognostic significance of interphase FISH detection of chromosome 13 abnormalities (Δ13) in multiple myeloma: An Eastern Cooperative Oncology Group (ECOG) Study. *Cancer Research, 62*, 715–720.

Fonseca, R., Harrington, D., Oken, M., Kyle, R., Dewald, G., Bailey, R., Van Wier, S., Henderson, K., Hoyer, J., Blood, E., Kay, N., Van Ness, B., and Greipp, P. (2002c). Myeloma and the t(11;14) (q13;q32) represents a uniquely defined biological subset of patients. *Blood, 99*, 3735–3741.

Fonseca, R., Oken, M., and Greipp, P. (2001b). The t(4;14)(p16.3;q32) is strongly associated with chromosome 13 abnormalities (Δ13) in both multiple myeloma and monoclonal gammopathies of undetermined significance. *Blood, 98*, 1271–1272.

Fonseca, R., Oken, M., Harrington, D., Bailey, R., Van Wier, S., Henderson, K., Kay, N., Van Ness, B., Greipp, P., and Dewald, G. (2001c). Deletions of chromosome 13 in multiple myeloma identified by interphase FISH usually denote large deletions of the q-arm or monosomy. *Leukemia, 15*, 981–986.

Fonseca, R., Witzig, T. E., Gertz, M. A., Kyle, R. A., Hoyer, J. D., Jalal, S. M., and Greipp, P. R. (1998b). Multiple myeloma and the translocation t(11;14)(q13;q32)—A report on 13 cases. *British Journal of Haematology*, 101, 296–301.

Gonzalez, M., Mateos, M. V., Garcia-Sanz, R., Balanzategui, A., Lopez-Perez, R., Chillon, M. C., Gonzalez, D., Alaejos, I., and San Miguel, J. F. (2000). De novo methylation of tumor suppressor gene p16/INK4a is a frequent finding in multiple myeloma patients at diagnosis. *Leukemia*, 14, 183–187.

Gould, J., Alexanian, R., Goodacre, A., Pathak, S., Hecht, B., and Barlogie, B. (1988). Plasma cell karyotype in multiple myeloma. *Blood*, 71, 453–456.

Greipp, P. R., Trendle, M. C., Leong, T., Oken, M. M., Kay, N. E., Van Ness, B., and Kyle, R. A. (1999). Is flow cytometric DNA content hypodiploidy prognostic in multiple myeloma? *Leukemia Lymphoma*, 35, 83–89.

Gutierrez, N. C., Hernandez, J. M., Garcia, J. L., Canizo, M. C., Gonzalez, M., Hernandez, J., Gonzalez, M. B., Garcia-Marcos, M. A., and San Miguel, J. F. (2001). Differences in genetic changes between multiple myeloma and plasma cell leukemia demonstrated by comparative genomic hybridization. *Leukemia*, 15, 840–845.

Hallek, M., Bergsagel, P. L., and Anderson, K. C. (1998). Multiple myeloma: Increasing evidence for a multistep transformation process. *Blood*, 91, 3–21.

Hanamura, I., Iida, S., Akano, Y., Hayami, Y., Kato, M., Miura, K., Harada, S., Banno, S., Wakita, A., Kiyoi, H., Naoe, T., Shimizu, S., Sonta, S. I., Nitta, M., Taniwaki, M., and Ueda, R. (2001). Ectopic expression of MAFB gene in human myeloma cells carrying (14;20)(q32;q11) chromosomal translocations. *Japanese Journal of Cancer Research*, 92, 638–644.

Harrison, C., Mazullo, H., Cheung, K., Mehta, A., Lachmann, H., Hawkins, P., and Orchard, K. (2001). Chromosomal abnormalities in systemic amyloidosis. In *Proceedings of the VIII International Myeloma Workshop*, p. P18; Banff, Alberta, Canada.

Hayman, S., Jalal, S., Bailey, R., Ahmann, G., Dispenzieri, A., Gertz, M., Greipp, P., Kyle, R., Lacy, M., Rajkumar, S., Witzig, T., Lust, J., and Fonseca, R. (2001). Translocations at the IgH locus are possible early genetic events in patients with primary systemic amyloidosis. *Blood*, 98, 2266–2268.

Hoyer, J. D., Hanson, C. A., Fonseca, R., Greipp, P. R., Dewald, G. W., and Kurtin, P. J. (2000). The (11;14)(q13;q32) translocation in multiple myeloma. A morphologic and immunohistochemical study. *American Journal of Clinical Pathology*, 113, 831–837.

Iida, S., Rao, P. H., Butler, M., Corradini, P., Boccadoro, M., Klein, B., Chaganti, R. S., and Dalla-Favera, R. (1997). Deregulation of MUM1/IRF4 by chromosomal translocation in multiple myeloma. *Nature Genetics*, 17, 226–230.

Intini, D., Baldini, L., Fabris, S., Lombardi, L., Ciceri, G., Maiolo, A. T., and Neri, A. (2001). Analysis of FGFR3 gene mutations in multiple myeloma patients with t(4;14). *British Journal of Haematology*, 114, 362–364.

Janssen, J. W., Vaandrager, J. W., Heuser, T., Jauch, A., Kluin, P. M., Geelen, E., Bergsagel, P. L., Kuehl, W. M., Drexler, H. G., Otsuki, T., Bartram, C. R., and Schuuring, E. (2000). Concurrent activation of a novel putative transforming gene, myeov, and cyclin D1 in a subset of multiple myeloma cell lines with t(11;14)(q13;q32). *Blood*, 95, 2691 2698.

Keath, E. J., Kelekar, A., and Cole, M. D. (1984). Transcriptional activation of the translocated c-myc oncogene in mouse plasmacytomas: Similar RNA levels in tumor and proliferating normal cells. *Cell*, 37, 521–528.

Konigsberg, R., Ackermann, J., Kaufmann, H., Zojer, N., Urbauer, E., Kromer, E., Jager, U., Gisslinger, H., Schreiber, S., Heinz, R., Ludwig, H., Huber, H., and Drach, J. (2000a). Deletions of chromosome 13q in monoclonal gammopathy of undetermined significance. *Leukemia*, 14, 1975–1979.

Konigsberg, R., Zojer, N., Ackermann, J., Kromer, E., Kittler, H., Fritz, E., Kaufmann, H., Nosslinger, T., Riedl, L., Gisslinger, H., Jager, U., Simonitsch, I., Heinz, R., Ludwig, H., Huber, H., and

Drach, J. (2000b). Predictive role of interphase cytogenetics for survival of patients with multiple myeloma. *Journal of Clinical Oncology*, 18, 804–812.

Krummel, K. A., Roberts, L. R., Kawakami, M., Glover, T. W., and Smith, D. I. (2000). The characterization of the common fragile site FRA16D and its involvement in multiple myeloma translocations. *Genomics*, 69, 37–46.

Kuehl, W. M., and Bergsagel, P. L. (2002). Multiple myeloma: Evolving genetic events and host interactions. *Nature Rev Cancer*, 2, 175–187.

Lai, J. L., Zandecki, M., Mary, J. Y., Bernardi, F., Izydorczyk, V., Flactif, M., Morel, P., Jouet, J. P., Bauters, F., and Facon, T. (1995). Improved cytogenetics in multiple myeloma: A study of 151 patients including 117 patients at diagnosis. *Blood*, 85, 2490–2497.

Latreille, J., Barlogie, B., Johnston, D., Drewinko, B., and Alexanian, R. (1982). Ploidy and proliferative characteristics in monoclonal gammopathies. *Blood*, 59, 43–51.

Liu, P., Leong, T., Quam, L., Billadeau, D., Kay, N. E., Greipp, P., Kyle, R. A., Oken, M. M., and Van Ness, B. (1996). Activating mutations of N- and K-ras in multiple myeloma show different clinical associations: Analysis of the Eastern Cooperative Oncology Group Phase III Trial. *Blood*, 88, 2699–2706.

Lo, Y. M., Wong, I. H., Zhang, J., Tein, M. S., Ng, M. H., and Hjelm, N. M. (1999). Quantitative analysis of aberrant p16 methylation using real-time quantitative methylation-specific polymerase chain reaction. *Cancer Research*, 59, 3899–3903.

Malgeri, U., Baldini, L., Perfetti, V., Fabris, S., Vignarelli, M. C., Colombo, G., Lotti, V., Compasso, S., Bogni, S., Lombardi, L., Maiolo, A. T., and Neri, A. (2000). Detection of t(4;14)(p16.3;q32) chromosomal translocation in multiple myeloma by reverse transcription-polymerase chain reaction analysis of IGH-MMSET fusion transcripts. *Cancer Research*, 60, 4058–4061.

Matozaki, S., Nakagawa, T., Nakao, Y., and Fujita, T. (1991). RAS gene mutations in multiple myeloma and related monoclonal gammopathies. *Kobe Journal of Medical Sciences*, 37, 35–45.

Mazars, G. R., Portier, M., Zhang, X. G., Jourdan, M., Bataille, R., Theillet, C., and Klein, B. (1992). Mutations of the p53 gene in human myeloma cell lines. *Oncogene*, 7, 1015–1018.

McClure, R., James, C., Kurtin, P., Winkler, J., Ahmann, G., Gonzalez-Paz, N., Greipp, P., and Fonseca, R. Methylation and deletion of the p16 gene in plasma cell neoplasms. Personal Communication.

Meeus, P., Stul, M. S., Mecucci, C., Cassiman, J. J., and Van den Berghe, H. (1995). Molecular breakpoints of t(11;14)(q13;q32) in multiple myeloma. *Cancer Genetics Cytogenetics*, 83, 25–27.

Moreau, P., Facon, T., Leleu, X., Morineau, N., Huyghe, P., Harousseau, J. L., Bataille, R., and Avet-Loiseau, H. (2002). Recurrent 14q32 translocations determine the prognosis of multiple myeloma, especially in patients receiving intensive chemotherapy. *Blood*, 100, 1579–1583.

Neri, A., Baldini, L., Trecca, D., Cro, L., Polli, E., and Maiolo, A. T. (1993). p53 gene mutations in multiple myeloma are associated with advanced forms of malignancy. *Blood*, 81, 128–135.

Neri, A., Murphy, J. P., Cro, L., Ferrero, D., Tarella, C., Baldini, L., and Dalla-Favera, R. (1989). Ras oncogene mutation in multiple myeloma. *Journal of Experimental Medicine*, 170, 1715–1725.

Ng, M. H., Wong, I. H., and Lo, K. W. (1999). DNA methylation changes and multiple myeloma. *Leukemia and Lymphoma*, 34, 463–472.

Nishida, K., Tamura, A., Nakazawa, N., Ueda, Y., Abe, T., Matsuda, F., Kashima, K., and Taniwaki, M. (1997). The Ig heavy chain gene is frequently involved in chromosomal translocations in multiple myeloma and plasma cell leukemia as detected by in situ hybridization. *Blood*, 90, 526–534.

Perez-Simon, J. A., Garcia-Sanz, R., Tabernero, M. D., Almeida, J., Gonzalez, M., Fernandez-Calvo, J., Moro, M. J., Hernandez, J. M., San Miguel, J. F., and Orfao, A. (1998). Prognostic value of numerical chromosome aberrations in multiple myeloma: A FISH analysis of 15 different chromosomes. *Blood*, 91, 3366–3371.

Perfetti, V., Coluccia, A., Intini, D., Malgeri, U., Colli Vignarelli, M., Casarini, S., Merlini, G., and Neri, A. (2001). Translocation t(4;14)(p16.3;q32) is a recurrent genetic lesion in primary amyloidosis. *Leukemia*, 158, 1599–1603.

Piccoli, S. P., Caimi, P. G., and Cole, M. D. (1984). A conserved sequence at c-myc oncogene chromosomal translocation breakpoints in plasmacytomas. *Nature*, 310, 327–330.

Preudhomme, C., Facon, T., Zandecki, M., Vanrumbeke, M., Lai, J. L., Nataf, E., Loucheux, L. M. H., Kerckaert, J. P., and Fenaux, P. (1992). Rare occurrence of P53 gene mutations in multiple myeloma. *British Journal of Haematology*, 81, 440–443.

Rajkumar, S. V., Fonseca, R., Dewald, G. W., Therneau, T. M., Lacy, M. Q., Kyle, R. A., Greipp, P. R., and Gertz, M. A. (1999). Cytogenetic abnormalities correlate with the plasma cell labeling index and extent of bone marrow involvement in myeloma. *Cancer Genetics Cytogenetics*, 113, 73–77.

Raynaud, S. D., Bekri, S., Leroux, D., Grosgeorge, J., Klein, B., Bastard, C., Gaudray, P., and Simon, M. P. (1993). Expanded range of 11q13 breakpoints with differing patterns of cyclin D1 expression in B-cell malignancies. *Genes, Chromosomes and Cancer*, 8, 80–87.

Richelda, R., Ronchetti, D., Baldini, L., Cro, L., Viggiano, L., Marzella, R., Rocchi, M., Otsuki, T., Lombardi, L., Maiolo, A. T., and Neri, A. (1997). A novel chromosomal translocation t(4;14)(p16.3;q32) in multiple myeloma involves the fibroblast growth-factor receptor 3 gene. *Blood*, 90, 4062–4070.

Ried, K., Finnis, M., Hobson, L., Mangelsdorf, M., Dayan, S., Nancarrow, J. K., Woollatt, E., Kremmidiotis, G., Gardner, A., Venter, D., Baker, E., and Richards, R. I. (2000). Common chromosomal fragile site FRA16D sequence: Identification of the FOR gene spanning FRA16D and homozygous deletions and translocation breakpoints in cancer cells. *Human Molecular Genetics*, 9, 1651–1663.

Ronchetti, D., Finelli, P., Richelda, R., Baldini, L., Rocchi, M., Viggiano, L., Cuneo, A., Bogni, S., Fabris, S., Lombardi, L., Maiolo, A., and Neri, A. (1999). Molecular analysis of 11q13 breakpoints in multiple myeloma. *Blood*, 93, 1330–1337.

Ronchetti, D., Greco, A., Compasso, S., Colombo, G., Dell'Era, P., Otsuki, T., Lombardi, L., and Neri, A. (2001). Deregulated FGFR3 mutants in multiple myeloma cell lines with t(4;14): Comparative analysis of Y373C, K650E and the novel G384D mutations. *Oncogene*, 20, 3553–3562.

Sawyer, J. R., Lukacs, J. L., Munshi, N., Desikan, K. R., Singhal, S., Mehta, J., Siegel, D., Shaughnessy, J., and Barlogie, B. (1998). Identification of new nonrandom translocations in multiple myeloma with multicolor spectral karyotyping. *Blood*, 92, 4269–4278.

Sawyer, J. R., Lukacs, J. L., Thomas, E. L., Swanson, C. M., Goosen, L. S., Sammartino, G., Gilliland, J. C., Munshi, N. C., Tricot, G., Shaughnessy, J. D., Jr., and Barlogie, B. (2001). Multicolour spectral karyotyping identifies new translocations and a recurring pathway for chromosome loss in multiple myeloma. *British Journal of Haematology*, 112, 167–174.

Sawyer, J. R., Waldron, J. A., Jagannath, S., and Barlogie, B. (1995). Cytogenetic findings in 200 patients with multiple myeloma. *Cancer Genetics Cytogenetics*, 82, 41–49.

Schultheis, B., Kramer, A., Willer, A., Hegenbart, U., Goldschmidt, H., and Hehlmann, R. (1999). Analysis of p73 and p53 gene deletions in multiple myeloma. *Leukemia*, 13, 2099–2103.

Seong, C., Delasalle, K., Hayes, K., Weber, D., Dimopoulos, M., Swantkowski, J., Huh, Y., Glassman, A., Champlin, R., and Alexanian, R. (1998). Prognostic value of cytogenetics in multiple myeloma. *British Journal of Haematology*, 101, 189–194.

Shaughnessy, J., Jr., Gabrea, A., Qi, Y., Brents, L., Zhan, F., Tian, E., Sawyer, J., Barlogie, B., Bergsagel, P. L., and Kuehl, M. (2001). Cyclin D3 at 6p21 is dysregulated by recurrent chromosomal translocations to immunoglobulin loci in multiple myeloma. *Blood*, 98, 217–223.

Sherr, C. J. (1996). Cancer cell cycles. *Science*, 274, 1672–1677.

Shou, Y., Martelli, M. L., Gabrea, A., Qi, Y., Brents, L. A., Roschke, A., Dewald, G., Kirsch, I. R., Bergsagel, P. L., and Kuehl, W. M. (2000). Diverse karyotypic abnormalities of the c-myc locus associated with c-myc dysregulation and tumor progression in multiple myeloma. *Proceedings of the National Academy of Sciences of the United States of America*, 97, 228–233.

Smadja, N. V., Bastard, C., Brigaudeau, C., Leroux, D., and Fruchart, C. (2001). Hypodiploidy is a major prognostic factor in multiple myeloma. *Blood*, 98, 2229–2238.

Smadja, N. V., Fruchart, C., Isnard, F., Louvet, C., Dutel, J. L., Cheron, N., Grange, M. J., Monconduit, M., and Bastard, C. (1998). Chromosomal analysis in multiple myeloma: Cytogenetic evidence of two different diseases. *Leukemia*, 12, 960–969.

Smith, L., Barlogie, B., and Alexanian, R. (1986). Biclonal and hypodiploid multiple myeloma. *American Journal of Medicine*, 80, 841–843.

Stanton, L. W., Watt, R., and Marcu, K. B. (1983). Translocation, breakage and truncated transcripts of c-myc oncogene in murine plasmacytomas. *Nature*, 303, 401–406.

Tabernero, D., San Miguel, J. F., Garcia-Sanz, M., Najera, L., Garcia-Isidoro, M., Perez-Simon, J. A., Gonzalez, M., Wiegant, J., Raap, A. K., and Orfao, A. (1996). Incidence of chromosome numerical changes in multiple myeloma: Fluorescence in situ hybridization analysis using 15 chromosome-specific probes. *American Journal of Pathology*, 149, 153–161.

Tahara, H., Smith, A. P., Gas, R. D., Cryns, V. L., and Arnold, A. (1996). Genomic localization of novel candidate tumor suppressor gene loci in human parathyroid adenomas. *Cancer Research*, 56, 599–605.

Tricot, G., Barlogie, B., Jagannath, S., Bracy, D., Mattox, S., Vesole, D. H., Naucke, S., and Sawyer, J. R. (1995). Poor prognosis in multiple myeloma is associated only with partial or complete deletions of chromosome 13 or abnormalities involving 11q and not with other karyotype abnormalities. *Blood*, 86, 4250–4256.

Tricot, G., Sawyer, J. R., Jagannath, S., Desikan, K. R., Siegel, D., Naucke, S., Mattox, S., Bracy, D., Munshi, N., and Barlogie, B. (1997). Unique role of cytogenetics in the prognosis of patients with myeloma receiving high-dose therapy and autotransplants. *Journal of Clinical Oncology*, 15, 2659–2666.

Uchida, T., Kinoshita, T., Ohno, T., Ohashi, H., Nagai, H., and Saito, H. (2001). Hypermethylation of *p16* INK4A gene promoter during the progression of plasma cell dyscrasia. *Leukemia*, 15, 157–165.

Vaandrager, J. W., Kluin, P., and Schuuring, E. (1997). The t(11;14)(q13;q32) in multiple myeloma cell line KMS12 has its 11q13 breakpoint 330 kb centromeric from the cyclin D1 gene [Letter]. *Blood*, 89, 349–350.

Vandenberghe, E., De Wolf-Peeters, C., van den Oord, J., Wlodarska, I., Delabie, J., Stul, M., Thomas, J., Michaux, J. L., Mecucci, C., Cassiman, J. J., and Van den Berghe, H. (1991). Translocation (11;14): A cytogenetic anomaly associated with B-cell lymphomas of non-follicle centre cell lineage. *Journal of Pathology*, 163, 13–18.

Vasef, M. A., Medeiros, L. J., Yospur, L. S., Sun, N. C., McCourty, A., and Brynes, R. K. (1997). Cyclin D1 protein in multiple myeloma and plasmacytoma: An immunohistochemical study using fixed, paraffin-embedded tissue sections. *Modern Pathology*, 10, 927–932.

Willis, T. G., and Dyer, M. J. (2000). The role of immunoglobulin translocations in the pathogenesis of B-cell malignancies. *Blood*, 96, 808–822.

Yoshida, S., Nakazawa, N., Iida, S., Hayami, Y., Sato, S., Wakita, A., Shimizu, S., Taniwaki, M., and Ueda, R. (1999). Detection of MUM1/IRF4-IgH fusion in multiple myeloma. *Leukemia*, 13, 1812–1816.

Zandecki, M. (1996). Multiple-myeloma—Almost all patients are cytogenetically abnormal. *British Journal of Haematology*, 94, 217–227.

Zandecki, M., Bernardi, F., Lai, J., Facon, T., Izydorczyk, V., Bauters, F., and Cosson, A. (1994). Image analysis in multiple myeloma at diagnosis. Correlation with cytogenetic study. *Cancer Genetics Cytogenetics*, 74, 115–119.

Zandecki, M., Lai, J. L., and Facon, T. (1996). Multiple myeloma: Almost all patients are cytogenetically abnormal. *British Journal of Haematology*, *94*, 217–227.

Zandecki, M., Lai, J. L., Genevieve, F., Bernardi, F., Volle-Remy, H., Blanchet, O., Francois, M., Cosson, A., Bauters, F., and Facon, T. (1997). Several cytogenetic subclones may be identified within plasma cells from patients with monoclonal gammopathy of undetermined significance, both at diagnosis and during the indolent course of this condition. *Blood*, *90*, 3682–3690.

Zandecki, M., Obein, V., Bernardi, F., Soenen, V., Flactif, M., Lai, J. L., Francois, M., and Facon, T. (1995). Monoclonal gammopathy of undetermined significance: Chromosome changes are a common finding within bone marrow plasma cells. *British Journal of Haematology*, *90*, 693–696.

Zhan, F., Hardin, J., Kordsmeier, B., Bumm, K., Zheng, M., Tian, E., Sanderson, R., Yang, Y., Wilson, C., Zangari, M., Anaissie, E., Morris, C., Muwalla, F., van Rhee, F., Fassas, A., Crowley, J., Tricot, G., Barlogie, B., and Shaughnessy, J., Jr. (2002). Global gene expression profiling of multiple myeloma, monoclonal gammopathy of undetermined significance, and normal bone marrow plasma cells. *Blood*, *99*, 1745–1757.

Zojer, N., Konigsberg, R., Ackermann, J., Fritz, E., Dallinger, S., Kromer, E., Kaufmann, H., Riedl, L., Gisslinger, H., Schreiber, S., Heinz, R., Ludwig, H., Huber, H., and Drach, J. (2000). Deletion of 13q14 remains an independent adverse prognostic variable in multiple myeloma despite its frequent detection by interphase fluorescence in situ hybridization. *Blood*, *95*, 1925–1930.

# CHAPTER 6

# Gene Expression Profiling and Multiple Myeloma

JOHN D. SHAUGHNESSY, JR.
A. KEITH STEWART

## Introduction

The recent completion of the human genome project, and the resulting advent of technologies allowing a global interrogation of the entire expressed human genome from very small starting tissue samples, promises to revolutionize medical diagnosis, prognosis, and treatment. The diagnosis and management of multiple myeloma (MM) will be no exception and will be changed irrevocably by the application of such technologies to this disease and its mysteries. Although the technology is young, dramatic progress is already being made. This chapter briefly describes the emerging genome-based technologies as they apply to myeloma and how use of these technologies has begun to impact thinking about this disease.

## Genomic Technologies

In as much as all cancer mutations appear to directly or indirectly affect gene transcription, the ability to follow these changes represents a powerful way in which to classify and study the molecular biology of malignancies. An important spin-off from the human genome project has been the capacity to rapidly acquire large datasets of DNA sequence (high throughput sequencing, express sequence tags [EST], SAGE libraries) at relatively low cost from target cells and subsequently to mine these libraries using gene expression technology. Changes in gene expression can be quantitatively monitored based on complementary base-pairing of nucleic acids. At its simplest level, gene expression profiling (GEP) uses microarrays of cDNAs spotted on nylon membranes or glass slides. The advantage of such microarrays is that they are relatively inexpensive and can be rapidly customized to contain only genes of interest. Alternatively, more sophisticated high-density oligonucleotide microarrays (HDA) were developed by exploiting technologies adapted from the semiconductor industry using photolithography and solid-phase chemistry to produce arrays containing hundreds of thousands of oligonucleotide probes packed at extremely high densities (Fodor et al., 1999). The probes are designed to maximize sensitivity, specificity, and reproducibility, allowing consistent discrimination between specific and background signals and between closely related target sequences (Lipshutz et al., 1999). Microarray technology was first used to study cancer in 1996 (DeRisi et al., 1996) and now has been used to identify disease subtypes in morphologically indistinguishable cancers (Alizadeh et al., 2000; Golub et al., 1999; Zhan et al., 2002) and to develop molecular predictors of response to therapeutic interventions (Shipp et al., 2002; Yeoh et al., 2002). HDAs can now simultaneously monitor the expression of nearly all of the estimated 35,000 human genes.

## Lessons from High Throughput Sequencing in Myeloma

Neoplastic transformation in multiple myeloma is thought to originate in illegitimate immunoglobulin heavy chain (IgH) switch recombinations. This seminal event results in the translocation of oncogenes to the IgH locus on 14q32. At least 5 genes had been identified as primary, nonrandom translocation partners. These genes include *Bcl-1/PRAD-1*/cyclin D1 (11q13) cyclin D3 (6p21) (Shaughnessy et al., 2001), *FGFR3-MMSET* (4p16.3) (Chesi et al., 1998a) *c-maf* (16q23) (Chesi et al., 1998b), and *mafB* (20q11) (Hanamura et al., 2001). Deletions of chromosome 13 are also common and appear early in the disease course. During the ensuing progression of the disease, additional karyotypic instability develops and mutations or dysregulation in expression of genes such as *c-myc*, *N-ras*, *K-ras*, *FGFR3*, and p53 occur (see Chapter 3). Nevertheless, little is understood about the progressive genetic events that result in the propagation of multiple myeloma.

Close to 60,000 3′ end single-pass gene sequences from cDNA libraries derived from normal and malignant human B cells have been deposited by the Cancer Genome Anatomy Project (Staudt and Brown, 2000). All of these gene sequences, however, were derived from lymphoma, germinal-center B cells, and chronic lymphocytic leukemia samples, and no sequences were derived from either normal or malignant plasma cells (PCs). cDNA libraries have therefore been obtained from myeloma patients and 5′ end single-pass sequence acquired from 6622 cDNA clones. To gain further insight into the transcriptional profile of myeloma cells, expressed genes were assigned functional categories using the SOURCE database (genome-www5.stanford.edu/cgibin/SMD/source/sourceSearch) and The Expressed Gene Anatomy Database (www.tigr.org/tdb/egad/egad.shtml) to classify known, named nuclear encoded genes. A notable proportion of expressed sequences (26.1%) were grouped as cell/organism defense and gene/expression categories (31.6%), whereas only 3.5% were catalogued as involved in cell structure/motility. Cell division/apoptosis genes, which include those involved in DNA synthesis/replication, programmed cell death, chromosome structure, and cell cycle, comprised 6.8% of all the expressed sequences (Fig. 6-1). Although subtraction with immunoglobulin and mitochondrial genes was performed before sequencing, immunoglobulin and mitochondrial genes still constitute the majority (21% and 13.6%, respectively) of genes sequenced. Thus, the overall frequency would naturally, in the absence of subtraction, be even higher. Taken together this initial functional classification of expressed genes demonstrated a high respiratory activity, low cell-cycle activity, CD138$^+$-expressing, immunoglobulin- and β2-microglobulin-producing cell population consistent with the known function of, and markers for, plasma cells. Thus, this sequencing effort seems representative of plasma cells and allows some confidence in mining this database for genes involved in myeloma/plasma cell growth and differentiation.

Further analysis of sequenced clones reveals some relevant findings of note in myeloma biology and reveals novel gene sequences of potential interest to the field. Genes that are highly expressed in myeloma cells were identified based on the number of times they were sequenced from randomly selected clones. Not surprisingly, genes with high expression include lymphoid genes such as MHC class I, β-2 microglobulin, immunoglobulin lambda light chain, kappa light chain, and heavy chain. Other highly expressed but less well characterized genes include protein tumor-related antigen 1 (*TRA1*) (Kasukabe et al., 1997), *TSC-22R/DSIPI* (Vogel et al., 1996), regulator of G protein signaling 1/(also called B cell activation gene [*BL34*]) (Hong et al., 1993), *DDX5* (DEAD/H p68 RNA helicase)

A

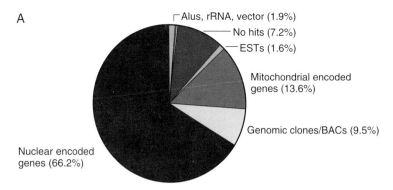

Nuclear encoded genes (66.2%)

Alus, rRNA, vector (1.9%)

No hits (7.2%)

ESTs (1.6%)

Mitochondrial encoded genes (13.6%)

Genomic clones/BACs (9.5%)

*Figure 6-1  Frequency analysis of expressed sequence tags (EST) from MM. Random cDNA clones from myeloma libraries were sequenced at the 5′ end. Sequence identities were determined using Blast algorithm against RefSeq, high throughput genomic sequence (htgs), dbEST, UniGene, and the nonredundant (nr) databases. Assignment of putative identities required a Blastn E value = 10⁻¹⁰. Each clone was classified based on nucleotide sequence database searches (A) or according to functional categories (B) using SOURCE (http://source.stanford.edu) and Expressed Gene Anatomy database (http://www.tigr.org/tdb/egad/egad.shtml). (Claudio, J. O., Masih-Khan, E., Tang, H., Goncalves, J., Voralia, M., Li, Z. H., Nadeem, V., Cokerman, E., Francisco-Pabalan, O., Liew, C. C., Woodgett, J. R., and Stewart, A. K. (2002). A molecular compendium of genes expressed in multiple myeloma. Blood, 100, 2175–2186.)*

B

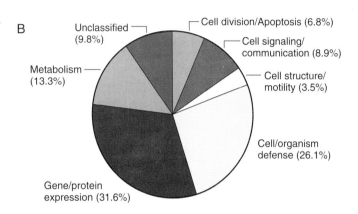

Unclassified (9.8%)

Metabolism (13.3%)

Gene/protein expression (31.6%)

Cell division/Apoptosis (6.8%)

Cell signaling/communication (8.9%)

Cell structure/motility (3.5%)

Cell/organism defense (26.1%)

(Dubey et al., 1997), and hypothetical protein MGC3178 (also annotated as UniGene Hs.6101; 58 kDa glucose regulated protein).

Previous reports indicated a possible viral involvement in the pathogenesis of multiple myeloma (Rettig et al., 1997). Nevertheless, excluding known oncogenes such as *c-fos, c-myc,* and *c-jun,* analysis of the myeloma sequences described here did not reveal any evidence of expressed viral genes that might support this hypothesis.

It is of interest to compare the sequencing effort with published GEP experiments (see subsequent paragraphs) in that genes identified by sequencing overlapped significantly with the genes upregulated in multiple myeloma described by GEP (Zhan et al., 2002). Indeed, 11 of 70 genes upregulated in myeloma GEP compared with normal plasma cells (*EIF3S9, LAMC1, SSA2, EWSR1, KIAA0020, PHB, EVI2A, CASP1, SNURF, ATF3,* and *MYC*) were also in the sequence dataset. Using both GEP and sequence information, a molecular resource of genes expressed in primary malignant plasma cells was created using a combination of cDNA library construction, 5′ end single-pass sequencing, bioinformatics, and microarray analysis. In total, this myeloma gene index houses 9732 nonredundant expressed genes (www.uhnres.utoronto.ca/akstewart_lab.mgi.html). This genetic catalogue should represent a valuable resource for investigators interested in further dissecting the molecular basis of this disease.

## The Molecular Portrait of Myeloma

Building on studies such as those described here, many groups have now attempted to better understand the heterogeneity of MM and perhaps identify new molecular targets by applying GEP technology to newly diagnosed MM. Commercially available Affymetrix oligo-based array system, glass slide-based arrays, and nylon membrane-spotted cDNAs have been used. Klein and colleagues were the first to use gene GEP to study MM 73. In this work the investigators used human MM cells lines and small-scale, filter-based cDNA arrays to identify key intercellular signaling genes expressed in malignant PCs. The investigators were able to distinguish MM cells from other B cell lineage cells and noted a significant alteration in gene expression of cell-cycle genes (cyclin D1, CDC34); c-myc and c-myc partners; apoptosis genes; genes involved in metastasis and bone remodeling (SPARC); and cellular signaling genes that include receptor tyrosine kinase Tyro3 and FRZB of the Wnt signaling pathway (De Vos et al., 2001, 2002). In another early paper, glass slide-based arrays, a myeloma-enriched 4.3K cDNA microarray, and a generic 19K array were used to interrogate MM cell lines and similar findings emerged (Claudio et al., 2002). Supervised cluster analysis of data from these arrays identified 52 and 13 genes, respectively, that

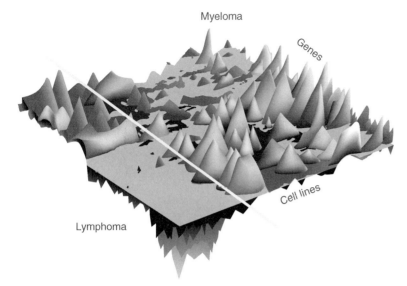

Myeloma

Genes

Cell lines

Lymphoma

**Figure 6-2** *Differentially expressed genes between myeloma and hematopoietic nonmyeloma cell lines. Supervised cluster analysis with a false-positive rate of 0.5% was used to identify genes showing differential expression between the 2 groups of cell lines. The genes showing statistically significant differences are shown as a 2-dimensional heat map. The dendrogram (top) indicates the 2 major branches corresponding to myeloma cell lines and nonmyeloma cell lines. Intensity of squares correlate with the degree of gene expression. (Claudio, J. O., Masih-Khan, E., Francisco-Pabalan, O., Liew, C. C., Woodgett, J. R., and Stewart, A. K. (2002). A molecular compendium of genes expressed in multiple myeloma.* Blood, 100, *2175–2186.)*

were differentially expressed between myeloma and nonmyeloma cell lines (Fig. 6-2, 3D heat map), whereas similar distinguishing gene sets differentiate healthy donor blood B cells from malignant plasma cells. This dataset includes genes known to be involved in plasma cell biology such as the multiple myeloma oncogene 1 (MUM/IRF4), BlyS/BAFF receptor BCMA, plasma cell marker CD138 (syndecan-1), serine threonine-protein kinase oncogene (PIM2), plasma cell transcription factor XBP1, and a gene involved in osteoclast formation and bone resorption (ANXA2). Such comparisons also revealed an upregulation of endoplasmic reticulum (ER) stress-response genes in MM cells, including the novel disulfide isomerase MGC3178, TRA1, heat shock 70 kDa protein 5 (HSPA5), and XBP-1. These genes are part of an adaptive pathway termed the unfolded protein response (UPR), a phenomenon suggested to be critical for B cell differentiation into plasma cells. This differentiation involves a 5-fold expansion of the ER to accommodate the high level of immunoglobulin secretion. Indeed, XBP-1 is the only factor identified to date that is absolutely required for plasma cell differentiation and is also identified as the key signaling molecule downstream of IRE1 and ATF6 in the UPR pathway (Yoshida et al., 2001).

One drawback of such studies is that MM cell lines and PC leukemias represent terminal stages of the disease; thus, it is important to put GEP data using these cells in the context of newly diagnosed disease so that gene expression events associated with initiation and those associated with progression might be more adequately defined. These early studies also demonstrated the need to establish corresponding gene expression profiles of normal plasma cells (PC). Given that PC typically make up less than 5% of the cells in normal human bone marrow, isolation of a sufficient number of cells for GEP without resorting to RNA amplification techniques required specialized methodologies. Two

different and complementary techniques have been used to accomplish this objective. The first and most commonly used is automated immunomagnetic bead sorting of PC from large-volume bone marrow aspirates using a monoclonal antibody, BB4, raised against syndecan-1/CD138 25. This technique has now been used to isolate highly homogenous populations of normal PC from both bone marrow and tonsil 75. Isolation of sufficient numbers of PC from normal human marrow for large-scale GEP experiments makes it an impractical endeavor for most laboratories. Thus, to create a source of polyclonal PC from normal donors, Tarte and colleagues developed a method for the in vitro differentiation of peripheral blood B cell 76. Global expression profiling of polyclonal PC and normal bone marrow PC derived from immunomagnetic sorting has revealed strong similarities, but also distinct differences, between the 2 populations and MM 76, 77.

More than 800 cases of MM, smoldering MM (SMM), monoclonal gammopathy of undetermined significance (MGUS), and other PC dyscrasias, as well as normal bone marrow PC, tonsil PC, and normal B cell populations, have been studied using the Affymetrix Genechip system, by far the largest dataset yet available. The first major MM study incorporating this technology interrogated 6800 genes in 74 newly diagnosed cases of MM, 7 MGUS, and 31 normal donors and showed that: (1) short-term longitudinal GEP reveal little intrapatient variability, suggesting that changes linked to progression, an unfortunate reality in MM, might eventually be identified; (2) microarray-derived gene expression levels and protein levels as determined by FACS analysis are tightly correlated; (3) spikes of CCND1, FGFR3, and other genes reflect the presence of 14q32 translocations involving these loci; (4) MM can be differentiated from normal PC on this array set by 120 genes, possibly representing fundamental genetic changes involved in, or a reflection of, neoplastic transformation; (5) MGUS, a benign PC dyscrasia, is currently indistinguishable from MM; and (6) 4 distinct molecular subgroups of MM can be identified with using unsupervised hierarchical clustering with the so-called MM4 subgroup being related to highly proliferative human myeloma cell lines (HMCL) and the MM1 subgroup being more similar to MGUS (Fig. 6-3).

Importantly, these data revealed that a subgroup of newly diagnosed MM has GEP features of HMCL and as such, HMCL appears to represent an appropriate model system for studying the biology of, and evaluation of preclinical drug efficacy for, at least, the HMCL-like subgroup of the disease.

Although the above series of studies present a medley of potential genes for further studies of myeloma biology, such studies also highlight a drawback of high throughput gene expression studies, either by sequencing or by microarray, which is the complexity of distinguishing genes of significance in MM biology from the cacophony of all upregulated genes. However, despite such obstacles, the new GEP-based portraits of MM described here have provided a platform on which to seek novel molecular targets that distinguish MM cells

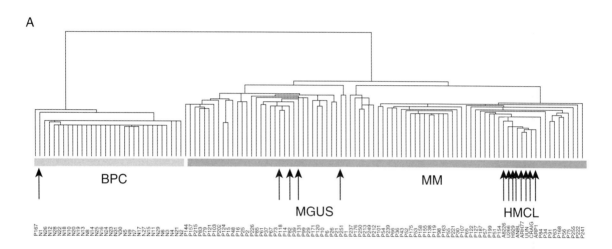

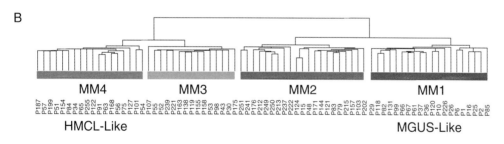

| Parameter | MM1 + MM2 | MM3 | MM4 | P |
|---|---|---|---|---|
| Abnormal cytogenetics | 22% | 53% | 72% | .0003 |
| β2M (mg/L) | 2.75 | 4.62 | 8.81 | .0005 |

***Figure 6-3*** *Global gene expression profiling distinguishes PC subgroups. (**A**) Two-dimensional hierarchical cluster analysis of 74 newly diagnosed MM, 31 normal bone marrow PC, 5 MGUS, and 6 human MM cell line samples clustered based on the correlation of 5483 genes (probe sets). The clustering is presented graphically as a shaded image. Along the vertical axis, the analyzed genes are arranged as ordered by the clustering algorithm. The genes with the most similar patterns of expression are placed adjacent to each other. Likewise, along the horizontal axis, experimental samples are arranged; those with the most similar patterns of expression across all genes are placed adjacent to each other. Both sample and gene groupings can be further described by following the solid lines (branches) that connect the individual components with the larger groups. The shade of each cell in the tabular image represents the expression level of each gene. (**B**) Enlarged view of patient sample cluster in Part **A**. Bars under samples indicate normal bone marrow PC and MM clusters. Note that no major subbranches in the MM samples contain MGUS or cell line samples. (**C**) Dendrogram of a hierarchical cluster analysis of 74 cases of newly diagnosed untreated MM (clustergram not shown). Two major branches contained 2 distinct cluster groups. The subgroups under the right branch, designated MM1 and MM2 were more related to the MGUS cases in Part **B**. The 2 subgroups under the left branch, designed MM3 and MM4, represent samples that were more related to the human MM cell lines in Part **C**. (Zhan, F., Hardin, J., Kordsmeier, B., Bumm, K., Zheng, M., Tian, E., Sanderson, R., Yang, Y., Wilson, C., Zangari, M., Anaissie, E., Moris, C., Muwalla, F., van Rhee, F., Fassas, A., Crowley, J., Tricot, G., Garlogie, B., Shaughnessy, J., Jr. (2002). Global gene expression profiling of multiple myeloma, monoclonal gammopathy of undetermined significance and normal bone marrow plasma cells. Blood, 99, 1745–1757.)*

from related cell types to determine a new prognostically relevant molecular classification of MM, to use pharmacogenomics for stratifying patients' responses to treatment regimens, and to further develop an understanding of the molecular mechanisms of chemotherapeutic agents as well as the progression of the disease. Early GEP-based studies exploring these topics are now explored in the rest of this chapter.

# Genomics and the Genesis for MM

Like many tumors of the B-cell lineage, MM harbors recurrent rearrangements of the IGH locus at 14q32.16. GEP can be used to identify these 14q32 translocations in MM. Briefly, some genes are expressed at particularly high levels on GEP, viewed as a spike on the histograms generated by array software. Such spikes noted on early GEP profiles include known translocation partners in MM, including FGFR3, CCND1, and CCND3. Subsequent studies demonstrate close to 100% correlation of these spikes with the presence of the t(11;14)(q13;q32), t(4;14)(p16;q32), or t(6;14)(p21;q32), respectively. Indeed, in 145 newly diagnosed cases of MM, CCND1 spikes were seen in 13%, FGFR3 spikes were seen in yet another 13%, MAF in 7.5%, and CCND3 in 4.1% of the cases, percentages almost identical to those derived by other technologies examining translocation frequency such as fluorescent in situ hybridization (FISH) or reverse transcriptase–polymerase chain reaction (RT-PCR). For example, a recent study by Avet-Loiseau and colleagues showed that 14q32 rearrangements are found in 73% ($n = 669$) of MM and that the translocation partners in 44% of these rearrangements are not known. A comparison of GEP spikes and the FISH data of Avet-Loiseau et al. demonstrate strong correlations with CCND1 (13% vs. 16%), FGFR3 (13% vs. 10%), and MAF (4.1% vs. 2%). GEP "spikes," including the 4 common translocation partner genes, were observed in 109 of 145 (75%) MM overall. We suspect that many of the 17 unclassified spike genes represent candidates for unknown 14q32 translocation partner genes. These observations suggest that GEP can be a powerful tool to study known and suspected MM-associated 14q32 translocations. Because such translocations appear to harbor prognostic significance and are potential molecular targets, GEP profiling might prove a simple and reliable means of simultaneously applying prognostic and therapeutically important information to individual patients.

In a comprehensive interphase FISH analysis of chromosome 13 ploidy, it was demonstrated that monosomy 13 is present in approximately 40% to 50% of myeloma patients, that 13q14 is a deletion hotspot, and that FISH deletion is linked to inferior overall survival in MM. In an effort to determine if GEP can be a surrogate for FISH and also aid in the identification of a putative tumor-suppressor gene, FISH deletion analysis was combined with GEP. In FISH analysis with 4 probes spanning the long arm of chromosome 13 performed on 112 patients, 74 were normal and 38 had monosomy of all 4 probes in >50% of the clonotypic PCs. A GEP comparison between the 2 groups revealed that 46 genes were differentially expressed. As expected, the top 14 differentially expressed genes mapped to chromosome 13. Although a total of 84 chromosome 13 genes were interrogated on the microarray, 34 were not expressed in PC, and 28 that were expressed showed no change across any comparison. A linear discriminate model using the expression levels of these 14 genes could predict, with 100% accuracy, the deletion status of MM (unpublished data). Overall, these data indicate that deletion of chromosome 13 results in loss or reduced expression of specific genes on the chromosome and that profiles of these genes can be used to accurately predict chromosome 13 deletion in primary MM.

Together, these studies demonstrate that GEP might eventually serve as a surrogate, single-platform analytic tool predicting the cytogenetic make-up of MM and providing the information required to make individually tailored therapeutic decisions.

# Molecular Diagnosis of Myeloma

Global GEP of malignant and normal cells can reveal tumor-specific gene expression patterns. These unique signatures can be used to develop highly sensitive quantitative RT–PCR-based molecular diagnostic assays for patient stratification and minimal residual disease detection. In a first attempt to develop such a test, statistical analysis, including chi-square, WRS, and SAM analysis, was used to compare the GEP of 12,000 genes in 150 cases of untreated MM and 33 normal bone marrow donors. Appropriate statistical analysis identified 14 genes (Table 6-1) capable of differentiating malignant from normal PCs with a high degree of accuracy in a training group of 150 MM and 26 normal PCs. When applied to a held-out validation group consisting of 78 MM cases and 3 normal bone marrow PC, the 14-gene model demonstrated an accuracy of classification of 98.8% (Shaughnessy, unpublished data). Importantly, the model was incapable of differentiating most MGUS from MM, because 15 of 19 cases of MGUS were classified as MM. An unsupervised cluster analysis with 33 normal bone marrow PCs, 19 MGUS, and 40 newly diagnosed MM using 6971 genes showed that 5 MGUS samples, including the 4 that were predicted to be normal in the model, were clustered with the normal bone marrow PC.

**TABLE 6-1**

Genes Whose Altered Expression Can Be Used to Differentiate Normal PC from MM

| Gene | Gene Function |
|------|---------------|
| CD24 | Modulation of B-cell activation responses |
| CD163 | Integral membrane protein and scavenger receptor cysteine-rich (SRCR) superfamily member: thought to play important role in regulating inflammatory response |
| ITGB2 | Cell surface adhesion glycoprotein that can interact with ICAM-1: expressed on tumor cells of low- and medium-grade malignant lymphomas, but characteristically absent on cells of high-grade malignant B cell lymphomas; absence results in escape from immunosurveillance in lymphoma |
| PF4V1 | CXC chemokine |
| PGYL | Allosteric enzyme in carbohydrate metabolism |
| PLA2G7 | Modulates the action of platelet-activating factor (PAF): PAF is a mediator of signaling, activation of proinflammatory cells, alteration of vascular permeability, and stimulation of glycogen metabolism |
| ABL1 | Cytoplasmic and nuclear protein tyrosine kinase: activated by certain DNA-damaging agents and involved in a mismatch repair-dependent apoptotic pathway |
| GMPS | De novo synthesis of guanine nucleotides |
| H2BHF | Replication-dependent histone |
| ILF3 | M-phase phosphoprotein that heterodimerizes with NF45 to form the NFAT DNA-binding complex; overexpressed in nasopharyngeal carcinoma cells |
| MTA1 | Subunit of NURD (nucleosome remodeling and histone deacetylation) complex |
| MVP | Implicated in multidrug resistance; confers a poor prognosis in MM |
| PTPRK | Regulates processes involving cell contact and adhesion; forms complexes with beta-catenin and gamma-catenin/plakoglobin |
| QSCN6 | Expressed at higher levels in quiescent cells than in logarithmically growing cells |

These data have potential important clinical implications in that a malignant signature can be observed in MGUS, even when PC are present at less than 10% frequency and likely mixed with normal PC. Such studies set the stage for the development of highly specific and sensitive diagnostic tests for MM which might be applied across a broad population base.

## Myeloma Biology Insights from Expression Profiling

By developing a method to differentiate normal peripheral blood B cells to polyclonal plasmablastic cells that maintains all morphologic, phenotypic, and functional characteristics, Klein and colleagues demonstrated by GEP that the limiting step in analyzing a control population of plasma cells can be overcome (Tarte et al., 2002). This study offers a more accurate means of comparing the expression profile of malignant plasma cells and their autologous normal counterpart. Follow-up studies comparing the expression profile of 5 cell populations representing the late stages of human B cell maturation (i.e., polyclonal plasmablastic cells, tonsil-derived plasma cells, bone marrow-derived plasma cells, peripheral blood B cells, and tonsil B cells) showed that 85 PC genes and 40 B cell genes, respectively, were overexpressed in the 3 PC subsets or in the 2 B cell subsets (Tarte et al., 2003). This gene dataset derived from the comparative expression profiling of these populations could be mined for genes involved in the molecular events that regulate survival, proliferation, differentiation, and commitment to PC both in normal physiology and in malignant disease.

Cells representing distinct stages of late stage B cell development such as CD19-enriched B cells (BC) from tonsils, CD138-enriched PC from tonsils, normal bone marrows, and MM bone marrows have also been studied by other groups (Zhan et al., 2003). In these studies, hierarchical cluster analysis with 3288 genes clearly segregated the 4 cell types. When genes expressed in tonsil BC were compared with tonsil PC, 359 genes defined a signature representing early differentiation (EDG), whereas 500 genes representing the signature for late differentiation (LDG) defined the difference between tonsil PC and bone marrow PC. Hierarchical cluster analysis using 30 and 50 most-variable EDG and LDG, respectively, revealed that MM cases could each be defined by gene expression subgroups that linked the MM to 1 of the 3 normal cell types. For example, 13 of 18 of the MM4 subgroup clustered with tonsil BC ($p = 0.00005$), 14 of 15 MM3 cases clustered with tonsil PC ($p = 0.000008$) and 14 of 20 MM2 cases clustered with bone marrow PC ($p = 0.00009$). MM1 showed no significant linkage with normal cell types studied. These studies demonstrate then that MM is a heterogenous disease that has its roots in normal physiological differentiation processes during plasma cell development, a finding that has implications in designing future therapies.

# Expression Profiles and Prognosis in Myeloma

The identification of multiple gene expression-based subgroups as described here is consistent with the variable clinical course of MM, with survival ranging from as short as 2 months to greater than 80 months after diagnosis. An important hope for GEP in this disease is therefore that this wide outcome variability, which cannot be accurately accounted for with current clinical parameters, might be better understood. With this in mind, bone marrow PCs from 74 patients with newly diagnosed MM, 5 with MGUS, and 31 healthy volunteers (normal PCs) were purified by CD138( + ) selection and gene expression of purified PCs and 7 MM cell lines were profiled using high-density oligonucleotide microarrays interrogating approximately 6800 genes. On hierarchical clustering analysis, normal and MM PCs were differentiated and 4 distinct subgroups of MM (MM1, MM2, MM3, and MM4) were identified. The expression pattern of MM1 was similar to normal PCs and MGUS, whereas MM4 was similar to MM cell lines. Clinical parameters linked to poor prognosis, abnormal karyotype ($p = 0.002$) and high-serum β2-microglobulin genes involved in DNA metabolism and cell-cycle control were overexpressed in a comparison of MM1 and MM4. An independent study of 45 multiple myeloma patients using a glass slide-based array has similar findings and suggested that 2 groups of MM can be distinguished based on expression signatures defined by peripheral blood CD19$^+$ B cells or normal CD138$^+$ plasma cells (Masih-Khan et al., unpublished data). One B cell-like (BL) group has characteristic expression most similar to CD19$^+$ B cells, with upregulation of unfolded protein response (UPR) genes. A second plasma cell-like (PL) group clusters with normal plasma cell controls. These data suggest that myeloma can be classified at the molecular level based on the developmental signature of B cells.

Long of interest to clinicians has been the apparent differences in outcome of MM patients based on the isotype expressed by the tumor with IgA MM usually reporting a worse prognosis than IgG. Interesting differences in molecular profile emerge when GEP is used in these isotypes defined MM subgroups, e.g., Minvielle and colleagues (Magrangeas et al., 2003) analyzed gene expression profiles of 92 primary tumors according to their Ig types and light chain subtypes. Several clusters of genes involved in various biologic functions such as immune response, cell-cycle control, signaling, apoptosis, cell adhesion, and structure significantly

discriminated IgA– from IgG-MM. Genes associated with inhibition of differentiation and apoptosis induction were upregulated, whereas genes associated with immune response, cell-cycle control, and apoptosis were downregulated in IgA-MM. According to the expression of the 61 most discriminating genes, BJ-MM represented a separate subgroup that did not express either the genes characteristic of IgG-MM or those of IgA-MM at a high level. Several genes whose products are known to stimulate bone remodeling discriminate between kappa and lambda MM (see subsequent paragraphs). The unifying theme in all these studies is that the highly variable outcomes of MM patients might in part be explained by unique genetic signatures that relate to the differentiation stage of the transformed plasma cell. Nevertheless, such hypotheses are speculative and all such studies require verification in prospective clinical correlative studies.

# Pharmacogenomics and Myeloma

Another promise inherent in the application of GEP to MM is the ability to use genomic information to predict response to therapy, or to use another term, pharmacogenomics. Although the data are, for now, limited by lack of prospective follow-up information, there is already some evidence to support the use of GEP in predicting initial response to chemotherapy. In one study, patients receiving VAD chemotherapy were placed in 1 of 2 subgroups based on expression of 11 cell-cycle genes. Seventy percent of patients with higher than median expression of at least 8 of the 11 cell-cycle genes showed a partial or complete response, whereas only 30% of the patients with lower than median expression of 8 of 11 of these genes responded. Although initial response to VAD is not necessarily an accurate predictor of overall response, this study does bode well for the use of GEP in patient risk stratification.

To evaluate the ability of gene expression profiling to predict response to single-agent drugs, GEP was performed on 30 patients before treatment with the proteasome inhibitor PS-341. After sufficient follow up, responders ($n = 15$) and nonresponders ($n = 15$) were identified and gene expression differences in baseline samples were examined. Of the 12,000 genes surveyed, 44 genes distinguished response from no response with $p$ values ranging from 0.0095 to 0.00046. A multivariate stepwise discriminant analysis revealed that 5 of the 44 genes could be used in a response predictor model. A leave-one-out crossvalidation analysis performed on a training group revealed the model was 96.7% accurate. Such studies are relatively early, but the immense promise of accurately predicting patients who will respond from those who will not is an exciting prospect.

# Molecular Target Identification

The molecular mechanisms of common chemotherapies for MM can be studied *in vitro* using GEP. For example, although it is known that a tumor's resistance to doxorubicin is often associated with the expression of the multidrug resistance (MDR1) gene, microarray analysis of the MM cell line RPMI 8226, including variants selected for a drug-resistant phenotype, demonstrated that gene expression profiles of drug-resistant subclones underwent a dramatic shift in the expression of apoptotic–response genes mediated by ceramide signaling and mitochondrial permeability (Watts et al., 2001). In other studies, Chauhan and colleagues showed that 2-Methoxyestradiol (2ME2), an estrogen-derivative, triggers an early but transient induction of genes known to trigger cell death, accompanied by repression of growth/survival-related genes (Chauhan et al., 2002). Likewise, GEP on the effects of PS-341 on myeloma demonstrated that this drug down-regulates the transcription of growth factor genes while simultaneously inducing apoptotic, ubiquitin/proteasome, and stress-response genes (Mitsiades et al., 2003a). Moreover, when combined with doxorubicin and melphalan, PS-341 downregulates several effectors mediating genotoxic stress response, consequently restoring sensitivity to DNA-damaging chemotherapeutic agents (Mitsiades et al., 2003b).

In other studies the mechanism of action of various single-agent compounds was studied *in vivo* on 56 patients before and after therapy with dexamethasone ($n = 16$), thalidomide ($n = 12$), IMiD ($n = 14$), or PS-341 ($n = 12$). A total of 60 pair-wise comparisons were performed, and induced changes greater than 2-fold in at least half the patients in each drug group was defined. As an example of the power of such analysis, it is instructive to examine the response of MM cells to the related compounds Thal and IMiD. IMiD or CC-5013, a potent thalidomide homolog, induced changes in 98 genes ($p < 0.001$; 41 up and 57 down), whereas thalidomide induced significant changes in 57 genes ($p < 0.001$; 29 up and 28 down). Given that IMiD and thalidomide are related molecules, it was speculated that consistent and common changes in gene expression influenced by both drugs might point to mechanisms of action. Six genes, *CROT, IL6, TPBG, ALB, PLSCR1*, and *DKK1* were activated by both drugs but upregulation after IMiD treatment was higher for all genes, attesting to the high potency of the derivative.

Importantly, Dickkopf1 (*DKK1*), a secreted antagonist of Wnt signaling, was hyperactivated a median 125% in 14 of 18 patients treated with thalidomide. Furthermore, DKK1 was upregulated a median of 315% in 13 of 15 cases treated with IMiD. Virtually all MM cases not showing a hyperactivation of *DKK1* after treatment with both drugs had little or no detectable expression in the baseline sample, suggesting that these cases had an inherent inability to activate *DKK1* expression.

Of 648 genes exhibiting >50% change in median expression levels (51–408%) after IMiD treatment, *DKK1*, at 315%, ranked as the fourth most significantly altered gene. In a similar analysis after thalidomide treatment, *DKK1* was ranked 13th out of 217 genes. Conversely, although activated in 14 of 20 patients treated with dexamethasone, *DKK1* only showed a median increase of 23%, was ranked 1426th, and not represented in the list of 280 genes exhibiting an upregulation of at least 50% (range, 51–470%) by this drug. The effects of PS-341 were even more skewed from the IMiD and thalidomide data in that only 7 of 15 patient samples exhibited increases in *DKK1* and the median change was essentially undetectable at −1.60%. *DKK1* ranked 7532 of 12,000 genes tested. Thus, these data provide the first *in vivo* evidence that thalidomide and IMiD have powerful upregulating effects on *DKK1* expression, that dexamethasone has an intermediate effect, and the proteasome inhibitor PS-341 has little or no effect on *DKK1* expression. It will be important to determine if the drug has a direct activating effect or whether the increase really reflects the rapid and preferential killing of cells not expressing *DKK1*, which would in turn create a virtual upregulation.

DKK1 has been shown to be critical for limb morphogenesis during vertebrate embryogenesis (*165, 168*). *DKK1*-null mutant embryos show duplications and fusions of limb digits (*168*), whereas forced overexpression of DKK1 in embryonic limb buds inhibits limb outgrowth (*165, 168*). The limb defects resulting from overexpression of *DKK1* have a strong resemblance to the limb defects seen in thalidomide embryopathy. Thus, an intriguing implication of the link between thalidomide and *DKK1* activation is that disruption of WNT signaling through *DKK1* activation by thalidomide might be the long-sought mechanism by which thalidomide causes such limb malformations. Interestingly, a link between *DKK1* expression and MM-specific bone defects has also become apparent through the use of microarray profiling (see subsequent paragraphs).

Thus, *in vivo* monitoring of gene expression after single-agent drug treatment appears to be feasible. This type of study has powerful advantages over *in vitro* models of the same design in that response can be taken into account in the final analysis, a variable that cannot be faithfully recapitulated in model systems. Short-term serial gene expression studies of tumor cells after single-agent drug treatment might provide insight into the mechanisms of action, especially when combined with clinical response data. This knowledge, if confirmed, can lead to the development of second-generation drugs with more effective responses and less toxicity. In addition, knowledge of pathways will allow development of drugs that target discrete points along pathways allowing use of complementary or synergistic drugs.

# The Microenvironment in MGUS and MM

It is now appreciated that MM growth, and probably growth of all cancers, partially relies on nontumor accessory cells providing growth and survival factors as well as a sanctuary from the effects of chemotherapy. Previous studies have identified the molecular signature of highly purified MM cells and their normal counterparts, yet the signature of the stromal component of the MM bone marrow microenvironment and whether this signature is qualitatively altered in disease is not known. These studies are of enormous clinical relevance, because it is becoming increasingly accepted that an important adjunct to current therapies, which target the tumor cell directly, depend on the manipulation of the microenvironment. This work is probably most clearly demonstrated by the effects of thalidomide and second-generation analogs that are thought to act through multiple mechanisms, ranging from direct tumoricidal activity to anti-angiogenesis and modulation of tumor necrosis factor-alpha (TNFα) signaling through direct and/or indirect effects on the tumor microenvironment [45].

GEP of the microenvironment component of MM and MGUS bone marrow with respect to normal counterparts can be studied using purified PC and biopsy pairs. Genes expressed in malignant cells are subtracted out leaving microenvironment genes behind for subsequent analysis. A pilot study using pair-wise comparisons of normal biopsies and MM biopsies has revealed 146 microenvironment genes with decreased and 86 genes with increased expression in the MM biopsies. Subtracting PC expressed genes revealed 75 microenvironment genes that were significantly different between MM and normal controls. These genes have been defined as microenvironment-associated genes (MAG). A total of 54 MAG showed decreased expression (range, 2- to 4-fold), and 21 MAG showed increased expression (range, 2- to 8-fold) in the MM biopsies.

Within the MAG upregulated genes, the most significantly altered gene was a voltage-gated K+ channel-related transcript. Two of the top 5 MAG, UMAG1, and UMAG2 code for adhesion proteins

implicated in MM PC stromal cell interactions. Interestingly, the expression of UMAG1 and UMAG2 was not elevated in MGUS biopsies. The apparent upregulation of 2 key adhesion molecules in cells of the microenvironment is consistent with studies suggesting that such molecules have a major influence on MM cell growth and drug resistance (Damiano et al., 1999; Ghia et al., 2002; Hazlehurst et al., 2000; Shain et al., 2000; Yaccoby et al., 2002). UMAG3, 1 of the 5 most upregulated MAG, is a member of the matrix metalloproteinase (MMP) family. The gene was essentially undetectable in purified PC. The overexpression of UMAG3 also has potential relevance, given the role of MMPs in various aspects of MM pathology, including angiogenesis and bone resorption (Barille et al., 1997; Vacca et al., 1999; Wahlgren et al., 2001). Further dissection of microenvironment genes in MM, particularly during therapy, might lead to new and innovative approaches to therapy.

# Gene Expression Profiling and Myeloma Bone Disease

Myeloma is the only hematologic malignancy consistently associated with debilitating lytic bone disease. To identify molecular determinants of lytic bone disease, the expression profiles of approximately 12,000 genes in CD138-enriched plasma cells from newly diagnosed MM exhibiting no radiologic evidence of lytic lesions on bone surveys (NoLL, $n = 28$) to those with ≥3 lytic lesions (LL) ($n = 47$) were compared. Genes distinguishing the 2 groups include the *RHAMM* proto-oncogene, *NCALD* (a calcium-binding protein involved in neuronal signal transduction), *FRZB* and DKK1 (2 secreted antagonists of Wnt signaling), *CBFA2/AML1B*, which has been linked to *MIP1α* expression, *PTTG1 (securin)*, involved in chromosome segregation and the *TSC-22* homologue *DSIPI*. In addition, 4 so-called "spike genes" that are more frequently found in LL versus NoLL ($p$ <0.05) were identified: *IL6*, Osteonidogen (*NID2*), regulator of G protein signaling (*RGS13*), and pyromidinergic receptor.

In other studies of MM bone disease, several genes whose products are known to stimulate bone remodeling discriminate between kappa and lambda MM. One of these genes, Mip-1α, was overexpressed in the kappa subgroup. In addition, a strong association ($p = 0.0001$) between kappa subgroup MM expressing high levels of Mip-1α and active myeloma bone disease was established. Together, these data suggest that gene expression patterns might provide valuable insight into MM bone disease. In addition to being potentially useful as predictors of the emergence of lytic bone disease and conversion from MGUS to overt

MM, they might also identify targets for potential intervention.

## Potential Problems and Pitfalls

Although it is clear that GEP is closer to becoming a relevant diagnostic and prognostic tool in the clinical management of hematologic malignancies, it is also important to point out some of the limitations of the technology.

### Nonstandardized System

One negative feature is that there is no universal standard microarray in use. Because "no microarray platform is alike" in either manufacturing standards or gene content, direct comparison of data derived from different laboratories can be difficult. Although it appears that more and more centers are shifting toward the use of the commercially available Affymetrix platform, in which lot-to-lot variability is minimal and other standards of manufacturing are imposed, many academic centers use cDNA microarrays that are produced in-house using internal standards. Even if a consensus on the use of a universal platform were adopted, cost for the foreseeable future will represent another prohibitive feature of microarray profiling.

### Sample Purity

A further problem with GEP involves the presence of cells other than the primary tumor in profiled tissue. As was pointed out previously, there is a distinct possibility that the tumor microenvironment might hold clues to tumor behavior in MM and thus its gene expression patterns might be informative; however, the ability to delineate from which cells individual signatures are derived can be virtually impossible in complex mixtures. Thus, if an experiment is designed to determine the tumor cell signature, the presence of nontumor cells has the potential of introducing nonspecific noise and must be taken into account. MM represents a good example of such a problem. The nature of MM results in dramatic intra- and interpatient variability in the percentage of PC in a given sample with inherent difficulties in subsequent interpretation of the data.

### Intratumor Variability

Even after purification, a potential limitation of GEP is that intratumor heterogeneity cannot be realized. By studying populations of cells, it is impossible to determine whether a detectable gene is active in all cells or in a subpopulation. This has important ramifications if the gene is, for example, associated with an aggressive subclone. However, recent elegant studies demonstrating the stochastic nature of gene expression suggest that studying mixtures of large populations, as is done in most microarray experiments, might be a more appropriate means of recognizing significant changes in patterns between 2 distinct sample types, e.g., normal versus malignant.

### Statistical Interpretation

Another potential problem with GEP is that unsupervised hierarchical classification schemes tend to show a low, but significant, degree of plasticity. That is to say that samples placed in one particular subgroup can shift to another group when additional patient samples or more genes are added to the analysis. This problem will become less of a concern when GEP incorporates all human genes and patient outcome is taken into consideration.

### Outcome Prediction

A clinically important drawback is that models predicting outcome based on GEP will likely be specific for distinct therapies, such that a model predicting outcome to high-dose therapy and transplant will be different from one that also incorporates thalidomide or one built on standard therapy or single agents, e.g., PS-341. An additional pitfall in development of prognostic models based on the use of first- and second-generation microarrays is that not all human genes are represented on most arrays, possibly resulting in the absence of genes whose inclusion could increase sensitivity and specificity of models. This lack of a complete genome survey also likely limits an understanding of the mechanisms of disease. It is certainly possible that critical genes not studied today could hold important clues to disease biology. Although GEP is revealing many new insights, changes in gene expression are liable to represent only one of many causes or effects of neoplastic development. For example, it is thought that the complexity of the human genome is magnified, possibly several-fold, by alternative splicing, a phenomenon not currently recognizable by GEP. Another level of complexity in eukaryotic cell systems involves posttranslational modification of proteins, e.g., glycosylation and phosphorylation, which is not appreciated directly with GEP. Furthermore, gene expression patterns do not always correlate with protein levels, and because the protein is the functional product of the mRNA blueprint, gene expression leads should be followed with complimentary and confirmatory studies. It is important to note, however, that although protein correlations are important for target validation and functional inferences, GEP patterns are sufficient for prognostic model development as long as the patterns are reproducible. A further variable not accounted for in GEP is allele variation that results in variations in functionality, e.g., drug metabolism, of gene products. Thus, even though a gene in 2 samples might be expressed at similar levels, the 2 patients could have inherited different alleles that have different functional capacities. Therefore, although gene expression is providing useful new information in both clinical and basic research, it does not provide a complete picture and is best used in the context of broad studies using other standard laboratory techniques.

# Summary

In this chapter we have highlighted the technologies of the genomics era and have illustrated how such technologies might change the way MM is diagnosed, treated, and monitored. We have also addressed the insights that gene expression profiling has already provided in characterizing MM biology. These are early days, technology is still evolving, and links to clinical outcomes are only now being made. The promise of genomics, informatics, and the emerging field of proteomics is clear, and time will tell whether such promise is realized.

## REFERENCES

Alizadeh, A. A., Eisen, M. B., Davis, R. E., Ma, C., Lossos, I. S., Rosenwald, A., et al. (2000). Distinct types of diffuse large B-cell lymphoma identified by gene expression profiling. *Nature, 403*, 503–511.

Barille, S., Akhoundi, C., Collette, M., Mellerin, M. P., Rapp, M. J., Harousseau, J. L., et al. (1997). Metalloproteinases in multiple myeloma: production of matrix metalloproteinase-9 (MMP-9), activation of proMMP-2, and induction of MMP-1 by myeloma cells. *Blood, 90*, 1649–1655.

Chauhan, D., Li, G., Auclair, D., Hideshima, T., Richardson, P., Podar, K., et al. (2003). Identification of genes regulated by 2-methoxyestradiol (2ME2) in multiple myeloma (MM) cells using oligonucleotide arrays. *Blood, 101*, 3606–3614.

Chesi, M., Bergsagel, P. L., Shonukan, O. O., Martelli, M. L., Brents, L. A., Chen, T., et al. (1998a). Frequent dysregulation of the c-maf proto-oncogene at 16q23 by translocation to an Ig locus in multiple myeloma. *Blood, 91*, 4457–4463.

Chesi, M., Nardini, E., Lim, R. S., Smith, K. D., Kuehl, W. M., and Bergsagel, P. L. (1998b). The t(4;14) translocation in myeloma dysregulates both FGFR3 and a novel gene, MMSET, resulting in IgH/MMSET hybrid transcripts. *Blood, 92*, 3025–3034.

Claudio, J. O., Masih-Khan, E., Tang, H., Goncalves, J., Voralia, M., Li, Z. H., Nadeem, V., Cukerman, E., Francisco-Pabalan, O., Liew, C. C., Woodgett, J. R., and Stewart, A. K. (2002). A molecular compendium of genes expressed in multiple myeloma. *Blood, 100*, 2175–2186.

Damiano, J. S., Cress, A. E., Hazlehurst, L. A., Shtil, A. A., and Dalton, W. S. (1999). Cell adhesion mediated drug resistance (CAM-DR): role of integrins and resistance to apoptosis in human myeloma cell lines. *Blood, 93*, 1658–1667.

DeRisi, J., Penland, L., Brown, P. O., Bittner, M. L., Meltzer, P. S., Ray, M., et al. (1996). Use of a cDNA microarray to analyse gene expression patterns in human cancer. *Nature Genetics, 14*, 457–460.

De Vos, J., Couderc, G., Tarte, K., Jourdan, M., Requirand, G., Delteil, M. C., et al. (2001). Identifying intercellular signaling genes expressed in malignant plasma cells by using complementary DNA arrays. *Blood, 98*, 771–780.

De Vos, J., Thykjaer, T., Tarte, K., Ensslen, M., Raynaud, P., Requirand, G., et al. (2002). Comparison of gene expression profiling between malignant and normal plasma cells with oligonucleotide arrays. *Oncogene, 21*, 6848–6857.

Dubey, P., Hendrickson, R. C., Meredith, S. C., Siegel, C. T., Shabanowitz, J., Skipper, J. C., et al. (1997). The immunodominant antigen of an ultraviolet-induced regressor tumor is generated by a somatic point mutation in the DEAD box helicase p68. *Journal of Experimental Medicine, 185*, 695–705.

Fodor, S. P., Read, J. L., Pirrung, M. C., Stryer, L., Lu, A. T., and Solas, D. (1991). Light-directed, spatially addressable parallel chemical synthesis. *Science, 251*, 767–773.

Ghia, P., Granziero, L., Chilosi, M., and Caligaris-Cappio, F. (2002). Chronic B cell malignancies and bone marrow microenvironment. *Semin Cancer Biol, 12*, 149–155.

Golub, T. R., Slonim, D. K., Tamayo, P., Huard, C., Gaasenbeek, M., Mesirov, J. P., et al. (1999). Molecular classification of cancer: class discovery and class prediction by gene expression monitoring. *Science, 286*, 531–537.

Hanamura, I., Iida, S., Akano, Y., Hayami, Y., Kato, M., Miura, K., et al. (2001). Ectopic expression of MAFB gene in human myeloma cells carrying (14;20)(q32;q11) chromosomal translocations. *Japanese Journal of Cancer Research, 92*, 638–644.

Hazlehurst, L. A., Damiano, J. S., Buyuksal, I., Pledger, W. J., and Dalton, W. S. (2000). Adhesion to fibronectin via beta1 integrins regulates p27kip1 levels and contributes to cell adhesion mediated drug resistance (CAM-DR). *Oncogene, 19*, 4319–4327.

Hong, J. X., Wilson, G. L., Fox, C. H., and Kehrl, J. H. (1993). Isolation and characterization of a novel B cell activation gene. *Journal of Immunology, 150*, 3895–3904.

Kasukabe, T., Okabe-Kado, J., and Honma, Y. (1997). TRA1, a novel mRNA highly expressed in leukemogenic mouse monocytic sublines but not in nonleukemogenic sublines. *Blood, 89*, 2975–2985.

Lipshutz, R. J., Fodor, S. P., Gingeras, T. R., and Lockhart, D. J. (1999). High density synthetic oligonucleotide arrays. *Nature Genetics, 21*, 20–24.

Magrangeas, F., Nasser, V., Avet-Loiseau, H., Loriod, B., Decaux, O., Granjeaud, S., et al. (2003). Gene expression profiling of multiple myeloma reveals molecular portraits in relation to the pathogenesis of the disease. *Blood, 101*, 4998–5006.

Mitsiades, N., Mitsiades, C. S., Richardson, P. G., McMullan, C., Poulaki, V., Fanourakis, G., et al. (2003a). Molecular sequelae of histone deacetylase inhibition in human malignant B cells. *Blood, 101*, 4055–4062.

Mitsiades, N., Mitsiades, C. S., Richardson, P. G., Poulaki, V., Tai, Y. T., Chauhan, D., et al. (2003b). The proteasome inhibitor PS-341 potentiates sensitivity of multiple myeloma cells to conventional chemotherapeutic agents: therapeutic applications. *Blood, 101*, 2377–2380.

Rettig, M. B., Ma, H. J., Vescio, R. A., Pold, M., Schiller, G., Belson, D., et al. (1997). Kaposi's sarcoma-associated herpesvirus infection of bone marrow dendritic cells from multiple myeloma patients. *Science, 276*, 1851–1854.

Shain, K. H., Landowski, T. H., and Dalton, W. S. (2000). The tumor microenvironment as a determinant of cancer cell survival: a possible mechanism for de novo drug resistance. *Current Opinions in Oncology, 12*, 557–563.

Shaughnessy, J., Jr., Gabrea, A., Qi, Y., Brents, L., Zhan, F., Tian, E., et al. (2001). Cyclin D3 at 6p21 is dysregulated by recurrent chromosomal translocations to immunoglobulin loci in multiple myeloma. *Blood, 98*, 217–223.

Shipp, M. A., Ross, K. N., Tamayo, P., Weng, A. P., Kutok, J. L., Aguiar, R. C., et al. (2002). Diffuse large B-cell lymphoma outcome prediction by gene-expression profiling and supervised machine learning. *Natural Medicine, 8*, 68–74.

Staudt, L. M., and Brown, P. O. (2000). Genomic views of the immune system. *Annual Review of Immunology, 18*, 829–859.

Tarte, K., De Vos, J., Thykjaer, T., Zhan, F., Fiol, G., Costes, V., et al. (2002). Generation of polyclonal plasmablasts from peripheral blood B cells: a normal counterpart of malignant plasmablasts. *Blood, 100*, 1113–1122.

Tarte, K., Zhan, F., De Vos, J., Klein, B., and Shaughnessy, J. (2003). Gene expression profiling of plasma cells and plasmablasts: toward a better understanding of the late stages of B-cell differentiation. *Blood, 100*, 1113–1122.

Vacca, A., Ribatti, D., Presta, M., Minischetti, M., Iurlaro, M., Ria, R., et al. (1999). Bone marrow neovascularization, plasma cell angiogenic potential, and matrix metalloproteinase-2 secretion parallel progression of human multiple myeloma. *Blood, 93*, 3064–3073.

Vogel, P., Magert, H. J., Cieslak, A., Adermann, K., and Forssmann, W. G. (1996). hDIP—a potential transcriptional regulator related to murine TSC-22 and Drosophila shortsighted (shs)—is expressed in a large number of human tissues. *Biochimica et Biophysica Acta, 1309*, 200–204.

Wahlgren, J., Maisi, P., Sorsa, T., Sutinen, M., Tervahartiala, T., Pirila, E., et al. (2001). Expression and induction of collagenases (MMP-8 and -13) in plasma cells associated with bone-destructive lesions. *Journal of Pathology, 194*, 217–224.

Watts, G. S., Futscher, B. W., Isett, R., Gleason-Guzman, M., Kunkel, M. W., and Salmon, S. E. (2001). cDNA microarray analysis of multidrug resistance: doxorubicin selection produces multiple defects in apoptosis signaling pathways. *Journal of Pharmacology and Experimental Therapeutics, 299*, 434–441.

Yaccoby, S., Pearse, R. N., Johnson, C. L., Barlogie, B., Choi, Y., and Epstein, J. (2002). Myeloma interacts with the bone marrow microenvironment to induce osteoclastogenesis and is dependent on osteoclast activity. *British Journal of Haematology, 116*, 278–290.

Yeoh, E. J., Ross, M. E., Shurtleff, S. A., Williams, W. K., Patel, D., Mahfouz, R., et al. (2002). Classification, subtype discovery, and prediction of outcome in pediatric acute lymphoblastic leukemia by gene expression profiling. *Cancer Cell, 1*, 133–143.

Yoshida, H., Matsui, T., Yamamoto, A., Okada, T., and Mori, K. (2001). XBP1 mRNA is induced by ATF6 and spliced by IRE1 in response to ER stress to produce a highly active transcription factor. *Cell, 107*, 881–891.

Zhan, F., Hardin, J., Kordsmeier, B., Bumm, K., Zheng, M., Tian, E., et al. (2002). Global gene expression profiling of multiple myeloma, monoclonal gammopathy of undetermined significance, and normal bone marrow plasma cells. *Blood, 99*, 1745–1757.

Zhan, F., Tian, E., Bumm, K., Smith, R., Barlogie, B., and Shaughnessy, J., Jr. (2003). Gene expression profiling of human plasma cell differentiation and classification of multiple myeloma based on similarities to distinct stages of late-stage B-cell development. *Blood, 101*, 1128–1140.

Zhan, F., Hardin, J., Kordsmeier, B., Bumm, K., Zheng, M., Tian, E., Sanderson, R., Yang, Y., Wilson, C., Zangari, M., Anaissie, E., Moris, C., Muwalla, F., van Rhee, F., Fassas, A., Crowley, J., Tricot, G., Garlogie, B., Shaughnessy, J., Jr. (2002). Global gene expression profiling of multiple myeloma, monoclonal gammopathy of undetermined significance, and normal bone marrow plasma cells. *Blood, 99*, 1745–1757.

# PART II

*Clinical Features*

# CHAPTER 7

## Multiple Myeloma: A History

ROBERT A. KYLE
DAVID P. STEENSMA

## Early Cases of Multiple Myeloma

Although multiple myeloma has almost certainly been present for centuries, the first well-documented case was the second patient described by Solly in 1844. Four years before her death, Sarah Newbury, a 39-year-old housewife, had developed fatigue and severe back pain while stooping. After a fall in February 1842, pain in her limbs increased, and she was confined to her room. Two months later, her femurs fractured when her husband lifted her and carried her to the bed. Fractures of the clavicles, right humerus, and right radius and ulna occurred (Fig. 7-1). She was hospitalized on April 15, 1844, at St. Thomas's Hospital, London. She was given wine and arrowroot, a mutton chop, and a pint of porter daily. Treatment consisted of an infusion of orange peel and a rhubarb pill as well as opiates at night. Arrowroot, an easily digestible starch extracted from the roots (rhizomes) of

Parts of this chapter have been previously published in Kyle, R. A. (2003). History of multiple myeloma. In P. H. Wiernik, G. P. Canellos, J. P. Dutcher, and R. A. Kyle (Eds.), *Neoplastic Diseases of the Blood*, ed 4. (pp. 415–423). Cambridge University Press; and Kyle, R. A., and Steensma, D. P. History of multiple myeloma. In G. Gahrton, B. G. M. Durie, and D. Samson (Eds.), *Multiple Myeloma*, ed 2. In press. Reprinted with permission.

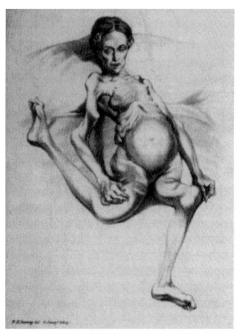

*Figure 7-1* Sarah Newbury. Fractures of femurs and right humerus. (From Solly, 1844.)

tubers such as *Maranta arundinacea*, was first imported from the West Indies to England in the 18th century (Stephens, 1994). In the 19th century it was considered a very bland food, appropriate mostly for convalescents who were in poor condition and had difficulty with digestion (Felter and Lloyd, 1898–1900).

Porter, a dark, bitter ale made from black malted barley, was a new substance in England in the early 19th century, an outgrowth of an 18th-century drinking fad. The beer was popular among working classes in London, especially among porters and draymen. In the early 19th century, when porter originated, three types of beer were widely available in London pubs: brown ale, strong ale, and a weak, marginally alcoholic beer sometimes called "two pence." Workmen in need of sustenance were fond of asking bartenders for a mellow mix of all three types of beer, a blend sometimes called "three threads" ("threads" could have been "thirds" with an East London accent). Eventually, breweries started premixing the drink to save bartenders time and end arguments over variability in the relative components; the new mix was first known as "entire" and later as "porter's beer." Because porter would have been an unlikely drink to offer an ailing high class woman, Sarah Newbury was probably part of the working class (Smith and Getty, 1998; Westemeier, 2001).

Rhubarb pills are a well-known purgative. Orange-based preparations such as *infusum aurantii*, a concoction made from oranges or peels, were often used to change the flavor of a medicine and make it more tolerable, but in their own right they were considered

carminatives, tonics, and stomachics. Opium compounds have been widely used since ancient times to provide pain relief, and this class of drugs also slows bowel motility, which might have been useful for Newbury's diarrhea (Felter and Lloyd, 1898–1900; *Pharmacopoeia of the United States of America*, 1820).

Sarah Newbury died suddenly on April 20, 1844, 2 years after the fractures of her femurs. Autopsy revealed that the cancellous portion of the sternum had been replaced by a red substance (Fig. 7-2). This red matter, similar to that seen in Mr. McBean, had also replaced much of the femur and ranged from Modena red to a bright scarlet crimson (Fig. 7-3). These cells, which were examined by Dr. Solly and Mr. Birkett of Guy's Hospital, London, were "very clear, their edge being remarkably distinct, and the clear oval outline enclosed one bright central nucleus, rarely two, never more." Solly thought that the disease was an inflammatory process and that it began with a "morbid action" of the blood vessels in which the "earthy matter of the bone is absorbed and thrown out by the kidneys in the urine." Little did he know that, 150 years later, antiangiogenesis drugs would be used for the treatment of multiple myeloma (Kyle, 2000). Newbury had a large quantity of phosphate of lime in her urine (Kyle, 1996).

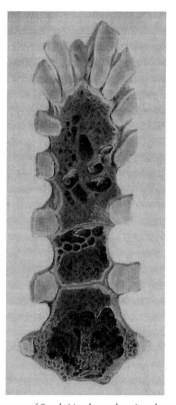

*Figure 7-2* Sternum of Sarah Newbury showing destruction of bone. (From Solly, 1844.)

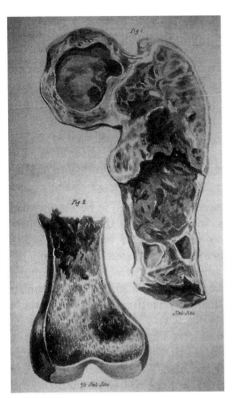

*Figure 7-3* Sarah Newbury. Destruction of femurs by myeloma tumor. (From Solly, 1844.)

## Case History of Thomas Alexander McBean

The best-known case of multiple myeloma is that of Thomas Alexander McBean, a "highly respectable tradesman," 45 years of age. His case was reported by William Macintyre, who was a 53-year-old Harley Street consultant and physician to the Metropolitan Convalescent Institution and to the Western General Dispensary, St. Marylebone (Clamp, 1967). Mr. McBean took a vacation in the country in September 1844 in an effort to regain his strength, which he felt had been impaired by work and a family illness. His father had died of complications of gout, and his mother had died suddenly after surgery for carcinoma of the breast. He had tired easily for the past year and appeared to stoop while walking. He noted that his "body linen was stiffened by his urine" despite the absence of a urethral discharge. While vaulting out of an underground cavern on his vacation, in September 1844 he "instantly felt as if something had snapped or given way within the chest, and for some minutes he lay in intense agony, unable to stir" (Macintyre, 1850).

The acute pain abated and he was able to walk to a neighboring inn. Soreness and stiffness of the chest persisted but was relieved by a "strengthening plaster to the chest" which gave temporary relief. The pain recurred 3 to 4 weeks later, and a pound of blood was removed and leeches were applied for "maintenance therapy." The phlebotomy was followed by considerable weakness for 2 or 3 months, but he had no nausea or vomiting and did not lose his hair.

Pleuritic pain developed in the spring of 1845 and was treated by cupping, which provided no benefit. Therapeutic phlebotomy produced greater weakness than before. Because of wasting, pallor, and slight puffiness of his face and ankles, McBean was seen in consultation by Dr. Thomas Watson, who later became a baronet and Physician-in-Ordinary to Queen Victoria. Watson was President of the Royal College of Physicians, and his popular book *Principles and Practice of Physics* earned him the title of the "British Cicero." Watson prescribed steel and quinine, which resulted in rapid improvement.

Quinine and iron have a long and storied history as therapeutic agents, and each continues to find use. The Germanic physician–alchemist Paracelsus (Philippus Aureolus Theophrastus Bombastus von Hohenheim, 1493–1541), the son of a chemist, is often given credit for being the first to use metallic compounds, such as iron, copper, antimony, and mercury, as medicines, supplementing the herbal remedies that had been used for millennia (Pagel, 1982). Quinine is an alkaloid of cinchona bark, used chiefly in the treatment of malaria. Jesuit missionaries brought cinchona, or "Jesuit's bark," to Europe from the Americas in the late 1630s after it purportedly cured malaria in the wife of the Peruvian viceroy. Quinine was purified from the powdered bark in the early 19th century. Iron was included in the influential first *London Pharmacopoeia* in 1618, and within a century cinchona bark had joined it in clinical practice (Royal College of Physicians of London, 1944).

By the 19th century, one or both of these remedies were used in a broad range of ailments, both well-characterized disorders such as cholera and typhoid and much murkier disorders; in the first American industrial cases of anthrax in the 1860s, the patients received iron and quinine mixed with iodine. Even a cursory review of 19th-century case records suggests that a trial of quinine was believed to be indicated in almost every febrile illness (in this role it was eventually replaced by salicylates). Iron was used as the base component of many tonics meant to give strength and vitality. This idea had nothing to do with knowledge about the composition of hemoglobin or the blood; however, because iron was the metal of Mars, the god of War, it was thought to give vigor and power. By the end of the 19th century, some of the dangers of the indiscriminate use of iron were beginning to be recognized; an 1877 article entitled "When Not to Use Iron" would have been much shorter if it had been written 50 years earlier (Stone, 1868; Fothergill, 1877).

During the summer of 1845, McBean was able to travel to Scotland, where on the seacoast "he was capable of taking active exercise on foot during the greater part of the day, bounding over the hills, to use his own expression, as nimbly as any of his companions" (Macintyre, 1850). His appetite became ravenous; he expressed it as being so much that he dreamed of eating dogs and cats (Jones, 1847). Unfortunately, diarrhea developed, and in September he returned to London in a debilitated state. The following month, lumbar and sciatic pain became severe. Warm baths, Dover's powder, acetate of ammonia, camphor julep, and compound tincture of camphor did not help.

Camphorated julep was commonly used for hysterical ailments and anxiety. Noted diarist Fanny Burney wrote in 1788 that a palace physician had prescribed camphor julep for use by Queen Charlotte whenever she became hysterical during George III's bouts of porphyria-induced madness (Burney, 1904–1905). In Charles Dickens' *The Pickwick Papers* (1837), camphor julep was recommended to an old woman for "nervousness" by Bob Sawyer, a medical student (Dickens, 1938).

Camphor preparations (from the *Cinnamomum camphora* and related plants in Asia) enjoyed a wide range of medicinal uses in the 19th century (Buchan, 1781). Camphor liniments were used topically for a wide range of rashes and superficial infections. Internally, camphor was used as a sedative in cases of insomnia, anxiety, or agitation and, paradoxically, as a stimulant–tonic for persons in a weakened state suspected to be the result of heart failure. It also seemed to relieve chills and slow the bowels. In addition, some physicians believed camphor had value for nonspecific "rheumatic pains," and therefore a camphor preparation would have been a logical choice for Thomas McBean with all of his troublesome bone pain, diarrhea, and the understandable attendant anxiety.

Acetate of ammonia and Dover's powder (an early patent medicine combining ipecac and opium, named after Thomas Dover [1660–1742]) were preparations with nearly identical therapeutic goals, producing diaphoresis and emesis. A vigorous sweat and a good purging were once considered therapeutic because "toxins" were expelled. The 19th century was the heyday of the theory of autointoxication (a term that appeared in the 1880s), a time when the belief that internal toxins contributed to illness and had to be expunged to bring about cure. The opium in Dover's powder probably was useful for McBean's diarrhea and bone pain (Felter and Lloyd, 1898).

McBean's pain became "fixed" in the left lumbar and iliac regions, causing him to assume a semi-bent posture because of the agony caused by every attempt at movement of the body (Macintyre, 1850). There was intermittent pain involving the chest and shoulders. He was only able to "get in and out of bed on all-fours"

because of the severe pain. He became weaker and was confined to his bed. Citrate of iron and quinine produced no benefit. His urine became thick and turbid, like pea soup. This change coincided with improvement characterized by sleeping well for 2 nights and the ability to get up and walk around the room with little or no pain. There was no change in the amount of "animal matter" in the urine. A cough and phlegm in the chest occurred, and severe pain developed. He had an episode of diarrhea that had been precipitated by a dose of rhubarb and soda, given to correct flatulence.

Dr. Macintyre saw him in consultation on October 30, 1845, and personally examined the urine because edema had been observed. The urine specimen had a specific gravity of 1.035. The urine was found to "abound in animal matter," but heating and the addition of nitric acid made it clear; after 1 hour a precipitate developed. The precipitate "underwent complete solution on the application of heat, but again consolidated on cooling."

Two days later, Macintyre sent a sample of urine and the following note to Henry Bence Jones, a 31-year-old physician at St. George's Hospital who was a well-recognized chemical pathologist: "Dear Dr. Jones, The tube contains urine of very high specific gravity. When boiled it becomes slightly opaque. On the addition of nitric acid, it effervesces, assumes a reddish hue, and becomes quite clear; but as it cools, assumes the consistence and appearance which you see. Heat reliquifies it. What is it?" (Jones, 1847).

Any movement of McBean's trunk produced excruciating pain. He became weaker and was confined to his bed. Flatulence, hardness in the region of the liver, and pronounced fullness occurred. Dr. Henry Bence Jones saw him on November 15, 1845, in consultation and recommended alum as treatment "with the view of checking the exhausting excretion of animal matter." McBean improved and was able to sit up and enjoy his food, but on December 7 "experienced a dreadful aggravation of lumbar pains" (Macintyre, 1850). He became weaker and died on January 1, 1846. The cause of death was recorded as "atrophy from albuminuria" (Fig. 7-4).

Emaciation was found on postmortem examination. The ribs were soft, brittle, readily broken, and easily cut with a knife. A soft "gelatiniform substance of a blood-red color and unctuous feel" filled the interior of the ribs. The sternum was soft and fragile and snapped when raised and turned back. "The liver was voluminous, but of healthy structure." The kidneys appeared to be normal on both gross and microscopic examination. The kidneys had "proved equal to the novel office assigned them" and "discharged the task without sustaining, on their part, the slightest danger." The thoracic and lumbar vertebrae had the same changes as found in the ribs and sternum.

The disease appeared to begin in the cancellous bone and then grew and produced irregularly sized

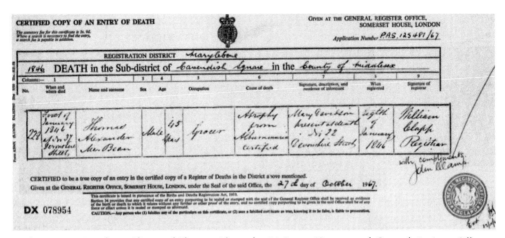

**Figure 7-4** *Death certificate of Thomas Alexander McBean. (Courtesy of General Register Office, London, England.) (From Kyle [1996] with permission.)*

round, dark-red projections that were visible through the periosteum. John Dalrymple, surgeon to the Royal Ophthalmic Hospital, Moorfields, examined two lumbar vertebrae and a rib. He reported that nucleated cells formed the bulk of the gelatiniform mass. Most of the cells were round or oval and were approximately one-half to two times as large as an average red blood cell. The cells contained one or two nuclei, each with a bright, distinct nucleolus. Woodcarvings made from the drawings of Mr. Dalrymple are consistent with the appearance of myeloma cells (Fig. 7-5). Dalrymple noted that the microscopic appearance of the bone marrow cells of Mrs. Newbury "accords very nearly" with the cells in McBean's marrow (Dalrymple, 1846).

The diarrhea, weakness, emaciation, hepatic enlargement, flatulence, ankle edema, and Bence Jones proteinuria suggest the possibility of amyloidosis in addition to multiple myeloma. However, the autopsy findings of the normal heart and kidneys and "voluminous liver of healthy structure" make the presence of amyloidosis unlikely. It is doubtful that amyloidosis would have been overlooked because the waxy changes of amyloidosis in the liver were commonly recognized at that time.

Macintyre stated that his "own share in this part of the inquiry, it must have been seen, was very humble." He went on to say that the examination and course of

the patient seemed to be "deserving of a detailed account" and that he "shall be content if I have succeeded in pointing out to future observers, gifted with the requisite qualifications for conducting researches of a higher order, certain definite and distinctive characters by which a peculiar and hitherto unrecorded pathological condition of the urine may be recognised and identified" (Macintyre, 1850). Dr. Jones corroborated the findings in the urine and calculated that the patient excreted more than 60 g per day. He concluded that the protein was an oxide of albumin, specifically "hydrated deutoxide of albumen" (Jones, 1848). He thought that chlorine caused this new protein to form from albumin.

There is some justification for changing the name "multiple myeloma" to McBean's disease with Macintyre's proteinuria. Although Macintyre described the heat properties of the urine, Jones emphasized their place in the diagnosis of myeloma, for he said "I need hardly remark on the importance of seeking for this oxide of albumin in other cases of mollities ossium" (softening of the bone) (Jones, 1847).

## Henry Bence Jones

### Early Life

Henry Bence Jones was born on December 31, 1813, at Thorington Hall in Yoxford, Suffolk, England, to Mathilda Bence and Lieutenant Colonel William Jones. The home was loaned to the family by Jones' maternal grandfather, Reverend Mr. Bence Sparrow, Rector of Beccles. Reverend Sparrow adopted the surname Bence in May 1804 and was thus known as Rev. Bence Bence (Jones, 1929). The Bence family was related to the Winthrops of colonial America, including John Winthrop, the first governor of Connecticut, and also to

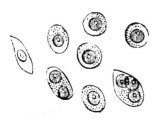

**Figure 7-5** *Plasma cells (wood engravings made from drawings by Mr. Dalrymple). (From Dalrymple, 1846.)*

the Bowdoins, including James Bowdoin, the first president of the American Academy of Arts and Sciences. Jones' father, William, originated from Cork, Ireland, and served in the Fifth Dragoon Guards and fought in the Peninsular War at Salamanca (Kyle, 2001).

Henry fell and fractured his left arm at the elbow at the age of 6 or 7 years. This injury required 1 year for recovery. At age 8 years, he went to school at Hingham, Norfolk, and then to a school in Putney in preparation for Harrow. He said that he learned little at Putney but enjoyed walking in Wimbledon Park. He entered Harrow in 1827 when it had fewer than 150 boys enrolled. In his words, he became a good "cricketer, football and racquet player, and in all games took an immense delight" (Jones, 1929). He became the best player in the school. He studied geometry and algebra under a tutor, Reverend Hartwell Horne, and did well in the former but not with algebra. He entered Trinity College, Cambridge, where he joined the second Trinity crew and rowed number 5. He placed in only the third class and took no first class honors despite his hard work. He made poor progress in Hebrew despite the help of a tutor. He attended the Divinity Lectures and obtained a certificate for ordination, but when he took his degree in January 1836 he decided not to pursue a career in the Church (Coley, 1973).

After graduation, Jones joined his father, who was living in London. Henry seriously considered immigrating to New Zealand and actually proceeded with the paperwork but did not go further. His father suggested he study medicine for 1 year with a general practitioner, Mr. Worthington, but George Babington, a surgeon at St. George's Hospital, introduced Henry to John Hammerton, an apothecary. Jones took two small rooms at Park Street, Grosvenor Square, and prepared medicines in the apothecary shop under Hammerton's direction for 6 months. He later said that this "was of the utmost use to me all my life" (Jones, 1929). He entered the medical school at St. George's Hospital on October 1, 1838, and began attending lectures in the dissecting room. He worked as a dresser in the surgeon's ward, but later returned to the physician's ward. He attempted to learn as much as possible about the stethoscope from Dr. James Hope, an assistant physician at St. George's. Jones also commented that "the glorious discoveries of Dr. Bright were not valued by any of our medical men" (Jones, 1929). He attended the lectures of Michael Faraday on electricity at the Royal Institution.

St. George's Hospital was established in 1733 in the village of Knightsbridge, which was noted for its clean air. Seven years before, its trustees commissioned William Wilkens (who designed the National Gallery in Trafalgar Square and University College) to design the hospital in a classic Greek style. The medical school had been founded in 1831, and its faculty included

John Hunter, Edward Jenner, Thomas Young, and Henry Gray (anatomist). During World War II, a 1,000-pound bomb fell on the lecture theater of the medical school, but fortunately, it did not explode. The hospital moved to Tooting in 1980 (Kyle, 2001). Currently, the Lanesborough Hotel is on the site, but the external features of the original building are preserved. Jones had rheumatic fever in the spring of 1839 and went home for 6 weeks and "recovered without complications of disease of the heart" (Jones, 1929). He returned to London but still felt very weak. He enrolled as a private pupil to Professor Thomas Graham, the father of colloid chemistry, at University College, but most of the teaching was done by his assistant, George Fownes (1815–1849). Fownes had studied with Justus von Liebig in Giessen, Germany. The cost of the year's "pupilage" was £50, which Jones had obtained as a small legacy. Fownes taught Jones the principles of organic analysis, which led to his analysis of the sulfur content in a cystine oxide calculus. This resulted in his first medical paper, which was awarded a "place" in the *Philosophical Transactions*.

Jones passed the examinations of the College of Physicians, which was competing with the new London University. He was admitted in the spring of 1841 as a licentiate of the college but had no university degree. He left London on Easter Sunday 1841 for Giessen, Germany, where he studied in Liebig's laboratory for 6 months. There he learned advanced analytical methods and analyzed the proteins in the brain and egg yolk, which led to a paper in Liebig's *Annalen* (Putnam, 1993). This experience resulted in a lifelong desire to apply chemistry to medicine. Jones was influenced by Liebig's teachings and remained in contact with him throughout his life. Interestingly, Liebig and Jones died 2 days apart in April 1873, and their obituaries were in the same issue of *Lancet*.

## Family History

Returning to London, Jones studied in the physicians' wards at St. George's Hospital and then went home to Lowestoft. He proposed to his second cousin, Lady Millicent Acheson, daughter of the Earl of Gosford. Lady Millicent was the third child and second daughter of Archibald Acheson (1776–1849), a prominent citizen of County Armagh in Northern Ireland. Millicent's father was the second Earl of Gosford, the Irish Representative to the British House of Lords (after 1811) and at one time Governor-in-Chief of Lower Canada in British North America (1835–1837) (*Columbia Encyclopedia*, 6th ed., 2001). The Achesons had maintained ties to Canada since an ancestor was named a Baronet of Nova Scotia in 1628, but Archibald Acheson resigned his Canadian governorship in 1837 when a policy of conciliation toward French Canadians alienated his English constituency. Archibald Acheson married Mary Sparrow Bence in 1805; Millicent's older brother Archibald (1806–1864), the third Earl of Gosford, was born in 1806 (Burke's Peerage and Gentry).

The Acheson family, originally from Scotland, were prominent in County Armagh in the Ulster region from the early 17th century onward. Their presence in Ireland originated with two brothers, Archibald and Henry Acheson (sometimes spelled "Atchison"), who were sent to Ireland in 1610 as "Planters" by King James I to take possession of Ulster land seized from Irish rebels against the hegemony of the British crown. This Irish land was likely a political reward, because the Acheson family was prominent in Scotland during the Jacobean period, and James I had been James VI of Scotland before succeeding Elizabeth to the throne of England. As a testament to the family's prominence in Scottish politics, there is an "Acheson House" along the elite Royal Mile in Edinburgh, built in 1633. In Ireland, the transplanted Achesons built a fortress that would eventually become Gosford Castle, just outside the Irish village of Markethill. A later version of the castle was constructed beginning in 1819 by Millicent's father; its Norman style is said to be inspired by the poet Lord Byron's "exotic and somewhat sinister brand of romanticism" (The Head Forester, Gosford Forest Park, Markethill, Co). The castle is still extant, although recently abandoned and no longer owned by the Achesons.

Mary Sparrow, Archibald Acheson's wife and Millicent's mother, was the daughter and heiress of Robert Sparrow, of Worlingham Hall, Beccles, Suffolk, very near where Henry Bence Jones was born. The Jones family has long maintained close ties to Ireland unrelated to the Achesons. Henry Bence Jones had an older brother, William (1812–1882), who was known as an Irish agriculturist and who wrote several books on Irish affairs. Like Henry, William Bence Jones was born in Beccles, Suffolk. William and Henry's grandfather had bought a moderate-sized estate at Lisselan in County Cork but never lived there. In the 1830s it became clear that the family's agent in Ireland was embezzling money, so William Bence Jones was sent to restore the family's fortune and he lived on the estate until 1880. Through shrewd business decisions, he dramatically enlarged the estate, but he was attacked by the Irish National Land League (formed in 1879 to achieve land reform) and was ostracized by his tenants. Although others, such as Captain Charles Boycott of County Mayo (who gave his name to the tactic) capitulated, Jones resisted successfully by bringing workers from Britain. Nevertheless, he left Ireland in 1881 and opposed Gladstone's Irish land reform policies in the last year of his life. His books included *Life's Work in Ireland* (1880) and *What Has Been Done in the Irish Church*

*Since Its Disestablishment* (1875) (Princess Grace Irish Library [Monaco], 2001).

After some difficulties, which were overcome with the aid of Lady Noel Byron (widow of the poet), Jones and Lady Millicent Acheson were married in May 1842. Lady Millicent's mother, Mary Sparrow, was a longtime friend of Lady Byron. Jones and his bride spent some months with Lady Olivia Sparrow at Brampton, and while there he went to Cambridge and took his MA degree. He returned to London on October 1, settling at 30 Grosvenor Square, and began his work at St. George's. He was asked to analyze and catalog the calculi in the Museum of University College Hospital. Working in a small laboratory in his home, he analyzed the calculi and published his second paper. Fownes had been asked to teach a course at Middlesex Hospital but was too busy, so he asked Jones to give the 100 lectures to the "six attentive pupils" (Jones, 1929). Beginning in the fall of 1843, Jones said that "in preparation for these lectures, I acquired more practical knowledge of chemistry than I could possibly have done in any other way" (Jones, 1929). In 1843 he began a systematic study of the chemical composition of the urine in health and disease. He became a member of the Council of the College of Chemistry, founded in 1845 by Sir James Clarke.

In December 1845, Jones obtained an assistant physicianship at St. George's. The following year another vacancy occurred, and he became a full physician at the hospital. He was elected a fellow of the College of Physicians that same year and delivered the Gouldstonian Lectures in 1846. He was elected a fellow of the Royal Society that same year with the help of Professors Fownes and Graham. He went to Cambridge and took his degree in medicine in 1846.

## Medical Practice and Research

Jones noted that "Each year my practice gradually increased and I endeavored to let no year pass without doing something original in natural science as applied to medicine" (Jones, 1929) (Fig. 7-6). He purchased a home near Folkestone, where he stayed in the summers, but he frequently went to the Continent for 3 to 4 weeks, visiting baths and spas, including Evian, France. He took his wife and two older children to Chamonix, France, in 1854, but his wife became very tired and barely got back to Paris. Consequently, in the future he traveled alone or with his eldest son. He and his wife had seven children but only one grandchild. In early 19th-century England, there was considerable interest in chemistry, and many believed that a knowledge of animal chemistry could be translated to humans and result in improved medical practice. Despite this, most medical schools neglected the physical scientists and students continued to be instructed

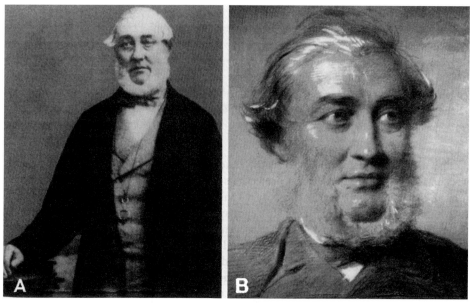

**Figure 7-6** *Portraits of Henry Bence Jones. (***A***, From Snapper, I., and Kahn, A. [1971].* Myelomatosis: Fundamentals and Clinical Features. *Baltimore: University Park Press.* **B***, From Kyle [1996], both with permission.)*

in the classics. William Prout, an animal chemist, advocated the study of physics and chemistry for medical students. From 1820 to 1850, Prout investigated the chemistry of the urine in health and disease. Henry Bence Jones continued in this direction and stated that he was indebted to the work of Prout and subsequently to the studies in physiological chemistry by Liebig. In fact, Jones believed that medicine would be better served if students spent more time acquiring knowledge of chemistry and physics than Latin and Greek. Michael Faraday, the London bookbinder, who became one of the world's greatest scientists, gave lectures on electricity for the medical students. It was difficult for the medical students to see the connection between Faraday's lectures and the action of drugs.

Jones published a series of journal articles on the sediment, uric acid, calcium oxalate, and the alkaline and earthy phosphates of urine. He gave a series of lectures at the conclusion of the course on chemistry at St. George's Hospital in 1849. The lectures were published the next year as a book "of animal chemistry." In 1851 to 1852, the *Medical Times and Gazette* printed 18 lectures on digestion, respiration, and secretion, which Jones had given at St. George's Hospital. Many of the lectures were printed in medical journals, and some of his papers were published in duplicate in several British journals. In addition, some of his articles were translated to German or French and published in European journals. Jones also translated and edited several books in German. His extensive obituary in the *Medical Times and Gazette* listed 34 papers and six additional articles. However, no accurate and complete bibliography exists.

Jones emphasized the frequency of diabetes in an older population. Eleven of his 29 patients with diabetes were older than 60 years (Jones, 1853). He noted that diabetes in the elderly frequently occurred without marked symptoms. He was aware that diabetes was detected far more frequently in the elderly than in any other age group. He advocated small meals, free of sugar and acid, as the best diet (Jones, 1853). He also noted that sugar was still found in the urine despite the withholding of sugar-containing foods (Rosenfeld, 1987). He was the first to describe xanthine crystals in the urine and differentiated them from uric acid crystals (Jones, 1862).

Jones believed that medications must diffuse throughout tissue before they could produce an effect. He thought that it would be worthwhile to know the rates of diffusion and the amount of time that a medication was present in the body. It occurred to him that spectrum analysis would allow him to determine when medications appeared in tissues or in the body excretions. Jones and August Dupré gave guinea pigs small doses of lithium carbonate orally or subcutaneously and sacrificed them at intervals of a few minutes to several days. Spectrum analysis detected lithium in vascular tissues, the cartilage of the hip joint, and the humors of the eye within 15 minutes. In 30 minutes, lithium appeared in the lens of the eye. The rate of diffusion was more rapid with subcutaneous injection than with oral administration. In humans, lithium carbonate appeared in the urine after only 10 minutes and in the lenses, obtained from cataract extraction, at 3.5 hours, but it took up to 18 hours to reach the fingernails and hair of the beard. Jones and Dupré extended their studies to quinine and noted that quinine had "passed into all of the vascular," and most probably into the extra-vascular tissues (Jones and Dupré, 1866), of guinea pigs within 15 minutes of ingestion of the drug. They extended their studies to humans and found that quinine was detectable in the urine 10 to 20 minutes after ingestion and attained a maximal level in tissues at 3 hours. They also noted a small amount of quinine in the lens of the eye at 2 hours. Thus, Jones introduced the use of biochemical tracers in medicine.

Jones began his laboratory work each day at 6:00 AM and arrived at the hospital at approximately 1:00 PM for ward rounds (Obituary, 1873a). According to Sir Clifford Allbutt, in a lecture to medical students at St. George's in 1922, few students sought a clerkship with Dr. Jones because of his "scandalous unpunctuality." As Allbutt, the medical student, was waiting at the stairhead, he saw Jones "bounding up the steps two or three at a time, and hour or an hour and a half too late . . . first appeared the silvery head, then the handsome presence, the sanguine and vivid countenance, the blue eyes; then came the bound towards the beds, and the sharp question—'Which are the worst cases, let me see?'" He frequently chided students with the phrase "O! Medical facts! Medical facts!" He was a skeptic in regard to therapeutics and, as a biochemist, believed in nothing that he could not separate, test, and measure. He scorned empiric experience, tradition, and authority. He concentrated on "medical facts." He would frequently bring foreign professors to the hospital, where lively discussions would occur (Allbutt, 1952). Another of Jones' students, E. L. Fox, was impressed with Jones' rapidity of diagnosis; however, he said that it was difficult for Jones to change his mind. He always taught students to "be as long as you like in forming your opinion on a case, but when you have thoroughly formed it, stick to it" (Obituary, 1873a). Fox stated that scientific truth, accuracy, and a dislike of empiricism were among Jones' chief characteristics as a hospital physician. His clinical lectures were clear and full of "matter" and his "Hearty, genial, kindliness won for him much affection from his pupils" (Obituary, 1873a). It was not enough for him to be a worthy and successful worker himself, but he sought to make others the same. No one could be more ready to encourage and aid every young aspirant than he. His chief aim in the wards was to make therapeutics scientific. His efforts to use scientific treatments made him unwilling to mix several remedies together. His prescriptions were simple and precise. Benjamin Disraeli is said to have used one of his prescriptions for his voice. In his autobiography, Herbert Spencer wrote "speaking of drugs, Bence Jones said that there is scarcely one which may not under different conditions produce opposite effects" (Rosenbloom, 1919).

Jones was described as energetic and as enthusiastic as a successful school boy. He was warm and generous. He was sensitive, irritable, and, at times, impetuous and intolerant of opposition and of the trammels of authority. However, he was most willing to acknowledge any error that he made. He was quick to show his resentment at anything that appeared to be spurious or artificial. His appreciation of studies, other than his own, was somewhat limited and led to hostile criticism on occasion. He mingled little in society, and most of his personal friends were scientists and a few physicians. He was frugal in his habits (Obituary, 1873a).

## Private Practice

In 1843, Jones' first private patient was sent by Dr. Latham, and the second, a nobleman, was referred by Justus von Liebig. His private medical practice grew slowly after his appointment to the staff at St. George's Hospital. After his appointment as Full Physician, his recognition as a "chemical" doctor and his lectures helped his medical practice become large and lucrative. In 1 year (April 5, 1864–April 5, 1865), his profits were £7,400 (Obituary, 1873a). He specialized in disorders of the genitourinary tract, gout, and rheumatism. He had many influential friends and important social contacts because of his reputation as a scientist, his position on hospital boards, his role as secretary of the Royal Institution, and family connections through his wife, Lady Millicent (Putnam, 1993).

His patients included Charles Darwin, the naturalist. Darwin's son later wrote that toward the end of 1865, his father began to recover under the care of Dr. Bence Jones, who dieted his father severely and, as he expressed it, "half starved him to death" (Rosenbloom, 1919). The following year, Jones wrote "My dear Mr. Darwin, I wished you had got over your flatulence but it is not easy and your progress must be slow," and he stated that he had "done famously so far" and that a trip abroad might be of value. Later that year, Jones wrote to Mrs. Darwin, stating that Darwin's temporary failure of memory was probably caused "by some irregularity of circulation arising from indigestion" (Putnam, 1993). Jones advised that all mental work be set aside for 1 month. Jones wrote to Darwin in 1870, stating that Darwin's nerve symptoms probably arose from indigestion and that he should take care of the quality and quantity of his food, get plenty of air, and take gentle exercise. Jones advised that if more nerve symptoms occurred, Darwin should stop work. On one occasion Jones invited Darwin to come to London for a meeting of the Royal Society, where Prince Albert was present. The Prince received only a few people and spent most of the time talking to Darwin. It is said that Jones consulted at Prince Albert's illness and death from typhoid (Putnam, 1993).

Michael Faraday was a patient and also was subjected to a strenuous diet. Other patients included the German chemist August Wilhelm Hoffmann and the English biologist Thomas Huxley. Hermann von Helmholtz, a physiologist and inventor of the ophthalmoscope, had a great deal of respect for Jones. On one occasion he dined with Dr. Jones and described him as a charming man, simple, harmless, cordial as a child, and extraordinarily kind. His friends included Willy Kühne, the celebrated chemist from Heidelberg and a former pupil of Dubois. Kühne described Bence Jones protein in a patient who died in 1869 (Kühne, 1883).

## Health Care

Bence Jones was well acquainted with Florence Nightingale and had a high opinion of her. He knew her because he was a consulting physician at the Institution for Invalid Ladies that she ran on Harley Street until she left for the Crimean War. After her return, he asked her to found a school for the training of nurses at St. George's Hospital, but she refused. He was an original member of the Nightingale Fund and served on several boards with her. She was not an easy person to get along with and had a number of disagreements with Dr. Jones. On one occasion she stated that Jones had written to her "for a plan." She retorted that people thought she had nothing to do but sit and form plans. On occasion she was critical of Jones and scoffed at his care of and advice to Sidney Herbert, who had renal insufficiency. She stated that the patient would do just as well if he would "consult a kitten."

Nevertheless, she stated that Bence Jones was "the best chemical doctor in London" (Putnam, 1993). She noted that he was a staunch supporter of nursing education and improvement of sanitation in the city. Nightingale did not believe in infection or contagion and thought that typhoid fever and smallpox arose spontaneously in filth. Consequently, she demanded a high standard of sanitation.

Jones played a role in the establishment of the Hospital for Sick Children on Great Ormond Street. Dr. Charles West, a physician to Waterloo Road Dispensary, which he had unsuccessfully tried to convert into a children's hospital, had approached him. The first meeting to discuss the problem took place in January 1850 in Jones' London home at 30 Lower Grosvenor Street. Bence Jones wrote "at that time I had many influential friends, and with their help I was able to form a provisional committee which had considerable influence" (Putnam, 1993). Jones served on the Committee of Management until March 1854, when he retired after a disagreement with West. The Hospital for Sick Children had opened in January 1852 (Coley, 1973).

## The Royal Institution

The Royal Institution of Great Britain was founded in 1799 by an American, Benjamin Thompson (Count Rumford). Its purpose was to promote research and teaching of science and to inform the public of scientific and technologic advances. The Royal Institution provided research laboratories for Thomas Young, who established the wave theory of light; Humphrey Davy, who isolated the first alkali and alkaline earth metals and invented the miner's lamp; John Tyndall, who explained the flow of glaciers and was the first to measure the absorption and radiation of heat by gases and vapors; and James Dewar, who liquefied hydrogen and invented the Dewar vessel, the forerunner of the vacuum bottle. W. H. Bragg and his son, W. L. Bragg, later used x-ray crystallography at the Royal Institution. The most famous scientist was Michael Faraday, who discovered electromagnetic induction. Jones published a two-volume biography on Faraday in 1870.

Jones became involved with the Royal Institution in 1851 when he gave a series of lectures. He subsequently was elected one of the managers, and in 1860 he became the honorary secretary. He also wrote an early history of the Royal Institution. He invited the leading scientists of the day, such as Emil du Bois-Reymond of Berlin, the founder of electrophysiology, and Helmholtz to lecture at the Institution. Queen Victoria became the patron of the Royal Institution, and Albert, the Prince Consort, was the vice patron. The scientific stars of the Royal Institution were Faraday and John Tyndall, who succeeded Faraday on the latter's death in 1867. Tyndall gave a series of lectures on light in the United States. His lecture in Washington, DC, was attended by President Grant and several members of the Cabinet and Congress. Jones was less successful in obtaining literary leaders such as Matthew Arnold. John Ruskin was a member and Alfred Lord Tennyson attended some of the lectures at the Royal Institution.

## Final Illness

In 1861 Jones experienced frequent heart palpitations and diagnosed rheumatic heart disease on hearing a mitral systolic murmur with his stethoscope. He had an episode of rheumatic fever in 1839 and now stated that chronic rheumatism had "done permanent damage to one of the valves" (Jones, 1929). He resigned as physician at St. George's Hospital in early 1862. He also gave up attending at the Institution for Invalid Ladies in Harley Street. One of his last pieces of extra work was his service on the Royal Commission regarding the cattle plague in 1865. In early 1866 his health began to fail and he again examined himself and stated "I fancied that one side was half-full of fluid" (Jones, 1929). Despite his illness, he went to

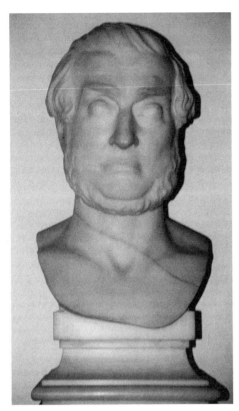

*Figure 7-7*   *Bust of Henry Bence Jones, Royal Institution. (From Kyle [1996] with permission.)*

Nottingham as the chairman of the Chemical Section of the British Association for the Advancement of Science. Jones was the first physician to hold this prestigious position. He returned to his home in Folkstone on September 1 and was taken "dangerously ill." He returned to London at the beginning of winter but his disease exacerbated and he almost died in January 1867. He improved slowly and was able to leave the house in May. The following year he delivered the Croonian Lectures on "Matter and Force" at the College of Physicians (Kyle, 2001). From then on, his energy decreased. He traveled to Oxford in 1870 to receive the honorary degree of Doctor of Civil Letters. In a letter to John Tyndall, in August 1870, he stated "I am very lazy and feel unfit for any work and as neither eating, drinking, or sleeping come pleasantly to me, I am a useless mortal and had better be helping the worms and the grass to grow faster than they otherwise would do . . ." (Putnam, 1993). He gave up his practice in early 1873 because of congestive hepatomegaly, ascites, and anasarca. He resigned as secretary of the Royal Institution on March 3, 1873. He wrote in his letter of resignation "I cannot end this letter without expressing to you again my report that I must cease to be your secretary, but my health forbids me to hope that I can no longer continue to be your most earnest servant," signed—Henry Bence Jones (Jones, 1929). His bust is in the Royal Institution (Fig. 7-7).

Jones died at his home (Fig. 7-8) at 84 Brook Street in London of congestive heart failure on April 20, 1873, at the age of 59 years and was buried at Kensall Green

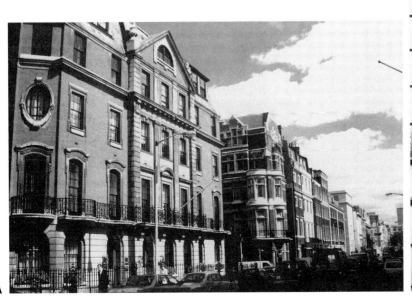

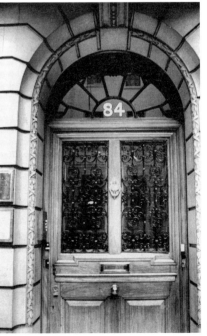

A     B

*Figure 7-8*   *(**A** and **B**) Henry Bence Jones' home at 84 Brook Street, London. (From Kyle [1996] with permission.)*

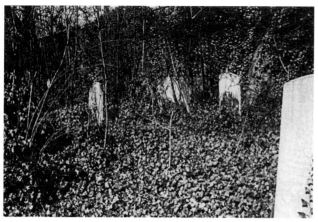

**Figure 7-9** *Gravesite of Henry Bence Jones at Kensall Green Cemetery, London. (From Kyle [1996] with permission.)*

Cemetery in grave 4327/59 (Fig. 7-9) (Obituary 1873a, 1873b). He had requested only a simple stone and, unfortunately, it has succumbed to the elements. He was survived by his wife and five of his seven children. The Bence Jones Ward exists at St. George's Hospital in Tooting, but it is devoted to gynecology patients (Fig. 7-10). Interestingly, although Jones' obituary described his work on renal stones, diabetes mellitus, and malignant and tuberculous involvement of the kidney and his emphasis on the value of microscopic analysis of the urine, there was no mention of his articles on the unique urinary protein that bears his name, except as a listing of the paper "On a new substance occurring in the urine of a patient with 'mollities osseum'" among his 40 publications (Obituary, 1873a). Incidentally, Henry Bence Jones did not hyphenate his name, and a hyphen is not used in any of his more than 40 papers and books; books published during his lifetime enter him under "Jones," as does the Royal

College of Physicians and the Dictionary of National Biography. He used H. Bence Jones and apparently did not like "Henry." His descendants added the hyphen more than a half century after his death (Rosenfeld, 1987).

## Other Contributions to Bence Jones Proteinuria

Several other persons were involved in the story of Bence Jones proteinuria. In 1846, J. F. Heller (Fig. 7-11) described a protein in the urine that precipitated when warmed above 50°C and then disappeared on further heating. He distinguished this from albumin and casein (Heller, 1846). Although he did not recognize the precipitation of the protein when the urine was cooled, it is almost certain that this was Bence Jones protein. The first use of the term "Bence Jones protein" was by Fleischer in 1880.

Kühne, in 1883, described a 40-year-old man from Amsterdam; Kühne thought the man had acute osteomalacia. There was marked tenderness of the cervical and thoracic spine, and the patient was unable to lie on his back because of pain and curvature of the spine. His head was flexed forward. During the last weeks of his life, dysphasia and paralysis of cranial nerve VII developed, probably from an extradural plasmacytoma. He died on August 27, 1869, 9 months after onset. There was no autopsy report. His brother was thought to have died of the same disease. The patient's urine precipitated on warming to between 40°C and 50°C and cleared at 100°C. Kühne isolated the protein and found

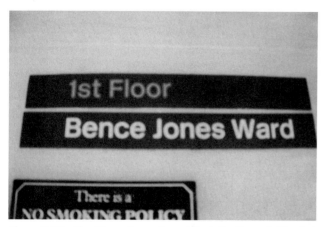

**Figure 7-10** *The Henry Bence Jones Ward, St. George's Hospital, Tooting. (From Kyle [1996] with permission.)*

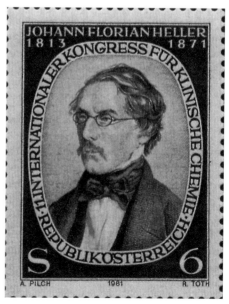

**Figure 7-11** *J. F. Heller. (From Kyle [1996] with permission.)*

that the carbon, hydrogen, and nitrogen levels were similar to those described by Jones. Kühne attributed any differences to the fact that his preparation was more pure than Bence Jones' preparation. He labeled the protein albumosurie. Bradshaw, in 1898, reported that there was no nocturnal variation and that meals had little or no influence on the amount of Bence Jones proteinuria. Walters (1921) also reported that the amount of protein in a patient's diet had no effect on the amount of Bence Jones protein in the urine.

Two distinct groups of Bence Jones proteins were recognized by Bayne-Jones and Wilson in 1922. In 1956, Korngold and Lipari demonstrated a relationship between Bence Jones protein and the serum proteins of multiple myeloma. As a tribute to Korngold and Lipari, the two major classes of Bence Jones protein have been designated κ and λ (Korngold and Lipari, 1956). Using $^{13}$C-labeled glycine, Putnam and Hardy (1955) demonstrated that synthesis of the serum globulin and synthesis of Bence Jones protein were independent processes. Bence Jones protein was synthesized directly from a nitrogen pool rather than from plasma protein.

One hundred seventeen years after the description of the unique heat properties, Edelman and Gally (1962) showed that the light chains prepared from an IgG myeloma protein and the Bence Jones protein from the same patient's urine had an identical amino acid sequence, similar spectrofluorometric behavior, identical appearance on chromatography with carboxymethyl cellulose, and, on starch gel electrophoresis after reduction and alkylation, the same ultracentrifugal pattern, identical thermal solubility, and the same molecular weight. These light chains precipitated when heated to between 40°C and 60°C, dissolved on boiling, and reprecipitated when cooled to between 40°C and 60°C, identical with the heat properties of Bence Jones protein.

# Early Cases of Multiple Myeloma

In 1867, Hermann Weber described a 40-year-old man who experienced pain, tenderness, and deformity of the sternum. Movement of his head produced pain in his neck and arms. The patient also had severe pain in the lumbar area. He died 3.5 months after the onset of pain. Postmortem examination revealed that the sternum was almost entirely replaced by a grayish-red substance that had the microscopic appearance of a sarcoma. There were two fractures of the sternum and several round defects in the skull. Many of the ribs, several vertebrae, and parts of the pelvis were involved. Amyloid was found in the kidneys and spleen. In 1872, William Adams described a patient with bone pain and fractures. The left humerus and

femur fractured while the body was being placed on the autopsy table. The cancellous portions of the bones had been replaced by a homogeneous, soft, gelatinous substance that consisted of small spherical and oval cells containing one oval nucleus (rarely two) with a bright nucleolus. Lardaceous changes were found in the liver and kidneys.

The term "multiple myeloma" was introduced by von Rustizky (working in von Recklinghausen's laboratory) in 1873 when he found eight separate tumors of bone marrow and designated them as multiple myelomas. The 47-year-old patient had presented with a tumor of the right temple and developed thickening of the manubrium and seventh rib, followed by paraplegia. An autopsy showed a fist-sized tumor in the right frontal region extending into the orbit and producing ophthalmoplegia, an apple-sized tumor in the right fifth rib, a tumor in the left seventh rib producing a fracture, tumors of the sternum and the sixth to the eighth thoracic vertebrae which produced the paraplegia, and three tumors of the right humerus. Although von Rustizky's description of the tumor cells is rather vague, he did describe cells whose nucleus was located in the periphery near the cell membrane. The presence of an eccentric nucleus is certainly suggestive of plasma cells. He did not mention albumosurie (Bence Jones protein). In Russia, the term "Rustizky's disease" is often used.

There was little further interest in the disease until 1889, when Otto Kahler described a striking case involving a 46-year-old physician named Dr. Loos, in whom sudden severe pain had developed in the right upper thorax in July 1879. The pain recurred 6 months later and was localized to the right third rib. During the next 2 years, intermittent pain aggravated by exercise occurred in the ribs, spine, left shoulder, upper arm, and right clavicle. Albuminuria was first noted in September 1881. Pallor was noted in 1883. In December 1885, Dr. Loos was first seen by Kahler, who noted anemia, severe kyphosis, tenderness of many bones, and albumosuria. Kahler recognized that the urinary protein had the same characteristics that Bence Jones had described. The kyphosis increased and his height decreased monthly. Kyphosis of the upper thoracic spine increased and his chin pressed against the sternum, producing a decubitus ulcer. When Dr. Loos stood, the lower ribs touched the iliac crest. He had recurrent bronchial infections and intermittent kyphosis. He became dwarf-like. Dr. Loos died on August 26, 1887, 8 years after the onset of symptoms. At autopsy, the ribs were soft and could be broken with minimal effort. Soft grey–reddish masses were noted in the ribs and thoracic vertebrae. Hepatosplenomegaly was noted. Microscopic examination showed large, round cells consistent with myeloma. Of interest, the patient had a high fluid intake and took sodium bicarbonate on

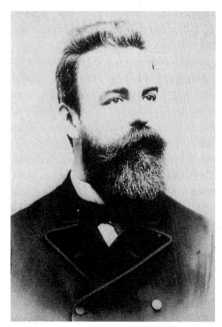

**Figure 7-12** *Otto Kahler. (Courtesy of Dr. Heinz Ludwig, Vienna.) (From Kyle [1996] with permission.)*

a regular basis. This regimen might have helped prevent renal failure.

Otto Kahler, born in 1849, was the son of a well-known physician in Prague (Fig. 7-12). After receiving his M.D. degree from the University of Prague in 1871, he worked as an assistant in Professor Halla's clinic. He studied in Paris, where he met two French neurologists, Jean Martin Charcot and G. B. A. Duchenne (Duchenne de Boulogne). He became interested in neurology and anatomy. Kahler contributed to the pathologic anatomy of the central nervous system and to the anatomy of tabes dorsalis, central oculomotor paralysis, and slow compression of the spinal cord. He became professor of medicine in Prague, and, after Halla's resignation, became head of the second Medical Clinic at the German University of Prague. In 1889 he succeeded Heinrich Bamberger as professor at the University of Vienna (Kraus, 1894). In his inaugural address in May 1889, Kahler finished his lecture with one of Bamberger's quotes: "Ars longa, vita brevis" (the art of medicine is long, life is short) (Sigmund, 1870). Little did he realize that the biopsy specimen of a tumor on his tongue in the summer of 1889 was malignant. His carcinoma of the tongue recurred, and a huge tumor developed, causing paralysis of the vagus nerve and compression of the esophagus and main bronchus. He died on January 24, 1893, shortly after his 44th birthday (Nothnagel, 1893). Kahler was extremely kind to his patients and was an excellent teacher. He emphasized that it was important to cover the entire field of general internal medicine. His obituaries and eulogies made no mention of his famous case report. Interestingly, the landmark contributions by Henry Bence Jones and Otto Kahler were not recognized during their lifetimes.

## Other Cases of Multiple Myeloma in the 19th and 20th Centuries

Probably the first reported case of multiple myeloma in the United States was published by Herrick and Hektoen in 1894. The patient, a 40-year-old white woman, had lumbar pain and a nodule on the lower end of the sternum. At autopsy, multiple nodules involved the sternum, right clavicle, and ribs. The sternum was thickened, irregular, and covered with tumor masses but was soft and flexible. Multiple nodules were found on the ribs, which bent readily without cracking. Fungoid masses were seen in the skull. Two of the dorsal vertebral bodies were largely replaced by soft tissue masses. Microscopic examination revealed round, lymphoid cells with large nuclei (Herrick and Hektoen, 1894).

Three years after the discovery of x-rays by Roentgen in 1895, Weber saw a patient with multiple myeloma and stated that the diagnosis of such cases would be greatly facilitated by the use of x-rays. He concluded that Bence Jones protein was produced by the bone marrow. He also believed that the presence of Bence Jones protein was of "fatal significance" and nearly always indicated that the patient had multiple myeloma (Weber et al., 1903). Weber and Ledingham (1909) later suggested that Bence Jones protein came from the cytoplasmic residua of karyolyzed plasma cells.

In 1900, Wright described a 54-year-old man with multiple myeloma and pointed out that the tumor consisted of plasma cells. He emphasized that the neoplasm originated not from red marrow cells collectively, but from only one type of cell, the plasma cell. This patient was the first in whom roentgenograms revealed changes in the ribs and thus contributed to the diagnosis. Geschickter and Copeland (1928) presented an analysis of all 425 cases of multiple myeloma reported since 1848. They emphasized six cardinal features, consisting of multiple involvement of the skeleton by tumors, pathologic fractures, Bence Jones protein, back pain, anemia, and renal insufficiency. Sternal aspiration of the bone marrow, described in 1929 by Arinkin, greatly increased the antemortem recognition of multiple myeloma (Rosenthal and Vogel, 1938). Bayrd and Heck (1947) described 83 patients with histologic proof of multiple myeloma seen at the Mayo Clinic through December 1945. The duration of survival ranged from 1 to 84 months (median, 15 mo).

The term "plasma cell" was coined by Waldeyer in 1875. The description is not characteristic of plasma cells, and he might have been describing tissue mast cells. Plasma cells were described accurately by Ramón y Cajal in 1896 during a study of syphilitic condylomas; he found that the unstained pernicular area (hof) contained the Golgi apparatus. In 1891, Unna used the term "plasma cells" while describing cells seen in the skin of patients with lupus erythematosus. However, it is not known whether he actually saw plasma cells. In 1895, Marschalkó described the essential characteristics of plasma cells, including blocked chromatin, eccentric position of the nucleus, a perinuclear pale area (hof), and a spherical or irregular cytoplasm.

Although Jacobson had reported Bence Jones protein in the serum in 1917, it was not until 1928 that Perlzweig et al. described hyperproteinemia when they described a patient with multiple myeloma who had 9 to 11 g of globulin in the serum. The patient also had Bence Jones proteinuria and probably a small amount of Bence Jones protein in the plasma. They also noted that it was almost impossible to obtain serum from the clotted blood because the clot failed to retract, even on prolonged centrifugation. Cryoglobulinemia was recognized by Wintrobe and Buell in 1933 and named cryoglobulin by Lerner and Watson in 1947. The patient described by Lerner and Watson had been previously reported as having allergic purpura with hypersensitivity to the cold (Peters and Horton, 1941). In 1938, Von Bonsdorff et al. described a patient with cryoglobulinemia in whom the globulins crystalized after exposure to cold for 24 hours.

In 1890, von Behring and Kitasato described a specific neutralizing substance in blood of animals immunized with diphtheria and tetanus toxin. These antibodies were found after the injection of most foreign proteins. Arnold Tiselius' (1902–1971) studies of the moving boundary method of electrophoresis led to his doctoral dissertation in 1930. His manuscript describing the apparatus for electrophoresis (Tiselius, 1968) was published in the *Transactions of the Faraday Society* (Tiselius, 1937a). Interestingly, this article, which led to his Nobel Prize and later to the presidency of the Nobel Foundation, was rejected initially by *The Biochemical Journal* (Putnam, 1983). Later that same year, Tiselius described the separation of serum globulins into three major protein components. Following the lead of his colleagues in the physical sciences (e.g., "alpha" particles, "beta" particles, and "gamma" rays), Tiselius designated these fractions $\alpha$, $\beta$, and $\gamma$ fractions according to their electrophoretic mobility (Tiselius, 1937b, c). Two years later, Tiselius and Kabat (1939) localized antibody activity to the $\gamma$ globulin fraction of the plasma proteins. They noted that antibodies to albumin or pneumococcus type I was found in the area of $\gamma$ mobility in rabbit serum, and antibodies to pneumococcal organisms migrated between $\beta$ and $\gamma$ in horse serum. Later it was recognized that some antibodies

migrate in the fast $\gamma$ region and others in the slow $\gamma$ region, and that some sediment in the ultracentrifuge as 7S and others as 19S molecules. The concept of a family of proteins with antibody reactivity was not proposed until late in the 1950s (Heremans, 1959). Before 1960, the term "gamma globulin" was used for any protein that migrated in the $\gamma$ mobility region of the electrophoretic pattern. Now these $\gamma$ globulins are referred to as immunoglobulins: IgG, IgA, IgM, IgD, and IgE.

In 1939, Longworth et al. applied electrophoresis to the study of multiple myeloma and demonstrated the tall, narrow-based "church spire" peak. The electrophoresis apparatus was cumbersome and difficult to use; the original commercial models were 20 feet long and 5 feet high and often occupied a separate laboratory room. A single electrophoresis run required a full day and the interpretation of an experienced operator (Putnam, 1993). The use of filter paper as a support permitted the separation of protein into discrete zones that could be stained with various dyes (Kunkel and Tiselius, 1951). Cellulose acetate-supplanted filter paper, and currently most laboratories use agarose electrophoresis.

In 1953, Grabar and Williams described immunoelectrophoresis, which facilitated the diagnosis of multiple myeloma. In 1964, Wilson reported immunofixation or direct immunoelectrophoresis, in which he applied antisera on the surface of the agarose immediately after completion of electrophoresis.

The immunoglobulins have acquired their names in a somewhat arbitrary fashion. Early naming practices for these proteins attempted to follow the 19th-century ideal of setting scientific terminology on a Greek linguistic foundation (Black, 1997). However, by 1964, when the World Health Organization system proposed a consistent isotype nomenclature (Ceppellini et al., 1964), this system had begun to unravel, and subsequent developments led to the irregular modern names IgG, IgM, IgA, IgD, and IgE and $\kappa$ and $\lambda$.

In 1944, Waldenström (1906–1996) described two patients with a novel syndrome of mucosal bleeding, diffuse lymphadenopathy, anemia, thrombocytopenia, hypoalbuminemia, hypofibrinogenemia, and bone marrow lymphocytosis. The sera of these patients contained a large protein that sedimented at the 19 and 20 Svedberg level, considerably heavier than the known gamma globulin protein that sedimented at 7. The new protein was found to be an immunoglobulin and became known as "macroglobulin." When the World Health Organization nomenclature was formalized, macroglobulin became IgM and "gamma" globulin was designated IgG, and the heavy components of these two proteins became known as $\mu$ and $\gamma$ chains, respectively (Ceppellini et al., 1964).

By the 1950s it was clear that the $\beta$ and $\gamma$ regions of human plasma contained an additional globulin protein that did not react with sera raised against gamma globulin or macroglobulin. To avoid confusion with the newly discovered $\beta_2$-macroglobulin, this protein was called provisionally $\beta$2A or $\gamma$1A globulin (Heremans et al., 1959). Later this substance became known simply as $\alpha$ immunoglobulin (IgA), despite the potential confusion that the name was chosen because the protein migrates in the $\alpha$ fraction on electrophoresis (it usually does not). The fourth immunoglobulin isotype to be discovered was IgD, which was named by the simple process of elimination (Black, 1997). When Rowe and Fahey isolated this protein in 1965, IgA had been designated. During that era it was anticipated that murine immunoglobulins would eventually be called $\beta$ globulins (IgB), so the investigators elected to steer clear of that term. The third letter of the Greek alphabet is $\gamma$, but gamma globulin had already been described and the Roman letter C has no Greek equivalent, so IgC was excluded. The obvious next choice was IgD ($\delta$ immunoglobulin).

The final immunoglobulin isotype to be described was IgE, characterized in 1966 (Ishizaka et al.). Although IgE ($\varepsilon$ globulin) was logically the next name choice after IgD from an alphabetical standpoint, this was only serendipitous. Because of the association of this protein with erythema and allergic disease (it had been known as "reaginic antibody" long before its 1966 description as a novel immunoglobulin), the antibody was already known as "fraction E" or "antigen E" and so the IgE name was a perfect fit.

Alwall, in 1947, reported that a patient with multiple myeloma had a reduction in globulin from 5.9 to 2.2 g/dL, an increase in the hemoglobin value from 60% to 87%, disappearance of proteinuria, and a reduction in bone marrow plasma cells from 33% to 0% when treated with urethane. For 20 years, urethane was commonly used for the treatment of multiple myeloma. Holland et al. (1966) randomized 83 patients with multiple myeloma to receive urethane or a placebo consisting of cherry- or cola-flavored syrup. There was no difference in objective improvement or in survival in the two treatment groups. In fact, the urethane-treated patients died earlier than those treated with placebo. This was ascribed to the increased mortality of urethane-treated patients who were azotemic. The patients with poorer prognostic features had a significantly shorter survival with urethane therapy.

In 1958, Blokhin et al. reported benefit in three of six patients with multiple myeloma who were treated with sarcolysin. Four years later, Bergsagel et al. (1962) found significant improvement in eight of 24 patients with multiple myeloma who were treated with L-phenylalanine mustard (melphalan, Alkeran). Six other patients obtained improvement in one or more objective factors. In another report, cyclophosphamide-treated patients who had myeloma had a median

survival of 24.5 months, and an ancillary myeloma group had a median survival of 9.5 months (Korst et al., 1964). Objective improvement occurred in 81 of 207 patients. Various combinations of alkylating agents have been used for the treatment of multiple myeloma, but no unequivocal evidence shows they are superior to melphalan and prednisone (Gregory et al., 1992; Myeloma Trialists' Collaborative Group, 1998).

# Acknowledgment

This work was supported in part by Research Grant CA 62242 from the National Institutes of Health, U.S. Public Health Service.

## REFERENCES

Adams, W. (1872). Mollities ossium. *Transactions of the Pathology Society of London, 23,* 186–187.

Allbutt, C. (1952). Cited in Dr. Bence Jones. In R. Coope (Ed.), *The Quiet Art: A Doctor's Anthology* (pp. 74–75). Edinburgh: Livingstone.

Alwall, N. (1947). Urethane and stilbamidine in multiple myeloma: Report on two cases. *Lancet, 2,* 388–389.

Arinkin, M. I. (1929). Die intravitale untersuchungsmethodik des Knochenmarks. *Folia Haematologica, 38,* 233–240.

Bayne-Jones, S., and Wilson, D. W. (1922). Immunological reactions of Bence-Jones proteins. II. Differences between Bence-Jones proteins from various sources. *Bulletin of Johns Hopkins Hospital, 33,* 119–125.

Bayrd, E. D., and Heck, F. J. (1947). Multiple myeloma: a review of 83 proved cases. *Journal of the American Medical Association, 133,* 147–157.

Bergsagel, D. E., Sprague, C. C., Austin, C., and Griffith, K. M. (1962). Evaluation of new chemotherapeutic agents in the treatment of multiple myeloma. IV. L-Phenylalanine mustard (NSC-8806). *Cancer Chemotherapy Report, 21,* 87–99.

Black, C. A. (1997). A brief history of the discovery of the immunoglobulins and the origin of the modern immunoglobulin nomenclature. *Immunology and Cell Biology, 75,* 65–68.

Blokhin, N., Larionov, L., Perevodchikova, N., Chebotareva, L., and Merkulove, N. (1958). Clinical experiences with sarcolysin in neoplastic diseases. *Annals of the New York Academy of Sciences, 68,* 1128–1132.

Bradshaw, T. R. (1898). A case of albumosuria in which the albumose was spontaneously precipitated. *Medico-Chirurgical Transactions of London, 81,* 259–271.

Buchan, W. (1781). *Domestic Medicine or A Treatise on the Prevention and Cure of Diseases by Regimen and Simple Medicines, With an Appendix, Containing a Dispensatory for the Use of Private Practitioners,* 7th ed (p. 61). London: W. Strahan.

*Burke's Peerage and Gentry.*

Burney, F. (1904–1905). *The Diary & Letters of Madame d'Arblay (1778–1840), as Edited by Her Niece Charlotte Barrett.* London: Macmillan.

Ceppellini, R., Dray, S., Edelman, G., et al. (1964). Nomenclature for the human immunoglobulins. *Bulletin of the World Health Organization, 30,* 447–450.

Clamp, J. R. (1967). Some aspects of the first recorded case of multiple myeloma. *Lancet, 2,* 1354–1356.

Coley, N. G. (1973). Henry Bence-Jones, M.D., F.R.S. (1813–1873). *Notes and Records of the Royal Society of London, 28,* 31–56.

*Columbia Encyclopedia,* 6th ed. 2001.

Dalrymple, J. (1846). On the microscopical character of mollities ossium. *Dublin Quarterly Journal of Medical Science, 2*, 85–95.

Dickens, C. (1938). *The Posthumous Papers of the Pickwick Club.* New York: For the Members of the Heritage Club.

Edelman, G. M., and Gally, J. A. (1962). The nature of Bence-Jones proteins: Chemical similarities to polypeptide chains of myeloma globulins and normal γ-globulins. *Journal of Experimental Medicine, 116*, 207–227.

Felter, H. W., and Lloyd, J. U. (1898–1900). *King's American Dispensatory.* Cincinnati: Ohio Valley Co.

Fleischer, R. (1880). XXIV. Ueber das Vorkommen des sogenannten Bence Jones'schen Eiweisskörpers im normalen Knochenmark. *Archiv für pathologische Anatomie und Physiologie und für klinishe Medicin, 80*, 842–849.

Fothergill, J. M. (1877). When not to use iron. *Practitioner (London), 2*, 183–188.

Geschickter, C. F., and Copeland, M. M. (1928). Multiple myeloma. *Archives of Surgery, 16*, 807–863.

Grabar, P., and Williams, C. A. (1953). Méthode permettant l'étude conjuguée des propriétés électrophorétiques et immunochimeques d'un mélange de protéines: Application au serum sanguin. *Biochimica et Biophysica Acta, 10*, 193–194.

Gregory, W. M., Richards, M. A., and Malpas, J. S. (1992). Combination chemotherapy versus melphalan and prednisolone in the treatment of multiple myeloma: An overview of published trials. *Journal of Clinical Oncology, 10*, 334–342.

The Head Forester: Gosford Forest Park, Markethill, Co. Armagh, Ireland.

Heller, J. F. (1846). Die mikroskopisch-chemisch-pathologische untersuchung. In G. Von Gaal (Ed.), *Physikalische Diagnostik und Deren Anwendung in der Medicin, Chirurgie, Oculistik Otiatrik und Geburtschilfe, enthaltend: Inspection, Mensuration, Palpation, Percussion und Auscultation, Nebst Einer Kurzen Diagnose der Krankheiten der Athmungs und Kreislaufsorgane* (pp. 576–597). Vienna: Braumüller and Seidel.

Heremans, J. F. (1959). Immunochemical studies on protein pathology: The immunoglobulin concept. *Clinica Chimica Acta, 4*, 639–646.

Heremans, J. F., Heremans, M. T., and Schultz, H. E. (1959). Isolation and description of a few properties of the β2A-globulin of human serum. *Clinica Chimica Acta, 4*, 96–102

Herrick, J. B., and Hektoen, L. (1894). Myeloma: Report of a case. *Medical News, Philadelphia, 65*, 239–242.

Holland, J. R., Hosley, H., Scharlau, C., et al. (1966). A controlled trial of urethane treatment in multiple myeloma. *Blood, 27*, 328–342.

Ishizaka, K., Ishizaka, T., and Hornbrook, M. M. (1966). Physicochemical properties of reaginic antibody. V. Correlation of reaginic activity with gamma-E-globulin antibody. *The Journal of Urology, 97*, 840–853.

Jacobson, V. C. (1917). A case of multiple myelomata with chronic nephritis showing Bence-Jones protein in urine and blood serum. *The Journal of Urology, 1*, 167–178.

Jones, H. B. (1847). Chemical pathology. *Lancet, 2*, 88–92.

Jones, H. B. (1848). On the new substance occurring in the urine of a patient with mollities ossium. *Philosophical Transactions of the Royal Society of London (Biology)*, 55–62.

Jones, H. B. (1853). On intermitting diabetes and the diabetes of old age. *Medico-Chirurgical Transactions London, 18*, 403–432.

Jones, H. B. (1862). On a deposit of crystallized xanthin in human urine. *Journal of the Chemistry Society of London, 15*, 78–80.

Jones, H. B. (1929). *An Autobiography (with elucidations at later dates by his son, A. B. Bence-Jones).* London: Crusha and Sons (privately printed).

Jones, H. B., and Dupré, A. (1866). On a fluorescent substance, resembling quinine, in animals; and on the rate of passage of quinine into the vascular and nonvascular textures of the body. *Proceedings of the Royal Society of London (Biology), 15*, 73.

Kahler, O. (1889). Zur Symptomatologie des multiplen myelomas: Boebachtung von Albumosurie. *Prager medizinische Wochenschrift, 14*, 33, 45.

Korngold, L., and Lipari, R. (1956). Multiple-myeloma proteins. III. The antigenic relationship of Bence Jones proteins to normal gamma-globulin and multiple-myeloma serum proteins. *Cancer, 9*, 262–272.

Korst, D. R., Clifford, G. O., Fowler, W. M., et al. (1964). Multiple myeloma. II. Analysis of cyclophosphamide therapy in 165 patients. *Journal of the American Medical Association, 189*, 758–762.

Kraus, F. (1894). Gedächtinisrede auf Otto Kahler. *Wiener klinische Wochenschrift, 27*, 1–10.

Kühne, W. (1883). Ueber Hemialbumose im Harn. *Zeitschrift für Biologie, 19*, 209–227.

Kunkel, H. G., and Tiselius, A. (1951). Electrophoresis of proteins on filter paper. *Journal of General Physiology, 35*, 89–118.

Kyle, R. A. (1996). History of multiple myeloma. In P. H. Wiernik, G. P. Canellos, J. P. Dutcher, et al. (Eds.), *Neoplastic Diseases of the Blood*, ed 3 (pp. 411–422). New York: Churchill Livingstone.

Kyle, R. A. (2000). Multiple myeloma: An odyssey of discovery. *British Journal of Haematology, 111*, 1035–1044.

Kyle, R. A. (2001). Henry Bence Jones: physician, chemist, scientist and biographer: A man for all seasons. *British Journal of Haematology, 115*, 13–18.

Lerner, A. B., and Watson, C. J. (1947). Studies of cryoglobulins. I. Unusual purpura associated with the presence of a high concentration of cryoglobulin (cold precipitable serum globulin). *American Journal of the Medical Sciences, 214*, 410–415.

Longworth, L. G., Shedlovsky, T., and MacInnes, D. A. (1939). Electrophoretic patterns of normal and pathological human blood serum and plasma. *Journal of Experimental Medicine, 70*, 399–413.

Macintyre, W. (1850). Case of mollities and fragilitas ossium, accompanied with urine strongly charged with animal matter. *Medico-Chirurgical Transactions of London, 33*, 211–232.

Marschalkó, T. (1895). Ueber die sogenannten Plasmazellen, ein Beitrag zur Kenntniss der Herkunft der entzündlichen Infiltrationszellen. *Archiv für Dermatologie und Syphilis, 30*, 241.

Myeloma Trialists' Collaborative Group. (1998). Combination chemotherapy versus melphalan plus prednisone as treatment for multiple myeloma: An overview of 6,633 patients from 27 randomized trials. *Journal of Clinical Oncology, 16*, 3832–3842.

Nothnagel. (1893). Hofrath Otto Kahler. *Wiener Klinische Wochenschrift, 6*, 79.

Obituary: Henry Bence Jones, MD, MA, FRCP, RFS. *Medical Times Gazette, 1*, 505–508, 1873a.

Obituary: Dr. Henry Bence Jones. *Lancet, 1*, 614–615, 1873b.

Pagel, W. (1982). *Paracelsus: An Introduction to Philosophical Medicine in the Era of the Renaissance*, ed 2. Basel: Karger.

Perlzweig, W. A., Delrue, G., Geschickter, C. (1928). Hyperproteinemia associated with multiple myelomas: Report of an unusual case. *Journal of the American Medical Association, 90*, 755–757.

Peters, G. A., and Horton, B. T. (1941). Allergic purpura with special reference to hypersensitiveness to cold. *Proceedings of the Staff Meetings of the Mayo Clinic, 16*, 631–636.

Pharmacopoeia of the United States of America. (1820). *By the Authority of the Medical Societies and Colleges.* Boston: Wells and Lilly for Charles Ewer.

Princess Grace Irish Library (Monaco). (2001).

Putnam, F. W. (1983). From the first to the last of the immunoglobulins: Perspectives and prospects. *Clinical Physiology and Biochemistry, 1*, 63–91.

Putnam, F. W. (1993). Henry Bence Jones: The best chemical doctor in London. *Perspectives in Biology and Medicine, 36*, 565–579.

Putnam, F. W., and Hardy, S. (1955). Proteins in multiple myeloma. III. Origin of Bence-Jones protein. *Journal of Biological Chemistry, 212*, 361–369.

Ramón y Cajal, S. (1896). Estudios histológicos sobre los tumores epiteliales. *Revue Trimestrielle, 1,* 83–111.

Rosenbloom, J. (1919). An appreciation of Henry Bence Jones, MD, FRS (1814–1873). *Annals of Medical History, 2,* 262–264.

Rosenfeld, L. (1987). Henry Bence Jones (1813–1873): The best 'chemical doctor' in London. *Clinical Chemistry, 33,* 1687–1692.

Rosenthal, N., and Vogel, P. (1938). Value of the sternal puncture in the diagnosis of multiple myeloma. *Journal of the Mount Sinai Hospital, 4,* 1001–1019.

Rowe, D. S., and Fahey, J. L. (1965). A new class of human immunoglobulin. I. A unique myeloma protein. *The Journal of Experimental Medicine, 121,* 171–184.

Royal College of Physicians of London. (1944). *Pharmacopoeia Londinensis of 1618,* reproduced in facsimile, with a historical introduction by George Urdang. Madison, WI: State Historical Society of Wisconsin.

Sigmund, C. L. (1870). Zur örtlichen Behandlung: syphilitischer Mund-, Nasen- und Rachenaffektionen. *Wiener medizinische Wochenschrift, 20,* 781.

Smith, G., and Getty, C. (1998). *The Beer Drinker's Bible: Lore, Trivia & History: Chapter & Verse.* Boulder, CO: Brewers Publication.

Solly, S. (1844). Remarks on the pathology of mollities ossium with cases. *Medico-Chirurgical Transactions of London, 27,* 435–461.

Stephens, J. L. (1994). 'Arrowroot—*Maranta arundinacea L.*' Fact Sheet HS-542. A series of the Horticultural Sciences Department, Florida Cooperative Extension Service, Institute of Food and Agricultural Sciences, University of Florida Gainesville.

Stone, S. E. (1868). Cases of malignant pustule. *Boston Medical and Surgical Journal, I,* 19–21.

Tiselius, A. (1937a). A new apparatus for electrophoretic analysis of colloidal mixtures. *Transactions of the Faraday Society, 33,* 524.

Tiselius, A. (1937b). Electrophoresis of serum globulin. II. Electrophoretic analysis of normal and immune sera. *Biochemical Journal, 31,* 1464–1477.

Tiselius, A. (1937c). Electrophoresis of serum globulin. *Biochemical Journal, 31,* 313–317.

Tiselius, A. (1968). Reflections from both sides of the counter. *Annual Review of Biochemistry, 37,* 1–24.

Tiselius, A., and Kabat, E. A. (1939). An electrophoretic study of immune sera and purified antibody preparations. *The Journal of Experimental Medicine, 69,* 119–131.

Unna, P. G. (1891). Über plasmazellen, insbesondere beim Lupus. *Monatsschrift für praktische Dermatologie, 12,* 296–317.

von Behring, S., and Kitasato, T. (1890). On the conditions under which immunity both from diphtheria and tetanus can be produced in animals [German]. *Deutsche medizinische Wochenschrift, 49,* 1113–1145.

Von Bonsdorff, B., Groth, H., and Packalén, T. (1938). On the presence of a high-molecular crystallizable protein in the blood serum in myeloma. *Folia Haematologica, 59,* 184–208.

von Rustizky, J. (1873). XXIV. Ueber das Vorkommen des sogenannten Bence Jones'schen Eiweisskorpers im normalen Knochenmark. *Archiv für pathologische Anatomie und Physiologie und für klinische Medicin, 80,* 482.

Waldenström, J. G. (1944). Incipient myelomatosis or 'essential' hyperglobulinemia with fibrinogenopenia: A new syndrome? *Acta Medica Scandinavica, 117,* 216–247.

Waldeyer, W. (1875). Ueber Bindegewebszeelen. *Archiv für mikroskopische Anatomie, 11,* 176–194.

Walters, W. (1921). Bence-Jones proteinuria: A report of three cases with metabolic studies. *Journal of the American Medical Association, 76,* 641–645.

Weber, H. (1867). Mollities ossium, doubtful whether carcinomatous or syphilitic. *Translations of the Pathology Society of London, 18,* 206–209.

Weber, F. P., Hutchinson, R., and Macleod, J. J. R. (1903). Multiple myeloma (myelomatosis), with Bence-Jones protein in the urine (myelopathic albumosuria of Bradshaw, Kahler's disease). *The American Journal of the Medical Sciences, 126,* 644–665.

Weber, F. P., and Ledingham, J. C. G. (1909). A note on the histology of a case of myelomatosis (multiple myeloma) with Bence-Jones protein in the urine (myelopathic albumosuria). *Proceedings of the Royal Society of Medicine, 2,* 193–206.

Westemeier, E. (2001). 'Porter Carries Robust History.' *The Cincinnati Enquirer.* September 2.

Wilson, A. T. (1964). Direct immunoelectrophoresis. *Journal of Immunology, 92,* 431–434.

Wintrobe, M. M., and Buell, M. V. (1933). Hyperproteinemia associated with multiple myeloma: With report of a case in which an extraordinary hyperproteinemia was associated with thrombosis of the retinal veins and symptoms suggesting Raynaud's disease. *Bulletin of Johns Hopkins Hospital, 52,* 156–165.

Wright, J. H. (1900). A case of multiple myeloma. *Johns Hopkins Hospital Report, 9,* 359–366.

# CHAPTER 8

# Epidemiology of Multiple Myeloma

ANNECLAIRE J. DE ROOS
DALSU BARIS
NOEL S. WEISS
LISA HERRINTON

Plasma cells, the final products of B-cell differentiation, synthesize and release immunoglobulin (Ig) and Ig subunits (light and heavy chains). Plasma cell malignancies, which are characterized by the presence of an elevated number of plasma cells in bone marrow and, very often, elevated levels of monoclonal protein in serum and urine, include the following: myeloma, in which there is production of IgA, IgD, IgE, IgG, or light chains; Waldenström's macroglobulinemia, in which there is production of IgM; and the heavy chain diseases, in which there is production of the heavy chains (gamma, mu, and delta) (Osserman et al., 1987). Because they occur relatively infrequently, descriptive and analytical studies of Waldenström's macroglobulinemia or the heavy chain diseases are not reported in this review.

Myeloma presently accounts for almost 10% of all hematologic malignancies and 1% of cancer deaths in Western countries (Kastrinakis et al., 2000). Although myeloma is a rare malignancy, there is a relatively high mortality, with a 5-year survival of 28% (Dalton et al., 2001). Nevertheless, disease prognosis has improved over the last decade, with treatments such as high-dose chemotherapy followed by autologous bone marrow transplantation proving more successful than conventional, non-intensive chemotherapy alone (Attal et al., 1996). Recent advances in the understanding of the molecular pathogenesis of the disease might prove useful in developing more effective therapies.

## Classification

There is strong evidence that the malignant transformation causing myeloma occurs not at the terminally differentiated B cell, but rather at the early B cell or lymphoid stem cell (Barlogie et al., 1989). B cell precursors express specific antigens during discrete stages of maturation, and early B cell and T cell antigens have been identified from tumor cells (Barlogie et al., 1989). Furthermore, cytogenetic abnormalities of transformed plasma cells from one myeloma patient were also evident in the patient's early B cells (MacKenzie and Lewis, 1985). The malignantly transformed B cell clone proliferates and accumulates in the bone marrow. Progression of the malignancy is then steered by various genetic events and factors regulating the growth of plasma cells.

The manifestations of myeloma are variable and the disease can be difficult to diagnose (Kyle, 1988). Excluding nonsecretory myeloma, the diagnosis is based on the presence of monoclonal protein in serum or urine and more than 10% atypical plasma cells in bone marrow (Kyle, 1988) with additional symptoms, which may include osteolytic lesions, renal insufficiency, hypercalcemia, anemia, and increased susceptibility to infections. Monoclonal protein can be detected using serum protein electrophoresis; however, in approximately 15% of patients, the only manifestation of disease is light chains (Bence Jones protein). Detection of heavy and light chains requires immunoelectrophoresis or immunofixation.

Nearly all myeloma cell lines harbor chromosome translocations involving the IgH locus (Avet-Loiseau et al., 1998, Fonseca et al., 2002a, Kuehl and Bergsagel, 2002), of which t(11;14)(q13;q32) is the most common, resulting in upregulation of the cyclin D1 oncogene (Fonseca et al., 2002a). Patients with this translocation exhibit an aggressive clinical course (Kastrinakis et al., 2000). Other common translocations involve several loci, including 4p16.3, 16q23, and 6p25, generally resulting in dysregulation of putative oncogenes including FGFR3 and MMSET (on 4p16.3), c-maf (on 16q23), and MUM-1 (on 6p25) (Fonseca et al., 2002a). Deletion of chromosome 13q is found in the majority of plasma cells in myeloma (Avet-Loiseau et al., 1999) and has been shown to be strongly associated with translocation t(4;14)(p16.3;q32) (Fonseca et al., 2001).

Methylation of chromosome p16 was common in a group of myeloma patients (42%) and was associated with shorter overall and progression-free survival, primarily as a result of its association with an increased proliferative rate of plasma cells (Mateos et al., 2002). Another study found high prevalences of both p16 (75%) and p15 (65%) methylation in a small group of myeloma patients (Ng et al., 1997). Silencing of the p73 tumor-suppressor gene by hypermethylation has also been observed in myeloma and other lymphoid neoplasms (Katusic et al., 1985). Research into the role of methylation in myeloma risk might provide some clues into chromosomal alterations unique to myeloma etiology.

## Incidence and Mortality

### Demographic Patterns

Internationally, the reported incidence of myeloma varies substantially, as shown in Table 8-1 for the years 1993 to 1995. The availability and use of serum protein electrophoresis, immunoelectrophoresis, and immunofixation, all relatively sensitive diagnostic methods, vary by location. This variation probably accounts for part of the geographic variability in the reported incidence of and mortality from the disease. The highest incidence rates have been reported for blacks; Europeans and North American Caucasians have intermediate rates; whereas generally low rates have been reported for Asians living in Asia and the United States. A nationwide evaluation of US myeloma mortality rates found higher rates in urban versus rural areas (Blattner et al., 1981), as did a study of myeloma incidence in Israel (Shapira and Carter, 1986), but a comprehensive review of studies from Europe, Japan, and the United States concluded that the urban and rural rates were similar (Doll, 1991).

Age-, sex-, and race-specific incidence rates from the US Surveillance, Epidemiology, and End Results (SEER) program are shown in Figure 8-1 for the time period 1975 to 1999, and corresponding graphs for mortality rates are shown in Figure 8-2 for 1970 to 1999. Myeloma incidence and mortality increased steeply with age during these time periods. Men had higher rates than women; this sex difference has been observed consistently in international comparisons (Cartwright et al., 2002; Levi et al., 1992). Blacks had higher rates than whites; the cumulative incidence (ages 0–74 y) in black men during the period from 1973 to 1990 was approximately 10 per 100,000; in black women, white men, and white women, the corresponding rates were 7, 4, and 3 per 100,000, respectively (Miller et al., 1993). Myeloma incidence among Asian Americans was lower still (Table 8-1). Racial differences in myeloma rates have also been observed internationally. British migrants from West Africa, East Africa, and the Caribbean had higher rates of mortality from myeloma than native-born British residents between 1970 and 1985 (Caribbean males relative risk [RR] = 2.2,

## TABLE 8-1

### Annual Age-Standardized* Incidence (per 100,000) Rates by Geographic Location (1993–1995)

| Location (Ethnicity) | Men | Women | Location (Ethnicity) | Men | Women |
|---|---|---|---|---|---|
| **America, Central and South** | | | **Europe** | | |
| Argentina | 3.0 | 2.1 | Austria | 2.4–2.7 | 2.3–2.9 |
| Brazil | 1.1–1.9 | 0.9–1.5 | Belarus | 1.4 | 1.1 |
| Colombia, Cali | 1.4 | 1.1 | Belgium | 3.4–4.3 | 2.8–2.9 |
| Costa Rica | 1.5 | 1.3 | Croatia | 2.1 | 1.6 |
| Cuba, Villa Clara | 1.2 | 1.4 | Czech Republic | 2.0 | 1.3 |
| Ecuador, Quito | 1.6 | 1.9 | Denmark | 3.3 | 2.1 |
| France, Martinique | 2.3 | 1.7 | Estonia | 1.7 | 1.1 |
| USA, Puerto Rico | 3.3 | 2.0 | Finland | 2.9 | 2.5 |
| Uruguay, Montevideo | 1.3 | 1.9 | France | 2.3–3.9 | 1.7–3.3 |
| **America, North** | | | Germany, Saarland | 3.0 | 2.5 |
| Canada | 4.0 | 2.7 | Iceland | 2.4 | 3.3 |
| USA, California | | | Ireland | 4.2 | 2.7 |
|   Non-Hispanic White | 3.9–4.0 | 2.5–2.6 | Italy | 2.7–6.2 | 2.0–3.7 |
|   Hispanic White | 4.2–5.6 | 2.1–3.3 | Latvia | 1.7 | 1.5 |
|   Black | 7.1–7.4 | 6.4–7.0 | Lithuania | 2.1 | 1.8 |
|   Chinese | 1.7 | 0.7 | The Netherlands | 3.3–4.1 | 2.3–2.4 |
|   Filipino | 3.3 | 2.3 | Norway | 3.5 | 2.1 |
|   Japanese | 2.9 | 0.8 | Poland | 2.0–2.6 | 1.2–1.6 |
|   Korean | 2.0 | 1.7 | Russia, St. Petersburg | 1.2 | 1.3 |
| USA, SEER | | | Slovakia | 2.4 | 2.2 |
|   White | 3.9 | 2.5 | Slovenia | 2.2 | 1.8 |
|   Black | 8.8 | 6.8 | Spain | 2.2–3.6 | 1.7–3.9 |
| **Asia** | | | Sweden | 3.6 | 2.4 |
| China | 0.2–1.9 | 0.2–1.3 | Switzerland | 3.0–4.9 | 1.6–3.0 |
| India | 0.7–1.9 | 0.5–1.1 | United Kingdom | 2.7–4.1 | 2.0–2.9 |
| Israel | | | Yugoslavia | 1.1 | 0.8 |
|   Jews | 3.3 | 2.5 | **Oceania** | | |
|   Jews born in Israel | 2.7 | 2.4 | Australia | 2.1–4.0 | 1.9–3.2 |
|   Jews born in Europe or America | 3.2 | 2.1 | New Zealand | 4.2 | 3.0 |
|   Jews born in Africa or Asia | 3.3 | 2.9 | USA, Hawaii | | |
|   Non-Jews | 2.7 | 1.9 |   White | 3.9 | 1.4 |
| Japan | 1.5–2.1 | 1.0–1.3 |   Filipino | 4.7 | 3.8 |
| Korea | 0.9–1.4 | 0.7–1.1 |   Hawaiian | 4.7 | 3.8 |
| Kuwait | | |   Japanese | 1.3 | 0.8 |
|   Kuwaitis | 2.4 | 0.8 | | | |
|   Non-Kuwaitis | 2.1 | 0.5 | | | |
| Philippines | 0.7–1.0 | 0.9–1.1 | | | |
| Singapore | 1.1–2.4 | 0.9–1.9 | | | |
| Thailand | 0.4–0.7 | 0.3–0.5 | | | |

*Standardized to the age distribution of the world population, ages 0–74

Adapted from Cancer Incidence in Five Continents, Volume VIII, Eds: D. M. Parkin, S. L. Whelan, J. Ferlay, L. Teppo and D. B. Thomas. *IARC Scientific Publications No. 155*, Lyon, France, 2002.

95% confidence interval [CI] = 1.7–2.7; Caribbean females, RR = 2.0, 95% CI = 1.5–2.7; East African males, RR = 1.9, 95% CI = 1.0–3.7; East African females, RR = 1.7, 95% CI = 0.7–4.1); West African males RR = 4.1, 95% CI = 2.2–7.6; West African females, RR = 1.6; 95% CI = 0.2–11.5) (Grulich et al., 1992). An epidemiologic study of healthy black and white Americans observed that the ratio of B to T cells was higher among blacks, and that blacks had a higher proportion of HLA-DR-positive cells and activated T cells (Tollerud et al., 1991); the investigators hypothesized that these differences could be related to the observed difference in myeloma incidence between these two groups.

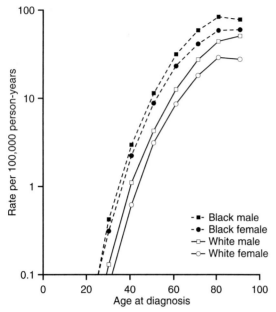

**FIGURE 8-1** *Age-specific multiple myeloma incidence rates in the United States (SEER areas) by race and sex, 1975–1999.*

## Time Trends

Trends in reported rates of myeloma incidence and mortality over time are likely to be misleading for a number of reasons related to improvements in case ascertainment (Velez et al., 1982). The availability and use of serum protein electrophoresis, immunoelectrophoresis, and immunofixation, all relatively sensitive diagnostic methods, have increased over time, likely resulting in more widespread and accurate identification of cases in later years. A unique International Classification of Diseases (ICD) code for multiple myeloma was first established in 1948, resulting in changes in reporting of the disease. Other factors influencing rates are changes in diagnostic criteria for myeloma, autopsy rates, and increased access to medical care across social and racial groups over time.

Increases in reported myeloma incidence in the United States have been observed for time periods from the mid-1900s through the 1970s, with little change in later years. Secular changes in myeloma incidence among white residents of four geographic areas of the United States who had participated in national cancer surveys or had established tumor registries (Atlanta, Connecticut, Detroit, San Francisco/Oakland) were examined by Devesa et al. for the period of 1947 through 1984 (Devesa et al., 1987). The reported annual incidence rates increased between 1947 and 1975 by approximately 150% to 3.8 per 100,000 in men and 2.6 per 100,000 in women (1950 US standard). However, no significant increases were observed between 1975 and 1985. The age-adjusted incidence of myeloma among blacks also did not change appreciably from 1973 to

1990 (Miller et al., 1993). Race- and sex- specific, age-adjusted, incidence rates from the US SEER program for the years 1975 to 1999 are shown in Figure 8-3, and corresponding graphs for mortality rates for 1950 to 1999 are shown in Figure 8-4. Both incidence and mortality rates appear to have increased slightly in each race- and sex-specific group between 1975 and 1990, leveling off in the most recent years after 1995, except for a continued increase in mortality among nonwhite females.

There have also been reports of increasing incidence through the 1970s in Denmark (Hansen et al., 1989), Australia (Nandakumar et al., 1988), New Zealand (Pearce et al., 1985), and Israel (Shapira and Carter, 1986). In Denmark, the reported annual incidence increased between 1943 and 1962 from 1.3 to 3.3 per 100,000 in men and from 1.2 to 2.5 per 100,000 in women (European standard); however, no increase was observed between 1963 and 1982. Increases in myeloma incidence in northeast Scotland were reported for a later time period, from 1973 through 1987; however, the observation that the increase was observed for registries with the lowest initial rates, but not among those with higher initial rates, argues for the role of improved surveillance in the increase (Soutar et al., 1996).

Three studies of time trends in myeloma incidence were conducted in areas where a particularly high level of case ascertainment would have been expected for the entire surveillance period: one in Olmsted County, Minnesota, where the Mayo Clinic is located and all major diagnoses are documented in a records-linkage system; another in Malmö, Sweden, where the relatively

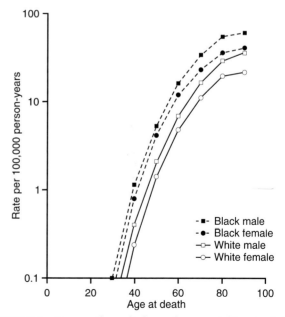

**FIGURE 8-2** *Age-specific multiple myeloma mortality rates in the United States by race and sex, 1970–1999.*

stable population has had access to comprehensive medical care since the 1950s; and the other in the Canton of Vaud, Switzerland, where close surveillance of incident cancers has occurred since the 1970s. In Olmsted County, the annual age-standardized rate (1950 US standard) of myeloma increased from 3.3 per 100,000 during 1945 through 1965, to 4.1 per 100,000 in 1978 through 1990, but the difference was not appreciable (Kyle et al., 1994). In Malmö, the incidence rate in men increased by 60% between 1950 and 1979 to an annual rate of 4.6 per 100,000 (1950 US standard) and all age groups were affected (Turesson et al., 1984). In contrast, no increase was observed in the rate among women (average annual incidence was 2.7 per 100,000) (Turesson et al., 1984). In the Canton of Vaud, no changes in incidence were noted between 1978 and 1987, with average annual incidence rates of 4.8 per 100,000 in men and 2.7 per 100,000 in women, European standard) (Levi and La Vecchia, 1990).

Several lines of evidence suggest that the reported secular increase in myeloma incidence was predominantly the result of changes in ascertainment of the disease, including the following:

1. There was no appreciable increase in Olmsted County or the Canton of Vaud, areas with good surveillance for myeloma;

2. In countries observing increases, rates generally stabilized since the 1970s;

3. When reported, increases were greatest among the elderly, a group in whom a laboratory

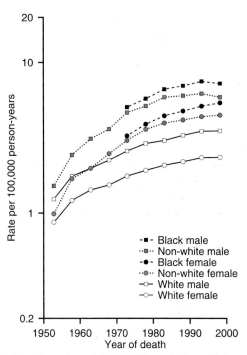

FIGURE 8-4 *Age-adjusted (1970 US standard) multiple myeloma mortality trends in the United States by race and sex, 1950–1954 to 1995–1999.*

diagnosis might have less commonly been sought in the past than in the present.

Thus, changes in case ascertainment, including the availability and use of serum protein electrophoresis, certainly account for much of the reported increases in incidence and mortality in some locations. Exceptions such as the finding of an increase in myeloma incidence in men, but not women, of all ages who resided in Malmö is consistent with the possible introduction of an occupational agent causing myeloma (Turesson et al., 1984).

### Socioeconomic Status

Positive associations of socioeconomic status indicators with myeloma were reported in several studies of myeloma mortality (Blattner et al., 1981; Cuzick et al., 1983; MacMahon, 1966; Velez et al., 1982). In a hospital-based case-control study conducted in North Carolina from 1976 to 1982, there was a 60% increased myeloma incidence associated with home ownership (odds ratio [OR] = 1.6, 95% CI = 1.0–2.6), and there was a suggested trend with increasing occupational rank; however, family income and education were unrelated to risk of the disease (Johnston et al., 1985). Conversely, a population-based case-control study found inverse associations between myeloma risk and occupation-based socioeconomic status, income, and education among both black and white subjects (Baris et al., 2000). Several additional studies that were

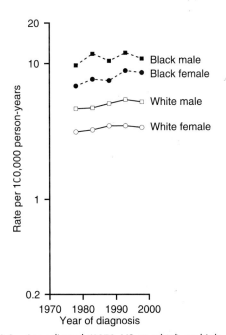

FIGURE 8-3 *Age-adjusted (1970 US standard) multiple myeloma incidence trends in the United States (SEER areas) by race and sex, 1975–1979 to 1995–1999.*

conducted in Europe, the United States, and Australia, with various study periods set between 1961 and 1986, observed little association between myeloma incidence and various indices of socioeconomic status (including occupational and educational level, income, and social class) (Boffetta et al., 1989; Cuzick and De Stavola, 1988; McWhorter et al., 1989; Miligi et al., 1999; Nandakumar et al., 1986, 1988; Vagero and Persson, 1986). The positive association of socioeconomic status with myeloma that was reported in earlier studies of mortality (Blattner et al., 1981; MacMahon, 1966; Velez et al., 1982) was possibly the result of better access to sensitive diagnostic methods by individuals of higher socioeconomic status.

## Host Factors

### Monoclonal Gammopathy of Undetermined Significance (MGUS)

MGUS is an asymptomatic disorder characterized by production of monoclonal protein (M-component) and proliferation of plasma cells in persons without evidence of a plasma cell proliferative disorder. Individuals with MGUS are predisposed to developing myeloma.

Sixty-four individuals with M-component, identified in a population-based survey in the Värmland district of Sweden, were followed for up to 20 years; two (3%) were diagnosed with myeloma and died from the disease (Axelsson, 1986), relating to an annual mortality rate of 2.1 per 1000 compared with approximately 0.02 per 1000 expected in similarly aged persons in Sweden during this time period (Cuzick et al., 1983). In a New Zealand rural community, six subjects (54%) were diagnosed with myeloma or Waldenström's macroglobulinemia from a series of 11 with M-component who were followed over a 31-year period, and five (46%) eventually died from their disease (Colls, 1999), relating to an annual mortality rate of approximately 42 per 1000. The higher rate of myeloma in the New Zealand study compared with the Swedish study might be attributable to the manner in which samples were stored and tested, possibly resulting in differences in the type of M-component identified (Colls, 1999). A rate of malignant transformation in persons with MGUS similar to that in the New Zealand study has also been observed in studies of patient populations (Kyle, 1993; Kyle et al., 2002; Pasqualetti et al., 1997; Van De Donk et al., 2001). This increased risk appears to continue even after 25 years or more of stable MGUS (Kyle et al., 2002).

The prevalence of M-component has been characterized in several large, population-based studies: the original Värmland study (Axelsson et al., 1966), and in studies conducted in the town of Thief River Falls, Minnesota (Kyle et al., 1972), the Finistère region of France (Saleun et al., 1982), and in a New Zealand

rural population (Colls, 1999). The studies were consistent in revealing an approximate 0.5% to 1.0% prevalence of M-component among adults, and an age-related increase in prevalence, which reached 4% to 5% among persons aged 80 years and over. There was also a sex differential, with men being 1.5 to 2.0 times more likely to have the condition. Each of these studies used either electrophoresis on paper or cellulose acetate, relatively insensitive methods to detect monoclonal proteins (Sinclair et al., 1986); the true prevalence could be higher by as much as 20% (Axelsson, 1986). The distribution of M-component in a French population was as follows: IgG, 68%; IgM, 24%; IgA, 6%; more than one component, 2%; light chains only, 1% (Saleun et al., 1982).

The age-specific prevalence of M-component in 1864 black veterans was higher than that in 857 white veterans (all ages: 5% in blacks compared with 2% in whites; age 70 years and older: 7% compared with 5%) (Schechter et al., 1991). There was also a difference in the prevalence of M-component between black and white elderly in North Carolina, using the more sensitive laboratory method of agarose gel electrophoresis and immunofixation (age >70 years: 8% in blacks compared with 4% in whites) (Cohen et al., 1998). The prevalence of M-component among adults aged 70 to 80 years was lower among Japanese persons presenting at a community center for a health screening (3%) than among white American residents of a retirement community (10%) (Bowden et al., 1993).

Several studies have found associations between clinical features of MGUS and progression to malignancy. The most consistent observation is that of the initial concentration of M-component at the time of MGUS diagnosis as a predictor of malignant progression (Baldini et al., 1996; Gregersen et al., 2001a, 2001b; Van De Donk et al., 2001); a recent study found a direct relation between the concentration of monoclonal protein in the serum and risk of malignant transformation (Kyle et al., 2002). Patients with IgA type M-component were found to be at increased risk of malignant transformation in some studies (Blade et al., 1992; Gregersen et al., 2001a; Kyle et al., 2002; Ogmundsdottir et al., 2002), but not others (Baldini et al., 1996; Kyle, 1993). Associations with other clinical features reported in some, but not all studies, include the plasma cell percentage (Van De Donk et al., 2001), total uninvolved immunoglobulin (Kyle et al., 2002), κ light chains (Van De Donk et al., 2001; van de Poel et al., 1995), hypogammaglobulinemia (Baldini et al., 1996; Gregersen et al., 2001a), and gammaglobulin (van de Poel et al., 1995).

Similar translocations are found in both MGUS and myeloma (Fonseca et al., 2002b), although aberrations involving two or more chromosomes are more common in myeloma (Feinman et al., 1997). Deletion of chromosome 13q is also common in MGUS, indicating a potential early event leading to malignancy, although its role for eventual progression to myeloma remains to be determined prospectively (Avet-Loiseau et al., 1999; Konigsberg et al., 2000). Comparison of MGUS and multiple myeloma patients showed that 42% of the myeloma patients had methylation of the p16 tumor-suppressor gene, whereas none of the MGUS patients did, indicating that methylation could be a relevant oncogenic event (Mateos et al., 2001).

## Prior Medical Conditions and Treatments

Certain prior medical conditions and treatments have been suspected to increase the risk of myeloma, either through chronic immune stimulation or through another biologic mechanism. When first put forth, the hypothesis that chronic immune stimulation could cause myeloma was based on the assumption that antigenic stimulation could increase the likelihood of a malignant transformation in a mature B cell. Since then, evidence has accumulated that the malignant transformation in myeloma occurs at the level of a pre-B or stem cell (Wolvekamp and Marquet, 1990); these cells are not stimulated by antigen. Nonetheless, chronic immune stimulation could have a promotional effect on myeloma, although there is no experimental evidence to support this hypothesis.

Table 8-2 lists the design of epidemiologic studies of the association between myeloma risk and prior medical conditions and treatments. Results from those studies are listed in Table 8-3. Interpretation of the

---

**TABLE 8-2**

### Design Characteristics of Studies That Have Assessed the Risk of Myeloma in Relation to Prior Medical Conditions and Treatments

| Study | Design | Population | Period |
|---|---|---|---|
| Bjornadal et al., 2002 | Cohort of patients with systemic lupus erythematosus | Sweden | 1964–95 |
| Boffetta et al., 1989 | Nested case-control, mortality | American Cancer Society members | 1982–86 |
| Bourguet and Logue, 1993 | Population-based case-control | NHANES I, US | 1971–86 |
| Brinton et al., 1989 | Cohort of patients with pernicious anemia | Veterans Administration institutions in US | 1969–85 |
| Cuzick and De Stavola, 1988 | Hospital-based case-control | Six areas in England and Wales | 1978–84 |
| Doody et al., 1992 | Population-based case-control | Kaiser Permanente, Oregon and California, US | 1956–82 |
| Eriksson et al., 1993 | Population-based case-control | Northern Sweden | 1982–86 |
| Gallagher et al., 1983 | Hospital-based case-control* | Vancouver, BC | 1972–81 |
| Gramenzi et al., 1991 | Hospital based case-control | Greater Milan area, northern Italy | 1983–89 |
| Goedert et al., 1998 | Cohort of patients with AIDS | US and Puerto Rico | 1985–89 |
| Gregersen et al., 2001 | Cohort of patients with pneumococcal infections | North Jutland, Denmark | 1981–96 |
| Gridley et al., 1993 | Population-based cohort | Sweden | 1965–84 |
| Grulich et al., 1999 | Cohort of patients with AIDS | New South Wales, Australia | 1980–93 |
| Isomaki et al., 1978 | Population based cohort | Finland | 1967–73 |
| Katusic et al., 1985 | Cohort of patients with rheumatoid arthritis | Rochester, Minnesota, US | 1950–74 |
| Kauppi et al., 1997 | Cohorts of patients with RA and Sjögren's syndrome | Finland | 1970–91 |
| Koepsell et al., 1987 | Population-based case-control | Four SEER areas, US | 1977–81 |
| Lewis et al., 1994 | Population-based case-control | Three metropolitan areas, US | 1986–89 |
| Linet et al., 1987, 1988 | Hospital-based case-control | Baltimore, MD, US | 1975–82 |
| Mellemkjaer et al., 1996a | Cohort of patients with pernicious anemia | Denmark | 1977–91 |
| Mellemkjaer et al., 1996b | Cohort of patients with rheumatoid arthritis | Denmark | 1977–87 |
| Mills et al., 1992 | Population-based cohort | California, US | 1977–82 |
| Montella et al., 2001 | Hospital-based case-control | Naples, Italy | 1997–99 |
| Pearce et al., 1986 | Tumor-registry-based case-control* | New Zealand | 1977–81 |
| Pickard et al., 2002 | Population-based cohort | Denmark | 1977–93 |
| Prior et al., 1984 | Cohort of patients with rheumatoid arthritis | Birmingham, UK | 1964–81 |
| Vesterinen et al., 1993 | Cohort of patients with asthma | Finland | 1970–87 |
| Vineis et al., 2000 | Population-based case-control | Italy | 1990–93 |

*Control subjects were registered with cancers other than multiple myeloma.

results shown in Table 8-3 is somewhat difficult for the following reasons:

1. Interviews of unknown and differing sensitivity and specificity were used in the various studies to measure prior conditions and treatments;

2. Because of the large number of factors examined, many comparisons were made, increasing the likelihood that spurious associations were identified;

3. Various studies categorized prior conditions and treatments in different ways, so it is not possible to make direct comparisons between studies;

4. Myeloma could have a prolonged prodromal period, and most studies did not account for such a period in their analyses. Therefore, for example, an association between a history of recent infection and myeloma could more plausibly be the result of myeloma leading to diminished immune competence than the result of a role of the infection in myeloma etiology.

Nonetheless, some limited inferences are possible.

### Autoimmune Disorders

A prospective analysis of the National Health and Nutrition Examination Survey (NHANES) I cohort found that myeloma risk increased with the number of autoimmune conditions reported, increasing to a 2.5-fold risk among those reporting two or more autoimmune conditions on the baseline questionnaire (Bourguet and Logue, 1993); however, this association was based on only 18 myeloma cases, and no association was observed when excluding myeloma cases diagnosed within 5 years after the NHANES interview. Two hospital-based case-control studies reported no association of any autoimmune disease with myeloma (Gramenzi et al., 1991; Linet et al., 1987); however, selecting control subjects from hospitalized patients might have introduced a bias that obscured an actual association. A population-based case-control study observed a modest increased myeloma risk with any autoimmune disease among blacks, but not whites (Lewis et al., 1994).

Elevated myeloma incidence (Isomaki et al., 1978; Katusic et al., 1985; Kauppi et al., 1997) and elevated incidence of all hematologic malignancies (Matteson et al., 1991) were observed in several cohorts of patients with rheumatoid arthritis, with relative risks ranging from 1.2 to 8. In other cohorts, there were small increased risk associated with a history of rheumatoid arthritis diagnosis, but higher risks associated with indications of more severe rheumatoid arthritis, namely, hospital visits or hospitalization for the condition (Gridley et al., 1993; Tennis et al., 1993). The results from Mellemkjaer et al. showed increased myeloma incidence only for the time period within 4 years since

hospitalization for rheumatoid arthritis, indicating a possible bias resulting from a prodromal period for myeloma (Mellemkjaer et al., 1996a). Case-control studies conducted in the United States (Doody et al., 1992), New Zealand (Pearce et al., 1986), and Sweden (Eriksson, 1993) found 1.2-fold to 8-fold myeloma risk associated with rheumatoid arthritis. Two other case-control studies found no association of myeloma risk with rheumatoid arthritis (Cuzick and De Stavola, 1989; Lewis et al., 1994), but the prevalence of rheumatoid arthritis was notably elevated in the two studies (6–14%, compared with 2% or less in the other studies), suggesting some degree of misclassification with osteoarthritis. Cytotoxic medications frequently used in treating rheumatoid arthritis, in particular azathioprine and cyclophosphamide, have been associated with increased risk of hematologic malignancy (Baker et al., 1987; Beauparlant et al., 1999; Georgescu et al., 1997; Matteson et al., 1991); nevertheless, several studies observed an increased risk of hematologic malignancies in patients with rheumatoid arthritis that could not be completely explained by the use of cytotoxic medications (Cibere et al., 1997; Symmons, 1985; Tennis et al., 1993).

Several other autoimmune diseases have been studied in relation to myeloma incidence. Three cohorts of patients with pernicious anemia, from Denmark (Mellemkjaer et al., 1996b), Sweden (Hsing et al., 1993), and the United States (Brinton et al., 1989), had an approximately 2-fold risk of myeloma. However, in Denmark the excess risk was restricted to within 5 years of follow up, indicating a possible bias (Mellemkjaer et al., 1996b). A modest association of prior pernicious anemia with myeloma was observed in black (OR = 1.5) but not white (OR = 0.8) persons in a population-based case-control study set in three metropolitan areas of the United States (Lewis et al., 1994). Sjögren's syndrome was associated with a 3.4-fold risk of myeloma (95% CI = 0.4–12.4) in a study of Finnish patients (Kauppi et al., 1997). In a cohort of patients with systemic lupus erythematosus, a 4.1-fold risk of hematologic cancers, including one case of Waldenström's macroglobulinemia, was observed (Abu-Shakra et al., 1996). A relatively large cohort of lupus patients in Sweden (n = 5715) found that myeloma risk was only slightly elevated (OR = 1.2), based on 7 cases (Blornadal et al., 2002). A 2-fold myeloma risk associated with lupus was also observed in a case-control study, but the estimate was very imprecise (Lewis et al., 1994). Some cohorts of patients with lupus did not observe any case of myeloma (Pettersson et al., 1992; Sweeney et al., 1995), but these studies were too small to reliably identify even a moderate increase in risk for such a rare malignancy. There has been some suggestion of increased myeloma risk associated with rare autoimmune conditions, including Graves disease and Hashimoto's disease (Lewis et al., 1994).

## TABLE 8-3

### Summary of Studies That Have Assessed the Risk of Multiple Myeloma in Relation to Prior Medical Conditions and Treatments*

| Category | Study | Prevalence of Exposure in Control Subjects (%) | Number of Exposed Cases[†] | Effect Estimate (95% CI) |
|---|---|---|---|---|
| **Autoimmune Diseases** | | | | |
| Autoimmune diseases | Gramenzi et al., 1991 | 9.2 | 17 | 1.3 (0.7–2.3) |
| | Lewis et al., 1994, whites | 4.5 | 15 | 1.0 (0.5–1.8) |
| | Lewis et al., 1994, blacks | 2.4 | 9 | 1.7 (0.7–3.7) |
| | Linet et al., 1987 | 8.0[‡] | 5[‡] | 1.0 (0.3–3.6) |
| Number of autoimmune conditions | Bourguet and Logue, 1993 | | | |
| 0 | | — | 7/14538 PY | 1.0 |
| 1 | | — | 7/10464 PY | 1.4 (1.0–2.0) |
| ≥2 | | — | 4/3717 PY | 2.5 (0.9–6.6) |
| Graves disease | Lewis et al., 1994, whites | 0.08 | 1 | 5.3 (0.2–114) |
| Hashimoto's disease | Lewis et al., 1994, whites | 0.08 | 2 | 6.9 (0.5–88.6) |
| Pernicious anemia | Brinton et al., 1989 | — | 9 O/4.3 E | 2.1 (1.0–4.0) |
| | Lewis et al., 1994, whites | 1.6 | 6 | 0.8 (0.3–2.2) |
| | Lewis et al., 1994, blacks | 1.2 | 5 | 1.5 (0.5–4.5) |
| | Mellemkjaer et al., 1996a | — | 7 O/5.3 E | 1.3 (0.5–2.7) |
| Psoriasis | Lewis et al., 1994, whites | 2.1 | 6 | 0.8 (0.3–2.0) |
| | Lewis et al., 1994, blacks | 0.8 | 1 | 0.5 (0.1–4.2) |
| | Vineis et al., 2000 | — | — | 0.4 (0.1–1.6) |
| Rheumatoid arthritis | Cuzick and De Stavola, 1989 | 5.8 | 22 | 1.0[§] |
| | Doody et al., 1992 | — | — | 1.2 |
| | Eriksson, 1993 | 0.9 | 9 | 8.0 (1.4–46.1) |
| | Gridley et al., 1993 | — | 16 | 1.2 (0.7–1.9) |
| | Isomaki et al., 1978, males | — | 7 O/3.3 E | 2.1[§] |
| | Isomaki et al., 1978, females | — | 21 O/9.5 E | 2.2[§] |
| | Katusic et al., 1985 | — | 4 O/0.8 E | 5.0 (1.4–12.8) |
| | Kauppi et al., 1997 | — | 8 | 1.2 (0.5–2.3) |
| | Lewis et al., 1994, whites | 9.3 | 38 | 0.9 (0.6–1.4) |
| | Lewis et al., 1994, blacks | 13.8 | 26 | 0.8 (0.5–1.3) |
| | Pearce et al., 1986 | 2.2 | 4 | 2.3 (0.6–8.0) |
| Rheumatoid arthritis patients with >2 hospital visits for RA | Gridley et al., 1993 | — | 7 | 1.6 (0.6–3.3) |
| Rheumatoid arthritis patients who were hospitalized | Mellemkjaer et al., 1996b | — | 21 O/19.0 E | 1.1 (0.7–1.7) |
| 1–4 years since hospitalization | | — | 16 O/9.5 E | 1.7 (1.0–2.7) |
| 5–15 years since hospitalization | | — | 5 O/9.5 E | 0.5 (0.2–1.2) |
| Scleroderma | Vineis et al., 2000 | — | — | 1.4 (0.2–11.9) |
| Sjögren's syndrome | Kauppi et al., 1997 | — | 2 | 3.4 (0.4–12.4) |
| Systemic lupus erythematosus | Bjornadal et al., 2002 | — | 7 O/5.9 E | 1.2 (0.5–2.5) |
| | Cuzick and De Stavola, 1989 | 0.0 | 2 | ∞[§] |
| | Lewis et al., 1994, blacks | 0.2 | 1 | 2.1 (0.2–24.2) |
| Thyroiditis | Cuzick and De Stavola, 1989 | 6.0 | 17 | 0.7[§] |
| **Asthma** | | | | |
| Asthma | Boffetta et al., 1989 | 4.1 | 5 | 1.0 (0.3–2.7) |
| | Cuzick and De Stavola, 1988 | 6.8 | 20 | 0.7 |
| | Lewis et al., 1994, whites | 5.4 | 22 | 1.2 (0.7–2.1) |
| | Lewis et al., 1994, blacks | 5.5 | 16 | 1.3 (0.7–2.3) |
| | Mills et al., 1992 | — | — | 0.8 (0.1–6.1) |
| | Pearce et al., 1986 | 9.2 | 9 | 1.3 (0.6–2.9) |
| | Vesterinen et al., 1993, men | — | 22 | 1.1 (0.7–1.6) |
| | Vesterinen et al., 1993, women | — | 16 | 0.5 (0.3–0.9) |
| Asthma medication | Pearce et al., 1986 | 6.0 | 8 | 1.8 (0.7–4.3) |

*Continued*

===== **TABLE 8-3** =====

## Summary of Studies That Have Assessed the Risk of Multiple Myeloma in Relation to Prior Medical Conditions and Treatments*—cont'd

| Category | Study | Prevalence of Exposure in Control Subjects (%) | Number of Exposed Cases[†] | Effect Estimate (95% CI) |
|---|---|---|---|---|
| **Allergies and Allergy Treatments** | | | | |
| Allergies | Cuzick and De Stavola, 1988 | 31.3 | 142 | 1.1 |
| | Eriksson, 1993 | 7.3 | 20 | 1.1 (0.5–2.3) |
| | Gallagher et al., 1983 | 11.3 | 24 | 3.1 (1.6–6.3) |
| | Gramenzi et al., 1991 | 20.5 | 17 | 0.6 (0.3–1.0) |
| | Lewis et al., 1994, whites | 47.3 | 153 | 1.1 (0.8–1.4) |
| | Lewis et al., 1994, blacks | 31.9 | 75 | 1.2 (0.9–1.7) |
| | Linet et al., 1987 | 17[‡] | 21[‡] | 1.0 (0.5–2.3) |
| | Mills et al., 1992 | 47.5 | — | 1.7 (0.7–4.0) |
| | Vineis et al., 2000 | — | — | 1.1 (0.6–1.8) |
| Number of allergies | Bourguet and Logue, 1993 | | | |
|   0 | | — | 11/20667 PY | 1.0[§] |
|   1 | | 5406 | 5 | 1.7 (0.3–10.6) |
|   ≥2 | | 2646 | 2 | 3.4 (0.1–286) |
| Number of allergies | Lewis et al., 1994, whites | | | |
|   1–2 vs. 0 | | 38.4 | 135 | 1.1 (0.8–1.4) |
|   3–4 vs. 0 | | 5.2 | 11 | 0.8 (0.4–1.6) |
|   ≥5 vs. 0 | | 3.7 | 7 | 0.7 (0.3–1.6) |
| Number of allergies | Lewis et al., 1994, blacks | | | |
|   1–2 vs. 0 | | 28.3 | 66 | 1.2 (0.9–1.7) |
|   3–4 vs. 0 | | 2.6 | 6 | 1.1 (0.4–2.8) |
|   ≥5 vs. 0 | | 1.0 | 3 | 1.5 (0.4–5.9) |
| Severe allergic reaction | Lewis et al., 1994, whites | 10.7 | 35 | 0.9 (0.6–1.4) |
| | Lewis et al., 1994, blacks | 5.9 | 18 | 1.1 (0.8–1.5) |
| Hayfever | Boffetta et al., 1989 | 7.4 | 14 | 1.6 (0.8–2.9) |
| | Cuzick and De Stavola, 1988 | 4.0 | 16 | 1.0[§] |
| | Doody et al., 1992 | 8.2 | 18 | 1.3 (0.6–2.7) |
| | Lewis et al., 1994, whites | 20.6 | 54 | 0.9 (0.7–2.0) |
| | Lewis et al., 1994, blacks | 17.7 | 40 | 1.1 (0.7–1.6) |
| | Mills et al., 1992 | 18.6 | — | 1.5 (0.5–4.6) |
| | Vineis et al., 2000 | — | — | 0.8 (0.4–1.5) |
| Allergy shots | Koepsell et al., 1987 | 7.4 | 43 | 0.8 (0.5–1.2) |
| | Lewis et al., 1994, whites | 7.6 | 18 | 0.7 (0.4–1.3) |
| | Lewis et al., 1994, blacks | 3.8 | 8 | 0.9 (0.4–2.0) |
| | Pearce et al., 1986 | 1.6 | 0 | — |
| Number of allergy desensitization shots | Koepsell et al., 1987 | | | |
|   1–99 vs. 0 | | 1.5 | 6 | 0.4 (0.1–1.1) |
|   ≥100 vs. 0 | | 2.0 | 14 | 0.9 (0.5–1.9) |
| Allergy treatment | Gallagher et al., 1983 | 4.2 | 11 | 3.5 (1.1–10.6) |
| Bee sting allergy | Mills et al., 1992 | 5.3 | — | 1.8 (0.4–7.7) |
| Drug allergies | Lewis et al., 1994, whites | 13.8 | 53 | 1.1 (0.8–1.5) |
| | Lewis et al., 1994, blacks | 5.4 | 18 | 1.6 (0.9–2.9) |
| | Mills et al., 1992 | 17.0 | — | 1.2 (0.4–3.6) |
| | Pearce et al., 1986 | 6.0 | 4 | 0.8 (0.3–2.5) |
| Dust allergy | Lewis et al., 1994, whites | 5.2 | 13 | 0.8 (0.4–1.5) |
| | Lewis et al., 1994, blacks | 3.5 | 9 | 1.2 (0.5–2.5) |
| Eczema | Cuzick and De Stavola, 1988 | 4.3 | 15 | 0.8[§] |
| | Doody et al., 1992 | 6.8 | 2 | 2.0 (1.1–4.0) |
| | Lewis et al., 1994, whites | 4.9 | 19 | 1.2 (0.7–2.0) |
| | Lewis et al., 1994, blacks | 2.6 | 6 | 1.1 (0.4–2.7) |
| | Pearce et al., 1986 | 5.7 | 4 | 0.9 (0.3–2.8) |
| | Vineis et al., 2000 | — | — | 0.6 (0.3–1.3) |

*Continued*

**TABLE 8-3**

## Summary of Studies That Have Assessed the Risk of Multiple Myeloma in Relation to Prior Medical Conditions and Treatments*—cont'd

| Category | Study | Prevalence of Exposure in Control Subjects (%) | Number of Exposed Cases† | Effect Estimate (95% CI) |
|---|---|---|---|---|
| Non-eczema skin allergy | Cuzick and De Stavola, 1988 | 20.1 | 93 | 1.1§ |
| Food allergies | Pearce et al., 1986 | 1.9 | 3 | 2.1 (0.5–8.5) |
| Household-product allergies | Lewis et al., 1994, whites | 1.8 | 21 | 0.9 (0.3–2.4) |
| | Lewis et al., 1994, blacks | 1.6 | 40 | 1.1 (0.7–1.6) |
| **Bacterial Infections** | | | | |
| Acute bacterial infections | Gramenzi et al., 1991 | 36.3 | 47 | 1.2 (0.8–1.8) |
| | Lewis et al., 1994, whites | 50.0 | 149 | 0.9 (0.7–1.1) |
| | Lewis et al., 1994, blacks | 36.3 | 71 | 1.0 (0.7–1.4) |
| Chronic bacterial infections | Gramenzi et al., 1991 | 13.6 | 26 | 1.8 (1.1–2.8) |
| | Lewis et al., 1994, whites | 2.8 | 10 | 1.1 (0.5–2.3) |
| | Lewis et al., 1994, blacks | 4.5 | 5 | 0.6 (0.2–1.4) |
| | Linet et al., 1987 | 11‡ | 16‡ | 0.8 (0.3–1.8) |
| Number of bacterial infections | Gramenzi et al., 1991 | | | |
| 1 vs. 0 | | 35.2 | 36 | 0.8 (0.5–1.6) |
| 2 vs. 0 | | 8.4 | 15 | 1.5 (0.7–3.0) |
| >2 vs. 0 | | 1.5 | 7 | 3.8 (1.3–10.8) |
| Number of bacterial infections | Bourguet and Logue, 1993 | | | |
| 1 vs. 0 | | 4734 | 2 | 0.4 (0.1–1.5) |
| ≥2 vs. 0 | | 2152 | 0 | 0.1 (0.01–2.3) |
| Number of bacterial infections | Koepsell et al., 1987 | | | |
| 1 vs. 0 | | 44.6 | 220 | 0.9 (0.7–1.1) |
| 2 vs. 0 | | 18.9 | 96 | 1.1 (0.8–1.5) |
| ≥3 vs. 0 | | 6.6 | 41 | 1.1 (0.7–1.8) |
| Number of acute bacterial infections | Lewis et al., 1994, whites | | | |
| 1–2 vs. 0 | | 20.1 | 71 | 1.0 (0.7–1.3) |
| 3–5 vs. 0 | | 8.7 | 31 | 1.0 (0.6–1.6) |
| ≥6 vs. 0 | | 20.8 | 47 | 0.7 (0.5–1.0) |
| Number of acute bacterial infections | Lewis et al., 1994, blacks | | | |
| 1–2 vs. 0 | | 19.8 | 46 | 1.3 (0.9–1.9) |
| 3–5 vs. 0 | | 6.8 | 12 | 0.9 (0.5–1.7) |
| ≥6 vs. 0 | | 9.7 | 13 | 0.6 (0.3–1.1) |
| Bronchitis | Doody et al., 1992 | 10.0 | 27 | 2.0 (1.0–3.9) |
| Chronic bronchitis | Gramenzi et al., 1991 | 10.7 | 15 | 1.3 (0.7–2.4) |
| | Koepsell et al., 1987 | 10.3 | 70 | 1.0 (0.7–1.3) |
| Ear infection | Lewis et al., 1994, whites | 8.9 | 22 | 0.7 (0.4–1.2) |
| | Lewis et al., 1994, blacks | 2.3 | 2 | 0.4 (0.1–1.6) |
| Gonorrhea | Koepsell et al., 1987 | 4.1 | 21 | 0.6 (0.4–1.0) |
| | Lewis et al., 1994, whites | 1.8 | 7 | 1.6 (0.6–3.9) |
| | Lewis et al., 1994, blacks | 12.0 | 2 | 0.4 (0.1–1.6) |
| Osteomyelitis | Koepsell et al., 1987 | 1.3 | 17 | 1.5 (0.7–3.0) |
| | Lewis et al., 1994, whites | 0.4 | 3 | 1.7 (0.4–7.5) |
| | Lewis et al., 1994, blacks | 0.6 | 3 | 2.3 (0.6–9.4) |
| Pancreatitis | Lewis et al., 1994, whites | 0.9 | 5 | 0.8 (0.3–2.2) |
| | Lewis et al., 1994, blacks | 0.8 | 2 | 0.3 (0.1–1.3) |
| Pneumonia | Koepsell et al., 1987 | 0.3 | 4 | 1.3 (0.3–5.1) |
| | Lewis et al., 1994, whites | 2.2 | 9 | 1.1 (0.5–2.4) |
| | Lewis et al., 1994, blacks | 0.7 | 4 | 2.6 (0.7–9.2) |
| Pyelonephritis | Gramenzi et al., 1991 | 0.8 | 3 | 2.0 (0.5–8.4) |
| Rheumatic fever | Doody et al., 1992 | 0.9 | 3 | 1.5 (0.3–9.0) |
| | Gramenzi et al., 1991 | 4.8 | 9 | 1.4 (0.6–3.2) |
| | Koepsell et al., 1987 | 3.1 | 32 | 1.7 (1.1–2.8) |
| | Lewis et al., 1994, whites | 2.7 | 15 | 1.4 (0.7–2.7) |
| | Lewis et al., 1994, blacks | 4.0 | 7 | 0.7 (0.3–1.6) |

*Continued*

**TABLE 8-3**

Summary of Studies That Have Assessed the Risk of Multiple Myeloma in Relation to
Prior Medical Conditions and Treatments*—cont'd

| Category | Study | Prevalence of Exposure in Control Subjects (%) | Number of Exposed Cases[†] | Effect Estimate (95% CI) |
|---|---|---|---|---|
| Scarlet fever | Cuzick and De Stavola, 1988 | 20.8 | 87 | 1.0[§] |
| | Gramenzi et al., 1991 | 8.2 | 17 | 2.0 (1.1–3.9) |
| | Koepsell et al., 1987 | 14.1 | 68 | 0.8 (0.6–1.0) |
| | Lewis et al., 1994, whites | 9.7 | 36 | 0.9 (0.6–1.4) |
| | Lewis et al., 1994, blacks | 3.0 | 6 | 1.0 (0.4–2.4) |
| Sinus infection | Koepsell et al., 1987 | 2.5 | 22 | 1.7 (1.0–3.1) |
| | Lewis et al., 1994, whites | 12.3 | 32 | 0.8 (0.5–1.2) |
| | Lewis et al., 1994, blacks | 7.3 | 12 | 0.6 (0.3–1.2) |
| Strep throat | Lewis et al., 1994, whites | 6.8 | 19 | 0.9 (0.5–1.5) |
| | Lewis et al., 1994, blacks | 2.6 | 1 | 0.2 (0.0–1.3) |
| Syphilis | Koepsell et al., 1987 | 0.8 | 12 | 1.9 (0.8–4.7) |
| | Lewis et al., 1994, whites | 0.09 | 2 | 11.6 (0.8–173) |
| | Lewis et al., 1994, blacks | 2.0 | 6 | 1.5 (0.6–4.0) |
| Throat, tonsil, or ear infection | Koepsell et al., 1987 | 1.6 | 18 | 1.6 (0.8–3.2) |
| Tonsillitis | Lewis et al., 1994, whites | 10.2 | 25 | 0.8 (0.5–1.2) |
| | Lewis et al., 1994, blacks | 5.3 | 7 | 0.6 (0.3–1.3) |
| Tooth abscess | Koepsell et al., 1987 | 49.1 | 341 | 1.0 (0.8–1.2) |
| Tuberculosis | Doody et al., 1992 | 5.0 | 11 | 2.0 (0.8–5.5) |
| | Eriksson, 1993 | 4.5 | 12 | 1.1 (0.4–2.8) |
| | Gramenzi et al., 1991 | 2.7 | 8 | 2.3 (0.9–5.7) |
| | Koepsell et al., 1987 | 2.1 | 20 | 1.3 (0.7–2.5) |
| | Vineis et al., 2000 | 2.0 | 5 | 0.7 (0.3–1.8) |
| Typhus | Gramenzi et al., 1991 | 5.9 | 9 | 1.2 (0.6–2.6) |
| Whooping cough | Cuzick and De Stavola, 1988 | 40.3 | 176 | 1.1[§] |
| | Gramenzi et al., 1991 | 28.3 | 35 | 1.1 (0.7–1.7) |
| Urinary tract infection | Koepsell et al., 1987 | 23.9 | 188 | 1.2 (1.0–1.5) |
| | Lewis et al., 1994, white men | 19.9 | 37 | 1.0 (0.7–1.5) |
| | Lewis et al., 1994, black men | 9.3 | 8 | 1.0 (0.4–2.3) |
| | Lewis et al., 1994, white women | 17.3 | 24 | 0.9 (0.5–1.5) |
| | Lewis et al., 1994, black women | 7.6 | 15 | 2.0 (1.1–3.8) |
| **Viral Infections** | | | | |
| Viral infections | Gramenzi et al., 1991 | 75.5 | 81 | 0.8 (0.5–1.3) |
| Number of viral diseases | Koepsell et al., 1987 | | | |
| 1 vs. 0 | | 8.4 | 25 | 0.7 (0.3–1.6) |
| 2 vs. 0 | | 19.0 | 76 | 0.9 (0.5–1.9) |
| 3 vs. 0 | | 37.8 | 169 | 1.1 (0.6–1.9) |
| 4 vs. 0 | | 31.2 | 161 | 1.2 (0.6–2.3) |
| AIDS | Fordyce et al., 2000 | — | 7 O/0.95 E | 7.4 (3.0–15.2) |
| | Goedert et al., 1998 | — | 3 | 4.5 (0.9–13.2) |
| | Grulich et al., 1999 | — | 3 | 12.1 (2.5–35) |
| Chickenpox | Cuzick and De Stavola, 1988 | 73.9 | 312 | 1.0[§] |
| | Gramenzi et al., 1991 | 47.4 | 42 | 0.7 (0.5–1.1) |
| | Koepsell et al., 1987 | 69.7 | 490 | 1.0 (0.8–1.3) |
| | Lewis et al., 1994, whites | 69.8 | 235 | 0.8 (0.6–1.1) |
| | Lewis et al., 1994, blacks | 67.6 | 235 | 0.9 (0.6–1.2) |
| | Vineis et al., 2000 | — | — | 0.8 (0.5–1.2) |
| Hepatitis | Koepsell et al., 1987 | 2.4 | 7 | 0.4 (0.2–1.0) |
| | Lewis et al., 1994, whites | 3.6 | 8 | 0.7 (0.3–1.6) |
| | Lewis et al., 1994, blacks | 1.0 | 3 | 1.5 (0.4–5.4) |
| | Vineis et al., 2000 | 6.3 | 23 | 1.5 (0.9–2.4) |
| Hepatitis C virus detected in blood | Montella et al., 2001 | 8.0 | 13 | 4.5 (1.9–10.7) |
| Herpes fever blisters | Koepsell et al., 1987 | 42.1 | 322 | 1.2 (1.0–1.4) |
| Herpes genitalis | Vineis et al., 2000 | — | — | 2.3 (0.8–6.5) |

*Continued*

═══ **TABLE 8-3** ═══

## Summary of Studies That Have Assessed the Risk of Multiple Myeloma in Relation to Prior Medical Conditions and Treatments*—cont'd

| Category | Study | Prevalence of Exposure in Control Subjects (%) | Number of Exposed Cases[†] | Effect Estimate (95% CI) |
|---|---|---|---|---|
| Herpes labialis | Vineis et al, 2000 | — | — | 0.8 (0.6–1.2) |
| Infectious mononucleosis | Cuzick and De Stavola, 1988 | 5.8 | 34 | 1.4[§] |
| | Gramenzi et al., 1991 | 0.6 | 2 | 0.4 (0.1–2.6) |
| | Koepsell et al., 1987 | 0.8 | 62 | 0.8 (0.2–3.1) |
| | Lewis et al., 1994, whites | 2.2 | 6 | 1.2 (0.5–3.0) |
| Measles | Cuzick and De Stavola, 1988 | 88.7 | 340 | 0.9[§] |
| | Gramenzi et al., 1991 | 59.7 | 69 | 1.0 (0.6–1.5) |
| | Koepsell et al., 1987 | 89.3 | 606 | 1.0 (0.7–1.4) |
| German measles | Cuzick and De Stavola, 1988 | 45.4 | 192 | 1.0[§] |
| Mumps | Cuzick and De Stavola, 1988 | 65.4 | 278 | 1.0[§] |
| | Gramenzi et al., 1991 | 40.9 | 45 | 1.0 (0.7–1.6) |
| | Koepsell et al., 1987 | 73.2 | 522 | 1.1 (0.9–1.5) |
| | Lewis et al., 1994, whites | 63.9 | 221 | 1.0 (0.8–1.3) |
| | Lewis et al., 1994, blacks | 69.3 | 134 | 0.8 (0.6–1.2) |
| Polio | Koepsell et al., 1987 | 1.2 | 5 | 0.7 (0.2–2.0) |
| | Lewis et al., 1994, whites | 1.6 | 5 | 0.9 (0.3–2.5) |
| Rubella | Gramenzi et al., 1991 | 14.3 | 15 | 0.8 (0.5–1.4) |
| Shingles (herpes zoster) | Cuzick and De Stavola, 1988 | 19.3 | 114 | 1.4[§] |
| | Eriksson, 1993 | 3.2 | 5 | 0.7 (0.2–2.3) |
| | Gramenzi et al., 1991 | 6.1 | 13 | 1.8 (0.9–3.5) |
| | Koepsell et al., 1987 | 8.3 | 71 | 1.2 (0.9–1.7) |
| | Lewis et al., 1994, whites | 9.7 | 39 | 1.0 (0.7–1.5) |
| | Lewis et al., 1994, blacks | 3.2 | 11 | 1.7 (0.8–3.6) |
| Shingles, by years before myeloma diagnosis | Cuzick and De Stavola, 1988 | | | |
| ≥10 years | | 7.5 | 36 | 1.2[§] |
| 5–10 years | | 1.5 | 16 | 2.7[§] |
| 3–5 years | | 0.8 | 6 | 1.9[§] |
| 1–3 years | | 1.5 | 14 | 2.3[§] |
| **Other Chronic Conditions** | | | | |
| Chronic inflammatory conditions | Gramenzi et al., 1991 | 11.9 | 21 | 1.6 (0.9–3.1) |
| Number of inflammatory conditions | Bourguet and Logue, 1993 | | | |
| 0 | | — | 10/21912 PY | 1.0[§] |
| 1 | | — | 1/3984 PY | 2.0 (1.2–3.3) |
| ≥2 | | — | 7/2823 PY | 4.3 (1.5–12.4) |
| Rheumatic diseases | Eriksson, 1993 | 10.0 | 37 | 1.9 (1.0–3.5) |
| Angina pectoris | Eriksson, 1993 | 4.5 | 6 | 0.8 (0.3–2.1) |
| Arthritis | Boffetta et al., 1989 | 32.0 | 39 | 0.9 (0.6–1.5) |
| | Doody et al., 1992 | 4.4 | 85 | 1.4 (0.9–2.2) |
| Chronic lung disease | Lewis et al., 1994, whites | 6.4 | 21 | 0.8 (0.5–1.4) |
| | Lewis et al., 1994, blacks | 3.9 | 8 | 1.0 (0.5–2.4) |
| Cirrhosis | Lewis et al., 1994, whites | 0.7 | 2 | 0.8 (0.2–4.1) |
| | Lewis et al., 1994, blacks | 1.4 | 1 | 0.3 (0.0–2.6) |
| Colitis or inflammatory bowel disease | Eriksson, 1993 | 5.9 | 9 | 0.6 (0.2–1.5) |
| | Lewis et al., 1994, whites | 5.2 | 18 | 0.9 (0.5–1.5) |
| | Lewis et al., 1994, blacks | 1.7 | 1 | 0.3 (0.1–2.1) |
| | Vineis et al., 2000 | | | 0.8 (0.3–2.1) |
| Diabetes | Boffetta et al., 1989 | 7.4 | 17 | 1.9 (1.1–3.8) |
| | Eriksson, 1993 | 14.1 | 22 | 0.7 (0.3–1.4) |
| | Lewis et al., 1994, whites | 8.5 | 38 | 1.1 (0.7–1.7) |
| | Lewis et al., 1994, blacks | 16.4 | 36 | 1.0 (0.6–1.4) |
| | Vineis et al., 2000 | | | 0.7 (0.4–1.1) |

*Continued*

## TABLE 8-3

### Summary of Studies That Have Assessed the Risk of Multiple Myeloma in Relation to Prior Medical Conditions and Treatments*—cont'd

| Category | Study | Prevalence of Exposure in Control Subjects (%) | Number of Exposed Cases[†] | Effect Estimate (95% CI) |
|---|---|---|---|---|
| Disc and other musculoskeletal disease | Doody et al., 1992 | 12.3 | 36 | 2.3 (1.2–4.1) |
| Embedded shrapnel | Koepsell et al., 1987 | 1.7 | 22 | 2.0 (1.1–3.5) |
| | Lewis et al., 1994, whites | 6.2 | 16 | 0.8 (0.4–1.4) |
| | Lewis et al., 1994, blacks | 4.1 | 3 | 0.4 (0.1–1.3) |
| Gallbladder disease | Eriksson, 1993 | 5.0 | 10 | 1.0 (0.4–2.7) |
| Gastric ulcer | Eriksson, 1993 | 4.5 | 14 | 1.5 (0.6–3.7) |
| Goiter | Lewis et al., 1994, whites | 0.4 | 1 | 0.9 (0.1–8.5) |
| | Lewis et al., 1994, blacks | 0.2 | 2 | 3.2 (0.4–23.0) |
| Hyperlipidemia | Eriksson, 1993 | 4.5 | 10 | 1.1 (0.4–3.0) |
| Hypertension | Eriksson, 1993 | 29.5 | 62 | 0.9 (0.6–1.4) |
| Hyperparathyroidism | Pickard et al., 2002 | — | 4/14703 PY | 2.2 (0.6–5.5) |
| Hyperthyroidism | Lewis et al., 1994, whites | 2.2 | 5 | 0.4 (0.2–1.1) |
| | Lewis et al., 1994, blacks | 1.8 | 7 | 1.5 (0.6–3.7) |
| Hypothyroidism and/or myxedema | Gallagher et al., 1983 | 1.2 | 6 | 5.0 (0.1–25.7) |
| | Lewis et al., 1994, whites | 4.4 | 18 | 1.1 (0.6–1.9) |
| | Lewis et al., 1994, blacks | 1.6 | 2 | 0.5 (0.1–2.3) |
| Kidney disease | Boffetta et al., 1989 | 2.7 | 5 | 1.4 (0.5–4.0) |
| Malaria | Gramenzi et al., 1991 | 3.6 | 7 | 1.8 (0.7–4.5) |
| | Koepsell et al., 1987 | 0.8 | 62 | 0.9 (0.3–2.5) |
| | Vineis et al., 2000 | 4.3 | 21 | 1.9[§] |
| Medical implant | Koepsell et al., 1987 | 7.0 | 46 | 1.0 (0.7–1.4) |
| Metabolic disorder | Eriksson, 1993 | 5.0 | 8 | 0.6 (0.3–1.6) |
| Nervous complaints | Eriksson, 1993 | 9.1 | 24 | 1.2 (0.6–2.3) |
| Skin infection | Koepsell et al., 1987 | 1.5 | 9 | 1.2 (0.5–2.5) |
| Thrombosis | Eriksson, 1993 | 9.0 | 169 | 0.8 (0.4–1.6) |
| **Other Acute Conditions** | | | | |
| Adenoidectomy | Vineis et al., 2000 | 10.1 | 21 | 1.2 (0.7–1.9) |
| Blood transfusion | Cuzick and De Stavola, 1988 | 20.0 | 65 | 0.8[§] |
| | Koepsell et al., 1987 | 25.1 | 182 | 1.1 (0.8–1.3) |
| | Lewis et al., 1994, whites | 18.6 | 83 | 1.1 (0.8–1.5) |
| | Lewis et al., 1994, blacks | 18.8 | 45 | 1.0 (0.7–1.5) |
| Horse serum injections | Koepsell et al., 1987 | 3.8 | 25 | 1.0 (0.6–1.8) |
| Insect sting | Koepsell et al., 1987 | 79.4 | 556 | 0.9 (0.7–1.2) |
| Lymphoid tissue surgery | Linet et al., 1987 | 19% | 25e | 1.2 (0.6–2.6) |
| Snakebite | Koepsell et al., 1987 | 2.8 | 10 | 0.5 (0.3–1.1) |
| Tonsillectomy | Cuzick and De Stavola, 1988 | 29.6 | 99 | 0.8[§] |
| | Lewis et al., 1994, whites | 54.1 | 166 | 0.8 (0.6–1.0) |
| | Lewis et al., 1994, blacks | 22.3 | 38 | 0.8 (0.5–1.1) |
| | Vineis et al., 2000 | 25.5 | 45 | 0.8 (0.6–1.2) |
| **Immunizations** | | | | |
| Childhood illness/vaccines | Lewis et al., 1994, whites | 98.1 | 339 | 0.7 (0.3–1.8) |
| | Lewis et al., 1994, blacks | 96.3 | 186 | 0.8 (0.4–1.6) |
| Number of diseases for which subject was immunized | Koepsell et al., 1987 | | | |
| 1 vs. 0 | | 14.0 | 99 | 0.8 (0.4–1.6) |
| 2 vs. 0 | | 24.0 | 137 | 0.7 (0.3–1.3) |
| 3 vs. 0 | | 32.9 | 153 | 0.7 (0.4–1.3) |
| 4 vs. 0 | | 26.2 | 127 | 0.8 (0.4–1.5) |
| BCG | Cuzick and De Stavola, 1988 | 6.5 | 28 | 1.0[§] |
| | Gramenzi et al., 1991 | 5.0 | 11 | 3.0 (1.4–6.4) |
| Cholera | Cuzick and De Stavola, 1988 | 9.5 | 46 | 1.2[§] |
| Diphtheria | Cuzick and De Stavola, 1988 | 4.0 | 29 | 1.8[§] |
| | Gramenzi et al., 1991 | 14.3 | 10 | 0.9 (0.4–1.8) |

*Continued*

**TABLE 8-3**

## Summary of Studies That Have Assessed the Risk of Multiple Myeloma in Relation to Prior Medical Conditions and Treatments*—cont'd

| Category | Study | Prevalence of Exposure in Control Subjects (%) | Number of Exposed Cases[†] | Effect Estimate (95% CI) |
|---|---|---|---|---|
| Influenza | Koepsell et al., 1987 | 60.2 | 393 | 0.9 (0.7–1.1) |
| | Lewis et al., 1994, whites | 59.1 | 220 | 1.1 (0.8–1.4) |
| | Lewis et al., 1994, blacks | 51.2 | 100 | 0.9 (0.7–1.2) |
| Polio | Cuzick and De Stavola, 1988 | 13.0 | 49 | 0.9[§] |
| | Gramenzi et al., 1991 | 23.7 | 28 | 0.9 (0.6–1.4) |
| | Koepsell et al., 1987 | 53.9 | 322 | 1.0 (0.8–1.3) |
| | Lewis et al., 1994, whites | 62.5 | 213 | 1.0 (0.8–1.4) |
| | Lewis et al., 1994, blacks | 45.7 | 82 | 0.8 (0.6–1.1) |
| Scarlet fever | Cuzick and De Stavola, 1988 | 0.8 | 7 | 2.3[§] |
| Smallpox | Cuzick and De Stavola, 1988 | 62.2 | 261 | 1.0[§] |
| | Cuzick and De Stavola, 1988 | 8.3 | 31 | 0.9[§] |
| | Gramenzi et al., 1991 | 83.4 | 91 | 0.7 (0.4–1.3) |
| | Koepsell et al., 1987 | 90.6 | 617 | 0.9 (0.7–1.3) |
| | Lewis et al., 1994, whites | 76.0 | 277 | 1.0 (0.7–1.4) |
| | Lewis et al., 1994, blacks | 66.0 | 138 | 1.1 (0.7–1.5) |
| Tetanus | Cuzick and De Stavola, 1988 | 46.6 | 182 | 1.0[§] |
| | Gramenzi et al., 1991 | 78.0 | 70 | 0.6 (0.4–1.0) |
| | Koepsell et al., 1987 | 59.2 | 386 | 0.9 (0.7–1.1) |
| | Lewis et al., 1994, whites | 75.7 | 262 | 1.0 (0.8–1.4) |
| | Lewis et al., 1994, blacks | 56.6 | 119 | 1.2 (0.8–1.7) |
| Tetanus ≥4 times | Cuzick and De Stavola, 1988 | 8.8 | 33 | 0.9[§] |
| Typhoid | Cuzick and De Stavola, 1988 | 14.8 | 63 | 1.0[§] |
| Typhus | Cuzick and De Stavola, 1988 | 6.3 | 29 | 1.1[§] |
| Whooping cough | Cuzick and De Stavola, 1988 | 1.8 | 12 | 1.7[§] |
| Yellow fever | Cuzick and De Stavola, 1988 | 7.0 | 36 | 1.3[§] |

* Comparison is ever vs. never unless otherwise specified.
[†] For cohort studies, the number of person years (PY), or observed (O) and expected (E) cases are presented, where available.
[‡] Based on the number of discordant pairs only.
[§] Unadjusted odds ratio.

## Allergies and Asthma

There appears not to be an association between myeloma risk and a history of asthma (Boffetta et al., 1989; Lewis et al., 1994; Pearce et al., 1986; Vesterinen et al., 1993), or with a history of allergies or allergy treatments (Boffetta et al., 1989; Cuzick and De Stavola, 1988; Doody et al., 1992, Friksson, 1993; Gramenzi et al., 1991; Koepsell et al., 1987; Lewis et al., 1994; Linet et al., 1987; Mills et al., 1992; Pearce et al., 1986; Vineis et al., 2000). A prospective analysis of the NHANES I cohort found that myeloma risk increased by the number of allergies reported in the interview, but the estimates were very imprecise (Bourguet and Logue, 1993), and this pattern was not observed in another study population (Lewis et al., 1994). In one study that found an overall association between a history of allergies and the risk of myeloma (OR = 3.1) (Gallagher et al., 1983), the authors noted that the character of reported allergies differed between cases and control subjects. Nearly half of the allergies reported by control subjects were described as breathing difficulties, whereas fewer than 20% of myeloma patients with allergies reported this symptom; myeloma patients described their symptoms mainly as skin rashes, swelling, and hives.

## Bacterial Infections

Three studies found no association of myeloma risk with the number of lifetime acute or chronic bacterial infections (Bourguet and Logue, 1993; Koepsell et al., 1987; Lewis et al., 1994). However, risk increased by the number of previous acute or chronic bacterial infections in a hospital-based case-control study in Italy, with a 3.8-fold risk for those reporting more than two infections (Gramenzi et al., 1991).

Osteomyelitis was associated with increased risk of myeloma in three study populations, with odds ratios ranging between 1.5 and 2.3 (Koepsell et al., 1987; Lewis et al., 1994). Four studies found an association between a history of rheumatic fever and myeloma risk, with odds ratios of 1.4 to 1.7 (Doody et al., 1992; Gramenzi et al., 1991; Koepsell et al., 1987; Lewis et al., 1994), although a fifth study reported no association (Eriksson, 1993). Other bacterial infections that have been associated with myeloma include bronchitis (Doody et al., 1992), pneumonia (Lewis et al., 1994), pyelonephritis (Gramenzi et al., 1991), scarlet fever (Gramenzi et al., 1991), sinus infection (Koepsell et al., 1987), syphilis (Lewis et al., 1994), tuberculosis (Doody et al., 1992; Gramenzi et al., 1991), and urinary tract infection (Lewis et al., 1994). Most of these associations were not confirmed in a second report.

## Viral Infections

Specific viruses might play a role in myeloma risk. Strong associations between myeloma incidence and AIDS (RR = 4.5–12.1) have been observed in studies linking AIDS patient registries to population cancer registries in the United States and Puerto Rico (Goedert et al., 1998), New York City (Fordyce et al., 2000), and Australia (Grulich et al., 1999). It is not known whether this excess of myeloma is attributable to AIDS-related immunosuppression or results from infection with viruses associated with other AIDS-related cancers, such as Kaposi sarcoma-associated herpesvirus, also known as human herpesvirus-8 (HHV-8) (Beral and Newton, 1998). HHV-8 viral sequences have been found in cultured nonmalignant bone marrow dendritic cells from myeloma patients and bone marrow biopsies (Beksac et al., 2001; Brousset et al., 1997; MacKenzie et al., 1997; Marcelin et al., 1997; Rettig et al., 1997; Said et al., 1997; Tedeschi et al., 2001). However, the role of HHV-8 in the pathophysiology of myeloma is controversial, and most investigators have failed to detect increased prevalence of HHV-8 in samples of blood, bone marrow, or bone marrow stromal cells from myeloma patients (Ablashi et al., 2000; Cathomas et al., 1998; Cull et al., 1999; Dominici et al., 2000; Drabick et al., 2002; Olsen et al., 1998; Parravicini et al., 1997; Patel et al., 2001; Rask et al., 2000; Sitas et al., 1999; Tarte et al., 1998; Tisdale et al., 1998; Yi et al., 1998). It has been suggested that HHV-8 sequence variation and differences in technique could account for discrepancies in results; for example, some studies found HHV-8 DNA in bone marrow stromal cells or biopsies, but no serologic responses to HHV-8 were present (Agbalika et al., 1998; Chauhan et al., 1999).

In three of five studies that ascertained a history of shingles, or herpes zoster, this condition was noted to be more prevalent among myeloma cases than controls (Cuzick and De Stavola, 1988; Gramenzi et al., 1991; Lewis et al., 1994). Some investigators suggested that because of the temporal proximity of the infection to the recognition of myeloma, it most likely was a manifestation of the as-yet undiagnosed malignancy; indeed, one analysis showing an overall increased myeloma risk associated with shingles indicated little association with shingles occurring 10 or more years before myeloma diagnosis (Cuzick and De Stavola, 1988).

Difficulties in recall could obscure associations between self-reported viral history and disease. Self-reported history of hepatitis infection has not been associated with myeloma risk (Koepsell et al., 1987; Lewis et al., 1994; Vineis et al., 2000), whereas hepatitis C virus (HCV) detected in blood was strongly associated (OR = 4.5) (Montella et al., 2001). A small seroprevalence study supported this finding, with an observed 11% anti-HCV positivity among myeloma cases and 0% among a rheumatoid arthritis patient control group (Gharagozloo et al., 2001).

## Other Chronic and Acute Conditions

A prospective analysis of the NHANES I cohort found that myeloma risk increased by the number of inflammatory conditions reported in the interview (including gout, gallstones, pleurisy, and recurrent or chronic enteritis), with the risk increasing from those reporting one condition (OR = 2.0, compared with those with 0 conditions) to those reporting two or more conditions (OR = 4.3); there was also a statistically significant increase in risk with increasing time since first exposure (RR = 1.6 for each additional 10 years since the start of the inflammatory condition) (Bourguet and Logue, 1993). Similarly, increased myeloma risk was associated with a history of chronic inflammatory conditions in a case-control study in Italy (Gramenzi et al., 1991), however, a different collection of diseases were included in their grouping (including rheumatic fever, ulcerative colitis, multiple sclerosis, glomerulonephritis, peptic ulcer, and Raynaud's disease) than in the NHANES study.

No consistent patterns emerge for specific chronic or acute conditions or treatments (Boffetta et al., 1989; Cuzick and De Stavola, 1988; Doody et al., 1992; Eriksson, 1993; Gallagher et al., 1983; Gramenzi et al., 1991; Koepsell et al., 1987; Lewis et al., 1994; Linet et al., 1987; Pickard et al., 2002; Vineis et al., 2000). Where elevated risks have been observed, they were usually not replicated in a subsequent study. There was some overlap of specific conditions examined in various studies with the groupings of inflammatory conditions examined in the studies by Bourguet et al. (Bourguet and Logue, 1993) and Gramenzi et al. (Gramenzi et al., 1991), with sometimes inconsistent results. For example, no association was observed between myeloma incidence and colitis or other inflammatory bowel disease in three studies (Eriksson, 1993; Lewis et al., 1994; Vineis et al., 2000). There were increased risks observed for undefined rheumatic conditions (OR = 1.9) (Eriksson, 1993), gastric ulcer (OR = 1.5) (Eriksson, 1993), disc and other musculoskeletal disease (OR = 2.3) (Doody et al., 1992), and kidney disease (OR = 1.5) (Boffetta et al., 1989).

*Summary*

The presence of some autoimmune diseases appears to increase myeloma risk, as do certain chronic inflammatory conditions. Specific viruses, particularly those that cause immunosuppression, likely contribute to the etiology of myeloma.

A possible underlying pathologic basis for the relation of certain autoimmune diseases, viruses, or other conditions with myeloma risk concerns the cytokine interleukin-6 (IL-6). IL-6 is a potent stimulator of B cell differentiation and a promoter of myeloma cell growth (Hirano, 1991; Wolvekamp and Marquet, 1990). IL-6 is produced by a wide variety of cell types in response to viruses, bacterial products, trauma, and other stimuli (Wolvekamp and Marquet, 1990). Hirano notes that IL-6 gene deregulation could occur from insertion of viral DNA in the promoter region of the IL-6 gene, by a cytokine cascade induced by an inflammatory reaction, or by other mechanisms (Hirano, 1991). IL-6 production has been noted to increase substantially in association with myeloma, rheumatoid arthritis and systemic lupus erythematosus, acute infectious neural diseases, trauma, cardiac myxoma, and transplantation (Wolvekamp and Marquet, 1990).

A second pathway by which certain medical conditions could contribute to myeloma risk is through an increased incidence of MGUS. The production of M-component as a response to chronic disease and infection has been studied epidemiologically only to a very limited extent. Autoimmune diseases are common in patients with monoclonal gammopathy (Youinou et al., 1996), and M-components have been observed to have autoimmune activity against self-antigens (Wang et al., 1992). Monoclonal and oligoclonal immunoglobulins were found in 24 of 27 patients with AIDS who had Kaposi's sarcoma, and 2 of 15 patients with AIDS who had opportunistic infections, suggesting that B cell activation might be operative in the malignant proliferation among patients with AIDS (Papadopoulos et al., 1985). A cohort of patients with infections found increased levels of M-component to be present in persons with leishmaniasis (80%) and cytomegalovirus (44%), but not in those with echinococcosis (6%) or infectious mononucleosis (0%) or among healthy control subjects (3%) (Haas et al., 1990). A second study also found a high prevalence of M-component in patients with cytomegalovirus (40%) compared to patients with Epstein-Barr virus (0%) (Buhler et al., 2002).

## Familial Aggregation

There have been numerous case reports of myeloma occurring in two or more members of a family and of myeloma occurring with MGUS in families (Maldonado and Kyle, 1974; Shoenfeld et al., 1982). Several case-control studies observed a relation between a first-degree family history of multiple myeloma with myeloma occurrence (OR = 2.3, 95% CI = 0.5–10.1, Bourguet et al., 1985; OR = 3.7, 95% CI = 1.2–2.0, Brown et al., 1999; OR = 5.6, 90% CI = 1.2–28, Eriksson and Hallberg, 1992). The increased risk of myeloma associated with family history of myeloma has been observed to be stronger in blacks (OR = 17.4, 95% CI = 2.4–348) than whites (OR = 1.5, 95% CI = 0.3–6.4), based on very small numbers (Brown et al., 1999). Such clustering of myeloma in families might arise from shared genetic factors or common environmental exposures. If familial myeloma cases derive from shared genetic or environmental factors, it is plausible that these tumors might differ from nonfamilial cases. Olshan (Olshan, 1991) compared the distributions of sex, age, immunoglobulin classes, and kappa-to-lambda ratios for familial myeloma cases reported in the literature with data from the SEER program and the Mayo Clinic. Kappa-to-lambda immunoglobulin ratios were higher in familial cases than in other cases, but other characteristics did not differ. Family aggregation of myeloma might be partially explained by familial aggregation of other medical conditions such as autoimmune diseases. Family members of myeloma patients have elevated levels of immunoglobulins, rheumatoid factor, and autoantibodies in blood (Festen et al., 1977; Linet et al., 1988; Youinou et al., 1996). Linet et al. investigated the relation between a history of autoimmune diseases in first-degree relatives and the occurrence of myeloma; they observed an odds ratio of 3.0 (95% CI = 1.3–7.1) (Linet et al., 1988). Familial aggregation of myeloma with degenerative central nervous system diseases in first-degree relatives has also been reported (OR = 4.4, 95% CI = 1.9–10.3) (Grufferman et al., 1989).

## Genetic Susceptibility

There have been several studies of common gene variants in the general population in relation to myeloma risk. Lines of investigation have primarily pursued polymorphisms in genes regulating immune response and inflammation.

Variations in human leukocyte antigen (HLA) were studied for many years before the ready availability of genotyping. Several studies have found associations between myeloma incidence and the B and C locus antigens. An analysis of pooled data on HLA-A and -B antigens showed a positive association between the presence of HLA B5 and the risk of myeloma (RR = 1.7, $p$ < 0.05) (Ludwig and Mayr, 1982). An association of myeloma with HLA B18 antigen was observed in both the pooled analysis (OR = 1.4, $p$ > 0.05) (Ludwig and Mayr, 1982) and a more recent study (OR = 6.3, 95% CI = 1.0–39.7) (Patel et al., 2002). A case-control study of 46 black men and 85 white men found a strong association between the HLA-Cw2 antigen and myeloma incidence in both racial groups (blacks, OR = 5.7, 95% CI = 1.0–7.2; whites, OR = 2.6, 95% CI = 1.0–7.2) (Pottern et al., 1992a), whereas two other studies noted associations with HLA-Cw2 that were more modest among African blacks (OR = 1.7, $p$ > 0.05) (Patel et al., 2002) and European whites (OR = 1.5, $p$ > 0.05) (Ludwig and Mayr, 1982). HLA-Cw5 and Cw6 antigens were associated with increased myeloma risk in blacks (Cw5, OR = 15.1, $p$ = 0.001; Cw6, OR = 6.5, $p$ = 0.007) (Leech et al., 1983), however, no association with Cw5 was observed among whites in another study (Ludwig and Mayr, 1982).

Several polymorphisms in proinflammatory cytokine genes have been investigated. IL-6 is an essential growth and survival factor for myeloma cells, and a polymorphism at position −174 is known to be functionally significant (Jeffery and Mitchison, 2001). However, two studies of IL-6 (−174) polymorphism have found no differences in genotype frequencies between cases and control subjects (Dring et al., 2001; Zheng et al., 2000). TNF-$\alpha$ and IL-1 are inducers of IL-6 production, and IL-1$\beta$ is mainly responsible for IL-6 production in the tumor environment. No differences have been observed in allele frequencies of the TNF-$\alpha$ (−308) (Zheng et al., 2000), IL-1$\beta$ TaqI (Zheng et al., 2000), or IL-1R$\alpha$ variable number tandem repeat (VNTR) polymorphisms (Demeter et al., 1996; Zheng et al., 2000) between myeloma cases and controls, or between MGUS patients and control subjects (Zheng et al., 2000). One study found that the haplotype of high-producer alleles TNF-$\alpha$ (−308) and lymphotoxin $\alpha$ (LT5.5/10.5) was associated with a 2-fold risk of myeloma (OR = 2.0, 95% CI = 1.3–3.4) (Davies et al., 2000); similar patterns were observed for MGUS patients compared with control subjects.

Myeloma and MGUS patients were compared with an ethnically matched control group for polymorphisms in the IL-10 gene, which is a gene implicated in growth and differentiation of normal B cells and in proliferation of myeloma cells (Zheng et al., 2001a). IL-10 production by stimulated peripheral blood mononuclear cells was significantly higher in subjects who were heterozygous or homozygous for the IL10.G allele 136 (Zheng et al., 2001a), demonstrating the functional significance of the variant. Myeloma risk was positively associated with the IL10.G genotype 136/136 (OR = 6.9, 95% CI = 2.6–18.2) and the IL10.R genotype 112/114 (OR = 3.1, 95% CI = 1.6–6.3), and negatively associated with the IL10.R genotype 114/116 (OR = 0.2, 95% CI = 0.1–0.5). Similar patterns were observed in comparisons of MGUS patients with control subjects.

Cytotoxic T lymphocyte antigen-4 (CTLA-4), which is involved in the regulation of immune responses, including mediating inhibitory signals to activated T cells, has a microsatellite polymorphism in the 3′ untranslated region of exon 3 which has been associated with an increased risk of certain autoimmune diseases (Kotsa et al., 1997). Of multiple CTLA-4 genotypes examined, the only association observed was presumably unpredicted inverse association of genotype 86/86 with a decreased risk of myeloma (OR = 0.5, 95% CI = 0.2, 1.0) and MGUS (OR = 0.1, 95% CI = 0.03, 0.6) (Zheng et al., 2001b).

NF-κB proteins act as transcription factors for many genes, the products of which have important roles in cell proliferation, the immune response, and inflammation. NF-κB activation is normally transient in most cells; during interim periods, NF-κB proteins remain bound to IκBα in the cytosol and are thus unable to act as transcription factors. Increased NF-κB activity has been observed in myeloma cell lines and is much higher in chemoresistant than chemosensitive cell lines. Because the presence of IκBα somewhat regulates NF-κB activity, polymorphisms in the IκBα gene have been investigated for their functional significance and association with malignancies. Certain variants of the IκBα gene have been shown to render the protein incapable of interacting with NF-κB (Cabannes et al., 1999). Increased risk of myeloma was associated in a small, hospital-based case-control study with polymorphisms in the IκBα gene, including sites 104149 (A → T) (OR = 7.8, 95% CI = 1.7–35.4), 101799 (T → C) (OR = 6.4, 95% CI = 1.2–34.0), and 101675 (A → G) (OR = 11, 95% CI = 1.9–64.6) (Parker et al., 2002).

Because chromosomal abnormalities are common in lymphoproliferative disorders, another line of investigation pursues variants in genes involved in maintaining error-free DNA. Given that folate availability is critical to DNA integrity, Gonzalez Ordonez et al. compared the frequency of polymorphisms in methylene tetrahydrofolate reductase (MTHFR), which plays a critical step in folate synthesis, between myeloma cases and control subjects (Gonzalez Ordonez et al., 2000). Variant alleles at nucleotides 677 and 1298 have been associated with a decrease in MTHFR activity (Skibola et al., 1999). The common MTHFR CC genotype, with homozygosity at nucleotide 677, was associated with a decreased risk of myeloma overall (19% vs. 46% in control subjects, OR = 0.3, 95% CI = 0.1–0.8) (Gonzalez Ordonez et al., 2000). A second study observed a similar association with the MTHFR nucleotide 677 genotype (common CC genotype: 34% in myeloma cases vs. 48% in control subjects, $p$ = 0.18), but no strong association with the nucleotide 1298 genotype (common AA genotype: 36% in cases vs. 43% in control subjects, $p = 0.61$) (Gonzalez-Fraile et al., 2002).

# Environmental Factors

## Ionizing Radiation

Two studies have been published of myeloma risk in Japanese survivors of the atomic bombs detonated in Hiroshima and Nagasaki in 1945 (Table 8-4). The study by Shimizu et al. (Shimizu et al., 1990) examined myeloma mortality during the period 1950 through 1985, whereas that of Preston et al. considered incidence from 1950 through 1987 (Preston et al., 1994). The design and methods differed appreciably between the two studies, as did the findings. Shimizu et al. ascertained 36 persons whose primary cause of death was myeloma and for whom DS86 revised doses had been estimated among the approximately 75,000 persons who were in the cities at the time of the bomb. They observed a slope in the relation of radiation dose and myeloma risk such that the RR was 3.3 (90% CI = 1.7–6.3) following exposure to 1 Gray (Gy) bone marrow dose (Shimizu et al., 1990). The mean bone marrow dose in the cohort was 0.14 Gy (corresponding RR of 1.2). Preston et al. identified 59 persons whose first cancer diagnosis was myeloma and whose DS86 kerma doses were estimated to be less than 4 Gy. After adjusting for age at diagnosis and age at the time of the bomb, they observed a relative risk of 1.3 ($p > 0.05$) per Sievert (Sv) (Preston et al., 1994). Including persons whose myeloma was a second primary or whose doses exceeded 4 Gy increased the RR to 1.9 ($p = 0.02$). More than 99% of the radiation from the atomic bomb was reported as gamma radiation, so the dose in Sv would be approximately equal to the dose in Gy in this study.

Radiation-exposed workers at three US nuclear weapons plants were found to be at increased risk of death from myeloma relative to their unexposed peers (Gilbert et al., 1989). A direct relation between dose and mortality was observed, with workers who received 0.050 to 0.099, 0.010 to 0.199, and 0.200 Sv or more of external radiation being at 3.3-fold ($n = 1$), 5.0-fold ($n = 1$), and 33-fold ($n = 1$) risk, respectively, relative to the general population. A case-control study of multiple myeloma at four US nuclear facilities did not show an association with lifetime cumulative whole-body ionizing radiation and myeloma risk; however, there was a significant effect of age at exposure indicating an association between multiple myeloma and doses received at older age (Wing et al., 2000). British radiation workers at major sites of the nuclear

industry were at lower risk of death from myeloma than the general population, with a standardized mortality ratio (SMR) of 0.7 (number of exposed cases = 40), but there was a trend ($p = 0.06$) of increasing risk with increasing level of exposure such that workers exposed to 0.400 or more Sv ($n = 2$) were at 2.5-fold risk compared with those exposed to less than 0.010 Sv ($n = 20$) (Kendall et al., 1992; Muirhead et al., 1999). A trend with dose for multiple myeloma risk was also observed in the IARC Canada/UK/US study (one-sided $p$ value = 0.037) (Cardis et al., 1995). A study conducted at the Sellafield nuclear fuels plant, in which there were seven deaths from myeloma, also showed a direct relation between dose and mortality, with workers receiving an external dose of 0.400 mSv or more being at a 2.0-fold ($n = 2$) risk relative to the general population (Smith and Douglas, 1986). Similar findings were observed when the followup of the study population was extended (Omar et al., 1999). A study of persons exposed occupationally to considerably lower levels of radiation (< 0.01 Sv) observed no excess risk (Beral et al., 1985). A combined analysis of mortality in three UK nuclear industry workforce showed a modest association between external radiation dose and risk of multiple myeloma (Carpenter et al., 1994). British workers who participated in atmospheric nuclear weapons testing were at 50% increased risk of death from myeloma (90% CI = 0.6–4.3); their radiation doses were not estimated (Darby, 1993). New Zealand subjects in the same testing were not at increased risk (SIR = 0 vs. 5.6 in unexposed workers, 90% CI = 0.0–3.1) (Pearce and Reif, 1990). Czech uranium miners with cumulative radon exposures of 210 to 329 and 330 or more "working level months" were at 1.9-fold ($n = 1$) and 4.4-fold ($n = 2$) risk of myeloma (Darby, 1993). In addition, the American Cancer Society case-control study noted a 1.9-fold risk of mortality (95% CI = 0.8–4.8) following occupational exposure to x-rays and radioactive materials (Boffetta et al., 1989).

Two cohort studies of medical radiology workers have been conducted. In China, no myeloma cases were diagnosed, although only 0.5 were expected, among 27,000 radiology workers (Wang et al., 1988). In the United States, physicians listed by the American Board of Radiologists in 1950 or 1960 were at a 5-fold risk of dying from myeloma (95% CI = 1.6–12) (Lewis, 1963).

Doses received during therapeutic irradiation can be high. However, both therapeutic and diagnostic irradiation are directed to a focal area, whereas the doses received by the atomic bomb survivors and by occupational cohorts were relatively uniform over the body. Three cohort studies and five case-control studies of the relation between myeloma and therapeutic irradiation have been reported. Risk of myeloma was

**TABLE 8-4**

## Summary of Studies That Have Assessed the Risk of Multiple Myeloma in Relation to Ionizing Radiation

| Study | Study Location and Design | Study Period | Comparison | No. of Exposed Cases | Effect Estimate | 95% CI |
|---|---|---|---|---|---|---|
| **A-Bomb Survivors** | | | | | | |
| Shimizu et al., 1990 | Japan, cohort mortality | 1950–85 | Increased risk per 1 Gy bone marrow dose | 23 | 3.3 | 1.7–6.3 |
| Preston et al., 1994 | Japan, cohort incidence | 1950–87 | Increased risk per Sv bone marrow dose | 59 | 1.3 | — |
| **Nuclear Workers** | | | | | | |
| Gilbert et al., 1989 | Three US nuclear weapons plants, cohort mortality | 1943–81 | External dose ≥10 years earlier, Sv | | | |
| | | | 0.001–0.009 vs. general population | 8 | 0.9 | — |
| | | | 0.010–0.049 | 1 | 0.4 | — |
| | | | 0.050–0.099 | 1 | 3.3 | — |
| | | | 0.100–0.199 | 1 | 5.0 | — |
| | | | ≥0.200 | 1 | 33.0 | — |
| Cardis et al., 1995 | Canada, UK, US study, nuclear industry workers, cohort mortality | 1944–88 | Nuclear industry workers vs. general population cumulative dose, mSv | | | |
| | | | 0–9 | 28 | 1.1 | 0.7–1.5 |
| | | | 10–19 | 3 | 0.6 | 0.1–1.7 |
| | | | 20–49 | 1 | 0.2 | 0.0–1.2 |
| | | | 50–99 | 5 | 1.9 | 0.6–4.3 |
| | | | 100–199 | 3 | 1.4 | 0.3–1.2 |
| | | | 200–399 | 2 | 1.1 | 0.1–3.8 |
| | | | 400+ | 2 | 2.5 | 0.3–9.0 |
| Muirhead et al., 1999 | National Registry for Radiation Workers, UK, cohort mortality | 1976–92 | Registered persons vs. general population, mSv | 40 | 0.7 | 0.5–1.0 |
| | | | <10 | 20 | 1.0 | 0.6–1.5 |
| | | | 10–19 | 4 | 0.8 | 0.2–2.1 |
| | | | 20–49 | 3 | 0.4 | 0.1–1.3 |
| | | | 50–99 | 8 | 2.3 | 1.0–4.6 |
| | | | 100–199 | 0 | 0.0 | 0.0–1.5 |
| | | | 200–399 | 3 | 1.8 | 0.4–5.2 |
| | | | 400+ | 2 | 2.5 | 0.3–9.1 |
| Kendall et al., 1992 | National Registry for Radiation Workers, UK, cohort mortality | 1976–83 | Registered persons vs. general population | 17 | 0.7 | — |
| Omar et al., 1999 | Sellafield plant, UK, cohort, mortality | 1947–92 | External dose, mSv | | | |
| | | | <10 | 0 | 0.0 | 0.0–16.1 |
| | | | 10–19 | 0 | 0.8 | 0.0–4.6 |
| | | | 20–49 | 2 | 1.3 | 0.2–4.8 |
| | | | 50–99 | 3 | 2.5 | 0.5–7.3 |
| | | | 100–199 | 1 | 0.9 | 0.0–5.1 |
| | | | 200–399 | 0 | 0.0 | 0.0–3.4 |
| | | | 400+ | 2 | 2.0 | 0.2–7.2 |
| Smith and Douglas, 1986 | Sellafield plant, UK, cohort, mortality | 1947–83 | External dose, mSv | | | |
| | | | <10 | 0 | 0.0 | 0.0–3.7 |
| | | | 10–19 | 0 | 0.0 | 0.0–6.1 |
| | | | 20–49 | 2 | 1.5 | 0.2–5.6 |
| | | | 50–99 | 3 | 1.8 | 0.2–6.6 |
| | | | 100–199 | 1 | 1.0 | 0.0–5.6 |
| | | | 200–399 | 0 | 0.0 | 0.0–27.6 |
| | | | 400+ | 2 | 2.2 | 0.3–8.0 |

*Continued*

**TABLE 8-4**

## Summary of Studies That Have Assessed the Risk of Multiple Myeloma in Relation to Ionizing Radiation—cont'd

| Study | Study Location and Design | Study Period | Comparison | No. of Exposed Cases | Effect Estimate | 95% CI |
|---|---|---|---|---|---|---|
| Carpenter et al., 1994 | Combined analyses of three UK nuclear industry workforce, cohort mortality | 1946–88 | Employed by three UK nuclear industry workforce vs. general population, cumulative whole body dose, mSv | | | |
| | | | <10 | 6 | 1.0 (ref.) | — |
| | | | 10–19 | 1 | 0.5 | — |
| | | | 20–49 | 2 | 0.6 | — |
| | | | 50–99 | 4 | 1.9 | — |
| | | | 100–199 | 2 | 1.4 | — |
| | | | 200–399 | 0 | 0.0 | — |
| | | | 400+ | 2 | 1.9 | — |
| Beral et. al., 1985 | UK Atomic Energy Authority, cohort mortality | 1946–79 | Employed by AEA vs. general population, median external dose <0.010 Sv | 8 | 0.8 | 0.4–1.6 |
| Pearce et al., 1990 | New Zealand, cohort mortality | 1957–87 | Nuclear weapons test workers vs. unexposed workers; doses not estimated | 0 | 0.0 | 0.0–3.1[†] |
| Iwasaki et al., | Nuclear industry workers in Japan | 1986–97 | Cumulative dose categories, mSv | | | |
| | | | <10 | 6 | 1.0 | 0.4–2.2 |
| | | | 10–20 | 0 | 0.0 | 0.0–4.7 (ref.) |
| | | | 20–50 | 0 | 0.0 | 0.0–4.6 |
| | | | 50–100 | 1 | 3.63 | 0.09–20.0 |
| | | | 100+ | 1 | 4.22 | 0.2–40.2 |
| Wing et al., 2000 | Three US nuclear weapons plants, case-control | 1979–90 | Cumulative dose categories, cumulative dose at ages 45 and above, 5-year lag, mSv | | | |
| | | | <10 | 83 | 1.0 (ref.) | — |
| | | | 10–49 | 5 | 0.8 | — |
| | | | 50–99 | 3 | 3.6 | — |
| | | | >100 | 7 | 5.2 | — |
| Darby et al., 1993 | UK, case-control | 1952–90 | Nuclear weapons test workers vs. unexposed workers; doses not estimated | 6 | 1.5 | 0.6–4.3 |
| Boffetta et al., 1989 | American Cancer Society, US, nested case-control | 1982–86 | Ever vs. never occupationally exposed to x-rays or radioactive materials | 7 | 1.9 | 0.8–4.8 |
| **Radiology Workers** | | | | | | |
| Wang et al., 1988 | China, cohort incidence | 1950–80 | Diagnostic x-ray workers vs. general population | 0 | 0.0 | 0.0–6.0 |
| Lewis, 1963 | US radiologist, cohort mortality | 1948–61 | Employed as radiologist vs. general population | 5 | 5.0 | 1.6–12.0 |

*Continued*

### TABLE 8-4

## Summary of Studies That Have Assessed the Risk of Multiple Myeloma in Relation to Ionizing Radiation—cont'd

| Study | Study Location and Design | Study Period | Comparison | No. of Exposed Cases | Effect Estimate | 95% CI |
|---|---|---|---|---|---|---|
| **Therapeutic Irradiation** | | | | | | |
| Boice et al., 1985 | International, cohort incidence | — | Exposed to cervical radiation ≥15 yr vs. unexposed; average bone marrow dose approximately 10 Gy | 33 | 2.0 | 1.1–3.2 |
| Darby et al., 1987 | England and N. Ireland ankylosing spondylitis patients, cohort mortality | 1935–83 | Single course of x-ray treatment ≥5 yr earlier vs. none; Skeletal dose approximately 3 Gy | 8 | 1.7 | — |
| Boice et al., 1988 | International, case-control study of cervical cancer patients | — | Bone marrow dose: | | | |
| | | | 2–4 vs. <2 Gy | 12 | 0.3 | 0.0–2.6[†] |
| | | | 5–9 vs. <2 Gy | 23 | 0.2 | 0.0–1.4[†] |
| | | | ≥10 vs. <2 Gy | 11 | 0.6 | 0.1–5.2[†] |
| Boffetta et al., 1989 | See above | | X-ray treatment vs. none | 14 | 1.6 | 0.8–3.0 |
| Darby et al., 1994 | Scotland, metropathia hemorrhagica patients cohort mortality | 1940–86 | Radiographic treatment 5 years earlier vs. general population, mean bone marrow dose = 1.3 Gy | 9 | 2.6 | 1.2–4.9 |
| Eriksson et al., 1993 | Northern Sweden, population-based case-control | 1982–86 | Ever vs. never received radiotherapy | 10 | 0.7 | 0.3–1.8 |
| Flodin et al., 1987 | Southeast Sweden, population-based case-control | 1973–83 | X-ray treatment vs. none | 4 | 0.9 | 0.3–2.7 |
| Friedman, 1986 | Kaiser Permanente, northern California, population-based case-control | 1969–82 | Ever vs. never exposed to x-ray therapy | 9[‡] | 1.9 | 0.9–4.2 |
| **Diagnostic Radiation** | | | | | | |
| Andersson and Storm, 1992 | Danish neurology patients, cohort mortality | 1946–88 | Throtrast injection vs. general population | 4 | 4.6 | 1.2–12.0 |
| Davis et al., 1989 | Massachusetts tuberculosis patients, cohort mortality | 1925–86 | Ever vs. never received x-ray fluoroscopy examination; mean dose = 0.09 Gy | 2 | 0.4 | 0.1–1.8 |
| Boffetta et al., 1989 | See above | See above | Diagnostic x-rays, above vs. below median number, median not reported | 62 | 0.9 | 0.6–1.4 |
| Hatcher et al., 2001 | Three areas of US | 1986–89 | Diagnostic x-rays | | | |
| | | | <5 | 106 | 1.0 (ref.) | — |
| | | | 5–9 | 104 | 0.9 | 0.7–1.2 |
| | | | 10–19 | 133 | 1.0 | 0.7–1.3 |
| | | | 20+ | 137 | 0.9 | 0.7–1.2 |
| Boice et al., 1991 | Kaiser Permanente, population-based case-control | 1956–82 | Bone marrow dose >2 years earlier: exposed to ≥0.01 Gy | 198 | | |
| | | | 0.01 vs. 0 Gy | | 1.3 | — |
| | | | 0.02 vs. 0 Gy | | 1.5 | — |
| | | | 0.03 vs. 0 Gy | | 1.3 | — |
| | | | 0.04 vs. 0 Gy | | 3.9 | — |

*Continued*

## TABLE 8-4
### Summary of Studies That Have Assessed the Risk of Multiple Myeloma in Relation to Ionizing Radiation—cont'd

| Study | Study Location and Design | Study Period | Comparison | No. of Exposed Cases | Effect Estimate | 95% CI |
|---|---|---|---|---|---|---|
| Cuzick and De Stavola, 1988 | England & Wales, hospital-based case-control | 1978–84 | Number of diagnostic x-rays: | | | |
| | | | 1–4 vs. 0 | 86 | 0.8[§] | — |
| | | | 5–8 vs. 0 | 79 | 0/7[§] | — |
| | | | ≥9 vs. 0 | 181 | 0/7[§] | — |
| Eriksson, 1993 | See above | See above | 5 vs. ≤4 | 65 | 0.6 | 0.3–11 |
| | | | 6–10 vs. ≤4 | 29 | 0.5 | 0.3–0.9 |
| | | | 11–20 vs. ≤4 | 20 | 0.8 | 0.4–1.5 |
| | | | ≥21 vs. ≤4 | 16 | 0.9 | 0.4–2.1 |
| Flodin et al., 1987 | See above | See above | Heavy vs. light x-ray examination 10–30 years earlier | 2 | 2.9 | 0.4–19.0 |

* Studies of ionizing radiation use various units of dose, including Sievert (Sv) and Gray (Gy), which are Standard International units, and rem (1 Sv = 100 rem) and rad (1 Gy = 100 rad). Sv is related to Gy as follows: Sv = Gy × Q, where Q is the "quality factor," i.e., the biologic potency of the specfic type of radiation relative to orthovoltage x-rays; although not standardized, gamma rays are often assigned a Q of 1, and fast neutrons a Q of 10. Dose can be expressed as external radiation dose (whole body dose, shielded kerma) or organ dose.

† 90% confidence interval.

‡ No. of discordant pairs in which only the case was exposed.

§ Unadjusted odds ratio.

increased among women who were estimated to have received a mean bone marrow dose of 10 Gy during therapy for cervical cancer; after 15 years, there was a 2.0-fold risk (95% CI = 1.1–3.2) (Boice et al., 1985). Boice et al. also conducted a nested case-control study using the cervical cancer cohort described previously, along with additional subjects, to obtain more precise information on radiation exposures (Boice et al., 1988). In the case-control study, no excess risk was noted among women who received an average marrow dose of 7.1 Gy compared with those who received less than 2.0 Gy (OR = 0.3, 90% CI = 0.1–1.4); no relation was observed even after excluding women who had been followed for less than 15 years. Furthermore, the investigators found no evidence that risk increased with increasing radiation dose above 2 Gy. The authors stated that the only differences between the case-control and cohort studies were the following:

1. The number of women with myeloma—34 in the cohort and 46 in the case-control study;

2. The comparison group—population rates were used for the cohort study, whereas patients with cervical cancer who did not undergo radiotherapy were used for the case-control study.

Compared with individuals who had never undergone x-ray therapy, myeloma mortality was modestly elevated in a cohort of patients receiving a single course of x-ray treatment for ankylosing spondylitis

(RR = 1.7, n = 8) (Darby et al., 1987) or metropathia hemorrhagica (RR = 2.6, 95% CI = 1.2–4.9) (Darby et al., 1994), among American Cancer Society subjects who had received x-ray treatment for any condition (OR = 1.6, 95% CI = 0.8–3.0) (Boffetta et al., 1989), and among Kaiser Permanente members who had received x-ray treatment for any condition (OR = 1.9, 95% CI = 0.9–4.2) (Friedman, 1986), but not among subjects who reported a history of radiotherapy for any condition in two Swedish population-based case-control studies (OR = 0.9, 95% CI = 0.3–2.7, Flodin et al., 1987; OR = 0.7, 95% CI = 0.3–1.8, Eriksson, 1993). Compared with the general population, myeloma incidence was elevated 4.6-fold (95% CI = 1.2–12) among 1095 Danish patients exposed to alpha-emitting Thorotrast used with cerebral arteriography (Andersson and Storm, 1992). A single diagnostic x-ray received by Massachusetts patients with tuberculosis did not increase their risk of myeloma (RR = 0.4, 95% CI = 0.1–1.8) (Davis et al., 1989). Having a relatively large number of diagnostic x-rays (more than the median) did not increase myeloma risk among American Cancer Society members (OR = 0.9, 95% CI = 0.6–1.4) (Boffetta et al., 1989), neither did having nine or more diagnostic x-rays in a UK case-control study (unadjusted OR = 0.7 relative to having no exams, number of exposed individuals = 81) (Cuzick and De Stavola, 1988). In a Swedish case-control study conducted between 1973 and 1983, individuals who received "heavy" levels of x-ray examinations had a 2.9-fold risk of myeloma (95% CI = 0.4–19) relative to individuals who received "light" levels (Flodin et al., 1987). In a later study set in northern Sweden, risk was reduced among persons who reported a history of five or more x-rays compared with those who reported a history of four or fewer; however, risk increased with increasing numbers of examinations such that exposure to 21 or more resulted in an odds ratio of 0.9 (95% CI = 0.4–2.1) compared with the odds ratio of 0.5 (95% CI = 0.3–0.9) for exposure to 6 to 10 examinations (Eriksson, 1993). At Kaiser Permanente, bone marrow doses of 0.04 Gy or more were related to a 3.9-fold increased risk of myeloma, and there was some evidence that increasing doses were related to increasing risk (see Table 8-4) (Boice et al., 1991). The authors remarked that categorizing the data on the basis of number of procedures resulted in substantial misclassification; for example, five or fewer x-ray procedures led to a range in the bone marrow dose of 0.00001 to 0.03 Gy, whereas the range for 15 or more x-ray procedures was 0.001 to 0.23 Gy. The discordance between the number of prior x-ray examinations and bone marrow dose was caused by differences in procedures; for example, an upper gastrointestinal procedure contributed 60 times more radiation to the bone marrow than a chest roentgenogram (Boice et al., 1991). Failure to take into account this source of misclassification might account for the negative findings in some studies (Boffetta et al., 1989; Cuzick and De Stavola, 1988; Eriksson, 1993). In a population-based case-control study in three US areas, there was no association between myeloma and the total number of reported x-rays of any type (OR = 2.0, 95% CI = 0.7–1.2) (Hatcher et al., 2001). There was no evidence of excess risk of myeloma among individuals who reported exposure to 10 or more diagnostic x-rays with high bone marrow dose, as compared with individuals reporting no such exposures (OR = 0.7, 95% CI = 0.4–1.3).

There is evidence from studies of atomic bomb survivors, occupational groups with exposure to approximately 0.05 Sv or more, persons exposed to therapeutic radiation, and from a carefully conducted study of diagnostic procedures (Boice et al., 1991) that ionizing radiation causes myeloma. It has also been reported that administration of ionizing radiation to rhesus monkeys was followed by an increased incidence of MGUS and myeloma (Radl et al., 1991). However, there are inconsistencies in the body of evidence, for example, from the two studies of the atomic bomb survivors and from the two studies of women who received radiotherapy for cervical cancer. There are also differences in the reported dose-response relations, but this could be due to differences in the quality and timing of exposure.

## Occupational Exposures

Because multiple myeloma is a relatively rare cancer, cohort studies of the relation between occupational exposures and myeloma have generally provided only limited information. The only cohort studies in which there were large numbers of myeloma cases have been those using census data; in such studies job title as recorded in the census was the only occupational exposure variable that could be reliably evaluated. Respondents in most interview-based case-control studies were asked whether they had ever been exposed to specific chemical and physical agents. However, it is possible that they knew the agents by different names, and self-reported occupational exposures are also subject to recall bias. The case-control studies generally were of limited power as well, in that only a small number of subjects had worked in the occupations and industries of interest. An exception is the case-control studies reported by Heineman et al. (Heineman et al., 1992) and Pottern et al. (Pottern et al., 1992b); they were based on work histories recorded in a national pension plan and included approximately 800 men and 600 women with myeloma. Characteristics of case-control studies that have evaluated the relation between occupation and myeloma are summarized in Table 8-4. Several studies have reported on cosmetologists and hairdressers as well; they are discussed in a later section in this chapter concerning personal and occupational exposure to hair coloring products.

### Agricultural Work and Pesticides

Numerous cohort (Cerhan et al., 1998; Lee et al., 2002; Nandakumar et al., 1988; Pukkala and Notkola, 1997; Stark et al., 1990; Steineck and Wiklund, 1986) and case-control studies (Alavanja et al., 1988; Boffetta et al., 1989; Brownson et al., 1989; Burmeister et al., 1983; Cantor and Blair, 1984; Costantini et al., 2001; Cuzick and De Stavola, 1988; Demers et al., 1993; Eriksson and Karlsson, 1992; Figgs et al., 1994; Flodin et al., 1987; Franceschi et al., 1993; Gallagher et al., 1983; Heineman et al., 1992; La Vecchia et al., 1989; Milham, 1971; Miligi et al., 1999; Nandakumar et al., 1986; Pasqualetti et al., 1990; Pearce and Howard, 1986; Pottern et al., 1992b; Reif et al., 1989a; Tollerud et al., 1985) of agricultural work in relation to myeloma occurrence have been conducted and most have observed relative risks exceeding 1.0 (Table 8-5), although some to only a very limited extent. One study that did not observe a positive relation was that of Tollerud et al. (Tollerud et al., 1985), which was one of several that ascertained occupational information from death certificates. A study in Italy found no increased risk for farmers, but did find a slight increased risk

## TABLE 8-5

### Design Characteristics of Case-Control Studies That Have Assessed the Risk of Multiple Myeloma in Relation to Job Title, Industry, or Specific Chemical and Physical Agents, Excluding Occupations and Exposures Related to Ionizing Radiation

| Study | Study Population and Period | Ascertainment of Exposure |
| --- | --- | --- |
| Alavanja et al., 1988 | Death certificates of persons who were employed at the US Department of Agriculture, 1970–79 | Employment as an agricultural extension agent ascertained from work records |
| Bethwaite et al., 1990 | Persons registered with the New Zealand tumor registry, 1981–84 | Most recent occupation at time of registration |
| Boffetta et al., 1989 | American Cancer Society members US, 1982–86 | Most recent occupation, occupation held for the longest period, and occupational and leisure-time exposure to 12 groups of agents |
| Brownson et al., 1989 | Persons registered with the Missouri tumor registry, US, 1984–88 | Most recent occupation at time of registration |
| Burmeister et al., 1983 | Death certificates, Iowa, US, 1964–78 | Most recent occupation as recorded on the death certificate |
| Cantor and Blair, 1984 | Death certificates, Wisconsin, US, 1968–76 | Most recent occupation as recorded on the death certificate |
| Costantini et al., 2001 | General population, Italy, 1991–93 | Occupational history ascertained during interview |
| Cuzick and De Stavola, 1988 | Hospital patients, six area in England and Wales, 1978–84 | Occupational history and occupational exposure to various agents ascertained during interview |
| Demers et al., 1993 | General population, four SEER areas, US, 1977–81 | Work history categorized by job title and industry ascertained during interview |
| Eriksson and Karlsson, 1992 | General population, northern Sweden, 1982–86 | Occupational history and occupational exposure to various agents ascertained during interview |
| Flodin et al., 1987 | General population, southeast Sweden, 1973–83 | Occupational history and occupational exposure to various agents ascertained from a mailed questionnaire |
| Franceschi et al., 1993 | Hospital patients, northeast Italy | Occupational history ascertained during interview |
| Friedman, 1986 | Kaiser Permanente members, northern California, US, 1969–82 | Occupation recorded on the medical chart 6 months or earlier prior to the reference date |
| Fritschi et al., 2002 | Myeloma cases recorded in the National Enhanced Cancer Surveillance System; General population controls, US, 1994–98 | Occupational history ascertained by mailed questionnaire |
| Gallagher et al., 1983 | Patients admitted to a Vancouver, BC cancer center, 1972–81 | Occupational history ascertained during interview |
| Heineman et al., 1992 | General population, Denmark, 1970–84 | Industrial history recorded since 1964 in the nationwide pension fund program; occupation recorded on the most recent tax records; job-exposure matrix developed by an industrial hygienist |
| Kawachi et al., 1989 | Persons registered with the New Zealand tumor registry, 1980–84 | Most recent occupation at time of registration |
| La Vecchia et al., 1989 | Hospital patients, Milan, 1983–88 | Occupational history and occupational exposures to various agents ascertained during interview |
| Linet et al., 1987 | Hospital patients, Baltimore, Maryland, US, 1975–82 | Occupational history and occupational exposure to various agents ascertained during interview |
| Milham, 1971 | Death certificates, Washington and Oregon, US, 1950–67 | Most recent occupation as recorded on the death certificate |

*Continued*

**TABLE 8-5**

Design Characteristics of Case-Control Studies That Have Assessed the Risk of Multiple Myeloma in Relation to Job Title, Industry, or Specific Chemical and Physical Agents, Excluding Occupations and Exposures Related to Ionizing Radiation—cont'd

| Study | Study Population and Period | Ascertainment of Exposure |
|---|---|---|
| Miligi et al., 1999 | General population, Italy, 1991–93 | Occupational history ascertained during interview |
| Morris et al., 1986 | General population, four SEER areas, US, 1977–81 | Formation of ever/never categories of exposure to various agents from responses to specific questions about a history of "high" exposures |
| Nandakumar et al., 1986 | Death certificates, Western Australia, 1975–84 | Most recent occupation as recorded on the death certificate |
| Pasqualetti et al., 1990 | Hospital patients resident in referral basin of Aquila and Avezzano, Italy, 1970–88 | Occupational history and ever exposure to classes of chemicals ascertained during interview |
| Pearce et al., 1986 | Persons registered with the New Zealand tumor registry, 1977–81 | Occupational history and occupational exposure to pesticides ascertained during interview |
| Pottern et al., 1992 | Women from the general population, Denmark, 1970–84 | Industrial history recorded since 1964 in the nationwide pension fund program; occupation recorded on the most recent tax records; job-exposure matrix developed by an industrial hygienist |
| Reif et al., 1989a | Persons registered with the New Zealand tumor registry, 1980–84 | Most recent occupation at time of registration |
| Schwartz et al., 1988 | General population, four SEER areas, US, 1977–81 | Probability and intensity of exposure to low, medium, and high levels of asbestos based on a job-exposure matrix from an occupational history |
| Tollerud et al., 1985 | Death certificates, North Carolina, US, 1956–80 | Most recent occupation as recorded on the death certificate |
| Wong et al., 1995 | Members of a cohort of petroleum workers, US | Estimated exposure to total hydrocarbons based on historical records |

(OR = 1.3) for agricultural and animal husbandry workers (Costantini et al., 2001; Miligi et al., 1999). No increased risk was associated with farming occupation among women in Denmark (Pottern et al., 1992b). However, any work in the agricultural products industry was associated with myeloma (OR = 1.5).

Four studies considered duration of employment as a farmer. A trend of increasing relative risk with duration was noted by Demers et al. (Demers et al., 1993) (less than 10 y, OR = 1.1; 10 y or longer, OR = 1.3), Alavanja et al. (Alavanja et al., 1988) (less than 15 y,

OR = 0.2; 15 y or longer, OR = 2.6), and Boffetta et al. (Boffetta et al., 1989) (20 y or less, OR = 0.0; 21–40 y, OR = 1.7; longer than 40 y, OR = 4.3), but not by Heineman et al. (Heineman et al., 1992)(employment in agricultural industry: 5 y or less, OR = 1.1; more than 5 y, OR = 0.8).

Following the observation that agricultural workers were at increased risk of myeloma, exposure to pesticides (i.e., insecticides, herbicides, fungicides) was hypothesized as the basis for the association. Two case-control studies that sought to estimate the risk of myeloma in relation to agricultural work and pesticide exposure as independent factors observed that myeloma risk was greater for individuals exposed to both factors than for individuals exposed to either factor alone. Boffetta et al. reported the following results for comparisons using persons with neither exposure as the referent: pesticides alone, OR = 1.0; farming alone, OR = 1.7; both pesticides and farming, OR = 4.3 (Boffetta et al., 1989). The results of Demers et al. were as follows: pesticides alone, OR = 2.1; farming alone, OR = 1.4; both pesticides and farming, OR = 7.9 (Demers et al., 1993). At an ecologic level, Burmeister et al. found that farming occupation was more strongly associated with myeloma mortality among residents of 33 Iowa counties with the highest herbicide and insecticide use, compared with the association among the counties with the lowest use (OR for mortality from myeloma associated with farming occupation for men born after the year 1900: counties with the highest herbicide use, OR = 2.4, $p < 0.05$; counties with the lowest herbicide use, OR = 1.2; counties with the highest insecticide use, OR = 2.0, $p < 0.05$, counties with the lowest insecticide use, OR = 1.2) (Burmeister et al., 1983).

Most of the studies of myeloma risk in relation to pesticide exposure had very limited exposure assessment, giving few leads to specific pesticides as potential risk factors. In a cohort study covering the period from 1965 to 1982 in which licensed Swedish agricultural pesticide applicators were compared with agricultural workers who had not been exposed to pesticides, Wiklund et al. (Wiklund et al., 1989) did not find an increased risk of myeloma (OR = 1.0, 95% CI = 0.5–1.9). Conversely, in a cohort study of Dutch licensed applicators that only applied herbicides, myeloma mortality was elevated by a factor of 8.2 (95% CI = 1.6–23) compared with the general population (Swaen et al., 1992). The most heavily used herbicides to which the applicators were exposed during the time period of interest were simazine, chlorothiamide, dalapon, dichlorbenil, and diuron. Myeloma mortality was significantly increased in a cohort of workers who applied the insecticide DDT during antimalarial campaigns in Italy between 1956 and 1992 (PMR = 3.4; 95% CI = 1.1–8.0) (Cocco et al., 1997), although no association was found between myeloma mortality and DDT residues in adipose tissue among the general US population from 22 states (Cocco et al., 2000). One study estimated the risk of myeloma associated with specific pesticide classes in a multivariable model while adjusting for other pesticides and farm animal exposures (Eriksson and Karlsson, 1992). Myeloma risk was associated with exposure to phenoxyacetic acids (OR = 1.9, 95% CI = 0.8–4.4) and DDT (OR = 1.4, 95% CI = 0.9–2.3), but not chlorophenols (OR = 0.9, 95% CI = 0.4–1.8). Evidence for a positive association

between pesticide exposure and myeloma was also provided by several case-control studies that did not take into account potential confounding by other aspects of agricultural work (Burmeister, 1990; Flodin et al., 1987; Morris et al., 1986; Pasqualetti et al., 1990; Pottern et al., 1992b). Besides the cohort study of Wiklund et al. (Wiklund et al., 1989), other studies that observed no relation between a history of pesticide exposure and myeloma risk were those of La Vecchia et al. (unadjusted OR = 0.9; number of exposed cases = 4) (La Vecchia et al., 1989), Pearce et al. (phenoxyherbicides, OR = 1.3, 95% CI = 0.8–2.5; chlorophenols, OR = 1.1, 95% CI = 0.4–2.7) (Pearce et al., 1986), and Heineman et al. (OR = 0.9, 95% CI = 0.5–1.5) (Heineman et al., 1992).

When interpreting results from these studies, it should be noted that dioxin (2,3,7,8-tetrachlorodibenzo-p-dioxin) has been a chemical contaminant in certain formulations of several commonly used herbicides, including phenoxyherbicides. In Seveso, Italy, where an industrial accident in 1976 exposed the local population to high levels of dioxin, myeloma incidence in the subsequent 10 years was elevated in both men (RR = 3.2, 95% CI = 0.8–13.3) and women (RR = 5.2, 95% CI = 1.2–22.6) (Bertazzi et al., 1993). Because dioxin has been a chemical contaminant of herbicides and has been associated with myeloma risk, epidemiologic studies of myeloma in relation to herbicide exposures should consider the possibility of dioxin as an etiologic agent in addition to the herbicide active ingredients.

Besides pesticides, other specific exposures common among farmers include paints, solvents, wood-treatment chemicals used for fencing, engine exhaust, welding fumes, dusts, animals, zoonotic infections, and pollen (Blair et al., 1985; Pearce and Reif, 1990). Efforts to identify myeloma risk in relation to animal exposures have been made in several studies (Eriksson and Karlsson, 1992; Pearce et al., 1986; Reif et al., 1989a). In the study by Pearce et al. conducted in New Zealand (Pearce et al., 1986), in which 36% of the control subjects reported having a history of employment as a farmer, the magnitude of the relation between farming and myeloma varied somewhat by type of farming (categories not mutually exclusive), as follows: orchard farmers (OR = 2.8), produce farmers (OR = 2.0), sheep farmers (OR = 1.9), mixed sheep and beef farmers (OR = 1.3), dairy farmers (OR = 1.4), and poultry farmers (OR = 0.9). Rather different results were obtained in another study conducted in New Zealand for orchard and crop farmers (OR = 0.5), livestock farmers (OR = 0.9), and dairy farmers (OR = 1.5) (Reif et al., 1989a).

Pearce et al. found little difference in the risk associated with exposure to specific animals, including sheep,

=== **TABLE 8-6** ===

## Summary of Studies That Have Assessed the Risk of Multiple Myeloma in Relation to Agricultural Work

| Study | Measure of Exposure | Prevalence of Exposure in Control Subjects (%) | Number of Exposed Cases* | Effect Estimate (95% Confidence Interval) |
|---|---|---|---|---|
| **Cohort Studies** | | | | |
| Cerhan et al., 1988 | Farmer as usual occupation listed on the death certificate | — | — | 1.2 (1.0–1.4) |
| Lee et al., 2002 | Farmer occupation in the crop or livestock industry as listed in the National Occupational Mortality Surveillance data system | — | 746 (crop farmer) | 1.1 (1.0–1.2) |
| | | | 186 (livestock Farmers) | 1.2 (1.0–1.4) |
| Nandakumar et al., 1988 | Farming occupation as recorded in the cancer registry | — | 15 | 1.3 (0.9–1.9) |
| Pukkala and Notkola, 1997 | Farmers registered in the Farm Register of Finland | — | — | 1.0 (0.8–1.1), men 0.9 (0.7–1.2), women |
| Stark et al., 1990 | Membership in New York State Farm Bureau | — | 11 O / 9 E | 1.1† |
| Steineck and Wiklund, 1986 | Agricultural occupations | — | 568/4330717 PY | 1.2 (1.1–1.3) |
| Vagero and Persson, 1986 | Self-employed in agriculture | — | 347 | 1.2 (1.0–1.3) |
| **Case-Control Studies** | | | | |
| Alavanja et al., 1988 | Agricultural extension agents | — | 7 | 1.1 (0.4–2.9) |
| Boffetta et al., 1989 | Farmers | 5.5 | 16 | 3.4 (1.5–7.5) |
| Brownson et al., 1989 | Farmers | 11 | 24 | 1.4 (0.9–2.2) |
| Burmeister et al., 1983 | Farmers | — | 550 | 1.5† |
| Cantor and Blair, 1984 | Farmers | 21.7 | 110 | 1.4 (1.0–1.8) |
| Costantini et al., 2001 | Farmers | — | 22 | 0.7 (0.5–1.2) |
| | Agricultural and animal husbandry workers | — | 30 | 1.3 (0.8–2.2) |
| Cuzick and De Stavola, 1988 | Farmers | 4.5 | 28 | 1.6† |
| | Food processing/agricultural industry | 10.3 | 72 | 1.8† |
| Demers et al., 1993 | Farmers | 3.3 | 26 | 1.2 (0.8–2.5) |
| | Farmworkers and gardeners | 8.2 | 57 | 1.0 (0.8–1.6) |
| | Agricultural industry | 10.8 | 19 | 1.2 (1.0–1.9) |
| Eriksson and Karlsson, 1992 | Farmers | 47.3 | 151 | 1.7 (1.2–2.3) |
| Figgs et al., 1994 | Farm worker supervisor | — | 5 | 2.5 (0.8–7.3) |
| Flodin et al., 1987 | Farmers | 12.3 | 29 | 1.4 (0.8–2.5) |
| Franceschi et al., 1993 | Farmers | 16.4 | 20 | 1.3 (0.7–2.3) |
| Gallagher et al., 1983 | Farmworkers | 22.6 | 31 | 2.2 (1.2–4.0) |
| Heineman et al., 1992 | Farm owners | 10.0 | 84 | 1.0 (0.8–1.3) |
| | Tenant farmers or agricultural garden workers | 10.4 | 98 | 1.1 (0.9–1.5) |
| | Herdsmen | 0.3 | 4 | 1.8 (0.5–6.6) |
| | Nurserymen | 0.3 | 3 | 1.3 (0.3–5.5) |
| | Other specialty farmworkers | 0.1 | 5 | 4.6 (1.1–20.3) |
| | Agricultural industry | 5.3 | 45 | 1.1 (0.8–1.5) |
| | Truck garden/orchard/nursery industry | 1.0 | 10 | 1.3 (0.6–2.8) |
| La Vecchia et al., 1989 | Agricultural occupations | — | — | 2.0 (1.1–3.5) |
| Milham, 1971 | Farmers | 7.3 | 60 | 1.8† |
| Miligi et al., 1999 | Farmers | — | 12 | 0.7 (0.4–1.5) |
| | Agricultural and animal husbandry workers | — | 21 | 1.3 (0.7–2.3) |
| | Orchard, vineyard, and related workers | — | 15 | 1.8 (0.9–3.5) |

*Continued*

===== **TABLE 8-6** =====

## Summary of Studies That Have Assessed the Risk of Multiple Myeloma in Relation to Agricultural Work—cont'd

| Study | Measure of Exposure | Prevalence of Exposure in Control Subjects (%) | Number of Exposed Cases* | Effect Estimate (95% Confidence Interval) |
|---|---|---|---|---|
| Nandakumar et al., 1986 | Farmers | 11.4 | 21 | 1.4 (0.8–2.5) |
| Pasqualetti et al., 1990 | Agricultural workers | 18.8 | 44 | 2.7 (1.9–4.4) |
| Pearce et al., 1986 | Farmers | 35.9 | 43 | 1.7 (1.0–2.9) |
| | Sheep farmers | 5.7 | 18 | 1.9 (1.0–3.6) |
| | Dairy farmers | 7.3 | 23 | 1.4 (0.8–2.5) |
| | Livestock farmers | 3.5 | 11 | 1.3 (0.6–2.6) |
| | Crop farmers | 1.0 | 5 | 2.0 (0.6–6.0) |
| | Poultry farmers | 0.3 | 1 | 0.9 (0.1–8.4) |
| | Orchard farmers | 0.6 | 2 | 2.8 (0.5–16.9) |
| Pottern et al., 1992b | Farm/land owner, farmer | 0.7 | 14 | 0.9 (0.3–3.0) |
| | Agricultural products industry | 2.7 | 14 | 1.5 (0.8–2.8) |
| | Orchards/nurseries industry | 2.0 | 11 | 1.5 (0.7–3.2) |
| Reif et al., 1989a | Farmers | 15.1 | 54 | 1.2 (0.9–1.6) |
| | General farmers | — | — | 1.3 (0.9–1.7) |
| | Dairy farmers | — | — | 1.5 (0.6–3.3) |
| | Livestock farmers | — | — | 0.9 (0.3–2.8) |
| | Orchard and crop farmers | — | — | 0.5 (0.1–1.9) |
| Tollerud et al., 1985 | Farmers | 19 | 39 | 0.6[†] |

* For cohort studies, the number of person years (PY), or observed (O) and expected (E) cases are presented, where available.
[†]Unadjusted odds ratio.

cows, beef cattle, poultry, and pigs, with odds ratios ranging from 1.3 to 1.7. Many of the respondents who did not report a history of agricultural employment nonetheless reported prior exposure to farm animals (for example, 23% of control subjects reported employment on a dairy farm, whereas 40% reported contact with dairy cows). In the study by Eriksson and Karlsson conducted in northern Sweden (Eriksson and Karlsson, 1992) in which 47% of respondents reported having a history of farming, the relation between exposure to specific farm animals and myeloma occurrence was evaluated after taking into consideration exposure to other farm animals, with the following results: horses, OR = 1.6 (number of exposed cases = 137); cattle, OR = 1.5 (number of exposed cases = 152); goats, OR = 1.5 (number of exposed cases = 24); hogs, OR = 0.9 (number of exposed cases = 124); and poultry, OR = 0.7 (number of exposed cases = 86). Little association with myeloma risk was found for exposure to beef or dairy cattle in a case-control study in Canada (Fritschi et al., 2002), but imprecise elevated risks were observed for poultry (OR = 1.6, 95% CI = 0.4–6.8) and horses (OR = 1.7, 95% CI = 0.2–13.9). Clearly, these contradictory results indicate that further investigation is needed to disentangle specific etiologic factors responsible for the increased risk of myeloma in agricultural occupations.

### Benzene and Other Organic Solvents

Rinsky et al. developed a job-exposure matrix for benzene using industrial hygiene data from an Ohio rubber plant and found a 2.5-fold risk of death from myeloma (95% CI = 0.7–4.8) associated with employment in benzene-exposed jobs (Rinsky et al., 2002). All of the myeloma cases were diagnosed 20 years or later after first exposure, but no patterns of risk with cumulative level of benzene exposure were apparent. Similar results of increased myeloma mortality (SMR = 2.3; 95% CI = 0.7–5.3) were observed in a cohort of chemical plant workers with low levels of benzene exposure, but there was no observed increased risk for maintenance workers suspected to have the highest benzene exposures (Ireland et al., 1997). No excess in myeloma incidence was observed in a large cohort of benzene-exposed workers in China (Hayes et al., 1997). There was also no association between occupational benzene exposure and myeloma occurrence in two case-control studies (Heineman et al., 1992; Linet et al., 1987), with exposures assigned based on self-report or according to occupation and industry.

The broad grouping of organic solvents, which includes benzene, has been investigated in two meta-analyses of cancer risk. In a meta-analysis of 55 cohort mortality studies across different industries with probable exposure to organic solvents, there was only a slightly increased risk for death from myeloma (SMR = 1.1, 95% CI = 8.3–15.6) (Chen and Seaton, 1996). A meta-analysis of case-control studies published from 1986 through 1994 found a slightly decreased risk of myeloma associated with exposure to organic solvents (OR = 0.7; 95% CI = 0.6–0.9) (Sonoda et al., 2001).

## Petroleum Refining and Distribution

Known carcinogens to which petroleum workers are exposed include polycyclic aromatic hydrocarbons and various solvents, which in the past might have included benzene. A meta-analysis of 22 cohort studies found that petroleum workers were at no increased risk of death from myeloma (SMR = 0.9; 95% CI = 0.8–1.1) (Wong, 1995). A cancer incidence study of a cohort of Australian petroleum industry workers found a 2.2-fold (95% CI = 0.6–5.6) risk for all men employed 5 years or longer in any department (Christie et al., 1991). The case-control study by Cuzick and De Stavola (Cuzick and De Stavola, 1988) noted that four cases but no controls had worked in the petroleum industry; however, three other case-control studies found no evidence for a relation (Demers et al., 1993; Eriksson and Karlsson, 1992; La Vecchia et al., 1989). Self-reported occupational exposure to petroleum was associated with increased myeloma risk in one case-control study (OR = 3.7, 95% CI = 1.3–10.3) (Linet et al., 1987).

## Rubber and Plastics Manufacturing

Rubber workers can be exposed to organic solvents, plastic monomers, rubber additives, and asbestos, and in the past, exposure to benzene was relatively high. Myeloma mortality was significantly increased among employees of a 1,3 butadiene monomer production facility who had worked 20 years or longer (SMR = 2.0, 95% CI = 0.5–50.3) (Divine and Hartman, 2001). Female workers from a cohort of rubber workers in the United States who were exposed between 1967 and 1973 were observed to be at increased risk of myeloma (RR = 2.3, n = 2 myeloma deaths) (Andjelkovich et al., 1978), but male members of the cohort were not (RR = 0.8, n = 5 myeloma deaths) (Andjelkovich et al., 1977). There was a greater than expected number of myeloma deaths in several cohorts of rubber workers,

but these elevations were based on small numbers of cases (Gustavsson et al., 1986; Wilczynska et al., 2001). No associations were found in a cohort of rubber workers in Great Britain followed from 1946 to 1985 (Sorahan and Cooke, 1989). Similarly, a meta-analysis of six case-control studies that evaluated myeloma risk associated with employment in workplaces producing rubber and/or plastic products (Demers et al., 1993; Figgs et al., 1994; Flodin et al., 1987; Heineman et al., 1992; Morris et al., 1986; Pottern et al., 1992b) found no association (OR = 1.1, 95% CI = 0.9–1.3) (Sonoda et al., 2001).

## Paint-Related Occupations

Painters are exposed to dyes and pigments, aromatic and aliphatic hydrocarbons, and low molecular weight solvents such as trichloroethylene and methylethyl ketone (Bethwaite et al., 1990). The majority of epidemiologic studies that have assessed it provide evidence for a relation between a history of paint-related occupation and myeloma risk. A cohort study of Swedish production workers in nine paint manufacturing companies who were employed for 5 years or longer from 1955 to 1975 observed a 5.5-fold risk (95% CI = 1.1–16) of myeloma; all of the workers who developed myeloma had received "high" exposures (RR = 10, n = 3) (Lundberg, 1986). A second Swedish cohort study using census information on occupation observed a 1.7-fold risk (n = 7) (McLaughlin et al., 1988). In six case-control studies, odds ratios of 1.6 to 3 were reported (Bethwaite et al., 1990; Cuzick and De Stavola, 1988; Demers et al., 1993; Friedman, 1986; Morris et al., 1986; Pasqualetti et al., 1990), but no association was observed in other studies conducted in Italy (unadjusted OR = 0.9, number of exposed cases = 5) (La Vecchia et al., 1989) or Denmark (women, OR = 0.7, 95% CI = 0.3–1.7) (Pottern et al., 1992b) (men, OR = 1.0, 95% CI = 0.5–2.1) (Heineman et al., 1992).

One study reported that myeloma risk increased with duration of employment as a painter (less than 10 y, OR = 1.4, 95% CI = 0.6–2.8; 10 y or longer, OR = 4.1, 95% CI = 1.8–10) and was stronger for individuals who reported relatively high exposure to paints or solvents (compared with low leisure-time exposure: high leisure-time exposure, OR = 1.6, 95% CI = 1.0–3.2; low occupational exposure, OR = 1.9, 95% CI = 0.6–5.5; high occupational exposure, OR = 3.1, 95% CI = 1.5–7.5) (Demers et al., 1993).

In terms of specific components of paint, a history of exposure to dyes and inks was associated with myeloma risk in studies conducted in the United States by Boffetta et al. (OR = 2.7, 95% CI = 0.9–8.6) (Boffetta et al., 1989) and Morris et al. (OR = 1.9, 95% CI = 0.7–5.3) (Morris et al., 1986), but not in studies conducted in the United Kingdom (Cuzick and De Stavola, 1988), Italy (La Vecchia et al., 1989), or Denmark (Heineman et al., 1992; Pottern et al., 1992b).

## Wood Products Industries

This category includes manufacturing of lumber, wood products, furniture, and fixtures, as well as the forestry industries, and could involve exposure to wood dust, chemicals used to treat wood, adhesives, paint, and stains. A pooled analysis of cohort studies in wood-related industries (Miller et al., 1989, 1994) suggested an increased risk of death from myeloma (SMR = 1.3, 95% CI = 0.9–1.9) (Demers et al., 1995). However, case-control studies of myeloma suggest little or no altered risk among workers in wood products industries (Cuzick and De Stavola, 1988; Figgs et al., 1994; Heineman et al., 1992; Kawachi et al., 1989; La Vecchia et al., 1989; McLaughlin et al., 1988; Nandakumar et al., 1986; Pottern et al., 1992b; Reif et al., 1989b; Tollerud et al., 1985), with some exceptions. Demers et al. reported a 2.5-fold (95% CI = 1.1–12) risk associated with forestry and logging occupations (Demers et al., 1993), whereas Eriksson and Karlsson reported a 1.5-fold risk (95% CI = 1.0–2.3) for lumberjacks (Eriksson and Karlsson, 1992). Myeloma mortality was associated with a 1.7-fold risk (95% CI = 0.8–3.9) for men in woodworking occupations in western Australia (Nandakumar et al., 1988). Some studies reported associations between myeloma risk and occupational exposure to wood dust (OR = 1.8, 95% CI = 0.7–4.3) (Boffetta et al., 1989, OR = 1.9, 95% CI = 0.4–8.4; Pottern et al., 1992b) and fresh wood (OR = 3.9, 95% CI = 1.9–7.6) (Flodin et al., 1987, OR = 1.5, 95% CI = 1.0–2.4; Eriksson and Karlsson 1992).

## Asbestos

Asbestos was postulated as a lymphoid system carcinogen following the publication of case reports of men with both asbestosis and B cell neoplasms, as well as animal and human studies that demonstrated increased production of M-component in relation to asbestos exposure and asbestosis (Kagan, 1985). A Danish cohort of all employees in an asbestos-cement plant, followed from their employment as early as 1928 through 1984, noted a 1.7-fold risk of myeloma (95% CI = 0.7–3.3) (Raffn et al., 1989). A meta-analysis of case-control studies conducted in the United States and Europe (Boffetta et al., 1989; Cuzick and De Stavola, 1988; Eriksson and Karlsson, 1992; Figgs et al., 1994; La Vecchia et al., 1989; Linet et al., 1987; Morris et al., 1986; Pasqualetti et al., 1990; Schwartz et al., 1988) found a slightly increased myeloma risk associated with asbestos exposure (OR = 1.2; 95% CI = 1.0–1.4) (Becker et al., 2001).

## Engine Exhaust

Myeloma risk was related to a history of occupational exposure to diesel or engine exhaust in one cohort and six case-control studies. Self-reported occupation as a truck driver in the 1970 Swedish census was related to myeloma mortality in the subsequent 10 years (standardized mortality ratio = 4.4, 95% CI = 1.4–10.2) (Hansen, 1993). In case-control studies, odds ratios for the association between myeloma risk and occupational exposure to engine exhaust ranged from 1.4 to 2.1 (Boffetta et al., 1989; Eriksson and Karlsson, 1992; Flodin et al., 1987; Heineman et al., 1992; Pottern et al., 1992b; Van den Eeden and Friedman, 1993). Boffetta et al. found an association for self-reported exposure to diesel exhaust (OR = 1.4, 95% CI = 0.7–2.7) but not gasoline exhaust (OR = 0.9, 95% CI = 0.5–1.6) (Boffetta et al., 1989). Risk was also related to prior carbon monoxide exposure in two studies, with odds ratios of 1.9 (95% CI = 1.1–3.2) (Morris et al., 1986) and 1.5 (95% CI = 1.2–2.2) (Pasqualetti et al., 1990). A meta-analysis found a slightly elevated summary odds ratio for the association between engine exhaust and myeloma risk (OR = 1.3, 95% CI = 1.1–1.6) (Sonoda et al., 2001).

## Metals

In a cohort study, Teta and Ott (Teta and Ott, 1988) noted that male hourly workers employed at a New York metal fabrication facility and followed from 1946 to 1981 were at slightly increased risk of myeloma (RR = 1.4, number of exposed cases = 3). A cohort study of metal workers found an increased myeloma risk among machinists (proportionate mortality ratio = 209) (Gallagher and Threlfall, 1983). In two case-control studies, a history of exposure to metals (not otherwise specified) was related to myeloma risk, with odds ratios of 1.8 (95% CI = 1.1–2.9) (Morris et al., 1986) and 1.5 (number of exposed cases = 81) (Cuzick and De Stavola, 1988). In four other reports, there was no relation (Heineman et al., 1992; La Vecchia et al., 1989; Pasqualetti et al., 1990; Pottern et al., 1992b). There is very limited information about exposure to specific metals in relation to the disease (Egedahl et al., 1993; Linet et al., 1987). However, one study found a significantly increased risk of myeloma mortality among workers of a nickel refinery in Canada (SMR = 12.6, 95% CI = 2.5–36.8) (Egedahl et al., 1993).

## Other Occupations and Exposures

Other occupations and exposures have not been extensively investigated, but have been associated with myeloma in several studies. Three cohort studies of firefighters observed increased myeloma mortality in Philadelphia, Pennsylvania (for 10-19 y employment: OR = 1.5, 95% CI = 0.5-4.7; for ≥20 y employment: OR = 2.3, 95% CI = 1.0-5.2) (Baris et al., 2001) in Seattle, Washington (for ≥20 y employment: SMR = 9.9, 2 cases) (Heyer et al., 1990), and in Canada (SMR = 10.0, 95% CI = 1.2-36.1); several proportionate mortality analyses in the United States have found similar results (Howe and Burch, 1990). Occupation as a welder was associated with myeloma incidence in several case-control studies (OR = 2.0, 95% CI = 0.6-5.7, Heineman et al., 1992; OR = 3.3, 95% CI = 1.3-8.5, Costantini et al., 2001; OR = 1.2, 95% CI = 0.7-2.0, Demers et al., 1993), and extremely low-frequency magnetic field exposure among welders was associated with myeloma incidence among women (high vs. low exposure, RR = 3.8, 95% CI = 0.9-15.6) (Hakansson et al., 2002). Myeloma risk was associated with occupation as an embalmer and funeral director (PMR = 1.4, 95% CI = 0.8-2.1) (Hayes et al., 1990) and formaldehyde exposure (OR = 1.8, 95% CI = 0.6-5.7) (Boffetta et al., 1989), but no association with formaldehyde was found in another case-control study (Heineman et al., 1992). Myeloma incidence and mortality were elevated in two cohorts of fishermen (RR = 2.5, 95% CI = 0.7-6.4) (Hagmar et al., 1992) (east coast of Sweden, SMR = 3.1, 95% CI = 1.2-6.4; west coast of Sweden, SMR = 3.2, 95% CI = 1.2-8.7) (Svensson et al., 1995), and a case-control study found a slight elevation associated with occupation as a fisherman (OR = 1.3, $p$ = 0.05) (McLaughlin et al., 1988).

## Summary

Multiple studies have provided evidence that agricultural work is associated with myeloma risk. Pesticide use might account for part of the association of agricultural work with myeloma, but there is also some evidence that other agricultural exposures could increase risk. Unfortunately, there are few data concerning the specific agricultural exposures that should be targeted for further investigation. There is fairly consistent evidence that exposures in paint-related occupations increase myeloma risk. Whether this increased risk results from dyes and pigments or from solvents used in paint formulations has not been discerned. Limited evidence from cohort studies that occupational exposure to benzene is associated with myeloma incidence is contradicted by largely negative results from studies of petroleum and rubber workers, arguing against a role of benzene as a strong risk factor for myeloma.

## Lifestyle Factors

### Alcohol Intake and Tobacco Use

Studies of the relation between alcohol intake and risk of myeloma have found no apparent association (Boffetta et al., 1989; Brown et al., 1992a; Linet et al., 1987; Tavani et al., 1997; Williams and Horm, 1977). Of many studies that have investigated the association between tobacco use and myeloma risk (Adami et al., 1998; Boffetta et al., 1989; Brown et al., 1992b; Brownson, 1991; Doll and Peto, 1976; Flodin et al., 1987; Friedman, 1993; Gallagher et al., 1983; Heineman et al., 1992; Herrinton et al., 1992; Linet et al., 1987; Miligi et al., 1999; Rogot and Murray, 1980; Stagnaro et al., 2001; Williams and Horm, 1977), only one found consistent evidence for an increased risk among smokers (Mills et al., 1990).

### Diet and Obesity

Obesity and overweight were associated with increased risk of myeloma in both whites (obesity vs. normal weight, OR = 1.9, 95% CI = 1.2-3.1) and blacks (obesity, OR = 1.5, 95% CI = 0.9-2.4) (Brown et al., 2001), corroborating observations from two previous cohorts of health maintenance organization patients (Friedman and Herrinton, 1994).

Dietary factors have been examined in relation to myeloma risk in only a handful of studies with some consistent results. Decreased risk of myeloma was observed in relation to certain vegetables, including cruciferous vegetable consumption (highest vs. lowest quartile, OR = 0.7, $p$ < 0.05) (Brown et al., 2001) and green vegetables (highest tertile, OR = 0.4, $p$ < 0.01) (Tavani et al., 1997). Inverse associations were also observed for high consumption of whole grain foods (> 3 days/wk, OR = 0.5, 95% CI = 0.2-1.1) (Chatenoud et al., 1998). In a US study, increased myeloma risk was associated with fruit and juice intake among blacks (highest quartile, OR = 1.5, $p$ for trend across quartiles < 0.05), but not whites (Brown et al., 2001). Intake of several meats and fats were associated with increased risk of myeloma, including liver (highest vs. lowest tertile, OR = 2.0, $p$ < 0.01), butter (highest tertile, OR = 2.8, $p$ < 0.01), and total seasoning fats (highest tertile, OR = 2.4, $p$ < 0.01) (Tavani et al., 1997), whereas fish intake was associated with decreased risk in two studies (highest vs. lowest quartile, OR = 0.6, $p$ < 0.05, Brown et al., 2001; ≥2 servings/wk, OR = 0.5, 95% CI = 0.3-0.9, Fernandez et al., 1999). Few specific nutrients have been evaluated in relation to myeloma. In a US study, vitamin C supplementation for 5 years or longer was associated with decreased risk among whites (OR = 0.6, 95% CI = 0.4-0.9), but not blacks (Brown et al., 2001). In an Italian study, β-carotene was inversely associated (highest tertile,

OR = 0.06, $p$ < 0.01), and retinol intake was positively associated (highest tertile, OR = 2.3, $p$ < 0.01) with myeloma risk. (Tavani et al., 1997), but neither nutrient was associated with myeloma in blacks or whites in the US study (Brown et al., 2001).

### Hair-Coloring Products

Some initial reports of an excess risk of myeloma among women working as cosmetologists or hair-dressers (Guidotti et al., 1982; Spinelli et al., 1984) led to a hypothesis of an association between exposure to hair-coloring products and myeloma risk. Observations in other study populations gave further indication of increased risk in occupations with exposure to hair-coloring products (Flodin et al., 1987; Herrinton et al., 1994; Miligi et al., 1999), although not all studies found such an association (Eriksson and Karlsson, 1992; Pottern et al., 1992b; Teta et al., 1984).

Personal use of permanent hair dyes for 20 years or longer was associated with a slightly increased risk of myeloma in the American Cancer Society cohort (RR = 1.4, 95% CI = 0.9–2.3) that was most apparent in women who had used black dyes (RR = 4.4, 95% CI = 1.1–18.3) (Thun et al., 1994). In case-control studies, personal use of hair dyes was associated with myeloma risk in both women (OR = 1.8, 95% CI = 0.9–3.7) (Zahm et al., 1992) and men (OR = 1.8, 95% CI = 0.5–5.7, Zahm et al., 1992; OR = 1.9, 95% CI = 1.0–3.6, Brown et al., 1992c; OR = 1.3, 95% CI = 0.7–2.3, Herrinton et al., 1994). No association between permanent hair dye use and myeloma risk was observed among women in a multicenter US study (Herrinton et al., 1994), or in a case-control study conducted in Italy (Miligi et al., 1999). In the Zahm et al. study, there was some indication of a higher increased risk among those using permanent hair coloring products compared with those using semi- or nonpermanent hair coloring products or products that change hair color gradually (Zahm et al., 1992).

### Medication Use

There are scant data on the use of specific medications in relation to myeloma risk. A study of members of the Kaiser Permanente Medical Care Program using computerized pharmacy records found increased myeloma risk associated with erythromycin use (14 observed cases, 5.1 expected; SMR = 2.72, $p$ < 0.002) (Selby et al., 1989). Diphenylhydantoin use was in excess among myeloma cases compared with control subjects in a hospital-based case-control study (3 vs. 0 discordant pairs) (Linet et al., 1987), but not in the Kaiser Permanente study (Selby et al., 1989). The same case-control study found a positive association with the use of laxatives (OR = 3.5; 95% CI = 1.1–11.1) and

imprecise increased risks (OR ≥ 2.0) associated with use of diazepam, ibuprofen, and diet pills or stimulants (Linet et al., 1987). A second case-control study found suggested positive associations with corticosteroids (OR = 2.3, 95% CI = 0.6–8.7) and salicylates or paracetamol (OR = 2.0, 95% CI = 0.7–5.7) (Eriksson, 1993).

## Future Directions

From the research completed to date, it appears that the question, "What causes myeloma?" will not be easy to answer. Within areas in which there are indicators, for example, associations with exposure to radiation or a history of farming, the difficulty of more precisely measuring potential etiologic factors has limited our understanding of the nature of the associations. One promising avenue for future research is based on the acceptance of MGUS as a strong predictor of myeloma risk, and would involve studying the causes of MGUS and the factors associated with malignant transformation of MGUS to myeloma.

Advances in the field of molecular biology have made research into genetic susceptibility feasible and affordable. Investigation into the role of common genetic polymorphisms in myeloma risk has just begun, with few promising leads so far. However, this line of research should be pursued, because an association with family history and racial differences in incidence strongly suggest a role of genetic factors. Genes of interest include those involved in immune function, growth factor genes (e.g., insulin growth factor [IGF] genes because of their influence on plasma cell growth), and metabolism genes responsible for biotransformation of toxic chemicals (e.g., cytochrome P-450 [CYP] gene family because of the possible effect of exogenous chemicals including pesticides on myeloma risk).

A promising area of research is investigation into risk factors for molecular changes (chromosomal translocations, gene silencing by methylation) that are commonly present in myeloma tumors, although the small numbers in patient subgroups will limit this research. It might be useful to look to differences between MGUS and myeloma for clues about other genes implicated in malignant transformation; for example, virtually all myeloma patients (95%) are positive for IL-1β production by monoclonal plasma cells, whereas the majority of patients with MGUS are negative for IL-1β expression (25%) (Lacy et al., 1999). Emerging technologies such as proteomics and DNA arrays might also be useful in further identifying proteins or genes that are overexpressed in myeloma cells (De Vos et al., 2001).

Targeting research toward demographic groups at increased risk of myeloma, such as blacks or farmers, might prove useful to investigate early biologic effects relevant to the development of myeloma. Investigations into the prevalence of MGUS, other immune system effects, or chromosomal alterations in these susceptible subgroups may provide clues into reasons for racial disparities and occupational risk factors among farmers.

## REFERENCES

Ablashi, D. V., Chatlynne, L., Thomas, D., Bourboulia, D., Rettig, M. B., Vescio, R. A., Viza, D., Gill, P., Kyle, R. A., Berenson, J. R., and Whitman, J. E. (2000). Lack of serologic association of human herpesvirus-8 (KSHV) in patients with monoclonal gammopathy of undetermined significance with and without progression to multiple myeloma. *Blood, 96,* 2304–2306.

Abu–Shakra, M., Gladman, D. D., and Urowitz, M. B. (1996). Malignancy in systemic lupus erythematosus. *Arthritis Rheumatism, 39,* 1050–1054.

Adami, J., Nyren, O., Bergstrom, R., Ekbom, A., Engholm, G., Englund, A., and Glimelius, B. (1998). Smoking and the risk of leukemia, lymphoma, and multiple myeloma (Sweden). *Cancer Causes Control, 9,* 49–56.

Agbalika, F., Mariette, X., Marolleau, J. P., Fermand, J. P., and Brouet, J. C. (1998). Detection of human herpesvirus-8 DNA in bone marrow biopsies from patients with multiple myeloma and Waldenström's macroglobulinemia. *Blood, 91,* 4393–4394.

Alavanja, M. C., Blair, A., Merkle, S., Teske, J., and Eaton, B. (1988). Mortality among agricultural extension agents. *American Journal of Industrial Medicine, 14,* 167–176.

Andersson, M., and Storm, H. H. (1992). Cancer incidence among Danish Thorotrast–exposed patients. *Journal of the National Cancer Institute, 84,* 1318–1325.

Andjelkovich, D., Taulbee, J., and Blum, S. (1978). Mortality of female workers in rubber manufacturing plant. *Journal of Occupational Medicine, 20,* 409–413.

Andjelkovich, D., Taulbee, J., Symons, M., and Williams, T. (1977). Mortality of rubber workers with reference to work experience. *Journal of Occupational Medicine, 19,* 397–405.

Attal, M., Harousseau, J. L., Stoppa, A. M., Sotto, J. J., Fuzibet, J. G., Rossi, J. F., Casassus, P., Maisonneuve, H., Facon, T., Ifrah, N., Payen, C., and Bataille, R. (1996). A prospective, randomized trial of autologous bone marrow transplantation and chemotherapy in multiple myeloma. Intergroupe Francais du Myelome. *New England Journal of Medicine, 335,* 91–97.

Avet-Loiseau, H., Li, J. Y., Facon, T., Brigaudeau, C., Morineau, N., Maloisel, F., Rapp, M. J., Talmant, P., Trimoreau, F., Jaccard, A., Harousseau, J. L., and Bataille, R. (1998). High incidence of translocations t(11;14)(q13;q32) and t(4;14)(p16;q32) in patients with plasma cell malignancies. *Cancer Research, 58,* 5640–5645.

Avet-Loiseau, H., Li, J. Y., Morineau, N., Facon, T., Brigaudeau, C., Harousseau, J. L., Grosbois, B., and Bataille, R. (1999). Monosomy 13 is associated with the transition of monoclonal gammopathy of undetermined significance to multiple myeloma. Intergroupe Francophone du Myelome. *Blood, 94,* 2583–2589.

Axelsson, U. (1986). A 20-year follow-up study of 64 subjects with M-components. *Acta Medica Scandinvica, 219,* 519–522.

Axelsson, U., Bachmann, R., and Hallen, J. (1966). Frequency of pathological proteins (M-components) om 6,995 sera from an adult population. *Acta Med Scand, 179,* 235–247.

Baker, G. L., Kahl, L. E., Zee, B. C., Stolzer, B. L., Agarwal, A. K., and Medsger, T. A., Jr. (1987). Malignancy following treatment of rheumatoid arthritis with cyclophosphamide. Long-term case-control follow-up study. *American Journal of Medicine, 83,* 1–9.

Baldini, L., Guffanti, A., Cesana, B. M., Colombi, M., Chiorboli, O., Damilano, I., and Maiolo, A. T. (1996). Role of different hematologic variables in defining the risk of malignant transformation in monoclonal gammopathy. *Blood, 87,* 912–918.

Baris, D., Brown, L. M., Silverman, D. T., Hayes, R., Hoover, R. N., Swanson, G. M., Dosemeci, M., Schwartz, A. G., Liff, J. M., Schoenberg, J. B., Pottern, L. M., Lubin, J., Greenberg, R. S., and Fraumeni, J. F. J. (2000). Socioeconomic status and multiple myeloma among US blacks and whites. *American Journal of Public Health, 90,* 1277–1281.

Baris, D., Garrity, T., Telles, J. L., Heineman, E. F., Olshan, A., and Zahm, S. H. (2001). A cohort mortality study of Philadelphia firefighters. *American Journal of Industrial Medicine, 39,* 463–476.

Barlogie, B., Epstein, J., Selvanayagam, P., and Alexanian, R. (1989). Plasma cell myeloma—new biological insights and advances in therapy. *Blood, 73,* 865–879.

Beauparlant, P., Papp, K., and Haraoui, B. (1999). The incidence of cancer associated with the treatment of rheumatoid arthritis. *Seminars in Arthritis and Rheumatism, 29,* 148–158.

Becker, N., Berger, J., and Bolm-Audorff, U. (2001). Asbestos exposure and malignant lymphomas—A review of the epidemiological literature. *International Archives of Occupational and Environmental Health, 74,* 459–469.

Beksac, M., Ma, M., Akyerli, C., DerDanielian, M., Zhang, L., Liu, J., Arat, M., Konuk, N., Koc, H., Ozcelik, T., Vescio, R., and Berenson, J. R. (2001). Frequent demonstration of human herpesvirus 8 (HHV-8) in bone marrow biopsy samples from Turkish patients with multiple myeloma (MM). *Leukemia, 15,* 1268–1273.

Beral, V., Inskip, H., Fraser, P., Booth, M., Coleman, D., and Rose, G. (1985). Mortality of employees of the United Kingdom Atomic Energy Authority, 1946–1979. *British Medical Journal (Clinical Research Edition), 291,* 440–447.

Beral, V., and Newton, R. (1998). Overview of the epidemiology of immunodeficiency-associated cancers. *Journal of the National Cancer Institute Monographs,* 1–6.

Bertazzi, A., Pesatori, A. C., Consonni, D., Tironi, A., Landi, M. T., and Zocchetti, C. (1993). Cancer incidence in a population accidentally exposed to 2,3,7,8-tetrachlorodibenzo-para-dioxin. *Epidemiology, 4,* 398–406.

Bethwaite, P. B., Pearce, N., and Fraser, J. (1990). Cancer risks in painters: Study based on the New Zealand Cancer Registry. *British Journal of Industrial Medicine, 47,* 742–746.

Blade, J., Lopez–Guillermo, A., Rozman, C., Cervantes, F., Salgado, C., Aguilar, J. L., Vives-Corrons, J. L., and Montserrat, E. (1992). Malignant transformation and life expectancy in monoclonal gammopathy of undetermined significance. *British Journal of Haematology, 81,* 391–394.

Blair, A., Malker, H., Cantor, K. P., Burmeister, L., and Wiklund, K. (1985). Cancer among farmers. A review. *Scandinavian Journal of Work, Environment, and Health, 11,* 397–407.

Blattner, W. A., Blair, A., and Mason, T. J. (1981). Multiple myeloma in the United States, 1950–1975. *Cancer, 48,* 2547–2554.

Bjornadal, L., Lofstrom, B., Yin, L., Lundberg, I. E., and Ekbom, A. (2002). Increased cancer incidence in a Swedish cohort of patients with systemic lupus erythematosus. *Scandinavian Journal of Rheumatology, 31,* 66–71.

Boffetta, P., Stellman, S. D., and Garfinkel, L. (1989). A case-control study of multiple myeloma nested in the American Cancer Society prospective study. *International Journal of Cancer, 43,* 554–559.

Boice, J. D., Jr., Day, N. E., Andersen, A., Brinton, L. A., Brown, R., Choi, N. W., Clarke, E. A., Coleman, M. P., Curtis, R. E., and Flannery, J. T. (1985). Second cancers following radiation treatment for cervical cancer. An international collaboration among cancer registries. *Journal of the National Cancer Institute, 74,* 955–975.

Boice, J. D., Jr., Engholm, G., Kleinerman, R. A., Blettner, M., Stovall, M., Lisco, H., Moloney, W. C., Austin, D. F., Bosch, A., and Cookfair, D. L. (1988). Radiation dose and second cancer risk in patients treated for cancer of the cervix. *Radiation Research, 116,* 3–55.

Boice, J. D., Jr., Morin, M. M., Glass, A. G., Friedman, G. D., Stovall, M., Hoover, R. N., and Fraumeni, J. F., Jr. (1991). Diagnostic x-ray procedures and risk of leukemia, lymphoma, and multiple myeloma. *Journal of the American Medical Association, 265*, 1290–1294.

Bourguet, C. C., Grufferman, S., Delzell, E., Delong, E. R., and Cohen, H. J. (1985). Multiple myeloma and family history of cancer. A case-control study. *Cancer, 56*, 2133–2139.

Bourguet, C. C., and Logue, E. E. (1993). Antigenic stimulation and multiple myeloma. A prospective study. *Cancer, 72*, 2148–2154.

Bowden, M., Crawford, J., Cohen, H. J., and Noyama, O. (1993). A comparative study of monoclonal gammopathies and immunoglobulin levels in Japanese and United States elderly. *Journal of the American Geriatric Society, 41*, 11–14.

Brinton, L. A., Gridley, G., Hrubec, Z., Hoover, R., and Fraumeni, J. F., Jr. (1989). Cancer risk following pernicious anaemia. *British Journal of Cancer, 59*, 810–813.

Brousset, P., Meggetto, F., Attal, M., and Delsol, G. (1997). Kaposi's sarcoma-associated herpesvirus infection and multiple myeloma. *Science, 278*, 1972–1973.

Brown, L. M., Everett, G. D., Burmeister, L. F., and Blair, A. (1992c). Hair dye use and multiple myeloma in white men. *American Journal of Public Health, 82*, 1673–1674.

Brown, L. M., Everett, G. D., Gibson, R., Burmeister, L. F., Schuman, L. M., and Blair, A. (1992b). Smoking and risk of non-Hodgkin's lymphoma and multiple myeloma. *Cancer Causes Control, 3*, 49–55.

Brown, L. M., Gibson, R., Burmeister, L. F., Schuman, L. M., Everett, G. D., and Blair, A. (1992a). Alcohol consumption and risk of leukemia, non-Hodgkin's lymphoma, and multiple myeloma. *Leukemia Research, 16*, 979–984.

Brown, L. M., Gridley, G,, Pottern, L. M., Baris, D., Swanson, C. A., Silverman, D. T., Hayes, R. B., Greenberg, R. S., Swanson, G. M., Schoenberg, J. B., Schwartz, A. G., and Fraumeni, J. F. J. (2001). Diet and nutrition as risk factors for multiple myeloma among blacks and whites in the United States. *Cancer Causes and Control, 12*, 117–125.

Brown, L. M., Linet, M. S., Greenberg, R. S., Silverman, D. T., Hayes, R. B., Swanson, G. M., Schwartz, A. G., Schoenberg, J. B., Pottern, L. M., and Fraumeni, J. F. J. (1999). Multiple myeloma and family history of cancer among blacks and whites in the U.S. *Cancer, 85*, 2385–2390.

Brownson, R. C. (1991). Cigarette smoking and risk of myeloma. *Journal of the National Cancer Institute, 83*, 1036–1037.

Brownson, R. C., Reif, J. S., Chang, J. C., and Davis, J. R. (1989). Cancer risks among Missouri farmers. *Cancer, 64*, 2381–2386.

Buhler, S., Laitinen, K., Holthofer, H., Jarvinen, A., Schauman, K. O., and Hedman, K. (2002). High rate of monoclonal gammopathy among immunocompetent subjects with primary cytomegalovirus infection. *Clinical Infectious Diseases, 35*, 1430–1433.

Burmeister, L. F. (1990). Cancer in Iowa farmers: recent results. *American Journal of Industrial Medicine, 18*, 295–301.

Burmeister, L. F., Everett, G. D., Van Lier, S. F., and Isacson, P. (1983). Selected cancer mortality and farm practices in Iowa. *American Journal of Epidemiology, 118*, 72–77.

Cabannes, E., Khan, G., Aillet, F., Jarrett, R. F., and Hay, R. T. (1999). Mutations in the IκBα gene in Hodgkin's disease suggest a tumour suppressor role for IkappaBalpha. *Oncogene, 18*, 3063–3070.

Cantor, K. P., and Blair, A. (1984). Farming and mortality from multiple myeloma: a case-control study with the use of death certificates. *Journal of the National Cancer Institute, 72*, 251–255.

Cardis, E., Gilbert, E. S., Carpenter, L., Howe, G., Kato, I., Armstrong, B. K., Beral, V., Cowper, G., Douglas, A., and Fix, J. (1995). Effects of low doses and low dose rates of external ionizing radiation: cancer mortality among nuclear industry workers in three countries. *Radiation Research, 142*, 117–132.

Carpenter, L., Higgins, C., Douglas, A., Fraser, P., Beral, V., and Smith, P. (1994). Combined analysis of mortality in three United Kingdom nuclear industry workforces, 1946–1988. *Radiation Research, 138*, 224–238.

Cartwright, R. A., Gurney, K. A., and Moorman, A. V. (2002). Sex ratios and the risks of haematological malignancies. *British Journal of Haematology, 118*, 1071–1077.

Cathomas, G., Stalder, A., Kurrer, M. O., Regamey, N., Erb, P., and Joller-Jemelka, H. I. (1998). Multiple myeloma and HHV8 infection. *Blood, 91*, 4391–4393.

Cerhan, J. R., Cantor, K. P., Williamson, K., Lynch, C. F., Torner, J. C., and Burmeister, L. F. (1998). Cancer mortality among Iowa farmers: recent results, time trends, and lifestyle factors (United States). *Cancer Causes and Control, 9*, 311–319.

Chatenoud, L., Tavani, A., La Vecchia, C., Jacobs, D. R., Negri, E., Levi, F., and Franceschi, S. (1998). Whole grain food intake and cancer risk. *International Journal of Cancer, 77*, 24–28.

Chauhan, D., Bharti, A., Raje, N., Gustafson, E., Pinkus, G. S., Pinkus, J. L., Teoh, G., Hideshima, T., Treon, S. P., Fingeroth, J. D., and Anderson, K. C. (1999). Detection of Kaposi's sarcoma herpesvirus DNA sequences in multiple myeloma bone marrow stromal cells. *Blood, 93*, 1482–1486.

Chen, R., and Seaton, A. (1996). A meta-analysis of mortality among workers exposed to organic solvents. *Occupational Medicine (London), 46*, 337–344.

Christie, D., Robinson, K., Gordon, I., and Bisby, J. (1991). A prospective study in the Australian petroleum industry. II. Incidence of cancer. *Br J Ind Med, 48*, 511–514.

Cibere, J., Sibley, J., and Haga, M. (1997). Rheumatoid arthritis and the risk of malignancy. *Arthritis Rheumatism, 40*, 1580–1586.

Cocco, P., Blair, A., Congia, P., Saba, G., Flore, C., Ecca, M. R., and Palmas, C. (1997). Proportional mortality of dichloro-diphenyl-trichloroethane (DDT) workers: a preliminary report. *Archives of Environmental Health, 52*, 299–303.

Cocco, P., Kazerouni, N., and Zahm, S. H. (2000). Cancer mortality and environmental exposure to DDE in the United States. *Environmental Health Perspects, 108*, 1–4.

Cohen, H. J., Crawford, J., Rao, M. K., Pieper, C. F., and Currie, M. S. (1998). Racial differences in the prevalence of monoclonal gammopathy in a community-based sample of the elderly. *American Journal of Medicine, 104*, 439–444.

Colls, B. M. (1999). Monoclonal gammopathy of undetermined significance (MGUS)—31-year followup of a community study. *Australian and New Zealand Journal of Medicine, 29*, 500–504.

Costantini, A. S., Miligi, L., Kriebel, D., Ramazzotti, V., Rodella, S., Scarpi, E., Stagnaro, E., Tumino, R., Fontana, A., Masala, G., Vigano, C., Vindigni, C., Crosignani, P., Benvenuti, A., and Vineis, P. (2001). A multicenter case-control study in Italy on hematolymphopoietic neoplasms and occupation. *Epidemiology, 12*, 78–87.

Cull, G. M., Carter, G. I., Timms, J. M., Thomson, B. J., Russell, N. H., and Haynes, A. P. (1999). Low incidence of human herpesvirus 8 in stem cell collections from myeloma patients. *Bone Marrow Transplantation, 23*, 759–761.

Cuzick, J., and De Stavola, B. (1988). Multiple myeloma—a case-control study. *British Journal of Cancer, 57*, 516–520.

Cuzick, J., and De Stavola, B. L. (1989). Autoimmune disorders and multiple myeloma. *International Journal of Epidemiology, 18*, 283.

Cuzick, J., Velez, R., and Doll, R. (1983). International variations and temporal trends in mortality from multiple myeloma. *International Journal of Cancer, 32*, 13–19.

Dalton, W. S., Bergsagel, P. L., Kuehl, W. M., Anderson, K. C., and Harousseau, J. L. (2001). Multiple myeloma. *Hematology (American Society of Hematology Education Program), 157*–177.

Darby, S. C., Doll, R., Gill, S. K., and Smith, P. G. (1987). Long term mortality after a single treatment course with x-rays in patients treated for ankylosing spondylitis. *British Journal of Cancer, 55*, 179–190.

Darby, S. C., Kendall, G. M., Fell, T. P., Doll, R., Goodill, A. A., Coquest, A. J., et al. (1993). Further followup of mortality and incidence of cancer in men from the United Kingdom who participated in the United Kingdom's atmospheric nuclear weapon tests and experimental programmes. *British Medical Journal, 307,* 1530–1535.

Darby, S. C., Reeves, G., Key, T., Doll, R., and Stovall, M. (1994). Mortality in a cohort of women given x-ray therapy for metropathia haemorrhagica. *International Journal of Cancer, 56,* 793–801.

Davies, F. E., Rollinson, S. J., Rawstron, A. C., Roman, E., Richards, S., Drayson, M., Child, J. A., and Morgan, G. J. (2000). High-producer haplotypes of tumor necrosis factor alpha and lymphotoxin alpha are associated with an increased risk of myeloma and have an improved progression-free survival after treatment. *Journal of Clinical Oncology, 18,* 2843–2851.

Davis, F. G., Boice, J. D., Hrubec, Z., and Monson, R. R. (1989). Cancer mortality in a radiation-exposed cohort of Massachusetts tuberculosis patients. *Cancer Research, 49,* 6130–6136.

Demers, P. A., Boffetta, P., Kogevinas, M., Blair, A., Miller, B. A., Robinson, C. F., Roscoe, R. J., Winter, P. D., Colin, D., and Matos, E. (1995). Pooled reanalysis of cancer mortality among five cohorts of workers in wood-related industries. *Scandinavian Journal of Work, Environment, and Health, 21,* 179–190.

Demers, P. A., Vaughan, T. L., Koepsell, T. D., Lyon, J. L., Swanson, G. M., Greenberg, R. S., and Weiss, N. S. (1993). A case-control study of multiple myeloma and occupation. *American Journal of Industrial Medicine, 23,* 629–639.

Demeter, J., Messer, G., Ramisch, S., Mee, J. B., di Giovine, F. S., Schmid, M., Herrmann, F., and Porzsolt, F. (1996). Polymorphism within the second intron of the IL-1 receptor antagonist gene in patients with hematopoietic malignancies. *Cytokines and Molecular Therapy, 2,* 239–242.

Devesa, S. S., Silverman, D. T., Young, J. L. J., Pollack, E. S., Brown, C. C., Horm, J. W., Percy, C. L., Myers, M. H., McKay, F. W., and Fraumeni, J. F. J. (1987). Cancer incidence and mortality trends among whites in the United States, 1947–84. *Journal of the National Cancer Institute, 79,* 701–770.

De Vos, J., Couderc, G., Tarte, K., Jourdan, M., Requirand, G., Delteil, M. C., Rossi, J. F., Mechti, N., and Klein, B. (2001). Identifying intercellular signaling genes expressed in malignant plasma cells by using complementary DNA arrays. *Blood, 98,* 771–780.

Divine, B. J., and Hartman, C. M. (2001). A cohort mortality study among workers at a 1,3 butadiene facility. *Chemico-Biological Interactions, 135–136,* 535–553.

Doll, R. (1991). Urban and rural factors in the aetiology of cancer. *International Journal of Cancer, 47,* 803–810.

Doll, R., and Peto, R. (1976). Mortality in relation to smoking: 20 years' observations on male British doctors. *British Medical Journal, 2,* 1525–1536.

Dominici, M., Luppi, M., Campioni, D., Lanza, F., Barozzi, P., Milani, R., Moretti, S., Nadali, G., Spanedda, R., Trovato, R., Torelli, G., and Castoldi, G. (2000). PCR with degenerate primers for highly conserved DNA polymerase gene of the herpesvirus family shows neither human herpesvirus 8 nor a related variant in bone marrow stromal cells from multiple myeloma patients. *International Journal of Cancer, 86,* 76–82.

Doody, M. M., Linet, M. S., Glass, A. G., Friedman, G. D., Pottern, L. M., Boice, J. D. J., and Fraumeni, J. F. J. (1992). Leukemia, lymphoma, and multiple myeloma following selected medical conditions. *Cancer Causes and Control, 3,* 449–456.

Drabick, J. J., Davis, B. J., Lichy, J. H., Flynn, J., and Byrd, J. C. (2002). Human herpesvirus 8 genome is not found in whole bone marrow core biopsy specimens of patients with plasma cell dyscrasias. *Annals of Hematology, 81,* 304–307.

Dring, A. M., Davies, F. E., Rollinson, S. J., Roddam, P. L., Rawstron, A. C., Child, J. A., Jack, A. S., and Morgan, G. J. (2001). Interleukin 6, tumour necrosis factor alpha and lymphotoxin alpha

polymorphisms in monoclonal gammopathy of uncertain significance and multiple myeloma. *British Journal of Haematology, 112,* 249–251.

Egedahl, R. D., Carpenter, M., and Homik, R. (1993). An update of an epidemiology study at a hydrometallurgical nickel refinery in Fort Saskatchewan, Alberta. *Health Reports, 5,* 291–302.

Eriksson, M. (1993). Rheumatoid arthritis as a risk factor for multiple myeloma: a case-control study. *European Journal of Cancer, 29A,* 259–263.

Eriksson, M., and Hallberg, B. (1992). Familial occurrence of hematologic malignancies and other diseases in multiple myeloma: A case-control study. *Cancer Causes Control, 3,* 63–67.

Eriksson, M., and Karlsson, M. (1992). Occupational and other environmental factors and multiple myeloma: A population based case-control study. *British Journal of Industrial Medicine, 49,* 95–103.

Feinman, R., Sawyer, J., Hardin, J., and Tricot, G. (1997). Cytogenetics and molecular genetics in multiple myeloma. *Hematology/Oncology Clinics of North America, 11,* 1–25.

Fernandez, E., Chatenoud, L., La Vecchia, C., Negri, E., and Franceschi, S. (1999). Fish consumption and cancer risk. *American Journal of Clinical Nutrition, 70,* 85–90.

Festen, J. J., Marrink, J., Waard-Kuiper, E. H., and Mandema, E. (1977). Immunoglobulins in families of myeloma patients. *Scandinavian Journal of Immunology, 6,* 887–896.

Figgs, L. W., Dosemeci, M., and Blair, A. (1994). Risk of multiple myeloma by occupation and industry among men and women: A 24-state death certificate study. *Journal of Occupational Medicine, 36,* 1210–1221.

Flodin, U., Fredriksson, M., and Persson, B. (1987). Multiple myeloma and engine exhausts, fresh wood, and creosote: A case-referent study. *American Journal of Industrial Medicine, 12,* 519–529.

Fonseca, R., Bailey, R. J., Ahmann, G. J., Rajkumar, S. V., Hoyer, J. D., Lust, J. A., Kyle, R. A., Gertz, M. A., Greipp, P. R., and Dewald, G. W. (2002b). Genomic abnormalities in monoclonal gammopathy of undetermined significance. *Blood, 100,* 1417–1424.

Fonseca, R., Blood, E. A., Oken, M. M., Kyle, R. A., Dewald, G. W., Bailey, R. J., Van Wier, S. A., Henderson, K. J., Hoyer, J. D., Harrington, D., Kay, N. E., Van Ness, B., and Greipp, P. R. (2002a). Myeloma and the t(11;14)(q13;q32); evidence for a biologically defined unique subset of patients. *Blood, 99,* 3735–3741.

Fonseca, R., Oken, M. M., and Greipp, P. R. (2001). The t(4;14) (p16.3;q32) is strongly associated with chromosome 13 abnormalities in both multiple myeloma and monoclonal gammopathy of undetermined significance. *Blood, 98,* 1271.

Fordyce, E. J., Wang, Z., Kahn, A. R., Gallagher, B. K., Merlos, I., Ly, S., Schymura, M., and Chiasson, M. A. (2000). Risk of cancer among women with AIDS in New York City. *AIDS Public Policy Journal, 15,* 95–104.

Franceschi, S., Barbone, F., Bidoli, E., Guarneri, S., Serraino, D., Talamini, R., and La Vecchia, C. (1993). Cancer risk in farmers: Results from a multi-site case-control study in north-eastern Italy. *International Journal of Cancer, 53,* 740–745.

Friedman, G. D. (1986). Multiple myeloma: Relation to propoxyphene and other drugs, radiation and occupation. *International Journal of Epidemiology, 15,* 424–426.

Friedman, G. D. (1993). Cigarette smoking, leukemia, and multiple myeloma. *Annals of Epidemiology, 3,* 425–428.

Friedman, G. D., and Herrinton, L. J. (1994). Obesity and multiple myeloma. *Cancer Causes and Control, 5,* 479–483.

Fritschi, L., Johnson, K. C., Kliewer, E. V., and Fry, R. (2002). Animal-related occupations and the risk of leukemia, myeloma, and non–Hodgkin's lymphoma in Canada. *Cancer Causes and Control, 13,* 563–571.

Gallagher, R. P., Spinelli, J. J., Elwood, J. M., and Skippen, D. H. (1983). Allergies and agricultural exposure as risk factors for multiple myeloma. *British Journal of Cancer, 48,* 853–857.

Gallagher, R. P., and Threlfall, W. J. (1983). Cancer mortality in metal workers. *Canadian Medical Association Journal, 129,* 1191–1194.

Georgescu, L., Quinn, G. C., Schwartzman, S., and Paget, S. A. (1997). Lymphoma in patients with rheumatoid arthritis: Association with the disease state or methotrexate treatment. *Seminars in Arthritis and Rheumatism, 26,* 794–804.

Gharagozloo, S., Khoshnoodi, J., and Shokri, F. (2001). Hepatitis C virus infection in patients with essential mixed cryoglobulinemia, multiple myeloma and chronic lymphocytic leukemia. *Pathology Oncology Research: POR, 7,* 135–139.

Gilbert, E. S., Fry, S. A., Wiggs, L. D., Voelz, G. L., Cragle, D. L., and Petersen, G. R. (1989). Analyses of combined mortality data on workers at the Hanford Site, Oak Ridge National Laboratory, and Rocky Flats Nuclear Weapons Plant. *Radiation Research, 120,* 19–35.

Goedert, J. J., Cote, T. R., Virgo, P., Scoppa, S. M., Kingma, D. W., Gail, M. H., Jaffe, E. S., and Biggar, R. J. (1998). Spectrum of AIDS-associated malignant disorders. *Lancet, 351,* 1833–1839.

Gonzalez-Fraile, M. I., Garcia-Sanz, R., Mateos, M. V., Balanzategui, A., Gonzalez, M., Vaquez, L., and San Miguel, J. F. (2002). Methylenetetrahydrofolate reductase genotype does not play a role in multiple myeloma pathogenesis. *British Journal of Haematology, 117,* 890–892.

Gonzalez Ordonez, A. J., Fernandez Carreira, J. M., Fernandez Alvarez, C. R., Martin, L., Sanchez, G. J., Medina Rodriguez, J. M., Alvarez, M. V., and Coto, E. (2000). Normal frequencies of the C677T genotypes on the methylenetetrahydrofolate reductase (MTHFR) gene among lymphoproliferative disorders but not in multiple myeloma. *Leukemia Lymphoma, 39,* 607–612.

Gramenzi, A., Buttino, I., D'Avanzo, B., Negri, E., Franceschi, S., and La Vecchia, C. (1991). Medical history and the risk of multiple myeloma. *British Journal of Cancer, 63,* 769–772.

Gregersen, H., Ibsen, J., Mellemkjoer, L., Dahlerup, J., Olsen, J., and Sorensen, H. (2001b). Mortality and causes of death in patients with monoclonal gammopathy of undetermined significance. *British Journal of Haematology, 112,* 353–357.

Gregersen, H., Mellemkjaer, L., Ibsen, J. S., Dahlerup, J. F., Thomassen, L., and Sorensen, H. T. (2001a). The impact of M-component type and immunoglobulin concentration on the risk of malignant transformation in patients with monoclonal gammopathy of undetermined significance. *Haematologica, 86,* 1172–1179.

Gridley, G., McLaughlin, J. K., Ekbom, A., Klareskog, L., Adami, H. O., Hacker, D. G., Hoover, R., and Fraumeni, J. F. J. (1993). Incidence of cancer among patients with rheumatoid arthritis. *Journal of the National Cancer Institute, 85,* 307–311.

Grufferman, S., Cohen, H. J., Delzell, E. S., Morrison, M. C., Schold, S. C. J., and Moore, J. O. (1989). Familial aggregation of multiple myeloma and central nervous system diseases. *Journal of the American Geriatric Society, 37,* 303–309.

Grulich, A. E., Swerdlow, A. J., Head, J., and Marmot, M. G. (1992). Cancer mortality in African and Caribbean migrants to England and Wales. *British Journal of Cancer, 66,* 905–911.

Grulich, A. E., Wan, X., Law, M. G., Coates, M., and Kaldor, J. M. (1999). Risk of cancer in people with AIDS. *AIDS, 13,* 839–843.

Guidotti, S., Wright, W. E., and Peters, J. M. (1982). Multiple myeloma in cosmetologists. *American Journal of Industrial Medicine, 3,* 169–171.

Gustavsson, P., Hogstedt, C., and Holmberg, B. (1986). Mortality and incidence of cancer among Swedish rubber workers, 1952–1981. *Scandinavian Journal of Work, Environment, and Health, 12,* 538–544.

Haas, H., Anders, S., Bornkamm, G. W., Mannweiler, E, Schmitz, H., Radl, J., and Schlaak, M. (1990). Do infections induce monoclonal immunoglobulin components? *Clinical and Experimental Immunology, 81,* 435–440.

Hagmar, L., Linden, K., Nilsson, A., Norrving, B., Akesson, B., Schutz, A., and Moller, T. (1992). Cancer incidence and mortality among Swedish Baltic Sea fishermen. *Scandinavian Journal of Work, Environment, and Health, 18,* 217–224.

Hakansson, N., Floderus, B., Gustavsson, P., Johansen, C., and Olsen, J. H. (2002). Cancer incidence and magnetic field exposure in industries using resistance welding in Sweden. *Occupational and Environmental Medicine, 59,* 481–486.

Hansen, E. S. (1993). A follow-up study on the mortality of truck drivers. *American Journal of Industrial Medicine, 23,* 811–821.

Hansen, N. E., Karle, H., and Olsen, J. H. (1989). Trends in the incidence of multiple myeloma in Denmark 1943–1982: A study of 5500 patients. *European Journal of Haematology, 42,* 72–76.

Hatcher, J. L., Baris, D., Olshan, A. F., Inskip, P. D., Savitz, D. A., Swanson, G. M., Pottern, L. M., Greenberg, R. S., Schwartz, A. G., Schoenberg, J. B., and Brown, L. M. (2001). Diagnostic radiation and the risk of multiple myeloma (United States). *Cancer Causes and Control, 12,* 755–761.

Hayes, R. B., Blair, A., Stewart, P. A., Herrick, R. F., and Mahar, H. (1990). Mortality of U.S. embalmers and funeral directors. *American Journal of Industrial Medicine, 18,* 641–652.

Hayes, R. B., Yin, S. N., Dosemeci, M., Li, G. L., Wacholder, S., Travis, L. B., Li, C. Y., Rothman, N., Hoover, R. N., and Linet, M. S. (1997). Benzene and the dose-related incidence of hematologic neoplasms in China. Chinese Academy of Preventive Medicine—National Cancer Institute Benzene Study Group. *Journal of the National Cancer Institute, 89,* 1065–1071.

Heineman, E. F., Olsen, J. H., Pottern, L. M., Gomez, M., Raffn, E., and Blair, A. (1992). Occupational risk factors for multiple myeloma among Danish men. *Cancer Causes and Control, 3,* 555–568.

Herrinton, L. J., Koepsell, T. D., and Weiss, N. S. (1992). Smoking and multiple myeloma. *Cancer Causes Control, 3,* 391–392.

Herrinton, L. J., Weiss, N. S., Koepsell, T. D., Daling, J. R., Taylor, J. W., Lyon, J. L., Swanson, G. M., Greenberg, R. S. (1994). Exposure to hair-coloring products and the risk of multiple myeloma. *American Journal of Public Health, 84,* 1142–1144.

Heyer, N., Weiss, N. S., Demers, P., and Rosenstock, L. (1990). Cohort mortality study of Seattle fire fighters: 1945–1983. *American Journal of Industrial Medicine, 17,* 493–504.

Hirano, T. (1991). Interleukin 6 (IL-6) and its receptor: their role in plasma cell neoplasias. *International Journal of Cell Cloning, 9,* 166–184.

Howe, G. R., and Burch, J. D. (1990). Fire fighters and risk of cancer: an assessment and overview of the epidemiologic evidence. *American Journal of Epidemiology, 132,* 1039–1050.

Hsing, A. W., Hansson, L. E., McLaughlin, J. K., Nyren, O., Blot, W. J., Ekbom, A., and Fraumeni, J. F., Jr. (1993). Pernicious anemia and subsequent cancer. A population-based cohort study. *Cancer, 71,* 745–750.

Ireland, B., Collins, J. J., Buckley, C. F., and Riordan, S. G. (1997). Cancer mortality among workers with benzene exposure. *Epidemiology, 8,* 318–320.

Isomaki, H. A., Hakulinen, T., and Joutsenlahti, U. (1978). Excess risk of lymphomas, leukemia and myeloma in patients with rheumatoid arthritis. *Journal of Chronic Diseases, 31,* 691–696.

Iwasaki, T., Murata, M., Ohshima, S., Miyake, T., Kudo, S., Inoue, Y., Narita, M., Yoshimura, T., Akiba, S., Tango, T., Yoshimoto, Y., Shimizu, Y., Sobue, T., Kusumi, S., Yamagishi, C., and Matsudaira, H. (2003). Second analysis of mortality of nuclear industry workers in Japan, 1986–1997. *Radiation Research, 159,* 228–238.

Jeffery, R., and Mitchison, N. A. (2001). IL-6 polymorphism, anti-IL-6 therapy and animal models of multiple myeloma. *Cytokine, 16,* 87.

Johnston, J. M., Grufferman, S., Bourguet, C. C., Delzell, E., Delong, E. R., and Cohen, H. J. (1985). Socioeconomic status and risk of multiple myeloma. *Journal of Epidemiology and Community Health, 39,* 175–178.

Kagan, E. (1985). Current perspectives in asbestosis. *Annals of Allergy, 54,* 464–473.

Kastrinakis, N. G., Gorgoulis, V. G., Foukas, P. G., Dimopoulos, M. A., and Kittas, C. (2000). Molecular aspects of multiple myeloma. *Annals of Oncology, 11,* 1217–1228.

Katusic, S., Beard, C. M., Kurland, L. T., Weis, J. W., and Bergstralh, E. (1985). Occurrence of malignant neoplasms in the Rochester, Minnesota, rheumatoid arthritis cohort. *American Journal of Medicine, 78,* 50–55.

Kauppi, M., Pukkala, E., and Isomaki, H. (1997). Elevated incidence of hematologic malignancies in patients with Sjögren's syndrome compared with patients with rheumatoid arthritis (Finland). *Cancer Causes and Control, 8,* 201–204.

Kawachi, I., Pearce, N., and Fraser, J. (1989). A New Zealand Cancer Registry-based study of cancer in wood workers. *Cancer, 64,* 2609–2613.

Kendall, G. M., Muirhead, C. R., MacGibbon, B. H., O'Hagan, J. A., Conquest, A. J., Goodill, A. A., Butland, B. K., Fell, T. P., Jackson, D. A., and Webb, M. A. (1992). Mortality and occupational exposure to radiation: First analysis of the National Registry for Radiation Workers. *British Medical Journal, 304,* 220–225.

Koepsell, T. D., Daling, J. R., Weiss, N. S., Taylor, J. W., Olshan, A. F., Lyon, J. L., Swanson, G. M., and Child, M. (1987). Antigenic stimulation and the occurrence of multiple myeloma. *American Journal of Epidemiology, 126,* 1051–1062.

Konigsberg, R., Ackermann, J., Kaufmann, H., Zojer, N., Urbauer, E., Kromer, E., Jager, U., Gisslinger, H., Schreiber, S., Heinz, R., Ludwig, H., Huber, H., and Drach, J. (2000). Deletions of chromosome 13q in monoclonal gammopathy of undetermined significance. *Leukemia, 14,* 1975–1979.

Kotsa, K., Watson, P. F., and Weetman, A. P. (1997). A CTLA-4 gene polymorphism is associated with both Graves's disease and autoimmune hypothyroidism. *Clinical Endocrinology (Oxford), 46,* 551–554.

Kuehl, W. M., and Bergsagel, P. L. (2002). Multiple myeloma: Evolving genetic events and host interactions. *Nature Reviews: Cancer, 2,* 175–187.

Kyle, R. A. (1988). Prognostic factors in multiple myeloma. *Hematological Oncology, 6,* 125–130.

Kyle, R. A. (1993). Monoclonal gammopathy—after 20 to 35 years of follow-up. *Mayo Clinic Proceedings, 68,* 26–36.

Kyle, R. A., Beard, C. M., O'Fallon, W. M., and Kurland, L. T. (1994). Incidence of multiple myeloma in Olmsted County, Minnesota: 1978 through 1990, with a review of the trend since 1945. *Journal of Clinical Oncology, 12,* 1577–1583.

Kyle, R. A., Finkelstein, S., Elveback, L. R., and Kurland, L. T. (1972). Incidence of monoclonal proteins in a Minnesota community with a cluster of multiple myeloma. *Blood, 40,* 719–724.

Kyle, R. A., Therneau, T. M., Rajkumar, S. V., Offord, J. R., Larson, D. R., Plevak, M. F., Melton, L. J., III. (2002). A long-term study of prognosis in monoclonal gammopathy of undetermined significance. *New England Journal of Medicine, 346,* 564–569.

La Vecchia, C., Negri, E., D'Avanzo, B., and Franceschi, S. (1989). Occupation and lymphoid neoplasms. *British Journal of Cancer, 60,* 385–388.

Lacy, M. Q., Donovan, K. A., Heimbach, J. K., Ahmann, G. J., and Lust, J. A. (1999). Comparison of interleukin-1 beta expression by in situ hybridization in monoclonal gammopathy of undetermined significance and multiple myeloma. *Blood, 93,* 300–305.

Lee, E., Burnett, C. A., Lalich, N., Cameron, L. L., and Sestito, J. P. (2002). Proportionate mortality of crop and livestock farmers in the United States, 1984–1993. *American Journal of Industrial Medicine, 42,* 410–420.

Leech, S. H., Bryan, C. F., Elston, R. C., Rainey, J., Bickers, J. N., and Pelias, M. Z. (1983). Genetic studies in multiple myeloma. 1. Association with HLA-Cw5. *Cancer, 51,* 1408–1411.

Levi, F., and La Vecchia, C. (1990). Trends in multiple myeloma. *International Journal of Cancer, 46,* 755–756.

Levi, F., La Vecchia, C., Lucchini, F., and Negri, E. (1992). Trends in cancer mortality sex ratios in Europe, 1950–1989. *World Health Statistics Quarterly, 45,* 117–164.

Lewis, D. R., Pottern, L. M., Brown, L. M., Silverman, D. T., Hayes, R. B., Schoenberg, J. B., Greenberg, R. S., Swanson, G. M., Schwartz, A. G., and Liff, J. M. (1994). Multiple myeloma among blacks and whites in the United States: The role of chronic antigenic stimulation. *Cancer Causes and Control, 5,* 529–539.

Lewis, E. B. (1963). Leukemia, multiple myeloma and aplastic anemia in American radiologists. *Science, 142,* 1492–1499.

Linet, M. S., Harlow, S. D., and McLaughlin, J. K. (1987). A case-control study of multiple myeloma in whites: Chronic antigenic stimulation, occupation, and drug use. *Cancer Research, 47,* 2978–2981.

Linet, M. S., McLaughlin, J. K., Harlow, S. D., and Fraumeni, J. F. (1988). Family history of autoimmune disorders and cancer in multiple myeloma. *International Journal of Epidemiology, 17,* 512–513.

Ludwig, H., and Mayr, W. (1982). Genetic aspects of susceptibility to multiple myeloma. *Blood, 59,* 1286–1291.

Lundberg, I. (1986). Mortality and cancer incidence among Swedish paint industry workers with long-term exposure to organic solvents. *Scandinavian Journal of Work, Environment, and Health, 12,* 108–113.

MacKenzie, J., Sheldon, J., Morgan, G., Cook, G., Schulz, T. F., and Jarrett, R. F. (1997). HHV-8 and multiple myeloma in the UK. *Lancet, 350,* 1144–1145.

MacKenzie, M. R., and Lewis, J. P. (1985). Cytogenetic evidence that the malignant event in multiple myeloma occurs in a precursor lymphocyte. *Cancer Genetics Cytogenetics, 17,* 13–20.

MacMahon, B. (1966). Epidemiology of Hodgkin's disease. *Cancer Research, 26,* 1189–1201.

Maldonado, J. E., and Kyle, R. A. (1974). Familial myeloma. Report of eight families and a study of serum proteins in their relatives. *American Journal of Medicine, 57,* 875–884.

Marcelin, A. G., Dupin, N., Bouscary, D., Bossi, P., Cacoub, P., Ravaud, P., and Calvez, V. (1997). HHV-8 and multiple myeloma in France. *Lancet, 350,* 1144.

Mateos, M. V., Garcia-Sanz, R., Lopez-Perez, R., Balanzategui, A., Gonzalez, M. I., Fernandez-Calvo, J., Moro, M. J., Hernandez, J., Caballero, M. D., Gonzalez, M., and San Miguel, J. F. (2001). p16/INK4a gene inactivation by hypermethylation is associated with aggressive variants of monoclonal gammopathies. *Hematology Journal, 2,* 146–149.

Mateos, M. V., Garcia-Sanz, R., Lopez-Perez, R., Moro, M. J., Ocio, E., Hernandez, J., Megido, M., Caballero, M. D., Fernandez-Calvo, J., Barez, A., Almeida, J., Orfao, A., Gonzalez, M., and San Miguel, J. F. (2002). Methylation is an inactivating mechanism of the p16 gene in multiple myeloma associated with high plasma cell proliferation and short survival. *British Journal of Haematology, 118,* 1034–1040.

Matteson, E. L., Hickey, A. R., Maguire, L., Tilson, H. H., and Urowitz, M. B. (1991). Occurrence of neoplasia in patients with rheumatoid arthritis enrolled in a DMARD Registry. Rheumatoid Arthritis Azathioprine Registry Steering Committee. *Journal of Rheumatology, 18,* 809–814.

McLaughlin, J. K., Malker, H. S., Linet, M. S., Ericsson, J., Stone, B. J., Weiner, J., Blot, W. J., and Fraumeni, J. F. J. (1988). Multiple myeloma and occupation in Sweden. *Archives of Environmental Health, 43,* 7–10.

McWhorter, W. P., Schatzkin, A. G., Horm, J. W., and Brown, C. C. (1989). Contribution of socioeconomic status to black/white differences in cancer incidence. *Cancer, 63,* 982–987.

Mellemkjaer, L., Gridley, G., Moller, H., Hsing, A. W., Linet, M. S., Brinton, L. A., and Olsen, J. H. (1996b). Pernicious anaemia and cancer risk in Denmark. *British Journal of Cancer, 73*, 998–1000.

Mellemkjaer, L., Linet, M. S., Gridley, G., Frisch, M., Moller, H., and Olsen, J. H. (1996a). Rheumatoid arthritis and cancer risk. *European Journal of Cancer, 32A*, 1753–1757.

Milham, S. J. (1971). Leukemia and multiple myeloma in farmers. *American Journal of Epidemiology, 94*, 507–510.

Miligi, L., Seniori, C. A., Crosignani, P., Fontana, A., Masala, G., Nanni, O., Ramazzotti, V., Rodella, S., Stagnaro, E., Tumino, R., Vigano, C., Vindigni, C., and Vineis, P. (1999). Occupational, environmental, and life-style factors associated with the risk of hematolymphopoietic malignancies in women. *American Journal of Industrial Medicine, 36*, 60–69.

Miller, B. A., Blair, A., and Reed, E. J. (1994). Extended mortality follow-up among men and women in a U.S. furniture workers union. *American Journal of Industrial Medicine, 25*, 537–549.

Miller, B. A., Blair, A. E., Raynor, H. L., Stewart, P. A., Zahm, S. H., and Fraumeni, J. F. J. (1989). Cancer and other mortality patterns among United States furniture workers. *British Journal of Industrial Medicine, 46*, 508–515.

Miller, B. A., Ries, L. A. G., Hankey, B. F., Kosary, C. L., Harras, A., Devesa, S. S., and Edwards, B. K. (1993). SEER Cancer Statistics: Review 1973–1990. NIH Pub. No. 93–2789,

Mills, P. K., Beeson, W. L., Fraser, G. E., and Phillips, R. L. (1992). Allergy and cancer: Organ site-specific results from the Adventist Health Study. *American Journal of Epidemiology, 136*, 287–295.

Mills, P. K., Newell, G. R., Beeson, W. L., Fraser, G. E., and Phillips, R. L. (1990). History of cigarette smoking and risk of leukemia and myeloma: Results from the Adventist health study. *Journal of the National Cancer Institute, 82*, 1832–1836.

Montella, M., Crispo, A., de Bellis, G., Izzo, F., Frigeri, F., Ronga, D., Spada, O., Mettivier, V., Tamburini, M., and Cuomo, O. (2001). HCV and cancer: A case-control study in a high-endemic area. *Liver, 21*, 335–341.

Morris, P. D., Koepsell, T. D., Daling, J. R., Taylor, J. W., Lyon, J. L., Swanson, G. M., Child, M., and Weiss, N. S. (1986). Toxic substance exposure and multiple myeloma: A case-control study. *Journal of the National Cancer Institute, 76*, 987–994.

Muirhead, C. R., Goodill, A. A., Haylock, R. G., Vokes, J., Little, M. P., Jackson, D. A., O'Hagan, J. A., Thomas, J. M., Kendall, G. M., Silk, T. J., Bingham, D., and Berridge, G. L. (1999). Occupational radiation exposure and mortality: Second analysis of the National Registry for Radiation Workers. *Journal of Radiological Protection, 19*, 3–26.

Nandakumar, A., Armstrong, B. K., and de Klerk, N. H. (1986). Multiple myeloma in Western Australia: A case–control study in relation to occupation, father's occupation, socioeconomic status and country of birth. *International Journal of Cancer, 37*, 223–226.

Nandakumar, A., English, D. R., Dougan, L. E., and Armstrong, B. K. (1988). Incidence and outcome of multiple myeloma in Western Australia, 1960 to 1984. *Australian and New Zealand Journal of Medicine, 18*, 774–779.

Ng, M. H., Chung, Y. F., Lo, K. W., Wickham, N. W., Lee, J. C., and Huang, D. P. (1997). Frequent hypermethylation of p16 and p15 genes in multiple myeloma. *Blood, 89*, 2500–2506.

Ogmundsdottir, H. M., Haraldsdottir, V., Johannesson, M., Olafsdottir, G., Bjarnadottir, K., Sigvaldason, H., and Tulinius, H. (2002). Monoclonal gammopathy in Iceland: A population-based registry and follow-up. *British Journal of Haematology, 118*, 166–173.

Olsen, S. J., Tarte, K., Sherman, W., Hale, E. E., Weisse, M. T., Orazi, A., Klein, B., and Chang, Y. (1998). Evidence against KSHV infection in the pathogenesis of multiple myeloma. *Virus Research, 57*, 197–202.

Olshan, A. F. (1991). Familial and genetic associations. In G. I. Obrams, and M. Potter (Eds.), *Epidemiology and Biology of Multiple Myeloma* (pp. 31–39). New York: Springer.

Omar, R. Z., Barber, J. A., and Smith, P. G. (1999). Cancer mortality and morbidity among plutonium workers at the Sellafield plant of British Nuclear Fuels. *British Journal of Cancer, 79*, 1288–1301.

Osserman, E. F., Merlini, G., and Butler, V. P., Jr. (1987). Multiple myeloma and related plasma cell dyscrasias. *Journal of the American Medical Association, 258*, 2930–2937.

Papadopoulos, N. M., Lane, H. C., Costello, R., Moutsopoulos, H. M., Masur, H., Gelmann, E. P., and Fauci, A. S. (1985). Oligoclonal immunoglobulins in patients with the acquired immunodeficiency syndrome. *Clinical Immunology and Immunopathology, 35*, 43–46.

Parker, K. M., Ma, M. H., Manyak, S., Altamirano, C. V., Tang, Y. M., Frantzen, M., Mikail, A., Roussos, E., Sjak-Shie, N., Vescio, R. A., and Berenson, J. R. (2002). Identification of polymorphisms of the IkappaBalpha gene associated with an increased risk of multiple myeloma. *Cancer Genetics and Cytogenetics, 137*, 43–48.

Parravicini, C., Lauri, E., Baldini, L., Neri, A., Poli, F., Sirchia, G., Moroni, M., Galli, M., and Corbellino, M. (1997). Kaposi's sarcoma–associated herpesvirus infection and multiple myeloma. *Science, 278*, 1969–1970.

Pasqualetti, P., Casale, R., Collacciani, A., and Colantonio, D. (1990). Work activities and the risk of multiple myeloma. A case-control study. *La Medicina del Lavoro, 81*, 308–319.

Pasqualetti, P., Festuccia, V., Collacciani, A., and Casale, R. (1997). The natural history of monoclonal gammopathy of undetermined significance. A 5- to 20-year follow-up of 263 cases. *Acta Haematologica, 97*, 174–179.

Patel, M., Mahlangu, J., Patel, J., Stevens, G., Stevens, W., Allard, U., and Mendelow, B. (2001). Kaposi sarcoma-associated herpesvirus/human herpesvirus 8 and multiple myeloma in South Africa. *Diagnostic Molecular Pathology, 10*, 95–99.

Patel, M., Wadee, A. A., Galpin, J., Gavalakis, C., Fourie, A. M., Kuschke, R. H., and Philip, V. (2002). HLA class I and class II antigens associated with multiple myeloma in southern Africa. *Clinical and Laboratory Haematology, 24*, 215–219.

Pearce, N., and Reif, J. S. (1990). Epidemiologic studies of cancer in agricultural workers. *American Journal of Industrial Medicine, 18*, 133–148.

Pearce, N. E., and Howard, J. K. (1986). Occupation, social class and male cancer mortality in New Zealand, 1974–78. *International Journal of Epidemiology, 15*, 456–462.

Pearce, N. E., Smith, A. H., and Fisher, D. O. (1985). Malignant lymphoma and multiple myeloma linked with agricultural occupations in a New Zealand Cancer Registry-based study. *American Journal of Epidemiology, 121*, 225–237.

Pearce, N. E., Smith, A. H., Howard, J. K., Sheppard, R. A., Giles, H. J., and Teague, C. A. (1986). Case-control study of multiple myeloma and farming. *British Journal of Cancer, 54*, 493–500.

Pettersson, T., Pukkala, E., Teppo, L., and Friman, C. (1992). Increased risk of cancer in patients with systemic lupus erythematosus. *Annals of the Rheumatic Diseases, 51*, 437–439.

Pickard, A. L., Gridley, G., Mellemkjae, L., Johansen, C., Kofoed-Enevoldsen, A., Cantor, K. P., and Brinton, L. A. (2002). Hyperparathyroidism and subsequent cancer risk in Denmark. *Cancer, 95*, 1611–1617.

Pottern, L. M., Gart, J. J., Nam, J. M., Dunston, G., Wilson, J., Greenberg, R., Schoenberg, J., Swanson, G. M., Liff, J., and Schwartz, A. G. (1992a). HLA and multiple myeloma among black and white men: Evidence of a genetic association. *Cancer Epidemiology, Biomarkers, and Prevention, 1*, 177–182.

Pottern, L. M., Heineman, E. F., Olsen, J. H., Raffn, E., and Blair, A. (1992b). Multiple myeloma among Danish women: Employment history and workplace exposures. *Cancer Causes and Control, 3*, 427–432.

Preston, D. L., Kusumi, S., Tomonaga, M., Izumi, S., Ron, E., Kuramoto, A., Kamada, N., Dohy, H., Matsuo, T., and Matsui, T. (1994). Cancer incidence in atomic bomb survivors. Part III. Leukemia, lymphoma and multiple myeloma, 1950–1987. *Radiation Research, 137*, S68–S97.

Pukkala, E., and Notkola, V. (1997). Cancer incidence among Finnish farmers, 1979–93. *Cancer Causes and Control, 8*, 25–33.

Radl, J., Liu, M., Hoogeveen, C. M., van den Berg, B. P., Minkman-Brondijk, R. J., Broerse, J. J., Zurcher, C., and van Zwieten, M. J. (1991). Monoclonal gammopathies in long-term surviving rhesus monkeys after lethal irradiation and bone marrow transplantation. *Clinical Immunology and Immunopathology, 60*, 305–309.

Raffn, E., Lynge, E., Juel, K., and Korsgaard, B. (1989). Incidence of cancer and mortality among employees in the asbestos cement industry in Denmark. *Brisith Journal of Industrial Medicine, 46*, 90–96.

Rask, C., Kelsen, J., Olesen, G., Nielsen, J. L., Obel, N., and Abildgaard, N. (2000). Danish patients with untreated multiple myeloma do not harbour human herpesvirus 8. *British Journal of Haematology, 108*, 96–98.

Reif, J., Pearce, N., and Fraser, J. (1989a). Cancer risks in New Zealand farmers. *International Journal of Epidemiology, 18*, 768–774.

Reif, J., Pearce, N., Kawachi, I., and Fraser, J. (1989b). Soft-tissue sarcoma, non-Hodgkin's lymphoma and other cancers in New Zealand forestry workers. *International Journal of Cancer, 43*, 49–54.

Rettig, M. B., Ma, H. J., Vescio, R. A., Pold, M., Schiller, G., Belson, D., Savage, A., Nishikubo, C., Wu, C., Fraser, J., Said, J. W., and Berenson, J. R. (1997). Kaposi's sarcoma–associated herpesvirus infection of bone marrow dendritic cells from multiple myeloma patients. *Science, 276*, 1851–1854.

Rinsky, R. A., Hornung, R. W., Silver, S. R., and Tseng, C. Y. (2002). Benzene exposure and hematopoietic mortality: A long-term epidemiologic risk assessment. *American Journal of Industrial Medicine, 42*, 474–480.

Rogot, E., and Murray, J. L. (1980). Smoking and causes of death among U.S. veterans: 16 years of observation. *Public Health Reports, 95*, 213–222.

Said, J. W., Rettig, M. R., Heppner, K., Vescio, R. A., Schiller, G., Ma, H. J., Belson, D., Savage, A., Shintaku, I. P., Koeffler, H. P., Asou, H., Pinkus, G., Pinkus, J., Schrage, M., Green, E., and Berenson, J. R. (1987). Localization of Kaposi's sarcoma-associated herpesvirus in bone marrow biopsy samples from patients with multiple myeloma. *Blood, 90*, 4278–4282.

Saleun, J. P., Vicariot, M., Deroff, P., and Morin, J. F. (1982). Monoclonal gammopathies in the adult population of Finistere, France. *Journal of Clinical Pathology, 35*, 63–68.

Schechter, G. P., Shoff, N., Chan, C., McManus, C. D., and Hawley, H. P. (1991). The frequency of monoclonal gammopathy of unknown significance in Black and Caucasian veterans in a hospital population. In G. I. Obrams, and M. Potter (Eds., *Epidemiology and Biology of Multiple Myeloma* (pp. 83–85). New York: Springer-Verlag.

Schwartz, D. A., Vaughan, T. L., Heyer, N. J., Koepsell, T. D., Lyon, J. L., Swanson, G. M., and Weiss, N. S. (1988). B cell neoplasms and occupational asbestos exposure. *American Journal of Industrial Medicine, 14*, 661–671.

Selby, J. V., Friedman, G. D., and Fireman, B. H. (1989). Screening prescription drugs for possible carcinogenicity: Eleven to fifteen years of follow-up. *Cancer Research, 49*, 5736–5747.

Shapira, R., and Carter, A. (1986). Multiple myeloma in Northern Israel, 1970–1979. *Cancer, 58*, 206–209.

Shimizu, Y., Kato, H., and Schull, W. J. (1990). Studies of the mortality of A-bomb survivors. 9. Mortality, 1950–1985: Part 2. Cancer mortality based on the recently revised doses (DS86). *Radiation Research, 121*, 120–141.

Shoenfeld, Y., Berliner, S., Shaklai, M., Gallant, L. A., and Pinkhas, J. (1982). Familial multiple myeloma. A review of thirty-seven families. *Postgraduate Medical Journal, 58*, 12–16.

Sinclair, D., Sheehan, T., Parrott, D. M., and Stott, D. I. (1986). The incidence of monoclonal gammopathy in a population over 45 years old determined by isoelectric focusing. *British Journal of Haematology, 64*, 745–750.

Sitas, F., Carrara, H., Beral, V., Newton, R., Reeves, G., Bull, D., Jentsch, U., Pacella-Norman, R., Bourboulia, D., Whitby, D., Boshoff, C., and Weiss, R. (1999). Antibodies against human herpesvirus 8 in black South African patients with cancer. *New England Journal of Medicine, 340*, 1863–1871.

Skibola, C. F., Smith, M. T., Kane, E., Roman, E., Rollinson, S., Cartwright, R. A., and Morgan, G. (1999). Polymorphisms in the methylenetetrahydrofolate reductase gene are associated with susceptibility to acute leukemia in adults. *Proceedings of the National Academy of Sciences of the United States of America, 96*, 12810–12815.

Smith, P. G., and Douglas, A. J. (1986). Mortality of workers at the Sellafield plant of British Nuclear Fuels. *British Medical Journal (Clinical Research Edition), 293*, 845–854.

Sonoda, T., Nagata, Y., Mori, M., Ishida, T., and Imai, K. (2001). Meta-analysis of multiple myeloma and benzene exposure. *Journal of Epidemiology, 11*, 249–254.

Sorahan, T., and Cooke, M. A. (1989). Cancer mortality in a cohort of United Kingdom steel foundry workers: 1946–85. *British Journal of Industrial Medicine, 46*, 74–81.

Soutar, R. L., Dawson, A. A., and Wilson, B. J. (1996). Multiple myeloma in northeast Scotland: A review of incidence and survival over three decades. *Health Bull (Edinb), 54*, 232–240.

Spinelli, J. J., Gallagher, R. P., Band, P. R., and Threlfall, W. J. (1984). Multiple myeloma, leukemia, and cancer of the ovary in cosmetologists and hairdressers. *American Journal of Industrial Medicine, 6*, 97–102.

Stagnaro, E., Ramazzotti, V., Crosignani, P., Fontana, A., Masala, G., Miligi, L., Nanni, O., Neri, M., Rodella, S., Costantini, A. S., Tumino, R., Vigano, C., Vindigni, C., and Vineis, P. (2001). Smoking and hematolymphopoietic malignancies. *Cancer Causes and Control, 12*, 325–334.

Stark, A. D., Chang, H. G., Fitzgerald, E. F., Riccardi, K., and Stone, R. R. (1990). A retrospective cohort study of cancer incidence among New York State Farm Bureau members. *Archives of Environmental Health, 45*, 155–162.

Steineck, G., and Wiklund, K. (1986). Multiple myeloma in Swedish agricultural workers. *International Journal of Epidemiology, 15*, 321–325.

Svensson, B. G., Mikoczy, Z., Stromberg, U., and Hagmar, L. (1995). Mortality and cancer incidence among Swedish fishermen with a high dietary intake of persistent organochlorine compounds. *Scandinavian Journal of Work, Environment, and Health, 21*, 106–115.

Swaen, G. M., van Vliet, C., Slangen, J. J., and Sturmans, F. (1992). Cancer mortality among licensed herbicide applicators. *Scandinavian Journal of Work, Environment, and Health, 18*, 201–204.

Sweeney, D. M., Manzi, S., Janosky, J., Selvaggi, K. J., Ferri, W., Medsger, T. A., Jr., and Ramsey-Goldman, R. (1995). Risk of malignancy in women with systemic lupus erythematosus. *Journal of Rheumatology, 22*, 1478–1482.

Symmons, D. P. (1985). Neoplasms of the immune system in rheumatoid arthritis. *American Journal of Medicine, 78*, 22–28.

Tarte, K., Olsen, S. J., Rossi, J. F., Legouffe, E., Lu, Z. Y., Jourdan, M., Chang, Y., and Klein, B. (1998). Kaposi's sarcoma–associated herpesvirus is not detected with immunosuppression in multiple myeloma. *Blood, 92*, 2186–2188.

Tavani, A., Pregnolato, A., Negri, E., Franceschi, S., Serraino, D., Carbone, A., and La Vecchia, C. (1997). Diet and risk of lymphoid neoplasms and soft tissue sarcomas. *Nutrition and Cancer, 27*, 256–260.

Tedeschi, R., Kvarnung, M., Knekt, P., Schulz, T. F., Szekely, L., De Paoli, P. D., Aromaa, A., Teppo, L., and Dillner, J. (2001). A prospective seroepidemiological study of human herpesvirus-8 infection and the risk of multiple myeloma. *British Journal of Cancer, 84,* 122–125.

Tennis, P., Andrews, E., Bombardier, C., Wang, Y., Strand, L., West, R., Tilson, H., and Doi, P. (1993). Record linkage to conduct an epidemiologic study on the association of rheumatoid arthritis and lymphoma in the Province of Saskatchewan, Canada. *Journal of Clinical Epidemiology, 46,* 685–695.

Teta, M. J., and Ott, M. G. (1988). A mortality study of a research, engineering, and metal fabrication facility in western New York State. *American Journal of Epidemiology, 127,* 540–551.

Teta, M. J., Walrath, J., Meigs, J. W., and Flannery, J. T. (1984). Cancer incidence among cosmetologists. *Journal of the National Cancer Institute, 72,* 1051–1057.

Thun, M. J., Altekruse, S. F., Namboodiri, M. M., Calle, E. E., Myers, D. G., and Heath, C. W., Jr. (1994). Hair dye use and risk of fatal cancers in U.S. women. *Journal of the National Cancer Institute, 86,* 210–215.

Tisdale, J. F., Stewart, A. K., Dickstein, B., Little, R. F., Dube, I., Cappe, D., Dunbar, C. E., and Brown, K. E. (1998). Molecular and serological examination of the relationship of human herpesvirus 8 to multiple myeloma: orf 26 sequences in bone marrow stroma are not restricted to myeloma patients and other regions of the genome are not detected. *Blood, 92,* 2681–2687.

Tollerud, D. J., Brinton, L. A., Stone, B. J., Tobacman, J. K., and Blattner, W. A. (1985). Mortality from multiple myeloma among North Carolina furniture workers. *Journal of the National Cancer Institute, 74,* 799–801.

Tollerud, D. J., Brown, L. M., Blattner, W. A., and Hoover, R. N. (1991). The influence of race on T-cell subset distributions. In G. I. Obrams, and M. Potter (Eds.), *Epidemiology and Biology of Multiple Myeloma* (pp. 45–49). New York: Springer-Verlag.

Tomasek, L., Darby, S. C., Swerdlow, A. J., Placek, V., and Kunz, E. (1993). Radon exposure and cancers other than lung cancer among uranium miners in West Bohemia. *Lancet, 341,* 919–923.

Turesson, I., Zettervall, O., Cuzick, J., Waldenstrom, J. G., and Velez, R. (1984). Comparison of trends in the incidence of multiple myeloma in Malmo, Sweden, and other countries, 1950–1979. *New England Journal of Medicine, 310,* 421–424.

Vagero, D., and Persson, G. (1986). Occurrence of cancer in socioeconomic groups in Sweden. An analysis based on the Swedish Cancer Environment Registry. *Scandinavian Journal of Social Medicine, 14,* 151–160.

Van De Donk, N., De Weerdt, O., Eurelings, M., Bloem, A., and Lokhorst, H. (2001). Malignant transformation of monoclonal gammopathy of undetermined significance: Cumulative incidence and prognostic factors. *Leukemia and Lymphoma, 42,* 609–618.

van de Poel, M. H., Coebergh, J. W., and Hillen, H. F. (1995). Malignant transformation of monoclonal gammopathy of undetermined significance among outpatients of a community hospital in southeastern Netherlands. *British Journal of Haematology, 91,* 121–125.

Van den Eeden, S. K., and Friedman, G. D. (1993). Exposure to engine exhaust and risk of subsequent cancer. *Journal of Occupational Medicine, 35,* 307–311.

Velez, R., Beral, V., and Cuzick, J. (1982). Increasing trends of multiple myeloma mortality in England and Wales; 1950–79: Are the changes real? *Journal of the National Cancer Institute, 69,* 387–392.

Vesterinen, E., Pukkala, E., Timonen, T., and Aromaa, A. (1993). Cancer incidence among 78,000 asthmatic patients. *International Journal of Epidemiology, 22,* 976–982.

Vineis, P., Crosignani, P., Sacerdote, C., Fontana, A., Masala, G., Miligi, L., Nanni, O., Ramazzotti, V., Rodella, S., Stagnaro, E., Tumino, R., Vigano, C., Vindigni, C., and Costantini, A. S. (2000). Haematopoietic cancer and medical history: A multicentre case control study. *Journal of Epidemiology and Community Health, 54,* 431–436.

Wang, C. R., Chuang, C. Y., Lin, K. T., Chen, M. Y., Lee, G. L., Hsieh, R. P., and Chen, C. Y. (1992). Monoclonal gammopathies and the related autoimmune manifestations in Taiwan. *Asian Pacific Journal of Allergy and Immunology, 10,* 123–128.

Wang, J. X., Boice, J. D., Jr., Li, B. X., Zhang, J. Y., and Fraumeni, J. F., Jr. (1988). Cancer among medical diagnostic x-ray workers in China. *Journal of the National Cancer Institute, 80,* 344–350.

Wiklund, K., Dich, J., Holm, L. E., and Eklund, G. (1989). Risk of cancer in pesticide applicators in Swedish agriculture. *British Journal of Industrial Medicine, 46,* 809–814.

Wilczynska, U., Szadkowska-Stanczyk, I., Szeszenia-Dabrowska, N., Sobala, W., and Strzelecka, A. (2001). Cancer mortality in rubber tire workers in Poland. *International Journal of Ocupational Medicine and Environmental Health, 14,* 115–125.

Williams, R. R., and Horm, J. W. (1977). Association of cancer sites with tobacco and alcohol consumption and socioeconomic status of patients: Interview study from the Third National Cancer Survey. *Journal of the National Cancer Institute, 58,* 525–547.

Wing, S., Richardson, D., Wolf, S., Mihlan, G., Crawford–Brown, D., and Wood, J. (2000). A case control study of multiple myeloma at four nuclear facilities. *Annals of Epidemiology, 10,* 144–153.

Wolvekamp, M. C., and Marquet, R. L. (1990). Interleukin-6: historical background, genetics and biological significance. *Immunology Letters, 24,* 1–9.

Wong, O. (1995). Risk of acute myeloid leukaemia and multiple myeloma in workers exposed to benzene. *Occupational and Environmental Medicine, 52,* 380–384.

Yi, Q., Ekman, M., Anton, D., Bergenbrant, S., Osterborg, A., Georgii-Hemming, P., Holm, G., Nilsson, K., and Biberfeld, P. (1998). Blood dendritic cells from myeloma patients are not infected with Kaposi's sarcoma–associated herpesvirus (KSHV/HHV-8). *Blood, 92,* 402–404.

Youinou, P., Le Corre, R., and Dueymes, M. (1996). Autoimmune diseases and monoclonal gammopathies. *Clinical and Experimental Rheumatology, 14,* S55–S58.

Zahm, S. H., Weisenburger, D. D., Babbitt, P. A., Saal, R. C., Vaught, J. B., and Blair, A. (1992). Use of hair coloring products and the risk of lymphoma, multiple myeloma, and chronic lymphocytic leukemia. *American Journal of Public Health, 82,* 990–997.

Zheng, C., Huang, D., Liu, L., Bjorkholm, M., Holm, G., Yi, Q., and Sundblad, A. (2001b). Cytotoxic T-lymphocyte antigen-4 microsatellite polymorphism is associated with multiple myeloma. *British Journal of Haematology, 112,* 216–218.

Zheng, C., Huang, D., Liu, L., Wu, R., Bergenbrant, G. S., Osterborg, A., Bjorkholm, M., Holm, G., Yi, Q., and Sundblad, A. (2001a). Interleukin-10 gene promoter polymorphisms in multiple myeloma. *International Journal of Cancer, 95,* 184–188.

Zheng, C., Huang, D. R., Bergenbrant, S., Sundblad, A., Osterborg, A., Bjorkholm, M., Holm, G., and Yi, Q. (2000). Interleukin 6, tumour necrosis factor alpha, interleukin 1beta and interleukin 1 receptor antagonist promoter or coding gene polymorphisms in multiple myeloma. *British Journal of Haematology, 109,* 39–45.

# CHAPTER 9

# Clinical Presentation, Laboratory Diagnosis, and Indications for Treatment

JAMES S. MALPAS
JAMIE D. CAVENAGH

## Introduction

Multiple myeloma (MM) is caused by a clonal proliferation of idiotypic B lymphoid cells characterized by infiltration of the bone marrow with malignant plasma cells causing suppression of normal hematopoiesis and bone destruction. Plasma cells have the ability to produce monoclonal "M" bands of immunoglobulin or the light chain moiety of immunoglobulin, which is present in serum, but because of its low molecular weight is excreted in the urine (known as Bence Jones protein).

The production of monoclonal immunoglobulins G, A, D, E, and (rarely) M, with or without a monoclonal kappa or lambda light chain is a major feature of the disease. It is not diagnostic because these paraproteins could be seen in a miscellaneous group of conditions, including amyloidosis, scleromyxoedema, heavy chain disease, lymphoplasmacytoid lymphoma, Waldenström's macroglobulinemia, and cold agglutinin disease.

In MM, IgG is the most common paraprotein in all series. The percentage distribution is shown in Table 9-1. The discrepancy in the proportion of rare forms between the two series probably is related to the fact that in the series collected since 1965 these forms were not recognized and were therefore not recorded.

# Epidemiology

The epidemiology of MM is discussed in Chapter 8. The main features that bear on diagnosis are reviewed.

## Incidence

Myeloma was once considered a rare disease (Atkinson, 1937; Geschicter and Copeland, 1928), but many series published in the 1960s commented on its frequency (Innes and Newall, 1961; Nordenson, 1966; Talerman, 1969). MM comprises approximately 1% of all malignant disease and 10% of hematologic malignancies (Kyle, 1990). The proportion of patients that present with MM as a hematologic malignancy increases with advancing age. Riggs (1995), in a study using United States mortality data, compared annual age-specific MM mortality rates from 1968 to 1989 in age groups over 60 years to annual age group population sizes. He was able to demonstrate that rising mortality rates in the United States were related to the increasing age group population size. The annual age-specific incidence of MM increases from less than 1 per 100,000 at 40 years of age to 40 per 100,000 at the age of 80 (Rodon, 2001). The median age of MM patients in the community who were referred for treatment in a general hospital was significantly higher at 70 years of age compared with the median age of patients referred to specialist hematology units at 64.5 years, significant at the $p = .0001$ level (Patriaca, 1997). In the context of other hematologic conditions, MM has an incidence of 3 per 100,000, compared with chronic lymphatic leukemia (6 per 100,000) or pernicious anemia (120 per 100,000). In elderly patients the proportion of patients presenting with MM is high and this must be considered in any primarily geriatric practice.

## Age

Myeloma is characteristically a disease of the late middle-aged and elderly. In most hospital series the median age is 65 years with the majority of patients falling within the 60- to 75-year age group. Fewer than 2% of Kyle's patients were under 40 years of age and approximately 3% were over the age of 80 at presentation. An analysis of the presenting features and survival of elderly patients with MM who were aged 70 or more (Blade et al., 1996) found that presenting features did not differ from younger patients but response to chemotherapy and survival was less satisfactory. The possibility of MM might be thought of in the elderly but it could be more difficult to remember as a differential diagnosis in the young in whom it is rare (Kyle, 1975). Six adolescents and young adults with features of MM have been reported (Maeda et al., 1973). All these patients showed unusual features, including nasopharyngeal and other soft tissue masses and nearly all had an IgA monoclonal band. One of the youngest classic MM patients was a 25-year-old man (De Coteau et al., 1992). Blade et al. (1992) studied the presenting clinical and laboratory features of 72 patients who were less than 40 years of age at presentation. MM is relatively infrequent in younger age groups with an incidence of 0.3% in patients under the age of 30 and 2.2% in patients under 40 years of age. Bone pain (66%), fatigue (26%), extramedullary plasmacytosis (19%), and bacterial infection were the leading presenting features, whereas impairment of renal function (29%) and hypercalcemia (30%) were common laboratory findings. Anecdotal reports of a more aggressive course in younger patients were not confirmed. In this series the presenting features of young patients were very similar to those of older populations, and in those with good prognostic features, survival tended to be better.

Recently the presence of acquired immunodeficiency syndrome (AIDS) in the community has begun to make an impression on disease incidence and age of first presentation (Fiorino and Atac, 1997). In a review of plasma cell tumors in patients with AIDS, there was an incidence of monoclonal or mono- and oligoclonal gammopathy in as high as 56% of patients with AIDS. AIDS patients with MGUS, plasmacytomas, or MM had a mean age of 33 years, significantly lower than the uninfected population.

## Sex

Most series (Hansen et al., 1989; Kapadia, 1980; Kyle, 1975; Talerman, 1969) show a slight male preponderance, with a male to female ratio varying from

---

## TABLE 9-1

### Distribution (in Percent) of Monoclonal Serum Proteins in MM

| Protein | St. Bart's Hospital (1968–2001) | Mayo Clinic (1982–1987) |
|---|---|---|
| IgG | 54 | 50 |
| IgA | 21 | 21 |
| Light chain | 19 | 17 |
| IgD | 1 | 2 |
| Non-secretory | 2 | 9 |

UK data, Malpas 2002
USA data, Kyle 1990

| TABLE 9-2 | |
|---|---|
| Sex Ratio Noted in Major Series | |
| **Male/Female Ratio** | **Authors** |
| 1.1:1 | Talerman, 1968 |
| 1.5:1 | Kyle, 1975 |
| 1.1:1 | Kapadia, 1980 |
| 1.2:1 | Hansen, 1989 |
| 1.5:1 | Malpas, 1995 |

1.1–1.5 to 1 (Table 9-2). Hansen et al. (1989) noted that between 1943 and 1963 there was an early and increased male incidence but that after 1963 the ratio remained stable.

## Race

There is a greater incidence of MM in both black males and females compared with the white population (Waterhouse et al., 1982). These authors estimate the incidence at more than double that in the white population in parts of the United States (Table 9-3). MM is said to be less common in Asian populations but this remains to be confirmed. Racial incidence should be considered in diagnosis.

## Familial Incidence

A retrospective study of related patients with MM showed that siblings were most frequently affected; 10 of 15 families were affected in this way (Grosbois et al., 1999). The clinical features were similar to unrelated patients with MM. In seven families the monoclonal component was IgG kappa. A familial history of MGUS was present in three families. Family cancer data in Sweden has enabled parental lineages in cancer to be examined. The sites of increased cancer risk in offspring included various solid tumors and MM (Hemminki and Vaittinen, 1998).

## Clinical Course

Myeloma in its classic form pursues a relentless course unless treated. Before the introduction of chemotherapy, the median survival was 6 to 9 months (Osgood, 1960). The use of alkylating agents with or without steroids produced responses in more than half the patients and increased median survival to 26 months in an unselected series of stage III patients (Durie and Salmon, 1975). The survival curve shown in Figure 9-1 is for an unselected series of patients at St. Bartholomew's Hospital and shows the inexorable attrition characteristic of the disease.

Currently the disease is thought to be incurable, although some series (Fuzibet et al., 1986; Kyle, 1983; Rosner et al., 1992) recorded patients surviving longer than 5 to 10 years. As shown in Figure 9-1, there are a small number of patients now surviving for more than 15 years and approximately 15% of patients are surviving 10 years. Good prognostic factors and an excellent response to chemotherapy were associated with a good outlook.

An unusual feature of MM is the phenomenon of the "plateau." The disease appears to become arrested and all measurements of the criteria of activity, such as the "M" band in the serum or urinary light chain, which show that although the disease is present, there is no progression. It would appear that although no further treatment is being given, the factors causing progression of the malignancy are temporarily down regulated, a feature uncommon in any other malignancy. The features of MM arising from previously established MGUS have been shown to differ in having a lower frequency of advanced stage disease, fewer high-risk characteristics such as anemia, renal failure, and bone lesions; and although responding to treatment equally well as de novo MM, had a significantly longer median duration of survival, 60 months versus 31 months $p = 0.05$ (Patriaca, 1998).

## Clinical Presentation

Before diagnostic criteria are discussed, it is important that the pace of development of a plasma cell malignancy is considered. This not only has importance for understanding and defining these conditions, but it is of practical value in determining when and how a patient should be treated. This is considered in more detail later in this chapter. The pace of the development of the disease is an expression of the malignancy of the B cell clone and underlies the spectrum from benign

| TABLE 9-3 | | |
|---|---|---|
| Incidence of MM in Black and White Communities in the United States (rates per 100,000) | | |
| | **Male** | **Female** |
| Bay Area | | |
| Blacks | 8.5 | 5.6 |
| Whites | 3.3 | 2.0 |
| Detroit | | |
| Blacks | 7.4 | 4.7 |
| Whites | 3.3 | 2.3 |
| Atlanta | | |
| Blacks | 4.8 | 4.3 |
| Whites | 2.7 | 2.5 |

## Overall Survival Myeloma Patients 1968 - 2001

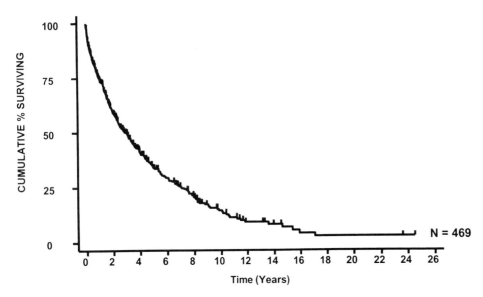

**Figure 9-1** *Survival of 469 consecutive patients admitted with multiple myeloma to St. Bartholomew's Hospital.*

monoclonal gammopathy (monoclonal gammopathy of undetermined significance [MGUS]) (Kyle, 1978) through indolent and smoldering myeloma to the familiar entity of overt clinical MM (Greipp, 1992). These monoclonal gammopathies should be defined.

### MGUS

This condition is described fully in Chapter 19. It must be considered in the differential diagnosis of MM. In MGUS the patient is well with no hematologic or renal symptoms; this good health is maintained for many years and the "M" component remains stable during this time. Approximately 18% of these patients progress to lymphoma or MM in 10 years, thus belying the original description of "benign monoclonal gammopathy." The diagnostic features are given in Table 9-4. It is detected in approximately 3% of elderly patients (Axelsson et al., 1966; Kyle et al., 1972, 1978) when conventional methods of electrophoresis are used. With the use of isoelectric focusing, the incidence rises to 11% (Sinclair et al., 1986).

Patients with MGUS need to be observed because they can be considered to have a premalignant condition. Approximately 25% of patients with MGUS go on to develop MM or related disorders. It is very difficult, if not impossible, to determine which patients with MGUS will progress (Fudenberg and Virella, 1980). Recent cytogenetic studies have not helped because chromosomal abnormalities are being found as frequently as in MM (Baldini et al., 1996) and have suggested that those patients with MGUS least likely to progress are those with no reduction in background immunoglobulin, no light chain proteinuria, bone marrow plasma cells less that 5%, and an IgG value of less than 1.5 g/dL.

### Smoldering Myeloma (SMM)

Patients with SMM, like those with MGUS, remain stable for many years. These patients resemble MM at presentation and diagnosis requires care. The criteria for diagnosis are given in Table 9-5. Kyle and Greipp (1980) first described patients fulfilling these criteria. They formed 2% of a series of patients with MM, and over 5 years these patients developed no signs or

| TABLE 9-4 | | |
|---|---|---|
| Criteria for the Diagnosis of MGUS | | |

| **Monoclonal Gammopathy** | | |
|---|---|---|
| "M" component | IgG < 35 g/L | |
| | IgA < 20 g/L | |
| Bence Jones protein | < 1.0 g/per 24 h | |
| Bone marrow infiltration with plasma cells | < 10% | |
| No bone lesions | | |
| No symptoms | | |
| No anemia, renal failure, or hypercalcemia | | |

| ═══════ TABLE 9-5 ═══════ |
| Criteria for the Diagnosis of SMM |

**Monoclonal Gammopathy**

| "M" component | IgG > 35 g/L |
| | IgA > 20 g/L |
| Bence Jones protein | > 1 g/per 24 h |
| Bone marrow infiltration with plasma cells | >10% but < 20% |
| No anemia, renal failure, or hypercalcemia | |
| No bone lesions on skeletal survey | |

| ═══════ TABLE 9-6 ═══════ |
| Diagnostic Criteria for MM |

**Durie (1986)**
**Major criteria**

| Plasmacytosis in tissue | |
| Bone marrow plasmacytosis >30% | |
| Monoclonal | IgG > 35 g/L |
| | IgA > 20 g/L |
| Bence Jones protein | > 1g/24h |
| Lytic bone lesions | |
| Suppression of normal immunoglobulins | |

**Greipp (1992)**
"M" band present in serum or urine
>10% plasma cells on aspirate or bone marrow biopsy
Increased beta2M
Thymidine labeling index >0.5%
Loss of light chain idiotype expression
Bone lesions

symptoms of MM. These patients need careful monitoring and if there is a change in their condition, a skeletal survey or MRI scan is indicated. Although the patients' "M" component might remain stable, it is "set" at a higher level.

### Indolent Multiple Myeloma (IMM)

IMM is very similar to SMM except that anemia and a few small lytic lesions do not preclude the diagnosis. The condition evolves slowly but there is usually a rise in the "M" component within 3 years, and this rise usually heralds the onset of overt MM. This is a difficult condition to diagnose and also needs careful monitoring. The importance of recognizing the previously mentioned conditions cannot be overemphasized because they do not require treatment. It is important that they are subject to careful followup.

None of the conditions described here should be confused with solitary plasmacytoma of bone (SPB) or extramedullary plasmacytoma (EMP), which are described in Chapter 20. In these conditions there is usually no evidence of systemic spread and disappearance of an "M" component or urinary light chain after therapy to the solitary lesion.

### Multiple Myeloma (MM)

Fully developed overt and symptomatic plasma cell dyscrasia (MM) is one of the most common plasma cell dyscrasias mentioned so far. It is characterized by numerous lytic bone lesions, bone marrow infiltration with more than 30% plasma cells and plasmablasts, overproduction of monoclonal immunoglobulin, and excretion of light chains in the urine. The excretion of light chains or Bence Jones protein might be the only abnormality and rarely, neither paraprotein nor light chain is present, the so-called "non-secretory MM." It is now possible to follow the course of this condition by new and sensitive methods for estimating serum-free light chains (Drayson et al., 2001). Several lists of criteria for the diagnosis of MM have been developed

(Durie, 1986; Greipp, 1992); these are given in Table 9-6. In a recent comparison of systems for defining MM, MM variants, and MGUS, Ong et al. (1995a) found little difference between currently used criteria, although they noted that a system used by the British Columbia Cancer Agency was easier to use. The diagnosis of MM is acceptable if one major and one minor criterion is present. Essential major criteria are either marrow plasmacytosis or an "M" component in the serum or urine.

# Staging

Staging and its effect on prognosis is dealt with in detail in Chapter 11, and reference will only be made to the well-tried staging system introduced by Durie and Salmon in 1975 in a study of 71 patients with MM. Their system is shown in Chapter 11.

### Presenting Features of MM

MM is a difficult disease to diagnose in the elderly, because so many symptoms, such as fatigue and pain, are common in this age group that presenting features might be easily missed. Support for this assertion comes from Ong et al. (1995b), who studied the case histories of 127 patients diagnosed with MM. They defined patients as "not immediately diagnosed" or "delayed diagnosis" when MM was not considered in the initial diagnosis. Thirty-seven percent of the patients belonged to this category. Surprisingly, more than half were found to have Durie and Salmon stage 111 disease on investigation. This emphasized how symptomatology secondary to other coincidental conditions might make diagnosis difficult.

## Bone Pain

One of the most common presenting features of MM is bone pain. This has been variously estimated at 87% (Talerman, 1969), 63% (Kapadia, 1980), 68% (Kyle, 1975), 55.3% (Oshima et al., 2001). The most common site is the back. Seventeen of 46 (34%) of Oshima et al.'s patients had backache or lumbago at presentation. Backache is usually exacerbated by standing and relieved by lying down. An exception is when rib lesions are present. When patients turn over in bed they experience severe chest pain; sudden severe pain across the front of the chest, which can mimic myocardial infarction, and can follow spontaneous fracture of the manubrium sterni. Pain can also occur in the extremities, and if severe or unresponsive to rest, might indicate that a pathologic fracture has occurred.

The pain of MM is usually of insidious onset but occasionally abrupt after lifting heavy weight while gardening, and so on. This is caused by compression collapse of the thoracic or lumbar vertebrae. Painful repeated compressions might lead to loss of height, thus it is worth asking the patient or spouse whether they have noted that height is being lost. It is of interest that skull deposits in MM are rarely if ever painful.

The more extensive the bone lesions, the greater the tumor mass (Durie, 1986). Excessive osteoclastic activity might result in lytic lesions, fractures, osteoporosis or various combinations of these features. The radiology of these features is reviewed in Chapter 10. Kyle (1975) noted that a combination of these features occurred in 57% of patients, whereas lytic lesions, osteoporosis, or fractures occurred as solitary features in 13%, 6%, and 3%, respectively. However, no radiologic changes are found in 20% of patients. Kapadia (1980) found mixed abnormalities in 63% of his patients, with 16% showing no radiologic abnormality. Riccardi et al. (1991), when reviewing the incidence of bone disease at presentation in three major series, studying patients in the three decades of the 1960s, 1970s, and 1980s, noted a fall in pain as a presenting feature from 68% to 37%, although the frequency and extent of the bone lesions on skeletal survey had not altered during that time. He attributed this to greater awareness of the disease and earlier diagnosis.

## Weakness and Fatigue

These are prominent symptoms in elderly patients with MM. Because of their age, many patients have come to expect some degree of loss of activity, so this might not be mentioned in the history. Although pain is a contributing factor, the main cause is anemia consequent on bone marrow suppression. Kyle (1975) found that 62% of patients showed a hemoglobin level of less than 12 g/dL at presentation. Talerman (1969) gives a similar figure but notes that in the Jamaican population at least 50% of the patients had hemoglobin levels below 9 g/dL. Kapadia (1980) reported anemia of some degree in 81%. In a Japanese study 17 of 48 patients (37.8%) had hemoglobin levels of less than 8.5 g/dL (Oshima et al., 2001). The proportion reporting fatigue and weakness correlates very closely with the level of anemia in most major series (Kyle, 1975; Riccardi et al., 1991). The anemia is usually the normochromic normocytic form associated with malignancy but occasionally can be the result of chronic bleeding, either as a result of thrombocytopenia or some rarer coagulation defect. Inquiry about the presence of purpura on the skin or bleeding from the mucous membranes is important, as Kyle (1975) noted that 10% to 13% of patients with MM presented with platelet counts below 100 $10^9$/L. Very rarely patients might be jaundiced as a result of a Coombs'-positive hemolytic anemia.

## Fever and Infection

Unlike other B cell neoplasms (low- and high-grade non-Hodgkin's lymphoma, for example), fever is rare in uncomplicated MM. Kyle (1975) records only 1% of patients with uncomplicated MM as having fever. Bacterial and viral infections are far more common, and again in his series in 1975 he noted that 12% presented with fever. In the review of three large series of MM already mentioned, Riccardi et al. (1991) noted a fall in most systemic symptoms over the three decades, with the exception of infection. Although the incidence of infection at presentation is similar in many series of patients presenting in the 55- to 65-year age group, it appears that infectious complications are less frequent in young patients with MM than in patients over 75. Blade et al. (1992) recorded an incidence of 11% in 72 patients under 40 years of age, whereas Rodon (2001), in a study of 130 patients over 75, noted 30 infections in 26 patients, an incidence of 20%, and pointed out that infection in elderly patients had a serious adverse effect on prognosis. It is possible that a greater awareness of infections in patients with MM who are leukopenic or immunocompromised has resulted in a greater success in diagnosing infections. Barasch et al. (1986) stressed the frequency of pneumococcemia as a presenting feature of MM, and a history of recurrent pneumonia is not unusual in this condition. Recurrent maxillary sinusitis might also occur; furthermore, uncommon infections such as pneumococcal septic arthritis (Graham et al., 1991), meningococcal arthritis (Miller et al., 1987), and recurrent urinary tract infections with *Escherichia coli* (Kapadia, 1980) might indicate that leukopenia and other causes of impaired response to infection are present.

# Less Common Presenting Features of MM

These are discussed under the system in which they present and will be confined to the presenting features alone.

## Presenting Neurologic Features

A full description of neurologic findings in MM is given in Chapter 17. This chapter concentrates on the presenting features only.

The first indication of the presence of MM could be neurologic. Although relatively uncommon with only 2% of patients evincing them at presentation, nonetheless their recognition is extremely important. A careful neurologic history and examination of a patient with MM is mandatory. The chief reason is that spinal cord compression might be recognized early and can be relieved, thus avoiding disastrous sequelae. With increasing awareness, an incidence of 12% presenting with compressive symptoms of the spinal cord has been recorded by Spiess et al. (1988). Neurologic symptoms were found in as many as 32% of 184 patients reported by Bisagni-Faure et al. (1991), and 10% of these patients were paraplegic at the time of presentation. Although delay in diagnosis might be inevitable (in rural areas, for example, 23% of 97 Chinese patients were paraplegic at the time of first admission (Woo et al., 1986), signs of an upper motor lesion should be an urgent indication for myelography, CT, or MRI scanning.

Another rare neurologic presentation is leptomeningeal MM (De Blay et al., 2000; Leifer et al., 1992). MM is increasingly reported to affect specific sites such as the eye with diplopia, proptosis, ptosis, or ophthalmoplegia as a result of local infiltration (De Smet and Rootman, 1987) or a very rare infiltration of the iris (Shakin et al., 1998). Meningeal involvement might even rarely give rise to hydrocephalus (Dennis et al., 2000). Progressive visual loss might occur as a result of bilateral optic neuropathy (Lieberman et al., 1999).

Neurologic symptoms might be the first manifestation of hyperviscosity syndrome. This syndrome is a group of symptoms and signs related to the increased blood viscosity produced by monoclonal immunoglobulin, particularly IgM, but also polymers of IgG and IgA (Chandy et al., 1981; Preston et al., 1978). Rarely, it might complicate light chain MM (Carter et al., 1989; Kahn et al., 1987). The neurologic features are headache, blurring of vision, drowsiness, pre-coma, coma, vertigo, ataxia, hemiparesis, and finally epileptiform seizures. Retinal venous engorgement and hemorrhages are seen in Figure 9-2. A common sequence is the onset of headache followed by blurring of vision,

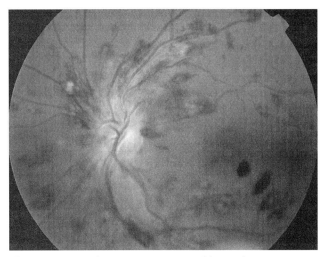

*Figure 9-2* Retinal vein engorgement and hemorrhage in a patient with hyperviscosity syndrome. Courtesy of Mr. R. A. F. Whitelocke.

lethargy, drowsiness, coma, and death. It is important to recognize the syndrome because it is rapidly relieved by plasmapheresis and the institution of specific therapy for MM.

## Presenting Ocular Features

In addition to the ocular features of hyperviscosity, some new presenting ocular features have been reported. Shami and Uy (1996) report the occurrence of isolated cotton-wool spots on examination of the retina in an elderly woman. The presenting symptoms were of a blurred circle in the right eye. The authors emphasize that in the absence of diabetes or hypertension, paraproteinemia should be considered. A description of exudative macular detachment is also reported in MM (Brody et al., 1995).

## Presenting Renal Symptoms

The renal complications of MM are discussed fully in Chapter 16. Presenting symptoms of thirst, polyuria, or nocturnal frequency are relatively uncommon, being found in only approximately 7% of patients (Riccardi et al., 1991). Studies on renal function in MM show a much higher incidence of dysfunction, with approximately one-third or more showing a raised serum creatinine or urea. In the MRC Third Myelomatosis Trial (Medical Research Council Working Party, 1980), 132 of 485 previously untreated patients with MM (27%) showed a blood urea concentration of more than 10 mM. In a smaller series, Kapadia (1980) noted blood urea levels greater than 40 mg/dL in 24 of 58 patients (41%) at presentation. The incidence of renal failure varies with the catchment area. Renal insufficiency with an elevated serum creatinine occurred in more than 50% of patients with plasma cell dyscrasias reviewed by Herrera (2000). Patients with MM might present to the nephrology department first where three-fourths of them are diagnosed as having MM after admission (Magee et al., 1998). Most patients were in the later stages, and 31 of 34 had severe renal failure at presentation (GFR <20 mL/min). Only one patient subsequently became independent of dialysis.

In some series, the level of blood urea or creatinine might be unduly high as a result of concomitant dehydration, which is a feature of MM. Increased recognition and earlier diagnosis of dehydration might be responsible for the gradual and significant fall noted over three decades by Riccardi et al. (1991). In a series of patients from St. Bartholomew's Hospital treated from 1981 to 1991, the incidence was 26%. Acute and chronic forms of renal failure are seen in MM at presentation. Renal failure might have an insidious onset and is commonly associated with Bence Jones proteinuria, the presence of IgD paraprotein, hypercalcemia, hyperuricemia, pyelonephritis, amyloidosis, and the use of nonsteroidal anti-inflammatory drugs.

Alexanian et al. (1990) studied 494 consecutive previously untreated patients with MM who had renal failure. For patients with a similar extent of disease, the presence or absence of renal failure did not greatly affect prognosis. Hypercalcemia and Bence Jones proteinuria explained the renal failure in 97% of cases. After treatment with hydration, specific chemotherapy, and measures to control the hypercalcemia, renal function returned to normal in more than 50% of patients. The authors concluded that control of MM was more important in prolonging survival than reversal of renal failure, and emphasized the importance of early and effective specific therapy. This is an important concept because, although the significance of renal failure as an adverse prognostic feature has been emphasized in many large series of MM patients, the excellent support now obtainable with renal dialysis and the arrest in decline, or even improvement, in renal function seen with more recent therapies underlines the necessity for a positive approach to this important presenting feature.

## Cardiopulmonary Presentation

### Cardiac Symptoms

Symptoms of heart failure are not uncommon as a presenting feature of illness in an elderly population and might be caused by concurrent ischemic heart disease, hypertension, or as a complication of infection. Specific causes for heart failure in MM might be anemia, hyperviscosity syndrome, amyloid, or the result of light chain cardiomyopathy in which fibrillary deposits of light chain are deposited (Gallo et al., 1996). These are relatively rare but important to recognize. Hyperviscosity is readily relieved by plasmapheresis and the fluid overload corrected at the same time. Suspicion of myocardial amyloid disease needs confirmation by ultrasonography, because administration of

chemotherapy can be lethal (Devoy and Tomson, 1992; Skadberg et al., 1988). High output cardiac failure in MM is being increasingly recognized (McBride et al., 1990).

In 36 patients with MM, with a high output state defined as a cardiac index of more than $41/m^2$, it was present in 8 of the 34 (23%). Four patients developed high output failure and two died. The patients who died had extensive bone disease leading to shunting; the authors concluded that this was a common finding in MM. Judson et al. (1989) reported their solution of high output failure in MM with therapy after reduction of the vascular bed. Sanchez et al. (1986) reported the successful treatment of high output failure by embolization of a highly vascular tumor.

### Pulmonary Symptoms

Pneumonia is one of the most common presenting symptoms with an incidence of up to 23%. Infection with *Streptococcus pneumoniae* and *Haemophilus influenzae* are more common early in the illness, with Gram-negative organisms and *Staphylococcus aureus* affecting the later course of the disease (Savage et al., 1982). The risk of pneumonia is greater during initial therapy and again at relapse. Opportunistic infections such as *Pneumocystis carinii* infection tend to occur later in the disease when the patient is most immuno-compromised.

Other manifestations of MM in the lung are rare as presenting features. Nodular mass lesions or reticulo-nodular infiltration have been reported (Shin et al., 1992). Pleural effusion in MM is uncommon. Makino et al. (1992) and Abbate et al. (1991) recorded this as a presenting phenomenon in IgD and Bence Jones MM, respectively. Myelomatous pleural effusion is rare. Meoli et al. (1997) reviewed the 57 cases reported. They found a predominance of IgG MM compared with the predominance of IgA reported in other series.

Cytology of the pleural effusion showed malignant plasma cells in 93% of the cases. Response to treatment was disappointing and the prognosis was poor, the median survival being only 4 months. It has been noted that eosinophils as well as immature plasma cells might be found in the effusion (Dhillon, 1988; Makino et al., 1992).

## Hematologic Presentation

Anemia and the frequency with which it can cause fatigue has already been mentioned as a common presenting feature. Less frequently, hematologic complications result from the hyperviscosity syndrome with purpura, ecchymoses, epistaxes, and bleeding from the gastrointestinal tract complicating the syndrome, which occurs in 4% to 19% of patients with MM. It is most frequently seen at presentation and should be suspected when persistent bleeding occurs in the absence of significant thrombocytopenia. The syndrome occurs most frequently with IgM paraprotein, but also occurs when IgG or IgA paraproteins polymerize. IgG is particularly likely to do this. Kahn et al. (1987), Carter et al. (1989), and Bachrach et al. (1989) have reported the syndrome in MM with a high degree of polymerization of light chain.

Impairment of platelet function with prolonged bleeding time, poor clot retraction, and poor platelet adhesion can be seen. Impairment of aggregation and release of platelet factor can be the result of paraprotein coating the surface of the platelets. As well as impairing platelet function, paraproteins can combine and interfere with coagulation factors. Richard et al. (1990) have reported a patient in whom von Willebrand's factor was selectively absorbed onto myeloma cells. They were able to show that von Willebrand's factor was progressively depleted from the plasma, giving rise to the acquired form of the disease.

## Association with Myelofibrosis

There is evidence of an association between proteinemias and myelofibrosis. Bartl et al. (1982) saw considerable bone marrow fibrosis in 11% of 220 patients with MM. Duhrsen et al. (1988), reviewing 199 patients with myelofibrosis, found three patients with MM among 46 with idiopathic myelofibrosis. They reviewed the literature and found an increased association of paraproteinemias, including MM, with myelofibrosis. The concurrence of these two conditions would suggest that bone marrow biopsy is justified because the implications for intensive chemotherapy in the presence of myelofibrosis are considerable.

## Symptoms of Metabolic Disorder

Although overt symptomatic metabolic disturbance is relatively uncommon at presentation, its recognition is important. The most common feature is hypercalcemia, but hyperuricemia, hyperphosphatemia, hyperparathyroidism, and hyperammonemia have all been reported.

## Hypercalcemia

Disturbances of calcium metabolism are discussed in detail in Chapter 15. The clinical manifestations of hypercalcemia are extremely variable. Patients presenting with a high serum calcium might be asymptomatic, whereas others with a more modest rise are comatose. Symptoms of hypercalcemia are rare in patients presenting with MM. However, it is probably the cause of the mild dehydration and increased fluid excretion seen in patients with MM.

Biochemical hypercalcemia was noted in 30% of Kyle's 1975 series. Defining hypercalcemia as a serum calcium level above 10.1 mg/dL, 28 patients had levels of 10.1 to 15 mg/dL; two patients had levels above 15 mg/dL. In a series from St. Bartholomew's Hospital, corrected calcium levels of above 2.67 mM/L were seen in 26% of patients. Riccardi et al. (1991) noted that in a recent series, the proportion of patients presenting with hypercalcemia had fallen to 20%, which could be the result of earlier recognition of MM, greater frequency of requests for serum calcium estimations, and the application of corrections necessary to give the true value. Albumin levels might be low in MM, so it is important to take this into consideration, otherwise hypercalcemia could be missed. An addition of 0.02 mM/L is made for every gram that the albumin level is below 40 g/L (Kanis, 1986). For example, in a patient with a plasma calcium level of 2.6 mM/L and an albumin of 30 g/L, $0.02 \times 10$ equals 0.2 mM/L and has to be added to the 2.6 mM/L, bringing the calcium to a corrected value of 2.8 mM/L, which is in the mild hypercalcemic range.

The mechanism whereby calcium is raised in MM is discussed in Chapter 14. Occasionally, primary hyperparathyroidism has been associated with hypercalcemia in MGUS and MM (Hoelzer and Silverberg, 1984; Leese et al., 1992; Mundis and Kyle, 1982; Stone et al., 1982). In the patient reported by Leese, serum parathyroid levels were raised and a large chief-cell parathyroid tumor was found and removed. They point out that dexamethasone given in the belief that the hypercalcemia was the result of MM did not suppress the calcium level and was an additional diagnostic factor. Rao et al. (1991), when reporting four cases of hyperparathyroidism in patients with MGUS and one in MM, noted that this occurred in 386 consecutive cases of hyperparathyroidism seen over a 12-year period. This gave an incidence of 1%, which they suggest had arisen by chance.

## Hyperuricemia

An elevated serum uric acid is a common presenting feature in patients with MM. It was seen in 30% of patients presenting at St. Bartholomew's Hospital. It is raised partly as a result of nucleic acid turnover associated with the increasing tumor mass and partly as a result of dehydration and renal failure. Except in patients with an established history of symptomatic hyperuricemia, it is very rare for patients with MM to present with gouty manifestations. The presence of biochemical hyperuricemia or its precipitation by therapy emphasizes the need for effective prophylaxis.

## Hyperphosphatemia

This condition is usually seen in patients with hyperparathyroidism, renal failure, or tumor lysis syndrome. Mandry et al. (1991) described its occurrence in an elderly lady with IgG MM. These authors differentiated the condition from the more frequent pseudohyperphosphatemia by showing that calcium, blood urea, and parathyroid levels were normal, but that serum 1,25-dihydroxyvitamin D levels were grossly subnormal; they were able to demonstrate that the IgG paraprotein bound phosphate and considered that the lower level of vitamin D might have a physiological significance. Pseudohyperphosphatemia is more common and results from interference of the monoclonal protein in the colorimetric assay for phosphorus (Busse et al., 1987). It has no clinical significance apart from alerting clinicians to the possible presence of paraproteinemia (McClure et al., 1992).

## Hyperammonemia

The rare metabolic disorder of hyperammonemia has been reported by Matsuzaki et al. (1990) in two patients with MM. The plasma cells from these patients produced ammonia. Although they had normal liver function, the hyperammonemia produced disturbances of consciousness with somnolence and pre-coma. One patient's symptoms were relieved by specific therapy.

## Skin Manifestations

In addition to the purpura associated with thrombocytopenia, hyperviscosity syndrome, cryoglobulinemia, and amyloidosis, a number of dermatologic disorders have been associated with monoclonal gammopathies. In an extensive review, Dhoud et al. (1999) divided these into four groups of gradually decreasing association. Group 1 included the conditions mentioned at the beginning of this paragraph, together with osteosclerotic myeloma (POEMS syndrome) and direct cutaneous extension by MM or plasmacytoma. Group 2 includes scleromyxoedema, scleroderma, necrobiotica xanthogranuloma, plane xanthoma, pyoderma gangrenosum, and Sweet syndrome in which the mechanism is not understood but there is a definite association with the gammopathies. Two of these are frequent enough to describe more fully.

### Scleroderma Adultorum

This is characterized by pigmented lesions that may become generalized. It is associated with hyperlipoproteinemia (McFadden et al., 1987).

### Sweet Syndrome

This is an acute febrile neurophilic dermatosis described by Sweet (1964). It was the presenting feature in three patients with MM described by Berth-Jones and Hutchinson (1989). The cardinal features are fever, polymorphonucleocytosis, and painful erythematous plaques. It has also been reported in association with MGUS. Groups 3 and 4 contain a multitude of dermatologic conditions in which it is likely that their joint occurrence with MM was coincidental.

## Musculoskeletal Presentations

Arthropathies are rare presenting features of MM. It is more common in elderly patients for pain to be ascribed to joints and diagnosed as arthritis when in fact the pain is the result of lytic lesions near the joints. Arthropathies, when present, are more likely to be the result of amyloid infiltration of the joint capsule and are difficult to distinguish from rheumatoid arthritis. However, arthropathies tend to occur later in the course of the disease. Polymyalgia has been recorded but is uncommon. Two of five patients with these symptoms were described by Kalra and Delamere (1987).

A series of patients with arthropathies occurring at or near the time of diagnosis has been described by Jorgensen et al. (1996). The cases had oligoarthritis or polyarthritis mimicking rheumatoid arthritis. They were all negative for rheumatoid factor. The joints affected were distal interphalangeal joints (two cases) and a sacroileitis (one case). Two patients had MM and the other seven MGUS. In another 12 cases reported in the literature and reviewed, three had MM and nine MGUS. Fifteen of these 21 cases had kappa light chain, three had lambda light chain, and three were not recorded. Cryoglobulinemia was present in four of the Jorgensen series. Specific therapy led to an improvement in two of the MM cases.

## Rare Types of Myeloma and Associated Syndromes

### IgD Myeloma

This form of MM is rare. Kyle (1975) noted only six patients in 537 with MM, giving an incidence of 1%. There is a predisposition in males and the mean age of presentation is younger than average for the disease. Extraosseous manifestations of the disease are more common and so is the frequency of acute and chronic renal failure. Blade et al. (1994) reviewed 53 patients with immunoglobulin D MM from a single institution. Bone pain occurred in 72%, fatigue in 36%, and weight loss in 32%. Extramedullary plasmacytosis occurred in 19% and amyloidosis in 19%. These were the major presenting features. Renal function was impaired in 33%, and this was associated with an incidence of Bence Jones proteinuria of 96%. Response to therapy was similar to other MM types but survival was shorter. Blade et al. (1999) consider that IgD MM is a variant of Bence Jones MM with an IgD paraprotein and lambda chain predominance.

### IgE Myeloma

This is one of the rarest forms of MM. The first case was reported by Johansson and Bennich (1967). Endo et al. (1981) described one case and reviewed another 10 noting the high male to female ratio, the younger age distribution, and that 3 of the 11 developed plasma cell leukemia. By 1999 35 patients with IgE MM had been reported; these are reviewed by Macro et al. (1999). They stress the frequency of Bence Jones proteinuria and confirm the increased incidence of plasma cell leukemia.

### IgM Myeloma

This is a very rare form of MM with an incidence of less than 0.5%. De Gramont et al. (1990) reviewed a total of 46 cases in the literature and added six of their own. The sex incidence and age of presentation was no different from classic MM.

### Nonsecretory Myeloma

This is another rare variant that is difficult to diagnose because a paraprotein is not found in the serum or light chain in the urine at presentation, although a small amount of paraprotein might develop during the course of the disease. More recently sensitive techniques have been developed to measure free light chains in the serum (Drayson et al., 2001). Immunoperoxidase or immunofluorescent studies should be done on plasma cells of patients suspected of having nonsecretory MM. Smith et al. (1986) recorded the features of 13 cases of nonsecretory MM. They noted a higher incidence of neurologic presentations, minimal lytic bone, a lower bone marrow infiltration with plasma cells, and less reduction in normal immunoglobulins. Blade and Kyle (1999), reviewing four of the largest series of this condition, consider that nonsecretory MM accounts for between 1% and 5% of all MM. The presenting features are similar to those of other forms of MM except for the absence of renal impairment. The response to therapy and survival of patients are similar to those with measurable M protein.

### Plasma Cell Dyscrasia with Polyneuropathy, Organomegaly, Endocrinopathy, M Protein, and Skin Changes (POEMS Syndrome)

The association of plasmacytoma with polyneuritis and endocrine disturbances was first described by Shimpo (1968). Bardwick et al. (1980) reviewed the literature and added two cases of their own. They proposed the acronym "POEMS" syndrome for the multisystem disorder whose cardinal feature was a severe progressive sensorimotor polyneuropathy. It was associated with osteosclerotic bone lesions, production of paraprotein, organomegaly, diabetes mellitus, amenorrhea in females, gynecomastia and impotence in males, and hyperpigmentation.

## Plasma Cell Leukemia

Plasma cell leukemia (PCL) forms 2% to 4% of plasma cell malignancies. It is therefore rare and is diagnosed on the basis of the presence of 20% of plasma cells in the peripheral blood and an absolute plasma cell count of more than $2 \times 10^9$/L. It might arise de novo or complicate 1% of MM cases. Woodruff et al. (1978) showed that PCL, when it relapsed, always reappeared in the leukemic phase. The biology of PCL has been reviewed by Blade and Kyle (1999).

Costello et al. (2000) reviewed 18 patients with primary PCL. Their median age was 51.5 years (range, 30–75 y). There were seven women and 11 men who presented with asthenia and bone pain. Five patients had splenomegaly and hepatomegaly. Bone lesions were observed in 11 patients, pleural effusions in two, and meningeal myelomatosis in one patient. Fifteen were anemic and 11 were thrombocytopenic. Half the patients had a creatinine level greater than 120 uM/L and half were hypercalcemic. Monoclonal protein was kappa IgG in three cases, kappa IgA in four cases, kappa IgM in one case, and lambda IgG in two. Kappa light chains only were present in four cases and lambda light chain in one. There were three nonsecretory cases. Eleven of 18 cases treated with an anthracycline-containing regimen achieved a partial remission, one patient had a complete remission, but six patients showed no response. The median survival time was seven months, which was slightly shorter than the 9.5 months in 16 patients, 7 with combination chemotherapy, as reported by Noel and Kyle (1987). The response rate and survival is better in patients treated with combination chemotherapy than with melphalan and prednisolone. Patients with secondary PCL rarely if ever respond. High-dose therapy with stem cell rescue is now recommended therapy in younger patients with PCL.

## Laboratory Findings in MM at Presentation and Diagnosis

MM is one of a wide variety of conditions in which the serum proteins are elevated. To distinguish between benign and malignant causes for this, it is essential to perform serum electrophoresis and demonstrate a monoclonal band. A monoclonal band indicates a clonal proliferation of plasma cells, which suggests that malignant or potentially malignant changes have taken place in the plasma cell series.

Serum electrophoresis should be done in all patients in whom a plasma cell dyscrasia is suspected or in whom laboratory findings have shown a high total protein, a raised erythrocyte sedimentation rate (ESR), a low serum protein level, or a reduced gap between the serum sodium and combined chloride with bicarbonate. This anion gap is normally above 12 meq/L, but if paraproteins are present it falls to less than 6 meq/L.

High-resolution agarose gel electrophoresis is the recommended method of detecting an M protein. M proteins are seen as discreet bands on electrophoresis or peaks on densitometry in the alpha, beta, or gamma regions. A polyclonal increase in immunoglobulin with multiple immunoglobulins appears as a broad band usually in the gamma region. Such increases are seen in infections, rheumatoid arthritis, sarcoid and other autoimmune diseases. The most common paraproteins are IgG followed by IgA and rarely, IgM. Klouch et al. (1995) showed that the most common subtype of IgG was IgG1 at 68%, with IgG2 and IgG3 at 13% and 16%, respectively, and IgG4 at 3%.

Approximately 10% of MM show a diminution of gamma globulin with no apparent spike. In these patients, it is important to look for free kappa or lambda light chain (FLC) in the serum or urine. Sensitive automated immunoassays have been developed. Using sheep antibodies that have been extensively absorbed against whole immunoglobulin, Bradwell et al. (2001) have developed a highly sensitive system for the detection of FLCs. This type of assay has been reported as having effectively detected FLCs in patients with nonsecretory MM (Drayson et al., 2001). Conditions that might give rise to problems in laboratory diagnosis have been reviewed by Kyle (1999).

Immunofixation should be carried out when a band is found on electrophoresis. M bands and FLCs give sharp bands and allow heavy and light chain analysis to be carried out.

Cryoglobulins are commonly seen with IgM paraproteins but occur with IgG3 and rarely IgA paraproteins. Blood needs to be taken into a syringe, warmed to 37°, and allowed to clot while warm. The cryoglobulins can then be separated and studied by immunofixation.

A marked increase in paraprotein can lead to hyperviscosity. This is most common with IgM paraprotein, but approximately 4% of hyperviscosity states are the result of polymers of IgG3 and IgG4. Viscosity should be measured using a machine that can perform at different sheer rates and variable temperature, and which gives a rapid answer. Viscosity is referred to in water ratios. A ratio of less than 4 is rarely associated with symptoms but symptoms occur frequently above 6.

Hyperviscosity should be monitored clinically and by plasma viscosity.

To complete the laboratory diagnostic assessment of a patient with MM, the Guidelines Working Group of the UK Myeloma Forum recommends a full blood count, serum urea electrolytes and creatinine, calcium, albumin, uric acid, electrophoresis followed by immunofixation as described previously, quantification of paraprotein and urinary light chain on a 24-hour collection, quantification on non-isotypic serum immunoglobulin, creatinine clearance, and plasma viscosity, B2-microglobulin (in the presence of normal renal function), lactate dehydrogenases (LDH), and C-reactive protein as prognostic markers. A bone marrow sample should be sent for cytogenetic studies whenever possible (UK Myeloma Forum, 2001).

# Management of MM and Indications for Treatment

Currently MM is an ultimately fatal disease. It is essential to distinguish conditions characterized by the presence of a paraprotein that need treatment from those that do not. Among those conditions needing no therapy are MGUS, smoldering MM, and indolent MM. These conditions should be monitored carefully until a 25% rise in the paraprotein level, an increase in light chain excretion in the urine, onset of anemia, hypercalcemia, appearance of bone lesions, or other symptoms of advancing disease make consideration of suitable therapy necessary.

The use of chemotherapy in conventional and high-dose regimens is dealt with in detail in Chapters 12 and 13, respectively, whereas the important supportive role of drugs affecting bone metabolism is considered in Chapter 15. This chapter gives a brief overview of therapy. Patients with MM at any age who have symptoms should be treated as there is a better than 50% chance that their symptoms can be relieved. In patients over 70 years of age, the specific therapy recommended will depend on the patient's physiological state and coincidental disease. With the improvement in supportive care, high-dose therapy can be considered in a few suitable patients, but the majority are best treated with melphalan and prednisolone or with a combination of drugs that the physician is conversant with. It is evident that elderly patients are not disadvantaged by having melphalan and prednisolone and might be saved from having unpleasant side effects (Gregory et al., 1992).

In patients under the age of 70, there are numerous options and these continue to increase as new classes of agents are introduced. Because of this, patients should be encouraged to enter trials of therapy. Combinations of chemotherapeutic agents have effectively relieved symptoms and improved overall response rate but have not improved survival. High-dose therapy with bone marrow or peripheral blood stem cell support was introduced with curative intent. The treatment relies on the premise that cell kill is proportional to the cytotoxic drug dose used. Randomized studies have shown that although relapse-free survival and quality of life is much improved when compared with standard combination regimens, it is doubtful if long-term cure is possible. Increasing the number of transplant procedures has yet to be shown to be curative, and the addition of total body irradiation increases morbidity and mortality. The role of targeted marrow irradiation using isotopes is currently under investigation.

Allogeneic bone marrow has been used successfully as a potential curative when suitable donors are available. It has the disadvantage that in the largely elderly population, suitable donors are not available and, when they are, the risk of graft-versus-host disease is considerable. Although this procedure has difficulties, the possibility of inducing a graft-versus-myeloma effect has prompted the exploration of mini-allografting with reduced intensity conditioning allografts. Maintenance therapy in MM has largely been with interferon after many attempts to find suitable chemotherapy. Although there is evidence that there is an improvement in disease-free survival and overall survival, the improvement is only modest (Myeloma Trialists Collaborative Group, 2001). With the introduction of new agents such as thalidomide and proteosome inhibitors such as PS-341, VEGF, and TNF inhibitors, a new era of possibly less toxic therapy is emerging. Just as the place of high-dose therapy has to be decided in the sequence of therapy for MM, so the place of these new drugs will need to be determined. It might well be that, for example, thalidomide or one of its analogues might be used to induce remission before consolidation with high-dose therapy. It is apparent that with all of these options available, patients with MM should be referred to centers specializing in their management.

## REFERENCES

Abbate, S. L., Jaff, M. R., Fishleder, A. J., and Meeker, D. P. (1991). Lambda light-chain myeloma with pleural involvement. *Cleveland Clinic Journal of Medicine, 58*, 235–239.

Alexanian, R., Barlogie, B., and Dixon, D. (1990). Renal failure in multiple myeloma-pathogenesis and prognostic implications. *Archives of Internal Medicine, 150*, 1693–1695.

Atkinson, F. R. B. (1937). Multiple myeloma. *Medical Press, 195*, 312–317.

Axelsson, U., Bachman, R., and Hallen, J. (1996). Frequency of pathological proteins (M-components in 6995 sera from an adult population. *Acta Medica Scandinavia, 179*, 235–247.

Bachrach, H. J., Myers, J. B., and Bartholomew, W. R. (1989). A unique case of Kappa light-chain disease associated with cryoglobulinaemia, pyroglobulinaemia, and hyperviscosity syndrome. *American Journal of Medicine, 86*, 596–602.

Baldini, L., Guffanti, A., Cesana, B. M. (1996). Role of different haematologic variables in defining the risk of malignant transformation in monoclonal gammopathy. *Blood, 87*, 912–915.

Barasch, E., Berger, S. A., Golan, E., and Siegman-Igra, Y. (1986). Pneumcoccaemia as a presenting sign in three cases of multiple myeloma. *Scandinavian Journal of Haematology, 36*, 228–231.

Bardwick, P. A., Zvaifler, N. J., Gill, G. N., Newman, D., Greenway, G. D., and Resnick, D. I. (1980). Plasma cell dyscrasia with polyneuropathy, organomegaly, endocrinopathy, M protein and skin changes—the POEMS syndrome. *Medicine (Baltimore), 59*, 311–322.

Bartl, R., Frisch, B., Burkhardt, R., Fateh-Moghadam, A., Mahl, G., Giester, P., Sund, M., and Kettner, G. (1982). Bone marrow histology in myeloma: its importance in diagnosis, prognosis, classification and staging. *British Journal of Haematology, 51*, 361–375.

Berth-Jones, J., and Hutchinson, P. E. (1989). Sweet's syndrome and malignancy: A case association with multiple myeloma and review of the literature. *British Journal of Dermatology, 121*, 123–127.

Bisagni-Faure, A., Ravaud, P., Amor, B., and Menkes, C. J. (1991). Myeloma and epidural invasiveness—clinical and therapeutic aspects (a study of 22 cases). *Revue Rheumatism, 58*, 301–306.

Blade, J., and Kyle, R. A. (1999). Nonsecretory myeloma, Immunoglobulin D myeloma and plasma cell leukaemia. *Haematology clinics of North America, 13*, 1259–1272.

Blade, J., Kyle, R. A., and Griepp, P. R. (1992). Presenting features and prognosis in 72 patients with multiple myeloma who were younger than 40 years. *British Journal of Haematology, 93*, 345–351.

Blade, J., Lust, J. A., and Kyle, R. A. (1994). Immunoglobulin D Multiple Myeloma: Presenting Features, Response to Therapy and survival in a series of 53 cases. *Journal of Clinical Oncology, 12*, 2398–2404.

Blade, J., Munoz, M., Fontanillas, M., San Miguel, J., Alcala, A., Maldonado, J., Besses, C., Moro, M. J., Garcia-Conde, J., Rozman, C., Montserrat, E., and Estape, J. (1996). Treatment of multiple myeloma in elderly people: long-term results in 178 patients. *Age and Ageing, 25*, 357–361.

Bradwell, A. R., Carr-Smith, D., Mead, G. P., Tang, L. X., Showell, P. J., Drayson, M. T., and Drew, R. (2001). Highly sensitive automated immunoassay for immunoglobulin free light-chains in serum and urine. *Clinical Chemistry, 47*, 673–680.

Brody, J. M., Butrus, S. I., Ashraf, M. F., Rabinowitz, A. I., and Whitmore, P. V. (1995). Multiple myeloma presenting with bilateral exudative macular detachments. *Acta Ophthalmologica Scandinavia, 73*, 81–83.

Busse, J. C., Gelbard, M. A., Byrnes, J. J., Hellman, R., and Vaamonde, C. A. (1987). Pseudohyperphosphataemia and dysproteinaemia. *Archives of Internal Medicine, 147*, 2045–2046.

Carter, P. W., Cohen, H. J., and Crawford, J. (1989). Hyperviscosity syndrome in association with kappa light-chain myeloma. *American Journal of Medicine, 86*, 591–595.

Chandy, K. G., Stockley, R. A., Leonard, R. C. F., Crockson, R. A., Burnett, D., and MacLennan, I.C.M. (1981). Relationships between serum viscosity and intravascular IgA polymer concentration in IgA myeloma. *Clinical and Experimental Immunology, 46*, 653–661.

De Blay, V., Misson, N., Dardenne, G., and Dupuis, M. J. (2000). Leptomeningeal myelomatosus mimicking a subdural haematoma. *Neuroradiology, 42*, 735–737.

De Couteau, J. F., Terrault, N. A., Reis, M. D., Senn, J. S., and Pinkerton, P. H. (1992). Multiple myeloma in children and young adults. *Diagnostic Radiology, 2*, 121–124.

De Gramont, A., Grosbois, B., Michaux, J. L., Peny, A. M., Pollet, J. P., Smadia, et al. (1990). IgM myeloma—Six cases and a review of the literature. *Revue Medicine Interne, 11*, 13–18.

Dennis, M., and Chu, P. (2000). A case of meningeal myeloma presenting as obstructive hydrocephalus. *A therapeutic challenge leukemia and lymphoma, 40*, 219–220.

De Smet, M. D., and Rootman, J. (1987). Orbital manifestations of plasmacytic lymphoproliferations. *Ophthalmology, 94,* 995–1003.

Devoy, M. A., and Tomson, C. R. (1992). Fatal cardiac failure after a single dose of doxorubicin in myeloma associated cardiac amyloid. *Postgraduate Medical Journal, 68,* 69.

Dhoud, M. S., Lust, J. A., and Kyle, R. A. (1999). Monoclonal gammopathies and associated skin disorders. *Journal of the American Academy of Dermatology, 40,* 507–531.

Drayson, M., Tang, L. X., Drew, R., Mead, L. P., Carr-Smith, H., and Bradwell, A. R. (2001). Serum free light-chain measurements for identifying and monitoring patients with non-secretory multiple myeloma. *Blood, 97,* 2900–2902.

Duhrsen, U., Uppenkamp, M., Mevser, P., Konig, E., and Brittinger, G. (1988). Frequent association of idiopathic myelofibrosis with plasma cell dyscrasia. *Blut, 56,* 97–102.

Durie, B. G. (1986). Staging and kinetics of multiple myeloma. *Seminars in Oncology, 13,* 300–309.

Durie, B. G., and Salmon, S. E. (1975). A clinical staging system for multiple myeloma. *Cancer, 36,* 842–854.

Endo, T., Okumura, H., Kikuchi, K., Monakata, J., Otake, M., Nomora, T., and Asakawa, H. (1981). Immunoglobulin E (IgE) multiple myeloma. *American Journal of Medicine, 70,* 1127–1132.

Fiorino, A. S., and Atac, B. (1997). Paraproteinaemia, plasmacytoma, myeloma, and HIV infection. *Leukemia, 11,* 2150–2156.

Fudenberg, H. H., and Virella, G. (1980). Multiple myeloma and Waldenström's macroglobulinaemia—Unusual presentations. *Seminars in Haematology, 17,* 63–79.

Fuzibet, J. G., Bataille, R., Bagarry, D., Sotto, J. J., Lepeu, G., Rossi, J. F., Cassuto, J. P., and Carcassonne, Y. (1986). Prolonged survival in multiple myeloma: Characteristics of presentation and response to treatment of 73 patients who survived 5 years or longer. *Presse Medicale, 15,* 1913–1916.

Gallo, G., Goni, F., Boctor, F., Vidal, R., Kumar, A., Stevens, F. J., Frangione, B., and Ghiso, J. (1996). Light-chain cardiomyopathy. Structural analysis of the light-chain tissue deposits. *American Journal of Pathology, 14,* 1397–1407.

Geschicter, C. F., and Copeland, M. M. (1928). Multiple myeloma. *Archives of Surgery, Chicago, 16,* 807–863.

Graham, M. P., Barzaga, R. A., and Cunha, B. A. (1991). Pneumococcal septic arthritis of the knee in a patient with multiple myeloma. *Heart/Lung, 20,* 416–418.

Gregory, W. M., Richards, M. A., and Malpas, J. S. (1992). Combination chemotherapy versus melphalan and prednisolone in the treatment of multiple myeloma. An overview of published trials. *Journal of Clinical Oncology, 10,* 334–342.

Greipp, P. R. (1992). Advances in the diagnosis and management of myeloma. *Seminars in Haematology, 29,* 24–45.

Grosbois, B., Jego, P., Attal, M., Payen, C., Rapp, M. J., Fuzibet, J. G., Maigre, M., and Bataille, R. (1999). Familial multiple myeloma: report of 15 families. *British Journal of Haematology, 105,* 768–770.

Hansen, N. E., Karle, H., and Olsen, H. H. (1989). Trends in the incidence of myeloma in Denmark 1943–1982—A study of 5,500 patients. *European Journal of Haematology, 42,* 72–76.

Hemminki, K., and Vaittinen, P. (1998). National Database of familial cancer in Sweden. *Genetic Epidemiology, 15,* 225–236.

Herrera, G. A. (2000). Renal manifestations of plasma cell dyscrasias: an appraisal from the patients bedside to the research laboratory. *Annals of Diagnostic Pathology, 4,* 174–200.

Hoelzer, R. D., and Silverberg, A. B. (1984). Primary hyperparathyroidism complicated by multiple myeloma. *Archives of Internal Medicine, 144,* 2069–2071.

Innes, J., and Newall, J. (1961). Myelomatosis. *Lancet, I,* 239–245.

Johansson, S. G. O., and Bennich, H. (1967). Immunological studies on an atypical (myeloma) immunoglobulin. *Immunology, 13,* 381–394.

Jorgensen, C., Guerin, B., Ferrazzi, V., Bologna, C., and Sany, J. (1996). Arthritis associated with monoclonal gammopathy: Clinical characteristics. *British Journal of Rheumatology, 35,* 241–243.

Judson, I. R., Gore, M. E., Tighe, J., Nicolson, M., and McElwain, T. J. (1989). Resolution of high-output cardiac failure following treatment of multiple myeloma. *New England Journal of Medicine, 321,* 1685–1686.

Kahn, P., Roth, M. S., Keren, D. F., and Foon, K. A. (1987). Light-chain disease associated with hyperviscosity syndrome. *Cancer, 60,* 2267–2268.

Kalra, L., and Delamere, J. (1987). Lymphoreticular malignancy and monoclonal gammopathy presenting as polymyalgia rheumatica. *British Journal of Rheumatology, 26,* 456–459.

Kanis, J. A. (1986). Disorders of calcium metabolism. In D. J. Weatherall, J. G. C. Ledingham, and D. A. Warrell (Eds.), *Oxford Textbook of Medicine* (vol 1, pp. 1051–1069). Oxford University Press.

Kapadia, S. B. (1980). Multiple myeloma: A clinicopathological study of 62 consecutively autopsied cases. *Medicine (Baltimore), 59,* 380–392.

Klouch, M., Bradwell, A. R., Wilhelm, D., and Kirchner, H. (1995). Subclass typing of IgG paraproteins by immunofixation electrophoresis. *Clinical Chemistry, 41,* 1475–1479.

Kyle, R. A. (1975). Multiple myeloma—Review of 869 cases. *Mayo Clinic Proceedings, 50,* 29–40.

Kyle, R. A. (1978). Monoclonal gammopathy of undetermined significance—Natural history in 241 cases. *American Journal of Medicine, 64,* 814–826.

Kyle, R. A. (1983). Long-term survival in multiple myeloma. *New England Journal of Medicine, 308,* 1347–1349.

Kyle, R. A. (1990). Multiple myeloma—An update on diagnosis and management. *Acta Oncologica, 29,* 1–8.

Kyle, R. A. (1999). Sequence of Testing for Monoclonal Gammopathies. Serum and Urine Assays. *Archives of Pathology and Laboratory Medicine, 123,* 114–118.

Kyle, R. A., Finkelstein, S., Elveback, L. R., and Kurland, L. T. (1972). Incidence of monoclonal proteins in a Minnesota community with a cluster of multiple myeloma. *Blood, 40,* 719–724.

Kyle, R. A., and Greipp, P. R. (1980). Smouldering multiple myeloma. *New England Journal of Medicine, 302,* 1347–1349.

Leese, G. P., Gunn, A., Jung, R. T., and Pippard, M. J. (1992). Primary hyperparathyroidism and monoclonal gammopathy. *Hospital Update, 18,* 750–751.

Leifer, D., Grabowski, T., Simonian, N., and Demirjian, Z. N. (1992). Leptomeningeal myelomatosis presenting with mental status changes and other neurologic findings. *Cancer, 70,* 1899–1904.

Lieberman, F. S., Odel, J., Hirsh, J., Heineman, M., Michaeli, J., and Posner, J. (1999). Bilateral optic neuropathy with IgG kappa multiple myeloma improved after myeloablative chemotherapy *Neurology, 52,* 414–416.

Macro, M. A., Andre, I., Comby, E., Cheze, S., Chapon, F., Ballet, J. J., Reman, O., Leporrier, M., and Troussand, X. (1999). IgE multiple myeloma. *Leukemia and Lymphoma, 32,* 587–603.

Maeda, K., Abesami, C. M., Kuhn, L. M., and Hyun, B. H. (1973). Multiple myeloma in childhood. *American Journal of Clinical Pathology, 60,* 552–558.

Magee, C., Vella, J. P., Tormey, W. P., and Walsh, J. J. (1998). Multiple myeloma and renal failure: one center's experience. *Renal Failure, 20,* 597–606.

Makino, S., Yamahara, S., Nagake, Y., and Kamura, J. (1992). Bence-Jones myeloma with pleural effusion: Response to alpha interferon and combined chemotherapy. *Internal Medicine, 31,* 617–621.

Mandry, J. M., Posner, M. R., Tucci, J. R., and Eil, C. (1991). Hyperphosphataemia in multiple myeloma due to a phosphate binding immunoglobulin. *Cancer, 68,* 1029–1024.

Matsuzaki, H., Uchiba, M., Yoshimura, M., Akahoshi, Y., Okazaki, K., et al. (1990). Hyperammonaemia in multiple myeloma. *Acta Haematologica, 84,* 130–134.

McBride, W., Jackman, J. D., and Grayborn, P. A. (1990). Prevalence and clinical characteristics of a high cardiac output state in multiple myeloma. *American Journal of Medicine, 89,* 21–24.

McClure, D., Lai, L. C., and Cornell, C. (1992). Pseudohyperphosphataemia in patients with multiple myeloma. *Journal of Clinical Pathology, 45,* 731–732.

McFadden, N., Ree, K., Syland, E., and Larsen, T. E. (1987). Scleroderma adultorum associated with a monoclonal gammopathy and generalised hyperpigmentation. *Archives of Dermatology, 123,* 629–632.

Medical Research Council Working Party. (1980). Report on the second myelomatosis trial after five years follow-up. *British Journal of Cancer, 42,* 813–822.

Meoli, I., Willsie, S., and Fiorella, R., (1997). Myelomatous pleural effusion. *Southern Medical Journal, 90,* 65–68.

Miller, M. I., Hoppman, R. A., and Pisko, E. J. (1987). Multiple myeloma presenting as primary meningococcal arthritis. *American Journal of Medicine, 82,* 1257–1258.

Mundis, R. J., and Kyle, R. A. Primary hyperparathyroidism and monoclonal gammopathy of undetermined significance. *American Journal of Clinical Pathology, 77,* 619–621.

Myeloma Trialists Collaborative Group. (2001). Combination chemotherapy vs. melphalan plus prednisolone in treatment for multiple myeloma. An overview of 6633 patients and 27 randomised trials. *Journal of Clinical Oncology, 16,* 3832–3842.

Noel, P., and Kyle, R. A. (1987). Plasma cell leukaemia an evaluation of response to therapy. *American Journal of Medicine, 83,* 1062–1065.

Nordenson, N. G. (1966). Myelomatosis: A clinical review of 310 cases. *Acta Medica Scandinavia, 445,* 178–186.

Ong, F., Hermans, J., Noordijk, E. M., and Kliun-Nelemans, J. C. (1995a). Is the Durie and Salmon classification system for plasma cell dyscrasias still the best choice? Application of three classification systems to a large population based registry of paraproteinaemias and multiple myeloma. *Annals of Haematology, 70,* 19–24.

Ong, F., Hermans, J., Noordijk, E. M., Wijermans, P. W., and Kliun-Nelemans, J. C. (1995b). Presenting signs and symptoms in multiple myeloma—High percentage of stage 111 among patients without apparent myeloma associated symptoms. *Annals of Haematology, 70,* 149–152.

Osgood, E. (1960). The survival time of patients plasmocytic myeloma. *Cancer Chemotherapy Reports, 9,* 1–10.

Oshima, K., Yoshinobu, K., Nannya, Y., Kaneko, M., Hamaki, T., Suguro, M., Yamamoto, R., Chizuka, A., Matsyama, T., Takezako, N., Miwa, A., Togawa, A., Niino, H., Nasu, M., Saito, K., and Morita, T. (2001). Clinical and pathological findings in 52 consecutive autopsied cases with multiple myeloma. *American Journal of Hematology, 67,* 1–5.

Patriaca, F., Fanin, R., Silvestri, F., Russo, D., and Baccarani, M. (1997). Multiple myeloma. Presenting features and survival according to hospital referral. *Leukemia and Lymphoma, 30,* 551–562.

Preston, F. E., Cooke, K. B., Foster, M. E., Winfield, D. A., and Lee, D. (1978). Myelomatosis and the hyperviscosity syndrome. *British Journal of Haematology, 38,* 517–530.

Rao, D. S., Antonelli, R., Kane, K. R., Kuhn, J. E., and Hetnal, C. (1991). Primary hyperparathyroidism and monoclonal gammopathy. *Henry Ford Hospital Journal, 39,* 41–44.

Riccardi, A., Gobbi, P. G., Ucci, G., Bertoloni, D., Luoni, R., Rutigliano, I., et al. (1991). Changing clinical presentation of multiple myeloma. *European Journal of Cancer, 27,* 1401–1405.

Richard, C., Cuadrado, M. A., Prieto, M., Batille, J., Lopez-Fernandez, M. F., Rodriguez-Salazar, M. L., et al. (1990). Acquired Von Willebrand disease in multiple myeloma secondary to absorption of Von Willebrand factor by plasma cells. *American Journal of Medicine, 35,* 114–117.

Riggs, J. E. (1995). Increasing multiple myeloma mortality rates in the elderly: Demonstration of increasing dependency with increasing age upon age group population size. *Mechanisms of Ageing and Development, 81,* 131–138.

Rodon, P., Linassier, C., Gauvain, J. B., Benbouker, L., Goupille, P., Maigre, M., Luthier, F., Dugay, J., Lucas, V., and Colombat, P. (2001). Multiple myeloma in elderly patients; presenting features and outcome. *European Journal of Haematology, 66,* 11–17.

Rosner, F., Grunwald, H. W., and Kalman, A. C. (1992). Ten-year survival in multiple myeloma: A report of two cases and review of the literature. *New York State Journal of Medicine, 92,* 316–318.

Sanchez, F. W., Chuang, V. P., and Skolkin, M. D. (1986). Transcatheter treatment of myelomatous AV shunting causing high-output failure. *Cardiovascular Interventional Radiology, 9,* 219–221.

Savage, D., Lindenbaum, J., and Garett, T. J. (1982). Biphasic pattern of bacterial infection in multiple myeloma. *Annals of Internal Medicine, 96,* 47–50.

Shakin, E. P., Augsburger, J. J., Eagle, R. C., Ehya, H., Shields, J. A., Fisher, D., et al. (1988). Multiple myeloma involving the iris. *Annals of Ophthalmology, 106,* 524–526.

Shami, M. J., and Uy, R. N. (1996). Isolated cotton-wool spots in a 67-year old woman. *Survey of Ophthalmology, 40,* 413–415.

Shimpo, S. (1968). Solitary plasmacytoma with polyneuritis and endocrine disturbances. *Japanese Journal of Clinical Medicine, 26,* 2444–2448.

Shin, M. S., Carcelen, M. F., and Ho, K. J. (1992). Diverse roentgenographic manifestations of the rare pulmonary involvement in myeloma. *Chest, 102,* 946–948.

Sinclair, D., Sheehan, T., Parrott, D. M. V., and Stott, D. I. (1986). The incidence of monoclonal gammopathy in a population over 45 years old determined by isoelectric focusing. *British Journal of Haematology, 64,* 745–750.

Skadberg, B. T., Bruserud, O., Karwinski, W., and Ohm, O. J. (1988). Sudden death caused by heart block in a patient with multiple myeloma and cardiac amyloidosis. *Acta Medica Scandinavica, 223,* 379–383.

Smith, D. B., Harris, M., Gowland, E., Chang, J., and Scarffe, J. H. (1986). Non-secretory multiple myeloma. A report of 13 cases with a review of the literature. *Haematology Oncology, 4,* 307–313.

Spiess, J. L., Adelstein, D. J., and Hines, J. D. (1988). Multiple myeloma presenting with spinal cord compression. *Oncology, 45,* 88–92.

Stone, M. J., Lieberman, Z. H., Chakmakjian, Z. H., and Matthews, J. L. (1982). Coexistent multiple myeloma and primary hyperparathyroidism. *Journal of the American Medical Association, 247,* 823–824.

Sweet, R. D. (1964). An acute febrile neutrophilic dermatosis. *British Journal of Dermatology, 76,* 340–356.

Talerman, A. (1969). Clinicopathological study of multiple myeloma in Jamaica. *British Journal of Cancer, 23,* 285–293.

UK Myeloma Forum. (2001). Guidelines on the diagnosis and management of multiple myeloma. *British Journal of Haematology, 115,* 522–540.

Waterhouse, J., Muir, C., Shan, M. U., Garath, A. M., and Powell, J. (Eds.). (1982). *Cancer Incidence in Five Continents.* IARC Scientific Publications, 42(4), 70.

Woo, E., Yu, Y. L., Ng, M., Huang, C. Y., and Todd, D. (1986). Spinal cord compression in multiple myeloma. Who gets it? *Australian New Zealand Journal of Medicine, 16,* 672–675.

Woodruff, R. K., Malpas, J. S., Paxton, A. M., and Lister, T. A. (1978). Plasma cell leukaemia (PLL) a report of 15 patients. *Blood, 52,* 839–848.

# CHAPTER 10

# Radiologic Features of Multiple Myeloma

LIA A. MOULOPOULOS
MELETIOS A. DIMOPOULOS

## Multiple Myeloma

### Plain Radiographs

Approximately 80% of patients with multiple myeloma have abnormal skeletal radiographs (Kyle, 1975). Today, despite the rapid development of new technology, a skeletal survey (i.e., conventional radiographs of the skull, central skeleton, proximal femurs, and proximal humeri) remains the initial imaging modality for the diagnosis and staging of multiple myeloma. Involvement of the peripheral skeleton is unusual.

Myeloma lesions are typically multiple, small, lytic, and well defined without perilesional sclerosis (Fig. 10-1). Autopsy studies have shown that these lesions are the result of nodular replacement of bone marrow by plasma cells (Kapadia, 1980). Lytic myeloma lesions might not be differentiated from lytic bone metastases. Sclerotic bone lesions are rare (less than 1%) and they are usually associated with POEMS syndrome (polyneuropathy, organomegaly, endocrinopathy, monoclonal gammopathy, and skin changes) (Fig. 10-2) (Resnick et al., 1981).

In approximately 10% of patients, generalized osteopenia without lytic lesions is the only finding on plain radiographs (Kyle, 1975). At autopsy, diffuse infiltration of the bone marrow by plasma cells is detected but the bone resorption is less

175

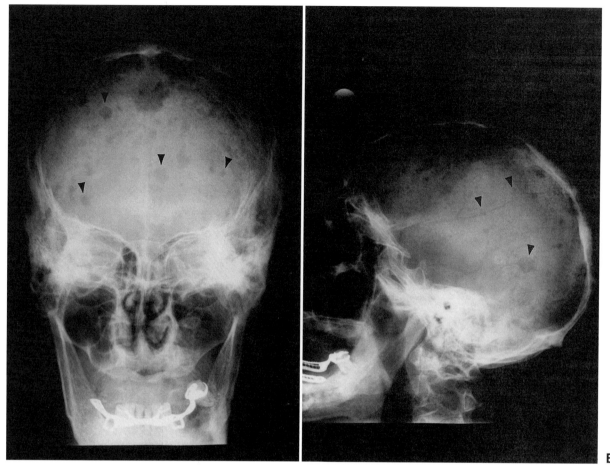

A                                                                                    B

**Figure 10-1**   *Anteroposterior (A) and lateral (B) skull radiographs show multiple, well-defined, lytic bone lesions (arrowheads) in a patient with multiple myeloma.*

severe when compared with that of lytic lesions (Kapadia, 1980). Osteopenia (and associated fractures) is found in many elderly patients without myeloma and in patients with other underlying disorders. In multiple myeloma, osteopenia might be the only manifestation of diffuse bone marrow infiltration by abnormal plasma cells and could account for reports of poor prognosis for myeloma patients without lytic lesions on skeletal surveys (Smith et al., 1988). Compression fractures in multiple myeloma might be related to osteopenia induced by osteoclast-activating factors or to bone destruction by underlying tumor. If there is no overt bone destruction, it is very difficult to distinguish fractures related to osteoporosis from those resulting from underlying tumor growth. Normal bone surveys are noted in 10% of myeloma patients.

### Radionuclide Imaging

Uptake on bone scans performed with technetium 99m depends on the degree of osteoblastic activity related to a bone lesion. Because this is typically absent in myelomatous lesions, the use of bone scans in this disease is limited, with reported sensitivity values of

this method ranging between 40% and 60% (Bataille et al., 1982). Bone scans of myeloma patients are either normal or might show areas of decreased uptake that correspond to sites of bone destruction. It is unusual for a radionuclide abnormality to precede a lytic lesion on plain films (Wahner et al., 1980). Bone scans might be reserved for areas that are difficult to evaluate with plain films, such as the ribs and sternum, even though CT and MRI can be used in such cases with more specific results.

Gallium-67 is less sensitive than plain radiographs in patients with myeloma. Increased gallium-67 uptake has been shown in patients with fulminant disease (Waxman et al., 1981). Thallium-201 scintigraphy has been investigated in myeloma patients with results comparable to those of bone scans (Watanabe et al., 1999). It has been shown to correlate with disease activity in occasional case reports (Ishibashi et al., 1998).

Technetium 99m 2-methoxy-isobutyl-isonitrile (99m Tc-MIBI) is a lipophilic cationic agent with gamma emission characteristics. It has been shown to differentiate active myeloma from disease in remission (Alexandrakis et al., 2001; Catalano et al., 1999; Pace et al., 1998; Tirovola et al., 1996). Pace et al. (1998)

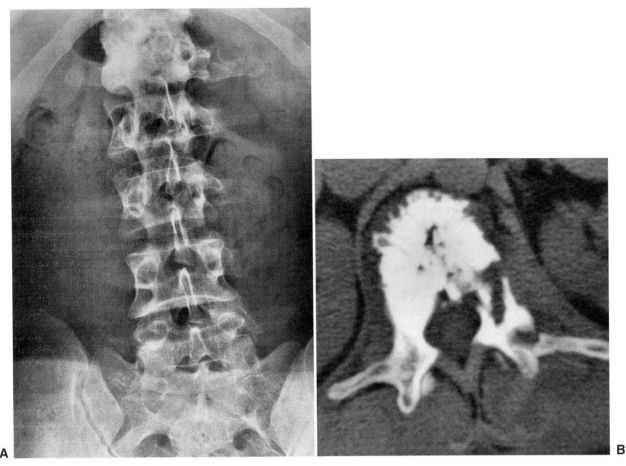

**Figure 10-2** *Plain radiograph (A) and CT scan of the spine (B) shows sclerotic lesion of the first lumbar vertebra in a patient with multiple myeloma and POEMS syndrome.*

observed that 91% of 32 myeloma patients with a positive 99m Tc-MIBI scan had active disease (Pace et al., 1998). In the study by Tirovola et al., four patients with active myeloma and negative 99m Tc-MIBI scans were resistant to chemotherapy, showing a potential for this radiopharmaceutical agent for *in vivo* testing of multidrug resistance (Tirovola et al., 1996). In a more recent study, 99m Tc-MIBI scans showed focal uptake in 25 of 55 patients with myeloma; all 25 patients had active myeloma (Catalano et al., 1999). In the same study, there was no uptake in 5 patients with MGUS, 6 patients with stage IA myeloma, 2 with stage IIA, and 6 patients with myeloma in early relapse. The authors suggested that the limitations of the method in detecting active myeloma lesions might be small lesion size (< 1 cm) or inadequate vascularization of lesions in collapsed bone.

There have been several promising reports on the investigation of patients with multiple myeloma with positron emission tomography using 2-[F-18] fluoro-2 deoxy-D-glucose (FDG-PET), a glucose analogue that accumulates at sites of increased glycolysis (Orchard et al., 2002; Schirrmeister et al., 2002). In a recent study of 43 patients with multiple myeloma or solitary bone plasmacytoma, Schirrmeister et al. reported a positive predictive value of 100% for active disease in patients with focal or mixed focal/diffuse skeletal FDG uptake and 75% in patients with diffuse marrow uptake (Schirrmeister et al., 2002).

## Computed Tomography

In patients with multiple myeloma, CT might show lytic bone lesions with discrete margins (Fig. 10-3). Computed tomography (CT) is not part of the staging for multiple myeloma. It is indicated when there is clinical suspicion of bony involvement and skeletal radiographs fail to show any findings. Before a lesion becomes apparent on plain radiographs, between 25% and 50% of bone loss must occur; computed tomography could, therefore, reveal small lytic lesions that are not seen on skeletal radiographs (Fig. 10-4). The appearance of myelomatous lesions is similar to that of lytic bone metastases. In the evaluation of the etiology of a vertebral fracture, computed tomography is of limited value unless frank bony lysis or mass is shown.

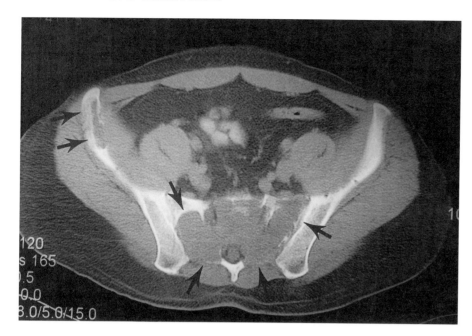

*Figure 10-3* *CT scan of the pelvis shows well-defined lytic myelomatous involvement of the sacrum and the right iliac bone (arrows).*

CT could help direct a needle for the establishment of histologic diagnosis. CT-guided percutaneous fine-needle aspiration bone biopsy of magnetic resonance-detected focal lesions provided highest detection rates of cytogenetic abnormalities and more accurate prognostic information in 31% of 78 patients with multiple myeloma (Avva et al., 2001).

## Magnetic Resonance Imaging

Magnetic resonance imaging (MRI) by directly visualizing a large volume of bone marrow is more sensitive than plain radiographs, CT, or bone scans in detecting myelomatous foci and is often part of the management of patients with multiple myeloma. Abnormal MR studies are found in the majority of symptomatic patients (Lecouvet et al., 1998; Rahmouni et al., 1993) and between 29% and 50% (Mariette et al., 1999; Moulopoulos et al., 1995; Vande Berg et al., 1996) of patients with asymptomatic myeloma. Approximately one-third of myeloma patients who have positive MR studies of the bone marrow do not have lytic lesions on skeletal surveys (Moulopoulos et al., 1994).

Magnetic resonance (MR) images of the bone marrow are obtained using T1-weighted and short inversion-time-inversion recovery (STIR) or T2-weighted

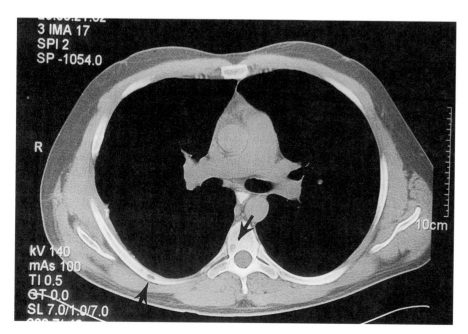

*Figure 10-4* *CT scan of the chest in a 60-year-old man with multiple myeloma shows small lytic lesions (arrows), which were not visible on plain radiographs (not shown).*

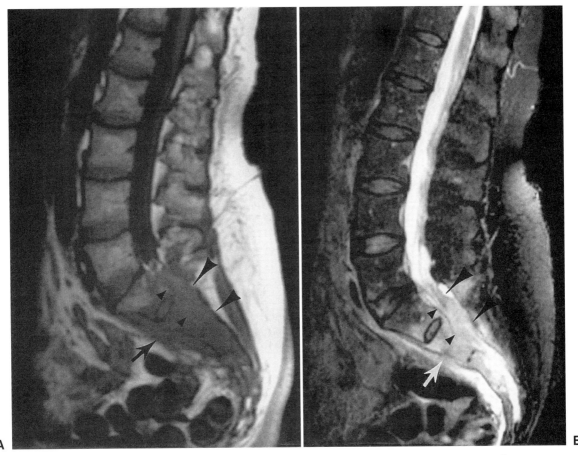

**Figure 10-5** *Focal MR pattern. Sagittal T1-weighted (**A**) image of the lumbosacral spine shows hypointense area of marrow replacement in the sacrum. On the T2-weighted image (**B**), tumor becomes hyperintense to uninvolved bone marrow. Both images show well anterior paraspinal (arrows) and epidural (arrowheads) soft tissue component.*

sequences. A screening examination of the bone marrow might include coronal images of the spine, pelvis, proximal humeri, and femurs and sagittal images of the spine. The presence of tumor extension in the spinal canal and the foramina can be easily and quickly assessed. Axial and contrast-enhanced T1-weighted images can be obtained as needed.

Myelomatous involvement on MR images can be focal, variegated, or diffuse (Moulopoulos et al., 1992). Focal patterns consist of well-defined foci of signal abnormality on a background of normal marrow (Fig. 10-5). Variegated MR patterns show innumerable small foci of disease (Fig. 10-6). In diffuse MR patterns of bone marrow involvement, there is almost complete absence of normal bone marrow (Fig. 10-7). Myeloma patients more frequently present with focal MR patterns.

Focal patterns are easily recognized with MRI; their signal intensity will be low on T1- and high on STIR or T2-weighted images. Difficulties arise when myelomatous involvement is diffuse. Diffuse patterns can mimic the appearance of hematopoietic marrow, which might be present in the central skeleton of younger patients or patients with underlying disorders that cause regeneration of red marrow. Contrast-enhanced images are helpful in this context; uninvolved red marrow enhances minimally. A greater than 40% increase of signal intensity following intravenous contrast medium injection has been shown to be indicative of a diffuse pattern of bone marrow infiltration (Stabler et al., 1996). Dynamic MRI (dMRI) consists of rapid (within seconds) acquisition of images after a bolus intravenous injection of paramagnetic contrast. Signal intensity to time curves obtained from bone marrow dMRI data differ significantly in patients with normal marrow from those with bone marrow malignancies (Fig. 10-8) (Moulopoulos et al., 2002). In- and opposed-phase gradient-echo images can also be used when diffuse infiltration of the bone marrow is suspected. On opposed-phase gradient echo images, the phases of water and fat protons are opposite, whereas on in-phase gradient echo images they are parallel. By acquiring images at the time point when water and fat proton magnetizations are in opposite directions (opposed-phase images), the signal of red marrow, which

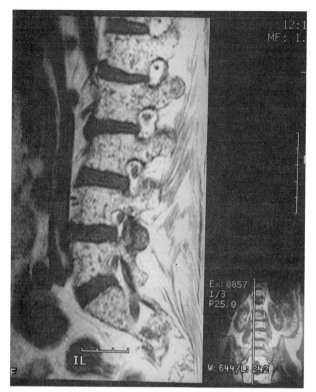

**Figure 10-6** *Variegated MR pattern. Sagittal T1-weighted image of the lumbar spine shows innumerable small focal lesions on a background of uninvolved fatty marrow.*

contains equivocal amounts of fat and water, is close to zero (Fig. 10-9). In fatty marrow, where fat outbalances water, and in infiltrated red marrow, where water outbalances fat, there will be no decrease in signal on opposed-phase images (Fig. 10-10).

Focal myeloma MR patterns are indistinguishable from bone metastases or other disorders that can affect the bone marrow in a similar manner (e.g., histiocytosis, lymphoma). Conversely, the MR appearance of diffuse myeloma patterns might not differ from other causes of diffuse bone marrow involvement (e.g., lymphoma, leukemia) (Moulopoulos and Dimopoulos, 1997).

### Prognostic Significance of MRI Findings

Findings on MRI of the bone marrow in patients with multiple myeloma have been correlated with several clinical parameters of tumor burden and have been found to be of prognostic value in this disease (Lecouvet et al., 1998; Moulopoulos et al., 1992). In one study, which included 57 patients with stage III multiple myeloma, 60-month survival rates differed significantly for patients with normal (70%) and abnormal (28%) MR studies (Lecouvet et al., 1998). Diffuse MR patterns have been associated with more advanced disease compared with focal MR patterns; patients with diffuse MR patterns have lower hemoglobin values, higher degrees of bone marrow plasmacytosis, and

higher β-2 microglobulin levels (Moulopoulos et al., 1992). In our study of 91 previously untreated symptomatic myeloma patients who had an abnormal baseline MRI, we found that the distribution of focal, variegated, and diffuse patterns was 53%, 16%, and 31%, respectively (Dimopoulos et al., 1999). We confirmed that the incidence of severe anemia, more extensive bone marrow plasmacytosis, and high tumor mass was higher in patients with diffuse MR patterns. Moreover, we found that the median survival was 23 months for patients with a diffuse pattern, 54 months for those with a focal pattern, and 51 months for those with variegated patterns ($p$ = 0.006) (Dimopoulos et al., 1999).

Asymptomatic multiple myeloma is diagnosed when the serum monoclonal protein is ≥30 g/L or when ≥10% clonal plasma cells are found in the bone marrow but there is no evidence of bone involvement on plain radiographs, anemia, hypercalcemia, or renal impairment, which could be explained by the underlying malignancy. Studies have shown that patients with asymptomatic myeloma who have an abnormal MRI of the bone marrow progress sooner (median, 10 or 16 mo) than those with a negative baseline MR study (median, 32 or 43 mo) (Moulopoulos et al., 1995; Vande Berg et al., 1996). Furthermore, MRI has been found to be independent from other established factors in the determination of prognosis in asymptomatic myeloma (Mariette et al., 1999; Moulopoulos et al., 1995; Vande Berg et al., 1996). MRI of the bone marrow has been found to be most helpful and cost effective in those patients with asymptomatic myeloma who are at intermediate risk for disease progression (i.e., patients with IgA myeloma or patients with serum peak ≥30g/L, or Bence Jones proteinuria > 50 mg/day); patients with a positive MRI develop symptomatic disease earlier (median, 21 mo) than those with normal MR studies (median, 57 mo) (Weber et al., 1997). It seems, therefore, justified to obtain a bone marrow MRI at diagnosis in all patients with asymptomatic multiple myeloma. Patients with positive MR studies should be followed more closely. Whether patients with an abnormal MRI will benefit from early institution of treatment has not been investigated.

### Posttreatment Followup

Patients with multiple myeloma are routinely followed with a bone survey. In those patients who respond to therapy, lytic bone lesions might decrease in size or show peripheral sclerosis (Fig. 10-11). However, usually no change between pre- and posttreatment bone surveys is seen. CT can better assess the soft tissue component and lesions that are not well seen on plain radiographs. MRI is the imaging modality of choice for assessing response to treatment in myeloma patients. In patients

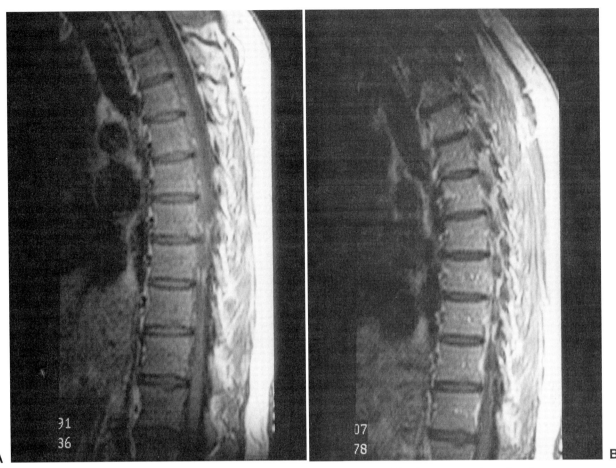

**Figure 10-7** *Diffuse MR pattern. T1-weighted (**A**) sagittal MR image of the thoracic spine shows low signal intensity throughout the spinal bone marrow. Contrast-enhanced T1-weighted MR image (**B**) shows diffuse contrast uptake by the abnormal marrow. Note that intervertebral discs, which should be hypointense to normal marrow, are isointense to the vertebral bodies in **A**, and become hypointense to abnormal, enhancing bone marrow in **B**.*

with nonsecretory disease, MRI of the bone marrow might be the only way to evaluate the effect of therapy apart from bone marrow aspiration and/or biopsy.

On posttherapy MR images, persistent active tumor must be differentiated from regenerating hematopoietic bone marrow, fibrosis and necrosis, or inflammation. Contrast-enhanced MR images are necessary in treated patients with multiple myeloma. T2-weighted MR images are not helpful because persistence of bright signal might be related to necrosis or inflammation of responding tumor (Rahmouni et al., 1993).

MR abnormalities might not entirely resolve, even in complete responders. In patients with focal MR patterns, absence of enhancement or rim enhancement of persistent bone marrow abnormalities on posttherapy MR studies are signs of complete response to therapy (Fig. 10-12) (Moulopoulos et al., 1994; Rahmouni et al., 1993). Persistent foci of abnormal homogeneous enhancement indicate the presence of active tumor. In patients with diffuse pretreatment MR patterns who

have responded to therapy, fatty marrow will reappear and gradually increase on follow-up studies (Moulopoulos et al., 1994). DMRI studies performed before and after treatment might show a change in pharmacokinetic parameters in those patients who achieve a response to therapy and help stage patients with equivocal static MRI findings (Fig. 10-8) (Moulopoulos et al., in press; Scherer et al., 2002). In- and opposed-phase gradient echo images might help the differential diagnosis of regenerating hematopoietic bone marrow from diffuse bone marrow infiltration in treated patients (Fig. 10-9).

Approximately 10 days after the initiation of radiotherapy there is an increase in signal intensity on T1-weighted images because of fatty cell migration from adjacent non-irradiated marrow (Stevens et al., 1990). The bright signal is sharply defined by the radiation portals and is irreversible for doses higher than 30 Gy. Lesions that have been radiated recently might show persistent enhancement, even in complete

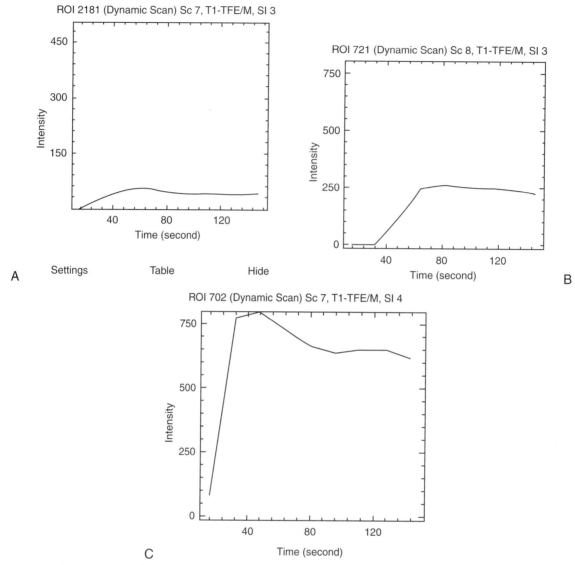

**Figure 10-8** *Signal intensity to time curves obtained from dMRI of the lumbar spine of a healthy individual (A) and a myeloma patient before (B) and after (C) treatment. Note steeper rise of signal intensity of abnormal bone marrow in B, which reaches a peak of 250 arbitrary units, compared with that of normal bone marrow (A), which reaches a peak of 70 units. After treatment the patient progressed; there is now an earlier and even steeper rise of contrast with a peak enhancement of 750 units (C).*

responders, because of an inflammatory reaction related to therapy. DMRI might be helpful in these cases by showing delayed and prolonged enhancement.

Often, patients treated for multiple myeloma experience new or more severe back pain because of new or progressive vertebral fractures (Moulopoulos et al., 1994). Such fractures might occur in patients who respond to therapy because when the tumor, which had replaced most of the vertebral bony trabeculae, resolves, the unsupported bony cortex collapses. In fact, 55% of 131 new vertebral fractures in 37 patients who were receiving treatment for stage III multiple myeloma were benign-appearing at MRI (Lecouvet,

1997a, 1997b). MRI can clearly differentiate such compression fractures from those resulting from progression of tumor and obviate the administration of unnecessary treatment, such as local irradiation.

## Compression Fractures

MRI is indicated for the evaluation of the etiology of a vertebral fracture when findings are unclear on plain film or CT. Findings suggestive of a fracture of malignant etiology include associated soft tissue mass, homogeneous abnormality involving almost the entire vertebral body, involvement of the pedicles, bulging of the

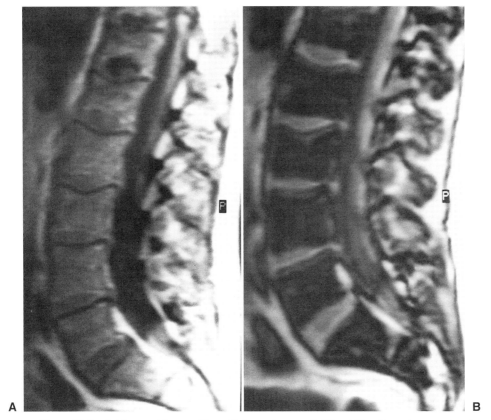

**Figure 10-9** *A 60-year-old man with multiple myeloma and diffuse MR pattern of marrow involvement. (**A**) Complete response to treatment. Posttreatment opposed-phase (**B**) sagittal MR image of the lumbar spine shows a diffuse drop in the signal intensity of normal red marrow.*

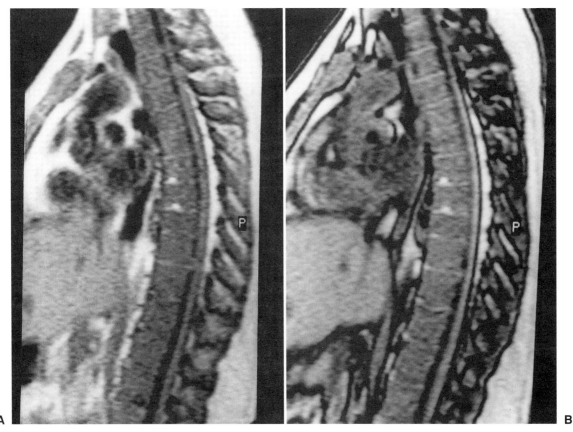

**Figure 10-10** *A 32-year-old patient with multiple myeloma and a diffuse MR pattern of bone marrow involvement. Progression of disease. Posttreatment in (**A**) and opposed (**B**) phase gradient-echo sagittal MR images of the thoracic spine show no change in signal intensity of infiltrated bone marrow.*

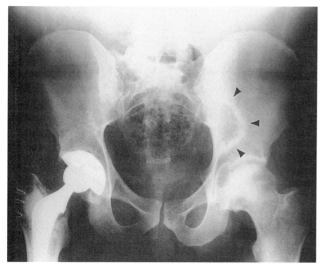

**Figure 10-11** *Anteroposterior view of the pelvis shows marginal sclerosis (arrows) of a lytic lesion of the left iliac bone in a patient who achieved complete response to treatment. Note right hip prosthesis and left hip subarticular sclerosis resulting from avascular necrosis.*

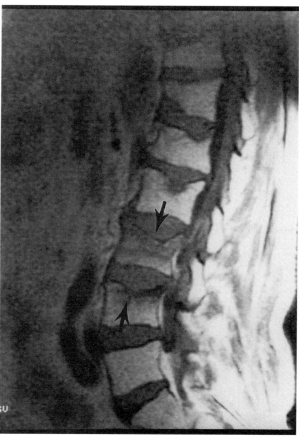

**Figure 10-13** *Sagittal T1-weighted MR image of the lumbar spine in a 60-year-old man shows benign L3 and L4 compression fractures with parallel band of low signal intensity (arrows).*

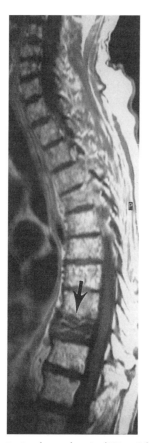

**Figure 10-12** *Contrast-enhanced sagittal T1-weighted MR image of the cervical and thoracic spine of a myeloma patient who has achieved a good response to therapy shows rim enhancement of treated vertebral body lesion (arrow).*

vertebral body contour, and a cervical or lumbosacral location (Moulopoulos et al., 1996; Yuh et al., 1989). A low signal intensity band parallel to a depressed vertebral end plate is highly specific of a benign fracture (Fig. 10-13). Inhomogeneous enhancement is highly specific for malignant vertebral fractures (Cuenod, 1996). More recently, diffusion-weighted MRI showed clearly different signal characteristics in benign and malignant fractures (Baur et al., 1998; Chan et al., 2002).

In multiple myeloma the mechanism of development of vertebral fractures is dual: osteoclastic resorption resulting from various osteoclast activating factors produced by the abnormal plasma cells, or bone destruction because of local growth of plasma cell aggregates. Therefore, vertebral fractures could have benign MR characteristics and still be related to the presence of multiple myeloma. In fact, 21% to 83% of vertebral fractures in patients with newly diagnosed myeloma had benign MR characteristics (Lecouvet et al., 1997a; Libshitz et al., 1992; Moulopoulos et al., 1992). Absence of MRI characteristics of malignancy does not justify classifying a vertebral compression fracture as benign in patients with suspected or known multiple myeloma.

In 50 patients diagnosed with stage III multiple myeloma, Lecouvet et al. found that the risk of vertebral fracture occurrence was higher (6 to 11 times) in patients with more than 10 focal lesions or in patients with diffuse marrow involvement compared with those with normal bone marrow or less than 10 focal lesions on pretreatment MRI (Lecouvet et al., 1997b). The issue of more intensive prophylactic treatment with antiresorptive medications (i.e., biphosphonates at higher doses or more frequent intervals) in patients at high risk for vertebral fractures has not, as yet, been addressed.

## Monoclonal Gammopathy of Undetermined Significance

Patients with monoclonal gammopathy of undetermined significance (MGUS) have a ≤30 g/L monoclonal protein in the serum and less than 10% plasma cells in the bone marrow, without any evidence of myeloma, macroglobulinemia, amyloidosis, or any related plasma cell or lymphoproliferative disorder. Risk of progression of MGUS to clinically malignant disease is 1% per year (Kyle et al., 2002). Many parameters of this disorder have been investigated in an attempt to identify those patients with MGUS who will develop a malignant transformation. Because MRI was very sensitive in demonstrating occult bone marrow lesions in patients with multiple myeloma, it seemed reasonable to investigate patients with MGUS with bone marrow MRI. Bellaiche et al. reported normal MR studies of the spinal bone marrow in all 25 patients with MGUS (Bellaiche et al., 1997). Vande Berg et al. found MRI abnormalities in 19% of 37 patients with a diagnosis of nonmyelomatous monoclonal gammopathy. The increased incidence of bone marrow abnormalities in Vande Berg's study might be the result of more extensive bone marrow sampling because they obtained MR images of the pelvis and femurs in addition to images of the spine. In addition, their patients had bone marrow plasmacytosis ranging from 0.5% to 23%; this means that some of their patients actually had asymptomatic myeloma (Vande Berg et al., 1997). In Vande Berg's study, all patients who had normal MRIs did not require specific treatment after a median followup of 30 months, whereas 7 patients with abnormal MRIs progressed within 58 months after the MR study (Vande Berg et al., 1997). An abnormal MRI in a patient with MGUS should strongly question this diagnosis.

## Solitary Plasmacytoma of Bone

Solitary plasmacytoma of bone (SBP) is the only disease feature in approximately 2% of patients with plasma cell dyscrasias. It is diagnosed when monoclonal plasma cells are found at a single bony site, no other lytic lesions are seen on skeletal surveys, and random bone marrow samples are normal. Monoclonal protein in the serum and/or urine is present in up to 70% of patients and uninvolved immunoglobulins are usually preserved (Dimopoulos et al., 2000). On plain radiographs and CT, SBP typically appears as a purely lytic, expansile bone lesion of the central skeleton and particularly the spine, often accompanied by a soft tissue mass (Fig. 10-14). MRI will show a bone marrow-replacing lesion with an intermediate signal intensity on T1-weighted images, high signal intensity on T2-weighted images, and evidence of enhancement after the intravenous administration of paramagnetic contrast. The soft tissue mass is more precisely delineated with MRI, and spinal cord or nerve root compression is easily depicted. The treatment for solitary bone plasmacytoma is local irradiation of the tumor. Despite local control in 95% of patients, 50% to 70% of patients with SBP develop multiple myeloma within 3 years from diagnosis, presumably because of growth of previously undetected occult disease (Dimopoulos et al., 2000).

MRI of the spine showed additional unsuspected lesions in 4 of 12 patients with SBP, 3 of whom developed systemic disease within 18 months from diagnosis

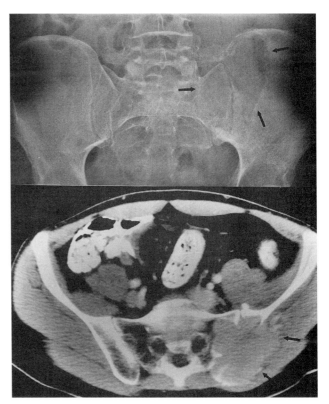

**Figure 10-14** *Anteroposterior radiograph (top) of the pelvis shows large lytic lesion of left iliac bone and sacral wing (arrows). Corresponding axial CT image (bottom) shows expansile lytic bone lesion with cortical destruction and associated soft tissue mass (arrows).*

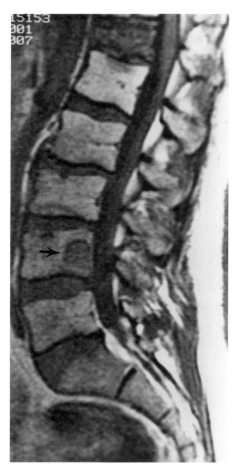

**Figure 10-15** *Patient with initial diagnosis of SBP of T12 who received local radiotherapy. Sagittal T1-weighted MR of the lumbosacral spine shows T12 lesion and a focal lesion at L4 (arrows), which was not shown on plain radiographs.*

(Moulopoulos et al., 1994) (Fig. 10-15). In another study, spinal MRI revealed occult lesions in 4 of 6 patients with SBP (Mathieu et al., 1993). Liebross et al. reported that 7 of 8 patients with SBP who were staged with conventional radiographs, but only 1 of 7 patients who were staged with both conventional radiographs and MRI developed multiple myeloma (Liebross et al., 1998). A recent update of the M.D. Anderson series showed that 26% of patients who were initially referred with the diagnosis of SBP were misdiagnosed because spinal MRI revealed additional bone lesions that were not present on skeletal surveys (Wilder et al., 2002).

Although the number of patients studied is small, there is enough evidence for MRI to become part of the staging for patients with SBP to better assess the extent of local tumor and to rule out occult lesions. Investigation of other skeletal parts besides the spine with MRI might increase the yield of occult lesions in patients with SBP.

## REFERENCES

Alexandrakis, M. G., Kyriakou, D. S., Passam, F., Koukouraki, S., and Karkavitsas, N. (2001). Value of TC-99m sestamibi scintigraphy in the detection of bone lesions in multiple myeloma: comparison with Tc-99m methylene diphosphonate. *Annals of Hematology, 80,* 349–353.

Avva, R., Vanhemert, R. L., Barlogie, B., Munshi, N., and Angtuaco, E. J. (2001). CT-guided biopsy of focal lesions in patients with multiple myeloma may reveal new and more aggressive cytogenetic abnormalities. *American Journal of Neuroradiology, 22,* 781–785.

Bataille, R., Chevalier, J., Rossi, M., and Sanny, J. (1982). Bone scintigraphy in plasma cell myeloma. A prospective study of 70 patients. *Radiology, 145,* 801–804.

Baur, A., Stabler, A., and Bruning, R. (1998). Diffusion-weighted MR imaging of the bone marrow: Differentiation of benign versus pathologic compression fractures. *Radiology, 207,* 349–356.

Bellaiche, L., Laredo, J. D., Liote, F., Koeger, A. C., Hamze, B., Ziza, J. M., Pertuiset, E., Bardin, T., Tubiana, J. M., and GRI Group. (1997). Magnetic resonance imaging of monoclonal gammopathies of unknown significance and multiple myeloma. *Spine, 22,* 2251–2257.

Catalano, L., Pace, L., Califano, C., Pinto, A. M., De Renzo, A., Di Gennaro, F., Del Vecchio, S., Fonti, R., Salvatore, M., and Rotoli, B. (1999). Detection of focal myeloma lesions by technetium-99m-sestaMIBI scintigraphy. *Haematologica, 84,* 119–124.

Chan, J. H., Peh, W. C., Tsui, E. Y., Chau, L. F., Cheung, K. K., Chan, K. B., Yuen, M. K., Wong, E. T., and Wong, P. T. (2002). Acute vertebral compression fractures: Discrimination between benign and malignant causes using apparent diffusion coefficients. *British Journal of Radiology, 75,* 207–214.

Cuenod, C. A., Laredo, J. D., Chevret, S., Hamze, B., Naouri, J. F., Chapaux, X., Bondeville, J. M., and Tubiana, J. M. (1996). Acute vertebral collapse due to osteoporosis or malignancy: appearance on unenhanced and gadolinium-enhanced MR images. *Radiology, 199,* 541–549.

Dimopoulos, M. A., Moulopoulos, L. A., Delasalle, K., Weber, D., Gika, D., and Alexanian, R. (1999). Prognostic significance of magnetic resonance imaging of bone marrow in previously untreated patients with multiple myeloma. *Blood, 15,* 563a (abstract 2398).

Dimopoulos, M. A., Moulopoulos, L. A., Maniatis, A., and Alexanian, R. (2000). Solitary plasmacytoma of bone and asymptomatic multiple myeloma. *Blood, 90,* 2037–2044.

Ishibashi, M., Nonoshita, M., Uchida, M., Kojima, K., Tomita, N., Matsumoto, S., Tanaka, K., and Hayabuchi, N. (1998). Bone marrow uptake of thallium-201 before and after therapy in multiple myeloma. *Journal of Nuclear Medicine, 39,* 473–475.

Kapadia, S. B. (1980). Multiple myeloma: A clinicopathologic study of 62 consecutively autopsied cases. *Medicine, 59,* 380–392.

Kyle, R. A. (1975). Multiple myeloma. Review of 869 cases. *Mayo Clinic Proceedings, 50,* 29–40.

Kyle, R. A., Therneau, T. M., and Rajkumar, S. V. (2002). A long-term study of prognosis in monoclonal gammopathy of undetermined significance. *New England Journal of Medicine, 346,* 564–569.

Lecouvet, F. E., Malghem, J., Michaux, L., Michaux, J. L., Lehmann, F., Maldague, B. E., Jamart, J., Ferrant, A., and Vande Berg, B. C. (1997b). Vertebral compression fractures in multiple myeloma. Part II. Assessment of fracture risk with MR imaging of spinal bone marrow. *Radiology, 204,* 201–205.

Lecouvet, F. E., Vande Berg, B. C., Maldague, B. E., Michaux, L., Laterre, E., Michaux, J. L., Ferrant, A., and Malghem, J. (1997a). Vertebral compression fractures in multiple myeloma. Part I. Distribution and appearance at MR imaging. *Radiology, 204,* 195–199.

Lecouvet, F. E., Vande Berg, B. C., Michaux, L., Malghem, J., Maldague, B. E., Jamart, J., Ferrant, A., and Michaux, J. L. (1998). Stage III multiple myeloma: clinical and prognostic value of spinal bone marrow MR imaging. *Radiology, 209,* 653–660.

Libshitz, H. I., Malthouse, S. R., Cunningham, D., Mac Vicar, A. D., and Husband, J. E. (1992). Multiple myeloma: appearance at MR imaging. *Radiology, 182,* 833–837.

Liebross, R. H., Ha, C. S., Cox, J. D., Weber, D., Delasalle, K., and Alexanian, R. (1998). Solitary bone plasmacytoma: outcome and prognostic factors following radiotherapy. *International Journal of Radiation Oncology, Biology, Physics, 41,* 1063–1067.

Mariette, X., Zagdanski, A. M., Guermazi, A., Bergot, C., Arnould, A., Frija, J., Brouet, J. C., and Fermand, J. P. (1999). Prognostic value of vertebral lesions detected by magnetic resonance imaging in patients with stage I multiple myeloma. *British Journal of Haematology, 104,* 723–729.

Mathieu, D., Rahmouni, A., Divine, M., Dao, T. H., Reyes, F., and Vasile, N. (1993). MR imaging of the spine in presumed solitary plasmacytoma [Abstract]. *Radiology, 189,* 119.

Moulopoulos, L. A., and Dimopoulos, M. A. (1997). Magnetic resonance imaging of the bone marrow in hematologic malignancies. *Blood, 90,* 2127–2147,

Moulopoulos, L. A., Dimopoulos, M. A., Alexanian, R., Leeds, N. E., and Libshitz, H. I. (1994). Multiple myeloma: MR patterns of response to treatment. *Radiology, 193,* 441–446.

Moulopoulos, L. A., Dimopoulos, M. A., Smith, T. L., Weber, D. W., Delasalle, K., Libshitz, H. I., and Alexanian, R. (1995). Prognostic significance of magnetic resonance imaging in patients with asymptomatic multiple myeloma. *Journal of Clinical Oncology, 13,* 251–256.

Moulopoulos, L. A., Dimopoulos, M. A., Weber, D., Fuller, L., Libshitz, H. I., and Alexanian, R. (1994). Magnetic resonance imaging in the staging of solitary plasmacytoma of bone. *Journal of Clinical Oncology, 11,* 1311–1315.

Moulopoulos, L. A., Varma, D. G. K., Dimopoulos, M. A., Leeds, N. E., Kim, E. E., Johnston, D. A., Alexanian, R., and Libshitz, H. I. (1992). Multiple myeloma: Spinal MR imaging in patients with untreated, newly diagnosed disease. *Radiology, 185,* 833–840.

Moulopoulos, L. A., Yoshimitsu, K., Johnston, D. A., Leeds, N. E., and Libshitz, H. I. (1996). MR prediction of benign and malignant vertebral compression fractures. *Journal of Magnetic Resonance Imaging, 6,* 667–674.

Orchard, K., Barrington, S., Buscombe, J., Hilson, A., Prentice, H. G., and Mehta, A. (2002). Fluoro-deoxyglucose positron emission tomography imaging for the detection of occult disease in multiple myeloma. *British Journal of Haematology, 117,* 133–135.

Pace, L., Catalano, L., Pinto, A. M., De Renzo, A., Di Gennaro, F., Califano, C., Del Vecchio, S., Rotoli, B., and Salvatore, M. (1998). Different patterns of technetium-99m sestamibi uptake in multiple myeloma. *European Journal of Nuclear Medicine, 25,* 714–720.

Rahmouni, A., Divine, M., Mathieu, D., Golli, M., Dao, T. H., Jazaerli, N., Anglade, M. C., Reyes, F., and Vasile, N. (1993). Detection of multiple myeloma involving the spine: efficacy of fat-suppression and contrast-enhanced MR imaging. *American Journal of Roentgenology, 160,* 1049–1052.

Rahmouni, A., Divine, M., Mathieu, D., Golli, M., Haioun, C., Dao, T., Anglade, M. C., Reyes, F., and Vasile, N. (1993). MR appearance of multiple myeloma before and after treatment. *American Journal of Roentgenology, 160,* 1053–1057.

Resnick, D., Dreenaway, G. D., Bardwick, P. A., Zvaifler, N. J., Gill, C. N., and Newman, D. R. (1981). Plasma cell dyscrasia with polyneuropathy, organomegaly, endocrinopathy, m-protein, and skin changes: The POEMS syndrome. *Radiology, 10,* 17–22.

Scherer, A., Strupp, C., Wittsack, H. J., Engelbrecht, V., Willers, R., Germing, U., Gattermann, N., Haas, R., and Modder, U. (2002). Dynamic contrast-enhanced MRI for evaluating bone marrow microcirculation in malignant hematological diseases before and after thalidomide therapy. *Radiologe, 42,* 222–230.

Schirrmeister, H., Bommer, M., Buck, A. K., Muller, S., Messer, P., Bunjes, D., Dohner, H., Bergmann, L., and Reske, S. N. (2002). Initial results in the assessment of multiple myeloma using 18F-FDG PET. *European Journal of Nuclear Medicine and Molecular Imaging, 29,* 361–366.

Smith, D. B., Scarffe, J. H., and Eddleston, B. (1988). The prognostic significance of x-ray changes at presentation and reassessment in patients with multiple myeloma. *Hematological Oncology, 6,* 1–6.

Stabler, A., Baur, A., Barti, R., Munker, R., Lamerz, R., and Reiser, M. F. (1996). Contrast enhancement and quantitative analysis in MR images of multiple myeloma: Assessment of focal and diffuse growth patterns in marrow correlated with biopsies and survival rates. *American Journal of Roentgenology, 167,* 1029–1036.

Stevens, S. K., Moore, S. G., and Kaplan, I. D. (1990). Early and late bone-marrow changes after irradiation: MR evaluation. *American Journal of Roentgenology, 154,* 745–750.

Tirovola, E. B., Biassoni, L., Britton, K. E., Kaleva, N., Kouykin, V., and Malpas, J. S. (1996). The use of 99mTc-MIBI scanning in multiple myeloma. *British Journal of Cancer, 74,* 1815–1820.

Vande Berg, B. C., Lecouvet, F. E., Michaux, L., Labaisse, M., Malghem, J., Jamart, J., Maldague, B. E., Ferrant, A., and Michaux, J. L. (1996). Stage I multiple myeloma: Value of MR imaging of the bone marrow in the determination of prognosis. *Radiology, 201,* 243–246.

Vande Berg, B. C., Michaux, L., Lecouvet, F. E., Labaisse, M., Malghem, J., Jamart, J., Malgague, B. E., Ferrant, A., and Michaux, J. L. (1997). Nonmyelomatous monoclonal gammopathy: Correlation of bone marrow MR images with laboratory findings and spontaneous clinical outcome. *Radiology, 202,* 247–251.

Wahner, H. W., Kyle, R. A., and Beabout, J. W. (1980). Scintigraphic evaluation of the skeleton in multiple myeloma. *Mayo Clinic Proceedings, 55,* 739–746.

Watanabe, N., Shimizu, M., Kageyama, M., Tanimura, K., Kinuya, S., Shuke, N., Yokoyama, K., Tonami, N., Watanabe, A., Seto, H., and Goodwin, D. A. (1999). Multiple myeloma evaluated with 201Tl scintigraphy compared with bone scintigraphy. *Journal of Nuclear Medicine, 40,* 1138–1142.

Waxman, A. D., Seimsen, J. K., Levine, A. M., Holdorf, D., Suzuki, R., Singer, F. R., and Bateman, J. (1981). Radiographic and radionuclide imaging of multiple myeloma: The role of gallium scintigraphy: Concise communication. *Journal of Nuclear Medicine, 22,* 232–236.

Weber, D. M., Dimopoulos, M. A., Moulopoulos, L. A., Delasalle, K. B., Smith, T., and Alexanian, R. (1997). Prognostic features of asymptomatic multiple myeloma. *British Journal of Haematology, 97,* 810–814.

Wilder, R. B., Ha, C. S., Cox, J. D., Weber, D., Delasalle, K., and Alexanian, R. (2002). Persistence of myeloma protein for more than one year after radiotherapy is an adverse prognostic factor in solitary plasmacytoma of bone. *Cancer, 94,* 1532–1537.

Yuh, W. T., Zachar, C. K., Barloon, T. J., Sato, Y., Sickels, W. J., and Hawes, D. R. (1989). Vertebral compression fractures: Distinction between benign and malignant causes with MR Imaging. *Radiology, 172,* 215–218.

# CHAPTER 11

## Prognostic Factors and Classification for Multiple Myeloma (Contribution to Clinical Management)

J. F. SAN MIGUEL
R. FONSECA
P. R. GREIPP

Myeloma is a disease with heterogeneous survival. For the past three decades many groups have sought to generate a prognostic set of factors capable of influencing clinical decisions. In fact, there has been dissociation between the generation of new data and the clinical application of the multiple factors available. The study of prognostic factors can be used to identify groups of patients in need of novel therapies, whereas some might benefit maximally from currently existing treatment protocols. Furthermore, all exiting prognostic factors and classifications will need to be evaluated in the context of novel therapeutic agents being tried for the treatment of myeloma.

In this two-part review, we discuss prognostic factors as they relate to patients treated with conventional therapy and high-dose chemotherapy (Kyle, 1994, 1995; San Miguel, 1998; Turesson, 1999). We also review classification schemes that consider several prognostic factors simultaneously.

In this chapter we focus on prognostic factors as they relate to (1) the host, (2) the specific characteristics of the malignant clone, and (3) a series of factors resulting from the interaction between the tumor clone and the host, which mainly reflect the tumor burden and disease complications.

## Host Factors

### General Demographic Factors

As is the case in other malignancies, in myeloma there is a favorable influence on prognosis when patients have a good performance status (PS) (Eastern Cooperative Oncology Group PS ≥ 2) and are young. In fact, an age lower than 70 years is associated with significantly improved overall survival. Moreover, it has been reported that very young patients (those under 40 years), when they also have a normal renal function and low $\beta_2$-microglobulin, have a median survival of over 8 years (Bladé, 1996). Ethnicity has not been thoroughly assessed as a prognostic factor for myeloma. The Southwest Oncology Group showed that survival is similar in blacks and whites (Modiano et al., 1996). We are not aware of any other similar studies comparing other ethnic groups.

### Immunity

It has long been suspected that permissive immunity allows emergence of malignant clones or the rapid progression of existing ones. Likewise, the immune status of the patient with myeloma could play an important role in tumor growth control. We have observed that the number of CD4 cells is significantly reduced in MM patients, particularly in those with advanced clinical stage, and the reduction is mainly the result of the memory and not to naive CD4 cells. This lower immunity seems to translate into meaningful clinical differences, as patients with low CD4 levels ( $< 700 \times 10^6$ cells/L) display a significantly lower survival in the univariate analysis (not an independent factor) (San Miguel et al., 1992). Similar observations have been made in the context of patients treated with conventional chemotherapy by ECOG (Kay et al., 2001). We have shown that a larger number of peripheral blood CD19$^+$ cells (B-lymphocytes) are associated with improvements in survival (Kay et al., 2001). Although less well explored, natural killer (NK) cells can also be important in the control of the malignant clone (Garcia-Sanz et al., 1996; Österborg et al., 1990). It appears that early in the process of the disease NK cells increase, probably in an attempt to control the tumor growth. In the advanced stages of the disease the number of peripheral blood mature NK cells decreases, whereas the relative number of immature NK cells increases (Garcia-Sanz et al., 1996).

The presence of anti-myeloma T cell clones has been well established. These cells can recognize the idiotypic Ig structures of the cell surface as tumor antigens. The functional significance or efficacy of these clones has not been thoroughly evaluated. However, the occurrence of expanded T cell clones (defined as a T cell β chain receptor detected by Southern blot) has been associated with an improved prognosis (Brown et al., 1997; Sze et al., 2001).

## Malignant Clone Factors

A number of prognostic factors that describe features intrinsic to the clone have been described. Some of these factors can be considered genotypic (e.g., cytogenetics, oncogenes, multidrug resistance) and others can be considered phenotypic (e.g., morphology, immunophenotyping, phenotype, and the proliferation rate).

### Genotype Factors

#### Cytogenetics

Cytogenetics are emerging as one of the most important prognostic factors in MM. Recent information suggests that a thorough investigation of chromosome abnormalities at the time of diagnosis should be undertaken to fully and accurately prognosticate patients. The group from the University of Arkansas (Tricot et al., 1995, 1997) has shown that partial or complete deletion of chromosome 13 are associated with short survival, event-free survivals, and decreased responsiveness to therapy among patients with MM treated with intensive chemotherapy. Several other groups, including ours, have subsequently confirmed this initial observation (Fonseca et al., 2001b; Perez-Simon et al., 1998; Zojer et al., 2000), applicable as well to patients treated with conventional chemotherapy. The method of detection has generated great controversy. The Arkansas Group has postulated that the prognostic influence of monosomy 13 detected by conventional cytogenetics is superior to that detected by fluorescent in situ hybridization (FISH). In the former situation, an abnormal test reflects both the biologic importance of chromosome 13 abnormalities plus an increased proliferative rate of the clone as shown by the documentation of abnormal metaphases. It is now well accepted that although all myeloma plasma cells harbor chromosome abnormalities, only a small fraction will exhibit abnormal metaphases (usually <30%). This is likely the result of the low proliferative rate of the myeloma clone. The information of other groups shows that this negative effect on prognosis is also apparent when FISH detects the abnormality. Several studies now show that monosomy

13 detected by FISH has prognostic relevance for both patients treated with conventional chemotherapy (Perez-Simon et al., 1998) and high-dose therapy with stem cell support (Worel et al., 2001). The specific immunoglobulin heavy-chain translocations are also associated with prognostic significance. t(4;14)(p16;q32) and t(14;16)(q32;q23) are both associated with an inferior outcome (Fonseca et al., 2001a). In contrast, t(11;14)(q13;q32) is not associated with a worse outcome and most likely has a favorable influence on prognosis (Fonseca et al., 2001a; Moreau et al., 2002). Mono-allelic deletions of the *p53* locus (17p13) are also associated with a shortened outcome (Drach, 1998; Fonseca et al., 2001a). Moreover, the presence of hypodiploidy as detected by karyotype analysis is also associated with treatment failure. Other potential adverse cytogenetic features are abnormalities of chromosome 1p/1q (Debes-Marun et al., 2002) and deletion of chromosome 22 (Segeren et al., 2002; Urbauer et al., 2002). Apart from t(11;14)(q13;q32), few chromosome abnormalities have been associated with an improved outcome, but the presence of hyperdiploidy is probably associated with an improved outcome. For instance, trisomies of chromosomes 9, 11, and 17 tend to have a favorable prognostic influence (Perez-Simon et al., 1998). In line with this latter observation, our results on DNA content analyzed by flow cytometry also show that cases with hyperdiploid DNA cell content have a significantly better prognosis than diploid myeloma, although the prognostic value of this parameter is lost in multivariate analysis (Greipp et al., 1999; San Miguel, 1996). Recent data suggest that karyotypic abnormalities of the c-*myc* locus are seen with advancing stages of the disease and are highly prevalent in human myeloma cell lines (Shou et al., 2000).

## Oncogenes

It has become increasingly evident that dysregulation of oncogenes not involved in structural chromosomal abnormalities could also contribute to the pathogenesis of MM. The process of clonal evolution is thought to be a consequence of a multistep process that requires the accumulation of sequential genetic changes. Some of these genetic abnormalities have been found, as well as associated with prognostic impact. Oncogenic events such as *p53* mutations (Corradini et al., 1994) are associated with progressive disease and relapse. The retinoblastoma *(Rb)* gene is located in chromosome 13, and accordingly the adverse prognostic impact of Rb deletions parallels that of monosomy 13 (Drach, 1998; Fonseca et al., 2001b; Perez-Simon et al., 1998). Patients treated with conventional chemotherapy and who harbor K-*ras* mutations have significantly shorter survival (2 vs. 3.7 y) (Liu et al., 1996). Another tumor suppressor inactivated by

methylation in myeloma is *p16*. We have observed that methylation of *p16* is associated with high proliferative activity of the plasma cells and poor prognosis, but it is not an independent prognostic factor because of its relationship with the number of plasma cells in S-phase (Mateos et al., 2001).

## Phenotype Factors

### Proliferation and Apoptosis Markers

The end result of the genetic and epigenetic abnormalities is the generation of an expanding clone primarily by cell proliferation. Accordingly, measurements of cell proliferation have been used for the prognostic assessment of patients with good success. Such measurements include the plasma cell labeling index (PCLI) with bromodeoxyuridine (Greipp et al., 1993) or by flow cytometry with PI (Orfao et al., 1994). The former is a slide-based technique that identifies the percent of clonotypic cells undergoing mitosis by virtue of the detection of bromodeoxyuridine incorporation. Both methods have shown that this is one of the most robust and reliable methods for establishing prognosis for myeloma patients. The combination of a proliferation factor with other variables such as those that reflect tumor burden (e.g., $\beta_2$-microglobulin) provide the basis for accurate prognostication of patients (Perez-Simon et al., 1998).

### Morphology

Morphologic features form the basis of classification and prognosis for many human neoplasias, but have been used only infrequently in the case of multiple myeloma. This is evident for those treating other hematologic malignancies, such as acute leukemias and lymphomas, in which the morphologic features of the malignant cells are quite significant for classification and prognosis. Several groups, including predominantly those from Germany and the Mayo Clinic, have shown negative prognostic implications for patients with immature/plasmablastic morphology (Bartl et al., 1982; Greipp et al., 1998). The presence of plasmablastic morphology is a powerful prognostic factor that retains its significance on the multivariate model (Greipp et al., 1985).

## Multidrug Resistance

Multidrug resistance has not yet been included in a large-scale multivariate analysis to determine its suspected negative influence for prognosis. Drug resistance resulting from expression of p-glycoprotein (also known as MDR-1) is usually observed in patients who have been exposed to anthracyclines and vinca alkaloids

(Grogan et al., 1993; Sonneveld et al., 1996), but with conflicting reports on prognosis (Gieseler and Nussler, 1997; Sonneveld et al., 1996). Novel information suggests that expression of lung-resistant protein is associated with a shorter survival. It is expressed in nearly one-half of patients and identifies patients with poor probability of response to melphalan chemotherapy, but this adverse influence disappears in patients treated with high-dose chemotherapy (Raaijmakers et al., 1998).

### Immunocytochemistry and Immunophenotyping

A study by the Southwest Oncology Group showed that low PC acid phosphatase levels are associated with worsening of survival (1.7 y for patients with low scores vs. 2.8 y for those with high scores) (Saaed et al., 1991). Likewise, the prognostic impact of influence of immunophenotyping characterization has been explored (Omede, 1993; Pellat-Deceunynck, 1995; Pellat-Deceunynck et al., 1994; San Miguel, 1991; San Miguel et al., 1995). Based on the experience of our group and others, it is suggested that expression of CD20 and surface immunoglobulin is associated with poor prognosis (Omede, 1993; San Miguel, 1991). A lower level of expression of CD56 and CD11a, two molecules that are critical for homing adhesion to the bone marrow, are associated with extramedullary spreading of malignant PC (Pellat-Deceunynck et al., 1994). Whether this reflects features of more aggressive cells or whether they actively contribute to the extramedullary expansion is unknown (Pellat-Deceunynck, 1995). The expression of CD28 is related with disease activity and is likely expressed by a component of highly proliferative cells (Pellat-Deceunynck et al., 1994; Robillard et al., 1998). Nevertheless, until further information becomes available, it seems that immunophenotyping does not confer independent prognostic significance and should not be routinely used for the prognostication of patients. Immunophenotyping seems to be more valuable for the differentiation between MGUS and MM (Harada et al., 1993) as well as to monitor changes in the plasma cells as a consequence of treatment (e.g., to assess tumor burden or minimal residual disease) (San Miguel et al., 2002). More recently the Nordic Myeloma Study Group reported that the serum levels of CD138 (syndecan-1) is useful as a prognostic marker. They reported that patients with increased serum concentrations of serum syndecan-1 (≥1170 units/mL) have a significantly shorter survival (20 mo vs. 44 mo) (Seidel et al., 2000).

### Treatment Modality

We cannot fail to mention the importance of response to first-line therapy as an important prognostic factor, but we should also be aware that patients with rapid response might have a shorter duration of response and survival. This was suggested by Hansen (Hansen et al., 1974) 25 years ago and confirmed by Boccadoro through kinetic studies (Boccadoro and Pileri, 1987).

# Prognostic Factors Associated with Tumor Burden and Disease Complications

There is more information available regarding the prognostic effect of factors that represent either tumor burden or disease complications. These factors can be considered as the end consequence of the host factors and clonal expansion. Among them are (1) those factors derived from the expansion of the malignant clone-tumor burden; (2) factors designated as "end organ damage" (e.g., anemia, renal insufficiency, skeletal lesions); and (3) a wide array of biochemical markers, including some cytokines that might reflect disease activity.

### Tumor Burden

Tumor burden is a consequence of clonal expansion and has immediate consequences on the host. One of the first widely accepted systems for estimation of tumor burden was proposed by the Durie-Salmon classification, which was specifically obtained from mathematical models for the evaluation of tumor mass. Estimating the proportion of plasma cells in the bone marrow, the histopathologic pattern of infiltration, and the presence of circulating plasma cells can be used to estimate tumor burden. Extensive infiltration of the bone marrow by the plasma cells, particularly with a diffuse pattern, is associated with a poor prognosis. These factors, however, have significant variability because of the heterogeneous distribution of the clonal plasma cells in the marrow (those areas with evidence of bone resorption are usually more heavily infiltrated). As tumor burden increases, plasma cells are thought to be more common in circulation. Accordingly, the detection of circulating plasma cells, identified either by morphology or immunophenotyping, is associated advanced disease (Witzig et al., 1996). It has been reported that the presence of a high number of circulating plasma cells (>4%) is an independent adverse prognostic factor (Witzig et al., 1996).

### End Organ Damage

It has been well established that disease complications such as anemia, thrombocytopenia, and particularly renal insufficiency have an important negative influence on outcome (San Miguel, 1989). In general, the presence of bone disease is associated with greater tumor burden. Bone disease, directly evaluated through imaging studies or indirectly by the measurements of markers of bone metabolism (e.g., pyridinoline [PyD], deoxy-pyridinoline [DPD], urinary NTX, and ICTP) are also associated with an inferior outcome. Although the urinary levels of PyD and DPD are increased in patients with advanced clinical stages and progressive disease, and they also correlate with other prognostic factors such as the C-reactive protein, serum creatinine, and albumin levels, and therefore the relation to survival is minimal (Pecherstorfer et al., 1997). Serum bone sialoprotein is another biochemical marker of bone turnover and affords similar results to DPD. Likewise, the serum levels of ICTP can have prognostic significance in myeloma patients but have not been shown to be independent predictors of survival. The use of markers indicative of bone disease is limited in that aggressive myeloma variants might have little bone resorption, such as might be seen in cases of plasma cell leukemia.

## $\beta_2$-microglobulin

The most important biochemical marker is serum concentration of the $\beta_2$-microglobulin. Its level is proportional to both tumor burden and renal filtering capacity. Several threshold values (range, 3–6 mg/dL) have been used to discriminate prognostic subgroups of patients (Bataille et al., 1984; Cuzick et al., 1990; Garewal et al., 1984; San Miguel et al., 1995). The marker can also be used as a continuous variable because the higher the $\beta_2$-M value, the shorter the survival. As a result of the important and reproducible effect on prognosis, measurement of the serum levels of $\beta_2$-microglobulin at the time of diagnosis should be done in all patients. The prognostic use of these markers is only well validated when determined at the time of diagnosis and is not thought to be useful for disease monitoring. For instance, patients might experience relapse without a concomitant increase in $\beta_2$-microglobulin (Boccadoro et al., 1989).

### Other Serum Markers

Other markers of disease activity, such as thymidine kinase (Brown et al., 1993), neopterin, and lactate dehydrogenase, do not usually remain independent prognostic factors in multivariate analysis (San Miguel et al., 1989). The serum concentration of interleukin-6 (IL-6) has been explored as a prognostic factor because it is the major plasma cell growth factor. Elevated serum levels of this cytokine are associated with a shorter survival (Bataille et al., 1989; Papadaki et al., 1997), and high levels of its soluble receptor (sIL-6R) correlate with poor prognosis (Pulkki et al., 1996; Turesson, 1999). A surrogate serum marker for IL-6 is

C-reactive protein, which is synthesized in the liver and is an "acute phase reactant protein." Therefore, the serum levels of the C-reactive protein (Bataille et al., 1992) can replace IL-6 as prognostic factors (Turesson, 1999), and in combination with the $\beta_2$-microglobulin can be used for the prognostic assessment of patients (Bataille et al., 1992). It should be noted that although CRP levels might be influenced by many factors different from myeloma activity, the presence at diagnosis of serum CRP values > 6 mg/L constitutes an independent prognostic factor.

# Prognostic Factors in Stem Cell Transplants

Because of the clinical benefit obtained by the application of high-dose chemotherapy, prognostic factors need to be separately validated for their use in patients treated with this modality in the same way as patients treated with standard chemotherapy doses. Fortunately, the preliminary data suggests that they are similar, although the magnitude of their effects is slightly different. The group from the University of Arkansas (Pulkki et al., 1996; Tricot et al., 1995) initially identified a low $\beta_2$-microglobulin, limited prior therapy, and non-IgA isotype as independent favorable variables for overall and disease-free survival. Other factors evident in the univariate analysis include age <50 years, performance status of <2, and Durie-Salmon stage I or II. As previously mentioned, they have observed that the presence of chromosome 13 and hypodiploidy were associated with poor outcome (Fassas et al., 2002; Tricot et al., 1997). The European Bone Marrow Transplant Registry (Bjorkstrand et al., 1995) has found that achieving a complete response before transplant, stage I, only one line of therapy, young age ( <45 y), and a low $\beta_2$-M were all favorable factors. Gertz and colleagues (Gertz et al., 1997) have recently shown that an elevated PCLI, as well as the presence of circulating monoclonal plasma cells in the blood stem cell harvest, were all associated with shortened survival after high-dose therapy with stem cell support.

The group from the Mayo Clinic (Rajkumar et al., 2000) has proposed that the ultimate outcome of patients undergoing high-dose chemotherapy is dependent more on biologic variables than on response to transplant (complete vs. partial response). However, other groups propose that achievement of a complete response is the most important prognostic factor (Alexanian et al., 2001; Barlogie et al., 1999; Lahuerta et al., 2000).

Previously in this chapter we discussed a large number of prognostic factors, but perhaps only a few of them have real independent value. A summary of the most important would include the following: (1) two host

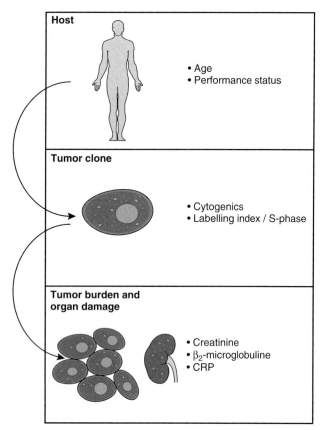

**Host**

- Age
- Performance status

**Tumor clone**

- Cytogenics
- Labelling index / S-phase

**Tumor burden and organ damage**

- Creatinine
- $\beta_2$-microglobuline
- CRP

*Figure 11-1*  *Prognostic factors in multiple myeloma.*

factors that reflect the ability of the patient to tolerate chemotherapy (*age and performance status*); and (2) two intrinsic characteristics of the malignant clone (*cytogenetics and proliferative activity LI*) together with two biochemical markers that reflect tumor burden/disease complications (*$\beta_2M$ and CRP*) (Fig. 11-1). The incorporation of these factors in classification schemes is of paramount importance.

# Classification Systems for Multiple Myeloma

Multiple myeloma can be classified according to a combination of several of the prognostic factors that have been mentioned before. Three major types of classification have been used: those that use simple clinical and laboratory values (e.g., the Durie-Salmon system, MRC); those that use combinations of markers of proliferation and tumor burden (e.g., Mayo and ECOG PCLI, Spanish); and those that classify the disease according to the underlying genomic aberrations of the cells (e.g., IFM and Mayo). Newer classification

systems are being proposed and based on some of the novel high-throughput technologies such as gene expression arrays (Zhan et al., 2002). These models have been proposed to discern several groups of patients with unique transcriptional profiles and are being validated. As such, they could result in future classification schemes that will be mostly focused on the transcriptional consequence of the clones. They are not further mentioned in this chapter.

## Clinical Staging Systems

Patients with MM display a very heterogeneous clinical course, their survival ranging from a few months to more than ten years (Kyle et al., 2002). Consequently, it is very important to have classification systems that will facilitate the categorization of patients and the evaluation of different protocols. These staging systems are usually based on prognostic clinical and biologic parameters obtained from multivariate analysis.

Two of the first staging systems were those developed by Costa et al. (1973) and the Southern Cancer Study Group (1975). Both established two risk groups: low and high. The first system considered as poor prognosis those patients with one or more of the following risk factors: (1) renal insufficiency, (2) hypercalcemia, (3) infections at diagnosis, and (4) low platelet or leukocyte counts. The second classification considered as poor risk those patients with anemia, hypercalcemia, or poor performance status. Interestingly, this latter system, although not including renal function, did provide very good risk discrimination. Carbone et al. (1967) grouped patients into four stages according to the presence of one to four of the following risk factors: hemoglobin < 9 g/dL, urea > 40 mg/dL, serum calcium > 12 mg/dL, and poor performance status. Based on our experience, this staging system does not allow good discrimination between stage 0 and I or between stage II and III/IV (San Miguel et al., 1989).

The classification that has been most widely accepted is that first proposed in 1975 by Durie and Salmon, which was designed from a mathematical model to evaluate cell tumor mass (1975). It established three stages based on those parameters that afford optimal correlation with tumor mass: level of monoclonal component, calcium, hemoglobin, and bone disease. Stage I patients have a low tumor mass (<0.6 × 10¹² cells/m²); stage II with 0.6 to 1.2 × 10¹² cells/m²; and stage III with >1.2 × 10¹² cells /mm². In addition, each stage is subclassified into two categories (A and B) according to renal function (creatinine lower or greater than 2 mg/dL, respectively) (Table 11-1). Unfortunately, this classification is only of moderate use and has been found inferior to other markers such as the $\beta_2$-microglobulin, and it does not

**TABLE 11-1**

Clinical Staging System for Multiple Myeloma Developed from Correlation of Measured Myeloma Cell Mass with Presenting Clinical Features, Response to Treatment, and Survival

| Stage | Criteria | Measured Myeloma Cell Mass (cells $\times 10^{12}/m^2$) |
|---|---|---|
| I. | *All* of the following:<br>1. Hemoglobin value >10 g/dL<br>2. Serum calcium value normal (≤12 mg/dL)<br>3. On radiograph, normal bone structure (scale 0) or solitary bone plasmacytoma only<br>4. Low M-component production rates<br>   a. IgG value <5 g/dL<br>   b. IgA value <3 g/dL<br>   c. Urine light chain M component on electrophoresis <4 g/24 h | <0.6<br><br>(low) |
| II. | Not fitting either stage I or stage II | 0.6–1.20 (intermediate) |
| III. | *One or more* of the following<br>1. Hemoglobin value <8.5 g/dL<br>2. Serum calcium value >12 mg/dL<br>3. Advanced lytic bone lesions (scale 3)<br>4. High M-component production rates<br>   a. IgG value >7 g/dL<br>   b. IgA value >5 g/dL<br>   c. Urine light chain M component on electrophoresis >12 g/24 h | >1.20<br>(high) |

Subclassification
  A. Relatively normal renal function (serum creatinine value <2.0 mg/dL)
  B. Abnormal renal function (serum creatinine value ≥2.0 mg/dL)
Examples
  Stage IA: Low cell mass with normal renal function
  Stage IIIB: High cell mass with abnormal renal function

From Durie, B. G. and Salmon, S. E. *Cancer 36*, 1975, 842–854. Copyright © 1975 American Cancer Society. Reprinted by permission of Wiley-Liss, Inc., a subsidiary of John Wiley & Sons, Inc.

provide accurate prediction of response to therapy. Associations among the elements of staging are common. Stage III without renal insufficiency, even with hypercalcemia, does not predictably lead to early mortality in MM. It is important for the clinician evaluating patient risk to be aware that patients who are stage III only because they meet the bone lesion criteria do not have a poorer prognosis.

The British Medical Research Council (MRC) proposed a three-category staging system (A, B, C) using only three parameters (hemoglobin, urea, and performance status) (1980). All three of these parameters should be normal for stage I patients, whereas the presence of one markedly abnormal factor (hemoglobin < 7.5 g/dL or urea > 40 mg/dL) would categorize the patient as stage III. Several other similar systems have been proposed. In an independent series of patients, San Miguel and colleagues have compared seven of these systems, and the best discrimination between risk patients was provided by the MRC classification (San Miguel et al., 1989).

## Classifications Based on Tumor Burden and Speed of Replication

With the growth of understanding of myeloma biology, it is not surprising that the prognostic significance of stage as a predictor of survival has been eclipsed by newer prognostic factors based on myeloma biology. As is the case for any other population dynamics studies, two factors are critical, burden and speed of replication. This knowledge was used to generate the Mayo–ECOG system that uses the combination of the PCLI (proliferation) and $\beta_2$-microglobulin (tumor burden) (Greipp et al., 1988). It is important to note, however, that $\beta_2$-microglobulin might measure other factors than tumor burden alone, because it is also elevated in the case of renal insufficiency and as-yet unknown

## TABLE 11-2
### Diagnostic Value of the Bone Marrow Plasma Cell Labeling Index

| Test | Reference | Year | No. of Cases | Mean LI (%) MGUS/SMM | MM | Discriminant (%) | p value |
|------|-----------|------|--------------|----------------------|-----|------------------|---------|
| ($^3$H)TdrLI | Greipp and Kyle | 1983 | 75 | 0.1/0.1 | 1.0 | 0.4 | <0.001* <0.001† |
| ($^3$H)TdrLI | Boccadoro et al. | 1984 | 52 | NA | NA | 1.0 | <0.001 |
| BrdUrdLI | Greipp et al. | 1987 | 52 | 0.3/— | 1.4 | 0.8 | <0.002 |
| BrdUrdLI | Boccadoro et al. | 1987 | 43 | 0.3/— | 1.4 | 1.0 | 0.004‡ |
| BrdUrdLI | Büchi et al. | 1990 | 43 | 0.6/0.8 | 2.5 | 1.0 | <0.05 |
| BrdUrdLI | Girino et al. | 1991 | 59 | 0.3/— | 1.9 | — | <0.05 |
| BrdUrdLI | Ahsmann et al. | 1992 | 28 | 0.4/— | 1.4 | — | — |
| BrdUrdLI | Leo et al. | 1992 | 53 | 0.3/— | 1.4 | — | — |
| BrdUrdLI | Büchi et al. | 1993 | 47 | 0.6/0.8 | 2.4 | 1.0 | <0.05 |
| BrdUrdLI | Witzig et al. | 1999 | 91 | NA | NA | 1.0 | <0.001 |

*For differences between MGUS (monoclonal gammopathy of undetermined significance) and MM (multiple myeloma).
†For differences between SMM (smoldering multiple myeloma) and MM.
‡For differences between MGUS and stage I MM (continuous variable).
BrdUrdLI, bromodeoxyuridine labeling index; ($^3$H) TdrLI, tritiated thymidine labeling index; LI, labeling index; NA, not available.

aspects of myeloma. Myeloma cell proliferation as measured by the bone marrow PCLI has repeatedly been shown to be a most significant and independent prognostic factor for patient survival (Table 11-2).

The combination of $\beta_2$-microglobulin with other parameters such as C-reactive protein, albumin, LDH, and PCLI or S-phase offers highly reliable classification systems. Based on the two aforementioned factors, Greipp et al. proposed a model based on $\beta_2$-microglobulin and PCLI that discriminates the following three risk categories: low risk ($\beta_2$-microglobulin < 4 g/mL and LI < 0.4%), intermediate risk ($\beta_2$-microglobulin > 4 g/mL and LI > 0.4%), and high risk ($\beta_2$-microglobulin > 4 g/mL, independently of LI) (Greipp et al., 1988). The median survivals for the three groups were 48, 29, and 12 months, respectively. San Miguel and colleagues (1995) proposed a similar scoring system but based on the following four variables: number of plasma cells in S-phase, $\beta_2$-microglobulin, age, and performance status (Table 11-3), which established three risk categories with median survivals of 80, 36, and 9 months, respectively).

## Cytogenetic Classifications

The prognostic impact of cytogenetics has been previously discussed in this chapter. It will be important, however, to incorporate all relevant cytogenetic information into a model that can discern prognostic groups of patients. Two models that incorporate molecular cytogenetic tests have been proposed. In the context of the ECOG study E9486/9487, a simple cytogenetic classification proposes three groups of patients: poor risk, intermediate risk, and good risk (Fonseca et al., 2001a, 2003). These patients were all treated with conventional chemotherapy. In this study, the poor risk category is composed of patients with t(4;14) (p16.3;q32), t(14;16)(q32;q23), and deletions of 17p13.1 (median survival, 25 mo; $p < 0.001$). Of those remaining patients, those with a chromosome 13 monosomy/deletion have an intermediate prognosis (median survival, 41 mo), whereas the remaining patients (including many with t[11;14][q13;q32]) have a better prognosis (median survival, 52 mo).

## TABLE 11-3
### Classification of MM Based on S-Phase, $\beta_2$M, PS, and Age

| Variable | Score |
|----------|-------|
| S-phase plasma cells | |
| <3% | 0 |
| ≥3% | 2 |
| $\beta_2$-M serum levels | |
| <6 mg/mL | 0 |
| ≥6 mg/mL | 1 |
| Performance status | |
| ECOG <3 | 0 |
| ECOG ≥3 | 1 |
| Age | |
| <69 y | 0 |
| ≥69 y | 1 |

The sum of scores gives 3 stages: stage I (score 0), stage II (score 1 to 3), stage III (score 4 to 5).
From San Miguel, et al., *Blood, 85*, 1995, 448–455.

A similar observation is made by the IFM in which patients treated with high-dose chemotherapy had their prognosis determined largely by the presence of the specific translocations (Moreau et al., 2002). Patients with t(4;14)(p16.3;q32) had a shorter survival whereas patients with t(11;14)(q13;q32) had the best outcome. Furthermore, of patients not fitting into any one of these two categories, chromosome 13 monosomy and/or deletion could separate them into two groups of patients. These models will need to be refined and validated. However, they provide the possibility of discerning patients for whom high-dose chemotherapy is associated with prolonged survival, whereas it also identified some for whom alternative treatment strategies must be sought.

# International Prognostic Index

Clinicians have a wide array of therapeutic options for myeloma patients, and it would be desirable to have an international classification system with widespread acceptance based on risk group categories. This classification would substitute the commonly used Durie and Salmon staging system that has limited PNC correlation with prognosis, and would allow clinicians to tailor treatments and clinical trial eligibility PNC according to patient characteristics, and could also serve as a basis for comparing the effectiveness of new treatment strategies.

In response to these needs, an International Staging System (ISS) derived from a total of 11,171 patients compiled from American, Asian, and European cooperative groups and large individual institutions has been recently reported (Greipp et al., 2003). The ISS is based on the levels of $\beta_2$-microglobulin and albumin (Table 11-4), and it discriminates three risk groups with median survivals of 62, 44, and 29 months, respectively. The capacity to discriminate three risk groups was independent of age, geographic region, or standard or transplant therapy. Further efforts should be carried out to improve the staging system with the inclusion of other parameters such as cytogenetics and molecular markers.

## REFERENCES

Alexanian, R., Weber, D., Giralt, S., Dimopoulos, M., Delasalle, K., Smith, T., et al. (2001). Impact of complete remission with intensive therapy in patients with responsive multiple myeloma. *Bone Marrow Transplantation, 27*, 1037–1043.

Barlogie, B., Jagannath, S., Desikan, K. R., Mattox, S., Vesole, D., Siegel, D., et al. (1999). Total therapy with tandem transplants for newly diagnosed multiple myeloma. *Blood, 93*, 55–65.

Bartl, R., Frisch, B., Burkhardt, R., Fateh-Moghadam, A., Mahl, G., Gierster, P., et al. (1982). Bone marrow histology in myeloma: Its importance in diagnosis, prognosis, classification and staging. *British Journal of Haematology, 51*, 361–375.

Bataille, R., Boccadoro, M., Klein, B., Durie, B., and Pileri, A. (1992). C-reactive protein and beta-2 microglobulin produce a simple and powerful myeloma staging system. *Blood, 80*, 733–737.

Bataille, R., Greiner, J., and Sany, J. (1984). Beta-2-microglobulin in myeloma: Optimal use for staging, prognosis and treatment: A prospective study of 160 patients. *Blood, 63*, 468–476.

Bataille, R., Jourdan, M., Zhang, X. G., and Klein, B. (1989). Serum levels of interleukin 6, a potent myeloma cell growth factor, as a reflection of disease severity in plasma cell dyscrasias. *Journal of Clinical Investigation, 84*, 2008–2011.

Bjorkstrand, B., Ljungman, P., Bird, J. M., Samson, D., Brandt, L., Alegre, A., et al. (1995). Autologous stem cell transplantation in multiple myeloma: Results of the European Group for Bone Marrow Transplantation. *Stem Cells, 13*(suppl 2), 140–146.

Bladé, J. (1996). Presenting features and prognosis in 72 patients with multiple myeloma who were younger than 40 years. *British Journal of Haematology, 93*, 345–351.

Boccadoro, M., Gavarotti, P., Fossati, G., Pileri, A., Marmont, F., Neretto, G., et al. (1984). Low plasma cell 3(H) thymidine incorporation in monoclonal gammopathy of undetermined significance (MGUS), smouldering myeloma and remission phase myeloma: A reliable indicator of patients not requiring therapy. *British Journal of Haematology, 58*, 689–696.

Boccadoro, M., Massaia, M., Dianzani, U., and Pileri, A. (1987). Multiple myeloma: Biological and clinical significance of bone marrow plasma cell labelling index. *Haematologica, 72*, 171–175.

Boccadora, M., Omede, P., Frieri, R., Battaglio, S., et al. (1989). Related articles, links: Multiple myeloma: beta-2-microglobulin is not a useful follow-up, parameter. *Acta Haematologica, 82*, 122–125.

Boccadoro, M., and Pileri, A. (1987). Cell kinetics of multiple myeloma. *Hematologic Pathology, 1*, 137–142.

Brown, R. D., Joshua, D. E., Nelson, M., Gibson, J., Dunn, J., and MacLennan, I. C. (1993). Serum thymidine kinase as a prognostic indicator for patients with multiple myeloma: Results from the MRC (UK) V trial. *British Journal of Haematology, 84*, 238–241.

Brown, R. D., Yuen, E., Nelson, M., Gibson, J., and Joshua, D. (1997). The prognostic significance of T cell receptor beta gene rearrangements and idiotype-reactive T cells in multiple myeloma. *Leukemia, 11*, 1312–1317.

Büchi, G., Girotto, M., Veglio, M., Clerico, M., Gario, S., Termine, G., et al. (1990). Kappa/lambda ratio on peripheral blood lymphocytes and bone marrow plasma cell labeling index in monoclonal gammopathies. *Haematologica, 75*, 132–136.

Carbone, P. P., Kellerhouse, L. E., and Gehan, E. A. (1967). Plasmacytic myeloma: a study of the relationship of survival to various clinical manifestations ans anomalous protein type in 112 patients. *American Journal of Medicine, 42*, 948.

## TABLE 11-4
### International Prognostic Index (IPI)

**Staging for Multiple Myeloma**

| | |
|---|---|
| STAGE 1 | $\beta2M < 3.5$ |
| | ALB $\geq 3.5$ |
| STAGE 2 | $\beta2M < 3.5$ |
| | ALB $< 3.5$ |
| | or |
| | $\beta2M$ 3.5–5.5 |
| STAGE 3 | $\beta2M > 5.5$ |

$\beta2M$ = serum $\beta_2$ microglobulin in mg/dL
ALB = serum albumin in g/dL

Corradini, P., Inghirami, G., Astolfi, M., Ladetto, M., Voena, C., Ballerini, P., et al. (1994). Inactivation of tumor suppressor genes, p53 and Rb1, in plasma cell dyscrasias. *Leukemia, 8*, 758–767.

Costa, G., Engle, R., and Schilling, A. (1973). Melphalan and prednisone: An effective combination for the treatment of multiple myeloma. *American Journal of Medicine, 54*, 589–597.

Cuzick, J., De Stavola, B. L., and Cooper, E. H. (1990). Long-term prognostic value of serum B-2-microglobulin in myelomatosis. *British Journal of Haematology, 75*, 506–510.

Debes-Marun, C., Dewald, G., and Bryant, E. (2002). Chromosome abnormalities clustering and its implications for pathogenesis and prognosis in myeloma. *Leukemia.*

Drach, J. (1998). Presence of a p53 gene deletion in patients with multiple myeloma predicts for short survival after conventional-dose chemotherapy. *Blood, 92*, 802–809.

Durie, B. G., and Salmon, S. E. (1975). A clinical staging system for multiple myeloma. Correlation of measured myeloma cell mass with presenting clinical features, response to treatment, and survival. *Cancer, 36*, 842–854.

Fassas, A. B., Spencer, T., Sawyer, J., Zangari, M., Lee, C. K., Anaissie, E., et al. (2002). Both hypodiploidy and deletion of chromosome 13 independently confer poor prognosis in multiple myeloma. *British Journal of Haematology, 118*, 1041–1047.

Fonseca, E., Harrington, D., and Blood, E. (2003). Clinical and biologic implications of recurrent chromosomes abnormalities in myeloma. *Blood, 101*, 4569–4575.

Fonseca, R., Harrington, D., Blood, E., Rue, M., Oken, M. M., Dewald, G. W., et al. (2001a). A molecular classification of multiple myeloma based on cytogenetic abnormalities detected by interphase FISH, is powerful in identifying discrete groups of patients with dissimilar prognosis [Abstract]. *Blood, 98*, 733a.

Fonseca, R., Oken, M. M., Harrington, D., Bailey, R. J., Van Wier, S. A., Henderson, K. J., et al. (2001b). Deletions of chromosome 13 in multiple myeloma identified by interphase FISH usually denote large deletions of the q arm or monosomy. *Leukemia, 15*, 981–986.

Garcia-Sanz, R., Gonzalez, M., Orfao, A., Moro, M. J., Hernández, J. M., Borrego, D., et al. (1996). Analysis of natural killer-associated antigens in peripheral blood and bone marrow of multiple myeloma patients and prognostic implications. *British Journal of Haematology, 93*, 81–88.

Garewal, H., Durie, B. G. M., Kyle, R. A., Finley, P., Bower, B., and Serokman, R. (1984). Serum B2-microglobulin in the initial staging and subsequent monitoring of monoclonal plasma cell disorders. *Journal of Clinical Oncology, 2*, 51–57.

Gertz, M. A., Witzig, T. E., Pineda, A. A., Greipp, P. R., Kyle, R. A., and Litzow, M. R. (1997). Monoclonal plasma cells in the blood stem cell harvest from patients with multiple myeloma are associated with shortened relapse-free survival after transplantation. *Bone Marrow Transplantation, 19*, 337–342.

Gieseler, F., and Nussler, V. (1997). Cellular resistance mechanisms with impact on the therapy of multiple myeloma. *Leukemia, 11*(suppl 5), S1–S4.

Greipp, P. R., Leong, T., Bennett, J. M., Gaillard, J. P., Klein, B., Stewart, J. A., et al. (1998). Plasmablastic morphology—An independent prognostic factor with clinical and laboratory correlates: Eastern Cooperative Oncology Group (ECOG) myeloma trial E9486 report by the ECOG Myeloma Laboratory Group. *Blood, 91*, 2501–2507.

Greipp, P. R., Lust, J. A., O'Fallon, W. M., Katzmann, J. A., Witzig, T. E., and Kyle, R. A. (1993). Plasma cell labeling index and beta 2-microglobulin predict survival independent of thymidine kinase and C-reactive protein in multiple myeloma. *Blood, 81*, 3382–3387.

Greipp, P. R., Raymond, N. M., Kyle, R. A., and O'Fallon, W. M. (1985). Multiple myeloma: Significance of plasmablastic subtype in morphological classification. *Blood, 65*, 305–310.

Greipp, P. R., San Miguel, J. F., Fonseca, R., Avet-Loiseau, H., Jacobson, J. L., Rasmussen, E., et al. (2003). Development of an international prognostic index (IPI) for myeloma. Report of the international myeloma working group. *The Hematology Journal, 4*, 542–544.

Greipp, P. R., Trendle, M. C., Leong, T., Oken, M. M., Kay, N. E., Van Ness, B., et al. (1999). Is flow cytometric DNA content hypodiploidy prognostic in multiple myeloma? *Leukemia and Lymphoma, 35*, 83–89.

Greipp, P. R., Witzig, T. E., Gonchoroff, N. J., Habermann, T. M., Katzmann, J. A., O'Fallon, W. M., et al. (1987). Immunofluorescence labeling indices in myeloma and related monoclonal gammopathies. *Mayo Clinic Proceedings, 62*, 969–977.

Grogan, T. M., Spier, C. M., Salmon, S. E., Matzner, M., Rybski, J., Weinstein, R. S., et al. (1993). P-glycoprotein expression in human plasma cell myeloma: correlation with prior chemotherapy. *Blood, 81*, 490–495.

Hansen, O. P., Jessen, B., and Videbaek, A. (1974). Prognosis of myelomatosis on treatment with prednisone and cytostatics [Abstract]. *Scand J Haematol, 10*, 282–290.

Harada, H., Kawano, M. M., Huang, N., Harada, Y., Iwato, K., Tanabe, O., et al. (1993). Phenotypic difference of normal plasma cells from mature myeloma cells. *Blood, 81*, 2658–2663.

Kay, N. E., Leong, T. L., Bone, N., Vesole, D. H., Greipp, P. R., Van Ness, B., et al. (2001). Blood levels of immune cells predict survival in myeloma patients: Results of an Eastern Cooperative Oncology Group phase 3 trial for newly diagnosed multiple myeloma patients. *Blood, 98*, 23–28.

Kyle, R. A. (1994). Why better prognostic factors for multiple myeloma are needed? *Blood, 83*, 1713–1716.

Kyle, R. A. (1995). Prognostic factors in multiple myeloma. *Stem Cells, 13*, 56–63.

Kyle, R. A., Therneau, T. M., Rajkumar, S. V., Offord, J. R., Larson, D. R., Plevak, M. F., et al. (2002). A long-term study of prognosis in monoclonal gammopathy of undetermined significance. *New England Journal of Medicine, 346*, 564–569.

Lahuerta, J. J., de la Serna, J., Blade, J., Grande, C., Alegre, A., Vazquez, L., et al. (2000). Remission status defined by immunofixation vs electrophoresis after autologous transplantation has a major impact on the outcome of multiple myeloma patients. *British Journal of Haematology, 109*, 438–446.

Liu, P., Leong, T., Quam, L., Billadeau, D., Kay, N. E., Greipp, P., et al. (1996). Activating mutations of N- and K-ras in multiple myeloma show different clinical associations: Analysis of the Eastern Cooperative Oncology Group Phase III Trial. *Blood, 88*, 2699–2706.

Mateos, M. V., Garcia-Sanz, R., Lopez-Perez, R., Balanzategui, A., Gonzalez, M. I., Fernandez-Calvo, J., et al. (2001). P16/INK4a gene inactivation by hypermethylation is associated with aggressive variants of monoclonal gammopathies. *The Hematology Journal, 3*, 146–149.

Modiano, M. R., Villar-Werstler, P., Crowley, J., and Salmon, S. E. (1996). Evaluation of race as a prognostic factor in multiple myeloma. An ancillary of Southwest Oncology Group Study 8229. *Journal of Clinical Oncology, 14*, 974–977.

Moreau, P., Facon, T., Leleu, X., Morineau, N., Huyghe, P., Harousseau, J. L., et al. (2002). Recurrent 14q32 translocations determine the prognosis of multiple myeloma, especially in patients receiving intensive chemotherapy. *Blood, 100*, 1579–1583.

Omede, P. (1993). Multiple myeloma: 'Early' plasma cell phenotype identifies patients with aggressive biological and clinical characteristics. *British Journal of Haematology, 85*, 504–513.

Orfao, A., Garcia-Sanz, R., Lopez-Berges, M. C., Belen, V. M., Gonzalez, M., Caballero, M. D., et al. (1994). A new method for the analysis of plasma cell DNA content in multiple myeloma samples using a CD38/propidium iodide double staining technique. *Cytometry, 17*, 332–339.

Österborg, A., Nilsson, B., and Björkholm, M. (1990). Natural killer cell activity in monoclonal gammapathies: Relation to disease activity. *European Journal of Immunology, 45*, 153–157.

Papadaki, H., Kyriakou, D., Foudoulakis, A., Markidou, F., Alexandrakis, M., and Eliopoulos, G. D. (1997). Serum levels of soluble IL-6 receptor in multiple myeloma as indicator of disease activity. *Acta Haematologica, 97*, 191–195.

Pecherstorfer, M., Seibel, M. J., and Woite, H. W. (1997). Bone resorption in multiple myeloma and in monoclonal gammopathy of undetermined significance: Quantification by urinary pyridinium cross-links of collagen. *Blood, 90*, 3743–3750.

Pellat-Deceunynck, C. (1995). Adhesion molecules on human myeloma cells: Significant changes in expression related to malignancy, tumor spreading, and immortalization. *Cancer Research, 55*, 3647–3653

Pellat-Deceunynck, C., Bataille, R., Robillard, N., Harousseau, J. L., Rapp, M J., Juge-Morineau, N., et al. (1994). Expression of CD28 and CD40 in human myeloma cells: A comparative study with normal plasma cells. *Blood, 84*, 2597–2603.

Perez-Simon, J. A., Garcia-Sanz, R., Tabernero, M. D., Almeida, J., Gonzalez, M., Fernandez-Calvo, J., et al. (1998). Prognostic value of numerical chromosome aberrations in multiple myeloma: A FISH analysis of 15 different chromosomes. *Blood, 91*, 3366–3371.

Pulkki, K., Pelliniemi, T. T., Rajamaki, A., Tienhaara, A., Laakso, M., and Lahtinen, R. (1996). Soluble interleukin-6 receptor as a prognostic factor in multiple myeloma. Finnish Leukaemia Group. *British Journal of Haematology, 92*, 370–374.

Raaijmakers, H. G., Izquierdo, M. A., Lokhorst, H. M., de Leeuw, C., Belien, J. A., Bloem, A. C., et al. (1998). Lung-resistance-related protein expression is a negative predictive factor for response to conventional low but not to intensified dose alkylating chemotherapy in multiple myeloma. *Blood, 91*, 1029–1036.

Rajkumar, S. V., Fonseca, R., Dispenzieri, A., Lacy, M. Q., Witzig, T. E., Lust, J. A., et al. (2000). Effect of complete response on outcome following autologous stem cell transplantation for myeloma. *Bone Marrow Transplantation, 26*, 979–983.

Robillard, N., Jego, G., Pellat-Deceunynck, C., Pineau, D., Puthier, D., Mellerin, M.P., et al. (1998). CD28, a marker associated with tumoral expansion in multiple myeloma. *Clin Cancer Res, 4*, 1521–1526.

Saeed, S. M., Stock-Novack, D., Pohlod, R., Crowley, J., and Salmon, S. E. (1991). Prognostic correlation of plasma cell acid phosphatase and beta-glucuronidase in multiple myeloma: A Southwest Oncology Group study. *Blood, 78*, 3281–3287.

San Miguel, J. F. (1991). Immunophenotypic heterogeneity of multiple myeloma: Influence on the biology and clinical course of the disease. Castellano-Leones (Spain) Cooperative Group for the Study of Monoclonal Gammopathies. *British Journal of Haematology, 77*, 185–190.

San Miguel, J. F. (1998). Overview of prognostic factors in multiple myeloma. *Cancer Research Therapy and Control, 6*, 97–99.

San Miguel, J. F., Almeida, J., Mateo, G., Blade, J., López-Berges, M. C., Caballero, M. D., et al. (2002). Immunophenotypic evaluation of the plasma cell compartment in multiple myeloma: A tool for comparing the efficacy of different treatment strategies and predicting outcome. *Blood, 99*, 1853–1856.

San Miguel, J F., Garcia-Sanz, R., Gonzalez, M., Moro, M. J., Hernández, J. M., Ortega, F., et al. (1995). A new staging system for multiple myeloma based on the number of S-phase plasma cells. *Blood, 85*, 448–455.

San Miguel, J. F., Garcia-Sanz, R., Gonzalez, M., and Orfao, A. (1996). DNA cell content studies in multiple myeloma. *Leukemia Lymphoma, 23*, 33–41.

San Miguel, J. F., Gonzalez, M., Gascon, A., Moro, M. J., Hernández, J. M., Ortega, F., et al. (1992). Lymphoid subsets and prognostic factors in multiple myeloma. Cooperative Group for the Study of Monoclonal Gammopathies. *British Journal of Haematology, 80*, 305–309.

San Miguel, J. F., Sanchez, I., and Gonzalez, M. (1989). Prognostic factors and classification in multiple myeloma. *British Journal of Cancer, 59*, 113–118.

Segeren, C., Beverloo, B., Poddighe, J., Slater, R., van der Holt, B., Steijaert, M., et al. (2002). Abnormal chromosomes 1p/q and 13/13q are adverse prognostic factors for the outcome of upfront high-dose therapy in patients with multiple myeloma. *Blood, 98*, 159a.

Seidel, C., Sundan, A., Hjorth, M., Turesson, I., Dahl, I. M., Abildgaard, N., et al. (2000). Serum syndecan-1: A new independent prognostic marker in multiple myeloma. *Blood, 95*, 388–392.

Shou, Y., Martelli, M. L., Garbea, A., Qi, Y., Brents, L. A., Roschke, A., et al. (2000). Diverse karyotypic abnormalities of the c-myc locus associated with c- myc dysregulation and tumor progression in multiple myeloma. *Proc Natl Acad Sci U S A, 97*, 228–233.

Sonneveld, P., Marie, J. P., Huisman, C., Vekhoff, A., Schoester, M., Faussat, A.M., et al. (1996). Reversal of multidrug resistance by SDZ PSC 833, combined with VAD (vincristine, doxorubicin, dexamethasone) in refractory multiple myeloma. A phase I study. *Leukemia, 10*, 1741–1750.

Southern Cancer Study Group. (1975). Treatment of myeloma: Comparison of melphalan, chlorambucil and azathioprine. *Archives of Internal Medicine, 135*, 157–162.

Sze, D. M., Giesajtis, G., Brown, R. D., Raitakari, M., Gibson, J., Ho, J., et al. (2001). Clonal cytotoxic T cells are expanded in myeloma and reside in the CD8(+)CD57(+)CD28(−) compartment. *Blood, 98*, 2817–2827.

Tricot, G., Barlogie, B., Jagannath, S., Bracy, D., Mattox, S., Vesole, D. H., et al. (1995). Poor prognosis in multiple myeloma is associated only with partial or complete deletions of chromosome 13 or abnormalities involving 11q and not with other karyotype abnormalities. *Blood, 86*, 4250–4256.

Tricot, G., Sawyer, J. R., Jagannath, S., Desikan, K. R., Siegel, D., Naucke, S., et al. (1997). Unique role of cytogenetics in the prognosis of patients with myeloma receiving high-dose therapy and autotransplants. *J Clin Oncol, 15*, 2659–2666.

Turesson, I. (1999). Prognostic evaluation in multiple myeloma: an analysis of the impact of new prognostic factors. *British Journal of Haematology, 106*, 1005–1012.

Urbauer, E., Kaufmann, H., Ackermann, J., Nösslinger, T., Weltermann, A., Jaeger, U., et al. (2002). Deletion of chromosome (del) 22q is a prognostic parameter in multiple myeloma in addition to (del) 13q, beta-2-microglobulin, and plasmablastic morphology. *Blood, 98*, 157a.

Witzig, T. E., Gertz, M., Lust, J. A., Kyle, R. A., O´Fallon, W., and Greipp, P. R. (1996). Peripheral blood monoclonal plasma cells as a predictor of survival in patients with multiple myeloma. *Blood, 88*, 1780–1787.

Worel, N., Greinix, H., Ackermann, J., Kaufmann, H., Urbauer, E., Hocker, P., et al. (2001). Deletion of chromosome 13q14 detected by fluorescence in situ hybridization has prognostic impact on survival after high-dose therapy in patients with multiple myeloma. *Annals of Hematology, 80*, 345–348.

Zhan, F., Hardin, J., Kordsmeier, B., Bumm, K., Zheng, M., Tian, E., et al. (2002). Global gene expression profiling of multiple myeloma, monoclonal gammopathy of undetermined significance, and normal bone marrow plasma cells. *Blood, 99*, 1745–1757.

Zojer, N., Konigsberg, R., Ackermann, J., Fritz, E., Dallinger, S., Kromer, E., et al. (2000). Deletion of 13q14 remains an independent adverse prognostic variable in multiple myeloma despite its frequent detection by interphase fluorescence in situ hybridization. *Blood, 95*, 1925–1930.

# PART III

# *Therapy of Myeloma*

# CHAPTER 12

# Conventional-Dose Chemotherapy of Myeloma

DANIEL E. BERGSAGEL
A. KEITH STEWART

## Introduction

Multiple myeloma (MM) is a chronic hematologic malignancy initiated by the malignant transformation of a B lymphocyte after immunoglobulin gene rearrangement (see Chapter 3). The originally transformed cell must proliferate extensively and form a clone of approximately $1 \times 10^9$ cells before enough of the idiotypic, monoclonal immunoglobulin (M-protein) is produced to be recognized as an M-peak in the serum electrophoresis pattern. The detection of an M-protein means that the subject has a sizeable monoclonal population of plasma cells, but does not indicate that a diagnosis of MM is justified or that treatment is required. Initially the growth of the plasma cell clone appears to be controlled, as judged by the M-protein level. The amount of M-protein gradually increases to a certain level and then forms a plateau. Subjects are usually asymptomatic during this phase and are labeled as having monoclonal gammopathy of undetermined significance (MGUS). Marrow plasmacytosis is modest (i.e., less than 10%) during the MGUS phase (see Chapter 18). If the subject continues to be asymptomatic with a stable M-protein, but marrow plasmacytosis increases to more than 10%, the diagnosis is changed to smoldering myeloma (SM). Treatment is delayed until the disease has progressed to cause symptoms as a result of bony lesions, anemia, a defective antibody, and neutrophil response leading to an increased susceptibility to infections, renal failure, the formation of soft tissue plasmacytomas, or weight loss. Bone pain is the most prominent symptom in patients with MM.

The median survival of newly diagnosed patients with MM treated with conventional-dose chemotherapy is approximately 30 months from the onset of treatment. The course of the disease, however, can be extremely variable. Patients who present with rapidly progressive MM, which does not respond to remission-induction chemotherapy, usually succumb within a few months. On the other hand, patients who present with asymptomatic SM, a labeling index of less than 1%, a normal serum $\beta$2-microglobulin level, and stable disease, do not require any treatment until they develop symptoms; some of these patients will survive for 20 years or more with no treatment. The management of patients with myeloma requires considerable skill and experience in the evaluation of the disease so that the right decisions are made about when treatment is started, how aggressive this treatment should be, the duration of remission-induction therapy, the use of appropriate supportive care, the management of complications, and the selection of appropriate alternate therapy for those who do not respond adequately.

The management policies described here for the treatment of patients with myeloma with conventional-dose chemotherapy are the best available today but are far from satisfactory. When a treatment plan for a patient is designed, one should first look for an organized study protocol testing some new approach to treatment. Enter patients in these studies whenever possible. Fall back on the conventional approaches to management described in this chapter only when the patient is not eligible or there are no suitable studies available. Solid advances in therapy require widespread participation in clinical trials.

# Choice of Therapeutic Agents

The most effective and useful drugs in the treatment of myeloma are alkylating agents, corticosteroids, irradiation, interferon $\alpha$, and thalidomide. Newer agents such as the proteasome inhibitor PS-341 (Orlowski et al., 2002; Richardson, et al., 2003) and the thalidomide analogue Revimid (Richardson et al., 2002) (see Chapter 14) also have single agent activity and can now be added to the therapeutic arsenal.

Many new agents for myeloma have been tested over the years. Indeed, a review of over 20 phase II trials testing the activity of single agents in the treatment of refractory myeloma (Buzaid and Durie, 1988) identified only 6 new agents, aside from doxorubicin and glucocorticoids, which induced responses in 10% of patients.

Some theoretically promising new agents have been added to other effective drug combinations without clear evidence that the new agent is effective as a single agent in the treatment of myeloma. For example, vincristine was added to the M2 protocol (Case et al., 1977), and to the vincristine, adriamycin, dexamethasone (VAD) combination (Barlogie et al., 1984), even though antimyeloma activity has not been demonstrated (see following paragraphs). Glucocorticoids are so useful in the treatment of patients with myeloma that they were often administered together with a new agent in phase II trials. The responses of patients with myeloma to the steroid-new-agent combination has occasionally been unwarrantedly attributed to the new agent, for example, with vindesine (Houwen et al., 1981) and hexamethylmelamine (Cohen and Bartolucci, 1982), when, in fact, the improvement was largely due to the result of the glucocorticoid (Alexanian et al., 1983; Oken et al., 1987). These problems have plagued our attempts to test the activity of new agents in the treatment of myeloma. As a result, our assessment of some agents has been incomplete. In the following review of the activity of chemotherapeutic agents we have tried to cover the principles that guide our treatment choices rather than attempting an exhaustively complete review of all agents.

## Alkylating Agents

Most alkylating agents show some activity in the treatment of mouse and human myeloma. Melphalan, cyclophosphamide, and the nitrosoureas (carmustine and lomustine) are the alkylating agents that have proven to be most useful. The sensitivity of a plasma cell neoplasm to different alkylating agents varies considerably. A BALB/c mouse plasmacytoma has been described, which is highly resistant to carmustine, moderately resistant to melphalan, and still very sensitive to cyclophosphamide (Bergsagel et al., 1975). Thus, resistance of a mouse plasma cell tumor to one alkylating agent does not mean that the tumor is resistant to all alkylating agents. The same phenomenon has been observed in human myeloma. We found that one-third of a group of patients, who were shown to be resistant to melphalan, achieved an objective response with cyclophosphamide therapy (Bergsagel et al., 1972). It would appear that intrinsic cellular factors determine whether a cell will be sensitive to an alkylating agent, rather than the proliferative state of the cell, or the alkylating function of the agent (Ogawa et al., 1973a, 1973b).

In the treatment of patients with myeloma, hematologic toxicity and metabolism of the alkylating agent have a strong influence on how and when the agent is used. For example, hematologic toxicity is cumulative with melphalan and the nitrosoureas, causing increasingly severe and prolonged neutropenia and thrombocytopenia with repeated courses; this could prevent the delivery of adequate chemotherapy to some patients. The hematologic toxicity following cyclophosphamide is not cumulative and it is less toxic to thrombopoiesis. For this reason cyclophosphamide is used for the treatment of patients who present with neutropenia or thrombocytopenia, or we switch to it if hematologic recovery is delayed following melphalan or carmustine.

### Glucocorticoids

Glucocorticoids are very useful in the management of patients with myeloma. In modern clinical trials, high-dose dexamethasone alone (40 mg each morning for 4 days, beginning on days 1, 9, and 17; repeated after a 7-day rest, with downward adjustments for side effects) has proven to be the most active single agent for inducing responses in previously untreated (Alexanian et al., 1992) and refractory myeloma patients (Alexanian et al., 1986). Dexamethasone alone induced responses in 51% of previously untreated myeloma patients with low tumor mass, and 37% of those with intermediate and high tumor mass, and in approximately one-fourth of refractory patients. Indeed, dexamethasone was judged to account for most of the responses to the vincristine, adriamycin, and dexamethasone (VAD) combination (Alexanian et al., 1992). The duration of the responses induced by prednisone alone is significantly shorter than those induced by an alkylating agent alone, or combinations of an alkylating agent and prednisone (McIntyre et al., 1985). Despite evidence of activity, glucocorticoids have not improved the survival of patients with myeloma in randomized trials of prednisone versus placebo (Mass, 1962), or melphalan/prednisone versus melphalan (Åhre et al., 1983), although the prednisone did increase the proportion of responders in these trials.

In a large trial, 685 previously untreated patients with myeloma were randomized to treatment with either Adriamycin, carmustine (BCNU), cyclophosphamide, melphalan, and prednisolone (ABCMP) or ABCM. The rate of M-protein decline was faster and the maximum response greater in the group receiving prednisolone, but the proportion reaching plateau and the duration of these responses was similar in the 2 groups. However, the survival of the ABCMP group was slightly shorter than for the ABCM group ($p = 0.06$) (Olujohungbe et al., 1996). This result was attributed to an excess of deaths from myeloma in the ABCMP arm. In an earlier study, Acute Leukemia Group B also noted that the survival of poor-risk myeloma patients treated with a combination of melphalan and prednisone (starting with a prednisone dose of 1.25 mg/kg

per day for 14 days and tapering to 0 over 70 days) was much shorter than for those treated with melphalan alone (Costa et al., 1973).

Intuitively, one would expect that agents like glucocorticoids, which are so active in inducing objective responses in patients with myeloma, would also prolong survival when combined with other effective agents. The failure of clinical trials to confirm this hypothesis is difficult to understand. We will have to add this conundrum to the long list of things we do not understand about the biology of myeloma.

### Cell-Cycle-Specific Agents

Agents that exert their antiproliferative effects against proliferating cells in cell cycle are known as cycle-active agents. These include antimetabolites such as methotrexate, 6-mercaptopurine, 6-thioguanine, 5-fluorouracil, hydroxyurea, and cytosine arabinoside, which inhibit DNA synthesis during the S-phase of the cell cycle; and the vinca alkaloids (vinblastine, vincristine, and vindesine), which arrest dividing cells in the metaphase of mitosis. None of these cell-cycle-active agents have shown significant activity as single agents in the treatment of plasma cell myeloma. Indeed, despite widespread adoption, none of the vinca alkaloids have demonstrated impressive activity as single agents in the treatment of human myeloma. The Eastern Cooperative Group in Solid Tumor Chemotherapy treated 17 patients with myeloma with vinblastine alone using doses of 0.1 to 0.3 mg/kg per week; no objective responses were observed (Costa et al., 1963). In the only phase II trial of vincristine as a single agent in the treatment of myeloma, Jackson et al. (Jackson et al., 1985) treated 21 refractory patients with a 0.5-mg intravenous bolus followed by 24-hour infusions of 0.25 to 0.5 mg/m$^2$ per day for 5 days. The M-protein fell below 50% of baseline briefly in 2 patients, for remissions of 1.2 and 2.2 months. These investigators conclude that vincristine infusions have limited activity in the treatment of refractory myeloma and are associated with appreciable neuralgic and hematologic toxicity. The value of adding vincristine (V) to a combination of melphalan (M) and prednisolone (P) was tested in the large IVth Medical Research Council (MRC) myelomatosis trial. In this study, 263 previously untreated patients with myeloma were randomly allocated treatment with MP and 267 received MVP. No significant difference in the survival of these 2 groups was detected at 5 years (MacLennan and Cusick, 1985). Despite the fact that vincristine is not active against mouse plasma cell tumors (Ghanta et al., 1981) and has shown only minimal activity as a single agent in the treatment of refractory myeloma, with no effect on survival when it is combined with MP, this drug is often included in drug combinations used in the treatment of myeloma (e.g., VBMCP, VMCP, VBAP, and VAD). This practice is surprising.

Vindesine was initially administered in combination with 100 mg prednisone per day for 5 days following each injection of vindesine; 6 of 11 refractory myeloma patients achieved a 50% or greater fall in the pretreatment M-protein (Houwen et al., 1981). Later, Alexanian et al. tested vindesine alone, prednisone alone, and a combination of vindesine and prednisone in the treatment of refractory myeloma patients. With vindesine alone, none of 11 patients responded, whereas 4 of 16 treated with vindesine and prednisone and 5 of 16 treated with prednisone alone responded. It would appear that vindesine by itself is inactive and that it does not enhance the action of prednisone against refractory myeloma.

The epipodophylotoxins, VP-16 (etoposide) and VM-26 (teniposide), are cycle-active agents, which bind to tubulin, like the vinca alkaloids do. Trials of these drugs as single agents have demonstrated good activity for teniposide in the treatment of refractory myeloma (4 of 12 responders) and for elderly, previously untreated patients (over age 70, 3 of 13 responders) with surprisingly little toxicity (Tirelli et al., 1985). Etoposide, however, did not induce any responses in 40 good-risk refractory patients, and only 1 response in 45 poor-risk refractory patients (Gockerman et al., 1986).

## Doxorubicin and Analogues

In one of the early phase II trials of doxorubicin, 3 of 20 patients with myeloma responded (O'Bryan et al., 1973). We can find only 2 other studies in which doxorubicin was tested as a single agent. Alberts et al. (Alberts and Salmon, 1975) treated 9 alkylator-resistant myeloma patients; only 1 achieved a response ( > 75% reduction in M-protein synthesis), which lasted for 3 months. In another study, only 1 of 17 resistant myeloma patients responded to doxorubicin; this response lasted less than 3 months (Bennett et al., 1978). Despite the sparse evidence of activity as a single agent, doxorubicin is widely used in the treatment of patients with myeloma, primarily in combination with vincristine and dexamethasone (VAD) and alkylating agents (e.g., VBAP, VCAP, and ABCM). We do not know whether doxorubicin adds anything to these drug combinations, because the effectiveness of the combination with and without doxorubicin has not been tested. In recent years a liposomal formulation of doxorubicin has entered clinical trials and is now in phase III testing (Hussein et al., 2002). It is hoped that this formulation might have less toxicity than the parent drug. Several anthracycline analogues of doxorubicin have been tested in the treatment of refractory myeloma. Although occasional objective responses

were observed, none of these analogues demonstrated encouraging activity in the treatment of these difficult, previously treated myeloma patients.

## Thalidomide

Initial reports of the efficacy of thalidomide in MM emerged with the description of a phase II trial of thalidomide in refractory MM, which used a dose schedule that escalated drug from 200 mg to 800 mg per day (Singhal et al., 1999). Response to treatment was noted in 37% of patients and 14% had either a complete remission (CR) or a near CR. The virtual absence of myelosuppressive toxicity suggests that thalidomide has potential for use in combination with cytotoxic agents and steroids and that this drug might also be suitable for maintenance therapy. Nevertheless, thalidomide exhibits dose-dependent toxicities. Common toxicities include neuropathy (54%), constipation (42%), fatigue (37%), dizziness (34%), infection (30%), sedation (22%), mouth dryness (22%), skin rash (20%), and edema (19%). Symptomatic DVT is observed in patients receiving thalidomide in combination with steroids and/or chemotherapy (Zangari et al., 2001). In earlier disease states thalidomide also has activity, for example, at the Mayo Clinic patients with smoldering or indolent multiple myeloma were studied. Thalidomide was initiated at a starting dose of 200 mg per day. Of the 29 eligible patients, 10 (34%) had a partial response to therapy with at least 50% or greater reduction in serum and urine monoclonal (M) protein. When minor responses (25% to 49% decrease in M-protein) were included, the response rate was 66%. Kaplan-Meier estimates of progression-free survival are 80% at 1 year and 63% at 2 years when it was given to 26 patients with active, previously untreated MM (Rajkumar et al., 2003). At the M.D. Anderson Cancer Center 28 patients with previously untreated asymptomatic myeloma were treated with thalidomide as tolerated to a maximum of 600 mg per day with a response rate of 36% (Weber et al., 2003). Although pilot studies reporting the results of thalidomide use at lower doses in the absence of dose escalation have been reported, no study has to date reported prospective dose-finding toxicity analysis.

Corticosteroids and thalidomide are being used in combination with increasing frequency in MM treatment. For example, at the Mayo Clinic 50 patients with newly diagnosed myeloma were given thalidomide at a dose of 200 mg per day orally along with high-dose dexamethasone. A response rate of 64% (95% confidence interval, 49–77%) was observed (Rajkumar et al., 2002). At the M.D. Anderson Cancer Center 40 previously untreated patients with symptomatic myeloma were treated with thalidomide (maximum dose, 400 mg) and received dexamethasone with a response rate of 72%.

Thalidomide, therefore, has a role to play in myeloma therapy, but the optimal timing and dose of drug to use still need to be defined, and the relative merits of this agent when compared with conventional alkylating agent-based therapy assessed.

### Interferon-α

Interferon-α is active as a single agent in the treatment of multiple myeloma. In a Swedish study, previously untreated myeloma patients were randomized to intermittent melphalan and prednisone (MP) versus leukocyte interferon (L-IFN-α), 3–6 × 10⁶ units intramuscularly per day. Only 10 of 74 (14%) in the L-IFN-α group achieved a response, compared with 24 of 54 (44%) of those treated with MP. A similar study comparing the vincristine, melphalan, cyclophosphamide, and prednisolone (VMCP) combination with recombinant interferon-α2c (rIFN-α2c) for untreated multiple myeloma also found a low response rate for rIFN-α2c (14%) in comparison with VMCP (57%) (Ludwig et al., 1986).

In a phase II trial of recombinant interferon-α2b (rIFN-α2b) for patients with myeloma resistant to previous therapy, Costanzi et al. (Costanzi et al., 1985) observed responses in 2 of 19 (11%) refractory patients and in 5 of 19 (26%) patients relapsing after a previous response. An extensive review of interferons in the treatment of myeloma (Ohno, 1987) showed that response rates of approximately 20% were achieved in both untreated and previously treated myeloma patients.

The observation that interferon inhibits the self-renewal capacity of myeloma stem cells (Bergsagel et al., 1986) suggested that this agent might be useful in prolonging the duration of remissions induced by other agents. The results of 7 clinical trials testing this hypothesis have been mixed. Most of these studies suggested that interferon-α maintenance therapy prolonged the duration of responses modestly (Browman et al., 1995; Mandelli et al., 1990; Westin et al., 1995), and 2 (Browman et al., 1995; Mandelli et al., 1990) noted that interferon-α maintenance therapy prolonged the survival of the patients with myeloma who achieved an objective response (i.e., a fall of 50% or more in the M-protein). Two groups found that interferon α maintenance treatment had no effect on remission durations or survival (Peest et al., 1995; Salmon et al., 1994). Two large meta-analyses of large numbers of patients with myeloma (Fritz and Ludwig, 2000) reached the same conclusions about the effectiveness of interferon-α, that treatment with interferon-α results in a slight, but definite improvement in overall survival and progression-free survival. The benefits to the patient, however, are not regarded as sufficient to warrant the toxicity of the interferon.

A randomized trial of interferon-α maintenance versus no treatment following high-dose melphalan (HDM) and autologous bone marrow transplantation at the Royal Marsden Hospital (Cunningham et al., 1998) demonstrated a median progression-free survival (PFS) in the 42 patients randomized to interferon-α of 46 months versus 27 months in the control subjects at a median 52-month follow up. Nevertheless, both overall survival and PFS ceased to be significant at 5.8 years' followup, because patients ultimately succumbed to their disease. A retrospective analysis of EBMT registry data also concluded that interferon prolonged remission duration when used as maintenance posttransplant (Bjorkstrand et al., 2001). Randomized trials addressing the role of interferon-α following high-dose therapy are ongoing.

### Phase I/II Trials of New Agents

Many other new agents have been tested, with negative results, in the treatment of patients with myeloma who are resistant to treatment. Only recently have some seemingly effective novel therapies emerged. In particular, the proteasome inhibitor Bortezomib (Orlowski et al., 2002; Richardson et al., 2003), the immunomodulator thalidomide (Kyle, 2002), and its analogue Revimid (Richardson et al., 2002) have recently emerged as drugs with single-agent activity. The clinical testing of thalidomide is described previously in this chapter. Data with the thalidomide analogue Revimid are even less mature and the results of phase I/II testing are only now emerging (Richardson et al., 2002). In a phase I trial, however, 17 (71%) of 24 patients demonstrated some response to the drug. Further clinical trials with this agent are required.

Bortezomib (PS-341) is a compound with unique activity functioning as a proteasome inhibitor. Impressive activity was noted in phase I testing in which all 9 patients with heavily pretreated myeloma who received a cycle of therapy responded (Orlowski et al., 2002). Phase II trials confirmed that 35% of otherwise refractory patients respond, albeit with side effects that may eventually limit the ability to administer drug (Adams, 2003). Phase III testing is ongoing.

## Combination Chemotherapy

With the discovery that resistance to one alkylating agent does not mean that a plasma cell neoplasm is resistant to other alkylating agents (Bergsagel et al., 1972, 1975), a study was designed by the National Cancer Institute of Canada Clinical Trials Group (NCI-C-CTG) to test the value of combining several alkylating agents in the treatment of myeloma (Bergsagel et al., 1979). Previously untreated, symptomatic myeloma patients were treated with melphalan (M), cyclophosphamide (C), and carmustine (B). Eligible patients were randomized to receive the drugs *sequentially* (group A), *alternately* (group B), or *concurrently* (group C). In the control group (group A), treatment started with M, increasing the dose until mild hematologic toxicity, or a response, resulted and continuing until there was evidence of progression, or relapse, when C was introduced; B was started if the disease progressed on both M and C. The three alkylating agents were given *alternately* to group B, beginning with M for 4 days in the first course, followed by C in the second course and B in the third. Group C received all 3 alkylating agents *concurrently*, in one-third of the dose used for each drug as a single agent. Prednisone (P), in a dose of 100 mg per day for 4 days, was given with each course of treatment to all 3 groups. There was no difference in the response rates or the survival of groups A, B, and C. We concluded that there was no advantage to administering these 3 alkylating agents alternately or concurrently, as compared with starting with M, and continuing with this agent until progression, or relapse, before switching to C or B.

Vincristine (V) and doxorubicin (adriamycin, A) have been added to alkylating agent combinations, such as the VMCP/VBAP alternating combination favored by SWOG (Salmon et al., 1983), and the ABCM combination explored in Great Britain (MacLennan et al., 1992). A meta-analysis of the results of 20 trials, involving 4930 patients with myeloma, comparing treatment with MP versus combination chemotherapy (CCT), revealed no significant difference in the survival of patients receiving these 2 forms of treatment (Myeloma Trialists' Collaborative Group, 1998). In retrospect we might wonder why we expected CCT, using several alkylating agents, which do not induce more responses or improved survival when combined, and agents such as V, which is inactive as a single agent, and A, which has only modest activity as a single agent in phase II trials on patients with myeloma, to be better than an effective alkylating agent and prednisone.

The MRC comparison of ABCM with M was not included in the Myeloma Trialists' (1998) meta-analysis because the control group was treated with M alone rather than MP. ABCM was compared with melphalan (7 mg/m$^2$ per day for 4 days), repeated at 3-week intervals (MacLennan et al., 1992); this might not be an optimal dosage schedule for M, because hematologic recovery sufficient to permit repeat courses of M requires intervals of 4 to 6 weeks between courses. In this large trial 314 patients were randomized to ABCM and 316 to M. The survival of the ABCM group was consistently longer than for those treated with M ($p = 0.003$) with a median survival of 24 months for M versus 32 months for ABCM. The survival of the M

group in this study was unusually short. The median survival for MP-treated patients in the 20 randomized trials analyzed by the Myeloma Trialists' Group (1998) ranged from 19 to 50 months, with a median of 32 months. The median survival for MP patients was 24 months, or less, in only 4 of the 18 trials. Although the survival of the ABCM-treated group was significantly better than for M-treated patients in this trial, the improvement was modest and not strikingly different from the survival values achieved by most other investigators with MP alone. The value of adding prednisolone (60 mg/m$^2$ for 5 days, repeated every 14 days for 4 courses) at the beginning of ABCM treatment was tested in the VIth MRC myelomatosis trial (MacLennan et al., 1988; Olujohungbe et al., 1996). The addition of prednisolone (P) to ABCM (ABCMP) induced greater early reduction in serum and urinary M-protein, but did not increase the proportion of patients achieving plateau, i.e., a state in which the serum or urine M-protein levels are stable or undetectable for 6 months and the patient had no or minimal symptoms and is transfusion-independent. The survival of patients treated with ABCMP was somewhat shorter than for those receiving ABCM ($p < 0.06$).

### A Management Plan

The discovery of an M-protein in the serum or urine does not mean that the patient has myeloma or that treatment is required. Many of these patients are asymptomatic and have either monoclonal gammopathy of unknown significance (MGUS) or smoldering, stable myeloma (see Chapter 18). They must be evaluated carefully and followed for a time on no therapy to determine whether the disease is stable or progressive before a decision about treatment can be made.

### Patient Evaluation

The evaluation of a patient with an M-protein is as follows:

1. Measure the M-protein
   a. Serum M-protein: measure the concentration (grams per liter) by serum protein electrophoresis. Urine M-protein: in a 24-hour urine collection, measure the total protein (grams per 24 h) excreted; determine the light-chain fraction (M-protein) by urine protein electrophoresis, and calculate the grams per 24 hours of M-protein.
2. Identify the light- and heavy-chain of the M-protein by immunoelectrophoresis or immunofixation. Measure the hemoglobin, leukocyte, platelet, differential and reticulocyte counts.

3. In the absence of other confirmatory diagnostic criteria, take needle aspirates of a solitary lytic bone lesion, extramedullary tumor(s), or enlarged lymph node(s) to determine whether these are plasmacytomas.

4. Evaluate renal function with serum creatinine and creatinine clearance. Electrophoresis of concentrated urine protein will differentiate proteinurea resulting from glomerular lesions (the urine contains an unselected mixture of all serum proteins, as in the nephrotoxic syndrome) from tubular lesions. Tubular lesions result in the excretion of mainly light chains, which cannot be resorbed by the damaged tubular cells, and albumin.

5. Measure serum levels of calcium, alkaline phosphatase, lactic dehydrogenase; and, when indicated by clinical symptoms, cryoglobulins and serum viscosity.

6. Obtain a formal skeletal survey.

7. Perform magnetic resonance imaging (MRI) if symptoms suggest spinal cord or nerve root compression. In patients with smoldering myeloma and back pain an MRI might also be prudent even when x-rays are normal.

8. If amyloidosis is suspected, examination of a needle aspiration of subcutaneous abdominal fat is the easiest and safest way to confirm the diagnosis, but stains of bone marrow could also be positive (Gertz et al., 1989).

9. Measurement of $\beta_2$-microglobulin and c-reactive protein is useful, because both are independent prognostic factors.

10. The marrow plasma cell labeling index, if available, is also useful as a prognostic indicator but is not performed by most centers.

11. Convincing evidence of the prognostic significance of cytogenetics supports use of marrow cytogenetics in staging. Deletion of chromosome 13 confers a particularly poor prognosis.

12. Emerging technologies, e.g., fluorescence in situ hybridization (FISH), allow definition of chromosome translocations, which have distinct prognostic outcome and, when available, should be used.

All of these initial studies should be done for a solid baseline evaluation. This database will be compared with subsequent values, when you will want to decide whether the patient is progressing or stable, responding to therapy or getting worse. The major challenge is to separate the stable asymptomatic group, who may not require immediate therapy, from those with progressive myeloma who should be started on treatment immediately.

## The Decision to Treat

Treatment is usually not given to asymptomatic patients until symptoms or signs announce that previously stable disease has entered the progressive phase.

Patients with MGUS, or asymptomatic, stable myeloma ("smoldering myeloma"), do not achieve remissions more frequently, or enjoy longer remissions, or improved survival if chemotherapy is started while they are still asymptomatic, as opposed to waiting for progression before starting therapy (Hjorth et al., 1993). If the indications for initiating treatment at the completion of the initial evaluation are not clear, patients should be followed carefully, measuring the serum and urinary M-protein at 1- to 2-month intervals, to make sure that these levels are stable. Therapy should not be started unless signs of progression, especially a sustained increase in the serum and/or urinary M-protein, or other significant manifestations of disease progression (for example, weight loss, bone pain, anemia, renal failure).

## General Measures

An important initial objective is to relieve bone pain so that the patient can be ambulated. Chemotherapy is more effective than radiation in relieving pain associated with extensive osteoporosis, whereas radiation might be needed for localized lytic lesions. This treatment should be supplemented with effective analgesia to control the frightening spasms of pain and allow the patient to relax and rest. Attempts should be made to ambulate the patient as soon as a measure of pain relief has been achieved. All patients should be encouraged to take long walks and to be as active as possible to avoid further demineralization of the skeleton. Routine bisphosphonates, and when risk of hypercalcemia subsides, oral calcium and vitamin D are all appropriate for patients with osteopenia or lytic disease. Lumbar corsets can improve back pain by stabilizing the spine and preventing rapid rotational movements, which may precipitate microfractures and muscle spasms. After eradication of the tumor, vertebroplasty or kyphoplasty should be considered at the site of painful vertebral compression fractures. Percutaneous vertebroplasty is a therapeutic, radiologic procedure that involves injection of bone cement into the vertebral body lesion. Results from 2 uncontrolled prospective studies and several case series reports, including 1 with 187 patients, indicate that percutaneous vertebroplasty can produce significant pain relief and increase mobility in 70% to 80% of patients with osteolytic lesions in the vertebrae from myeloma or with osteoporotic compression fractures. Pain relief was apparent within 1 to 2 days after injection, and persisted for at least several months up to several years (Levine et al., 2000).

Patients should be encouraged to increase their fluid intake to 3000 mL per day to maintain the increased urine output required for the excretion of light chains, calcium, uric acid, urea, and other metabolites (MacLennan et al., 1984). All infections must be investigated and treated as emergencies.

Routine antibiotic prophylaxis is recommended in patients receiving high-dose steroids, which predispose to recurrent infection. Symptomatic anemia can be effectively relieved through effective use of erythropoietin (Osterborg et al., 2002). In one double-blind trial, erythropoietin significantly decreased the incidence of transfusion compared with placebo (28% vs. 47%) and increased mean Hb (1.8 g/dL vs. 0.0 g/dL) (Dammacco et al., 2001). Treated patients showed significant improvement in quality of life and performance status. Adverse events were similar between treatment groups. This agent should be used in the face of symptomatic anemia.

## Chemotherapy

The choice of chemotherapeutic agents for the treatment of multiple myeloma was reviewed previously in this chapter. Patients aged less than 70 years are generally treated with nonalkylating agent regimens, thus preserving hematopoiesis for future autologous stem cell transplant in support of high-dose therapy (see subsequent paragraphs). In the remaining patients, generally those older than age 70 and those who do not want or are otherwise unsuitable for high-dose therapy, conventional-dose chemotherapy is appropriate. Because drug combinations have not been shown to be better than MP in a large meta-analysis (Myeloma Trialists' Collaborative Group, 1998), and the results of treating patients with ABCM are reported to be similar to the results of treatment with optimal schedules of MP, we initiate therapy (in patients not destined for future high-dose melphalan and stem cell support) with either M or C and P. Dosage schedules for these drugs are:

1. Melphalan + Prednisone (MP)
   a. M: 9 mg/m$^2$ per day (or 0.25 mg/kg per day) by mouth on an empty stomach, for example, 1 hour before breakfast, for 4 days
   b. P: 100 mg per day with breakfast for 4 days
   c. Repeat MP every 4 to 6 weeks, as soon as neutrophils have recovered to more than $1.0 \times 10^9$/L and platelets to more than $100 \times 10^9$/L. Increase M by 2.0 mg per day for 4 days if there is no objective response, or neutrophils

and platelets do not fall below $1.0 \times 10^9$/L or $100 \times 10^9$/L, respectively

2. Cyclophosphamide + Prednisone (CP)
   a. CP every 3 weeks
   b. C: 1.0 g/m$^2$ intravenously or 0.25 g/m$^2$ by mouth per day for 4 days
   c. P: 100 mg per day with breakfast for 4 days
   d. Repeat every 3 weeks
   e. Weekly C and alternate day P
   f. C: 300 mg/m$^2$ intravenously, or by mouth, in the morning, every 7 days
   g. P: 100 mg by mouth in the morning on alternate days

3. ABCM
   a. Day 1: Adriamycin: 30 mg/m$^2$ intravenously
   b. BCNU (carmustine): 30 mg/m$^2$ intravenously
   c. Day 22: C: 100 mg/m$^2$ per day by mouth for 4 days
   d. M: 6 mg/m$^2$ per day by mouth for 4 days
   e. Day 42: Repeat the cycle every 6 weeks

M is chosen if there is no neutropenia or thrombocytopenia. Blood counts are repeated weekly. The initial dose of MP is repeated in the fourth to sixth week and should be increased if the neutrophil count does not fall below $0.5 \times 10^9$/L or platelets below $70 \times 10^9$/L during the posttreatment blood count nadir. Retreatment is usually possible at 4 to 6 weeks but should be delayed until the counts rise again above $1.0 \times 10^9$/L and $100 \times 10^9$/L, respectively. The dose of M should be reduced if neutrophils and/or platelets fall below these limits. Alternatively, if no hematologic toxicity is observed, the dose of M should be increased by 2.0 mg per day (not per m$^2$) for 4 days in the next course. The dose of M is increased again in subsequent courses until some evidence of toxicity, or objective response, indicates that adequate amounts of M have been absorbed. Blood counts are repeated at weekly intervals until the dose of M, which causes moderate decreases in leukocytes and platelets, has been determined. Thereafter, counts need be repeated only once, just before the next course is to begin.

The absorption of M from the gastrointestinal tract varies from person to person (Bacigalupo, 1994; Bosanquet and Gilby, 1982, 1984; Ehrsson et al., 1989; Taha et al., 1982). Because administering M with food reduces the amount absorbed by approximately 50% (Bosanquet and Gilby, 1984), the drug should be administered on an empty stomach, for example, 60 minutes before breakfast.

If the patient presents with neutropenia or thrombocytopenia, or if cumulative melphalan toxicity develops after repeated courses of M, and marrow recovery is delayed beyond 6 weeks, therapy is changed to weekly C and alternate day P, which is much less toxic to thrombopoiesis. It is advisable to monitor hematologic toxicity in patients with myeloma with renal failure very carefully during treatment with oral M. Despite the fact that administering M intravenously is more reliable in achieving consistent M blood levels, a clinical trial of intravenous and oral M did not show any advantage for the intravenous route, in either response or survival (Cornwell et al., 1982a).

Most alkylating agents are equally toxic for resting and proliferating cells, cause delayed recovery from hematologic toxicity after intermittent administration for 4 to 6 weeks, and lead to cumulative hematologic toxicity after repeated courses. In these respects, C is unique, because proliferating cells are much more sensitive than resting. Leukocytes fall to a nadir at 10 to 12 days and recover by 17 to 21 days after an intravenous dose of 1.0 g/m$^2$ (Bergsagel et al., 1968) and cumulative toxicity is unknown. If the neutrophil nadir does not fall below $0.5 \times 10^9$/L after a dose of 0.25 g/m$^2$ per day for 4 days by mouth, or 1.0 g/m$^2$ intravenously, the same dose can be repeated in 3 weeks, but should be reduced if the nadir is lower than this.

Patients who present with pancytopenia are better treated with weekly C and alternate-day P. If there is a possibility that the low counts might be caused by prior chemotherapy, marrow cellularity should be evaluated. The low counts are probably not the result of drug toxicity if the marrow is cellular. The pancytopenia probably results from the inhibition of hemotopoiesis that occurs in patients with myeloma and becomes more marked as the disease progresses. When this occurs, treatment is indicated to reduce the myeloma cell infiltration of the marrow and improve hemotopoiesis, like we do with patients with acute leukemia. Weekly C and alternate-day P is well tolerated by most patients. This therapy often results in a marked rise in hemoglobin, leukocytes, and platelets. Alternate-day P can be continued for months without causing unacceptable hypercorticism, but the dose can be reduced in those who are bothered by the hyperstimulation associated with this hormone.

Cyclophosphamide should be given in the morning so that most of the drug is cleared from the bladder before the patient goes to sleep. Patients should maintain a fluid intake of at least 3000 mL on the day before, the day they receive C, and the day after, to ensure prompt clearance of the drug from the bladder and to reduce the incidence of hemorrhagic cystitis.

M and C are equally effective in the treatment of myeloma (Working Party for Therapeutic Trials in Leukaemia, 1971). When combined with P, these agents induce objective responses in approximately 50% of patients with myeloma. Successful chemotherapy relieves bone pain, leads to weight gain, occasionally initiates skeletal healing, and improves survival. This therapy alleviates complications such as anemia, hypercalcemia, hyperviscosity, and renal failure, and

controls the disease during the chronic phase, but does not cure patients.

Although high-dose steroids alone or combinations of chemotherapy that use high-dose steroids are no more effective than the use of alkylating agents, concerns about the leukemogenic potential of alkylating agents and the toxic effects of M in particular on hematopoietic cells have swayed many to adopt high-dose steroids alone or in combination with infusional Adriamycin and vincristine (VAD) as primary therapy for patients who might later be considered for high-dose therapy and autologous blood stem cell collection. It is unknown if dexamethasone gives an equivalent response to VAD because the 2 have never been tested statistically in valid prospective trials. Dexamethasone with or without thalidomide (Rajkumar et al., 2002; Weber et al., 2003) might be a better choice in view of the equivalent response rates, lack of known efficacy of vincristine, and need for central venous access with the VAD regimen. In patients receiving steroid-based induction therapy, careful attention must be paid to the unique side effects of high-dose steroids, which include infection, diabetes, agitation, gastrointestinal irritation, and myopathy among others. Routine monitoring and prophylaxis against gastrointestinal bleeding, oral candidiasis, and *Pneumocystis* are strongly recommended. In patients who receive thalidomide with dexamethasone, antithrombotic therapies should be considered (Zangari et al., 2001).

# The Response of Patients with Myeloma to Chemotherapy

The following tests are used to follow the response to therapy:

1. On each visit record date, weight, height, temperature, symptoms, signs, and the treatment prescribed.

2. Take blood counts once a week until an acceptable pattern of toxicity is established, then only before each treatment

3. Measure the M-protein every 1 to 2 months.
   a. Serum M-protein: If a serum M-peak is visible, electrophoresis is more reliable than quantitative immunoassays. Immunofixation (IF) can measure much smaller amounts of M-protein than electrophoresis; the modern definition of a "complete response" requires that no M-protein can be detected in the serum by IF.
   b. Urine protein: The total protein excreted per 24 hours (gram per 24 h) is usually sufficient once electrophoresis of concentrated urine

protein has established that most of the urine protein is M-protein light chains. When the urine protein falls below 1.0 grams per 24 hours, the electrophoresis pattern of concentrated urine protein should be done so that the fraction of urine protein that is M-protein light chains can be determined. Again, the definition of a "complete response" requires that no urinary M-protein can be detected by IF.

4. Serum calcium and creatinine should be checked with a frequency determined by the clinical status. For example, check the calcium whenever the patient reports nausea, vomiting, polydipsia, polyuria, constipation, somnolence, or confusion.

5. Bone radiographs are required to investigate new sites of bone pain. Lateral skull films are useful for deciding whether skeletal disease is healing, stable, or progressing.

6. MRI should be used in preference to plain radiographs for the evaluation of vertebral lesions and suspected spinal cord compression.

7. Marrow aspiration and/or biopsy should be done if pancytopenia develops. A hypocellular marrow suggests that the cytopenias might be the result of treatment and that further therapy should be withheld until recovery occurs. A cellular marrow, however, suggests that the cytopenias might be secondary to progressive myeloma and indicates a need for additional treatment. Look for ringed sideroblasts and other signs of the myelodysplastic syndrome, or an increase in blasts indicating progression to acute leukemia.

The most useful indices of response and relapse are measurements of serum and urine M-proteins. A flow sheet that lists the date, weight, blood counts, serum and urinary M-protein values, serum calcium and creatinine, complications, and treatment in chronological sequence is essential. The response of patients with myeloma to treatment, the duration and status of the response, and the onset of relapse can be recognized by checking this record.

## Criteria of Response

The criteria for a response to treatment are as follows:

1. Objective response: One or more of the following, together with improvement in pain, other symptoms, and performance status:
   a. Plasmacytomas decrease by at least 50% on 2 measurements at least 4 weeks apart.
   b. Serum M-protein falls to less than 50% of the pretreatment value on 2 measurements at least 4 weeks apart.

   c. Urine total protein falls to less than 10% of the pretreatment value on 2 measurements at least 4 weeks apart.
   d. A stable response is achieved when serum and urinary M-protein values fall below the levels indicated above and remain stable for at least 4 months.

2. Progression during initial treatment: One or more of the following:
   a. Serum M-protein increases, or might fall initially, but does not achieve a stable response level and increases progressively by at least 10 g/L above baseline.
   b. Total urine protein increases, or might fall transiently initially, and then increases by at least 100% above baseline; urine electrophoresis confirms that the increase is the result of light-chain proteinuria.
   c. Hypercalcemia.
   d. Progressive enlargement of plasmacytomas.
   e. An increase in the number or size of lytic bone lesions. Collapse of osteoporotic vertebrae is not regarded as progression.

3. No change: No change in the serum or urine M-proteins, or a slight fall that fails to satisfy the criteria of an objective response.

The M-protein changes associated with various types of response are illustrated in Figure 12-1. The criteria outlined previously were used to classify the responses of 460 patients with myeloma treated in the NCI-C MY-2 trial of maintenance MP (Belch et al., 1988). The initial treatment for these patients was MP. Of the 460 eligible patients registered, 202 (44%) progressed, 211 (46%) achieved a stable response, and 47 (10%) were classified as "no change" because the M-protein did not fall sufficiently to qualify as a response, but was stable, and did not qualify as a progression. The survival of these groups of patients is shown in Figure 12-2. As expected, the survival of the progressors was poor, with a median of only 15 months. The surprise was that the survival of the "no change" group matched the survival of the stable response group. In a retrospective study, Joshua et al. (Joshua et al., 1991) also found that 11% of patients with myeloma were in the plateau phase at diagnosis, and that the percent fall in M-protein levels following treatment did not correlate with the duration of the plateau phase or survival. The Edmonton group (Palmer et al., 1989), similarly, did not find a significant correlation between the percent M-protein decrement and the survival of 134 patients with myeloma. Thus, the percent fall in the M-protein following treatment is not a critical determinant of survival in myeloma; what is important is the achievement of a stable plateau.

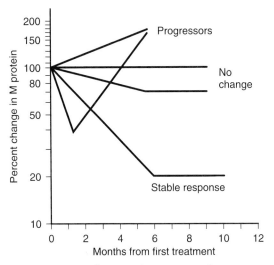

**Figure 12-1** *Patterns of M-protein response after treatment for myeloma.*

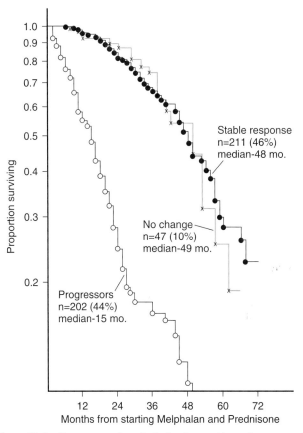

**Figure 12-2** *Response and survival of patients with myeloma treated with melphalan and prednisone in the NCI-C MY-2 trial (Belch et al., 1988). Patients were classified as stable responders, no change, or progressors by the criteria shown on pages 285–286 illustrated in Figure 12-1. The actuarial survival of these groups of patients from the onset of treatment is shown.*

## Treatment of Refractory Myeloma

As mentioned previously, we must be careful about how we define "refractory myeloma." Patients who do not respond with a 50% fall in the M-protein, but have disease that remains stable (the "no change" group), account for 10% of all myelomas (Bergsagel, 1988; Joshua et al., 1991). These patients have "refractory" but not progressive myeloma and survive as well as those who achieve a stable response. These patients do not require treatment as long as they remain asymptomatic; they are referred to as having *nonprogressive refractory* myeloma. There are 2 types of patients with progressive refractory myeloma who do need to be treated:

1. Those with *primary refractory* myeloma who progress while receiving adequate doses of primary therapy.

2. Those with *relapsing refractory* myeloma who have responded but are now relapsing despite continuation of previously effective treatment.

Most authors have not recognized the different natures of these groups in reports of trials of new approaches for the treatment of refractory myeloma. In a large review of the treatment of refractory myeloma, Buzaid and Durie (Buzaid and Durie, 1988) did indicate the effectiveness of treatments for 2 groups, "resistant" (primary refractory) and "relapsing" (relapsing refractory). In this review, patients with nonprogressive refractory myeloma were probably included with the resistant group, reducing the response rate but improving the survival of the group. Primary refractory groups of patients tend to have somewhat lower response rates than the relapsing group with all forms of second-line therapy.

Patients with progressive refractory myeloma are a frequent challenge. Many of these patients are in poor shape, often with marrow failure and pancytopenia. The object of treatment is to relieve symptoms and restore disease stability without causing unacceptable drug toxicity. There are 4 basic approaches to the treatment of primary refractory and relapsing refractory myeloma patients, as described subsequently.

## High-Dose Glucocorticoids

An objective response can be obtained in approximately 25% of primary and relapsing refractory myeloma patients treated with 40 mg dexamethasone (D) per day on days 1 through 4, 9 through 12, and 17 through 20, repeated every 28 days (Alexanian et al., 1986) or 100 mg prednisone (P) every other morning (Buzaid and Durie, 1988). This approach is especially useful as a temporary measure for delicate patients with advanced disease and marrow failure. Alternate-day P is much better tolerated than D.

## Thalidomide

As discussed previously in this chapter, thalidomide is active in 37% of patients with refractory myeloma (Barlogie et al., 2001) and appears to be synergistic when applied in conjunction with dexamethasone. Although randomized trials are lacking, use of steroids and thalidomide in combination is becoming very prevalent in relapsed disease.

## Vincristine, Adriamycin, and Dexamethasone (VAD)

This drug combination became the most popular for treating myeloma during the 1990s predominantly as a result of the rapid response rate and lack of stem cell toxicity that was observed. Nevertheless, there are many problematic issues relevant to this regimen. It was designed as a 4-day infusion of V and A, which was assumed to be more effective than single injections. In fact, such studies that exist suggest this might be true (Browman et al., 1992). VAD is, however, complicated by the requirement for a central line with its inherent complications, and by the use of V which has not been shown to have any activity as a single agent against myeloma, thus adding only toxicity to the combination. Most of the activity of the combination is likely to be the result of the industrial-sized dose of D, 40 mg day given for 4 days beginning on days 1, 9, and 17 (Alexanian et al., 1992). As mentioned previously, it is not known whether the VAD regimen is superior to D alone because this has not been tested.

Although VAD became popular as an alternative to melphalan, which had earned its reputation for knocking out hematopoietic stem cells, other agents, such as cyclophosphamide and thalidomide, are available, which are nontoxic to these cells.

## Weekly Cyclophosphamide and Alternate-Day Prednisone

This form of treatment has been adapted from the regimen introduced in 1982 (Brandes and Israels, 1982). The original regimen, using a lower dose of C (150–250 mg/m$^2$), induced responses in 7 of 28 (25%) primary refractory and 10 of 29 (35%) relapsing refractory myeloma patients. The mean response duration was approximately 10 months (Wilson et al., 1987). The advantages of this regimen are the convenience of oral administration and the reduced myelotoxicity and hypercorticism. It is well tolerated by most patients. Much of the initial response is probably the result of the P, which can be tolerated for months without causing hypercorticism when given on alternate days. This approach to the treatment of progressive refractory myeloma is widely used in Canada and the United Kingdom.

It is not possible to compare the effectiveness of these 3 approaches (dexamethasone, VAD, or cyclophosphamide and prednisone) in the treatment of progressive refractory myeloma. Each of the regimens has been tested in single-arm studies. These studies were not done on comparable groups of patients. Prospective, randomized comparisons of the different regimens have not been done.

## Summary

Treatment for myeloma should only be initiated in symptomatic patients and care should be taken not to treat patients with MGUS or smoldering myeloma. Once a decision to treat has been made, treatment options can be divided into patients destined for future stem cell collection and those who will not be transplant candidates. For the former, melphalan and prednisone remains the standard of care. For patients heading to transplant, a steroid-based regimen such as high-dose dexamethasone is recommended. Although VAD combination chemotherapy is widely used, the rationale for inclusion of vincristine and Adriamycin has never been well established; nevertheless, this regimen is among the most common used today. Preliminary results suggest that a combination of dexamethasone and thalidomide is effective in newly diagnosed patients, but further studies and comparison with traditional regimens will be required before widespread adoption of this regimen. In relapsed patients, high-dose dexamethasone, oral cyclophosphamide, and alternate-day prednisone or use of thalidomide alone or in combination with steroids is recommended. Beyond such checkpoints, investigational drugs should be explored such as PS-341 and the ImiDs, both of which hold promise. Supportive care is critical and includes regular fluid intake, bisphosphonates and other antiosteoporosis measures, effective pain relief, erythropoietin, and a high index of suspicion for infection. Overall, better supportive care, high-dose melphalan, and the introduction of new drugs seem to be gradually yet steadily improving the outlook for patients with myeloma.

## REFERENCES

Adams, J. (2003). Preclinical development of velcade (bortezomib; formerly PS-341) for multiple myeloma. *European Journal of Haematology, 70,* 265.

Åhre, A., Björkholm, M., Mellstedt, H., Holm, G., Brenning, G., Engstedt, L., Gahrton, G., Hällen, J., Johansson, B., Johansson, S. G. O., Karlström, L., Killander, A., Lerner, R., Lockner, D., Lönnqvist, B., Simonsson, B., Stalfelt, A. M., Ternsted, B., and Wadman, B. (1983). Intermittent high-dose melphalan/prednisone vs. continuous low-dose melphalan treatment in multiple myeloma. *European Journal of Cancer Clinical Oncology, 19,* 499–506.

Alberts, D. S., and Salmon, S. E. (1975). Adriamycin in the treatment of alkylator-resistant multiple myeloma: a pilot study. *Cancer Chemotherapy Reports, 59,* 345–350.

Alexanian, R., Barlogie, B., and Dixon, D. (1986). High-dose gluco-corticoid treatment of resistant myeloma. *Annals of Internal Medicine*, 105, 8–11.

Alexanian, R., Dimopoulos, M. A., Delasalle, K., and Barlogie, B. (1992). Primary dexamethasone treatment of multiple myeloma. *Blood*, 80, 887–890.

Alexanian, R., Yap, B. S., and Bodey, G. P. (1983). Prednisone pulse therapy for refractory myeloma. *Blood*, 62, 572–577.

Bacigalupo, A. (1994). The clinical benefits of recombinant human granulocyte-colony-stimulating factor in the treatment of cancer patients. *European Journal of Cancer*.

Barlogie, B., Desikan, R., Eddlemon, P., Spencer, T., Zeldis, J., Munshi, N., Badros, A., Zangari, M., Anaissie, E., Epstein, J., Shaughnessy, J., Ayers, D., Spoon, D., and Tricot, G. (2001). Extended survival in advanced and refractory multiple myeloma after single-agent thalidomide: identification of prognostic factors in a phase 2 study of 169 patients. *Blood*, 98, 492–494.

Barlogie, B., Smith, L, and Alexanian, R. (1984). Effective treatment of advanced multiple myeloma refractory to alkylating agents. *New England Journal of Medicine*, 310, 1353–1356.

Belch, A., Shelley, W., Bergsagel, D., Wilson, K., Klimo, P., White, D., and Willan, A. (1988). A randomized trial of maintenance versus no maintenance melphalan and prednisone in responding multiple myeloma patients. *British Journal of Cancer*, 57, 94–99.

Bennett, J. M., Silber, R., Ezdinli, E., Levitt, M., Oken, M., Bakemeier, R. F., Bailer, J. C., and Carbone, P. P. (1978). Phase II study of Adriamycin and bleomycin in patients with multiple myeloma. *Cancer Chemotherapy Reports*, 62, 1367–1369.

Bergsagel, D. E. (1979). Treatment of plasma cell myeloma. *Annual Review of Medicine*, 30, 431–443.

Bergsagel, D. E. (1988). Use a gentle approach for refractory myeloma patients [Editorial]. *Journal of Clinical Oncology*, 6, 757–758.

Bergsagel, D. E., Bailey, A. J., Langley, G. R., MacDonald, R. N., White, D. F., and Miller, A. B. (1979). The chemotherapy of plasma-cell myeloma and the incidence of acute leukemia. *New England Journal of Medicine*, 301, 743–748.

Bergsagel, D. E., Cowan, D. H., and Hasselback, R. (1972). Plasma cell myeloma: response of melphalan-resistant patients to high-dose intermittent cyclophosphamide. *Canadian Medical Association Journal*, 107, 851–855.

Bergsagel, D. E., Haas, R. H., and Messner, H. A. (1986). Interferon alpha-2b in the treatment of chronic granulocytic leukemia. *Seminars in Oncology*, 13, 29–34.

Bergsagel, D. E., Ogawa, M., and Librach, S. L. (1975). Mouse myeloma: a model for studies of cell kinetics. *Archives of Internal Medicine*, 135, 109–113.

Bergsagel, D. E., Robertson, G. L., and Hasselback, R. (1968). Effect of cyclophosphamide on advanced lung cancer and the toxicity of large, intermittent intravenous doses. *Canadian Medical Association Journal*, 98, 532–538.

Bjorkstrand, B., Svensson, H., Goldschmidt, H., et al. (2001). Alpha-interferon maintenance treatment is associated with improved survival after high-dose treatment and autologous stem cell transplantation in patients with multiple myeloma: a retrospective registry study from the European Group for Blood and Marrow Transplantation (EBMT). *Bone Marrow Transplantation, 27*, 511–515.

Bosanquet, A. G., and Gilby, E. D. (1982). Pharmacokinetics of oral and intravenous melphalan during routine treatment of multiple myeloma. *European Journal of Cancer Clinical Oncology*, 18, 355–362.

Bosanquet, A. G., and Gilby, E. D. (1984). Comparison of the fed and fasting states on the absorption of melphalan in multiple myeloma. *Cancer Chemotherapy and Pharmacology*, 12, 183–186.

Bramwell, V., Calvert, R. T., Edwards, G., Scarffe, H., and Crowther, D. (1979). The disposition of cyclophosphamide in a group of myeloma patients. *Cancer Chemotherapy and Pharmacology*, 3, 253–259.

Brandes, L. J., and Israels, L. G. (1982). Treatment of advanced plasma cell myeloma with weekly cyclophosphamide and alternate-day prednisone. *Cancer Treatment Reports*, 66, 1413–1415.

Browman, G. P., Belch, A., Skillings, J., Wilson, K., et al. (1982). Modified adriamycin-vincristine-dexamethasone (m-VAD) in primary refractory and relapsed plasma cell myeloma: an NCI (Canada) pilot study. *The National Cancer Institute of Canada Clinical Trials Group, 82*, 555–559.

Browman, G. P., Bergsagel, D., Sicheri, D., O'Reilly, S., Wilson, K. S., Rubin, S., Belch, A., Shustik, C., Barr, R., Walker, I., James, K., Zee, B., and Johnston, D. (1995). Randomized trial of interferon maintenance in multiple myeloma: a study of the National Cancer Institute of Canada Clinical Trials Group. *Journal of Clinical Oncology*, 13, 2354–2360.

Buzaid, A. C., and Durie, B. G. (1988). Management of refractory myeloma: a review. *Journal of Clinical Oncology*, 6, 889–905.

Case, D. C., Jr., Lee, B. J., and Clarkson, B. D. (1977). Improved survival times in multiple myeloma treated with melphalan, prednisone, cyclophosphamide, vincristine and BCNU: M-2 protocol. *American Journal of Medicine*, 63, 897–903.

Cohen, H. J., and Bartolucci, A. A. (1982). Hexamethylmelamine and prednisone in the treatment of refractory myeloma. *American Journal of Clinical Oncology*, 5, 21–27.

Cornwell, G. G. III, Pajak, T. F., Kochwa, S., McIntyre, O. R., Glowienka, L. P., Brunner, K., Rafla, S., Silver, R. T., Cooper, M. R., Henderson, E., Kyle, R. A., Haurani, F. I., and Cuttner, J. (1982a). Comparison of oral melphalan, CCNU, and BCNU with and without vincristine and prednisone in the treatment of multiple myeloma. Cancer and Leukemia Group B experience. *Cancer, 50*, 1669–1675.

Costa, G., Carbone, P. P., Gold, G. L., Owens, A. H., Jr., Miller, S. P., Krant, M. J., and Bono, V. H., Jr. (1963). Clinical trial of vinblastine in multiple myeloma. *Cancer Chemotherapy Reports*, 27, 87–89.

Costa, G., Engle, R. L., Jr., Schilling, A., Carbone, P., Kochwa, S., and Glidewell, O. (1973). Melphalan and prednisone: an effective combination for the treatment of multiple myeloma. *American Journal of Medicine*, 54, 589–599.

Costanzi, J. J., Cooper, M. R., Scarffe, J. H., Ozer, H., Grubbs, S. S., Ferraresi, R. W., Pollard, R. B., and Spiegel, R. J. (1985). Phase II study of recombinant alpha-2 interferon in resistant multiple myeloma. *Journal of Clinical Oncology*, 3, 654–659.

Cunningham, D., Powles, R., Malpas, J., Raje, N., Milan, S., Viner, C., Montes, A., Hickish, T., Nicolson, M., Johnson, P., Treleaven, J., Raymond, J., and Gore, M. (1998). A randomized trial of maintenance interferon following high-dose chemotherapy in multiple myeloma: long-term follow-up results. *British Journal of Haematology, 102*, 495–502.

Dammacco, F., Castoldi, G., and Rodjer, S. (2001) Efficacy of epoetin alfa in the treatment of anaemia of multiple myeloma. *British Journal of Haematology, 3*, 172–179.

Ehrsson, H., Eksborg, S., Osterborg, A., Mellstedt, H., and Lindfors, A. (1989). Oral melphalan pharmacokinetics–relation to dose in patients with multiple myeloma. *Medical Oncology and Pharmacotherapeutics, 6*, 151–154.

Fritz, E., and Ludwig, H. (2000). Interferon-alpha treatment in multiple myeloma: meta-analysis of 30 randomised trials among 3948 patients. *Annals of Oncology*, 11, 1427–1436.

Gertz, M. A., Lacy, M. Q., Dispenzier, A. (1999). Amyloidosis: Recognition, confirmation, prognosis, and therapy. *Mayo Clinic Proceedings, 5*, 490–494.

Ghanta, V. K., Cohen, H. J., Silberman, H. R., Durant, J. R., and Hiramoto, R. N. (1981). Assessment of myeloma maintenance regimen of prednisone, Adriamycin, Imuran and vincristine in a murine plasmacytoma model. *Cancer Clinical Trials, 4*, 135–141.

Gockerman, J. P., Bartolucci, A. A., Nelson, M. O., Silberman, H., Velez-Garcia, E., and Stein, R. (1986). Phase II evaluation of etoposide in refractory multiple myeloma: a Southeastern Cancer Study Group trial. *Cancer Treatment Reports, 70*, 801–802.

Hjorth, M., Hellquist, L., Holmberg, E., Magnusson, B., Rodjer, S., and Westin, J. (1993). Initial versus deferred melphalan-prednisone therapy for asymptomatic multiple myeloma stage I: a randomized study. *European Journal of Haematology, 50,* 95–102.

Houwen, B., Ockhuizen, T., Marrick, J., and Nieweg, H. O. (1981). Vindesine therapy in melphalan-resistant multiple myeloma. *European Journal of Cancer, 17,* 227–231.

Hussein, M. A., Wood, L., Hsi, E., Srkalovic, G., Karam, M., Elson, P., and Bukowski, R. M. (2002). A phase II trial of pegylated liposomal doxorubicin, vincristine, and reduced-dose dexamethasone combination therapy in newly diagnosed multiple myeloma patients. *Cancer, 95,* 2160–2168.

Jackson, D. V., Case, E. K., Pope, D. R., White, D. R., Spurr, C. L., Richards, F. II, Stuart, J. J., Muss, H. B., Cooper, M. R., Black, W. R., Wortman, J. E., Herring, W. B., Caldwell, R. D., and Capizzi, R. L. (1985). Single agent vincristine by infusion in refractory multiple myeloma. *Journal of Clinical Oncology, 3,* 1508–1512.

Joshua, D. E., Snowdon, L., Gibson, J., Iland, H., Brown, R., Warburton, P., Vincent, P., Basten, A., and Kronenberg, H. (1991). Multiple myeloma: plateau phase revisited. *Hematology Reviews and Communications, 5,* 59–66.

Kyle, R. A. (2002). Current therapy of multiple myeloma. *Internal Medicine, 41,* 175–180.

Ludwig, H., Cortelezzi, A., Scheithauer, W., Van Camp, B. G. K., Kuzmits, R., Fillet, G., Peetermans, M., Polli, E., and Flener, R. (1986). Recombinant interferon alpha-2C versus polychemotherapy (VMCP) for treatment of multiple myeloma: a prospective randomized trial. *European Journal of Cancer Clinical Oncology, 22,* 1111–1116.

Levine, S. A., Perin, L. A., Hayes, D., and Hayes, W. S. (2000). An evidence-based evaluation of percutaneous vertebroplasty. *Managed Care, 9,* 56–60.

MacLennan, I. C., Chapman, C., Dunn, J., and Kelly, K. (1992). Combined chemotherapy with ABCM versus melphalan for treatment of myelomatosis. The Medical Research Council Working Party for Leukaemia in Adults. *Lancet, 339,* 200–205.

MacLennan, I. C., and Cusick, J. (1985). Objective evaluation of the role of vincristine in induction and maintenance therapy for myelomatosis. Medical Research Council Working Party on Leukaemia in Adults. *British Journal of Cancer, 52,* 153–158.

MacLennan, I. C. M., Falconer Smith, J. F., Crockson, R. A., Cooper, E. H., Knight, F. R., Cuzik, J., and Hardwicke, J. (1984). Analysis and management of renal failure in fourth MRC myelomatosis trial. MRC working party on leukaemia in adults. *British Medical Journal, 288,* 1411–1416.

MacLennan, I. C. M., Kelly, K., Crockson, R. A., Cooper, E. H., Cuzik, J., and Chapman, C. (1988). Results of the MRC myelomatosis trials for patients entered since 1980. *Hematologic Oncology, 6,* 145–158.

Mandelli, F., Avvisati, G., Amadori, S., Boccadoro, M., Gernone, A., Lauta, V. M., Marmont, F., Petrucci, M. T., Tribalto, M., Vegna, M. L., Dammacco, F., and Peleri, A. (1990). Maintenance treatment with recombinant interferon alfa-2b in patients with multiple myeloma responding to conventional induction chemotherapy. *New England Journal of Medicine, 322,* 1430–1434.

Mass, R. E. (1962). A comparison of the effect of prednisone and a placebo in the treatment of multiple myeloma. *Cancer Chemotherapy Reports, 16,* 257–259.

McIntyre, O. R., Pajak, T. F., Kyle, R. A., Cornwell, G. G. III, and Leone, L. (1985). Response rate and survival in myeloma patients receiving prednisone alone. *Medical and Pediatric Oncology, 13,* 239–243.

Myeloma Trialists' Collaborative Group. (1998). Combination chemotherapy versus melphalan plus prednisone as treatment for multiple myeloma: an overview of 6,633 patients from 27 randomized trials. *Journal of Clinical Oncology, 16,* 3832–3842.

O'Bryan, R. M., Luce, J. K., Talley, R. W., Gottlieb, J. A., Baker, L. H., and Bonnadonna, G. (1973). Phase II evaluation of Adriamycin in human neoplasia. *Cancer, 32,* 1–8.

Ogawa, M., Bergsagel, D. E., and McCulloch, E. A. (1973a). Chemotherapy of mouse myeloma: quantitative cell cultures predictive response in vivo. *Blood, 41,* 7–15.

Ogawa, M., Bergsagel, D. E., and McCulloch, E. A. (1973b). Studies of nitrogen mustard transport by mouse myeloma and hemotopoietic precursor cells. *Cancer Research, 33,* 3172–3175.

Ohno, R. (1987). Interferons in the treatment of multiple myeloma. *International Journal of Cancer, Supplement 1,* 14–20.

Oken, M. M., Lenhard, R. E., Jr., Tsiatis, A. A., Glick, J. H., and Silverstein, M. M. (1987). Contribution of prednisone to the effectiveness of hexamethylmelamine in multiple myeloma. *Cancer Treatment Reports, 71,* 807–811.

Olujohungbe, A. B., Dunn, J. A., Drayson, M. T., and MacLennan, I. C. M. (1996). Prednisolone added to the ABCM as treatment for multiple myeloma increases serological responses but not overall survival or the number of stable clinical responses. *British Journal of Haematology, 93,* 77 (abstract 296).

Orlowski, R. Z., Stinchcombe, T. E., Mitchell, B. S., et al. (2002). Phase I trial of the proteasome inhibitor PS-341 in patients with refractory hematologic malignancies. *Journal of Clinical Oncology, 20,* 4420–4427.

Osterborg, A., Brandberg, Y., Molostova, V., Iosava, G., Abdulkadyrov, K., Hedenus, M., and Messinger, D. (2002). Randomized, double-blind, placebo-controlled trial of recombinant human erythropoietin, epoetin Beta, in hematologic malignancies. *Journal of Clinical Oncology, 15,* 2486–2494.

Palmer, M., Belch, A., Hanson, J., and Brox, L. (1989). Reassessment of the relationship between M-protein decrement and survival in multiple myeloma. *British Journal of Cancer, 59,* 110–112.

Peest, D., Deicher, H., Coldewey, R., Leo, R., Bartl, R., Bartels, H., Braun, H. J., Fett, W., Fischer, J. T., Gobel, B., Harms, P., Henke, R., Hoffmann, L., Kreuser, E. D., Maier, W. D., Meier, C. R., Oertel, J., Petit, M., Planker, M., Platzeck, C., Respondek, M., Schafer, E., Schumacher, K., Stennes, M., Stenzinger, W., Tirier, C., Wagner, H., Weh, H. J., Vonwussow, P., and Wysk, J. (1995). A comparison of polychemotherapy and melphalan prednisone for primary remission induction, and interferon-alpha for maintenance treatment, in multiple myeloma—a prospective trial of the German Myeloma Treatment Group. *European Journal of Cancer, 31A,* 146–151.

Rajkumar, S. V., Dispenzieri, A., Fonseca, R., et al. (2003). Thalidomide for previously untreated indolent or smoldering multiple myeloma. *Leukemia, 15,* 1274–1276.

Rajkumar, S. V., Hayman, S., Gertz, M. A., Dispenzieri, A., Lacy, M. Q., Greipp, P. R., Geyer, S., Iturria, N., Fonseca, R., Lust, J. A., Kyle, R. A., and Witzig, T. E. (2002). Combination therapy with thalidomide plus dexamethasone for newly diagnosed myeloma. *Journal of Clinical Oncology, 20,* 4319–4323.

Richardson, P. G., Barlogie, B., Berenson, J., Singhal, S., Jagannath, S., et al. (2003). A phase 2 study of Bortezomib in relapsed, refractory myeloma. *New England Journal of Medicine, 26,* 2597–2598.

Richardson, P. G., Schlossman, R. L., Weller, E., et al. (2002). Immunomodulatory drug CC-5013 overcomes drug resistance and is well tolerated in patients with relapsed multiple myeloma. *Blood, 100,* 3063–3067.

Salmon, S. E., Crowley, J. J., Grogan, T. M., Finley, P., Pugh, R. P., and Barlogie, B. (1994). Combination chemotherapy, glucocorticoids, and interferon-alfa in the treatment of multiple myeloma: a Southwest Oncology Group Study. *Journal of Clinical Oncology, 12,* 2405–2414.

Salmon, S. E., Haut, A., Bonnet, J. D., Amare, M., Weick, J. K., Durie, B. G., and Dixon, D. O. (1983). Alternating combination chemotherapy and levamisole improves survival in multiple myeloma: a Southwest Oncology Group Study. *Journal of Clinical Oncology, 1,* 453–461.

Singhal, S., Mehta, J., Desikan, R., et al. (1999). Antitumor activity of thalidomide in refractory multiple myeloma *New England Journal of Medicine, 341,* 1565–1571.

Taha, I. A., Ahmad, R. A., Gray, H., Roberts, C. I., and Rogers, H. J. (1982). Plasma melphalan and prednisolone concentrations during oral therapy for multiple myeloma. *Cancer Chemotherapy and Pharmacology, 9,* 57–60.

Tirelli, U., Zagonel, V., Veronesi, A., Volpe, R., Carbone, A., Brema, F., and Grigoletto, E. (1985). Phase II study of teniposide (VM-26) in multiple myeloma. *American Journal of Clinical Oncology, 8,* 329–331.

Weber, D., Rankin, K., Gavino, M., Delasalle, K., and Alexanian, R. (2003). Thalidomide alone or with dexamethasone for previously untreated multiple myeloma. *Journal of Clinical Oncology, 21,* 16–19.

Wilson, K., Shelley, W., Belch, A., Brandes, L., Bergsagel, D., Klimo, P., White, D., and Willan, A. (1987). Weekly cyclophosphamide and alternate-day prednisone: an effective secondary therapy in multiple myeloma. *Cancer Treatment Reports, 71,* 981–982.

Working Party for Therapeutic Trials in Leukaemia, M.R.C. (1971). Myelomatosis: comparison of melphalan and cyclophosphamide therapy. *British Medical Journal, i,* 640–641.

Zangari, M., Anaissie, E., Barlogie, B., et al. (2002). Increased risk of deep-vein thrombosis in patients with multiple myeloma receiving thalidomide and chemotherapy. *Blood, 98,* 1614–1615.

# CHAPTER 13

———

# High-Dose Therapy in Multiple Myeloma

FAITH E. DAVIES
J. ANTHONY CHILD

## Introduction and Background

The early studies of dose escalation of melphalan, which were initiated by McElwain and Powles (1983), demonstrated that the dose of melphalan could be escalated to as high as 140 mg/m$^2$ without stem cell or growth factor support with the achievement of high complete response (CR) rates of approximately 30%. There were limitations in applicability because of toxicity, but the later availability of growth factors and the development of autologous stem cell–supported treatment subsequently encouraged the progressive introduction of myeloablative high-dose therapy (HDT). Such approaches, adopted initially as second-line treatment in younger patients, were soon applied to previously untreated patients as a component of therapy and many centers developed programs for HDT (chemotherapy or chemoradiotherapy) with supporting autograft (Attal, 1992; Bensinger et al., 1996a; Bjorkstrand et al., 1997; Cunningham et al., 1994; Fermand et al., 1993; Gore et al., 1989; Harousseau et al., 1995; Marit et al., 1996; Schiller et al., 1995; Selby et al., 1987; Vesole et al., 1996). Complete remissions, as defined by the disappearance of paraprotein from serum and urine on conventional electrophoresis and reduction of the bone marrow plasma cell population to less than 5%, was achievable in approximately one-half of the patients treated (Gore et al., 1989). The heterogeneity of treatment and the patient populations in these studies made comparisons difficult. Despite the apparent improvement in responses, there was a clear need to determine whether HDT conferred a survival advantage in comparison with conventional dose treatment with more systematic investigations, and, in particular, randomized trials.

Allogeneic bone marrow transplantation (BMT), which had been widely adopted in the treatment of other hematologic disorders, notably the acute leukemias, in conjunction with high-dose chemoradiotherapy, was another approach. The collective experience of many centers, some carrying out very few transplants, was collated through the European Bone Marrow Transplant Group (EBMT). Data on 690 patients showed that approximately one-half of the patients achieved a complete response, some of these enduring in the long term (Gahrton et al., 1995, 2001). Both EBMT and larger single-center experience, exemplified by Seattle (Bensinger et al., 1996b) was of high procedure-related mortality, which inhibited wider application. However, over the last two decades there appears to have been a clear trend to improved overall survival and reduction in treatment-related mortality. Because of the assumption that this mode of treatment is most likely to eradicate myeloma cells and the possibility of a significant graft versus myeloma effect, there is continuing interest in allogeneic procedures in the treatment of multiple myeloma, most recently in the development of reduced intensity conditioning, nonmyeloablative "mini-allogeneic" transplantation. Currently, both autologous and allogeneic transplants, in conjunction with predominantly chemotherapy, are the subject of a wide variety of investigations and trials.

## Comparison of Conventional-Dose Therapy with High-Dose Therapy (HDT)

The increasing application of HDT supported initially by autologous bone marrow transplantation and then by the use of peripheral blood stem cells was encouraged by reports of reasonable safety margins, high response rates, and improved survival in relapsed, "previously refractory" and newly diagnosed patients with multiple myeloma. Comparisons with historical controls (Barlogie et al., 1997; Lenhoff et al., 2000) or population-based studies (Bladé et al., 1996, 2000) are liable to bias in patient selection, and the emerging data suggesting improved responses and outcomes when HDT is incorporated in first-line treatment clearly required substantiation in prospective randomized trials (Table 13-1).

The first such trial to be reported was carried out by the Intergroupe Francais du Myelome (IFM) in which 200 patients under the age of 65 with previously untreated myeloma were randomized to receive either conventional-dose chemotherapy with VMCP/VBAP or VMCP/VBAP followed by melphalan at 140 mg/m$^2$ with TBI supported with unpurged autologous bone marrow collected after two cycles of the induction chemotherapy (Attal et al., 1996). Patients in both arms of the study received maintenance interferon-$\alpha$. In this study, 74 of the 100 patients in the planned intensive treatment arm went on to receive HDT. The IFM group reported significant benefit for the intensively treated patients in terms of response rate, duration of response, and survival. A recent update gave an overall median survival of 44 months in the standard group and 56 months in the intensive group (Attal, personal communication, 2000).

Another randomized study in which a direct comparison between conventional-dose and treatment incorporating HDT was made was reported by the Myeloma Autograft Group (MAG) (Fermand et al., 1999). Patients either received VMCP or VAD followed by melphalan at 200 mg/m$^2$ (or 140 mg/m$^2$ melphalan plus 16 mg/m$^2$ busulphan). One hundred ninety patients between the ages of 55 and 65 were randomized with 94 allocated to intensive treatment, but 25% did not actually proceed to the HDT module. Patients in the intensive group had a median overall survival of 55.3 months compared with 50.4 months in the conventional-dose treatment group, a difference that

=== **TABLE 13-1** ===

Autologous Transplantation Versus Conventional Chemotherapy for Newly Diagnosed Myeloma

| | Patients (*n*) | | CR (%) | | EFS (median mo) | | OS (median mo) | |
|---|---|---|---|---|---|---|---|---|
| | Con | HDT | Con | HDT | Con | HDT | Con | HDT |
| Barlogie et al., 1997* | 116 | 123 | — | 40 | 22 | 49 | 48 | 62 |
| Lenhoff et al., 2000* | 274 | 274 | — | 34 | — | 27 | 46% at 4 y | 61% at 4 y |
| Attal et al., 1996 | 100 | 100 | 5 | 22 | 18 | 27 | 37 | 52% at 5 y |
| Fermand et al., 1999 | 96 | 94 | — | — | 18.7 | 24.3 | 50.4 | 55.3 |
| Blade et al., 2000* | 83 | 81 | 11 | 30 | 34.3 | 42.5 | 66.9 | 67.4 |
| Child et al., 2003 | 200 | 201 | 8.5 | 44 | 19.6 | 31.6 | 42.3 | 54.8 |

*Historical controls.
Con, Conventional; HDT, high-dose treatment; CR, complete response; EFS, event-free survival; OS, overall survival.

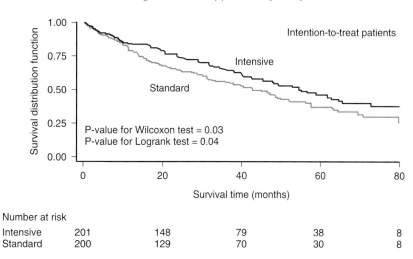

**FIGURE 13-1** *Kaplan-Meier survival curve of overall survival in the MRC Myeloma VII trial according to treatment group (intention-to-treat population). Overall, there was an improvement in median survival of 12 months in the intensive group, median survival 54.1 months (95% confidence interval, 44.9–65.2) compared with 42.3 months (95% confidence interval, 33.1–51.6) in the standard group (p = 0.04 log-rank test, p = 0.03 Wilcoxon test).*

was not statistically significant. Patients in the conventional group crossed over to receive HDT at disease progression at the physician's discretion.

The third and largest comparable trial was the Medical Research Council (MRC) Myelomatosis Therapy Trial, Myeloma VII (Child et al., 2003). Four hundred seven previously untreated patients under 65 years of age were randomized to receive either ABCM (adriamycin, BCNU, cyclophosphamide, melphalan) the previous MRC standard or treatment that included HDT: C-VAMP (cyclophosphamide, vincristine, adriamycin, methylprednisolone) followed by HDT (200 mg/m² melphalan or 140 mg/m² melphalan plus TBI). Patients in both arms of the study received interferon-α maintenance therapy. In 401 patients available for analysis, response rates for the intensive group were higher than for the standard group (CR 44.3% vs. 8.5%, PR 42.3% vs. 40.5%, and MR 3.5% vs. 17.5%). Intention-to-treat (ITT) analysis also showed significantly better overall survival and progression-free survival for the intensive group. Intensive treatment improved the median survival by approximately 1 year from 42.3 to 54.1 months (Fig. 13-1).

A fourth randomized trial also addressed this question by comparing patients receiving VBMCP/VBAD with HDT (200 mg/m² melphalan or 140 mg/m² melphalan plus TBI) (Bladé et al., 2001). However, in this trial, patients were only randomized to further chemotherapy or HDT after response to initial induction chemotherapy. Despite an improvement in response rates in the HDT arm (CR 30% vs. 11%), there was no statistical difference in progression-free or overall survival.

In a systematic review of the literature, three trials were identified as addressing the question of conventional-dose chemotherapy versus treatment incorporating a module of HDT with supporting autologous transplantation with randomization at diagnosis (Attal et al., 1996; Child et al., 2003; Fermand et al., 1999). Although meta-analysis of the two French trials did not confirm survival benefit from HDT, when data from all three studies were combined, the estimate of treatment effect as illustrated by the Forest Plot was consistent with a significant survival benefit (odds ratio, 0.70; 95% confidence interval, 0.53–0.93; *p* = 0.01) (Fig. 13-2). It seems unlikely that further trials

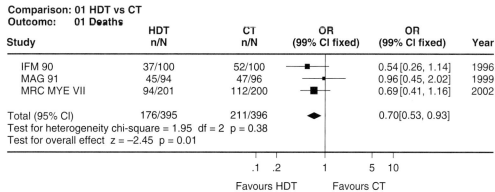

**FIGURE 13-2** *Forest plot showing the odds ratio and 99% confidence limits for the current study with the other two published studies comparing conventional with high-dose treatment in myeloma. The odds ratio for all of the studies combined is consistent with a beneficial effect for patients receiving the high-dose treatment option.*

addressing this particular issue will be pursued, and the incorporation of HDT in first-line treatment of younger, fitter patients might be regarded as a standard approach. There are, however, a range of other studies that have examined or are currently investigating other aspects of the role of HDT in the treatment of myeloma.

# Early versus Late High-Dose Therapy (HDT)

The issue of the timing of HDT and the differences in responses and outcome when given in the relapsed disease setting as compared with its incorporation in first-line therapy has been the subject of several studies, the largest of which from the US Intergroup has yet to be reported. To date two trials have been reported. An MAG trial showed no difference in overall survival between patients receiving either early or late (relapse) HDT; however, the Time Without Symptoms and Toxicity (TwisTT) study favored the early transplant cohort (Fermand et al., 1998). The IFM have also addressed this issue of timing in the setting of more intensive approaches in the CIAM trial by randomizing patients following induction chemotherapy with conventional chemotherapy and 140 mg/m$^2$ melphalan with no PBSCT support to either additional HDT as part of front-line therapy or at relapse (Harousseau et al., 1998). Preliminary results suggested that after a first course of HDT without PBSCT support, consolidation with a second course of HDT with BM support did not confer a clear survival advantage over HDT at the time of relapse.

Taking this data in the context of the HDT versus conventional trials, the results to date would suggest that all eligible patients should receive HDT. Although the optimum timing of this in the disease course remains unclear, it would be prudent to collect sufficient stem cells in all such cases to support a subsequent high-dose procedure.

# Multiple High-Dose Therapies (HDT)

The response data emerging from the early studies on the use of HDT vindicating pursuit of dose escalation in the treatment of myeloma encouraged exploration of the use of further courses of intensification therapy after the initial high-dose procedure. Individual centers, and notably the Arkansas group, have been able to demonstrate that this is feasible and effective (Barlogie et al., 1997, 1999). However, the question of whether there is indeed an improved outcome from such approaches requires substantiation in the randomized trial setting. To date, three randomized trials comparing single HDT versus double (or "tandem") HDT have been reported (Attal et al., 2002; Cavo et al., 2002; Fermand et al., 2001). Conditioning regimens for the HDT included 140 mg/m$^2$ melphalan, 200 mg/m$^2$ melphalan, 140 mg/m$^2$ melphalan plus TBI, or 140 mg/m$^2$ melphalan plus 12 mg/m$^2$ busulphan. The approach appears to be feasible with the second HDT being delivered in a timely fashion in approximately 75% of patients with a low transplanted related mortality (TRM). One group reported that despite similar response rates between the two arms, there was prolonged progression-free survival (20% vs. 10% at 7 y) and overall survival (42% vs. 21% at 7 y) in the double HDT arm (Attal et al., 2002). Interim analysis reports from the other two trials have shown similar response rates and overall survival rates in the two arms (Cavo et al., 2002; Fermand et al., 2001). Drawing firm conclusions about overall survival benefit from these studies is difficult at present and more follow-up data are required.

# Comparison of High-Dose Therapy (HDT) with Intermediate-Dose Therapy

A number of groups have explored the use of intermediate doses of melphalan as a way of reducing the toxicity of HDT and avoiding the requirement for PBSCT. In one randomized trial, patients aged <70 years received a VAD-based regimen before randomization to either intermediate-dose melphalan (80 mg/m$^2$) with G-CSF or high-dose melphalan (200 mg/m$^2$) plus PBSCT (Singer et al., 2001). An interim analysis demonstrated that although a higher proportion of patients achieved a CR in the HDT arm, there was no difference in the overall survival between the two groups. As a result of the decreased toxicity of such a regimen, this approach has also been explored in an older population of patients (Boccadoro et al., 2002) and results compared with an historical group of younger patients who received HDT. Despite the difference in age between the two groups, progression-free and overall survival were similar. This work has recently been updated by comparing 90 patients receiving 100 mg/m$^2$ melphalan × 2 plus PBSCT with "matched" patients receiving 200 mg/m$^2$ melphalan × 2 plus PBSCT. Despite similar CR rates, progression-free survival was longer in the 200 mg/m$^2$ melphalan group, although overall survival was the same in both groups (Boccadoro et al., 2002). A further trial has examined the effect of additional HDT following intermediate-dose melphalan (Segeren et al., 2003). Newly diagnosed myeloma patients aged <65 years initially received VAD chemotherapy and then were randomized to receive intermediate-dose melphalan (70 mg/m$^2$) × 2 or the same regimen followed by cyclophosphamide (120 mg/kg), TBI, plus PBSCT. There appeared to be no additional effect of this HDT with progression-free and overall survival being similar between the two groups.

## Prognostic Factors for High-Dose Therapy

A number of prognostic factors have been identified as important in predicting survival post-HDT. To date, nearly all centers have identified beta2-microglobulin (β2m) as the single most important prognostic variable with patients with a high β2m at diagnosis having a shorter survival post-HDT (Attal et al., 1996; Barlogie et al., 1997; Child et al., 2003). Importantly, patients with a high β2m still benefit from HDT, with the HRC Myeloma VII trial reporting a median survival of 41.9 months in patients receiving HDT with a high presenting β2m ( > 8 mg/L) compared with 13.1 months in a similar group of patients receiving conventional combination chemotherapy (Child et al., 2003). Patients with 11q breakpoints or partial/complete deletions of chromosome 13 also fare worse following HDT (Barlogie et al., 1999). When both β2m and chromosome 13 abnormalities are taken into account, a group of patients with a particularly poor outlook can be identified (Barlogie et al., 1999; Facon et al., 2001).

The majority of studies have demonstrated that having chemosensitive disease at the time of transplant is also an important prognostic factor (Attal et al., 1996; Barlogie et al., 1997). The introduction of HDT has resulted in more patients attaining complete remissions, and conceptually attaining a CR can be seen as the first step to achieving a cure. It has been suggested that the level of response after HDT might influence outcome and that patients who achieve a CR could have an improved survival. A number of studies have shown improved progression-free and overall survival in patients with CR critically defined by negative immunofixation (Barlogie et al., 1999; Child et al., 2003; Davies et al., 2001; Lahuerta et al., 2000). Even in patients who attain a CR, there is a suggestion that the level of minimal residual disease (MRD) post-HDT measured by PCR or flow cytometry can have prognostic significance. Using a sensitive ASO-PCR, which can detect one normal cell in 10$^6$ tumor cells, PCR-positive patients have a shorter progression-free survival compared with those patients who become PCR negative (Corradini et al., 1999; Martinelli et al., 2000). In another study using a less sensitive consensus fluorescent IgH PCR method, with a sensitivity of 1 in 10$^4$,

there was little additional benefit over serum immunofixation (Davies et al., 2001). Flow cytometry offers an alternative method for the detection of MRD. A recent study suggests that patients who are immunofixation negative and consistently produce plasma cells with a normal phenotype post-HDT have an improved survival compared with patients who are immunofixation negative yet have plasma cells with malignant phenotype (Rawstron et al., 2002).

A number of groups are now investigating the potential for gene expression analysis to add additional prognostic information to conventional criteria. In diffuse large B cell lymphoma and acute myeloid leukemia, cases at presentation have been split into groups of patients with gene expression patterns that have differing overall survivals. Although such studies are still in their infancy in myeloma, preliminary results are promising (Davies et al., 2002; Zhan et al., 2002) and suggest the possibility of future use in stratification for different treatment approaches.

## The Role of Purging in High-Dose Therapy

A particular concern surrounding the reinfusion of autologous progenitor cells following a high-dose procedure has been the contamination of the harvest with myeloma cells, with the potential to proliferate in the marrow leading to disease relapse. In the majority of myeloma cases (70%), the contamination as measured by flow cytometry and polymerase chain reaction is less than one tumor cell in 10$^{3-4}$ normal cells. The cases with high tumor contamination tend to be those with persistent disease within the bone marrow at the time of mobilization (Owen et al., 1996). Using a more sensitive oligospecific PCR, which is able to detect one tumor cell in 10$^6$ normal cells, there is evidence of contamination in almost 100% of cases (Corradini et al., 1995). Whether these cells are clonogenic is a difficult question to address. However, sensitive immunophenotypic tests have suggested that the cells within apheresis products have a similar phenotype to myelomatous plasma cells from the bone marrow but express lower levels of syndecan-1 (Rawstron et al., 1997). There is no definitive evidence from mouse studies regarding this matter but it seems likely that if such cells are reinfused, they could result in or contribute to relapse.

A number of groups have tried to reduce/eliminate the tumor contamination of harvests by either depleting tumor cells or selecting normal hematopoietic progenitor cells by virtue of CD34 expression from autologous bone marrow or peripheral blood stem cells before transplantation (Johnson et al., 1996;

Vescio et al., 1999). Although these methods can achieve up to a 5 log depletion of tumor cells without affecting engraftment, their clinical benefit is unproven because residual tumor cells can still be detected within both the graft and the patient. For purging to be effective, the major source of contamination must be considered to be from the graft with the patient being tumor free, which is unlikely in the majority of cases. A large multicenter randomized study assessing the clinical benefits of CD34 selection in myeloma showed that purging conferred no significant benefit in either progression-free or overall survival (Stewart et al., 2001).

# High-Dose and Reduced Intensity Conditioning Allogeneic Transplantation

Allogeneic bone marrow transplantation has not been widely adopted in the treatment of multiple myeloma because of the high morbidity and mortality (up to 40%) associated with the procedure, especially in older patients. Experience drawn from the European Group for Bone Marrow Transplantation (EBMT; 1983–1993 and 1994–1998) on data from 690 patients showed approximately 50% of patients achieve a complete response, with some of the responses durable (Gahrton et al., 1995, 2001). Important prognostic factors include disease stage, serum β2 microglobulin, extent of previous treatment, and preconditioning remission status (Gahrton et al., 1995). Over the two time periods, the overall survival at 3 years rose from 35% to 56% and treatment-related mortality (TRM) fell from 40% to 30%. This might be presumed to be the result of better patient selection and improved supportive care with a major reduction in bacterial and fungal infections and interstitial pneumonitis. However, the development of both acute and chronic graft versus host disease (GvHD) still accounts for significant morbidity and mortality with incidences of up to 50%. The recently reported SWOG experience supports these findings with many patients experiencing good responses and evidence of long-term disease control. However, 13 of 38 patients in this series died within 6 months of transplantation from a combination of infections and acute GvHD (Kee Lee et al., 2002). The use of peripheral blood stem cell (PBSC) support rather than bone marrow (BM) support has had an impact on survival following allogeneic transplantation for myeloma. The more rapid engraftment associated with PBSC has resulted in a reduced infection rate and the suggestion that this rapid engraftment translates into an improved overall survival (Bensinger et al., 2001; Gahrton et al., 2001). A number of groups have also reported the use of donor lymphocyte infusion (DLI)

following allogeneic BMT for the treatment of relapse (Alyea et al., 2001; Lokhust et al., 1997). Although many patients responded, providing further support for a graft versus myeloma (GvM) effect, GvHD occurred in approximately one-half of the patients, resulting in significant morbidity.

Despite the high TRM of conventional high-dose allogeneic transplantation in myeloma, the assumption that this mode of treatment is most likely to eradicate the myeloma cells and the possibility of a significant GvM effect has encouraged its further consideration. Non-myeloablative or reduced intensity conditioning (RIC) transplantation approaches are currently undergoing evaluation, with the goal of reducing the conditioning regimen-related toxicity while retaining the putative GvM effect of allogeneic transplantation. Immunosuppression rather than cytoreduction is used to induce donor engraftment with minimal toxicity. The approach can be considered in older individuals or patients who would otherwise not be eligible for conventional high-dose allogeneic transplantation because of impaired performance status. This is particularly important in myeloma patients because less than 10% of patients prove eligible for a conventional allograft. A number of conditioning regimens are being investigated using various combinations of low-dose radiotherapy, chemotherapy, and immunosuppressive agents. Initial reports using radiotherapy with mycophenolic acid (MMF) and cyclosporine in end-stage myeloma patients were disappointing because of poor engraftment and poor response rates, which was thought to be the result of the high tumor burden at the time of transplantation (Storb et al., 1999). More recent studies have included low-dose chemotherapy and these studies are more encouraging. The Arkansas group reports such an approach in 31 heavily pretreated patients with myeloma (Badros et al., 2002). Melphalan at a dose of 100 mg/m² was used for sibling RIC allografts and 100 mg/m² melphalan combined with TBI and fludarabine for unrelated RIC allografts. Donor lymphocytes were administered to induce full chimerism or to eradicate residual disease. TRM was 29%, with 58% of patients having acute GvHD and 32% chronic GvHD. Response rates were encouraging given the nature of the patients group, with 61% of patients achieving at least a near complete response. The EBMT have assembled data from 34 European centers on 204 patients receiving RIC allogeneic transplants (Crawley et al., 2002). TRM at 1 year was 13.4% with acute GvHD occurring in 10.5% of patients. Overall survival at 2 years was 49.6%, suggesting the approach is feasible with a lower TRM than conventional allogeneic transplantation. To reduce the tumor burden before the RIC allograft procedure, a number of groups have been investigating its effects following high-dose melphalan and autologous stem cell transplant (Bruno et al., 2002; Kroger et al., 2002; Maloney

=== **TABLE 13-2** ===

## Representative Studies of Mini-Allogeneic Transplantation in Myeloma

| | No. | TRM | Complete Responses | Acute GVHD | Chronic GVHD | PFS | OS |
|---|---|---|---|---|---|---|---|
| Badros et al., 2002 | 31 | 10% early, 20% late | CR 61% PR 10% | 58% | 32% | 1 year 86% | 1 year 86% |
| Kroger et al., 2002 | 17 | 18% | CR 73% PR 20% | 63% | 40% | 2 year 56% | 2 year 74% |
| Maloney et al., 2001 | 31 | 16% | CR 43% PR 31% | 45% | 55% | — | 1 year 81% |
| Crawley et al., 2002 | 204 | 13% | — | 32% | — | | 2 year 50% |
| Hoepfner et al., 2002 | 19 | 32% | — | 37% | — | | 3 year 50% |
| Bruno et al., 2002 | 25 | 0 (early) | CR 56% PR 31% | 48% | — | | 1 year 84% |
| Beltrami et al., 2002 | 17 | 5% | CR 30% | 46% | 29% | | ~1 year 70% |

TRM, transplant-related mortality; GVHD, graft versus host disease; PFS, progression-free survival; OS, overall survival; CR, complete response; PR, partial response.

et al., 2001). The procedure is evidently well tolerated with a TRM of 16% to 18% and all patients achieving full donor chimerism. Response rates are reported as good with a high number of patients achieving a CR (up to 73% using stringent criteria); however, the incidence of GvHD is over 50%, and fungal infections and reactivation of cytomegalovirus were significant complications.

All of these studies have relatively short followup and the possible survival benefit is not yet apparent (Table 13-2). The approach retains the antitumor effect of conventional allogeneic transplantation, is able to induce complete responses, and appears less toxic with less early transplant-related complications and mortality. Conditioning regimens continue to be an important aspect of evaluation with respect to chemotherapy, TBI, and GvHD prophylaxis. The need is to reduce the incidence and intensity of GvHD, which is currently the major complication of the procedure, while retaining the GvM effect.

## Future Directions

Although HDT with autologous stem cells and allogeneic transplantation have been shown to be of benefit for patients with myeloma, these approaches are not appropriate for all patients. The survival curves show no obvious plateau, and the treatments are not curative. Overview of the results of trial data would suggest that the incorporation of HDT in first-line treatment might now be regarded as a standard approach. Although primarily assessed in younger patients, a strict age cutoff is probably not appropriate, and decisions about suitability should be determined by performance status and assessment of individual cases. A "framework" treatment strategy would include HDT to achieve maximal cytoreduction. If a donor was available, an allogeneic procedure would also need to be considered. Further treatment would be aimed at the maintenance of minimal residual disease states, and there would also need to be effective strategies for "refractory" and relapsed disease. The framework approach should have flexibility to allow incorporation of new agents in due course and, ideally, allow critical evaluation in the randomized trial setting. Many of the newer agents are non-cytotoxic-based therapies targeting specific pathways involved in myeloma biology (thalidomide, IMiDs, proteasome inhibitors, Holmium, anti-IL-6, and anti-CD138), or aimed at enhancing allogeneic and autologous anti-myeloma immunity (vaccination strategies using patient-specific idiotype, RNA, and DNA, or pulsed dendritic cells). Early reports are promising but whether they will complement or replace components of current induction/intensification therapies or have roles in maintenance remains to be determined.

## REFERENCES

Alyea, E., Weller, E., Schlossman, R., Canning, C., Webb, I., Doss, D., et al. (2001). T cell depleted allogeneic bone marrow transplantation followed by donor lymphocyte infusion in patients with multiple myeloma: induction of graft versus myeloma effect. *Blood 98*, 934–939.

Attal, M., Harousseau, J. L., Facon, T., Guilhot, F., Doyen, C., Fuzibet, J. G., Monconduit, M., Hullen, C., Caillot, D., Bouabdallah, R., Voillat, L., Sotto, J. J., Grosbois, B., and Bataille, R. (2002). Double autologous transplantation improves survival of multiple myeloma patients: Final analysis of a prospective randomized study of the Intergroupe Francophone du Myelome (IFM 94). *Blood, 100*, abstract 7.

Attal, M., Harousseau, J. L., Stoppa, A. M., Sotto, J. J., Fuzibet, J. G., Rossi, J. F., et al. (1996). Autologous bone marrow transplantation versus conventional chemotherapy in multiple myeloma: A prospective randomized trial. *New England Journal of Medicine, 335*, 91–97.

Attal, M., Huguet, F., Schlaifer, D., Payen, C., Laroche, M., Fournie, B., Mazieres, B., Pris, J., and Laurent, G. (1992). Intensive combined therapy for previously untreated aggressive myeloma. *Blood, 79*, 1130–1136.

Badros, A., Barlogie, B., Siegel, E., Cottler-Fox, M., Zangari, M., Fassas, A., et al. (2002). Improved outcome of allogeneic transplantation in high risk multiple myeloma patients after nonmyeloablative conditioning. *Journal of Clinical Oncology, 20*, 1295–1303.

Barlogie, B., Jagannath, S., Desikan, K. R., Mattox, S., Vesole, D. H., Siegel, G., et al. (1999). Total therapy with tandem transplants for newly diagnosed multiple myeloma. *Blood, 93*, 55–65.

Barlogie, B., Jagannath, S., Vesole, D. H., Naucke, S., Cheson, B., Mattox, S., et al. (1997). Superiority of tandem autologous transplantation over standard therapy for previously untreated multiple myeloma. *Blood, 89*, 789–793.

Beltrami, G., Corsetti, M. T., Musto, P., Carella, A. M., Scalzulli, P. R., Greco, M. M., Lerma, E., and Carella, A. M. (2002). Autografting followed by non-myeloablative allografting (NST) induces high complete remissions in high risk multiple myeloma. *Blood, 100*, 2452.

Bensinger, W. I., Buckner, C. D., Anasetti, C., Clift, R., Storb, R., Barnett, T., et al. (1996b). Allogeneic marrow transplantation for multiple myeloma: Analysis of risk factors on outcome. *Blood, 88*, 2787–2793.

Bensinger, W. I., Rowley, S. D., Demirer, T., Lilleax, K., Schiffman, K., Clift, R. A., et al. (1996a). High dose therapy followed by autologous haemopoietic stem cell infusion in patients with multiple myeloma. *Journal of Clinical Oncology, 14*, 1447–1456.

Bensinger, W. I., Martin, P. J., Storer, B., Clift, R., Forman, S. J., Negrin, R., et al. (2001). Transplantation of bone marrow as compared with peripheral blood cells from HLA identical relatives in patients with hematologic cancers. *New England Journal of Medicine, 334*, 175–181.

Bjorkstrand, B., Ljungham, P., Svensson, H., Hermans, J., Alegre, A., Apperley, J., et al. (1997). Allogeneic bone marrow transplantation versus autologous stem cell transplantation in multiple myeloma—A retrospective case-matched study from the European group for Blood and Marrow Transplantation (EBMT). *Blood, 88*, 4711–4718.

Bladé, J., Esteve, J., Rives, S., Martinez, C., Rovira, M., Urbano-Ispizua, A., Marin, P., Carreras, E., and Montserrat, E. (2000). High-dose therapy autotransplantation/intensification vs. continued standard chemotherapy in multiple myeloma in first remission. Results of a non-randomized study from a single institution. *Bone Marrow Transplantation, 26*, 845–849.

Bladé, J., San Miguel, J. F., Fontanillas, M., Alcala, A., Maldonado, J., Garcia-Conde, J., et al. (1996). Survival of multiple myeloma patients who are potential candidates for early high-dose therapy intensification/autotransplantation and who are conventionally treated. *Journal of Clinical Oncology, 7*, 21667–21673.

Bladé, J., Sureda, A., Ribera, J. M., Diaz-Mediavilla, J., Palomera, L., Fernandez-Calvo, J., et al. (2001). High-dose therapy autotransplantation/intensification vs. continued conventional chemotherapy in multiple myeloma patients responding to initial treatment chemotherapy. Results of a prospective randomized trial from the Spanish Cooperative Group PETHEMA. *Blood, 98*, abstract 3386.

Boccadoro, M., Bringhen, S., Cavallo, F., Falco, P., Bertola, A., Barbui, A., Caravita, T., Musto, P., Pescosta, N., Vignetti, M., and Palumbo, A. (2002). Two dose-intensive melphalan regimens (100 mg/m$^2$ versus 200 mg/m$^2$) in multiple myeloma patients. *Blood, 100*, abstract 1669.

Bruno, B., Patriarca, F., Maloney, D., Mordini, N., Casini, M., Rambaldi, A., Carnevale, F., Allione, B., Soligo, D., Bavaro, P., Aitoro, G., Corradini, P., Fanin, R., Gallamini, A., Coser, P., Levis, A., Aglietta, M., Massaia, M., Palumbo, A., Sandmaier, B., Storb, R.,

and Boccadoro, M. (2002). Autografting followed by non myelo-ablative TBI-based allografting for treatment of multiple myeloma: A multi-center trial. *Blood, 100*, abstract 1642.

Cavo, M., Tosi, P., Zamagni, E., Ronconi, S., Cellini, C., Ronconi, S., De Vivo, A., Cangini, D., Bassarani, M., and Sante, T. (2002). The Bologna 96 clinical trial of single vs. double autotransplants for previously untreated multiple myeloma. *Blood, 100*, abstract 669.

Child, J. A., Morgan, G. J., Davies, F. E., Bell, S. E., Hawkins, K., Brown, J., et al. (2003). High dose therapy improves the outcome of patients with multiple myeloma: The MRC Myeloma VII randomized study. *New England Journal of Medicine, 348*, 1875–1883.

Corradini, P., Voena, C., Astolfi, M., Ladetto, M., Tarella, C., Boccadoro, M., et al. (1995). High dose sequential chemoradiotherapy in multiple myeloma: Residual tumor cells are detectable in bone marrow and peripheral blood cell harvests and after autografting. *Blood, 85*, 1596–1602.

Corradini, P., Voena, C., Tarella, C., Astolfi, M., Ladetto, M., Palumbo, A., et al. (1999). Molecular and clinical remissions in multiple myeloma: Role of autologous and allogeneic transplantation of haematopoietic cells. *Journal of Clinical Oncology, 17*, 208–215.

Crawley, C., Lalanacette, M., Szydlo, R., Gilleece, M., Juliusson, G., Michallet, M., Mackinnon, S., Einsele, H., Reiffers, J., Zander, A. R., Carreras, E., Carella, A., Gratwohl, A., Sotto, J. J., Cavenagh, J. D., Niederweiser, D., Ciceri, F., and Apperley, J. F. (2002). Reduced intensity conditioned allografts for myeloma: A study from the Chronic Leukaemia Working Party of the EBMT. *Blood, 100*, abstract 542.

Cunningham, D., Paz-Ares, L., Milan, S., Powles, R., Nicolson, M., Hiekish, T., et al. (1994). High dose melphalan and autologous bone marrow transplantation as consolidation in previously untreated myeloma. *Journal of Clinical Oncology, 12*, 759–763.

Davies, F. E., Dring, A. M., Rawstron, A. C., Shammas, M., Fenton, J. A. L., Hideshima, T., Chauhan, D., Tai, I. T., Robinson, E., Auclair, D., Rees, K., Gonzalez de Castro, D., Ashcroft, A. J., Dasgupta, R., Mitsiades, C., Mitsiades, N., Chen, L. B., Wong, W., Munshi, N. C., Morgan, G. J., and Anderson, K. C. (2002). Presentation myeloma patients with a normal plasma cell gene expression pattern have a trend towards an improved survival. *Blood, 100*, abstract 1511.

Davies, F. E., Forsyth, P. D., Rawstron, A. C., Owen, R. G., Pratt, G., Evans, P. A., et al. (2001). The impact of attaining a minimal disease state following high dose melphalan and autologous transplantation for multiple myeloma. *British Journal of Haematology, 112*, 814–820.

Facon, T., Avet-Loiseau, H., Guillerm, G., Moreau, P., Genevieve, F., Zandecki, M., et al. (2001). Chromosome 13 abnormalities identified by FISH analysis and serum B2 microglobulin produce a powerful myeloma staging system for patients receiving high dose therapy. *Blood, 97*, 1566–1571.

Fermand, J. P., Chevret, S., Ravaud, P., Divine, M., Leblond, V., Dreyfus, F., et al. (1993). High dose chemoradiotherapy and autologous blood stem cell transplantation in multiple myeloma: Results of a phase II trial involving 63 patients. *Blood, 82*, 2005–2009.

Fermand, J. P., Marolleau, J. P., Alberti, C., Divine, M., Leblond, V., Macro, M., Jaccard, A., Belanger, C., Maloisel, F., Dreyfus, F., Royer, B., McIntyre, E., and Brouet, J. C. (2001). Single versus tandem high dose therapy supported with autologous blood stem cell transplantation using unselected or CD34 enriched ABSC: Preliminary results of a two by two designed randomized trial in 230 young patients with multiple myeloma. *Blood, 98*, abstract 3387.

Fermand, J. P., Ravaud, P., Chevret, S., Divine, M., Leblond, V., Belanger, C., et al. (1998). High dose therapy and autologous blood stem cell transplantation in multiple myeloma: Up front or rescue treatment? Results of a multicenter sequential randomized clinical trial. *Blood, 92*, 3131–3136.

Fermand, J. P., Ravaud, P., Katsahian, S., Divine, M., Leblond, V., Belanger, C., et al. (1999). High dose therapy and autologous blood stem cell transplantation versus conventional treatment in multiple myeloma: results of a randomized trial in 190 patients 55–65 years of age. *Blood, 94,* abstract 1754.

Gahrton, G., Svensson, H., Cavo, M., Apperly, J., Bacigalupo, A., Bjorkstrand, B., et al. (2001). Progress in allogenic bone marrow and peripheral blood stem cell transplantation for multiple myeloma: A comparison between transplants performed 1983–1993 and 1994–1998 at European Group for Blood and Marrow Transplantation centers. *British Journal of Haematology, 113,* 209–216.

Gahrton, G., Tura, S., Ljungman, P., Blade, J., Brandt, L., Cavo, M., et al. (1995). Prognostic factors in allogeneic bone marrow transplantation for multiple myeloma. *Journal of Clinical Oncology, 13,* 1312–1322.

Gore, M. E., Selby, P. J., Viner, C., Clark, P. I., Meldrum, M., Millar, B., et al. (1989). Intensive treatment of multiple myeloma and criteria for complete remission. *Lancet, 2,* 879–882.

Harousseau, J. L., Attal, M., Divine, M., Marit, G., Leblond, V., Stoppa, A. M., et al. (1995). Autologous stem cell transplantation after first remission induction treatment in multiple myeloma: A report of the French Registry on autologous transplantation in multiple myeloma. *Blood, 85,* 3077–3085.

Harousseau, J. L., Facon, T., Mary, J. Y., Attal, M., Bosly, A., Michaux, J. L., Maloisel, F., and Sadoun, A. (1998). What is the optimal timing of autologous transplantation in multiple myeloma. *Cancer Research Therapy and Control, 6,* 255–256.

Hoepfner, S., Probst, S. M., Breitkreutz, I., Moehler, T., Benner, A., Goldschmidt, H., Ho, A. D., and Gorner, M. (2002). Non-myeloablative allogeneic transplantation as part of salvage therapy for relapse of multiple myeloma after autologous transplantation. *Blood, 100,* abstract 3387.

Johnson, R. J., Owen, R. G., Smith, G. M., Child, J. A., Galvin, M., Newton, L. J., et al. (1996). Peripheral blood stem cell transplantation in myeloma using CD34 selected cells. *Bone Marrow Transplantation, 17,* 723–727.

Kee Lee, C., McCoy, J., Anderson, K. C., Kyle, R., Crowley, J., Tricot, G., and Barlogie, B. (2002). Long term follow-up of previously symptomatic myeloma patients treated with myeloablative therapy and sibling-matched allogeneic transplantation of the SWOG study 9321. *Blood, 100,* abstract 1644.

Kroger, N., Schwerdtfeger, R., Kiehl, M., Gottfried, S., Renges, H., Zabelina, T., et al. (2002). Autologous stem cell transplantation followed by a dose-reduced allograft induces high complete remission rate in multiple myeloma. *Blood, 100,* 755–760.

Lahuerta, J. J., Martinez-Lopez, J., Serna, J. D., Blade, J., Grande, C., Algere, A., et al. (2000). Remission status defined by immunofixation vs. electrophoresis after autologous transplantation has a major impact on the outcome of multiple myeloma. *British Journal of Haematology, 109,* 438–446.

Lenhoff, S., Hjorth, M., Holmberg, E., Turesson, I., Westin, J., Nielsen, J. L., et al. (2000). Impact on survival of high dose therapy with autologous stem cell support in patients younger than 60 years with newly diagnosed multiple myeloma: A population based study. *Blood, 95,* 7–11.

Lokhust, H. M., Schattenberg, A., Cornelissen, J. J., Thomas, L. L., Verdonck, L. F. (1997). Donor leucocyte infusions are effective in relapsed multiple myeloma after allogeneic bone marrow transplantation. *Blood, 90,* 4206–4211.

Maloney, D. G., Sahebi, F., Stockerl-Goldstein, K. E., Sandmaier, B. M., Mlina, A. J., Bensinger, W., et al. (2001). Combining an allogeneic graft vs. myeloma effect with high dose autologous stem cell rescue in the treatment of multiple myeloma. *Blood, 98,* abstract 1822.

Marit, G., Faberes, C., Aco, J. L., Boiron, J. M., Bourmis, J. H., Brault, P., et al. (1996). Autologous peripheral blood progenitor cell support following high dose chemotherapy or chemoradiotherapy in patients with high risk multiple myeloma. *Journal of Clinical Oncology, 14,* 1306–1313.

Martinelli, G., Terragna, C., Zamagni, E., Ronconi, S., Tosi, P., Lemoli, R. M., et al. (2000). Molecular remission after allogeneic or autologous transplantation of haematopoietic stem cells for multiple myeloma. *Journal of Clinical Oncology, 18,* 2273–2281.

McElwain, T. J., and Powles, R. L. (1983). High dose intravenous melphalan for plasma-cell leukaemia and myeloma. *Lancet, ii,* 822–824.

Owen, R. G., Johnson, R. J., Rawstron, A. C., Evans, P. A. S., Jack, A., Smith, G. M., et al. (1996). Assessment of IgH PCR strategies in multiple myeloma. *Journal of Clinical Pathology, 49,* 672–675.

Rawstron, A. C., Davies, F. E., Dasgupta, R., Ashcroft, A. J., Patmore, R., Drayson, M. T., et al. (2002). Flow cytometric disease monitoring in multiple myeloma: The relationship between normal and neoplastic plasma cells predicts outcome post-transplantation. *Blood, 100,* 3095–3100.

Rawstron, A. C., Owen, R. G., Davies, F. E., Johnson, R. J., Jones, R. A., Richards, S. J., et al. (1997). Circulating plasma cells in multiple myeloma: Characterisation and correlation with disease stage. *British Journal of Haematology, 97,* 46–55.

Schiller, G., Vescio, R., Frettes, C., Stizer, G., Sahebi, F., Lee, M., et al. (1995). Transplantation of CD34+ peripheral blood progenitor cells after high dose chemotherapy for patients with advanced multiple myeloma. *Blood, 86,* 390–397.

Segeren, C. M., Sonneveld, P., Van der Holt, B., et al. (2003). Overall and event-free survival are not improved by the use of myeloablative therapy following intensifies chemotherapy in previously untreated patients with multiple myeloma: a prospective randomized phase 3 study. *Blood, 101,* 2144–2151.

Selby, P. J., McElwain, T. J., Nandi, A. C., Perren, T. J., Powles, R. L., Tillyer, C. R., Osborne, R. J., Slevin, M. L., and Malpas, J. S. (1987). Multiple myeloma treated with high dose intravenous melphalan. *British Journal of Haematology, 66,* 55–62.

Singer, C. R. J., Cavenagh, J., Mills, M., et al. (2001). Preliminary report of a multicenter randomized study of high dose or intermediate dose melphalan after initial VAD/VAMP therapy of myeloma. VIIIth International Workshop on Multiple Myeloma, May 4–8; Banff, Canada.

Stewart, A. K., Vescio, R., Schiller, G., Ballester, O., Noga, S., Rugo, H., et al. (2001). Purging of autologous peripheral blood stem cells using cell selection does not improve overall or progression free survival after high dose chemotherapy for multiple myeloma: Results of a multicenter randomized controlled trial. *Journal of Clinical Oncology, 19,* 3771–3779.

Storb, R., Yu, C., Sandmaier, B., McSweeney, P., Georges, G., Nash, R., et al. (1999). Mixed haematopoietic chimerism after haematopoietic stem cell allografts. *Transplantation Proceedings, 31,* 677–678.

Vescio, R., Schiller, G., Stewart, A. K., Ballester, O., Noga, S., Rugo, H., et al. (1999). Multicenter phase III trial to evaluate CD34+ selected versus unselected autologous peripheral blood progenitor cell transplantation in multiple myeloma. *Blood, 93,* 1858–1868.

Vesole, D. H., Tricot, G., Jagannath, S., Desikan, K. R., Siegel, D., Bracy, D., et al. (1996). Autotransplantation in multiple myeloma: What have we learned? *Blood, 88,* 838–847.

Zhan, F., Hardin, J., Lordsmeier, B., et al. (2002). Global gene expression profiling of multiple myeloma monoclonal gammopathy of undetermined significance and normal bone marrow plasma cells. *Blood, 99,* 1745–1757.

# CHAPTER 14

# Novel Therapies for Multiple Myeloma

TERU HIDESHIMA
PAUL G. RICHARDSON
KENNETH C. ANDERSON

## Introduction

The conventional therapies, including alkylating agents, anthracyclines, and corticosteroids, have not achieved long-term benefit in multiple myeloma (MM) (Grogan et al., 1993; Salmon et al., 1983; Sonneveld et al., 1997) as a result of the inevitable development of tumor cell resistance. In this chapter, we describe recent preclinical studies and early clinical trials of novel agents targeting not only MM cells, but also their bone marrow (BM) milieu (Table 14-1), which demonstrate great promise to overcome classic drug resistance and improve patient outcome.

## Novel Agents Targeting Both MM Cells and Interactions of MM Cells with the Bone Marrow Microenvironment

### Thalidomide (Thal) and Its Analogs

Thalidomide (Thal; alpha-N[phthalimido]glutarimide), a derivative of glutamic acid pharmacologically classified as an immunomodulatory agent (IMiD) (Tseng et al., 1996), inhibits tumor necrosis factor (TNF)α production (Moreira et al.,

## TABLE 14-1
### Novel Agents for Myeloma

**Targeting both MM cells and interaction of MM cells with the bone marrow microenvironment**
Thalidomide and its analogs (lMiDs, S-3APG)
Proteasome inhibitor (PS-341)
Arsenic trioxide
2-Methoxyestradiol (2-ME2)
Lysophosphatidic acid acyltransferase-β inhibitor

**Targeting circuits mediating MM cell growth and survival**
VEGF receptor tyrosine kinase inhibitor (PTK787/ZK 222584)
Farnesyltransferase inhibitor
Histone deacetylase inhibitor (SAHA, LAQ824)
Heat shock protein-90 inhibitor (Geldanamycin)
Telomerase inhibitor (Telomestatin)
Non-taxane microtubule stabilizing agent (Epothilone B)
bcl-2 antisense oligonucleotide (Genasense)

**Targeting the bone marrow microenvironment**
IκB kinase (IKK) inhibitor (PS-1145)
p38 MAPK inhibitor (VX-745)
Neovastat (AE-941)

**Targeting cell surface receptors**
TNF-related apoptosis-inducing ligand/Apo2 ligand
IGF-1 receptor inhibitor (ADW)
HMG-CoA reductase inhibitor (Statins)
Anti-CD20 antibody (Rituximab)

1993; Sampaio et al., 1991, 1993) and angiogenesis by blocking basic fibroblast growth factor (bFGF) and/or vascular endothelial growth factor (VEGF) (D'Amato et al., 1994b; Kenyon et al., 1997; Kotoh et al., 1999). Although Thal was withdrawn from clinical use in the 1960s as a result of reports of teratogenicity and phocomelia associated with its use, Thal and IMiDs have been more recently used to treat inflammatory and malignant diseases.

Potential anti-MM activities of Thal and IMiDs are multiple. First, Thal/IMiDs have a direct effect on MM cells to induce G1 growth arrest or apoptosis, even of drug-resistant cells (Hideshima et al., 2000; Mitsiades et al., 2002d). Thal inhibits DNA binding activity of the p50/p65 NF-κB heterodimer triggered by TNFα and IL-1β in Jurkat cells (Keifer et al., 2001), and we have shown that IMiDs inhibit NF-κB activity in MM cells (Mitsiades et al., 2002d). Because NF-κB plays an essential role in cell survival, antiapoptosis, and cytokine production not only in MM (Hideshima et al., 2001a, 2002a), but also in other cancers, inhibition of NF-κB activation by Thal/IMiDs might enhance sensitivity to other chemotherapeutic agents. Moreover, our studies in MM show that Thal/IMiD-induced apoptosis is caspase-8 mediated, suggesting the benefit of coupling these agents with agents triggering caspase-9-mediated apoptosis (i.e., dexamethasone [Dex]) to induce dual apoptotic signaling (Chauhan et al., 1997; Hideshima

et al., 2000; Mitsiades et al., 2002d). Second, Thal/IMiDs inhibit adhesion of MM cells to BM stromal cells (SCs), and thereby can overcome cell adhesion-mediated drug resistance (CAM-DR) (Damiano et al., 1999; Hazlehurst et al., 2000). Third, Thal/IMiDs inhibit bioactivity and/or secretion in MM cells and/or BMSCs of cytokines, which augment MM cell growth, survival, drug resistance, and migration. Fourth, these agents demonstrate antiangiogenic activity, at least in part by inhibiting βFGF and/or VEGF (D'Amato et al., 1994b; Kenyon et al., 1997; Kotoh et al., 1999). Finally, Thal/IMiDs might be acting against MM through immunomodulatory effects, such as induction of a Th1 T cell response with secretion of interferon gamma (IFN γ) and IL-2 (Haslett et al., 1999). Most recently, we have shown that NK cell anti-MM immunity can also be induced both *in vitro* and *in vivo* by Thal and IMiDs (Fig. 14-1) (Davies et al., 2001).

Recently, a new derivative of thalidomide, S-3-[3-amino-phthalimido]-glutarimide (S-3APG) with dual activity against B-cell neoplasias has been reported (Lentzsch et al., 2002). S-3APG inhibits the proliferation of MM and Burkitt's lymphoma cell lines *in vitro* without toxicity to normal BMSCs or hematopoietic progenitor cells. *In vivo*, S-3APG treatment of drug-resistant MM in mice achieved complete and sustained regressions without toxicity. S-3APG also inhibits angiogenesis more potently than Thal (Lentzsch et al., 2002; Treston et al., 2002).

These preclinical observations have been translated to the bedside in derived clinical trials. Thal therapy has been reported from the University of Arkansas in a large phase II clinical trial in patients with relapsed and refractory MM (Singhal et al., 1999). In this study, the serum or urine levels of paraprotein were reduced by at least 90% in 8 patients, at least 75% in 6 patients, at least 50% in 7 patients, and at least 25% in 6 patients, for an overall 32% response rate. Reductions in paraprotein levels were apparent within 2 months in 78% of patients, and were associated with decreased numbers of BM plasma cells and increased hemoglobin levels. This clinical trial, therefore, demonstrated for the first time that Thal can achieve marked durable responses in some patients with relapsed and/or refractory MM. Another phase II trial of Thal in 45 patients with MM resistant to conventional therapies has been reported from M.D. Anderson Cancer Center. In this study, partial response or greater (defined by ≥50% reduction of serum MM protein and/or ≥75% reduction of Bence-Jones protein) was achieved in 26% of patients (Alexanian and Weber, 2000). At the Mayo Clinic, 16 patients, 25% of whom had failed stem cell transplants and 88% who had received 2 or more prior chemotherapy regimens, received 200 mg Thal per day for 2 weeks, which was escalated by 200 mg per day every 2 weeks to a maximum of 800 mg per day as tolerated (Rajkumar et al., 2000). Four (25%) patients

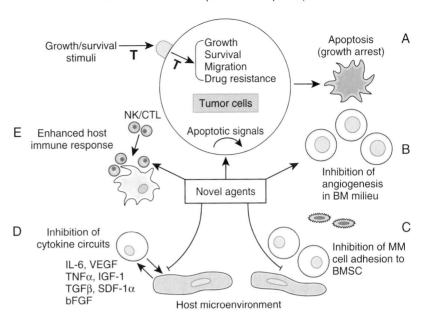

*Figure 14-1 Novel MM therapies induce apoptosis (A), inhibit angiogenesis in MM BM milieu (B), inhibit MM cell adhesion to BMSC (C), inhibit cytokine circuits in MM BM milieu and (D), enhance host immune response (E).*

achieved partial response, defined as ≥50% reduction in serum and urine protein level of 2 to 10 months' duration. These studies confirm the activity of Thal in MM and further suggest that it should be evaluated in combination with other drugs or as maintenance therapy. Finally, the combination of Dex and Thal has recently been reported in 50 patients with newly diagnosed MM; 64% of patients responded (Rajkumar et al., 2002). This study suggests that response rates to Thal combined with Dex in newly diagnosed patients are twice as high as those achieved after Thal treatment of relapsed refractory MM. Thal/Dex did not preclude subsequent stem cell collection and autotransplantation, and Thal/Dex therefore represents a novel effective induction regimen (Richardson, 2002a).

Most recently, we have completed a phase I study of Revimid (IMiD3, CC-5013) in patients with relapsed, refractory MM (Richardson et al., 2002). In these patients with progressive MM and rising paraproteins despite conventional therapy, remarkable anti-MM clinical activity, evidenced by >25% decrease in MM serum paraprotein, was achieved in two-thirds of patients; stabilization or a decrease in MM paraprotein was evident in 79% of patients. Based on this promising anti-MM activity and very favorable side effect profile, phase II trials are either ongoing or will begin soon to define the clinical use of Revimid in patients with newly diagnosed MM, at the time of first relapse, and as a maintenance therapy post-autografting in MM.

## Proteasome Inhibitor PS-341

The ubiquitin-proteasome pathway (UPP) is a proteolytic system in both the cytosol and nucleus, which regulates cyclin and cyclin-dependent kinase (CDK) inhibitor proteins, thereby regulating cell cycle progression (King et al., 1996). PS-341 (pyrazylcarbonyl-Phe-Leu-boronate, Velcade) represents a class of peptide boronate proteasome inhibitors that inhibit 26S proteasome activity (Kisselv and Goldberg, 2001). The initial rationale to use proteasome inhibitor in MM was its inhibitory effect on nuclear factor (NF)-κB activation, because NF-κB regulates transcription of IL-6 in BMSCs, adhesion molecule (CD54, CD106) expression on MM cells and BMSCs, cell cycle (cyclin D1), and antiapoptotic protein (IAPs, Bcl-xL) expression in MM cells. Importantly, our previous studies in MM demonstrated that NF-κB activation confers drug resistance; regulates adhesion molecule expression on MM cells and BMSCs with related binding and drug resistance; and regulates both constitutive and MM cell adhesion-induced cytokine transcription and secretion in BMSCs (Chauhan et al., 1996; Hideshima et al., 2001a, 2001c). Specifically, PS-341 blocks the degradation of IκBα, an inhibitory protein constitutively bound to cytosolic NF-κB, and thereby inhibits IκBα degradation, related nuclear translocation, and binding of NF-κB to its binding consensus in DNA. PS-341 was therefore of great interest as a novel therapeutic agent to overcome drug resistance in MM cells, inhibit binding of MM cells in BM, and abrogate transcription and secretion of cytokines in the BM microenvironment. Our *in vitro* studies to date have confirmed that PS-341 induces apoptosis through caspase-8 and -9 followed by caspase-3 activation in drug-resistant MM cell lines and patient cells (Hideshima et al., 2001c, in press; Mitsiades et al., 2002c); downregulates expression of adhesion molecules on MM cells and BMSCs and related binding (Hideshima et al., 2001a, 2001c); blocks constitutive and MM cell adhesion-induced

NF-κB-dependent cytokine secretion in BMSCs (32); and inhibits angiogenesis (Fig. 14-1) (LeBlanc et al., 2002).

Although PS-341 inhibits NF-κB activation, the molecular mechanisms of its anti-MM activity are not fully defined. Our gene microarray profiling demonstrates that PS-341 downregulates growth and survival gene transcription; with an associated induction of apoptotic, ubiquitin/proteasome, and stress response gene transcripts in MM cells (Mitsiades et al., 2002c). These studies define molecular targets conferring sensitivity and resistance to PS-341; provide the molecular rationale for combination strategies with conventional or novel agents; and provide for the development of next-generation targeted more potent, selective, and less toxic agents. Importantly, our most recent studies show that PS-341 also inhibits DNA repair by cleavage of DNA-dependent protein kinase catalytic subunit (DNA-PKcs) (Hideshima et al., 2003). This bioactivity might have important clinical application, because treatment of MM cell lines resistant to DNA damaging agents (melphalan, anthracycline) with those agents to which they are resistant, followed 12 to 24 hours later with sublethal doses of PS-341, can inhibit repair of DNA damage and thereby overcome drug resistance, restoring sensitivity to DNA damaging agents (Mitsiades et al., 2002g). Most recently, we showed that PS-341 induces caspase-dependent cleavage of gp130 (CD130), the β-subunit of IL-6 receptor (Hideshima et al., submitted), thereby blocking IL-6 mediated downstream Raf/MEK/p42/44 MAPK, JAK2/STAT3, and PI3-K/Akt signaling pathways. Therefore, PS-341-induced cleavage of gp130 blocks both IL-6-induced and cell adhesion-mediated MM cell growth, survival, and drug resistance in the BM microenvironment.

PS-341 also has remarkable *in vivo* anti-MM activity. In a dose-dependent manner, it inhibits human MM cell growth, decreases tumor-associated angiogenesis, and prolongs host survival in SCID mice bearing human MM cells (LeBlanc et al., 2002). These preclinical studies have already translated to the bedside. Phase I trials in humans have established the safety profile and dose regimen for phase II trials. Most importantly, preliminary analysis of a recently completed phase II trial of PS-341 treatment of patients with refractory relapsed MM achieved 35% responses, including 10% complete and near-complete responses. Responses were durable (median, 12 mo) and associated with clinical benefit, including improvement in quality of life; increased hemoglobin and decreased transfusions; improved renal function; and increase in normal immunoglobulin levels (Richardson et al., 2002). Drug-related gastrointestinal toxicity and fatigue were in most cases manageable; thrombocytopenia and neuropathy occurred primarily in patients in whom these conditions were preexistent. Based on this promising clinical activity and tolerable toxicity profile in patients with advanced disease, PS-341 is now undergoing evaluation in phase II trials to treat patients with MM at earlier stages (newly diagnosed, at first relapse), and is being compared with Dex in a multicenter international phase III trial of patients with relapsed MM.

## Arsenic Trioxide (As$_2$O$_3$)

Our studies show that As$_2$O$_3$ also induces apoptosis in drug-resistant MM cell lines and patient cells through caspase-9 activation; inhibits activation of JAK/STAT3 and upregulation of Mcl-1 triggered by IL-6; and inhibits NF-κB activation in BMSCs, thereby downregulating CD54 expression and tumor cell-BM stromal cell binding as well as inhibiting paracrine IL-6 and VEGF transcription and secretion in BMSCs (Hayashi et al., 2002). Deaglio and colleagues have reported that As$_2$O$_3$ increases killing of MM cells mediated by lymphokine-activated killer (LAK) cells through selective upregulation of CD38 and CD54 on MM cells, as well as CD31 and CD11a on LAK cells (Fig. 14-1) (Deaglio et al., 2001). Preliminary analysis of phase I/II clinical trials of As$_2$O$_3$ in patients with refractory or relapsed MM shows minor decreases or stabilization in MM-paraprotein; side effects include leukopenia, anemia, abdominal pain and diarrhea, fever, and fatigue (Hussein et al., 2001). Moreover, As$_2$O$_3$-induced MM cell cytotoxicity might be enhanced by ascorbic acid (Grad et al., 2001). Based on *in vitro* studies showing that Dex enhances MM cell apoptosis induced by As$_2$O$_3$ (Hayashi et al., 2002), a clinical trial of this combination therapy is ongoing.

## 2-Methoxyestradiol (2ME2)

2ME2 is a natural metabolite of estradiol with potent antitumor and antiangiogenic activity in leukemia *in vitro* and *in vivo* (D'Amato et al., 1994a; Klauber et al., 1997). Although a natural derivative of estradiol (E2), 2ME2 binds poorly to the estrogen receptor and mediates its antiproliferative effects independent of either estrogen receptor expression or responsiveness. We have demonstrated that 2ME2 inhibits growth and induces apoptosis in drug-resistant MM cell lines and patient cells; enhances Dex-induced apoptosis; overcomes the protective effect of IL-6 and IGF-1; as well as decreases secretion of VEGF and IL-6 in BM stromal cells triggered by MM cell binding (Fig. 14-1) (Chauhan et al., 2002a). In our study, 2ME-induced MM cell apoptosis through release of mitochondrial cytochrome-c and second mitochondria-derived activator of caspases (Smac), followed by activation of caspases-8, -9, and -3. We further delineated the molecular mechanisms of anti-MM activity of 2ME2 using gene microarray profiling (Chauhan et al., 2002b). Based on these preclinical studies, 2ME2 is presently under evaluation in a phase II clinical trial in MM.

## Lysophosphatidic Acid Acyltransferase (LPAAT)-β Inhibitor

Lysophosphatidic acid (LPA) and phosphatidic acid (PA) are 2 phospholipids involved in signal transduction and in lipid biosynthesis. We have recently examined the effects of isoform specific functional inhibitors (Cell Therapeutic Inc., Seattle, WA) of the enzyme lysophosphatidic acid acyltransferase (LPAAT), which converts lysophosphatidic acid (Lyso-PA) to PA, on MM cell growth and survival. These compounds demonstrate potent cytotoxicity against MM cell lines and patient MM cells with IC50 of 50–100 nM. LPAAT-β inhibitors trigger apoptosis in MM cells through PARP cleavage, and IL-6 and IGF-1 do not inhibit LPAAT-β inhibitor-induced apoptosis. Furthermore, LPAAT-β inhibitors induce cytotoxicity even in the presence of BMSCs (Hideshima et al., 2002b), suggesting that they can overcome CAM-DR (Fig. 14-1). Our data therefore provides the framework for clinical trials of these novel agents in MM.

# Novel Agents Targeting Circuits Within the Cell Mediating MM Cell Growth and Survival

## PTK787/ZK222584

Because of the increased angiogenesis in MM BM, we and others have characterized the role of VEGF in MM (Bellamy et al., 1999; Podar et al., 2001, 2002). VEGF is expressed and secreted by MM cells and BMSCs; moreover, VEGF secreted by MM cells augments IL-6 secretion in BMSCs (Bellamy et al., 1999; Dankbar et al., 2000; Gupta et al., 2001). High-affinity VEGF receptor (VEGFR) Flt-1 is expressed in MM cells and plasma cell leukemia (PCL) cells; VEGF triggers phosphorylation of this receptor and downstream p42/44 MAPK activation and proliferation, which can be inhibited by anti-VEGF antibody or MEK inhibitor PD98059 (Podar et al., 2001). VEGF also induces migration of MM cells, which can be abrogated by the PKC inhibitor bisindolylmaleimide I hydrochloride (BIM). In addition, VEGF triggers activation of PI3-K/Akt; coupled with β1-integrin–mediated binding to fibronectin, PI3-K triggers recruitment and activation of PKCα, and thereby further enhances migration of MM cells (Podar et al., 2001). Importantly, VEGF receptor tyrosine kinase inhibitor PTK787/ZK222584 blocks VEGF-induced tyrosine phosphorylation of Flt-1, MEK/MAPK activation, and proliferation, as well as PKC activation-dependent migration (Fig. 14-1) (Lin et al., 2002). These studies both define VEGF as a novel therapeutic target and provide the basis for a clinical trial of PTK787/ZK222584 in patients with relapsed MM.

## Farnesyltransferase Inhibitors (FTIs)

The cytosolic enzyme farnesyltransferase transfers the farnesyl group from farnesyl diphosphate to the CAAX motif of Ras, thereby facilitating its attachment to the inner plasma cell membrane and related signal transduction (Kato et al., 1992). Inhibition of farnesylation is therefore a strategy for blocking Ras activity, and several farnesyltransferase inhibitors (FTI) inhibit tumor cell growth both *in vitro* and *in vivo* (Karp et al., 2001a). We have demonstrated that cytokine (IL-6, VEGF, IGF-1)-induced proliferation or MM cells is mediated through Ras/Raf/MAPK signaling (Fig. 14-1) (Adjei et al., 2001; Mitsiades et al., 2002e; Ogata et al., 1997; Podar et al., 2001), providing the preclinical rationale for ongoing phase I/II clinical trials of 2 FTIs, SCH-66336 (Adjei et al., 2001) and R115777 (Karp et al., 2001b).

## Histone Deacetylase (HDAC) Inhibitors

Histone acetylation modulates gene expression, cellular differentiation, and survival; it is regulated by histone acetyltransferases (HATs) and histone deacetylases. Novel hydroxamic acid-based hybrid polar compounds, such as suberoylanilide hydroxamic acid (SAHA), are histone deacetylase inhibitors; they induce accumulation of acetylated core nucleosomal histones, with related induction of differentiation and/or apoptosis in transformed and neoplastic cells. We have demonstrated that SAHA induces growth arrest and apoptosis in MM patient cells and cell lines, even those resistant to Dex or conventional chemotherapy. We also recently reported the effect of new cinnamyl hydroxamic acid HDAC inhibitor LAQ824 in MM cells (Catley et al., 2002). LAQ824 induces caspase-dependent MM cell apoptosis, and inhibits both 20S proteasome activity and constitutive activation of NF-κB in MM (Fig. 14-1). Phase I clinical testing of LAQ824 is underway.

## Heat Shock Protein-90 (Hsp90) Inhibitors

Hsp90 is a molecular chaperone that facilitates intracellular protein trafficking, conformational maturation, and 3-dimensional folding required for protein function. The Ansamycin antibiotic Geldanamycin (GA) and its analogs bind to the critical ATP-binding site of Hsp90, thereby abrogating its chaperoning activity in the MM BM milieu; decreasing IGF-1R and IL-6R expression on MM cells; depleting growth kinases (e.g., Akt, IKK, Raf) and antiapoptotic proteins (FLIP, XIAP, cIAP, telomerase); as well as inhibiting both constitutive and cytokine-induced activation of NF-κB and telomerase (hTERT) in the BM milieu (Fig. 14-1) (Mitsiades et al., 2001a). GA and other Hsp90 inhibitors induce apoptosis of MM cell lines and patient cells that are resistant to Dex, anthracyclines, Thal or IMiDs, TRAIL/Apo2L, and PS-341. Importantly, our gene microarray profiling shows that PS-341 induces Hsp90 in MM cells; conversely, blocking this response with GA enhances PS-341-triggered MM cell apoptosis (Mitsiades et al., 2002c). These data, coupled with *in vivo* anti-MM activity of GA in an SCID mouse model of human MM, provide the framework for a derived clinical trial in MM.

## Telomestatin (Telomerase Inhibitor)

Telomestatin is a natural product isolated from Streptomyces anulatus 3533-SV4, which has antitelomerase activity. Its structural similarity to G-tetrad suggests that its telomerase inhibition might be the result of its ability to selectively facilitate the formation of or to stabilize intramolecular G-quadruplexes (Kim et al., 2002; Shin-ya et al., 2001). We have recently shown that treatment of MM cell lines with Telomestatin induces apoptosis after 3- to 4-week cultures associated with telomere shortening (Shammas et al., 2002). Our results therefore identify telomerase as another novel therapeutic target in MM.

## Epothilone B (EPO906)

The epothilones are non-taxane microtubule-stabilizing agents obtained from the fermentation of the cellulose degrading myxobacteria, Sorangium cellulosum. A novel epothilone B analogue BMS-247550 induces cell cycle arrest at the G(2)-M phase transition and subsequent apoptotic cell death of MDA-MB-468 (468) in breast cancer cells (Yamaguchi et al., 2002); our recent study has shown that EPO906 (Novartis Pharmaceuticals, Summit, NJ) also directly inhibits growth and survival of MM cells (IC90 between 1 and 10 nM), including drug-resistant MM cells, and that IL-6 and IGF-1 do not block this effect (Fig. 14-1). EPO906 also prolongs the median survival of SCID mice transplanted with human MM cells (Lin et al., 2002a). These *in vitro* and *in vivo* studies provide the basis for clinical studies.

## Genasense (G3139, bcl-2 Antisense Oligonucleotide)

Members of Bcl-2 family of proteins (i.e., Bcl-2, Bcl-X$_L$, Bcl-X$_S$, Bax, and so on) regulate apoptosis and drug resistance in MM. Overexpression of Bcl-2 has

also been correlated with resistance to interferon (Sangfelt et al., 1995). Dex-induced apoptosis in ARP-1 and RPMI 8226 MM cell lines is correlated with the level of Bcl-2 expression; specifically, resistance to Dex, but not melphalan, is associated with overexpression of Bcl-2 (Gazitt et al., 1998). Genasense (Genta, Inc., Berkeley Heights, NJ) is a bcl-2 antisense oligonucleotide that reduces both bcl-2 mRNA and protein levels in MM cell lines and MM patient cells, reducing Bcl-2 protein by 75% in 4 days (Klasa et al., 2002). Phase I-II trials of this agent in hematologic and solid tumors have shown that Genasense downregulates Bcl-2 protein and has an acceptable toxicity profile; a phase III trial comparing Dex versus Dex plus Genasense is nearly completed.

# Novel Agents Targeting Tumor Cell Interactions with the Bone Marrow Microenvironment

## IκB Kinase (IKK) Inhibitor PS-1145

We have recently used the novel-specific IκB kinase (IKK) inhibitor PS-1145 to delineate the selective effect of NF-κB blockade in the MM BM milieu. PS-1145 only partially inhibits MM cell proliferation, suggesting that NF-κB blockade cannot account for all of the anti-MM activity of proteasome inhibitor PS-341. Importantly, however, PS-1145 blocks NF-κB activation in MM cells and BMSCs, as well as sequelae, including adhesion molecule expression and MM cell-BMSC binding; proliferation of adherent MM cells; as well as IL-6 transcription and secretion in BMSCs (Fig. 14-1) (Hideshima et al., 2002a). These studies highlight the importance of examining the effects of novel therapeutics on MM cells in their BM microenvironment, and demonstrate that specific targeting of NF-κB can overcome the growth and survival advantage conferred both by MM cell binding to BM stromal cells and cytokine secretion in the BM milieu.

## p38 MAPK Inhibitor

p38 mitogen-activated protein kinase (MAPK) is activated by cytokines and growth factors; and activation of p38 MAPK is associated with IL-6 gene expression and/or protein secretion in Sertoli cells (De Cesaris et al., 1998), myocardial cells (Craig et al., 2000), and osteoblasts (Chae et al., 2001). We have recently demonstrated that the specific p38 MAPK inhibitor VX-745 (Vertex Pharmaceuticals Inc, Cambridge, MA) inhibits IL-6 and VEGF secretion in BMSCs, without affecting their viability. TNF-α-induced IL-6 secretion in BMSCs is also inhibited by VX-745. Importantly,

VX-745 inhibits both MM cell proliferation and IL-6 secretion in BMSCs triggered by adherence of MM cells to BMSCs, suggesting that it can both inhibit paracrine MM cell growth in the BM milieu and overcome cell adhesion-related drug resistance (Fig. 14-1) (Hideshima et al., 2003). These studies therefore identify p38 MAPK as a novel therapeutic target to overcome drug resistance and improve patient outcome in MM.

### Neovastat (AE-941)

Neovastat (AE-941) is a shark cartilage extract, which inhibits blood vessel formation in the chicken embryo vascularization assay and blocks endothelial cell proliferation (Beliveau et al., 2002; Falardeau et al., 2001). It also inhibits *in vivo* formation of blood vessels in Matrigel implants containing bFGF (Beliveau et al., 2002). Phase I clinical trials have established that Neovastat is well tolerated, and a phase II clinical trial in early relapsed and refractory MM is ongoing.

# Novel Agents Targeting Cell Surface Receptors

### Tumor Necrosis Factor (TNF)-Related Apoptosis-Inducing Ligand/Apo2 Ligand (TRAIL/Apo2L)

We have shown that TRAIL/Apo2L, a member of TNF superfamily of death-inducing ligands which includes TNFα and Fas ligand (FasL), induces downstream caspase 8-mediated apoptosis of human MM cell lines and patient MM cells, including those resistant to conventional therapies (Mitsiades et al., 2001b, 2002b). TRAIL/Apo2L also inhibits growth of S6B45 human MM cells in SCID mice (Mitsiades et al., 2001b). Our preclinical studies provide the rationale for inducing TRAIL apoptotic signaling to overcome drug resistance in MM.

### Insulin-Like Growth Factor (IGF)-1 Receptor Inhibitors

We have recently shown that IGF-1 receptor tyrosine kinase inhibitor ADW (Novartis AG, Basel, Switzerland) mediates anti-MM activity in both *in vitro* and *in vivo* SCID/NOD mouse models of human MM (Mitsiades et al., 2002a). Because IGF-1 is a major survival and antiapoptotic factor in MM (Mitsiades et al., 2002f; Ogawa et al., 2000; Tu et al., 2000), blockade of IGF-1-mediated signaling cascades is a promising therapeutic option for MM cell.

### Statins

Statins (lovastatin, fluvastatin) are irreversible inhibitors of HMG-CoA reductase, which block production of mevalonate, a critical compound in the synthesis of cholesterol and isoprenoids. Isoprenylation of target proteins, including GTP-binding protein Ras, is essential for their membrane localization and intracellular signaling. Lovastatin effectively induces apoptosis in MM cell lines and MM patients' tumor cells, and is effective in combination with other therapeutic drugs (van De Donk et al., 2002). Importantly, we have recently shown that lovastatin induces apoptosis in patient MM cells, even those resistant to both conventional and novel (IMiD3, PS-341) chemotherapeutic agents (Mitsiades et al., 2002c).

### Anti-CD20 Ab (Rituximab)

Serotherapy directed against CD20 targets only a minority of MM patients, because CD20 expression is uncommon in MM (20% CD20+). We have recently evaluated the effect of the anti-CD20 monoclonal antibody Rituximab in 19 previously treated MM patients. Six of 19 (32%) patients had either a partial response or stable disease, with a median time to treatment failure of 5.5 months. All 6 patients who responded had CD20+ MM cells (Treon et al., 2002).

# Conclusions and Future Directions

Although conventional and high-dose therapy can modestly improve outcome in MM, few, if any, patients are cured. However, a new treatment paradigm is evolving in MM using novel agents that target not only the MM cell, but also the MM cell–host interaction and BM milieu. These novel agents, used alone or in combination with conventional or other novel agents, offer great promise to improve patient outcome in MM. Importantly, gene array and proteomic evaluation of MM and BM samples from patients treated with these novel agents on clinical protocols will define molecular mechanisms of tumor cell sensitivity versus resistance, thereby providing the framework for developing next-generation more potent, selective, and less toxic targeted MM therapies.

## REFERENCES

Adjei, A. A., Davis, J. N., Bruzek, L. M., Erlichman, C., and Kaufmann, S. H. (2001). Synergy of the protein farnesyltransferase inhibitor SCH66336 and cisplatin in human cancer cell lines. *Clinical Cancer Research, 7,* 1438–1445.

Alexanian, R., and Weber, D. (2000). Thalidomide for resistant and relapsing myeloma. *Seminars in Hematology, 37,* 22–25.

Beliveau, R., Gingras, D., Kruger, E. A., Lamy, S., Sirois, P., Simard, B., Sirois, M. G., Tranqui, L., Baffert, F., Beaulieu, E., Dimitriadou, V., Pepin, M. C., Courjal, F., Ricard, I., Poyet, P., Falardeau, P., Figg, W. D., and Dupont, E. (2002). The antiangiogenic agent Neovastat (AE-941) inhibits vascular endothelial growth factor-mediated biological effects. *Clinical Cancer Research, 8,* 1242–1250.

Bellamy, W. T., Richter, L., Frutiger, Y., and Grogan, T. M. (1999). Expression of vascular endothelial growth factor and its receptors in hematopoietic malignancies. *Cancer Research, 59,* 728–733.

Catley, L., Weisberg, E., Tai, Y. T., Lin, B., Mitsiades, N., Hideshima, T., LeBlanc, R., Shringapurne, R., Burger, R., Mitsiades, N., Chauhan, D., Schlossman, R., Munshi, N., Richardson, P., Griffin, J., and Anderson, K. (2002). LAQ824 is a novel histone deacetylase inhibitor with significant activity against multiple myeloma: results of a pre-clinical evaluation *in vitro* and *in vivo. Blood,* 106a.

Chae, H. J., Chae, S. W., Chin, H. Y., Bang, B. G., Cho, S. B., Han, K. S., Kim, S. C., Tae, K. C., Lee, K., Kim, D. E., Im, M. K., Lee, S. J., Chang, J. Y., Lee, Y. M., Kim, H. M., Kim, H. H., Lee, Z. H., and Kim, H. R. (2001). The p38 mitogen-activated protein kinase pathway regulates interleukin-6 synthesis in response to tumor necrosis factor in osteoblasts. *Bone, 28,* 45–53.

Chauhan, D., Catley, L., Sattler, M., Li, G., Hideshima, T., LeBlanc, R., Gupta, D., Richardson, P., Schlossman, R. L., Podar, K., Munshi, N., and Anderson, K. (2002a). 2-methoxyestradiol (2ME2) acts directly on tumor cells and in the bone marrow microenvironment to overcome drug resistance in multiple myeloma. *Blood, 100,* 2187–2194.

Chauhan, D., Li, G., Hideshima, T., Auclair, D., Richardson, P., Schlossman, R. L., Podar, K., Li, C., Kim, R. S., Li, W. W., and Anderson, K. C. (2002b). Identification of genes regulated by 2-methoxyestradiol (2ME2) in multiple myeloma (MM) cells using oligonucleotide arra. *Blood, 101,* 3606–3614.

Chauhan, D., Pandey, P., Ogata, A., Teoh, G., Treon, S., Urashima, M., Kharbanda, S., and Anderson, K. C. (1997). Dexamethasone induces apoptosis of multiple myeloma cells in a JNK/SAP kinase independent mechanism. *Oncogene, 15,* 837–843.

Chauhan, D., Uchiyama, H., Akbarali, Y., Urashima, M., Yamamoto, K., Libermann, T. A., and Anderson, K. C. (1996). Multiple myeloma cell adhesion-induced interleukin-6 expression in bone marrow stromal cells involves activation of NF-κB. *Blood, 87,* 1104–1112.

Craig, R., Larkin, A., Mingo, A. M., Thuerauf, D. J., Andrews, C., McDonough, P. M., and Clembotski, C. C. (2000). p38 MAPK and NF-κB collaborate to induce interleukin-6 gene expression and release. *Journal of Biological Chemistry, 275,* 23814–23824.

D'Amato, R. J., Loughnan, M. S., Flynn, E., and Folkman, J. (1994a). Thalidomide is an inhibitor of angiogenesis. *Proceeding of the National Academy of Science of the United States of America, 91,* 4082–4085.

D'Amato, R. J., Lin, C. M., Flynn, E., Folkman, J., and Hamel, E. (1994b). 2-Methoxyestradiol, an endogenous mammalian metabolite, inhibits tubulin polymerization by interacting at the colchicine site. *Proceeding of the National Academy of Science of the United States of America, 91,* 3964–3968.

Damiano, J. S., Cress, A. E., Hazlehurst, L. A., Shtil, A. A., and Dalton, W. S. (1999). Cell adhesion-mediated drug resistance (CAM-DR): role of integrins and resistance to apoptosis in human myeloma cell lines. *Blood, 93,* 1658–1667.

Dankbar, B., Padro, T., Leo, R., Feldmann, B., Kropff, M., Mesters, R. M., Serve, H., Berdel, W. E., and Kienast, J. (2000). Vascular endothelial growth factor and interleukin-6 in paracrine tumor-stromal cell interactions in multiple myeloma. *Blood, 95,* 2630–2636.

Davies, F. E., Raje, N., Hideshima, T., Lentzsch, S., Young, G., Tai, Y. T., Lin, B., Podar, K., Gupta, D., Chauhan, D., Treon, S. P., Richardson, P. G., Schlossman, R. L., Morgan, G. J., Muller, G. W., Stirling, D. I., and Anderson, K. C. (2001). Thalidomide and immunomodulatory derivatives augment natural killer cell cytotoxicity in multiple myeloma. *Blood, 98,* 210–216.

Deaglio, S., Canella, D., Baj, G., Arnulfo, A., Waxman, S., and Malavasi, F. (2001). Evidence of an immunologic mechanism behind the therapeutical effects of arsenic trioxide (As$_2$O$_3$) on myeloma cells. *Leukemia Research, 25,* 227–325.

De Cesaris, P., Starace, D., Riccioli, A., Padula, F., and Filippin, A. (1998). Tumor necrosis factor-α induces interleukin-6 production and integrin ligand expression by distinct transcription pathways. *Journal of Biological Chemistry, 273,* 7566–7571.

Falardeau, P., Champagne, P., Poyet, P., Hariton, C., and Dupont, E. (2001). Neovastat, a naturally occurring multifunctional antiangiogenic drug, in phase III clinical trials. *Seminars in Oncology, 28,* 620–625.

Gazitt, Y., Rothenberg, M. L., Hilsenbeck, S. G., Fey, V., Thomas, C., and Montegomery, W. (1998). Bcl-2 overexpression is associated with resistance to paclitaxel, but not gemcitabine, in multiple myeloma cells. *International Journal of Oncology, 13,* 839–848.

Grad, J. M., Bahlis, N. J., Reis, I., Oshiro, M. M., Dalton, W. S., and Boise, L. H. (2001). Ascorbic acid enhances arsenic trioxide-induced cytotoxicity in multiple myeloma cells. *Blood, 98,* 805–813.

Grogan, T. M., Spier, C. M., Salmon, S. E., Matzner, M., Rybski, J., Weinstein, R. S., Scheper, R. J., and Dalton, W. S. (1993). P-glycoprotein expression in human plasma cell myeloma: correlation with prior chemotherapy. *Blood, 81,* 490–495.

Gupta, D., Treon, S. P., Shima, Y., Hideshima, T., Podar, K., Tai, Y. T., Lin, B., Lentzsch, S., Davies, F. E., Chauhan, D., Schlossman, R. L., Richardson, P., Ralph, P., Wu, L., Payvandi, F., Muller, G., Stirling, D. I., and Anderson, K. C. (2001). Adherence of multiple myeloma cells to bone marrow stromal cells upregulates vascular endothelial growth factor secretion: therapeutic applications. *Leukemia, 15,* 1950–1961.

Haslett, P. A., Klausner, J. D., Makonkawkeyoon, S., Moreira, A., Metatratip, P., Boyle, B., Kunachiwa, W., Maneekarn, N., Vongchan, P., Corral, L. G., Elbeik, T., Shen, Z., and Kaplan, G. (1999). Thalidomide stimulates T cell responses and interleukin 12 production in HIV-infected patients. *AIDS Research and Human Retroviruses, 15,* 1169–1179.

Hayashi, T., Hideshima, T., Akiyama, M., Richardson, P., Schlossman, R. L., Chauhan, D., Munshi, N. C., Waxman, S., and Anderson, K. C. (2002). Arsenic trioxide inhibits growth of human multiple myeloma cells in the bone marrow microenvironment. *Molecular Cancer Therapeutics, 1,* 851–860.

Hazlehurst, L. A., Damiano, J. S., Buyuksal, I., Pledger, W. J., and Dalton, W. S. (2000). Adhesion to fibronectin via β1 integrins regulates p27kip1 levels and contributes to cell adhesion-mediated drug resistance (CAM-DR). *Oncogene, 19,* 4319–4327.

Hideshima, T., Akiyama, M., Hayashi, T., Richardson, P., Schlossman, R., Chauhan, D., and Anderson, K. C. (2003). Targeting p38 MAPK inhibits multiple myeloma cell growth in the bone marrow milieu. *Blood, 101,* 703–705.

Hideshima, T., Chauhan, D., Hayashi, T., Akiyama, M., Mitsiades, N., Mitsiades, C., Podar, K., Munshi, N. C., Richardson, P. G., and Anderson, K. C. Caspase-dependent cleavage of gp130/interleukin-6 receptor β-subunit in multiple myeloma: therapeutic implications. *Cancer Research.* Submitted.

Hideshima, T., Chauhan, D., Richardson, P., Mitsiades, C., Mitsiades, N., Hayashi, T., Munshi, N., Dang, L., Castro, A., Palombella, V., Adams, J., and Anderson, K. C. (2002). NF-κB as a therapeutic target in multiple myeloma. *Journal of Biological Chemistry, 277,* 16639–16647.

Hideshima, T., Chauhan, D., Schlossman, R., Richardson, P., and Anderson, K. C. (2001). The role of tumor necrosis factor α in the pathogenesis of human multiple myeloma: therapeutic applications. *Oncogene, 20,* 4519–4527.

Hideshima, T., Chauhan, D., Shima, Y., Raje, N., Davies, F. E., Tai, Y. T., Treon, S. P., Lin, B., Schlossman, R. L., Richardson, P., Muller, G., Stirling, D. I., and Anderson, K. C. (2000). Thalidomide and its analogs overcome drug resistance of human multiple myeloma cells to conventional therapy. *Blood, 96,* 2943–2950.

Hideshima, T., Hayashi, T., Akiyama, M., Chauhan, D., Richardson, P. G., Mitsiades, N., Mitsiades, C., Podar, K., Munshi, N., Singer, J. W., and Anderson, K. C. (2002). Induction of apoptosis by lysophosphatidic acid acyltransferase (LPAAT)-β inhibitors in multiple myeloma (MM). *Blood, 100,* 813a.

Hideshima, T., Mitsiades, C., Akiyama, M., Hayashi, T., Chauhan, D., Richardson, P., Schlossman, R., Munshi, N., Mitsiades, N., and Anderson, K. C. (2003). Molecular mechanisms mediating anti-myeloma activity of proteasome inhibitor PS-341. *Blood, 101,* 1530–1534

Hideshima, T., Nakamura, N., Chauhan, D., and Anderson, K. C. (2001). Biologic sequelae of interleukin-6 induced PI3-K/Akt signaling in multiple myeloma. *Oncogene, 20,* 5991–6000.

Hideshima, T., Richardson, P., Chauhan, D., Palombella, V. J., Elliot, P. J., Adams, J., and Anderson, K. C. (2001). The proteasome inhibitor PS-341 inhibits growth, induces apoptosis, and overcomes drug resistance in human multiple myeloma. *Cancer Research, 61,* 3071–3076.

Hussein, M. A. (2001). Arsenic trioxide: a new immunomodulatory agent in the management of multiple myeloma. *Medical Oncology, 18,* 239–242.

Karp, J. E., Kaufmann, S. H., Adjei, A. A., Lancet, J. E., Wright, J. J., and End, D. W. (2001a). Current status of clinical trials of farnesyltransferase inhibitors. *Current Opinions in Oncology, 13,* 470–476.

Karp, J. E., Lancet, J. E., Kaufmann, S. H., End, D. W., Wright, J. J., Bol, K., Horak, I., Tidwell, M. L., Liesveld, J., Kottke, T. J., Ange, D., Buddharaju, L., Gojo, I., Highsmith, W. E., Belly, R. T., Hohl, R. J., Rybak, M. E., Thibault, A., and Rosenblatt, J. (2001b). Clinical and biologic activity of the farnesyltransferase inhibitor R115777 in adults with refractory and relapsed acute leukemias: a phase 1 clinical-laboratory correlative trial. *Blood, 97,* 3361–3369.

Kato, K., Cox, A. D., Hisaka, M. M., Graham, S. M., Buss, J. E., and Der, C. J. (1992). Isoprenoid addition to Ras protein is the critical modification for its membrane association and transforming activity. *Proceeding of the National Academy of Science of the United States of America, 89,* 6403–6407.

Keifer, J. A., Guttridge, D. C., Ashburner, B. P., and Baldwin, A. S., Jr. (2001). Inhibition of NF-κB activity by thalidomide through suppression of IκB kinase activity. *Journal of Biological Chemistry, 276,* 22382–22387.

Kenyon, B. M., Browne, F., and D'Amato, R. J. (1997). Effects of thalidomide and related metabolites in a mouse corneal model of neovascularization. *Experimental Eye Research, 64,* 971–978.

Kim, M. Y., Vankayalapati, H., Shin-Ya, K., Wierzba, K., and Hurley, L. H. (2002). Telomestatin, a potent telomerase inhibitor that interacts quite specifically with the human telomeric intramolecular g-quadruplex. *Journal of the American Chemistry Society, 124,* 2098–2099.

King, R. W., Deshaies, R. J., Peters, J. M., and Kirschner, M. W. (1996). How proteolysis drives the cell cycle. *Science, 274,* 1652–1959.

Kisselv, A. F., and Goldberg, A. L. (2001). Proteasome inhibitors: from research tools to drug candidates. *Chemistry and Biology, 21,* 1–20.

Klasa, R. J., Gillum, A. M., Klem, R. E., and Frankel, S. R. (2002). Oblimersen Bcl-2 antisense: facilitating apoptosis in anticancer treatment. *Antisense Nucleic Acid Drug Dev, 12,* 193–213.

Klauber, N., Parangi, S., Flynn, E., Hamel, E., and D'Amato, R. J. (1997). Inhibition of angiogenesis and breast cancer in mice by the microtubule inhibitors 2-methoxyestradiol and Taxol. *Cancer Research, 57,* 81–86.

Kotoh, T., Dhar, D. K., Masunaga, R., Tabara, H., Tachibana, M., Kubota, H., Kohno, H., and Nagasue, N. (1999). Anti-angiogenic therapy of human esophageal cancers with thalidomide in nude mice. *Surgery, 125,* 536–544.

LeBlanc, R., Catley, L. P., Hideshima, T., Lentzsch, S., Mitsiades, C. S., Mitsiades, N., Neuberg, D., Goloubeva, O., Pien, C. S., Adams, J., Gupta, D., Richardson, P. G., Munshi, N. C., and Anderson, K. C. (2002). Proteasome inhibitor PS-341 inhibits human myeloma cell growth in vivo and prolongs survival in a murine model. *Cancer Research, 62,* 4996–5000.

Lentzsch, S., Rogers, M. S., LeBlanc, R., Birsner, A. E., Shah, J. H., Treston, A. M., Anderson, K. C., and D'Amato, R. J. (2002). S-3-amino-phthalimido-glutarimide inhibits angiogenesis and growth of B-cell neoplasias in mice. *Cancer Research, 62,* 2300–2305.

Lin, B. K., Catley, L. P., LeBlanc, R., Gupta, D., Burger, R., Tai, Y.-T., Podar, K., Wartmann, M., Griffin, J. D., and Anderson, K. C. (2002). EPO906 (Epothilone B) inhibits cell growth and survival of multiple myeloma cells in the bone marrow microenvironment, *in vitro* and *in vivo. Blood, 100,* 818a.

Mitsiades, C. S., Mitsiades, N., Kung, A. L., Shringapurne, R., Poulaki, V., Richardson, P. G., Libermann, T. A., Munshi, N. C., Loukopoulos, D., and Anderson, K. C. (2002a). The IGF/IGF-1R system is a major therapeutic target for multiple myeloma, other hematologic malignancies and solid tumors. *Blood, 100,* 170a.

Mitsiades, C. S., Mitsiades, N., Poulaki, V., Akiyama, M., Treon, S. P., and Anderson, K. C. (2001a). The HSP90 molecular chaperone as a novel therapeutic target in hematologic malignancies. *Blood, 98,* 377a.

Mitsiades, N., Mitsiades, C. S., Poulaki, V., Anderson, K. C., and Treon, S. P. (2002b). Intracellular regulation of tumor necrosis factor-related apoptosis-inducing ligand-induced apoptosis in human multiple myeloma cells. *Blood, 99,* 2162–2171.

Mitsiades, N., Mitsiades, C. S., Poulaki, V., Chauhan, D., Gu, X., Bailey, C., Joseph, M., Libermann, T. A., Treon, S. P., Munshi, N. C., Richardson, P. G., Hideshima, T., and Anderson, K. C. (2002c). Molecular sequelae of proteasome inhibition in human multiple myeloma cells. *Proceeding of the National Academy of Science of the United States of America, 99,* 14374–14379.

Mitsiades, N., Mitsiades, C. S., Poulaki, V., Chauhan, D., Richardson, P. G., Hideshima, T., Munshi, N. C., Treon, S. P., and Anderson, K. C. (2002d). Apoptotic signaling induced by immunomodulatory thalidomide analogs in human multiple myeloma cells: therapeutic implications. *Blood, 99,* 4525–4530.

Mitsiades, C. S., Mitsiades, N., Poulaki, V., Schlossman, R., Akiyama, M., Chauhan, D., Hideshima, T., Treon, S. P., Munshi, N. C., Richardson, P. G., and Anderson, K. C. (2002e). Activation of NF-κB and upregulation of intracellular anti-apoptotic proteins via the IGF-1/Akt signaling in human multiple myeloma cells: therapeutic implications. *Oncogene, 21,* 5673–5683.

Mitsiades, N., Mitsiades, C. S., Richardson, P. G., Poulaki, V., Tai, Y. T., Chauhan, D., Gu, X., Bailey, C., Joseph, M., Libermann, T. A., Schlossman, R., Munshi, N. C., Hideshima, T., and Anderson, K. C. (2002f). The proteasome inhibitor PS-341 potentiates sensitivity of multiple myeloma cells to conventional chemotherapeutic agents: therapeutic applications. Submitted.

Mitsiades, C. S., Treon, S. P., Mitsiades, N., Shima, Y., Richardson, P., Schlossman, R., Hideshima, T., and Anderson, K. C. (2001b). TRAIL/Apo2L ligand selectively induces apoptosis and overcomes drug resistance in multiple myeloma: therapeutic applications. *Blood, 98,* 795–804.

Moreira, A. L., Sampaio, E. P., Zmuidzinas, A., Frindt, P., Smith, K. A., and Kaplan, G. (1993). Thalidomide exerts its inhibitory action on tumor necrosis factor α by enhancing mRNA degradation. *Journal of Experimental Medicine, 177,* 1675–1680.

Ogata, A., Chauhan, D., Teoh, G., Treon, S. P., Urashima, M., Schlossman, R. L., and Anderson, K. C. (1997). Interleukin-6 triggers cell growth via the *ras*-dependent mitogen-activated protein kinase cascade. *Journal of Immunology, 159,* 2212–2221.

Ogawa, M., Nishiura, T., Oritani, K., Yoshida, H., Yoshimura, M., Okajima, Y., Ishikawa, J., Hashimoto, K., Matsumura, I., Tomiyama, Y., and Matsuzawa, Y. (2000). Cytokines prevent dexamethasone-induced apoptosis via the activation of mitogen-activated protein kinase and phosphatidylinositol 3-kinase pathways in a new multiple myeloma cell line. *Cancer Research, 60,* 4262–4269.

Podar, K., Tai, Y. T., Davies, F. E., Lentzsch, S., Sattler, M., Hideshima, T., Lin, B. K., Gupta, D., Shima, Y., Chauhan, D., Mitsiades, C., Raje, N., Richardson, P., and Anderson, K. C. (2001). Vascular endothelial growth factor triggers signaling cascades mediating multiple myeloma cell growth and migration. *Blood, 98,* 428–435.

Podar, K., Tai, Y. T., Lin, B. K., Narsimhan, R. P., Sattler, M., Kijima, T., Salgia, R., Gupta, D., Chauhan, D., and Anderson, K. C. (2002). Vascular endothelial growth factor-induced migration of multiple myeloma cells is associated with β1 integrin- and phosphatidylinositol 3-kinase-dependent PKCα activation. *Journal of Biological Chemistry, 277,* 7875–7881.

Rajkumar, S. V., Fonseca, R., Dispenzieri, A., Lacy, M. Q., Lust, J. A., Witzig, T. E., Kyle, R. A., Gertz, M. A., and Greipp, P. R. (2000). Thalidomide in the treatment of relapsed multiple myeloma. *Mayo Clinic Proceedings, 75,* 897–901.

Rajkumar, S. V., Hayman, S., Gertz, M. A., Dispenzieri, A., Lacy, M. Q., Greipp, P. R., Geyer, S., Iturria, N., Fonseca, R., Lust, J. A., Kyle, R. A., and Witzig, T. E. (2002). Combination therapy with thalidomide plus dexamethasone for newly diagnosed myeloma. *Journal of Clinical Oncology, 20,* 4319–4323.

Richardson, P., Jagannath, S., Schlosman, R., Weller, E., Zeldenrust, S., Rajkumar, S. V., Alsina, M., Desikan, R. K., Mitsiades, C., Kelly, K., Doss, D., McKenny, M., Shepard, T., Rich, R., Warren, D., Freman, A., Deocampo, R., Doucet, K., Knight, R., Balinski, K., Zeldis, J., Dalton, W. S., Hideshima, T., and Anderson, K. (2002a). A multi-center randomized, phase II study to evaluate the efficacy and safety of two CDC-5013 dose regimens when used alone or in combination with dexamethasone (Dex) for the treatment of relapsed and refractory multiple myeloma. *Blood, 100,* 104a.

Richardson, P., Schlosman, R., Weller, E., Hideshima, T., Mitsiades, C., Davies, F., LeBlanc, R., Catley, L., Doss, D., Kelly, K. A., McKenney, M., Mechlowicz, J., Freeman, A., Decampo, R., Rich, R., Ryoo, J., Chauhan, D., Balinski, K., Zeldis, J., and Anderson, K. C. (2002). Immunomodulatory derivative of thalidomide CC-5013 overcomes drug resistance and is well tolerated in patients with relapsed multiple myeloma. *Blood, 100,* 3063–3067.

Salmon, S. E., Haut, A., Bonnet, J. D., Amare, M., Weick, J. K., Durie, B. G., and Dixon, D. O. (1983). Alternating combination chemotherapy and levamisole improves survival in multiple myeloma: a Southwest Oncology Group Study. *Journal of Clinical Oncology, 1,* 453–461.

Sampaio, E. P., Kaplan, G., Miranda, A., Nery, J. A., Miguel, C. P., Viana, S. M., and Sarno, E. N. (1993). The influence of thalidomide on the clinical and immunologic manifestation of erythema nodosum leprosum. *Journal of Infectious Diseases, 168,* 408–414.

Sampaio, E. P., Sarno, E. N., Galilly, R., Cohn, Z. A., and Kaplan, G. (1991). Thalidomide selectively inhibits tumor necrosis factor α production by stimulated human monocytes. *Journal of Experimental Medicine, 173,* 699–703.

Sangfelt, O., Osterborg, A., Grander, D., Anderbring, E., Ost, A., Mellstedt, H., and Einhorn, S. (1995). Response to interferon therapy in patients with multiple myeloma correlates with expression of the Bcl-2 oncoprotein. *International Journal of Cancer, 63,* 190–192.

Shammas, M. A., Shmookler Reis, R. J., Koley, H., Goyal, R. K., Hurley, L. H., Anderson, K. C., and Munshi, N. C. (2002). Telomerase inhibition and apoptotic cell death following Telomestatin treatment of multiple myeloma. *Blood, 100,* 810a.

Shin-ya, K., Wierzba, K., Matsuo, K., Ohtani, T., Yamada, Y., Furihata, K., Hayakawa, Y., and Seto, H. (2001). Telomestatin, a novel telomerase inhibitor from Streptomyces annulatus. *Journal of the American Chemistry Society, 123,* 1262–1263.

Singhal, S., Mehta, J., Desikan, R., Ayers, D., Roberson, P., Eddlemon, P., Munshi, N., Anaissie, E., Wilson, C., Dhodapkar, M., Zeldis, J., and Barlogie, B. (1999). Antitumor activity of thalidomide in refractory multiple myeloma. *New England Journal of Medicine, 341,* 1565–1571.

Sonneveld, P., Lokhorst, H. M., and Vossebeld, P. (1997). Drug resistance in multiple myeloma. *Seminars in Hematology, 34,* 34–39.

Treon, S. P., Pilarski, L. M., Belch, A. R., Kelliher, A., Preffer, F. I., Shima, Y., Mitsiades, C. S., Mitsiades, N. S., Szczepek, A. J., Ellman, L., Harmon, D., Grossbard, M. L., and Anderson, K. C. (2002). CD20-directed serotherapy in patients with multiple myeloma: biologic considerations and therapeutic applications. *Journal of Immunotherapy, 25,* 72–81.

Treston, A. M., Swartz, G. M., Conner, B., Shah, J., and Pribluda, V. S. (2002). Pre-clinical evaluation of a thalidomide analog with activity against multiple myeloma and solid tumors–ENMD-0995 (S-[-]-3-[3-amino-phthalimido]-glutarimide). *Blood, 100,* 816a.

Tseng, S., Pak, G., Washenik, K., Pomeranz, M. K., and Shupack, J. L. (1996). Rediscovering thalidomide: a review of its mechanism of action, side effects, and potential uses. *Journal of the American Academy of Dermatology, 35,* 969–979.

Tu, Y., Gardner, A., and Lichtenstein, A. (2000). The phosphatidylinositol 3-kinase/AKT kinase pathway in multiple myeloma plasma cells: roles in cytokine-dependent survival and proliferative responses. *Cancer Research, 60,* 6763–6770.

van de Donk, N. W., Kamphuis, M. M., Lokhorst, H. M., and Bloem, A. C. (2002). The cholesterol lowering drug lovastatin induces cell death in myeloma plasma cells. *Leukemia, 16,* 1362–1371.

Yamaguchi, H., Paranawithana, S. R., Lee, M. W., Huang, Z., Bhalla, K. N., and Wang, H. G. (2002). Epothilone B analogue (BMS-247550)-mediated cytotoxicity through induction of Bax conformational change in human breast cancer cells. *Cancer Research, 62,* 466–471.

# CHAPTER 15

## Management of Skeletal Complications

### JAMES R. BERENSON

## Introduction

The major clinical manifestation of multiple myeloma is related to the osteolytic bone destruction (Mundy et al., 1986). Even patients responding to chemotherapy could have progression of skeletal disease (Belch et al., 1991; Kyle et al., 1975) and recalcification of osteolytic lesions is rare. The bone disease can lead to pathologic fractures, spinal cord compression, hypercalcemia, and pain, and is a major cause of morbidity and mortality in these patients (Kyle, 1975). These patients frequently require radiation therapy or surgery. These complications result from asynchronous bone turnover in which increased osteoclastic bone resorption is not accompanied by a comparable increase in bone formation. The increase in osteoclast activity in multiple myeloma is mediated by the release of osteoclast-stimulating factors (Mundy, 1991; Stashenko et al., 1987). These factors are produced locally in the bone marrow microenvironment by cells of both tumor and nontumor origin (Bataille et al., 1995). The enhanced bone loss results from the interplay among the osteoclasts, tumor cells, and other nonmalignant cells in the bone marrow microenvironment.

Bisphosphonates are specific inhibitors of osteoclastic activity and are effective in the treatment of hypercalcemia associated with malignancies (Coleman and Purohit, 1993; Fleisch, 1989; Kanis et al., 1991). These agents have been evaluated alone and as adjunctive therapy to primary anticancer treatment in patients with cancers involving the bone, including multiple myeloma (Lahtinen et al., 1992; Man et al., 1990; Menssen et al., 2002; Purohit et al., 1994; Thiebaud et al., 1991; van Holten-Verzantvoort et al., 1993). Bisphosphonates have been evaluated in several large randomized trials in patients with myeloma also receiving chemotherapy. Oral etidronate given daily showed no clinical benefit (Kyle et al., 1975), whereas the use of oral clodronate daily has produced variable clinical results in 2 randomized trials (Man et al., 1990; McCloskey et al., 1998). Oral administration of pamidronate was ineffective in reducing the skeletal complications of these patients (Brincker et al., 1998). A large randomized, double-blind study was conducted in which stage III patients with multiple myeloma received 90 mg of either pamidronate or placebo as a 4-hour infusion every 4 weeks for 21 cycles in addition to antimyeloma chemotherapy (Berenson et al., 1998). This intravenously administered bisphosphonate significantly reduced the development of skeletal complications and improved the survival of patients who had failed first-line chemotherapy. Recent studies show the efficacy and increased convenience of the newer, more potent imidazole-containing bisphosphonate zoledronic acid in the management of the skeletal complications of myeloma. A number of other types of new anti-bone resorptive agents are also in early clinical development. Recent new surgical techniques such as kyphoplasty offer the opportunity to greatly improve the quality of life of patients with myeloma with vertebral compression fractures.

# Assessment of Myeloma Bone Disease

## Plain Radiographs and Bone Scans

Because the major clinical manifestations of myeloma are related to bone disease, the importance of assessing its status cannot be overestimated. A variety of techniques have been used to evaluate myeloma patients' bone disease. Early detection of lesions at risk to fracture or leading to cord compression allows prompt use of prophylactic surgery or radiotherapy. In addition, determination of changes in bone disease is an important part of assessing the patient's response to systemic treatment. The gold standard has been the use of plain radiographs of the skull, spine, pelvis, and long bones of the upper and lower extremities. One study has suggested that patients without either osteoporosis or lytic bone disease have the worst survival, whereas patients with minimal lytic changes have the longest survival (Smith et al., 1988). Although older studies suggest that the lytic lesions that make up myeloma bones are not well demonstrated using bone scans (Bataille et al., 1982; Woolfenden et al., 1980), recent studies suggest that this modality might be useful, especially in lesions in the ribs, vertebral bodies, and sternum (Agren et al., 1997). On the other hand, the

skull, the extremities, and the pelvic bones were better evaluated with plain radiographs in this study. In most cases, bone scans are really unnecessary as part of the routine evaluation of myeloma bone disease.

## Bone Histomorphometry

Although bone histomorphometry might be effective in assessing the extent of bone loss at individual sites (Coleman and Purohit, 1993), its usefulness is limited by both the invasiveness of the procedure and the heterogeneous nature of bone involvement in these patients. The expertise of an experienced bone pathologist is required for interpretation of the results.

## Bone Densitometry

To gain a better idea of general bone status in these patients, use of dual-energy z-ray absorptiometry (DEXA) has now been evaluated in some centers (Abildgaard et al., 1996; Diamond et al., 1997). This technique has clearly provided important information in patients with osteoporosis with respect to risk of fractures and response to therapeutic interventions (Cummings et al., 1998). Early studies in patients with myeloma have shown marked bone loss, and suggested changes in bone density correlate with clinical stage and risk of fractures (Shipman et al., 1998; Tassone et al., 2000). Although treatment with oral glucocorticoids effectively lowers tumor burden in these patients, its use has also been shown to be associated with loss of bone mineral density (Tassone et al., 2000). DEXA has recently been used to assess changes in bone density in patients with myeloma treated with bisphosphonates and shows marked increases in patients receiving intravenous pamidronate alone as their antimyeloma therapy in an ongoing phase II trial (Berenson et al., 1998). Whether it will be predictive of the efficacy of bisphosphonate treatment or of the risk of developing skeletal complications during the course of an individual's disease remains to be determined.

## Magnetic Resonance Imaging (MRI)

MRI techniques have become increasingly used in assessing patients with myeloma. These procedures are much more sensitive in detecting lesions that are not identified by plain radiographs. In the small subset of patients (approximately 20%) with normal MRI scans, the clinical features suggest earlier-stage disease and the prognosis appears to be better (Kusumoto et al., 1997). When the MRI scan is abnormal, it generally demonstrates 3 patterns, including diffuse involvement without the appearance of normal marrow signal, nodular or focal areas of replacement of normal marrow, or multiple tiny areas of replacement (Moulopoulos and Dimopoulos, 1997). Studies demonstrate that patients with diffuse involvement have the worst outlook with decreased hemoglobin and increased plasma cell loads (Singhal et al., 1999). Recent studies by Moulopoulos et al. show that MRI might be particularly useful in determining which patients with early myeloma will develop active disease (Moulopoulos et al., 1995). Approximately 2% of patients with plasma cell dyscrasias present with a solitary bony lesion. Although radiotherapy might effectively eliminate this tumor, most patients eventually develop multiple myeloma (Frassica et al., 1989). It is in these patients that MRI might be especially useful in predicting outcome. The presence of other bone lesions on the MRI scan is associated with an earlier progression to multiple myeloma than in those patients with normal MRI scans (Moulopoulos et al., 1993). However, no studies have shown that additional interventions at the time of diagnosis in this subset of patients change the clinical outcome for these individuals.

In patients with more advanced myeloma, MRI is particularly useful in the evaluation of spinal cord compression, but its role as a routine procedure in these patients has not been well established. However, the presence of more than 10 focal lesions or diffuse involvement in the spine predicted the earlier development of vertebral compression fractures in these patients (Agren et al., 1998; Rahmouni et al., 1993). However, other studies show a lack of correlation between MRI-identified lesions and risk of vertebral fractures (Lecouvet et al., 1998).

With the increasing use of MRI in evaluating patients with myeloma at diagnosis, the modality has also been used to assess response to treatment. Despite effective chemotherapy, most MRI scans remain abnormal, although there does appear to be an improvement in their appearance in responding patients (Greipp et al., 2001; Moulopoulos et al., 1994; Rahmouni et al., 1993). However, until the cost of this procedure is reduced, it is unlikely to gain widespread use in the routine followup of patients with myeloma.

### Other Radionuclide Scans

Recently, a new radionuclide tracer has been shown to predict overall disease status in these patients. Patterns of uptake of a new radionuclide tracer, technetium-99m 2-methoxyisobutylisonitrile ($^{99m}$Tc-MIBI), have been shown useful in predicting the stage of disease and current clinical status of patients with myeloma (Pace et al., 1998; Tirovola et al., 1996). The recent development of PET scans has led to the use of this modality among patients with myeloma. Whether this newer technique will prove useful in following patients with myeloma remains unknown.

### Markers of Bone Resorption and Bone Formation

A variety of markers of bone resorption and formation have been used to assess bone disease in patients with myeloma. These individuals show the expected increases in bone resorption markers such as C-terminal telopeptide of type I collagen, pyridinoline, and deoxypyridinoline and decreases in bone formation markers such as osteocalcin (Abildgaard et al., 1997; Berenson et al., 1998; Cummings et al., 1998; Nawawi et al., 1996). In addition, a decrease in osteocalcin level or higher ICTP concentrations predicts a shortened survival in myeloma. In a recent placebo-controlled, randomized Finnish clinical trial involving oral clodronate (Elomaa et al., 1996), higher baseline levels of the amino-terminal propeptide of type I procollagen (PINP), a product of growing osteoblasts, ICTP, and alkaline phosphatase (AP), were associated with a worse survival. PINP and ICTP levels decreased dramatically during clodronate treatment. Similarly, treatment with oral risedronate reduced urinary pyridinoline/creatinine and deoxypyridinoline/creatinine ratios as well as the bone formation markers AP and osteocalcin plasma levels (Roux et al., 1994). Monthly administration of intravenous pamidronate is also associated with a decrease in both bone resorption and bone forma-tion markers (Menssen et al., 2002). In the Finnish clodronate trial, a decrease in these markers during clodronate therapy was associated with a better survival. In current clinical trials evaluating newer bisphosphonates, it is being determined whether baseline values or changes in these markers predict for either the development of new skeletal complications or whether these agents will be clinically effective in individual cases. A recent study suggests that bone resorption markers show normalization after high-dose therapy followed by autologous hematopoietic support (Clark et al., 2000).

# Treatment of Myeloma Bone Disease

Until the early 1950s, radiotherapy and surgery were the only treatment modalities available to the myeloma patient. Although both modalities could effectively palliate the majority of patients, these interventions had little impact on the overall course of the disease. With the development of effective chemotherapy, the role of these other modalities became of secondary importance in the overall management of the myeloma patient. With the recent use of hemibody irradiation, total body irradiation, and bone-seeking radionuclides as part of high-dose therapy regimens, radiation treatment might become recognized as an important part of the systemic management of these patients' disease. The recent development of the minimally invasive surgical technique kyphoplasty for the treatment of patients with vertebral compression fractures (VCFs) has led to a major improvement in the quality of their lives.

## Radiation Therapy

Early studies showed the exquisite sensitivity of myeloma cells to irradiation (Rowell and Tobias, 1991). This treatment modality might be curative in some patients with solitary plasmacytoma of bone or extramedullary sites, although the majority of these patients will eventually progress to multiple myeloma. Most patients with multiple myeloma will require radiotherapy at some time in the course of their disease. The most common indication for radiotherapy is a painful lesion (Adamietz et al., 1991; Bosch and Frias, 1988). The vast majority of patients achieve pain relief with local radiotherapy at a dose of approximately 3000 cGy given in 10 to 15 fractions. Occasional patients with more extensive bone pain might benefit from more extensive hemibody irradiation (Giles et al., 1992; Rostom, 1988). Other indications for radiotherapy might include treatment of impending or actual pathologic fractures, spinal cord compression, tumor causing local neurologic problems, and large soft tissue plasma cell tumors. Approximately 10% of patients with multiple myeloma will develop spinal cord compression, and the immediate use of systemic glucocorticosteroids and radiotherapy are important to prevent the development of a permanent neurologic deficit. Radiotherapy has also been evaluated in preventing the development of new vertebral fractures in patients with myeloma with neurologic complications (Lecouvet et al., 1997). In this small nonrandomized study, there was some suggestion that less vertebral fractures occurred in irradiated vertebrae than in nonirradiated ones as assessed by MRI. However, caution must be used in the application of radiotherapy because this will result in permanent bone marrow damage in the treated areas. The importance of this point cannot be overemphasized in a patient whose overall clinical status depends on chemotherapeutic agents, which cause loss of bone marrow function. A recently published study showed that radiation of the entire shaft of the long bone is probably not necessary in most cases (Catell et al., 1998). Even in the few cases showing recurrence outside the previously irradiated field, palliation with radiotherapy was effective.

## Surgery

Surgical intervention might be required in patients with an impending or actual fracture or a destabilized spine. Several recent reports suggest that this modality is underused in patients with myeloma with either long bone or vertebral fractures. In some patients, the presence of myeloma not evident radiographically in areas adjacent to the surgical site could impede the success of the procedure. Most patients also require radiotherapy in conjunction with the surgical procedure. Importantly, consideration must be given to the patient's overall clinical status in decisions regarding the timing of surgery.

Although previous attempts to reduce the morbidity of vertebral compression fractures through techniques such as vertebroplasty were met with limited success, the recent development of a new minimally invasive surgical procedure known as kyphoplasty has made a major change in the quality of lives of patients with myeloma with VCFs. Specifically, a small surgical needle is implanted into the collapsed vertebral body and a balloon contained within the needle is inflated to reverse the compression. The balloon is withdrawn and methylmethacrylate cement is placed within the cavity. A recent study from the Cleveland clinic confirms the safety and efficacy of this procedure for patients with myeloma with VCFs.

# Drug Therapy

Earlier attempts to reduce the skeletal complications of myeloma involving large randomized trials with sodium fluoride either alone or in combination with calcium and androgenic steroids proved unsuccessful (Acute Leukemia Group B, Eastern Cooperative Oncology Group B, 1972; Cohen et al., 1984; Kyle, 1975). In addition, gallium nitrate was evaluated in one published study, which suggested both a decrease in bone pain and loss of total body calcium with this treatment, but this trial was open-label involving only 13 patients (Warrell et al., 1993).

## Bisphosphonates

Most of the recent studies have evaluated whether a variety of bisphosphonates administered either orally or intravenously have an impact on skeletal disease as well as its clinical manifestations. Bisphosphonates are specific inhibitors of osteoclastic activity and are effective in the treatment of hypercalcemia associated with malignancies (Fleisch, 1989; Major et al., 2001).

## Pharmacology of Bisphosphonates

Pyrophosphates are natural compounds that contain 2 phosphonate groups bound to common oxygen and are potent inhibitors of bone resorption *in vitro*. However, when used *in vivo*, this compound is readily hydrolyzed and ineffective at reducing bone resorption (Fleisch, 1989). By simply substituting the oxygen with a carbon, the molecule becomes resistant to hydrolysis and yet remains active as an inhibitor of bone resorption. With the carbon substitution, these synthetic compounds known as bisphosphonates contain 2 additional chains of variable structure (called R1 and R2) that have given rise to a large number of different drugs. Most bisphosphonates contain a hydroxyl group at R1 that allows high affinity for calcium crystals and bone mineral. Marked differences in antiresorptive potency result from differences at the R2 site.

These drugs are poorly absorbed orally (usually less than 1%) and are also poorly tolerated orally with significant gastrointestinal toxicity particularly esophagitis and esophageal ulcers. The bisphosphonates are almost exclusively eliminated through renal excretion and significant nephrotoxicity can occur with these compounds. Because bisphosphonates have high affinity for bone mineral, the drug is highly concentrated in bone. Once the drug becomes a part of the bone, which is not remodeling, it is biologically inactive. As a result, continued administration of bisphosphonates is required to achieve the desired lasting inhibition of bone resorption.

## Bisphosphonates in Myeloma Bone Disease

These agents have been evaluated alone and as adjunctive therapy to primary anticancer treatment in patients with cancers involving the bone, including multiple myeloma. Recent large placebo-controlled clinical trials have shown the efficacy of bisphosphonates in reducing skeletal complications in patients with myeloma, and suggested that these agents might also alter the overall course of the disease.

Although early studies involving bisphosphonates in patients with myeloma suggested a reduction in bone pain and healing of lytic lesions, the trials involved relatively few patients (Man et al., 1990; Thiebaud et al., 1991). Nine large randomized trials of long-term bisphosphonate use have now been published and involved the use of etidronate, clodronate, pamidronate, ibandronate, or zoledronic acid.

## Etidronate

In the Canadian study involving etidronate (Belch et al., 1991), 173 newly diagnosed patients all received intermittent oral melphalan and prednisone as primary chemotherapy, and 166 were then randomized to receive either 5 mg/kg oral etidronate per day or placebo until death or stopping the treatment as a result of side effects. Although significant height loss occurred in both placebo- and etidronate-treated patients, no difference was found between the 2 arms. Similarly, the other outcome measures (new fractures, hypercalcemic episodes, and bone pain) showed no differences between the 2 arms.

## Clodronate

In a small study involving only 13 patients, use of daily oral clodronate was associated with a reduction in bone pain and lack of progression of bone lesions in contrast to the clinical deterioration that occurred in the patients treated with placebo (Delmas et al., 1982). Histomorphometric analysis of bone biopsies showed decreases in osteoclast numbers with clodronate treatment, whereas patients receiving placebo showed a slight increase in these cells. Intravenously administered clodronate was evaluated in a randomized Italian study that involved only 30 patients with active bone disease (Merlini et al., 1990). There was a reduction in new lytic lesions and pathologic fractures with the bisphosphonate therapy.

Three large randomized trials have been published using oral clodronate in patients with myeloma. In the Finnish trial (Lahtinen et al., 1992), 350 previously untreated patients were entered and 336 randomized to receive either 2.4 g clodronate or placebo daily for 2 years. All patients were also treated with intermittent oral melphalan and prednisolone. Only a little more than half of the patients had radiographs completed at both study entry and 2 years. Given this limitation, the proportion of patients with progression of lytic lesions was less in the clodronate treated group (12%) than in the placebo group (24%). However, the progression of overall pathologic fractures, as well as both vertebral and nonvertebral fractures, was no different between the arms. In addition, the number of patients developing hypercalcemia was similar in the 2 arms. Changes in pain index and use of analgesics were similar in both arms.

Clodronate has also been evaluated in an open-label randomized German trial (Heim et al., 1995). In this study, 170 previously untreated patients were randomized to receive either no bisphosphonate or oral clodronate (1.6 g) daily for 1 year. All patients were also treated with intermittent intravenous melphalan and oral prednisone. Unfortunately, premature termination occurred in more than half of the patients despite the short length of the study (1 y). The results showed no difference in progression of bone disease as assessed by plain radiographs in the 2 arms. However, there was a trend toward a reduction in the number of new progressive sites in the clodronate-treated group after 6 and

12 months, although this did not reach statistical significance. Although patients without pain and those not using analgesics were higher in the clodronate group, the open-label design of this trial makes it difficult to interpret these findings.

Recently, the Medical Research Council has published the results of a large randomized trial involving 536 recently diagnosed patients with myeloma randomized to receive either 1.6 g oral clodronate or placebo daily in addition to alkylator-based chemotherapy (McCloskey et al., 1998). After combining the proportion of patients developing either nonvertebral fractures or severe hypercalcemia, including those leaving the trial because of severe hypercalcemia, there were less clodronate-treated patients experiencing these combined events than placebo patients. However, the number of patients developing hypercalcemia was similar between the 2 arms. The number of patients experiencing nonvertebral fractures was lower in the clodronate group. Although vertebral fractures reportedly occurred in significantly fewer clodronate-treated patients than placebo patients, only half of patients obtained at least one post-baseline radiograph. Back pain and poor performance status were not significantly different between the 2 groups except at one time point (24 mo). The proportion of patients requiring radiotherapy was similar between the 2 arms. There was no difference in time to first skeletal event or overall survival.

## Pamidronate

In patients with multiple myeloma, results of small open-label trials lasting up to 24 months suggested that pamidronate disodium might be effective in reducing skeletal complications of multiple myeloma (Man et al., 1990; Thiebaud et al., 1991). Thus, a large randomized, double-blind study was conducted to determine whether monthly 90-mg infusions of pamidronate compared with placebo for 21 months reduced skeletal events in patients with multiple myeloma who were receiving chemotherapy (Berenson et al., 1996, 1998). This study included patients with Durie-Salmon stage III multiple myeloma and at least one osteolytic lesion. Unlike the etidronate and clodronate trials, which involved untreated patients, patients were required to receive an unchanged chemotherapy regimen for at least 2 months before enrollment. Patients were stratified according to their antimyeloma therapy at trial entry: stratum 1, first-line chemotherapy; stratum 2, second-line or greater chemotherapy. The primary end point, skeletal events (pathologic fractures, spinal cord compression associated with vertebral compression fracture, surgery to treat or prevent pathologic fracture or spinal cord compression associated with vertebral compression fracture, or radiation to bone) and

secondary end points (hypercalcemia, bone pain, analgesic drug use, performance status, and quality of life) were assessed monthly. Importantly, although the chemotherapeutic regimen was not uniform at study entry, the types and numbers of chemotherapeutic regimens in the 2 groups were similar at study entry and during the trial.

At the preplanned primary end point after 9 cycles of therapy (Berenson et al., 1996), the proportions of patients with myeloma having any skeletal event was 41% in patients receiving placebo but only 24% in pamidronate-treated patients. In addition, the number of skeletal events per year was half in the patients treated with pamidronate. The proportion of pamidronate-treated patients with skeletal events was lower in both stratum 1 (first-line therapy) and stratum 2 (≤ second-line therapy). The patients who received pamidronate also had significant decreases in bone pain, no increase in analgesic use, and showed no deterioration in performance status and quality of life at the end of 9 months. Similar to the results after 9 cycles of therapy, the proportions of patients developing any skeletal event and the skeletal morbidity rate continued to remain significantly lower in the pamidronate group than in the placebo group during the additional 12 cycles of treatment (Berenson et al., 1998). However, there were no differences between the treatment groups in the percentage of patients with healing or progression of osteolytic lesions. Although overall survival in all patients was not significantly different between the 2 treatment groups, in stratum 2, the median survival time was 21 months for pamidronate patients compared with 14 months for placebo patients.

In a double-blind, randomized trial, a Danish–Swedish cooperative group evaluated daily oral pamidronate (300 mg per day) compared with placebo in 300 newly diagnosed patients with myeloma also receiving intermittent melphalan and prednisone (Brincker et al., 1998). After a median duration of 18 months, there was no significant reduction in the primary end point defined as skeletal-related morbidity (bone fracture, surgery for impending fracture, vertebral collapse, or increase in number and/or size of lytic lesions), hypercalcemic episodes, or survival between the arms. Fewer episodes of severe pain and less height loss were observed in the oral pamidronate-treated patients, however.

## Ibandronate

Ibandronate is a nitrogen-containing bisphosphonate that in preclinical models shows more antibone resorptive potency than pamidronate and the other non-nitrogen-containing bisphosphonates. The results of a phase III placebo-controlled trial of 214 stage II or III patients with myeloma with osteolytic bone disease were recently published (Menssen et al., 2002). Patients either received monthly injections of 2 mg of ibandronate or placebo in addition to their antineoplastic therapy. Ninety-nine patients were evaluable in each arm for efficacy. The mean number of events per patient year on treatment was similar in both groups (ibandronate 2.13 vs. placebo 2.05). In addition, there was no difference in pain, analgesic use, or quality of life between the arms. However, among patients treated with ibandronate who showed a sustained and marked reduction in bone resorption markers, fewer skeletal complications occurred. There was no difference in overall survival. Thus, this monthly dose of intravenous ibandronate did not show significant benefits in reducing skeletal complications in patients with myeloma with lytic bone disease.

### Zoledronic Acid

Zoledronic acid is an imidazole-containing bisphosphonate that shows more potency in preclinical studies than any other bisphosphonate currently available (Green et al., 1994). Two small phase I trials established the safety and marked sustained reduction in bone resorption markers for patients with myeloma and other cancers associated with metastatic bone disease with monthly infusions of small doses given over several minutes (Berenson et al., 2001a, 2001b). A large randomized phase II study compared this newer bisphosphonate with pamidronate in 280 patients with lytic bone metastases from either multiple myeloma ($n = 108$) or breast cancer ($n = 172$). Patients were randomized to 9 monthly infusions of 0.4 mg, 2.0 mg, or 4.0 mg of zoledronic acid, or to 90 mg of pamidronate as a 2-hour infusion. The primary end point was to determine a dose of zoledronic acid that reduced the need for radiation therapy to less than 30% of treated patients, although all skeletal events were also analyzed similar to those determined in the previously reported phase III pamidronate trials. Radiation therapy was required in a similar proportion of patients receiving pamidronate and zoledronic acid at 2.0 and 4.0 mg (18%–21%), whereas more patients receiving the lowest dose of zoledronic acid underwent radiotherapy (24%). Similarly, the proportion of patients with any skeletal event was lower (30%–35%) in these same groups compared with patients receiving 0.4 mg of zoledronic acid. Interestingly, significant increases in bone density (over 6% in the lumbar spine) and inhibition of bone resorption markers were observed in this latter cohort, but this failed to translate to any clinical benefit. Although the results of this study suggested that 0.4 mg was an inadequate monthly dose of zoledronic acid to be of clinical use in the prevention of skeletal complications for patients with myeloma or breast cancer metastatic to bone, the small size of this phase II trial

did not allow for a complete assessment of the efficacy of higher doses of zoledronic acid compared with pamidronate.

Thus, a larger phase III trial evaluated 2 doses of zoledronic acid (4 and 8 mg) compared with pamidronate (90 mg) infused every 3 to 4 weeks for treatment of myeloma or breast cancer patients with metastatic bone disease (Rosen et al., 2001). The doses and infusion time (5 min) of zoledronic acid were selected based on the safety and superiority of these doses in reversing hypercalcemia of malignancy compared with pamidronate (90 mg) (Major et al., 2001).

Importantly, the primary efficacy end point of this trial was designed to show the noninferiority of zoledronic acid compared with pamidronate in reducing skeletal complications for patients with myeloma or breast cancer metastatic to bone. The trial involved 1643 patients who were stratified among individuals with myeloma ($n = 513$) or breast cancer on either hormonal therapy or chemotherapy ($n = 1130$). The proportion of patients with any skeletal event did not differ among the 3 treatment arms. In addition, the time to first skeletal event was similar in the 3 groups (12–13 mo). The effects of these treatments on pain and analgesic use were similar to those observed in prior studies. Importantly, during the clinical trial, rises in creatinine were more frequently observed in the zoledronic acid arms, and the infusion time was increased to 15 minutes. Despite this increase in infusion time, patients receiving the 8-mg dose continued to be at a higher risk of developing rises in serum creatinine, and these patients were subsequently changed to the 4-mg dose for the remainder of the trial. Long-term follow-up data is now available and shows no difference in the renal profile between patients receiving 4 mg zoledronic acid infused over 15 minutes compared with 90 mg pamidronate infused over 120 minutes. Following the change in infusion time, zoledronic acid was well tolerated with changes in serum creatinine observed in a similar proportion of patients receiving 90 mg pamidronate 90 mg over 2 hours compared with 4 mg zoledronic acid infused over 15 minutes.

### ASCO Clinical Practice Guidelines on the Role of Bisphosphonates in Multiple Myeloma

Recently, the American Society of Clinical Oncology published guidelines based on the recommendations of the ASCO Bisphosphonates Expert Panel (Berenson et al., 2002). The panel recommended that for patients with multiple myeloma who have on plain radiographs evidence of lytic bone disease either 4 mg of intravenous zoledronic acid infused over 15 minutes or 90 mg pamidronate delivered over 120 minutes every

3 to 4 weeks. The panel also believes it is reasonable to start these agents for patients with osteopenia but without evidence of lytic bone disease. Once initiated, the panel recommended that the intravenous bisphosphonate be continued until there was a substantial decline in the patient's performance status.

The panel also recommended intermittent monitoring of renal function as well as urinary protein evaluation to assess possible renal dysfunction that could occur from these agents. It is important to recognize that when renal dysfunction occurs with pamidronate, it is more often associated with a glomerular lesion so that albuminuria is often found, whereas zoledronic acid usually causes tubular dysfunction so that albumin in the urine is uncommon in patients with renal problems from the newer bisphosphonate.

For patients with either solitary plasmacytoma or indolent myeloma, no data exists to suggest their efficacy. In addition, although clinical studies would be interesting to conduct for patients with monoclonal gammopathy of undetermined significance, because many of these individuals show significant amounts of bone loss, the panel did not recommend treatment of these patients with bisphosphonates.

### Antimyeloma Effects of Bisphosphonates

The role of bisphosphonates for patients with myeloma may go beyond simply inhibiting bone resorption and the resulting skeletal complications. Some studies suggest that these drugs might have antitumor effects both directly and indirectly (Mundy, 1999). Using the murine 5T2 multiple myeloma model, Radl and colleagues suggested that pamidronate might reduce tumor burden in treated mice (Radl et al., 1985). *In vitro* studies also suggest pamidronate might possess antimyeloma properties as demonstrated by its ability to induce apoptosis of myeloma cells (Aparicio et al., 1998) and suppress the production of IL-6, an important myeloma growth factor, by bone marrow stromal cells from myeloma patients (Savage et al., 1996). A recent *in vitro* study might help explain the induction of apoptosis by these compounds (Shipman et al., 1998). These drugs inhibit the mevalonate pathway, and, as a result, decrease the isoprenylation of proteins such as *ras* and other GTPases. The antitumor effects of these agents appear to be synergistic with glucocorticoids (Tassone et al., 2000). Several recent studies show that bisphosphonates are markedly antiangiogenic (Fournier et al., 2002; Wood et al., 2002), and the recent demonstration of the marked antimyeloma clinical effects of the antiangiogenic agent thalidomide in patients with myeloma (Singhal et al., 1999) suggests another putative mechanism by which bisphosphonates might possess antimyeloma effects. In addition to the effects on the tumor cells and the

tumoral microenvironment, recent studies suggest that nitrogen-containing bisphosphonates might stimulate γδT lymphocytes and induce antiplasma cell activity in myeloma patients (Kunzmann et al., 2000). Several recent murine models of human myeloma show that the administration of pamidronate or zoledronic acid both reduces the development of lytic bone disease and tumor burden (Yaccoby et al., 1998, 2000). In addition to the survival advantage observed in relapsing patients in the large randomized Berenson et al. trial (1998), 2 recent patients with myeloma treated with pamidronate alone were recently reported to show reductions in myeloma tumor cell burden (Dhodapkar et al., 1998). Attempts to increase the dose of pamidronate to more clearly show the antimyeloma effect of this agent were accompanied by the development of albuminuria and azotemia. However, because 4 mg of zoledronic acid could be administered safely over 15 minutes, it might be possible to increase the dose of this newer agent with longer infusion times and clearly show the hoped-for antimyeloma effects clinically that have been suggested from the preclinical studies mentioned previously.

### Other Antiresorptive Agents

An analog of the natural inhibitor of RANK signaling known as OPG has recently completed a phase I trial with promising results in terms of suppression of bone resorption markers (Greipp et al., 2001). In addition, inhibitors of src activity show marked antiresorptive capability and might enter clinical trials soon. The statin drugs have shown the potential to increase bone density by their stimulatory effects on specific bone morphogenetic proteins (BMPs) involved in stimulating bone formation as well as their inhibitory effects on mevalonic acid biosynthesis, which results in the lack of prenylation of critical cellular proteins.

## Summary

The results of 2 large phase III clinical trials show the benefit of adjunctive use of intravenously administered monthly zoledronic acid or pamidronate in addition to chemotherapy is superior to chemotherapy alone in patients with advanced multiple myeloma with respect to safely reducing bone complications. Bisphosphonate treatment should now be considered for all patients with multiple myeloma and evidence of bone loss. The 3 large randomized studies with clodronate show inconsistent results with oral administration of this first-generation bisphosphonate. Curiously, the Finnish trial using a larger daily dose shows less effect than the MRC trial using a smaller amount of clodronate. In addition, in the latter trial, although the drug had some effect on reducing fractures and severe hypercalcemia in these patients, the drug did not affect the time to first skeletal event or use of radiotherapy. Similarly, oral pamidronate has not been effective either. Given the clinical results and the poor tolerability of oral agents, this route of administration for bisphosphonates is unlikely to be of much benefit in these patients. Clearly, both intravenously administered pamidronate and zoledronic acid reduce the skeletal complications as well as improve the quality of life of these patients. Whether these drugs are effective in earlier stages of disease or for patients without bone loss is unknown. The possibility of antitumor effects of these agents as suggested from preclinical studies is now being evaluated in trials evaluating higher doses of zoledronic acid infused over several hours.

## REFERENCES

Abildgaard, N., Bentzen, Nielsen, et al. (1997). Serum markers of bone metabolism in multiple myeloma: prognostic significance of the carboxy-terminal telopeptide of type 1 collagen (ICTP). *British Journal of Haematology, 96*, 103–110.

Abildgaard, N., Brixen, K., Kristensen, J. E., et al. (1996). Assessment of bone involvement in patients with multiple myeloma using bone densitometry. *European Journal of Haematology, 57*, 370–376.

Acute Leukemia Group B, Eastern Cooperative Oncology Group B. (1972). Ineffectiveness of fluoride therapy in multiple myeloma. *New England Journal of Medicine, 286*, 1283–1288.

Agren, B., Lonnqvist, B., Bjorkstrand, B., et al. (1997). Radiography and bone scintigraphy in bone marrow transplant multiple myeloma patients. *Acta Radiologica, 38*, 144–150.

Agren, B., Rudberg, U., Isberg, B., et al. (1998). MR Imaging of multiple myeloma patients with bone-marrow transplants. *Acta Radiologica, 39*, 36–42.

Adamietz, I. A., Schober, C., Schulte, R. W. M., et al. (1991). Palliative radiotherapy in plasma cell myeloma. *Radiotherapy and Oncology, 20*, 111–116.

Aparicio, A., Gardner, A., Tu, Y., Savage, A., Berenson, J., et al. (1998). In vitro cytoreductive effects on multiple myeloma cells induced by bisphosphonates. *Leukemia, 12*, 220–229.

Bataille, R., Chappard, D., and Basle, M. (1995). Excessive bone resorption in human plasmacytomas: direct induction by tumor cells *in vivo. British Journal of Haematology, 90*, 721–724.

Bataille, R., Chevalier, J., Rossi, M., et al. (1982). Bone scintigraphy in plasma-cell myeloma. *Radiology, 145*, 801–804.

Belch, A. R., Bergsagel, D. E., Wilson, K., et al. (1991). Effect of daily etidronate on the osteolysis of multiple myeloma. *Journal of Clinical Oncology, 9*, 1397–1402.

Berenson, J., Hillner, B., Kyle, R., et al. (2002). American Society of Clinical Oncology Clinical Practice Guidelines: the role of bisphosphonates in multiple myeloma. *Journal of Clinical Oncology, 20*, 3719–3736.

Berenson, J., Lichtenstein, A., Porter, L., et al. (1998). Long-term pamidronate treatment of advanced multiple myeloma patients reduces skeletal events. *Journal of Clinical Oncology, 16*, 593–602.

Berenson, J., Vescio, R., Rosen, L. S., et al. (2001b). A phase I dose-ranging trial of monthly infusions of zoledronic acid for the treatment of metastatic bone disease. *Clinical Cancer Research, 7*, 478–485.

Berenson, J., Webb, I., et al. (1998). A phase II dose-ranging trial of single-agent pamidronate for relapsed/refractory multiple myeloma. *Blood, 92*, 107a.

Berenson, J. R., Lichtenstein, A., Porter, L., et al. (1996). Efficacy of pamidronate in reducing the skeletal events in patients with advanced multiple myeloma. *New England Journal of Medicine, 334*, 488–493.

Berenson, J. R., Vescio, R., Henick, K., et al. (2001a). A phase I open label, dose-ranging trial of intravenous bolus zolderonic acid, a novel bisphosphonate, in cancer patients with metastatic bone disease. *Cancer, 91*, 144–154.

Bosch, A., and Frias, Z. (1988). Radiotherapy in the treatment of multiple myeloma. *International Journal of Radiation Oncology Biology Physics, 15*, 1363–1369.

Brincker, H., Westin, J., Abildgaard, et al. (1998). Failure of oral pamidronate to reduce skeletal morbidity in multiple myeloma: a double-blind placebo-controlled trial. *British Journal of Haematology, 101*, 280–286.

Catell, D., Kogen, Z., Donahue, B., et al. (1998). Multiple myeloma of an extremity: must the entire bone be treated? *International Journal of Radiation Oncology Biology Physics, 40*, 117–119.

Clark, R. E., Flory, A. J., Ion, E. M., et al. (2000). Biochemical markers of bone turnover following high-dose chemotherapy and autografting in multiple myeloma. *Blood, 96*, 2697–2702.

Cohen, H. J., Silberman, H. R., Tornyos, K., et al. (1984). Comparison of two long-term chemotherapy regimens, with or without agents to modify skeletal repair, in multiple myeloma. *Blood, 63*, 639–648.

Coleman, R. E., and Purohit, O. P. (1993). Osteoclast inhibition for the treatment of bone metastases. *Cancer Treatment Reviews, 19*, 79–103.

Cummings, S. R., Black, D. M., Thompson, D. E., et al. (1998). Effect of alendronate on risk of fracture in women with low bone density but without vertebral fractures. *Journal of the American Medical Association, 280*, 2077–2082.

Delmas, P. D., Charhon, S., Chapuy, M. C., et al. (1982). Long-term effects of dichloromethylene diphosphonate (C12MDP) on skeletal lesions in multiple myeloma. *Metabolic Bone Disorders and Related Research, 4*, 163–168.

Dhodapkar, M. V., Singh, J., Mehta, J., et al. (1998). Antimyeloma activity of pamidronate in vivo. *British Journal of Haematology, 103*, 530.

Diamond, T., Levy, S., Day, P., et al. (1997). Biochemical, histomorphometric and densitometric changes in patients with multiple myeloma: effects of glucocorticoid therapy and disease activity. *British Journal of Haematology, 97*, 641–648.

Elomaa, I., Risteli, L., Laakso, M., et al. (1996). Monitoring the action of clodronate with type I collagen metabolites in multiple myeloma. *European Journal of Cancer, 32A*, 1166–1170.

Fleisch, H. (1989). Bisphosphonates: a new class of drugs in diseases of bone and calcium metabolism. In K. W. Brunner, H Fleisch, and H.-J. Senn (Eds.), *Recent Results in Cancer Research, vol 116: Bisphosphonates and Tumor Osteolysis* (pp. 1–28). Berlin-Heidelberg: Springer-Verlag.

Fournier, P., Boissier, S., Filleur, S., et al. (2002). Bisphosphonates inhibit angiogenesis in vitro and testosterone-stimulated vascular regrowth in the ventral prostate in castrated rats. *Cancer Research, 62*, 6538–6544.

Frassica, D. A., Frassica, F. J., Schray, M. F., et al. (1989). Solitary plasmacytoma of bone: Mayo clinic experience. *International Journal of Radiation Oncology Biology Physics, 16*, 43–48.

Giles, F. J., McSweeney, E. N., Richards, J. D. M., et al. (1992). Prospective randomised study of double hemibody irradiation with and without subsequent maintenance recombinant alpha 2b interferon on survival in patients with relapsed multiple myeloma. *European Journal of Cancer, 28A*, 1392–1395.

Green, J. R., Muller, K., and Jaeggi, K. A. (1994). Preclinical pharmacology of CGP 42'446, a new, potent, heterocyclic bisphosphonate compound. *Journal of Bone and Mineral Research, 9,* 745–751.

Greipp, P., Facon, T., Williams, C. D., et al. (2001). A single subcutaneous dose of an osteoprotegerin (OPG) construct (AMGN-0007) causes a profound and sustained decrease in bone resorption comparable to standard intravenous bisphosphonate in patients with multiple myeloma. *Blood, 98,* 775a.

Heim, M. E., Clemens, M. R., Queisser, W., et al. (1995). Prospective randomized trial of dicloromethylene bisphosphonate (clordronate) in patients with multiple myeloma requiring treatment: a multicenter study. *Onkologie, 18,* 439–448.

Kanis, J. A., McCloskey, E. V., Taube, T., et al. (1991). Rationale for the use of bisphosphonates in bone metastases. *Bone, 12* (suppl 1):S13–S18.

Kunzmann, V., Bauer, E., Feurle, J., et al. (2000). Stimulation of gdT cells by aminobisphosphonates and induction of antiplasma cell activity in multiple myeloma. *Blood, 96,* 384–392.

Kusumoto, S., Jinnai, I., and Itoh, K. (1997). Magnetic resonance imaging patterns in patients with multiple myeloma. *British Journal of Haematology, 99,* 649–655.

Kyle, R. A. (1975). Multiple myeloma, review of 869 cases. *Mayo Clinic Proceedings, 50,* 29–40.

Kyle, R. A., Jowsey, J., Kelly, P. J., et al. (1975). Multiple myeloma bone disease. The comparative effect of sodium fluoride and calcium carbonate or placebo. *New England Journal of Medicine, 293,* 1334–1338.

Lahtinen, R., Laakso, M., Palva, I., et al. (1992). Randomised, placebo-controlled multicentre trial of clodronate in multiple myeloma. *Lancet, 340,* 1049–1052.

Lecouvet, F., Richard, F., Vande Berg, B., et al. (1997). Long-term effects of localized spinal radiation therapy on vertebral fractures and focal lesions appearance in patients with multiple myeloma. *British Journal of Haematology, 96,* 743–745.

Lecouvet, F. E., Vande Berg, B. C., and Michaux, L. (1998). Development of vertebral fractures in patients with multiple myeloma: does MRI enable recognition of vertebrae that will collapse? *Journal of Computer Assisted Tomography, 22,* 430–436.

Major, P., Lortholary, A., Hon, J., et al. (2001). Zoledronic acid is superior to pamidronate in the treatment of hypercalcemia of malignancy: a pooled analysis of two randomized, controlled clinical trials. *Journal of Clinical Oncology, 19,* 558–567.

Man, Z., Otero, A. B., Rendo, P., et al. (1990). Use of pamidronate for multiple myeloma osteolytic lesions. *Lancet, 335,* 663.

McCloskey, E. V., MacLennan, C. M., Drayson, M. T., et al. (1998). A randomized trial of the effect of clodronate on skeletal morbidity in multiple myeloma. *British Journal of Haematology, 101,* 317–325.

Menssen, H. D., Sakalova, A., Fontana, A., et al. (2002). Effects of long-term intravenous ibandronate therapy on skeletal-related events, survival, and bone resorption markers in patients with advanced multiple myeloma. *Journal of Clinical Oncology, 20,* 2353–2359.

Merlini, G., Parrinello, G. A., Piccinini, L., et al. (1990). Long-term effects of parenteral dichloromethylene bisphosphonate (C12MDP) on bone disease of myeloma patients treated with chemotherapy. *Hematological Oncology, 90,* 2127–2147.

Moulopoulos, L. A., and Dimopoulos, M. A. (1997). Magnetic resonance imaging of the bone marrow in hematologic malignancies. *Blood, 90,* 2127–2147.

Moulopoulos, L. A., Dimopoulos, M. A., Alexanian, R., et al. (1994). Multiple myeloma: MR patterns of response to treatment. *Radiology, 193,* 441–446.

Moulopoulos, L. A., Dimopoulos, M. A., Smith, T. L., et al. (1995). Prognostic significance of magnetic resonance imaging in patients with asymptomatic multiple myeloma. *Journal of Clinical Oncology, 13,* 251–256.

Moulopoulos, L. A., Dimopoulos, M. A., Weber, D., et al. (1993). Magnetic resonance imaging in the staging of solitary plasmacytoma of bone. *Journal of Clinical Oncology, 11,* 1311–1315.

Mundy, G. R. (1999). Bisphosphonates as cancer drugs. *Hospital Practice (Office Edition), 34,* 81–84.

Mundy, G. R., and Bertoline, D. R. (1986). Bone destruction and hypercalcemia in plasma cell myeloma. *Seminars in Oncology, 13,* 291–299.

Mundy, G. R. (1991). Mechanisms of osteolytic bone destruction. *Bone, 12*(suppl 1), S1–S6.

Nawawi, H., Samson, D., Apperley, J., et al. (1996). Biochemical bone markers in patients with multiple myeloma. *Clinica Chimica Acta, 253,* 61–77.

Pace, L., Catalano, L., Pinto, A., et al. (1998). Different patterns of technetium-99m sestamibi uptake in multiple myeloma. *European Journal of Nuclear Medicine, 25,* 714–720.

Purohit, O. P., Anthony, C., Radstone, C. R., et al. (1994). High-dose intravenous pamidronate for metastatic bone pain. *British Journal of Cancer, 70,* 554–558.

Radl, J., Croese, J. W., Zircher, C., et al. (1985). Influence of treatment with APD-bisphosphonate on the bone lesions in the mouse 5T2 multiple myeloma. *Cancer, 55,* 1030–1040.

Rahmouni, A., Divine, M., Mathieu, D., et al. (1993). Appearance of multiple myeloma of the spine before and after treatment. *American Journal of Roentgenology, 160,* 1053–1057.

Rahmouni, A., Divine, M., Mathieu, D., et al. (1993). MR appearance of multiple myeloma of the spine before and after treatment. *American Journal of Roentgenology, 160,* 1053–1057.

Rosen, L. S., Gordon, D., Antonio, B. S., et al. (2001). Zoledronic acid versus pamidronate in the treatment of skeletal metastases in patients with breast cancer or osteolytic lesions of multiple myeloma: a phase III, double-blind, comparative trial. *Cancer Journal, 7,* 377–387.

Rostom, A. Y. (1988). A review of the place of radiotherapy in myeloma with emphasis on whole body irradiation. *Hematological Oncology, 6,* 193–198.

Roux, C., Ravaud, P., Cohen-Solal, M., et al. (1994). Biologic, histologic and densitometric effects of oral risedronate on bone in patients with multiple myeloma. *Bone, 15,* 41–49.

Rowell, N. P., and Tobias, J. S. (1991). The role of radiotherapy in the management of multiple myeloma. *Blood Reviews, 5,* 84–89.

Savage, A. D., Belson, D. J., Vescio, R. A., et al. (1996). Pamidronate reduces IL-6 production by bone marrow stroma from multiple myeloma patients. *Blood, 88,* 105a.

Shipman, C. M., Croucher, P. I., Russell, R. G., et al. (1998). The bisphosphonate incandronate (YM175) causes apoptosis of human myeloma cells in vitro by inhibiting the mevalonate pathway. *Cancer Research, 58,* 5294–5297.

Singhal, S., Mehta, J., Desikan, R., et al. (1999). Antitumor activity of thalidomide in refractory multiple myeloma. *New England Journal of Medicine, 341,* 1565–1571.

Smith, D. B., Scarffe, J. H., and Eddleston, B. (1988). The prognostic significance of x-ray changes at presentation and reassessment in patients with multiple myeloma. *Hematological Oncology, 6,* 1–6.

Stashenko, P., Dewhirst, F. E., Peros, W. J., et al. (1987). Synergistic interactions between interleukin 1, tumor necrosis factor, and lymphotoxin in bone resorption. *Journal of Immunology, 138,* 1464–1468.

Tassone, P., Forciniti, S., Galea, E., et al. (2000). Growth inhibition and synergistic induction of apoptosis by zoledronate and dexamethasone in human myeloma cell lines. *Leukemia, 14,* 841–844.

Thiebaud, D., Leyuraz, S., Von Fliedner, V., et al. (1991). Treatment of bone metastases from breast cancer and myeloma with pamidronate. *European Journal of Cancer, 27,* 37–41.

Tirovola, E. B., Biassoni, L., Britton, K. E., et al. (1996). The use of 99mTc-MIBI scanning in multiple myeloma. *British Journal of Cancer, 74,* 1815–1820.

van Holten-Verzantvoort, A. A. T. M., Kroon, H. M., Bijvoet, O. L. M., et al. (1993). Palliative treatment in patients with bone metastases from breast cancer. *Journal of Clinical Oncology, 11*, 491–498.

Warrell, R. P., Lovett, D., Dilmanian, A., et al. (1993). Low-dose gallium nitrate for prevention of osteolysis in myeloma: results of a pilot randomized study. *Journal of Clinical Oncology, 11*, 2443–2450.

Wood, J., Bonjean, K., Ruetsz, S., et al. (2002). Novel antiangiogenic effects of the bisphosphonate compound zoledronic acid. *The Journal of Pharmacology and Experimental Therapeutics, 302*, 1055–1061.

Woolfenden, J. M., Pitt, M. J., Durie, B. G. M., et al. (1980). Comparison of bone scintigraphy and radiography in multiple myeloma. *Radiology, 134*, 723–728.

Yaccoby, S., Barlogie, B., and Epstein, J. (1998). Pamidronate inhibits growth of myeloma in vivo in the SCID-hu system. *Blood, 92*, 106a.

Yaccoby, S., Pearse, R., Epstein, J., et al. (2000). Reciprocal relationship between myeloma-induced changes in the bone marrow microenvironment and myeloma cell growth. *Blood*, 96, 549a.

# CHAPTER 16

―――――

# Management of Renal, Hematologic, and Infectious Complications

JOAN BLADÉ

## Renal Complications

### Incidence

Between 20% and 25% of patients with multiple myeloma (MM) seen in a tertiary hospital have a serum creatinine equal to or higher than 2 mg/dL (Alexanian et al., 1990; Bernstein et al., 1982; Bladé et al., 1998; Cohen et al., 1984; DeFronzo et al., 1975; Kyle, 1975) (Table 16-1). In 2 large multicenter studies, in which renal failure was defined by a serum creatinine higher than 1.5 mg/dL, the frequency of renal failure was 31% and 29%, respectively (Knudsen et al., 1994, 2000). Although the degree of renal failure is usually moderate with a serum creatinine lower than 4 mg/dL (Alexanian et al., 1990; Bernstein et al., 1982; Bladé et al., 1998; Cohen et al., 1984; DeFronzo et al., 1975; Knudsen et al., 1994, 2000; Kyle, 1975), in a series from a tertiary hospital the proportion of patients with newly diagnosed MM and renal failure requiring dialysis can be higher than 10% (Torra et al., 1995). In contrast, in large reference centers receiving a high proportion of outpatients, the proportion requiring dialysis is between 2% and 3% (Alexanian et al., 1990; Johnson et al., 1990). A lower proportion of patients develop renal insufficiency during the course of their disease. In these patients, renal function impairment is usually the result of episodes of hypercalcemia or the use of nephrotoxic antibiotics used in the treatment of bacterial infections.

## TABLE 16-1
### Renal Failure in Multiple Myeloma

|  | Percent |
| --- | --- |
| Frequency (creatinine ≥ 2 mg/dL) | 20–25 |
| Dialysis requirement | 10 |
| Reversibility rate | < 50 |
| Mortality within the first 2 mo | 30 |

## Pathogenesis of Renal Failure

The causes of renal insufficiency in patients with MM are summarized in Table 16-2. The excretion of light chains causes renal tubular damage with cast nephropathy (myeloma kidney) leading to progressive renal failure that might be worsened by precipitating factors. The clinical picture of tissue deposition of light chains is a nephrotic syndrome with or without renal failure. The structural differences in the light chains might cause different toxicity for specific organ structures (i.e., glomerular basement membranes, distal tubules) (Hill et al., 1983; Verroust et al., 1982).

### Light Chain Excretion

As already mentioned, the main cause of renal failure in patients with MM is the "myeloma kidney" resulting from light chain tubular damage. Light chains are filtered through the glomerulus and catabolized by proximal tubular renal cells. The characteristic feature of the myeloma kidney is the presence of myeloma casts consisting of eosinophilic material composed of light chains within renal tubule lumens surrounded by multinucleated giant cells of foreign body type in the distal tubules and collecting ducts (Boege et al., 1994; Hill et al., 1983; Sanders, 1994; Verroust et al., 1982). Tubular atrophy is usually present. No glomerular abnormalities are generally observed. In addition, by immunofluorescence or ultrastructural studies, the Tamm-Horsfall protein, a mucoprotein synthesized by the distal tubular cells, is also identified in the tubular casts (Hill et al., 1983). Although the Tamm-Horsfall

## TABLE 16-2
### Causes of Renal Failure in Multiple Myeloma

Light chain excretion
  Cast nephropathy (myeloma kidney)
Immunoglobulin tissue deposition
  Amyloid (AL)
  Immunoglobulin deposition disease (IMDD)
Tubular dysfunction
  Fanconi syndrome

protein and light chains within the tubules can lead to precipitation with subsequent cast formation, the role of Tamm-Horsfall protein in myeloma cast formation is not well understood. There is a correlation between the degree of cast formation and the severity of renal failure (Boege et al., 1994; Hill et al., 1983; Johnson et al., 1990; Pozzi et al., 1987; Verroust et al., 1982).

The reasons why some light chains are nephrotoxic while others not are unknown. It was suggested that the isoelectric point could play an important role in the light chain toxicity (Pasqualli et al., 1990; Rota et al., 1987). However, in several studies no relationship between the light chain isoelectric point and nephrotoxicity was observed (Coward et al., 1984; Johns et al., 1986; Melcion et al., 1984; Palant et al., 1986). Of interest, there are patients who never develop renal failure despite having a high light chain urine protein excretion. Thus, Kyle and Greipp reported a series of 7 patients with "idiopathic" light chain proteinuria who had been excreting large amounts of Bence Jones proteinuria for many years without developing nephropathy (Kyle and Greipp, 1982). Patients with MM and renal failure are usually diagnosed simultaneously with both conditions, with only few patients developing light chain nephropathy later in the course of the disease. Thus, when the light chains are nephrotoxic, they cause renal failure from the beginning, even before other clinical manifestations of myeloma emerge (Bladé et al., 1998; Torra et al., 1995). In fact, many patients who develop renal failure during the course of the disease have precipitating factors such as hypercalcemia, infection, or nephrotoxic antibiotics.

### Light Chain Tissue Deposition

Light chain tissue deposition consists of glomerular deposits of immunoglobulins, usually light chains, leading to amyloid or non-amyloid glomerular involvement. The clinical consequence is the development of nephrotic syndrome.

The amyloid deposits consist of fibrillar structures composed of light chains, characterized by positive staining with Congo red (Hill et al., 1983; Verroust et al., 1982). Amyloid deposition is found in mesangial and/or glomerular basement membranes. In a report from the Mayo Clinic (Bladé et al., 1994), including 1705 patients with MM, the frequency of associated AL varied according to the M-protein type: 5% in IgG, 2% in IgA, 13% in light chain (Bence Jones), and 19% in IgD myeloma. The finding of an M-protein in serum or urine in an adult with nephrotic syndrome is highly suspicious of AL (Gertz et al., 1999).

Light-chain deposition disease (LCDD), characterized by the deposition of nonfibrillar (Congo red–negative) material has been more recently recognized (Randall et al., 1976). However, in some patients the tissue deposits might also contain immunoglobulin heavy chain fragments. For this reason, the term monoclonal immunoglobulin deposition disease (MIDD) seems more appropriate (Dhodapkar et al., 1997; Preudhomme et al., 1994). In contrast with AL, the light chain in MIDD is usually of the kappa type. Renal involvement, resulting in nephrotic syndrome, is usually a characteristic feature in MIDD. In contrast with AL, in which renal serum creatinine remains normal in most cases, in MIDD renal function might rapidly deteriorate, resembling a picture of glomerulonephritis. These patients might have heart, liver, or other organ involvement, mimicking primary systemic amyloidosis (Dhodapkar et al., 1997). Nodular glomerulosclerosis, resembling diabetic lesions or membranoproliferative glomerulonephritis, is the most typical histologic feature of MIDD. In early phases of the disease, the glomerular lesions might be minimal. In these cases, the demonstration of monoclonal immunoglobulins along the outer part of the tubular basement membrane could be a diagnostic clue (Preudhomme et al., 1994). Interstitial fibrosis is constantly seen.

## Tubular Dysfunction

Acquired Fanconi's syndrome is a rare condition characterized by a failure in the reabsorption capacity of the proximal renal tubules, resulting in glucosuria, aminoaciduria, hypouricemia, and hypophosphatemia (Lacy and Gertz, 1999). The renal damage seems to be caused by imcompletely digested light chains, which form crystalline inclusions within the proximal tubular cells interfering with membrane transporters. In more than 90% of the cases the light chain is of the kappa type. Most patients are asymptomatic and the findings of glycosuria, proteinuria, hypokalemia, renal tubular acidosis, mild renal failure, or unexplained hypouricemia lead to the diagnosis of acquired Fanconi's syndrome. Mild renal insufficiency and bone pain from osteoporosis are the most common clinical features (Lacy and Gertz, 1999).

## Is a Kidney Biopsy Necessary in Patients with Multiple Myeloma?

In patients with symptomatic MM and renal failure in whom proteinuria mainly consists of light chains, the histopathologic picture of myeloma kidney is so likely that renal biopsy is not helpful and should be avoided. In cases in which the clinical finding consists of a nephrotic syndrome with or without renal failure, the first diagnostic possibility is associated AL and less likely IMDD. In this situation, a subcutaneous fat aspirate should be done and if negative for amyloid a rectal biopsy might be helpful. If there is no demonstration of amyloid in these locations, a renal biopsy would be the next step in the search for AL, IMDD, or unrelated glomerular nephropathy.

## Reversibility of Renal Function Impairment

The reversibility rate of renal failure in patients with MM varies from 20% to 60% (Alexanian et al., 1990; Bernstein et al., 1982; Bladé et al., 1998; Cavo et al., 1986; Cohen et al., 1984; Knudsen et al., 1994, 2000; Medical Research Council, 1984; Misiani et al., 1987; Pozzi et al., 1987). Approximately 50% of patients with serum creatinine levels lower than 4 mg/dL completely recover their renal function (Alexanian et al., 1990; Bladé et al., 1998; Knudsen et al., 2000). In contrast, in patients with a serum creatinine greater than 4 mg/dL, the recovery rate is less than 10% (Bladé et al., 1998). In the author's experience, the factors associated to renal function recovery are a serum creatinine level lower than 4 mg/dL, a 24-hour urine protein excretion lower than 1 g, and a serum calcium level higher than 11.5 mg/dL (Bladé et al., 1998) (Table 16-3). However, other studies reported no significant correlation between the serum creatinine levels and reversibility of renal failure (Cavo et al., 1986; Cohen et al., 1984). The improvement of renal function in patients with severe renal failure requiring renal replacement with dialysis is very low (Torra et al., 1995) (see "Dialysis" section).

## Chemotherapy Approaches

### Conventional Chemotherapy

In patients with MM and renal failure, the response rate to chemotherapy ranges from 40% to 50% (Bladé et al., 1998; Iggo et al., 1989; Knudsen et al., 2000; Korzets et al., 1990; Medical Research Council, 1984; Misiani et al., 1987). In our experience, the response rate in patients with renal function impairment is lower than in those with normal renal function (39% vs. 56%). Nevertheless, the lower response rate is because of the early mortality rate in patients with renal failure as compared with those with normal renal function (30% vs. 7%) (Bladé et al., 1998). If patients who die

---

=== **TABLE 16-3** ===

## Renal Failure in Multiple Myeloma

Predictors of reversibility*
  Serum creatinine <4 mg/dL
  Serum calcium ≥11.5 mg/dL
  Urine excretion <1 g/24 h

From Bladé, J., Fernández-Llama, P., Bosch, F., et al. (1998). Renal failure in multiple myeloma. Presenting features and predictors of outcome in 94 patients from a single institution. *Archives of Internal Medicine, 158,* 1889–1893.

within the first 2 months of initiation of treatment are excluded, the response to therapy is similar regardless of their renal function status (Bladé et al., 1998). Of interest, in patients on chronic hemodialysis program who survive the first 2 months on dialysis, the response rate is similar to that of those with normal renal function (Torra et al., 1995).

In patients with renal failure, conventional chemotherapy with melphalan and prednisone appears not to be the most appropriate treatment approach because the need for dose adjustment of melphalan to avoid excessive myelosuppression could lead to suboptimal treatment. On the other hand, combination chemotherapy could produce a more rapid response with a faster reduction in the light-chain protein production. In this regard, it has been suggested that chemotherapy with a 4-day continuous infusion of adriamycin and vincristine plus high-dose dexamethasone (VAD) (Barlogie et al., 1984) or high-dose methylprednisolone (VAMP) (Aitchison et al., 1990) could be more effective than more conventional approaches in patients with MM and renal failure. Although this has not been prospectively investigated, it seems to be the best approach for patients with severe renal failure. For patients in whom treatment with VAD is not feasible (associated cardiac disorders, poor clinical condition), treatment with pulse cyclophosphamide (800–1000 mg every 3 wk), which produces only a transient granulocytopenia, plus high-dose dexamethasone on days 1 through 4 also at 3-week intervals, would be the most appropriate therapy.

### High-Dose Therapy/Stem Cell Transplantation

A number of case reports and small series have shown the feasibility of high-dose therapy/stem cell transplantation (HDT/SCT) in patients with MM and renal failure (Ballester et al., 1997; Rebibou et al., 1997; Reiter et al., 1999; Tosi et al., 2000). The Spanish Registry reported a series of 14 patients with nonreversible renal failure undergoing HDT/SCT and compared the results with those achieved in patients with normal renal function at transplantation (San Miguel et al., 2000). The transplant-related mortality (TRM) was significantly higher in patients with renal function impairment (29% vs. 4%). The factors significantly associated to TRM were a serum creatinine level > 5 mg/dL, a hemoglobin level < 9.5 mg/dL, and poor performance status (ECOG > 2). The overall event-free and overall survival were not significantly different in patients with or without renal failure. From this study it was concluded that patients with MM and renal failure with a serum creatinine level > 5 mg/dL and poor performance status should be excluded from HDT/SCT programs. Badros et al. (2001) reported the results of HDT/SCT with melphalan 200 mg/m$^2$ (MEL-200) or melphalan 140 mg/m$^2$ (MEL-140) in 81 patients with

nonreversible renal failure (38 on dialysis) at the time of transplant. The TRM was 6% and 13% after a single or double transplant, respectively. In addition, nonhematologic toxicity, particularly in dialysis-dependent patients receiving MEL-200, was really high. In this regard, serious bacterial infections were documented in 48% of the patients. Other frequent complications were pneumonia (8 patients required mechanic ventilation) and atrial dysrhythmias (Badros et al., 2001). Encephalopathy was observed in several patients with renal failure, particularly in those on dialysis. The cause of encephalopathy was unclear. Low serum albumin and a high serum concentration of melphalan increased toxicity and mortality and significantly influenced overall survival. The incidence of complications was significantly higher in patients receiving MEL-200 than in those given MEL-140. Interestingly enough, patients given MEL-140 had a similar outcome (complete remission [CR], event-free survival [EFS], and overall survival [OS]) than those receiving MEL-200. Chemoresistant disease, low serum albumin, and older age were associated with a significantly shorter overall survival. Considering these results, in patients with renal failure, HDT/SCT should be individually considered and only performed in relatively younger patients with chemosensitive disease and good general condition, being the best intensification regimen MEL-140.

When MIDD or AL is associated to overt MM, the treatment approach must be the same as for patients with myeloma. In the treatment of AL in patients younger than 65 years with less than 3 organs involved and no symptomatic cardiopathy, HDT/SCT should be considered. This approach might be particularly helpful when nephrotic syndrome is the prominent feature of AL. In patients with AL who have a serum creatinine level higher than 1.5 mg/dL or a creatinine clearance lower than 50 mL/min, the dose of melphalan should be reduced from 200 mg/m$^2$ to 140 mg/m$^2$, because these patients with AL and renal function impairment, even if it is moderate, are at high risk for developing severe renal failure requiring dialysis with the usual high-dose regimen (Comenzo and Gertz, 2002). Importantly, the mortality rate of patients with AL requiring dialysis during the peritransplant period is almost 80% (Comenzo and Gertz, 2002). In patients with MIDD with no symptomatic cardiac involvement, HDT/SCT should also be considered. Of interest, patients with no overt myeloma in whom the plasma cell burden is low and the organ dysfunction is the result of tissue deposition (AL, MIDD, POEMS), the likelihood of response to high-dose therapy is high because the tumor burden at the time of transplant is low (Comenzo and Gertz, 2002; Dhodapkar et al., 1997; Jaccard et al., 2002; Rovira et al., 2001). In addition, in these circumstances there is no need for tumor reduction before stem cell mobilization.

In patients with nonreversible renal failure requiring chronic dialysis who achieve complete remission (disappearance of malignant bone marrow plasma cells with no evidence of serum/urine M-protein on immunofixation) after conventional or high-dose therapy, the possibility of a kidney transplant might be considered. However, most patients will end up with recurrence of their nephropathy at relapse (Gerlag et al., 1986).

## Supportive Measures

### Plasma Exchange

It has been suggested that the removal of light chains with plasma exchange could prevent irreversible renal failure by avoiding further renal damage (Cavo et al., 1986; Pasqualli et al., 1990; Pozzi et al., 1987; Vhalin et al., 1987). Misiani et al. (1987) reported that 9% (2 of 23) patients treated with chemotherapy and plasma exchange recovered from their acute renal failure. In a non-controlled study including 50 patients, Pozzi et al. (1987) showed that in patients treated with chemotherapy and plasma exchange, the recovery of renal function was significantly higher than in those treated with chemotherapy alone (61% vs. 27%). Zucchelli et al. (1988) reported the results of a randomized trial comparing chemotherapy plus plasma exchange versus chemotherapy alone in 29 patients with MM and severe renal failure (24 of them on dialysis) and light chain urine protein excretion higher than 1 g/24 hours. Importantly, in 13 of the 15 patients of the plasma exchange arm the serum creatinine level decreased to less than 2.5 mg/dL, whereas only 2 of the 14 patients treated with chemotherapy alone could discontinue dialysis. Finally, the 1-year survival rate was 66% in the plasma exchange arm versus 28% in the control group. In a small randomized trial, the Mayo Clinic group compared forced diuresis and chemotherapy (10 patients) versus forced diuresis, chemotherapy, and plasma exchange (11 patients) (Johnson et al., 1990). They only found a statistical trend in favor of the plasma exchange group. In our experience, patients with renal failure severe enough to require dialysis do not benefit from plasma exchange (Torra et al., 1995). This is in agreement with the findings by Johnson et al. (1990) and Pozzi et al. (1987) who recognized the severity of myeloma cast formation as the major factor associated with nonreversible renal failure, even in patients undergoing plasma exchange (Johnson et al., 1990; Pozzi et al., 1987; Torra et al., 1995). In fact, the Oxford Renal Unit group (Winearls, 1995) treated 16 patients whom they thought had reversible renal damage with plasma exchange achieving significant renal function improvement in 6 with dialysis

discontinuation in 3. In contrast, only 1 of 26 patients not treated with plasma exchange improved. We treated 8 patients with severe non-oliguric renal failure (median serum creatinine of 5.5 mg/dL; range, 4.6–7.5 mg/dL) with VAD chemotherapy and plasma exchange. One patient required dialysis, in 3 patients renal failure was basically unchanged, 2 had a significant improvement with serum creatinine levels between 2 and 3 mg/dL, and the remaining 2 patients reached serum creatinine levels lower than 2 mg/dL (Bladé, unpublished results). This compares favorably with the less than 10% reversibility rate in our population not undergoing plasma exchange (Bladé et al., 1998), but the number of patients is too low to draw consistent conclusions.

It is our practice to perform plasma exchange with 5% albumin in saline solution with a total volume of approximately 100% to 120% of the total plasma volume in each session in patients with MM and non-oliguric severe renal failure. Serum and urine M-protein are measured before and after each plasma exchange procedure and the sessions are repeated every 2 or 3 days until a maximum of 4 or 5. With this approach, replacement with coagulation factors is usually not necessary. As a result of the background immunoglobulin removal with plasma exchange, intravenous inmunoglobulins are given after the end of plasma exchange program to prevent bacterial infections in these high-risk patients (multiple myeloma with severe renal failure receiving their initial chemotherapy and undergoing plasma exchange with uninvolved normal immunoglobulin depletion). Also, the use of a number 9F flexible silicone catheter, which produces less local lesion with a lower incidence of thrombophlebitis, is recommended.

### Dialysis

The frequency of patients with MM and renal failure severe enough to require dialysis varies from 2% to 13% depending on the characteristics of the institutions where the patients are seen (Alexanian et al., 1990; Johnson et al., 1990; Sharland et al., 1997; Torra et al., 1995). It is of interest that in between 70% and 80% of the patients, the diagnosis of both conditions is simultaneous (Cohen et al., 1984; Cosio et al., 1981; Pozzi et al., 1987; Rota et al., 1987; Torra et al., 1995). Severe renal failure is most commonly seen in light chain and IgD myeloma than in IgG and IgA myeloma types. Thus, in patients with renal failure the frequency of light chain myeloma ranges from 20% to 62%, whereas in the general myeloma series the incidence of Bence Jones myeloma is approximately 15% (Cohen et al., 1984; Cosio et al., 1981; Iggo et al., 1989; Johnson et al., 1980, 1990; Lazarus et al., 1983; Misiani et al., 1987; Pasqualli et al., 1990; Pozzi et al., 1987; Rota et al., 1987; Sharland et al., 1997).

The response rate to chemotherapy in patients with MM on long-term dialysis program ranges from 40% to 60% (Iggo et al., 1989; Korzets et al., 1990; Torra et al., 1995). At our institution we found a response rate of 40% in patients on dialysis versus 43% in our population of patients with stage III myeloma who did not require dialysis and who had survived the first 2 months from the initiation of chemotherapy (Torra et al., 1995). Thus, renal failure does not per se influence the response to chemotherapy.

In patients requiring dialysis, the reversibility of renal failure is usually less than 10% (Cosio et al., 1981; Coward et al., 1983; Iggo et al., 1989; Johnson et al., 1980, 1990; Korzets et al., 1990; Lazarus et al., 1983; Torra et al., 1995) and the recovery rarely occurs after 4 months on dialysis. In contrast with most series, 2 studies reported that 75% (12 of 16) and 43% (13 of 30) of patients were able to discontinue dialysis, respectively (Misiani et al., 1987; Pasqualli et al., 1990).

The mortality rate among patients with MM and renal failure during the first 2 months from diagnosis is still approximately 30% (Bladé et al., 1998; Cohen et al., 1984; Johnson et al., 1980; Pasqualli et al., 1990; Torra et al., 1995). Concerning patients not dying during the initiation of dialysis, the Mayo Clinic group (Johnson et al., 1980) reported that 5 of 11 patients on long-term dialysis had a prolonged survival. In another 2 series the median survival was approximately 2 years, with one-third of patients surviving for more than 3 years (Korzets et al., 1990; Torra et al., 1995). The need for hospitalization, in patients with MM and long-term dialysis program, has been assessed in several studies. In the series by Korzets et al. (1990), the number of hospital admissions was 6.1 per year and the total number of days in hospital was 75 per patient per year. In contrast, in 2 series the average of hospitalization was 12 and 19 days per patient year, respectively (Johnson et al., 1980; Torra et al., 1995). In the author's experience patients who survive for more than 1 year spend less than 10 days per year in the hospital, a figure similar to that observed in patients on chronic dialysis because of diabetic nephropathy (Torra et al., 1995). Considering all this, long-term dialysis is a worthwhile treatment for patients with myeloma and severe non-reversible renal failure.

## Treatment Approach in Patients with Multiple Myeloma and Renal Failure

The treatment approaches for patients with MM and renal function impairment are summarized in Table 16-4. Patients with a moderate increase in serum creatinine levels or reversible renal failure should receive the standard chemotherapy followed (or not) by HDT/SCT according to age and patient clinical condition. Patients with a serum creatinine higher than

---

**TABLE 16-4**

### Treatment Approaches in Patients with Multiple Myeloma and Renal Failure

MP: not recommended (myelosuppression, need for dose adjustments)

VAD or Cyclo/Dexa: best initial therapy

HDT/SCT intensification: in selected patients (<60 y, chemosensitive disease, good PS)

MP, melphalan and prednisone; VAD, infusional vincristine and adriamycin plus high-dose dexamethasone; HDT/SCT, high-dose therapy/stem cell transplantation.

---

4 mg/dL should be treated with VAD or cyclophosphamide plus dexamethasone. High-dose therapy should only be performed in selected patients and the intensification regimen should consist of MEL-140 or MEL-100. In non-oliguric patients, still not requiring dialysis, an early plasma exchange program along with forced diuresis and chemotherapy is likely to be of benefit. However, in patients with advanced myeloma kidney already requiring dialysis, plasma exchange does not seem to be beneficial. Renal replacement with dialysis is a worthwhile palliative measure for patients with myeloma with end-stage renal failure (Table 16-5).

# Hematologic Complications

## Anemia

### Incidence

Anemia is the most common hematologic complications in patients with multiple myeloma. Thus, in the first Mayo Clinic series reported by Kyle (1975), the median hemoglobin level was 11.1 g/dL and 8% of the patients had a hemoglobin level lower than 8 g/dL. Similar results have been observed in the most recent Mayo Clinic series, including 1027 patients (Kyle et al., 2003). In the Spanish PETHEMA series, composed of 914 patients, the mean hemoglobin level was 10 g/dL, with 37% of the patients having an Hb level lower than

---

**TABLE 16-5**

### Renal Failure in Multiple Myeloma, Supportive Measures

Plasma exhange
  Likely of benefit: severe non-oliguric renal failure
  Limited or no efficacy: severe myeloma kidney (patients already on dialysis)
Dialysis replacement
  Worthwhile palliative measure

9 g/dL (Bladé et al., 2001). Anemia is associated to a loss in quality of life and is a prognostic factor in most studies. In fact, an Hb level of less than 8.5 g/dL defines per se in stage III disease (high tumor mass), according to the Durie and Salmon staging system (Durie and Salmon, 1975). In addition to the patients presenting with anemia at diagnosis, many patients develop anemia severe enough to require red cell transfusions later in the course of the disease because of progressive myeloma unresponsive to chemotherapy with increasing plasma cell bone marrow infiltration.

## Etiology

In patients with multiple myeloma, the cause of anemia is likely multifactorial (Meharchand, 1998) (Table 16-6).

Considering that the median proportion of bone marrow plasma cells in patients with symptomatic MM is between 50% and 60%, bone marrow replacement by myeloma cells is one major cause of anemia. Nevertheless, some patients with MM and significant anemia have only a discrete increase in bone marrow plasma cells. On the other hand, it is of note that, despite the heavy bone marrow involvement by plasma cells, only 13% and 7% of patients with MM have WBC and platelet counts lower than $4 \times 10E^9/L$ and $100 \times 10E^9/L$, respectively (Bladé et al., 2001). These facts support that there is an important role for other mechanisms of anemia in patients with myeloma.

When treatment with chemotherapy, particularly when using alkylating agents, is started in patients with significant bone marrow involvement and "borderline" Hb level, the Hb can drop during the first courses of chemotherapy until malignant plasma cells are cleared from the bone marrow and a response is achieved. Thus, it is not unusual that patients with an initial Hb level between 9 and 10 g/dL will require transfusion because of worsening of anemia during the first 2 or 3 months of treatment. Usually, the response to chemotherapy is associated with an increase in the Hb level after the first months of treatment.

Patients with cancer do not respond to anemia through the common increase in erythropoietin

production observed in other patient populations (Means and Kranz, 1992). Concerning MM, Beguin et al. (1992) found a decreased erythropoiesis, even in patients with no extensive bone marrow involvement by plasma cells. Thus, 25% of 62 patients with MM had an inadequate erythropoietin production according to the degree of anemia. Furthermore, a reduction in erythropoietin production was noted in up to 50% of patients with stage III myeloma. Although the role of cytokines in the anemia associated with MM is unclear, it has been suggested the interleukin-1 and tumor necrosis factor might impair the use of reticuloendothelial iron, playing a role in the anemia of MM and other chronic disorders (Denz et al., 1990; Faquin et al., 1992). It has been recently reported that disregulated myeloma cell apoptosis might contribute to progressive destruction of the erythroid matrix through the induction of erythroblast cytotoxicity. Thus, the upregulated expression of several apoptogenic receptors, including both Fas-L and 1g tumor necrosis factor-related apoptosis-inducing ligand (TRAIL), is a critical factor in the pathogenesis of anemia in MM (Tucci et al., 2002).

Patients with very high serum IgG or IgA M-protein level apparently could have a higher degree of anemia as a result of hemodilution. This should be taken into account in patients with smoldering multiple myeloma in whom a moderate degree of anemia should not be an indication for initiation of treatment with chemotherapy agents per se. Occasionally, folate or $B_{12}$ vitamin deficiencies can be observed. In cases of $B_{12}$ deficiency, it should be excluded that it is the result of associated amyloidosis with malabsorption. Autoimmune hemolytic anemia is very rare (Kyle et al., 2003).

In patients heavily pretreated with alkylating agents, particularly with melphalan, the development of an unexplained anemia, while in response of MM, might be the first feature of myelodysplasia. Megaloblastic changes, dysgranulo- and dysmegakaryopoiesis as well as the presence of ring-sideroblasts in the bone marrow, should be carefully investigated. Cytogenetic abnormalities might be the diagnostic key of myelodysplasia.

## Management

Blood transfusion has been the only available treatment for cancer-associated severe anemia until recently. The main problems with blood transfusion are its temporary effect and the risk of adverse effects, particularly immunologic reactions and infections (hepatitis, HIV). With FDA approval for the use of recombinant human erythropoietin (rHuEPO) for the treatment of anemia of renal failure slightly more than a decade ago, this growth factor has been used in an attempt to improve anemia in different cancer patient populations. The results of the seminal report by Ludwig et al. (1990) showing in a small series of patients with

═══════ **TABLE 16-6** ═══════

## Mechanisms of Anemia in Multiple Myeloma

Plasma cell bone marrow replacement
Relative EPO deficiency
Renal insufficiency
Decreased erythropoiesis (cytokine mediated-TNFα and IL-1)
Chemotherapy/radiation therapy
Disregulated cell apoptosis
Others ($B_{12}$ or folate deficiency, hemolytic autoimmune—rare)

**TABLE 16-7**

## Clinical Trials with rHu-EPO in Multiple Myeloma

| Author | EPO | No. | Response Criteria | Response Rate |
|--------|-----|-----|-------------------|---------------|
| Ludwig et al., 1994 | α | 18 | ≥2 g/dL | 76 |
| Barlogie et al., 1993 | α | 41 | ≥2 g/dL | 78 |
| Garton et al., 1995 | α | 21 | >38% Ht* | 60 vs 0 |
| Musto et al., 1997 | β | 37 | No transf | 35 |
| Cazzola et al., 1995 | β | 84 | ≥2 g/dL* | 61 vs 7 |
| Österborg et al., 1996 | β | 65 | ≥2 g/dL* | 55 vs 20 |
| Littlewood et al., 2001 | α | 58 | No transf* | 55 vs 11 |
| Dammacco et al., 2001 | α | 145 | No transf* | 47 vs 23 |
| Österborg et al., 2002 | β | 116 | ≥2 g/dL | 76 vs 23 |

*Randomized trials.

MM, the beneficial effect of rHuEPO have been confirmed in a number of trials. The results of rHuEPO versus placebo in several randomized studies are summarized in Table 16-7 (Barlogie and Beck, 1993; Cazzola et al., 1995; Dammacco et al., 2001; Garton et al., 1995; Littlewood et al., 2001; Ludwig et al., 1994; Musto et al., 1997; Osterborg et al., 2002). Patients given rHuEPO had a significant increase in Hb level and a decrease in transfusion requirement along with an improvement in quality of life. Of interest, the greatest improvement in quality of life has been particularly found when the Hb level was increased from 11 to 12 g/dL (Cleeland et al., 1999). In addition, several factors have been recognized as critical in the use of rHuEPO therapy: (1) dose/schedule and type of rHuEPO, (2) importance of baseline endogenous erythropoietin level, (3) predictors of response, and (4) role of iron repletion. In this regard, the American Society of Clinical Oncology and the American Society of Hematology have recently provided evidence-based guidelines for the use of rHuEPO in patients with cancer (Rizzo et al., 2002a; Rizzo et al., 2002b). Furthermore, a panel of experts have also made recommendations for management of disease-related anemia in patients with MM and chronic lymphocytic leukemia (Ludwig et al., 2002). Both groups essentially agree in the recommendations of rHuEPO use (Table 16-8).

It has been reported that rHuEPO can also be useful in patients resistant to the initial chemotherapy when given in association with rescue regimens (Silvestris et al., 1995). In addition, a randomized trial showed that rHuEPO was useful in patients refractory to standard chemotherapy (Dammacco et al., 1998). However, I assume that in patients with refractory relapse with extensive bone marrow involvement and a short life expectancy, who usually do not enter

**TABLE 16-8**

## Recommendations for rHuEPO Therapy in Cancer Patients*

Patients with Hb level <10 g/dL
Restricted to certain clinical circumstances if Hb is between 10–12 g/dL
Starting dose: 10,000 IU 3 times per week; dose escalation to 20,000 IU if no response at 4 wk (Hb ⇑ <1 g/dL) or
Starting dose: 40,000 IU once a week with increase to 60,000 IU if no response
Discontinue therapy if there is no response at 8 wk (Hb ⇑ 1–2 g/dL)
Dose tritiation to maintain Hb around 12 g/dL
   If Hb >12 g/dL: reduce dose by 25%
   If Hb >14 g/dL: discontinue EPO and re-start at reduced dose if it falls <12 g/dL
Iron repletion

Data from Ludwig, H., Rai, K., Bladé, J., et al. (2002). Management of disease-related anemia in patients with multiple myeloma or chronic lymphocytic leukemia: epoetin alfa treatment recommendations. *The Hematology Journal, 3,* 121–130. Rizzo, J. D., Lichtin, A.E., Woolf, S. H., Seidenfeld, J., Bennett, C. L., Cella, D., et al. (2002a). Use of epoietin in patients with cancer: evidence-based clinical practice guidelines of the American Society of Clinical Oncology and the American Society of Hematology. *Blood, 100,* 2303–2320.

clinical trials, the likelihood of response to rHuEPO is very low. In consequence, I would not favor the administration of rHuEPO in patients with advanced refractory myeloma.

The "novel erythropoiesis-stimulating protein" (NESP), or darbepoietin alpha, has a longer half-life and a greater erythropoietic activity than rHuEPO. It has been shown to be effective and safe in patients with cancer and needs to be given only once a week. There are several ongoing clinical trials aimed at fully establishing its safety and optimal dose-response effect (Beguin, 2002).

In most studies, patients with a relatively low EPO level or a decreased observed/medicated EPO ratio are the most likely to respond. In fact, the most powerful predictors of response are the initial endogenous EPO level along with an absolute increase in Hb level ($> 0.5$ g/dL) after 2 weeks of therapy or changes in other indicators of erythropoietic activity such as reticulocyte count $>40,000$ µL or increase in soluble transferrin receptor (sTfR) $>25\%$ (Beguin, 2002; Cazzola et al., 1995; Ludwig et al., 1994). The direct relationship between the number of erythroid precursors and the sTfR has made its measurement a useful parameter to assess the erythropoietic response to EPO. In fact, patients with $< 0.5$ g/L in Hb level and a $<25\%$ increase in sTfR at 3 weeks from initiation of EPO therapy are very unlikely to respond (Beguin, 2002).

The most common causes of failure to respond or loss of rHuEPO efficacy are listed in Table 16-9. The most frequent cause of limitation in rHuEPO therapy is functional iron deficiency. Iron supplementation should be given when iron deficiency is suspected in patients with anemia of chronic disease (serum ferritine $< 100$ µg/L) or functional iron deficiency (transferrin saturation $<20\%$) (Beguin, 2002). In patients with anemia or chronic renal failure, oral iron supplementation was proven to be of limited value, whereas intravenous iron was proven to be useful (Beguin, 2002). Thus, weekly intravenous administration of 100 to 300 mg of iron saccharate is likely the best supplementation therapy (Table 16-10).

## TABLE 16-9

### Causes of rHuEPO Failure in Patients with Multiple Myeloma

Functional iron deficiency
Infection
Surgery
Bleeding/hemolysis
Folate or B$_{12}$ deficiency
Extensive plasma cell bone marrow involvement

## TABLE 16-10

### rHuEPO Treatment, Iron Repletion

Indications
 Suspected iron deficiency
  (i.e., serum ferritin $<100$ mg/L in ACD)
 Functional iron deficiency
  Transferrin saturation $<20\%$
  Soluble transferrin receptor ⇑
Iron administration
 Oral: limited efficacy
 Intravenous iron saccharate
  (100–300 mg/wk)

ACD, anemia of chronic disease.

## Granulocytopenia and Thrombocytopenia

Severe granulocytopenia at the time of diagnosis is extremely unusual in patients with MM. Moderate degrees of leukopenia/granulocytopenia have been reported in less than 10% of the patients and are not generally associated with serious infections. The proportion of patients with a platelet count lower than $100 \times 10E^9$/L was 8% of a large series from the Spanish Group PETHEMA (Bladé et al., 2001). Platelet counts lower than $20 \times 10^9$/L with risk of severe bleeding is very rare. Conventional chemotherapy with MP, BVMCP, or alternating VCMP/VBAP produce a variable but usually moderate degree of neutropenia. In one study using VCMP/VBAP at higher doses, cyclophosphamide and doxorubicin produced a higher degree of transient granulocytopenia; it was associated with a significantly higher probability of early death, particularly in patients older than 60 years and in an advanced stage of the disease (Bladé et al., 2001). It seems that in elderly patients with advanced disease a modest increase in the conventional doses can result in early death as a result of granulocytopenia and infection. In contrast, MP resulted in a significantly higher degree of thrombocytopenia than VCMP/VBAP, both at standard and higher doses. These different patterns of toxicity resulted in a significantly higher need for dose reduction on melphalan in the MP arm. Thus, in elderly patients with extensive plasma cell bone marrow involvement and low or borderline platelet count, full doses of melphalan should be avoided to prevent the development of more severe thrombocytopenia precluding subsequent chemotherapy. For these patients, cyclophosphamide/prednisone or alternating VCMP/VBAP are better options (Bladé et al., 2001; MacLennan et al., 1992).

## Myelodysplasia and Secondary Acute Leukemia

The development of an unexplained pancytopenia in a patient who has received melphalan should raise the possibility of myelodysplasia (MDS) or acute leukemia

(AL) (Bergsagel et al., 1979). In this situation a bone marrow aspirate in the search of dyshemopoietic features, ring-sideroblasts, and cytogenetic abnormalities is mandatory. The expected incidence of AL in patients with MM treated with alkylating agents is 100 to 230 times higher than expected in a normal population (Bergsagel, 1982). In a series from the National Cancer Institute of Canada including 364 patients treated with alkylating agents, a total of 15 cases of AL were recognized (Bergsagel et al., 1979). In this study the actuarial probability of AL at 5 and 10 years of followup was 14% and 25%, respectively (Bergsagel, 1988). In a recent study by the Finish Leukemia Group Study, including 432 patients treated with conventional chemotherapy, the incidence of AL was analyzed after a median followup of 16 years (range, 11–19 y) (Finish Leukaemia Group, 2000) with only 19 of the patients still alive. Fourteen of the 432 patients developed AL with an actuarial risk of almost 10% at 9 years. Of interest, in the Finish study, no cases of AL were observed among the 53 patients who survived beyond 9 years from initiation of treatment. The Medical Research Council (MRC) reported an actuarial risk of AL or MDS of 3% and 10% at 5 and 8 years of followup, respectively (Cuzick et al., 1987). This study showed that melphalan was much more leukemogenic than cyclophosphamide. Although the development of AL might be part of the natural history of plasma cell dyscrasias (Anderson et al., 1999; Bergsagel, 1982; Rosner and Grünwald, 1984), the exposure to alkylating agents, particularly melphalan, is crucial. The dose of melphalan during the years preceding the development of acute leukemia seems important. However, the role of the cumulative dose of melphalan remains controversial (Finish Leukaemia Group, 2000).

A high incidence of MDS and AL has been reported in patients with follicular lymphoma undergoing high-dose therapy followed by stem cell support (HDT/SCS) (Miller et al., 1994). This fact raised the question on the role of HDT itself or conventional chemotherapy preceding HDT as the crucial cause of secondary leukemia. This issue has been investigated in patients with MM who underwent HDT/SCS at the University of Arkansas (Govindarajan et al., 1996). The authors of this study showed that a previous standard dose of alkylating agents before transplant is the cause of MDS/AL rather than the myeloablative therapy.

## Hyperviscosity Syndrome

The hyperviscosity syndrome is a characteristic manifestation of Waldenström's macroglobulinemia that can also be seen in patients with MM. However, although serum viscosity is usually elevated, symptomatic hyperviscosity requiring plasmapheresis is exceedingly rare in patients with MM (Kyle, 1975).

The main mechanisms of hyperviscosity involve total serum protein concentration, physicochemical characteristics of the M-protein, and the degree of aggregation of the monoclonal protein. Thus, the protein more frequently associated with hyperviscosity is IgM, followed by IgA and IgG or even aggregates of light chains, particularly of the kappa type (Meharchand, 1998).

The clinical picture of the hyperviscosity syndrome can include: (1) mucosal bleeding (epistaxis, postsurgical hemorrhage); (2) ocular manifestations (retinopathy, loss of vision); (3) neurologic symptoms (headaches, vertigo); and (4) congestive heart failure. The clinician should be aware that the manifestations of hyperviscosity can be extremely variable.

The management of symptomatic hyperviscosity syndrome should consist of plasmapheresis. This procedure results in a prompt decrease in the serum M-protein concentration. Although plasmapheresis is used with relative frequency in patients with Waldenström's macroglobulinemia, in the author's experience it is very rarely required in patients with MM.

## Bleeding Disorders

Significant bleeding disorders are uncommon in patients with MM, except in the terminal phase of the disease when heavy plasma cell bone marrow replacement and the effect of salvage chemotherapy can result in severe thrombocytopenia. Severe thrombocytopenia can also be the consequence of secondary leukemia or myelodysplasia. Both renal failure and the hyperviscosity syndrome can result in abnormal platelet function. When the abnormal platelet function is associated with thrombocytopenia the risk of severe bleeding is significantly increased. Patients with primary amyloidosis (AL) or multiple myeloma with associated AL usually have an increased bleeding tendency as a result of the amyloid vascular involvement. Clinicians should be aware that these patients are at risk of massive hemorrhage or bleeding from unusual locations with surgical procedures. In addition, approximately 10% of patients with systemic AL have a factor X below 50% of normal values as a result of the factor adsorption on amyloid deposits (Choufani et al., 2001). Approximately 50% of these patients have bleeding complications, which are more frequent and severe in those who have factor X levels below 25% of normal. Occasionally the bleeding episodes are fatal (Choufani et al., 2001). Of interest, most patients responding to therapy have an improvement in their factor X deficiency. In case of factor X deficiency and severe bleeding, reposition with plasma is necessary until hemorrhage stops. In cases of severe recurrent bleeding, splenectomy might be helpful (Rosenstein et al., 1983).

# Infectious Complications

## Incidence

Infectious complications remain the major cause of morbidity and mortality in patients with MM (Kelleher and Chapel, 2002). The susceptibility of patients with myeloma to bacterial infections was recognized almost 50 years ago, when the importance of Gram-positive infections, particularly recurrent pneumococcal pneumonia, was noted (Glenchur et al., 1959; Zinneman and Hall, 1954). Subsequent studies reported that the frequency of infectious episodes in MM ranges from 0.80 to 2.22 per patient year, which is 7 to 15 times higher than that observed in patients hospitalized from other causes (Table 16-11) (Kelleher and Chapel, 2002). Finally, infection is often the cause of death in patients with MM, usually in the late phase of the disease (Bladé et al., 2001).

## Causes of Infection

Although the increased susceptibility to infection in MM is multifactorial (Table 16-12), it is very likely that the major cause is the impaired specific antibody production (Jacobson and Zolla-Pazner, 1986). In fact, three-fourths of patients with MM have a decreased synthesis of uninvolved immunoglobulins, thus resulting in a low level of polyclonal immunoglobulins (Broder et al., 1975; Fahey et al., 1963; Kyle et al., 2003). Decreased serum levels of uninvolved IgG and IgA have been significantly associated with an increased risk of serious infections in MM. In addition, the antibody response following immunization is severely impaired (Hargreaves et al., 1995).

It has been reported that imbalances of CD4/CD8 T cells might play an important role in the immune suppression in MM (Jacobson and Zolla-Pazner, 1986; Kelleher and Chapel, 2002; Mills and Cawley, 1983).

### TABLE 16-11
#### Serious Infections in Multiple Myeloma

| Overall incidence | 0.8–2.22 per patient-year |
| | During active disease: 1.9 patient-year |
| | Plateau phase: 0.49 patient-year* |
| | 1 every 22 plateau-year[†] |
| Highest risk | First 2 months of initiation of therapy |
| | Patients with renal failure |

*Hargreaves, R. M., Lea, J. R., Griffiths, H., Faux, J. A., Holt, J. M., Bunch, C., et al. (1995). Immunological factors and risk of infection in plateau phase myeloma. *Journal of Clinical Pathology, 48,* 260–266.
[†]Snowdon, L., Gibson, J., and Joshua, D. E. (1994). Frequency of infection in plateau-phase multiple myeloma [Letter]. *Lancet, 344,* 262.

### TABLE 16-12
#### Causes of Infection in Multiple Myeloma

Decreased synthesis of uninvolved immunoglobulins
CD4/CD8 imbalances
Defective opsonization
Decreased granulocyte adhesiveness
Impaired leukocyte migration
Renal function impairment
Chemotherapy-induced granulocytopenia
Glucocorticoid treatment (particularly high-dose dexamethasone)

However, infections related to cell-mediated immunity, except those caused by herpes virus, are very unusual in patients with myeloma.

Non-immune mechanisms such as defective opsonization (Cheson et al., 1980; Kansu et al., 1986), decreased granulocyte adhesiveness (Hopen et al., 1984; MacGregor et al., 1978), and impaired leukocyte migration (Hopen et al., 1984) can contribute to increase the susceptibility to infections. Most patients with MM have a normal granulocyte count, and conventional chemotherapy usually produces granulocytopenia of a moderate degree not associated with a significant risk of serious infection. When chemotherapy results in severe granulocytopenia, this constitutes an additional risk factor for infection. This is particularly true in older patients with advanced-stage disease, especially during the first courses of combination chemotherapy (Bladé et al., 2001). Treatment with glucocorticoids, in particular with high-dose dexamethasone, also increase the risk of infection. High-dose therapy followed by autologous stem cell rescue produces transient but severe granulocytopenia, which usually results in infection. However, the risk of infection after autologous transplantation in MM is not higher than in other diseases undergoing the procedure.

It is uncertain whether renal insufficiency is an independent risk factor of infection in patients with MM, because this subset of patients constitutes by itself a poor prognosis group (Jacobson and Zolla-Pazner, 1986). In any event, renal function impairment is associated with a higher incidence of infectious complications (Hoen et al., 1995). In fact, one-third of patients with MM and renal failure die within the first 2 months from diagnosis, most of them from serious infections (Bladé et al., 1998).

## Timing of Infection

There is a close relationship between disease activity and infection rate (Table 16-11). Thus, the highest risk falls within the first months of initiation of therapy and in patients with relapsed/refractory disease, whereas patients responding to chemotherapy, in the so-called plateau phase, are at low risk of infectious complications. As mentioned, the overall frequency of infection in patients with MM ranges from 0.8 to 2.22 per patient per year (Kelleher and Chapel, 2002). Hargreaves et al. (1995) reported that the incidence of serious infections was 4 times higher during active disease compared with the plateau phase (1.9 vs. 0.49 episodes per patient per year). However, even the frequency of 0.49 episodes per patient/year in the plateau phase seems higher than the one usually seen in clinical practice. In fact, Snowdon et al. (1994) in a series of 114 patients in the plateau phase followed for 241 plateau-years reported a frequency of a serious or life-threatening infection every 22 plateau-years. The discrepancy between the last 2 studies has been attributed to differences in patient selection and plateau definition (Snowdon et al., 1994). Regarding timing of infection, the highest risk group is constituted by patients with renal failure (serum creatinine > 2 mg/dL) during the first 2 months of chemotherapy with a mortality rate within the first 2 months of approximately 30%. Another fragile group is constituted by refractory/relapsed patients who are given conventional chemotherapy at higher doses than the usual, with or without growth factors. These rescue chemotherapy regimens are usually given to quickly reduce the tumor burden as a previous step for a subsequent HDT/SCT approach. These combinations usually produce transient but severe granulocytopenia with a real increase incidence of serious infections.

Considering patients who receive HDT followed by autologous stem cell support as consolidation or intensification of the response achieved with chemotherapy, the episodes of fever with or without clinical or bacteriologic evidence of infection is very high. However, these infections are easily controlled with broad-spectrum antibacterial antibiotics because the patients are usually in good clinical condition and the period of granulocytopenia is short. When dealing with patients who undergo autologous transplantation for refractory disease, the incidence of severe infections increase (poorer clinical condition with active disease and usually heavier previous chemotherapy, all of this resulting in severely impaired immunosurveillance). Patients with MM undergoing allogeneic transplantation develop all the infectious complications associated with the allogeneic procedure, particularly those derived from graft-versus-host disease (GVHD) and its immunosuppressive therapy, including viral (CMV), fungal (*Aspergillus* sp. and other filamentous fungi, *Candida* sp.), *Pneumocystis carinii,* and bacterial (Gram-negative and Gram-positive).

## Sites of Infection and Microbiology

The main sites of infection are the respiratory and the urinary tracts as well as septicemia. *Streptococcus pneumoniae, Staphylococcus aureus,* and *Haemophilus*

---

**TABLE 16-13**

### Microbiology of Infections in Multiple Myeloma

**Gram-positive bacteria** *(Streptococcus pneumoniae)*
  All throughout the course of active disease
**Gram-negative bacilli**
  Renal failure
  Chemotherapy-induced severe granulocytopenia
  Advance phases of the disease (relapsed/refractory
    disease, previous hospitalization, granulocytopenia)

---

*influenzae* are the main causes of respiratory tract infections whereas *Escherichia coli, Pseudomonas* sp., *Proteus* sp., and *Klebsiella* mainly cause urinary tract infections and septicemia. Currently, Gram-negative bacilli have become more common than Gram-positive cocci. However, Gram-positive organisms continue to cause serious infections in patients with MM in all the active phases of the disease (Table 16-13). In fact, the main cause of respiratory tract infections is *S. pneumoniae* and some patients still develop recurrent pneumonia. In approximately 15% of patients with MM the presenting feature is a bacterial infection. In these still untreated patients, *S. pneumoniae* is the most common pathogen. This population of patients is at particular risk of new infections within the first 2 months of initiation of therapy and all throughout the phases of active disease. Although Gram-positive bacteria, particularly *S. pneumoniae,* was the most common reported cause of initial reports on infections in patients with MM, an increasing infectious rate by Gram-negative bacteria has been recognized (Meyers et al., 1972; Savage et al., 1982; Shaikh et al., 1982). A temporal biphasic microbial pattern was recognized by Savage et al. (1982). Most infections in untreated newly diagnosed patients and during the first courses of chemotherapy are the result of *S. pneumoniae* and *H. influenzae.* In fact, in the Savage et al. (1982) series the occurrence of Gram-negative infections in the early phase was very unusual. In this phase, the impaired immunoglobulin synthesis would be the main predisposing factor. In responding patients the incidence of infections is low and rarely caused by Gram-negative bacilli in the absence of severe chemotherapy-induced granulocytopenia. In contrast, in patients with initial renal failure as well as in those with advanced disease receiving salvage chemotherapy, more than 90% of infectious episodes are caused by Gram-negative bacilli or *S. aureus.* In these situations, additional factors to hypogammaglobulinemia such as hospitalization, previous antibiotic therapy, chemotherapy, glucocorticoids, intravenous lines, and eventually granulocytopenia from heavy bone marrow myeloma involvement and/or rescue chemotherapy as well as corticosteriod treatment are contributory factors enhancing the incidence of Gram-negative infections. Bacteremia is documented in more than 50% of patients with myeloma with serious infections (Savage et al., 1982). Of interest, and contrasting with patients with acute leukemia, bacteremia usually occurs in the absence of granulocytopenia. Active disease is a critical risk factor for infection in MM (Hargreaves et al., 1995; Perri et al., 1981; Savage et al., 1982; Snowdon et al., 1994). This is enforced by the fact that there are patients who develop recurrent severe infections, particularly pneumococcal sepsis, as presenting feature during the first courses of chemotherapy and at the time of relapse when chemotherapy is restarted, whereas they do not develop a single episode of severe infection during the periods while they are on response to chemotherapy (plateau phase).

## Treatment of Infections

In patients with MM, infectious episodes should be considered as potential serious complications and require immediate therapy. In a given patient with MM who develops fever, a careful anamnesis and physical examination in the search for a possible site of infection are mandatory. Fever from myeloma mimicking an active infection is exceedingly rare (Mueller et al., 2002). Blood and urine cultures plus pneumococcal antigen determination in the urine should be done. Before the causal agent is identified, treatment should cover both encapsulated bacteria and Gram-negative microorganisms. In case the patient is not granulocytopenic, it is our practice to start treatment with cefotaxime or ceftriaxone. In case the patient is neutropenic, we use cefotaxime plus amikacin or an antipseudomonal agent such as cefepime or carbapenem. Of course, the antibiotic choice will be determined by the local flora and by the pattern of antibiotic resistance at each institution.

## Infection Prophylaxis

Oken et al. (1996) reported that antibiotic prophylaxis with trimethoprim-sulphametoxazol (TMP-SMX), administered during the first 2 months of initiation of chemotherapy, significantly decreased the number of infections. Thus, 28 patients were assigned to TMP-SMX and 26 to no prophylaxis. Eleven patients in the control group developed bacterial infections during the 3-month study period compared with only 2 patients given TMP-SMX. In addition, 8 severe infections were seen in the control group versus only 1 in the group receiving prophylactic antibiotics, this leading to 4 and 1 deaths from infection, respectively. The bacterial infection rate was 2.43 versus 0.29 per patient/year for the control and prophylactic groups, respectively (Oken et al., 1996). Although the results of this study are worthwhile to take into account, the number of

patients is too small to establish definitive conclusions and need confirmation in larger trials.

A trial of intramuscular immunoglobulins did not result in a significant decrease in severe infections (Salmon et al., 1967). A randomized study showed that intravenous immunoglobulins (IVIG) significantly decreased the number of serious/recurrent infections in patients with MM (Chapel et al., 1994). Eighty-two patients with stable MM were given monthly infusions of IVIG at a dose of 0.4 g/kg or placebo. No episodes of pneumonia or sepsis were seen in patients receiving IVIG compared with 10 episodes in the placebo group. Concerning serious infections, there were 38 episodes in 470 patient/months in the placebo arm versus 19 in 449 patient/months in the IVIG group. Interestingly, a poor pneumococcal antibody response identified the patients more likely to benefit from IVIG. However, and as previously highlighted, patients in the plateau phase have a low rate of infectious episodes because there is a close relationship between disease activity and infection. In fact, even in the study patients we have mentioned with a bone marrow compromised reserve as well as those receiving chemotherapy did not benefit from IVIG (Chapel et al., 1994). In terms of cost effectiveness, it does not seem appropriate to give prophylactic immunoglobulins to patients with MM.

As already emphasized, patients with MM have an impaired immunoglobulin and antibody-specific synthesis. Thus, it is not surprising that pneumococcal vaccination yields a suboptimal antibody response with a significant increase in antibody against pneumococcal strains in only 30% to 40% of the patients (Birgens et al., 1983; Hargreaves et al., 1995; Lazarus et al., 1980; Schmid et al., 1981; Shildt et al., 1981). Patients with IgG M-protein seem to have lower antipneumococcal IgG antibody titers compared with those of IgA or light chain only (Bence Jones) myeloma (Hargreaves et al., 1995). This poor immunologic response to pneumococcal vaccination is clinically relevant because there is an association between poor responders to pneumococcal immunization and septicemic episodes (Hargreaves et al., 1995). Pneumococcal vaccination is usually given every 3 to 5 years in immunocompetent patients who have an increased risk of pneumococcal infections. Reimmunization has not been studied in patients with low preimmunization antibodies. However, even after a response to immunization, patients with MM usually show a quick decrease in their antibody level. In fact, in one study, 18 months after immunization, the antibody concentration returned to preimmunization levels (Birgens et al., 1983). In consequence, even in responders to vaccination, the efficacy of reimmunization every 3 to 5 years is uncertain. It seems likely that patients with myeloma could benefit from more frequent immunization.

The low cost, the absence of toxicity, and the possible benefit, at least in some patients, makes

## TABLE 16-14

### Infection Prophylaxis in Multiple Myeloma

Immunoglobulin: not recommended
Pneumococcal vaccination: recommended, particularly in
   IgG myeloma with high-serum M-protein levels
Antibiotic:
   Likely of benefit: first 2 months of therapy
   Recommended in patients at high risk (initiation of therapy
      in patients with history of serious infections,
      particularly recurrent pneumoniae, renal failure)

pneumococcal vaccination a recommended prophylactic measure in patients with MM, particularly in those with a very high IgG M-protein with low background IgG immunoglobulins (Table 16-14). However, the patients who are more likely to benefit, the possible usefulness of postimmunization antibody serial measurements to try to maintain adequate antibody levels by more frequent vaccination, and whether the new protein-conjugate vaccine is more effective than the classical pneumococcal vaccine remain to be determined.

Of particular concern is the subset of patients who develop recurrent pneumococcal infections. Although it seems of no doubt that they should receive pneumococcal vaccination, the administration of prophylactic antibiotics is more controversial. The use of prophylactic penicillin is of uncertain efficacy because of the increasing emergence of resistant strains and should be used only in geographic areas where the proportion of penicillin-resistant pneumococcus is lower than 10%. In selected patients at very high risk of serious pneumoccocal infections (i.e., history of recurrent pneumonia at initiation of chemotherapy either as front-line or rescue chemotherapy), antibiotic prophylaxis with new macrolides such as telitromicine or new fluoroquinolones such as levofloxacin until a response to chemotherapy is achieved should be considered.

## REFERENCES

Aitchison, R. G., Reilly, I. A. G., Morgan, A. G., and Russell, N. H. (1990). Vincristine, adriamycin and high dose steroids in myeloma complicated by renal failure. *British Journal of Cancer, 61,* 765–766.

Alexanian, R., Barlogie, and Dixon, D. (1990). Renal failure in multiple myeloma: pathogenesis and prognostic implications. *Archives of Internal Medicine, 150,* 1693–1695.

Anderson, C. M., Bueso-Ramos, C. E., Wallner, S. A., Albitar, M., Rosenzweig, T. E., and Koller, C. A. (1999). Primary myeloid leukemia presenting concomitantly with primary multiple myeloma: two cases and an update of the literature. *Leukemia & Lymphoma, 32,* 385–390.

Badros, A., Barlogie, B., Siegel, E., et al. (2001). Autologous stem cell transplantation in elderly multiple myeloma patients over the age of 70 years. *British Journal of Haematology, 114,* 600–607.

Ballester, O. F., Tummala, R., Janssen, W. E., et al. (1997). High-dose chemotherapy and autologous peripheral blood stem cell transplantation in patients with multiple myeloma and renal failure. *Bone Marrow Transplantation, 20,* 653–656.

Barlogie, B., and Beck, T. (1993). Recombinant human erythropoietin and the anemia of multiple myeloma. *Stem Cells, 11,* 88–94.

Barlogie, B., Smith, L., and Alexanian, R. (1984). Effective treatment of advanced myeloma refractory to alkylating agents. *New England Journal of Medicine, 310,* 1353–1356.

Beguin, Y. (2002). Prediction of response and other improvements on the limitations of recombinant human erythropoietin therapy in anemic cancer patients. *Haematologica, 87,* 1209–1221.

Beguin, Y., Yerna, M., Loo, M., Weber, M., and Fillet, G. (1992). Erythropoiesis in multiple myeloma: defective red cell production due to inappropriate erythropoietin production. *British Journal of Haematology, 82,* 648–653.

Bergsagel, D. E. (1982). Plasma cell neoplasms and acute leukemia. *Clinical Hematology, 11,* 221–234.

Bergsagel, D. E. (1988). Chemotherapy of myeloma: drug combinations versus single agents, an overview, and comments on acute leukemia in myeloma. *Hematologic Oncology, 6,* 159–166.

Bergsagel, D. E., Bailey, A. J., Langley, G. R., MacDonald, R. N., White, D. F., and Miller, A. B. (1979). The chemotherapy of plasma-cell myeloma and the incidence of acute leukemia. *New England Journal of Medicine, 301,* 743–748.

Bernstein, S. P., and Humes, H. D. (1982). Reversible renal insufficiency in multiple myeloma. *Archives of Internal Medicine, 142,* 2083–2086.

Birgens, H. S., Espersen, F., Hertz, J. B., Pedersen, F. K., and Drivsholm, A. (1983). Antibody response to pneumococcal vaccination in patients with myelomatosis. *Scandinavian Journal of Haematology, 30,* 324–330.

Bladé, J., Esteve, J., Rosiñol, L., et al. (2001). Thalidomide in refractory and relapsing multiple myeloma. *Seminars in Oncology, 28,* 588–592.

Bladé, J., Fernández-Llama, P., Bosch, F., et al. (1998). Renal failure in multiple myeloma. Presenting features and predictors of outcome in 94 patients from a single institution. *Archives of Internal Medicine, 158,* 1889–1893.

Bladé, J., Lust, J. A., and Kyle, R. A. (1994). Immunoglobulin D multiple myeloma: presenting features, response to therapy, and survival in a series of 53 cases. *Journal of Clinical Oncology, 12,* 2398–2404.

Bladé, J., San Miguel, J. F., Fontanillas, M., et al. (2001). Initial treatment of multiple myeloma: long-term results in 914 patients. *The Hematology Journal, 2,* 272–278.

Boege, F., Merkle, M., Werle, E., and Rückle, H. (1994). Structural features related to the nephropathogenicity of Bence Jones protein. *Kidney International, 46,* S93–S96.

Broder, S., Humphrey, R., Durm, M., Blackman, M., Meade, B., Goldman, B. S., et al. (1975). Impaired synthesis of polyclonal (non-paraprotein) immunoglobulins by circulating lymphocytes from patients with multiple myeloma. *New England Journal of Medicine, 193,* 887–892.

Cavo, M., Baccarani, M., Galieni, P., Gobbi, M., and Tura, S. (1986). Renal failure in multiple myeloma: a study of the presenting findings, response to treatment and prognosis in 26 patients. *Nouvelle Revue Français d' Hematology, 28,* 147–152.

Cazzola, M., Messinger, D., Battistel, V., Brun, D., Cimino, R., Enller-Ziegler, L., et al. (1995). Recombinant human erythropoietin in the anemia associated with multiple myeloma or non-Hodgkin's lymphoma: dose finding and identification of predictors of response. *Blood, 86,* 4446–4453.

Chapel, H. M., Lee, M., Hargreaves, R., Pamphilon, D. H., and Prentice, A. G. (1994). Randomised trial of intravenous immunoglobulin as prophylaxis against infection in plateau-phase multiple myeloma. *Lancet, 343,* 1059–1063.

Cheson, B., Plass, R. R., and Rothstein, G. (1980). Defective opsonization in multiple myeloma. *Blood, 55,* 602–606.

Choufani, E. B., Sanchorawala, U., Ernst, T., Quillen, K., Skinnar, M., Wright, D. G., et al. (2001). Acquired factor X deficiency in patients with amyloid light-chain amyloidosis: incidence, bleeding manifestations and response to high-dose chemotherapy. *Blood, 97,* 1885–1887.

Cleeland, C. S., Demetri, G. D., Glaspy, J., et al. (1999). Identifying hemoglobin level for optimal quality of life: results from an incremental analysis. *Journal of Clinical Oncology, 8,* 574a.

Cohen, D. J., Sherman, W., Osserman, E. F., and Appel, G. B. (1984). Acute renal failure in patients with multiple myeloma. *American Journal of Medicine, 76,* 247–256.

Comenzo, R. L., and Gertz, M. A. (2002). Autologous stem cell transplantation for primary systemic amyloidosis. *Blood, 99,* 4276–4282.

Cosio, F. G., Pence, T. V., Shapiro, F. L., and Kjellstrand, C. M. (1981). Severe renal failure in multiple myeloma. *Clinical Nephrology, 15,* 206–210.

Coward, R. A., Delamore, I. W., Mallick, N. P., and Robinson, E. L. (1984). The importance of urinary immunoglobulin light chain isoelectric point (pI) in nephrotoxicity in multiple myeloma. *Clinical Science, 66,* 229–232.

Coward, R. A., Mallick, N. P., and Delamore, I. W. (1983). Should patients with renal failure associated to multiple myeloma be dialysed? *British Medical Journal, 287,* 1575–1578.

Cuzick, J., Erskine, S., Edelman, D., and Galton, D. A. G. (1987). A comparison of the incidence of myelodysplastic syndrome and acute myeloid leukemia following melphalan and cyclophosphamide treatment for myelomatosis. *British Journal of Cancer, 55,* 523–529.

Dammacco, F., Castoldi, G., and Rödjer, S. (2001). Efficacy of epoetin alfa in the treatment of anaemia of multiple myeloma. *British Journal of Haematology, 113,* 172–179.

Dammacco, F., Silvestris, F., Castoldi, G. L., et al. (1998). The effectiveness and tolerability of epoetin alfa in patients with multiple myeloma refractory to chemotherapy. *International Journal of Clinical and Laboratory Research, 28,* 127–134.

DeFronzo, R. A., Humphrey, R. L., Wright, J. R., and Cooke, C. R. (1975). Acute renal failure in multiple myeloma. *Medicine (Baltimore), 54,* 209–223.

Denz, H., Fuchs, D., Huber, H., et al. (1990). Correlation between neopterin, interferon gamma and haemoglobin in patients with haematologic disorders. *European Journal of Haematology, 44,* 186–189.

Dhodapkar, M. V., Merlini, G., and Solomon, A. (1997). Biology and therapy of immunoglobulin deposition diseases. *Hematology Oncology Clinics of North America, 11,* 89–110.

Durie, B. G. M., and Salmon, S. E. (1975). A clinical staging system for multiple myeloma. *Cancer, 36,* 842–854.

Fahey, J. L., Scoggins, R., Utz, J. P., and Szwed, C. F. (1963). Infection, antibody response and gammaglobulin components in multiple myeloma and macroglobulinemia. *American Journal of Medicine, 35,* 698–707.

Faquin, W. C., Schneider, T. J., and Goldberg, M. A. (1992). Effect of inflammatory cytokines on hypoxia-induced erythropoietin production. *Blood, 79,* 1987–1994.

Finnish Leukaemia Group. (2000). Acute leukemia and other secondary neoplasms in patients treated with conventional chemotherapy for multiple myeloma: a Finnish Leukaemis Group study. *European Journal of Haematology, 65,* 123–127.

Garton, J. P., Gertz, M. A., Witzig, T. E., Greipp, P. R., Lust, J. A., Schroeder, G., et al. (1995). Epoetin alfa for the treatment of the anemia of multiple myeloma. A prospective, randomized, placebo-controlled, double-blind trial. *Archives of Internal Medicine, 155,* 2069–2074.

Gerlag, P. G. G., Koene, R. A. P., and Berden, J. H. M. (1986). Renal transplantation in light chain nephropathy: case report and review of the literature. *Clinical Nephrology, 25,* 101–104.

Gertz, M. A., Lacy, M. Q., and Dispenzieri, A. (1999). Amyloidosis. *Hematology Oncology Clinics of North America, 13,* 1211–1234.

Glenchur, H., Zinneman, H. H., and Hall, W. H. (1959). A review of 51 cases of multiple myeloma: emphasis on pneumonia and other infections as complications. *Archives of Internal Medicine, 103,* 173–183.

Govindarajan, R., Jagannath, S., Flick, J. T., Vesole, D. H., Sawyer, J., Barlogie, B., et al. (1996). Preceding standard therapy is the likely cause of MDS after autotransplants for multiple myeloma. *British Journal of Haematology, 95,* 349–353.

Hargreaves, R. M., Lea, J. R., Griffiths, H., Faux, J. A., Holt, J. M., Bunch, C., et al. (1995). Immunological factors and risk of infection in plateau phase myeloma. *Journal of Clinical Pathology, 48,* 260–266.

Hill, G. S., Morel-Maroger, L., Méry, J. P., Brouet, J. C., and Mignon, F. (1983). Renal lesions in multiple myeloma: their relationship to associated protein abnormalities. *American Journal of Kidney Diseases, 4,* 423–438.

Hoen, B., Kessler, M., Hestin, D., and Mayeux, D. (1995). Risk factors for bacterial infections in chronic haemodialysis adult patients: a multicentre prospective survey. *Nephrology, Dialysis, and Transplantation, 10,* 377–381.

Hopen, G., Glette, J., and Matre, R. (1984). Mechanisms of decreased leucocyte adhesiveness and migration in plasma from patients with IgG myelomatosis. *Scandinavian Journal of Haematology, 32,* 88–94.

Iggo, N., Palmer, A. B. D., Severn, A., et al. (1989). Chronic dialysis in patients with multiple myeloma and renal failure: a worthwhile treatment. *Quarterly Journal of Medicine, 270,* 903–910.

Jaccard, A., Royer, B., Dordessoule, D., Brouet, J. C., and Fermand, J. P. (2002). High-dose therapy and autologous stem cell transplantation in POEMS syndrome. *Blood, 99,* 3057–3059.

Jacobson, D. R., and Zolla-Pazner, S. (1986). Immunosuppression and infection in multiple myeloma. *Seminars in Oncology, 13,* 282–280.

Johns, E. A., Turner, R., Cooper, E. H., and MacLennan, I. C. M. (1986). Isoelectric points of urinary light chains in myelomatosis: analysis in relation to nephrotoxicity. *Journal of Clinical Pathology, 39,* 833–837.

Johnson, W. J., Kyle, R. A., and Dahlberg, P. J. (1980). Dialysis in the treatment of multiple myeloma. *Mayo Clinic Proceedings, 55,* 65–72.

Johnson, W. J., Kyle, R. A., Pineda, A. A., O'Brien, P. C., and Holley, K. E. (1990). Treatment of renal failure associated to multiple myeloma. *Archives of Internal Medicine, 150,* 863–869.

Kansu, E., Akalin, E., Civelek, C., Tekesin, O., Lalely, Y., and Firat, D. (1986). Serum bactericidal and opsonic activities in chronic lymphocyic leukemia and multiple myeloma. *American Journal of Hematology, 23,* 191–196.

Kelleher, P., and Chapel, H. (2002). Infections: principles of prevention and therapy. In J. Metha, and S. Singhal (Eds.), *Myeloma* (pp. 223–239). London: Martin Dunitz Ltd.

Knudsen, L. M., Hippe, E., Hjorth, M., Holmberg, E., and Westin, J. (1994). Renal function in newly diagnosed multiple myeloma. A demographic study of 1353 patients. *European Journal of Haematology, 53,* 207–212.

Knudsen, L. M., Hjorth, M., and Hippe, E. (2000). Renal failure in multiple myeloma: reversibility and impact on prognosis. *European Journal of Haematology, 65,* 175–181.

Korzets, A., Tam, F., Russell, G., Feehally, J., and Walls, J. (1990). The role of continuous ambulatory peritoneal dialysis in end-stage renal failure due to multiple myeloma. *American Journal of Kidney Diseases, 6,* 216–223.

Kyle, R. A. (1975). Multiple myeloma: review of 869 cases. *Mayo Clinic Proceedings, 50,* 29–40.

Kyle, R. A., Gertz, M. A., Witzig, T. E., Lust, J. A., Lacy, M. Q., Dispenzieri, A., et al. (2003). Review of 1027 patients with newly diagnosed multiple myeloma. *Mayo Clinic Proceedings, 78,* 21–33.

Kyle, R. A., and Greipp, P. R. (1982). "Idiopathic" Bence Jones proteinuria: long-term follow-up in seven patients. *New England Journal of Medicine, 306,* 564–567.

Lacy, M. Q., and Gertz, M. A. (1999). Acquired Fanconis syndrome associated with monoclonal gammopathies. *Hematology Oncology Clinics of North America, 13,* 1273–1280.

Lazarus, H. M., Adelstein, D. J., Herzig, R. H., and Smith, M. C. (1983). Long-term survival of patients with multiple myeloma and acute renal failure at presentation. *American Journal of Kidney Diseases, 2,* 521–525.

Lazarus, H. M., Lederman, M., Lubin, A., Herzig, R. H., Schiffman, G., Jones, P., et al. (1980). Pneumoccocal vaccination: the response of patients with multiple myeloma. *American Journal of Medicine, 69,* 419–424.

Littlewood, T. J., Fajetta, E., Nortier, J. W., et al. (2001). Effects of epoetin alfa on haematologic parameters and quality of life in cancer patients receiving non-platinum chemotherapy: results of a randomized, double-blind, placebo-controlled trial. *Journal of Clinical Oncology, 19,* 2865–2874.

Ludwig, H., Fritz, E., Kotzmann, H., Höcker, P., Gisslinger, H., and Barnas, U. (1990). Erythropoietin treatment of anemia associated with multiple myeloma. *New England Journal of Medicine, 322,* 1693–1699.

Ludwig, H., Fritz, E., Leitgeb, C., Pecherstorfer, M., Samonigg, H., and Schuster, J. (1994). Prediction of response to erythropoietin treatment in chronic anemia of cancer. *Blood, 84,* 1056–1063.

Ludwig, H., Rai, K., Bladé, J., et al. (2002). Management of disease-related anemia in patients with multiple myeloma or chronic lymphocytic leukemia: epoetin alfa treatment recommendations. *The Hematology Journal, 3,* 121–130.

MacGregor, R. R., Negendank, W. G., and Schreiber, A. D. (1978). Impaired granulocytic adherence in multiple myeloma: relationship to complement system, granulocyte delivery, and infection. *Blood, 51,* 591–599.

MacLennan, I. C., Chapman, C., Dunn, J., and Kelly, K. (1992). Combined chemotherapy with ABCM versus melphalan for treatment of myelomatosis. *Lancet, 339,* 200–205.

Means, R. T., and Kranz, S. B. (1992). Progress in understanding the pathogenesis of the anemia of chronic disease. *Blood, 80,* 1639–1647.

Medical Research Council Working Party on Leukemia in Adults. (1984). Analysis and management of renal failure in the fourth myelomatosis trial. *British Medical Journal, 288,* 1411–1416.

Meharchand, J. (1998). Management of haematological complications of myeloma. In J. S. Malpas, D. E. Bergsagel, R. A. Kyle, and K.C. Anderson (Eds.). *Myeloma: Biology and Management,* 2nd ed (pp. 332–357). Oxford: Oxford University Press.

Melcion, C., Mougenot, B., Baudouin, B., et al. (1984). Renal failure in myeloma: relationship with isoelectric point of immunoglobulin light chains. *Clinical Nephrology, 22,* 138–143.

Meyers, B. R., Hirschman, S. Z., and Axelrod, J. A. (1972). Current pattern of infection in multiple myeloma. *American Journal of Medicine, 52,* 87–92.

Miller, J. S., Arthur, D. C., Litz, C. E., Neglia, J. P., Miller, W. J., and Weisdorf, D. J. (1994). Myelodysplastic syndrome after autologous bone marrow transplantation: an additional complication of curative cancer therapy. *Blood, 82,* 3780–3786.

Mills, H. G., and Cawley, J. C. (1983). Abnormal monoclonal antibody-defined helper/suppressor T-cell subpopulations in multiple myeloma: relationship to treatment and clinical stage. *Scandinavian Journal of Haematology.*

Misiani, R., Tiraboschi, G., Mingardi, G., and Mecca, G. (1987). Management of myeloma kidney: an anti-light-chain approach. *American Journal of Kidney Diseases, 10,* 28–33.

Mueller, P. S., Terrell, C. L., and Gertz, M. A. (2002). Fever of unknown origin caused by multiple myeloma. A report of nine cases. *Archives of Internal Medicine, 162,* 1305–1309.

Musto, P., Falcone, A., D'Arena, G., Scalzulli, P. R., Matera, R., Minervini, M. M., et al. (1997). Clinical results of recombinant erythropoietin in transfusion-dependent patients with refractory multiple myeloma: role of cytokines and monitoring of erythropoiesis. *European Journal of Haematology, 58,* 314–319.

Oken, M. M., Pomeroy, C., and Weisdorf, D. (1996). Prophylactic antibiotics for the prevention of early infection in multiple myeloma. *American Journal of Medicine, 100,* 624–628.

Österborg, A., Boogaerts, M. A., Cimino, R., Essers, U., Holoowiecki, J., Juliusson, G., et al. (1996). Recombinant human erythropoietin in transfusion-dependent anemic patients with multiple myeloma and non-Hodgkin's lymphoma: a randomized multicentric study. *Blood, 87,* 2675–2682.

Österborg, A., Brandbeg, Y., Molostova, V., et al. (2002). Randomized, double-blind, placebo-controlled trial of recombinant human erythropoietin, epoetin beta, in hematologic malignancies. *Journal of Clinical Oncology, 20,* 2486–2494.

Palant, C. E., Bonitati, J., Bartholomew, W. R., Brentjens, J. R., Walshe, J. J., and Bentzel, C. J. (1986). Nodular glomerulosclerosis associated with multiple myeloma. Role of light chain isoelectric point. *American Journal of Medicine, 80,* 98–102.

Pasqualli, Casanova, S., Zuchelli, A., and Zuchelli, P. (1990). Long-term survival in patients with acute and severe renal failure due to multiple myeloma. *Clinical Nephrology, 34,* 247–254.

Perri, R. T., Hebbel, R. P., and Oken, M. M. (1981). Influence of treatment and response status on infection in multiple myeloma. *American Journal of Medicine, 71,* 935–940.

Pozzi, C., Pasquali, S., Donini, U., et al. (1987). Prognostic factors and effectiveness of treatment in acute renal failure due to multiple myeloma: review of 50 cases. *Clinical Nephrology, 28,* 1–9.

Preudhomme, J. L., Aucouturier, P., Touchard, G., et al. (1994). Monoclonal immunoglobulin deposition disease (Randall type). Relationship with structural abnormalities of immunoglobulin chains. *Kidney International, 46,* 965–972.

Randall, R. E., Williamson, W. C., Mullinax, F., Tung, M. Y., and Still, W. J. S. (1976). Manifestations of systemic light chain deposition. *American Journal of Medicine, 60,* 293–299.

Rebibou, J. M., Caillot, D., Casasnovas, R. O., et al. (1997). Peripheral blood stem cell transplantation in a myeloma patient with end-stage renal failure. *Bone Marrow Transplantation, 20,* 63–65.

Reiter, E., Kalhs, P., Keil, F., et al. (1999). Effects of high-dose melphalan and peripheral blood stem cell transplantation on renal function in patients with multiple myeloma and renal insufficiency: a case report and review of the literature. *Annals of Hematology, 78,* 189–191.

Rizzo, J. D., Lichtin, A. E., Woolf, S. H., Seidenfeld, J., Bennett, C. L., Cella, D., et al. (2002a). Use of epoetin in patients with cancer: evidence-based clinical practice guidelines of the American Society of Clinical Oncology and the American Society of Hematology. *Blood, 100,* 2303–2320.

Rizzo, J. D., Lichtin, A. E., Woolf, S. H., Seidenfeld, J., Bennet, C. L., Cella, D., et al. (2002b). Use of epoetin in patients with cancer: evidence-based clinical practice guidelines of the American Society of Clinical Oncology and the American Society of Hematology. *Journal of Clinical Oncology, 20,* 40–83.

Rosenstein, E. D., Itzkowitz, S. H., Penziner, J. I., et al. (1983). Resolution of factor X deficiency in primary amyloidosis following splenectomy. *Archives of Internal Medicine, 143,* 597–599.

Rosner, F., and Grünwald, H. W. (1984). Simultaneous occurrence of multiple myeloma and acute myeloblastic leukemia: fact or myth? *American Journal of Medicine, 76,* 891–899.

Rota, S., Mougenot, B., Baudouin, B., et al. (1987). Multiple myeloma and severe renal failure: a clinicopathologic study of outcome and prognosis in 34 patients. *Medicine, 66,* 126–137.

Rovira, M., Carreras, E., Rovira, M., et al. (2001). Dramatic improvement of POEMS syndrome following haematopoietic cell transplantation. *British Journal of Haematology, 115,* 373–375.

Salmon, S. E., Samal, B. A., Hayes, D. M., et al. (1967). Role of gamma globulin for immunoprophylaxis in multiple myeloma. *New England Journal of Medicine, 277*, 1336–1340.

Sanders, P. W. (1994). Pathogenesis and treatment of myeloma kidney. *Journal of Laboratory and Clinical Medicine, 124*, 484–488.

San Miguel, J. F., LaHuerta, J. J., García-Sanz, R., et al. (2000). Are myeloma patients with renal failure candidates for autologous stem cell transplantation?. *The Hematology Journal, 1*, 28–36.

Savage, D. G., Lindenbaum, J., and Garret, T. J. (1982). Biphasic pattern of bacterial infection in multiple myeloma. *Annals of Internal Medicine, 96*, 47–50.

Schmid, G. P., Smith, R. P., Baltch, A. L., Hall, C. A., and Schiffman, G. (1981). Antibody response to pneumococcal vaccine in patients with multiple myeloma. *Journal of Infectious Diseases, 143*, 590–597.

Shaikh, B. S., Lombard, R. M., Appelbaum, P. C., and Bentz, M. S. (1982). Changing patterns of infections in patients with multiple myeloma. *Oncology, 39*, 78–82.

Sharland, A., Snowdon, L., Joshua, D. E., Gibson, J., and Tiller, D. J. (1997). Hemodialysis: an appropriate therapy in myeloma-induced renal failure. *American Journal of Kidney Diseases, 30*, 786–792.

Shildt, R. A., Rubin, R. R., Schiffman, G., and Giolma, P. (1981). Polyvalent pneumococcal immunization of patients with plasma cell dyscrasias. *Cancer, 48*, 1377–1380.

Silvestris, F., Romito, A., Fanelli, P., Vacca, A., and Dammacco, F. (1995). Long-term therapy with recombinant human erythropoietin (rHu-EPO) in progressing multiple myeloma. *Annals of Hematology, 70*, 313–318.

Snowdon, L., Gibson, J., and Joshua, D. E. (1994). Frequency of infection in plateau-phase multiple myeloma [Letter]. *Lancet, 344*, 262.

Torra, R., Bladé, J., Cases, A., et al. (1995). Patients with multiple myeloma and renal failure requiring long-term dialysis: presenting features, response to therapy, and outcome in a series of 20 cases. *British Journal of Haematology, 91*, 854–859.

Tosi, F., Zamagni, E., Ronconi, S., et al. (2000). Safety of autologous hematopoietic stem cell transplantation in patients with multiple myeloma and chronic renal failure. *Leukemia, 14*, 1310–1313.

Tucci, M., Grinello, D., Cafforio, P., Silvestris, F., and Dammacco, F. (2002). Anemia in multiple myeloma: role of deregulated plasma cell apoptosis. *Leukemia & Lymphoma, 43*, 1527–1530.

Verroust, P., Morel-Maroger, L., and Preudhomme, J. L. (1982). Renal lesions in dysproteinemia. *Seminars in Immunopathology, 5*, 333–356.

Vhalin, A., Löfvenberg, E., and Holm, J. (1987). Improved survival in multiple myeloma with renal failure. *Acta Medica Scandinavica, 221*, 205–209.

Winearls, C. G. (1995). Acute myeloma kidney. *Kidney International, 48*, 1347–1361.

Zinneman, H. H. and Hall, W. H. (1954). Recurrent pneumonia in multiple myeloma and some observations on immunological response. *Annals of Internal Medicine, 41*, 1152–1163.

Zucchelli, P., Pasquali, S., Cagnoli, L., and Ferrari, G. (1988). Controlled plasma exchange trial in acute renal failure due to multiple myeloma. *Kidney International, 33*, 1175–1180.

# CHAPTER 17

# Neurological Manifestations of Myeloma and Their Management

JEFFREY GAWLER

## Introduction

Plasma cell dyscrasias often present with neurologic symptoms. These might be a direct manifestation of the disease (for example, lower limb weakness resulting from spinal cord compression from myelomatous involvement of the vertebral column) or be caused by the immunologic effects of monoclonal proteins, which might be directed against neural structures (particularly peripheral nerves). Nonspecific neurologic symptoms, such as fatigue and weakness, might be features of systemic complications like anemia, uremia, or hypercalcemia, which frequently develop in patients with multiple myeloma.

Neurologists should consider myeloma in their differential diagnosis of back pain, particularly if simple investigations such as blood count reveal anemia or elevation of the erythrocyte sedimentation rate (ESR); they should remember that plain x-rays of the spine might suggest only osteoporosis, and isotope bone scans might be negative in patients with this condition. Oncologists need an understanding of the neurologic manifestations of the plasma cell disorders; this chapter will deal principally with such conditions. Although the direct effects of multiple myeloma on the nervous system are usually easy to understand, the causation of paraneoplastic manifestations like the peripheral nerve disorders is complex and our understanding of these conditions is still evolving.

# Vertebral Myeloma and Intraspinal Plasmacytoma

Multiple myeloma has a special predilection for the spinal column; indeed, Henson and Urich (1982, p. 290) concluded that "few patients with myeloma escape lesions in this region" and spinal pain is often stated to be the most frequent presenting symptom of the disease (Parker and Malpas, 1979). The dorsal spine is most often affected; lumbar involvement is common, but cervical and sacral disease are less frequent (Benson et al., 1979; Clarke, 1956; Heisner and Schwartzman, 1952; McKissock et al., 1961). Multiple vertebral involvement and evidence of bone disease elsewhere is usual, but solitary vertebral myeloma (often without hematologic abnormalities or paraprotein) occurs in less than 10% of all patients with myeloma; such solitary tumors might have an indolent course and they are sometimes associated with a paravertebral mass, which can calcify (Currie and Henson, 1971). Among patients presenting with vertebral and extradural tumors of all types, the proportion with myeloma has varied from 2% to 21% (Auld and Bueman, 1966; Brice and McKissock, 1965) with figures between 5% and 10% being most representative (Gilbert et al., 1978; Svien et al., 1953; Veith and Odom, 1965), the relative rarity of myeloma balancing the high incidence of its spinal involvement. Myeloma usually involves the bone of the vertebral body and then spreads into the extradural space forming a collarlike mass that does not penetrate the dura (Russell and Rubinstein, 1989). Patients with extradural myeloma without vertebral involvement have been reported (Benson et al., 1979), and an intradural plasmacytoma causing cord compression has also been described (Sod and Wiener, 1959). Spinal cord and cauda equina compression, seen in patients with myeloma, might be caused by vertebral collapse with the extrusion of bony fragments into the spinal canal or by spinal subluxation, in addition to the direct extradural spread of tumor.

Vertebral involvement by myeloma causes local pain that might be exacerbated by coughing or straining and by movement, especially if there is vertebral collapse or instability. Pain is often worse when patients are supine and they might be awakened at night. Radicular pain is caused by compression of nerve roots within the spinal canal or their exit foraminae by tumor extension, vertebral collapse, or spinal instability. The term referred pain is used to describe pain felt in an area that is remote from the site of the causative lesion, the area where the pain is perceived being innervated by nerve fibers that arise from the same segmental level as the lesion but where there is no direct nerve root involvement (Hockaday and Whitty, 1967). Funicular pain arises from spinal cord involvement and is caused by compression of ascending sensory pathways (Posner, 1995, p. 120). Currie and Henson (1971), in their study of 125 patients with myeloma, found that local spinal pain was the only symptom in 23%, and 15% experienced radicular pain without evidence of spinal cord involvement. Patients with dorsal spinal disease usually present with dorsal back pain, which may be associated with radicular pain radiating around the chest or abdomen on one or both sides. There may be associated radicular sensory disturbance with a band of numbness or paresthesia reflecting involvement of the dorsal root at the level of the lesion. Some patients with dorsal cord compression go on to develop paraparesis, which usually evolves over weeks, although the onset can be abrupt with severe paralysis developing within a few hours. In patients with mild paraparesis, weakness of hip flexion often develops first, followed by weakness of knee flexion, dorsiflexion, and eversion of the feet (an upper motor neurone or "pyramidal" distribution of weakness). Some patients present with unsteadiness or stiffness, reflecting ataxia, or spasticity rather than weakness. Impairment of sensation is usually present below the level of the lesion; severe cord lesions might show a sensory level appropriate to the site of cord compression, but the localizing value of a sensory level with partial cord lesions is imprecise and tends to rise as the cord lesion becomes more complete. Early cervical spinal cord compression might be missed if the patient presents with lower limb weakness and sensory disturbance confined to the legs or thoracic dermatomes (Jamieson et al., 1996). Disturbance of bladder control and, in men, impotence might also occur.

When lumbar vertebral involvement leads to cauda equina compression (the spinal cord usually terminates at the disc between the L1 and L2 vertebrae), pain in the low back radiates into the buttocks and legs (particularly posteriorly). Weakness of the legs is lower motor neuron in type and often associated with wasting. In general, the lower the level of lumbar vertebral involvement, the more distal the weakness of the legs. Sensory disturbance tends to involve the saddle area, the posterior thighs, and the legs distally. If examination is conducted only in the supine position, distal weakness of the legs and sensory impairment involving the L4 and L5 dermatomes might be misinterpreted as indicating a peripheral neuropathy; it is important to examine the patients prone to see whether the sensory disturbance involves the buttocks and posterior thighs (sacral dermatomes). Spinal cord or cauda equina syndromes develop in 10% to 20% of patients with myeloma (Clarke, 1956; Henson and Urich, 1982, p. 293; Silverstein and Doniger, 1963). In Clarke's series (1956) only 6% of patients with spinal myeloma developed cord dysfunction of severity sufficient to warrant active intervention.

Plain x-rays of the spine might reveal lytic lesions in the vertebral body, pedicles, laminae, or spines, sometimes associated with collapse. Scalloping of the vertebral body anteriorly (fishtail vertebra) is said to be suggestive of myeloma. Bone changes might, however, be subtle; nonspecific loss of bone might mimic osteoporosis and honeycomb formation can lead to the erroneous diagnosis of a benign vertebral hemangioma. Sclerosis of the vertebral body is usually a feature of solitary, vertebral myeloma, which is often associated with peripheral neuropathy from POEMS syndrome. Magnetic resonance (MR) scanning with gadolinium enhancement provides the most reliable method of displaying the degree of vertebral involvement and any associated intraspinal or paraspinal soft tissue mass. The degree of spinal cord or cauda equina involvement by intraspinal tumor is best appreciated by this technique, which also shows whether individual nerve roots are compressed by bone expansion or collapse in relation to their exit foraminae. Isotope bone scans might fail to demonstrate myelomatous involvement of the vertebrae. Spinal cord compression in patients with spinal myeloma is more likely to develop when the vertebral cortex is more extensively involved than the medulla (Woo et al., 1986).

When patients present with vertebral collapse and spinal cord dysfunction, a diagnosis of myeloma might be suggested by the presence of anemia, uremia, hypercalcemia, M-protein in the blood, or Bence Jones protein in the urine. A computed tomogram (CT) or MR-guided needle biopsy of an affected vertebra can be undertaken to achieve a histologic diagnosis. Spinal fluid analysis is relatively insensitive; cytologic examination only rarely reveals malignant cells, but M-protein is sometimes detected in the spinal fluid (Hansotia et al., 1983).

The management of patients with vertebral myeloma, which causes neurologic deficit, is evolving (Byrne, 1992; Johnson, 1993). When spinal pain is the predominant problem, a conservative approach with radiotherapy and chemotherapy might be appropriate, even when MR imaging shows that there is extradural spread of tumor involving the spinal cord or cauda equina. When radiotherapy is given in this situation, it might be necessary to cover treatment with dexamethasone because neurologic deterioration sometimes complicates radiotherapy (Brenner et al., 1982). Similarly, patients with radicular pain without cord compression are usually treated conservatively (occasionally intractable pain or progressive motor deficit requires

neurosurgical decompression of the affected root). When patients present with spinal cord or cauda equina compression, steroids are usually given as the first line of treatment, particularly if the neurologic deficit has been evolving rapidly or is profound. Dexamethasone is usually given, but the dose is controversial (Byrne, 1992). Some authors recommend 4 mg dexamethasone 4 times a day (Weissman, 1988). However, because there is some evidence that the beneficial effect of dexamethasone is dose related, other authors (Posner, 1987) use a loading dose of 100 mg followed by 24 mg 4 times a day. Using high doses of dexamethasone requires consideration of toxicity (Weissman, 1988). A number of studies (Findlay, 1984; Gilbert et al., 1978; Posner, 1987; Siegal and Siegal, 1989; Young et al., 1980) have failed to demonstrate a difference in the neurologic outcome following radiotherapy as opposed to laminectomy in patients with myeloma or metastatic carcinoma involving the spine. Furthermore, decompression of the spinal cord posteriorly by laminectomy (which involves removing the posterior arch of the vertebral canal) may contribute to spinal instability (Findlay, 1984) and 20% of patients may deteriorate neurologically (Johnson, 1993). For this reason, dexamethasone and radiotherapy followed by chemotherapy have been advocated for patients with myeloma, which is generally sensitive to this form of treatment. However, when the myeloma has already caused vertebral collapse or spinal instability, and spinal cord compression has this basis, rather than reflecting extradural extension of tumor alone, surgical management to decompress the cord may be required urgently. In selected patients, anterior decompression, which usually involves resection of the affected vertebral body or bodies, might be undertaken, followed by the insertion of vertebral prostheses supported by bone grafting or methyl methacrylate. This technique, which involves major surgery (i.e., thoracotomy to approach the dorsal spine), is clearly inappropriate for patients with very widespread bone disease or serious systemic complications of myeloma. Nonetheless, excellent neurologic results have been reported in selected cases (Harrington, 1984). It might be possible to avoid surgical intervention in patients with spinal cord compression caused by vertebral collapse or subluxation by the short-term use of a halo vest to stabilize the cervical spine while healing and mechanical stability are restored using chemotherapy and radiotherapy (Abitbol et al., 1989).

The results of surgical treatment and radiotherapy in patients with myeloma involving the spine are generally better than those who have metastatic carcinoma. The best prognosis relates to patients who undergo removal of solitary extradural plasmacytomas followed by radiotherapy. Although the prognosis must relate to the extent of disease elsewhere (Cohen et al., 1964), it has been observed that patients who have dorsal spinal disease fair far better than those with cervical or lumbar involvement (Benson et al., 1979). Despite an excellent response to surgery and radiotherapy, recurrent disease with vertebral collapse is not infrequent, and patients should be followed closely (Dahlstrom and Lindstrom, 1979). Although management of spinal cord compromise in patients with myeloma usually involves radiotherapy with or without surgery, dramatic resolution of neurologic disability has been reported after treatment with chemotherapy alone (melphalan and prednisolone) (Sinoff and Blumsohn, 1989).

Berenson et al. (1996) advised treatment of advanced multiple myeloma with bisphosphonates (monthly infusions of pamidronate) to protect against the skeletal complications of the disease, in particular bone pain, spinal collapse, and spinal cord compression.

Although the majority of patients who present with apparently solitary plasmacytoma affecting a single vertebral body will be shown to have, or will soon develop, multiple myeloma, there would appear to be a discrete group of patients who have solitary vertebral plasmacytomas, which pursue a relatively benign course. McLain and Weinstein (1989), in their review, defined solitary plasmacytoma as a solitary osseous lesion of the spinal column that was shown to be myelomatous on biopsy. The absence of disseminated disease was documented by negative skeletal survey, negative marrow aspiration, normal serum and urine electrophoresis (although they included patients with M-protein that resolved on treatment of the single vertebral lesion), and a documented absence of dissemination for a period in excess of 2 years after the presentation (because the vast majority of patients who have typical multiple myeloma will manifest progressive disease within 24 mo of diagnosis). The 84 patients from the literature who fulfilled these criteria had a mean disease-free interval of 76 months; 44% developed disseminated disease 2 to 13 years after the diagnosis. The 5-year disease-free survival was 60%. However, after dissemination, survival was limited to a mean of 17 months; once dissemination became apparent, the course was typical for that of multiple myeloma. They advised treatment of solitary lesions with radiotherapy and lifelong followup.

# Cranial Myeloma and Intracranial Plasmacytoma

The skull is frequently involved by myeloma; multiple osteolytic lesions from diploic involvement are often seen on plain skull x-rays. Curiously, these lesions are frequently asymptomatic (Clarke, 1954), although they can cause local pain. Solitary plasmacytoma of the skull is relatively rare; Christopherson and Millar (1950) found only 4 cases of solitary myeloma involving the cranium in a survey of 52 patients with solitary myeloma of bone. Myeloma of the skull might grow externally; less often there is intracranial expansion but this rarely involves the brain. It has been suggested that the dura forms a reliable barrier to the intracranial extension of myeloma within the skull (Clarke, 1954). When skull lesions arise in the context of generalized myeloma, local treatment is rarely required, but isolated lesions may require biopsy for diagnosis. If there is pain, an enlarging external mass, or intracranial extension of the disease, radiotherapy is usually the treatment of choice.

Myelomatous involvement of the skull floor might extend into the orbits, paranasal sinuses, or nasopharynx. Conversely, primary extramedullary plasmacytoma may spread into the skull, particularly the skull base. Extramedullary plasmacytomas are most often found in the head and neck; 50% of these tumors occur in the nose, paranasal sinuses, and nasopharynx (Woodruff et al., 1979). However, even when there is extensive myelomatous involvement of the skull floor, the basal dura is rarely involved (Henson and Urich, 1982). Nonetheless, the cranial nerves are not infrequently involved by myeloma of the skull floor, which encroaches on their exit foraminae. The cranial nerves may also be affected in their extracranial course by soft tissue tumor in the orbit or nasopharynx. Clarke (1954) found that the sixth, eighth, and fifth cranial nerves were most often affected, whereas Spaar (1980) reported involvement of the sixth, seventh, eighth, fifth, and optic nerves, on one or both sides, in order of decreasing frequency. The distribution of cranial nerve palsies seems likely to reflect the frequent involvement of sphenoid and petrous temporal bones by myeloma. Such patients often report headache in addition to symptoms caused by their cranial nerve palsies.

When the orbit is affected, either by extension of skull base myeloma or a solitary plasmacytoma arising in the orbital fat, muscle, or lacrimal gland, patients present with orbital pain, ocular protuberance, periorbital swelling, and double vision. Diplopia is caused by both the mechanical effects of the tumor and ophthalmoplegia resulting from involvement of cranial nerves within the orbit. Visual impairment is usually the result of optic nerve compression, but can be caused by mechanical distortion of the globe, with secondary consequences such as retinal detachment. Patients who have cranial nerve palsies or visual symptoms caused by myeloma within the orbit might also respond well to radiotherapy.

Rarely, myeloma of the skull breeches the dura where it might spread along the leptomeninges or infiltrate the surface of the brain. In addition, there are infrequent reports of isolated extradural, intradural, or subdural plasmacytoma, myelomatous infiltration of the leptomeninges, and even parenchymal cerebral plasmacytoma (without attachment to the skull or meninges).

Henson and Urich (1982, p. 219) were able to trace only 10 patients with primary intracranial plasmacytoma. Such tumors occurred predominantly in women; they arose from the dura and superficially resembled meningiomas. A patient reported by Adams and Plank (1973) had plasmacytoma spread diffusely through the leptomeninges, and Spaar (1980) noted a resemblance between such tumors and nodular or plaque-like meningiomas; he commented on their dural origin at sites of duplication of the venous sinuses. Further reports of meningeal myelomatosis include Oda et al. (1991), Schulman et al. (1980), Spiers et al. (1980), Truong et al. (1982), and Woodruff and Ireton (1982).

Isolated intracerebral plasmacytomas without a dural attachment are extremely rare (French, 1947; Krumholz et al., 1982; Mancardi and Mandybur, 1983; Russell and Rubinstein, 1989; Spaar, 1980). Multiple cerebral plasmacytomas associated with spontaneous intratumoral hemorrhage were reported by Husain et al. (1987). Henson and Urich (1982, p. 221) concluded that patients with generalized myeloma and an intracranial tumor were likely to have dual malignancy; the intracranial tumor was likely to be either a primary cerebral tumor or a metastasis from carcinoma (Sohier and Richardson, 1971).

# Hyperviscosity Syndrome

Central nervous system dysfunction in patients with multiple myeloma or Waldenström's macroglobulinemia was originally referred to as the Bing-Neel syndrome following the clinical description given by these authors (Bing et al., 1937; Bing and Neel, 1936); they attributed focal or diffuse cerebral impairment to a "toxic-infectious" cause. Subsequently, Wuhrmann (1956) used the term "coma paraproteinemicum" to describe mental deterioration and impairment of consciousness in patients with myeloma or macroglobulinemia. Although metabolic complications of myeloma (for example, uremia or hypercalcemia) and opportunistic infections can cause central nervous system dysfunction, the hyperviscosity syndrome might well have been responsible for some of these cases, and the term Bing-Neel syndrome is best avoided in favor of stating the likely cause for compromised cerebral function (bearing in mind that more than one pathologic process and the side effects of treatment might be operating).

Hyperviscosity develops in less than 10% of patients with multiple myeloma (it is detectable at presentation in 3% to 4% of patients with IgG myeloma and 5% to 10% of those with IgA myeloma) (Bergsagel and Rider,

1985), but a higher proportion of patients who have Waldenström's macroglobulinemia and an IgM paraproteinemia (10% to 30% of cases). Nonetheless, because myeloma occurs 10 times more often than Waldenström's macroglobulinemia, the hyperviscosity syndrome may be seen more often as a manifestation of multiple myeloma (Pruzanski and Watt, 1972), in particular when there is an IgA paraprotein (Freel et al., 1972; Preston et al., 1978). This reflects the greater tendency of an IgA paraprotein to form polymers; approximately one-third of patients with an IgA myeloma will develop the hyperviscosity syndrome (Chandy et al., 1981). In patients who have myeloma and an IgG paraprotein, those expressing the IgG$_3$ immunoglobulin subtype are most likely to develop the hyperviscosity syndrome (Capra and Kunkel, 1970). The clinical picture, which was first attributed to hyperviscosity by Waldenström in 1944, involves hemorrhage diathesis, disturbance of vision, and impairment of cerebral function. In general, symptoms do not occur until the serum viscosity is greater than 4 in comparison to the viscosity of water (normal range, 1.4–1.8) (Bergsagel and Rider, 1985). Bleeding involves the mucous membranes of the mouth and nose in particular; gastrointestinal bleeding might also occur. A decline in visual acuity is associated with distension, tortuosity, and segmentation of the retinal veins, punctate or flame-shaped retinal hemorrhages, and papilloedema. The changes in retinal circulation and associated hemorrhage can cause blindness. It might be possible to see sludging in the conjunctival vessels. Patients usually report malaise, anorexia, lethargy, generalized weakness, and weight loss. More specific neurologic symptoms include headache, lightheadedness, syncope, seizures, vertigo, impairment of hearing, gait ataxia, somnolence, and coma; some patients have psychologic symptoms (Somer, 1987). Hyperviscosity has also been reported to present with reversible dementia (Mueller et al., 1983). Pseudohyponatremia and pseudohypoglycemia should lead to suspicion of serum hyperviscosity. The mechanisms and measurement of blood viscosity were reviewed by Patterson et al. (1990). The symptoms and signs caused by hyperviscosity are responsive to treatment with plasmapheresis or plasma exchange, which leads to improvement in the retinal appearances and the disappearance of sludging from the conjunctival capillaries (Kopp et al., 1967; Smith et al., 1965). Plasmapheresis in the treatment of dysproteinemias has recently been renewed by Drew (2002). Cytotoxic chemotherapy should be started for the underlying myeloproliferative disease but maintenance plasma exchange of 1 to 2 liters once or twice a week can be continued, if need be, to prevent recurrence of symptoms caused by hyperviscosity (Buskard et al., 1977).

# Neuropathies Associated with Myeloma, Waldenström's Macroglobulinemia, and Monoclonal Gammopathy of Undetermined Significance (MGUS)

The classification of neuropathies associated with plasma cell dyscrasias is complex and confusing because our understanding of their cause remains under scientific evaluation and researchers have approached the disorders from different standpoints (clinical, immunologic, and therapeutic). Most neuropathies are seen in association with monoclonal gammopathy of undetermined significance (MGUS); neuropathy is relatively uncommon in patients with myeloma, except for those who have the osteosclerotic variant (POEMS syndrome).

In some of the neuropathic syndromes, the paraprotein appears to have a pathogenic role, for example, the neuropathy associated with IgM antimyelin-associated glycoprotein (anti-MAG) antibodies, whereas in others it is uncertain whether paraproteinemic antibodies directed against neural elements are pathogenic or coincidental. Many of the patients with paraproteinemic neuropathy have no demonstrable antibody activity against neural structures.

When considering peripheral neuropathies in general (rather than those specifically associated with paraproteinemia), the majority are axonal in type; it is presumed that Wallerian degeneration of the distal axon reflects metabolic derangement within the neurone, which "dies back." Clinically there is symmetric distal sensory and motor impairment that begins in the legs and spreads proximally; weakness is associated with muscular atrophy and loss of reflexes. Neurophysiologically the axonopathies lead to reduction or loss of sensory action potentials and compound muscle action potentials, but nerve conduction velocity is maintained or only mildly slowed. Electromyography of affected muscles shows denervation. Demyelinating neuropathies imply injury to either the Schwann cell or the myelin sheath, which is often immunologically determined. Clinically there is often sparing of pain and temperature perception (which are subserved by small, lightly myelinated or unmyelinated fiber). Position and vibration sense, which are transmitted in more heavily myelinated fibers, are more markedly impaired; tremor and ataxia might be present as a manifestation of impaired proprioceptive input. Muscle weakness might be proximal as well as distal, and muscle bulk might be preserved despite marked weakness and areflexia. Motor and sensory conduction studies showed velocities reduced below 70% of normal, often in association with localized conduction block, dispersion of the compound muscle action potentials, and prolongation of distal latencies.

The following classification provides an overview of neuropathies associated with plasma cell dyscrasias.

1. Paraproteinemic neuropathy
    a. Neuropathy associated with an IgM paraprotein
        i. Demyelinating sensorimotor neuropathy with antimyelin-associated glycoprotein (anti-MAG antibodies)
        ii. Demyelinating sensory neuropathy associated with antidisialosyl antibodies
        iii. Neuropathies associated with antisulphatide antibodies
        iv. Motor neuropathy associated with anti-GM1 antibodies
        v. Neuropathy associated with antibodies directed against other neural antigens
        vi. Neuropathy associated with IgM monoclonal proteins that have no recognizable autoimmune effect
    b. Neuropathy associated with an IgG or IgA paraprotein
        i. Demyelinating neuropathy associated with an IgG or IgA paraprotein
        ii. Axonal neuropathy associated with an IgG or IgA paraprotein
        iii. Neuropathy associated with myeloma
        iv. POEMS syndrome (polyneuropathy, organomegaly, endocrinopathy, M-protein, and skin changes)
    c. Cryoglobulinemic neuropathy
2. Amyloid neuropathy
3. Neuropathy caused by diffuse malignant infiltration of peripheral nerves
4. Neuropathy caused by associated metabolic diseases
5. Neuropathy by chance association

## Paraproteinemic Neuropathy

The neuropathies seen in association with paraproteinemia have been extensively reviewed during the past decade (Kyle and Dyck, 1993, pp. 1275–1287; Latov, 1995; Latov and Steck, 1995; Miescher and Steck, 1996; Nobile-Orazio and Carpo, 2001; Notermans, 1996; Ropper and Gorson, 1998; Simmons, 1999).

A monoclonal serum protein (M-protein or paraprotein) might be an expression of a malignant process (multiple or solitary osteosclerotic myeloma, Waldenström's macroglobulinemia, B-cell lymphoma, or chronic lymphatic leukemia), but when these conditions and amyloidosis have been excluded, there remain a majority of patients in whom the M-protein appears "benign." However, the term benign monoclonal gammopathy is best avoided because a proportion of these patients will eventually develop a malignant condition, and the term monoclonal gammopathy of undetermined significance (MGUS) is presently preferred. A follow-up study of patients with MGUS showed the risk of progression to multiple myeloma or a related disorder was in the order of 1% per year (Kyle et al., 2002). An association between MGUS and peripheral neuropathy is well established, and a pathogenic relationship is suspected in some but not all patients.

MGUS is characterized by a serum M-protein concentration less than 3 g/dL, fewer than 5% plasma cells in the bone marrow, little if any M-protein in the urine, an absence of lytic bone lesions, anemia, hypercalcemia or renal insufficiency, together with stability of the M-protein, and a failure to develop a malignant process; MGUS accounts for two-thirds of patients with a serum M-protein (Kyle and Dyck, 1993, pp. 1275–1287).

Monoclonal proteins are found in 0.1% of the population over the age of 25 years, but they increase with age so that 1% of patients over 50, 3% over 75, and 19% over 95 years have serum M-proteins. M-proteins in the elderly are usually IgG or IgA (88%); IgM paraprotein is uncommon (12%). However, more than half the patients who have neuropathy associated with MGUS have an IgM paraprotein, approximately one-third an IgG paraprotein, and the minority an IgA paraprotein.

Although cellulose acetate electrophoresis is satisfactory when screening for paraproteinemia, high-resolution agarose gel electrophoresis is a more sensitive method for detecting small amounts of monoclonal protein; immunoelectrophoresis or immunofixation should be used for confirmation to distinguish the immunoglobulin type and light chain class. Serum protein electrophoresis and electrophoresis of urine for Bence Jones protein should be routine investigations for adult patients presenting with peripheral neuropathy. When common causes of neuropathy such as diabetes, alcoholism, and connective tissue disorders are excluded, 10% of patients will be found to have a paraprotein: MGUS 6%, amyloid and malignant disease 4% (Kyle and Dyck, 1993, pp. 1275–1287).

The clinical picture of neuropathies associated with MGUS is generally that of a slowly progressive sensory and motor neuropathy evolving in older patients and affecting males more often than females. Sensory symptoms with distal paresthesia and pain might be prominent at the outset, tremor and ataxia are common, and weakness might evolve at a later stage. The reflexes are diminished or absent. The cranial nerves are generally spared and autonomic function is usually normal.

Most authorities agree that there are important differences between the neuropathies associated with

an IgM paraprotein on the one hand and those seen with an IgG or IgA paraprotein on the other. In particular, many authors think patients with demyelinating neuropathies associated with IgM MGUS differ significantly from those associated with IgG or IgA MGUS (Gosselin et al., 1991, 1993; Kyle and Dyck, 1993, pp. 1275–1287; Nobile-Orazio and Carpo, 2001; Saperstein et al., 2001; Suarez and Kelly, 1993; Vital et al., 2000). Patients with IgM MGUS neuropathies show more marked sensory impairment, more obvious sensory ataxia, and greater neurophysiological abnormalities, although they might pursue a more benign course. Anti-MAG antibodies are demonstrable in half the patients with IgM MGUS neuropathies, but the response to immunomodulating therapies is often modest or poorly sustained. The neuropathies associated with IgG and IgA paraproteinemia may resemble chronic inflammatory demyelinating peripheral neuropathy (CIDP) and are generally more responsive to treatment.

When M-proteins act as antibodies, they might be directed against components of the myelin sheath or the axon, although some can be directed at both structures. Antibodies directed against myelin-associated glycoprotein (MAG) are believed by most authors to exert a pathogenic role in the development of demyelinating neuropathy in patients with IgM MGUS. Myelin-associated glycoprotein is concentrated in periaxonal Schwann cell membranes and perinodal loops of myelin, where it appears to act as an adhesion molecule between the Schwann cell and axon. It has 5 immunoglobulin-like domains, which lie outside the cell where they are accessible to antibodies, a transmembrane domain, and a cytoplasmic tail. MAG shares antigens with the main P0 protein of myelin, peripheral myelin protein 22 (PMP22), and several glycolipids, of which the most relevant to neuropathy is sulphoglucuronylparagloboside (SGPG). Gangliosides are complex glycolipids that form part of the membrane of neurones and Schwann cells. Gangliosides (GM1, GM2, GB1A, GD1B, GT1B, GQ1B, LM1), sulphated glycolipids (SGPG), and galactosylceramide 3-O-Sulphate (sulphatide) can all serve as antigens in immune-mediated peripheral neuropathy. Antibodies directed against specific antigens might be responsible for a characteristic clinical picture, for example, anti-GM1 antibodies are associated with motor neuropathy (GM1 being located predominantly in motor nerves). Conversely, other antibodies, like anti-sulphatide antibodies, have been associated with more than one type of neuropathy (Ropper and Gorson, 1998).

Neuropathies in patients who are shown to have a paraprotein might also be caused by amyloid deposition in the peripheral nerves, cryoglobulinemia, vasculitis and, in those with an underlying malignant disease, direct tumorous infiltration of the peripheral nerves. Finally, because idiopathic neuropathies are increasingly common in older patients, the association with paraproteinemia is likely to be coincidental in a significant number. The relationship between CIDP and the demyelinating neuropathies that occur in patients with paraproteinemia remains uncertain; some studies have suggested significant differences (Simmons et al., 1993, 1995).

Nonetheless, some patients who present with idiopathic CIDP will go on to develop MGUS, whereas others with idiopathic CIDP or CIDP/MGUS eventually develop myeloma or other malignant lymphoproliferative disorders (Simmons et al., 1995).

## Neuropathy Associated with IgM Paraprotein

Patients with neuropathy and an IgM paraprotein usually have MGUS; rarely is Waldenström's macroglobulinemia, B-cell lymphoma, or chronic lymphatic leukemia identified. Neuropathy has been reported in 5% to 50% of patients with an IgM paraprotein (Harbs et al., 1987; Kyle and Garton, 1987; Logothetis, 1960; Nobile-Orazio et al., 1987).

### Demyelinating Sensorimotor Neuropathy and Anti-Myelin-Associated Glycoprotein (anti-MAG) Antibodies

In 50% to 65% of those with neuropathy and an IgM monoclonal paraprotein, the M-protein can be shown to bind to a carbohydrate (oligosaccharide) determinant that is shared by myelin-associated glycoprotein (MAG), the Po glycoprotein, myelin protein PMP22, and the glycolipids sulphoglucuronyl paragloboside (SGPG) and sulphoglucuronyl lactosaminyl paragloboside (SGLPG) (Latov et al., 1988a; Nobile-Orazio et al., 1989; van den Berg et al., 1992). Latov et al. (1988a) estimated the incidence of this type of neuropathy to be 1 to 5 per 10,000 of the adult population, with symptoms beginning in later life, although onset as early as the fourth decade has been described. Men are affected more often than women. A distinctive clinical, neurophysiological, and pathologic syndrome has been suggested (Nobile-Orazio et al., 1994). The clinical presentation involves a slowly progressive symmetric, distal, sensorimotor neuropathy involving the arms and legs. At the outset, sensory symptoms usually predominate, with numbness, paresthesia, and pain in stocking and glove distribution. Weakness often evolves later, and there might be significant ataxia with an intention tremor and unsteadiness when walking. The ataxia is thought to have a peripheral basis related to the slowness of nerve conduction rather than reflecting central nervous system (cerebellar) involvement (Sindic et al., 1989). Upper limb tremor of postural type and distal distribution is frequently apparent; rest tremor and intention tremor have also been described.

Tremor of the legs is rare and titubation is generally absent. Bain et al. (1996) suggested that the postural tremor is generated centrally, probably in the cerebellum, because the central system receives a faulty input from the sensory nerves. The cranial nerves and autonomic function are spared. Only rarely have predominantly motor neuropathies been reported in patients with anti-MAG antibodies (van den Berg et al., 1992), and very rapidly progressive weakness with fatal outcome has been described (Antoine et al., 1993). Examination of the cerebrospinal fluid (CSF) reveals no excess of cells but the protein value is often elevated. Neurophysiological studies show slowing of motor and sensory conduction together with dispersal of action potentials, indicative of demyelination (Kelly, 1990). Disproportionate prolongation of the distal motor latency, in comparison with relatively preserved proximal motor conduction velocity, might be a specific feature of this syndrome (Kaku et al., 1994). Visual evoked potentials might be prolonged (Barbieri et al., 1987). The demonstration of a high titer of IgM antibodies reacting with the 100 kDa MAG band on Western blot analysis, using crude myelin protein preparations, provides a reliable diagnostic procedure for routine purposes (Miescher and Steck, 1996). Although the affinity of the IgM paraprotein for MAG is variable and the paraprotein level correlates poorly with disease activity (Brouet et al., 1992), M-proteins are thought to cause the neuropathy because pathologic studies show demyelination associated with the deposition of anti-MAG M-protein plus complement on the affected myelin sheath (Monaco et al., 1990). Serum from affected patients injected intraneurally into cat nerves induce demyelination (Hayes et al., 1987; Willison et al., 1988), and the systemic administration of anti-MAG antibodies to chickens causes a demyelinating neuropathy whose pathology resembles the human disease (Tatum, 1993). It remains uncertain how anti-MAG antibodies cross the blood-nerve barrier to trigger a chronic demyelinating neuropathy when the central nervous system is spared.

Some authors have drawn attention to the relatively benign course of the predominantly sensory neuropathy associated with IgM anti-MAG antibodies (Nobile-Orazio et al., 2000), whereas others have been unable to confirm that the demonstration of antibodies directed against antigens such as MAG influence the long-term prognosis (Eurelings et al., 2001).

Pathologically, the neuropathy is characterized by segmental demyelination associated with widening of the outer myelin lamellae at the intraperiod line, corresponding to the outer leaflets of the Schwann cell plasma membrane (Vital et al., 1989). The myelin lamellae might also show widening at the Schmidt-Lanterman incisures and paranodal loops (Jacobs and Scadding, 1990). Granular material might be deposited at these areas of abnormal myelin architecture.

Pathologic spiraling of the myelin sheath, tomaculous bodies, and onion bulbs may develop (Jacobs and Scadding, 1990). However, nerve biopsy is not needed when there is a characteristic presentation of slowly progressive, predominantly sensory peripheral neuropathy, which proves to be demyelinating in type on neurophysiological studies, and the patient has an IgM paraproteinemia and demonstrable anti-MAG antibodies.

Improvement in the demyelinating neuropathies associated with anti-MAG antibodies has been reported following a variety of immunomodulating therapies, including plasma exchange (Dyck et al., 1991; Haas and Tatum, 1988; Sherman et al., 1994); intravenous immunoglobulin (IVIG) (Cook et al., 1990; Ellie et al., 1996; Leger et al., 1994); chemotherapy using chlorambucil, cyclophosphamide, and fludarabine (Latov, 1988a; Leger et al., 1993; Nobile-Orazio et al., 1988; Oksenhendler et al., 1995; Sherman et al., 1994; Wilson et al., 1999); and rituximab, a monoclonal antibody directed against the B-cell surface membrane marker CD20 (Latov and Sherman, 1999; Levine and Pestronk, 1999). A preliminary phase two open study of interferon alpha suggested a beneficial effect (Mariette et al., 1997), but this was not confirmed (Mariette et al., 2000).

Studies that have compared the response to immunomodulating therapies in patients with paraproteinemic neuropathy have almost invariably shown a more favorable response to treatment in those with IgG/IgA-associated neuropathies as compared with those having an IgM paraprotein.

A long-term follow-up study of 25 patients with neuropathy associated with IgM anti-MAG antibodies confirmed a generally favorable long-term prognosis with disability rates (caused principally by hand tremor and gait ataxia) at 5, 10, and 15 years from onset of symptoms to be 16%, 24%, and 50%, respectively. None of the 8 patients who died during the course of followup succumbed to the effect of the neuropathy, but in 3 patients there may have been a relation to treatment given for the neuropathy. The findings led the authors to recommend caution in respect of introducing immunomodulating therapies, given the side effects associated with their long-term use and limited efficiency. They advised that treatment should be reserved for patients who were significantly impaired in their daily life or who showed an aggressive form of the disease (Nobile-Orazio et al., 2000).

## Demyelinating Sensory Neuropathy with Antidisialosyl Antibodies

Ilyas et al. (1985) reported a patient with a predominantly sensory neuropathy of demyelinating type who had monoclonal IgM antibodies that reacted with gangliosides containing disialosyl groups. Similar cases were reported in patients with monoclonal antibodies that reacted strongly with GD1b (Arai et al., 1992; Daune et al., 1992; Obi et al., 1992; Yucki et al., 1992). Four of the patients showed strong crossreactivity with disialosyl-containing gangliosides (Latov and Steck, 1995). The clinical picture was that of a demyelinating sensory neuropathy with ataxia and areflexia. The CSF protein was elevated. Neurophysiological studies supported a demyelinating neuropathy, and improvement with plasma exchange and steroids was reported (Arai et al., 1992; Obi et al., 1992). In 1996 a patient with sensory ataxic neuropathy in association with ophthalmoplegia was reported under the acronym CANOMAD (chronic ataxic neuropathy with ophthalmoplegia, M-protein, agglutination, and disialosyl antibodies). Eighteen patients defined by the presence of IgM antibodies reacting principally with NEUAc (alpha 2-8), NEUAc (alpha 2-3), Gal-configured disialosyl epitopes common to many gangliosides, including GD1b, GD3, GT1b, and GQ1b, were reported; 17 of the patients had benign IgM paraproteinemia and cold agglutinins were present in 50% of cases. The clinical picture was that of sensory ataxia with preservation of motor function, whereas, in addition, 16 of the 18 patients had weakness involving ocular motor and bulbar muscles, either in a relapsing/remitting or persistent form. Similarity to the Miller-Fisher variant of the Guillain-Barré syndrome in which antibodies to GQ1b and GT1a may be detected, was underlined. Some patients showed a partial response to treatment with plasma exchange or intravenous immunoglobulin (Willison et al., 2001).

## Neuropathies Associated with Antisulphatide Antibodies

A predominantly sensory neuropathy has been described in association with monoclonal or polyclonal IgM antibodies directed against sulphatide (galactosyl-ceramide-3-0-sulphate) (Nemni et al., 1993; Pestronk et al., 1991; Quattrini et al., 1992; van den Berg et al., 1993). The clinical picture is usually that of distal sensory disturbance (in particular, pain and paresthesia, which may be predominantly nocturnal), beginning in the feet, usually associated with neuro-physiological changes, suggesting either an axonal neuropathy or dorsal/root ganglionitis. However, van den Berg et al. (1993) described patients with more marked sensory impairment, tremor, and ataxia who showed a predominantly demyelinating picture neurophysiologically, and Nobile-Orazio et al. (1994) reported abnormal spacing of the myelin lamellae on electron microscopy and deposits of IgM on the myelin sheaths in the biopsied cases. Sulphatide is present not only in peripheral nerve myelin, but also on neurones in the dorsal roots; antibodies from patients with ganglionitis can be shown to bind to the surface of dorsal root ganglia neurones rather than peripheral myelin (Quattrini et al., 1992).

In a study of 19 patients with polyneuropathy and high titers of IgM antisulphatide antibodies, a distinction was made between patients without a paraprotein who were most likely to have an axonal neuropathy with a pure sensory syndrome frequently associated with neuropathic pain or dysesthesia, whereas those with an IgM paraprotein had a demyelinating neuropathy with more prominent motor involvement and sensory loss but an absence of pain (Lopate et al., 1997). A further study of 25 patients with significantly elevated antisulphatide antibodies confirmed their association with several different types of neuropathy; although the majority showed either sensory or sensorimotor axonal neuropathy, a smaller group had demyelinating neuropathies that resembled CIDP. Seven patients had an IgM paraprotein that was associated with either axonal or demyelinating neuropathies (although not small-fiber axonal neuropathies, the type most often encountered in patients who do not have a paraprotein) (Dabby et al., 2000). It is unclear why antisulphatide antibodies are associated with neuropathies of different types, and the role that these antibodies play in pathogenesis is uncertain. They are, however, probably the second most frequently encountered antineural reactivity in patients with IgM monoclonal gammopathy (Nobile-Orazio and Carpo, 2001).

## Motor Neuropathy Associated with Anti-GM1 Antibodies

Freddo et al. (1986a) reported a progressive lower motor neurone syndrome associated with antibodies that bound to GM1 gangliosides in a patient with IgM monoclonal gammopathy. Subsequently, an association between elevated monoclonal or polyclonal anti-GM1 antibodies and lower motor neurone syndromes has been confirmed. Immunologically mediated motor neuropathies have an average age of onset in the fifth decade and occur twice as often in men than women. The time course varies from 1 to 25 years (Pestronk et al., 1990). The clinical picture is that of slowly progressive muscle weakness associated with wasting and fasciculation, which is often asymmetric. At the outset weakness might be remarkably focal, involving muscles that are innervated by a single motor nerve. There may be little wasting at the onset, and marked weakness of muscles that are not wasted (as a manifestation of motor conduction block) is a helpful diagnostic feature of the disease. The arms tend to be more severely affected than the legs. Muscles innervated by the cranial nerves might also be involved; ophthalmoplegia and unilateral weakness with hemiatrophy of the tongue have been described (Kaji et al., 1992). The deep reflexes are reduced or absent. Sensory symptoms

are rare. There are no upper motor neurone features. Nonetheless, the clinical presentation might be difficult to distinguish from a lower motor neurone presentation of motor neurone disease. Typically, nerve conduction studies reveal one or more segments of motor conduction block along the course of affected peripheral nerves whereas sensory conduction is quite normal, including those segments of the nerves that show motor conduction block (Parry and Clark, 1988). Less often there is diffuse slowing of motor conduction and, occasionally, motor conduction appears normal. The CSF is normal or shows an elevated protein value. The IgM anti-GM1 antibodies in patients with multifocal motor neuropathy are most often polyclonal, but might be monoclonal in up to 20% of cases.

The anti-GM1 antibodies usually recognize the Gal (β1-3) Gal Nac determinant, which is shared by asialo GM1 and the ganglioside GD1b. GM1 gangliosides are in high concentration at the nodes of Ranvier and might therefore represent the antigenic target, which triggers the demyelinating process in the motor nerves. Postmortem examination of a patient with multifocal motor neuropathy and conduction block with high anti-GM1 antibodies (Adams et al., 1993) showed degeneration of the anterior roots, which were affected more markedly than the distal aspect of the nerves. There was also chromatolysis involving the spinal motor neurones. The involvement of the anterior roots might explain why there is a poor correlation between the distribution and degree of weakness and the demonstration of motor conduction block in many patients. It is uncertain whether anti-GM1 antibodies cause the motor neuropathy, but the binding of anti-GM1 antibodies to motor but not sensory nerves supports a pathogenic role. Furthermore, a favorable response to treatment with intravenous immunoglobulin has been described (Azulay et al., 1994; Chaudhry et al., 1993; Kaji et al., 1992; Nobile-Orazio et al., 1993), and chemotherapy with chlorambucil, cyclophosphamide, or fludarabine may be of value (Feldman et al., 1991; Latov et al., 1988b; Shy et al., 1990; reviewed by Kornberg and Pestronk, 1995).

## Neuropathy Associated with Antibodies to Other Neural Structures

A small number of patients with monoclonal or polyclonal IgM antichondroitin sulphate antibodies, and predominantly axonal neuropathy, have been described (Freddo et al., 1986b; Nemni et al., 1993; Nobile-Orazio et al., 1994; Quattrini et al., 1991; Sherman et al., 1983; Yee et al., 1989). Clinically, the neuropathies were mixed sensorimotor in type, although some patients had predominantly sensory or motor neuropathy. In some patients deposits of IgM were demonstrable in the endoneurium by immunofluorescence. Some patients with antibodies to chondroitin sulphate C also show reactivity to sulphatide (Nemni et al., 1993).

Isolated cases of neuropathy have been associated with monoclonal IgM antibodies to a number of further glycolipids, for example, Miyatani et al. (1987) reported a patient with an IgM paraproteinemia and a polyradicular syndrome associated with antibodies to sialosyllactosaminylparagloboside, and Bollensen et al. (1989) reported a patient with a motor neuropathy associated with IgM antibodies to the ganglioside GD1a.

In 1982 Dellagi et al. reported patients with IgM antibodies to intermediate filaments. In 1997 Connolly et al. reported 5 patients with IgM monoclonal antibodies that bound to tubulin. Three of their patients, who showed IgM binding to tubulin amino acids 301–314, had slowly progressive weakness, hyporeflexia, and neurophysiological studies suggesting CIDP. The 2 other patients had different clinical pictures, one a polyradiculopathy and the other a lower motor neurone form of motor neurone disease; neither had evidence of peripheral nerve demyelination. They concluded that IgM monoclonal antitubulin antibodies could be associated with a spectrum of neurological syndromes, but a CIDP picture was likely if the antibodies recognized the 301–314 amino acid epitope on tubulin.

### Neuropathy Associated with IgM Monoclonal Proteins That Have No Autoimmune Effect

In a substantial number of patients who have a peripheral nerve disorder associated with IgM monoclonal proteins, the antibody does not appear to react with neural antigens. However, the neuropathy in such patients may improve after treatment with immunosuppressant drugs or plasma exchange, suggesting that the neuropathy may be immunologically mediated. There may be further neural antigens that have not yet been identified with which these antibodies cross-react. Alternatively, it is possible that the monoclonal antibodies are causing neural damage by alternative means, for example, inducing vasculitis by acting as cryoglobulins.

### Neuropathy Associated with an IgG or IgA Paraprotein

Patients with IgG or IgA paraproteinemia are less likely to develop neuropathy than those with IgM M-protein. Nonetheless, patients with IgG or IgA MGUS may develop either a demyelinating or an axonal neuropathy. The demyelinating neuropathies resemble CIDP, although some authors think there are important differences between idiopathic CIDP (CIDP-I) and CIDP associated with MGUS (CIDP-MGUS) (Simmons et al., 1995). The axonal neuropathy seen in patients with IgG or IgA paraproteinemia resembles chronic idiopathic axonal polyneuropathy (CIAP) (Notermans et al., 1996).

### Demyelinating Neuropathy Associated with an IgG or IgA Paraprotein

The demyelinating neuropathy seen in association with IgG and IgA paraproteinemia resembles CIDP, a chronic disorder of peripheral nerve function, which may have a relapsing or chronic progressive course over a period in excess of 2 months. The majority of patients have symmetric motor and sensory neuropathy. Weakness of proximal muscles is generally as severe as that seen in distal groups; there is equivalent involvement of the upper and lower limbs. Wasting is rarely pronounced; the reflexes are depressed or absent. Sensory disturbance involves numbness and paresthesia in stocking and glove distribution; pain is less frequently reported. Additional features include postural tremor, facial weakness, bulbar involvement, and papilloedema. The peripheral nerves might be palpably thickened. Nerve conduction studies show a reduction in motor velocity below 70% of normal; distal latencies are prolonged and multifocal conduction block is demonstrable (Albers and Kelly, 1989). The CSF protein is elevated; levels above 100 mg/dL are frequently encountered. CSF pleocytosis is rare. In their initial comparison of CIDP-I and CIDP-MGUS, Simmons et al. (1993a) noted that patients with CIDP associated with a paraprotein had a more indolent course, less marked weakness (although there was no difference in motor conduction velocities), and more marked sensory loss (with greater abnormalities of sensory conduction). Their long-term followup of 69 patients with CIDP-I and 25 patients with CIDP-MGUS (Simmons et al., 1995) showed that patients with CIDP associated with a paraprotein were likely to have a chronic progressive course rather than showing the monophasic or relapsing pattern that may be encountered with CIDP-I. Functional impairment evolved more slowly in patients with CIDP-MGUS and was less marked than those with CIDP-I. The cause of functional impairment in many of the CIDP-MGUS patients was sensory, whereas in those with CIDP-I, weakness was the principal cause. Patients with CIDP-MGUS were less likely to improve, either spontaneously or with immunomodulating therapies. (It should be noted that Simmons et al. [1995] included patients with IGM as well as IgG and IgA MGUS neuropathies; they were unable to demonstrate significant clinical, neurophysiological, or therapeutic differences between those with IgM MGUS on the one hand and those with IgG or IgA MGUS on the other.) They went on to underline the difficulties with classifying this group of demyelinating neuropathies, because reclassification was required in 7 of their patients: 2 of the CIDP-I patients developed

MGUS, one a plasmacytoma (without demonstrating a monoclonal protein in blood or urine), and one Castleman disease (again without demonstrating monoclonal proteins). Three CIDP-MGUS patients required reclassification because they were shown to have a plasmacytoma, multiple myeloma, and myelogenous leukemia, respectively.

Mygland and Monstad (2003) subdivided patients with chronic acquired demyelinating neuropathy into those with proximal and distal weakness (CIDP) and those with only distal involvement, which they termed "distal acquired demyelinating symmetric polyneuropathy" (DADS). An M-protein was found in 20% of CIDP and 36% of DADS. Most patients with DADS had a slowly progressive course and half had only sensory symptoms. Those with CIDP were significantly more likely to respond to treatment than those with DADS irrespective of the presence of an M-protein.

Patients fulfilling the criteria for CIDP should be treated by plasma exchange or intravenous immunoglobulin, supported by prednisolone or a cyclophosphamide (Gorson et al., 1997). Waterston et al. (1992) reported a patient with severe IgG paraprotein-associated neuropathy causing respiratory failure who responded dramatically to cyclosporine when standard treatment failed.

### Axonal Neuropathy Associated with an IgG or IgA Paraprotein

Although any of the plasma cell dyscrasias may be associated with an axonal rather than a demyelinating neuropathy, little is known about the role of paraproteins in causing axonal damage. Even in patients with IgM paraproteins, antibodies to glycoconjugates such as GM1, sulphatide, or chondroitin sulphate have been detected in only a tiny number of patients with axonal neuropathies. Furthermore, in contrast to the anti-MAG antibodies seen with demyelinating neuropathy, there has been little evidence to support their pathogenic role. A CIAP has been defined by Notermans et al. (1993), and it might be that this condition, which is not uncommon, occurs coincidentally in patients who have MGUS. In a study to determine whether axonal polyneuropathies associated with MGUS were distinct from CIAP, Notermans et al. (1996) prospectively studied 71 patients with CIAP and 16 patients with CIAP plus MGUS (this study included 11 patients with IgG and 5 patients with IgM paraproteins). Clinically, those with CIAP-MGUS were more likely to have upper limb involvement, and their overall disability was worse. On neurophysiological study, denervation was more marked in patients with CIAP-MGUS, but otherwise the patients demonstrated no difference in clinical symptoms, signs, neurophysiological parameters, or

nerve-biopsy findings. Notermans et al. (1996) were unable to demonstrate antibodies against MAG, GM1, or chondroitin sulphate. A single patient showed IgM antibodies to sulphatide. They concluded that the axonal polyneuropathy seen in patients with and without MGUS is indistinguishable, rather than significantly different, and that many of these patients may have coincidental neuropathies. Although antisulphatide antibodies can be associated with axonal neuropathies, the studies undertaken by Lopate et al. (1997) and Dabby et al. (2000) failed to reveal any patients with axonal neuropathy in the presence of paraproteinemic antisulphatide antibodies.

### Neuropathy Associated with Myeloma

Peripheral neuropathy is uncommon in patients with myeloma; the frequency has been estimated to be between 1% and 13% of cases (Diego Mirales et al., 1992; Driedger and Pruzanski, 1988; Kelly et al., 1981), except in those who have the uncommon osteosclerotic myeloma, in which most of the patients develop neuropathy (it is often the presenting symptom). Some patients develop a multisystem illness characterized by hyperpigmentation, hirsutism, hepatic or splenic enlargement, and anasarca (Crow Fukase or POEMS syndrome). Although the POEMS syndrome is most often seen with osteosclerotic myeloma, it could rarely develop in patients with osteolytic myeloma, extramedullary plasmacytoma, and monoclonal gammopathies. In addition, a similar syndrome has been described in patients who have polyclonal rather than monoclonal paraproteins. The neuropathy that develops in patients with myeloma may be caused by amyloidosis (the amyloid neuropathies are discussed in detail later in this section). Other patients may have a paraneoplastic neuropathy that resembles carcinomatous neuropathy (Kelly et al., 1981). The neuropathy seen with myeloma is usually progressive, symmetric, and distal in distribution with motor and sensory involvement. The serum paraprotein is nearly always IgG or IgA in type. Neurophysiological studies usually reveal an axonal neuropathy. Improvement of neurologic function has been reported to follow radiotherapy given to solitary lesions and chemotherapy given in the context of multiple myeloma (Alexanian and Dimopoulos, 1994; Donofrio et al., 1984).

### POEMS Syndrome—Polyneuropathy, Organomegaly, Endocrinopathy, M-protein and Skin Changes

POEMS syndrome is frequently associated with osteosclerotic myeloma. Patients with osteosclerotic myeloma differ in many ways from those with multiple myeloma; there is a male preponderance and onset is at a younger age, with a peak incidence during the fourth decade (Takatsuki and Sanada, 1983). Bone pain, fractures, anemia, hypercalcemia, and renal failure are infrequent in osteosclerotic myeloma; the level of M-protein in the serum is low; Bence Jones protein is usually absent from the urine; and bone marrow examination generally shows less than 5% of plasma cells. Osteosclerotic myeloma tends to pursue a relatively benign course and neurologic manifestations might cause the predominant disability.

Scheinker (1938) reported a 39-year-old man with a solitary osteosclerotic myeloma in the sternum in association with sensorimotor neuropathy. He also noted that the patient had localized patches of thickened, deeply pigmented skin over the anterior chest. Crow (1956) described 2 cases of osteosclerotic myeloma associated with neuropathy and diffuse skin hyperpigmentation. The CSF protein was elevated. A syndrome, characterized by polyneuropathy, anasarca, skin abnormalities, endocrine disturbance, dysglobulinemia, and organomegaly associated with extramedullary plasmacytoma, was presented in Japan at a conference directed by Professor Fukase (Shimpo et al., 1968). Subsequently, many similar cases were reported from Japan, but it soon became clear that the condition was not confined to that country; and Bardwick et al. (1980) suggested the acronym POEMS to reflect the combination of polyneuropathy, organomegaly, endocrinopathy, M-protein, and skin changes. Some authors (Nakanishi et al., 1984) used the eponymous title Crow-Fukase syndrome to describe the multisystem presentation seen in patients with a variety of plasma cell dyscrasias; of their 102 cases, half had myeloma (31 sclerotic, 17 sclerotic and lytic, and 8 lytic), 2 had extramedullary plasmacytoma, 33 M-paraprotein in isolation, and 11 a polyclonal increase in plasma proteins. The features of the multisystem illness were similar in the myeloma and nonmyeloma groups (except for splenomegaly and impotence, which were more often seen in those without bone lesions). Their series showed male predominance of 2:1, an age range of 27–80 years with an average of 46 years; 25% were under 40.

Peripheral neuropathy is the cardinal feature of the multisystem illness; it is usually sensorimotor in type (although predominantly motor neuropathy has been described) (Miralles et al., 1992), symmetric in distribution, and distal in onset. Numbness, paresthesia, and coldness spread proximally from the feet; later the upper limbs are affected but the cranial nerves are usually spared. Examination reveals loss of touch position and vibration sensation with relative sparing of pain and temperature perception. The cranial nerves are usually spared, although some patients develop papilloedema. Weakness is usually predominant and associated with loss of reflexes; more than half of patients become unable to walk. Hepatomegaly is more frequent than splenomegaly, and some patients develop lymphadenopathy. Endocrinologic manifestations include diabetes in as many as 50% of patients (Stewart et al., 1989); impotence in males is associated with testicular atrophy and gynecomastia. Females develop amenorrhea. Hypothyroidism and adrenal failure may occur, although serum T3, T4, and cortisol levels are usually normal or only slightly diminished. Males often show a low testosterone level, sometimes associated with high estrogen values (Takatsuki and Sanada, 1983). Hyperprolactinemia has been described (Bardwick et al., 1980). The most frequently encountered skin abnormality is diffuse hyperpigmentation, but many patients develop hypertrichosis with stiff, coarse, dark hairs involving the limbs. The skin may become thickened and hyperhidrosis occurs. Whitening of the nails and clubbing of the fingers may be seen. Cutaneous angiomas have been reported (Puig et al., 1985). Viard et al. (1988) described skin changes reminiscent of scleroderma. Peripheral edema involving the legs is common, and some patients develop ascites and pleural effusions. Low-grade fever may be recorded.

When POEMS syndrome is associated with myeloma, lesions are most often seen in the spine, pelvis, and ribs; the skull tends to be spared. Lesions may be single or few in number. They may be sclerotic throughout, there could be mixed sclerotic and lytic lesions; cyst-like lytic lesions with only a tiny rim of sclerosis have been described. The changes may be subtle and easily misinterpreted as benign sclerosis, fibrous dysplasia, and vertebral hemangioma. CT scanning may be helpful in defining the bone lesions. Radiologic abnormalities have been reviewed by Resnick et al. (1981).

Neurophysiological investigation reveals that the neuropathies are associated with moderate slowing of conduction in motor and sensory nerves: electromyography shows denervation. A study of nerve biopsy (Ono et al., 1985) suggested axonal degeneration with secondary segmental demyelination. Inflammatory changes were minimal and there was no evidence of amyloid. Adams and Said (1998) reported deposition of immunoglobulins in the endoneurial space and myelin sheath (but not the axon) and suggested a pathogenic role for the M-protein. Spinal fluid analysis usually shows a normal cell count but significant elevation of the protein value. The blood count is often normal but sometimes there is polycythemia and thrombocytosis (Kelly et al., 1983). The erythrocyte sedimentation rate may be high. The enlarged lymph nodes seen in patients with osteosclerotic myeloma might show changes reminiscent of Castleman disease (angiofollicular lymph node hyperplasia), a condition that may also be associated with aggressive neuropathy.

The cause of this multisystem illness is unknown, although it has been suggested that plasma cells secrete immunoglobulins or other toxins, which are responsible for the syndrome. The possible pathogenic role of monoclonal light chains has been reviewed by Kyle and Dyck (1993, pp. 1288–1293); they also discuss the significance of hormonal abnormalities. Cytokines may be pathogenic: Gherardi et al. (1994) has reported elevated levels of tumor necrosis factor $\alpha$ (TNF-$\alpha$) in patients with POEMS syndrome, but not in controlled patients with multiple myeloma and Waldenström's macroglobulinemia; they postulate a nonimmuno-globulinemic pathogenesis of the POEMS syndrome, perhaps mediated by TNF-$\alpha$ (which has been implicated in autoimmune peripheral nerve demyelination). Watanabe et al. (1998) reported very high levels of vascular endothelial growth factor/vascular permeability factor and suggested its overproduction may account for the vasculopathy and increased vascular permeability seen with the disorder.

The prognosis of patients with osteosclerotic myeloma and POEMS syndrome is relatively good when compared with typical multiple myeloma; Miralles et al. (1992) estimated a 5-year survival of 60% in comparison to 20% in those with multiple myeloma. They also concluded that the differentiation of POEMS syndrome from osteosclerotic myeloma with neuropathy had little clinical value. Single osteosclerotic lesions should be treated by radiotherapy; isolated plasmacytoma should be removed or treated with radiotherapy. In both cases there may be substantial recovery from the neuropathy. Multiple osteosclerotic lesions may be treated with radiotherapy if they are in close proximity, otherwise chemotherapy (usually melphalan and prednisolone) is required. Steroids alone may have a beneficial effect on the manifestations of the POEMS syndrome, but generally they are ineffective and the small experience with plasma exchange is not encouraging (Silberstein et al., 1985). Responsiveness to intravenous immunoglobulin has varied (Benito-Leon et al., 1998; Henze and Krieger, 1995; Huang et al., 1996). Barrier et al. (1989) and Enevoldson and Harding (1992) reported dramatic improvement in POEMS syndrome on treatment with tamoxifen. Kuwabara et al. (1997) found long-term treatment with melphalan and prednisolone the most effective therapy. If the patient has widespread osteosclerotic lesions, autologous stem cell transplantation after high-dose melphalan therapy is a consideration for younger patients. The stem cells should be collected before the patient is exposed to alkylating agents because they will damage the hematopoietic stem cells.

## Cryoglobulinemic Neuropathy

Cryoglobulins are proteins that precipitate on cooling and redissolve when warmed. They may be composed of isolated monoclonal immunoglobulin (type 1), a mixture of monoclonal and polyclonal immunoglobulin (type 2), or only polyclonal immunoglobulin (type 3) (Brouet et al., 1974). Cryoglobulins might be idiopathic (essential mixed cryoglobulinemia [EMC]) or seen as a manifestation of other diseases, such as the lympho-proliferative diseases, connective tissue disorders, and chronic infections. An association between peripheral neuropathy and cryoglobulinemia (particularly types 2 and 3) has long been recognized, and several different pathogenic mechanisms have been suggested. Clinically, patients may present with individual peripheral nerve lesions or a multifocal neuropathy of acute or subacute onset, suggesting vasculitis. With time, such multifocal neuropathies may acquire a more symmetric distribution. Other patients show a more typical mixed motor and sensory neuropathy with distal onset. Gemignani et al. (1992), in their study of 37 patients with EMC, found that generalized neuropathy was most often seen with type 2 cryoglobulinemia, whereas multifocal neuropathy, often in association with more generalized neuropathy, was the common form in type 3 cryoglobulinemia. They suggested that the 2 clinical pictures may reflect different types of vascular change. It is usually suggested that the intravascular deposition of cryoglobulin or vasculitis induced by circulating immune complexes causes the vascular damage seen with cryoglobulinemia. Cream et al. (1974) considered that vasculitis involving the vasa nervorum was the cause of peripheral nerve dysfunction in the patients they reported. Konishi et al. (1982) described a patient with multifocal neuropathy and mixed cryoglobulinemia in which there was vasculitis, associated with inflammatory change, involving the perineurium. Chad et al. (1982) also attributed neuropathy in EMC to vasculitis. Other authors (Dayan and Lewis, 1966) have suggested demyelination as a possible mechanism of neuropathy in patients with cryoglobulinemia. Clemmensen et al. (1986) reported a patient with IGM$\lambda$ monoclonal essential cryoglobulinemia with antibodies directed against type 1 collagen. Nemni et al. (1988) described 8 patients with peripheral neuropathies associated with type 2 or type 3 cryoglobulinemia, most of whom presented with multifocal neuropathy suggesting vasculitis. Nerve biopsy supported vasculitis involving the vasa nervorum, supporting an ischemic basis for the peripheral nerve dysfunction. They were unable to demonstrate immunoglobulin reacting with myelin or axons, and they did not encounter cryoglobulin aggregates occluding the lumen of capillaries. They suggested that these mechanisms of peripheral nerve damage may occur with type 1 cryoglobulinemia but attributed the neuropathy in types 2 and 3 cryoglob-ulinemia to ischemic damage caused by inflammatory vascular destruction. Treatment with plasma exchange, immunosuppressant drugs, such as cyclophosphamide and steroids, may arrest the progression of neuropathy (Cavaletti et al., 1990; Steck, 1998).

## Amyloid Neuropathy

Weber (1867) drew attention to the association of amyloidosis with myeloma and, in 1931 Magnus-Levy suggested there may be a relationship between Bence Jones protein and the development of amyloid. Osserman et al. (1964) showed that Bence Jones proteins were directly involved in the production of amyloid, and Glenner (1980) was able to demonstrate that the fibrillar material of primary amyloid was identical to monoclonal light chains. In primary amy-loidosis (AL) λ light chains are more frequently repre-sented than κ (ratio of 2:1), but the reverse is true with myeloma or MGUS. In patients with primary amyloido-sis, 89% have a monoclonal protein in serum or urine (Kyle and Gertz, 1995). The distinction between primary amyloidosis and amyloidosis associated with myeloma is based on the number and appearance of plasma cells in the marrow, the presence of monoclonal protein in the blood or urine, and the development of myeloma-tous skeletal lesions. The manifestations of amyloidosis in these conditions are identical and should be distin-guished from those of secondary amyloidosis (AA), which complicates chronic infective or inflammatory processes (and in which neuropathy does not occur). Distinction is also required from the rapidly expanding group of genetically determined or familial amyloidoses (AS), many of which are associated with peripheral neuropathy; however, here, the amyloid fibers are often composed of transthyretin (pre-albumin) generated by mutations that involve the gene on chromosome 18, which codes for transthyretin. Amyloidosis is generally seen in elderly patients, and it is more common in males than females.

Presentation usually involves fatigue, malaise, and weight loss; on examination patients may show hepatomegaly (20%), macroglossia (10%), dependent edema, and purpura. Neuropathy might be present for a long time before the diagnosis of amyloid is made (Rajkumar et al., 1998), it is apparent at the time of diagnosis in 17% of patients (Kyle and Gertz, 1995). Sensory symptoms are usually predominant at the outset, with numbness, paresthesia, and pain, which generally begins distally in the limbs, the legs being affected before the arms (with the exception of those patients who present with carpal tunnel syndrome). Pain might involve superficial burning associated with hypersensitivity of the skin, lightening pain, or deep aching. Some patients describe unpleasant coldness of the extremities. Examination characteristically reveals loss of sensory modalities conveyed by non-myelinated or lightly myelinated sensory fibers (in particular, pain and temperature perception) (Dyck and Lambert, 1969), but the other sensory modalities may also be involved (Kyle and Dyck, 1993, pp. 1294–1309). Autonomic features are present in 65% of those with primary amyloidosis who have neuropathy as the dominant presenting feature (Rajkumar et al., 1998), with postural hypotension, syncope (which might also be caused by amyloid cardiomyopathy), impotence, constipation/diarrhea, nocturia, and alacrima (amyloid infiltration of the lachrymal glands might contribute to the last symptom) (Mathias, 1995). Weakness evolves as the neuropathy advances. There may be palpable enlargement of the peripheral nerves. A motor neurone disease-like syndrome with fibrillation of the tongue, fasciculation, atrophy of limb muscles, and brisk reflexes has been described as a manifestation of amyloid neu-ropathy (Abarbanel et al., 1986); Quattrini et al. (1998) described a lower motor neurone syndrome. Cranial nerve palsies might develop; the facial, trigeminal, and oculomotor nerves have been most frequently affected (Traynor et al., 1991). Nerve conduction studies usually show small or absent sensory potentials, and there might be mild slowing of motor conduction velocities. Electromyogram examination might reveal denervation of peripheral muscles.

Pathologic examination reveals axonal degeneration involving unmyelinated and lightly myelinated fibers (Thomas and King, 1974). Amyloid is deposited, often focally but sometimes diffusely, within the epineurial and endoneurial connective tissues; the peripheral nerves, limb girdle plexuses, sensory and autonomic ganglia might all be affected (Davies-Jones and Esiri, 1971). Electron microscopy shows that the amyloid fibrils in the endoneurium might be closely related to the basal laminae of the Schwann cells and sometimes with exposed axons (Thomas et al., 1997). Endoneurial and epineurial blood vessels are frequently involved by amyloid. The nerve itself usually shows loss of myelinated fibers; the changes involve axonal degener-ation with a lesser degree of segmental demyelination and remyelination. The mechanism of peripheral nerve damage in patients with amyloidosis (AL) is uncertain. Amyloid deposits might indent or compress nerve fibers causing local demyelination and axonal degeneration, but this is thought to be an unlikely explanation for the development of generalized peripheral neuropathy. Some authors (Kernohan and Woltman, 1942) have suggested that the neuropathy is a reflection of ischemic neural damage caused by the amyloid involvement of endoneurial vessels. The absence of a blood–nerve barrier in the dorsal root and sympathetic ganglia might allow amyloid protein to cause local damage (Verghese et al., 1983). The neuropathies certainly appear to be distinct from the demyelinating neuropathies, which are thought to be a consequence of pathogenic monoclonal antibody formation. The neuropathies associated with amyloid were reviewed by Kyle and Dyck (1993, pp. 1294–1309), who also drew attention to the high incidence of carpal tunnel syndrome, which was the presenting symptom in no less than one-fourth of their patients with primary amyloidosis (AL). The median nerve is entrapped by deposits of amyloid involving either the tendon sheaths or the transverse carpal ligament. Nerve conduction studies allow confirmation of the diagnosis, showing a small or absent median sensory potential and prolonged distal motor latency to the median innervated small hand muscles. Electromyography might show denervation in abductor pollicis brevis. Kyle et al. (1989) reported 152 patients with amyloid detected in the tenosynovium at the time of carpal tunnel decompression. Twenty-four were primary amyloid, 3 secondary amyloid, and 1 familial amyloid; the remaining 124 patients had local amyloid deposition without evidence of systemic disease, and only 2 of these patients developed systemic amyloidosis after an interval of nearly a decade. Twelve patients had paraprotein in the serum or urine. Nonetheless, none of the other patients have developed myeloma or systemic amyloidosis over a median follow-up period of 14 years.

The possibility of primary amyloidosis must be considered in patients presenting with neuropathy, especially if this is predominantly sensory and autonomic in type, and particularly if a paraprotein is present in the serum or urine. Diagnosis can be made by abdominal fat aspiration (70%), marrow examination (50%), or rectal biopsy (80%) (Kyle and Dyck, 1993, pp. 1294–1309). Sural nerve biopsy is not infrequently undertaken, whereas amyloid deposits can be demonstrated in the peripheral nerves using Congo red staining (apple green birefringence is apparent under polarized light). It is also possible to demonstrate the immunoglobulin components (light chains) by staining with the appropriate antisera (Linke et al., 1986; Sommer and Schroder, 1989). Biopsies show axonal degeneration with predominant involvement of unmyelinated or lightly myelinated fibers (Kyle and Gertz, 1995). Nerve biopsy might, however, fail to achieve a diagnosis (Simmons et al., 1993b). The benefit of treatment in patients with primary amyloid is uncertain, but treatment with a combination of melphalan and prednisolone, with or without colchicine, has been advocated; such treatment appears to have no effect on the progression of the neuropathy. High-dose intravenous melphalan with autologous stem cell transplantation (Comenzo et al., 1996; Moreau et al., 1998) and allogenic bone marrow transplantation (Gillmore et al., 1998) might prove more effective. Pain might be troublesome at the outset, but resolves as sensory impairment becomes more dense. Symptomatic treatment with amitriptyline or carbamazepine is often helpful. Patients with carpal tunnel syndrome should have the benefit of decompression, although this does not always result in resolution of the sensory symptoms. In patients with autonomic neuropathy causing postural hypotension, support stockings, blocking the head of the bed at night, and fludrocortisone might be helpful (Li et al., 1992).

### Neuropathy Caused by Diffuse Malignant Infiltration of Peripheral Nerves

Diffuse malignant infiltration of the peripheral nerves is usually included as one of the possible causes for generalized peripheral neuropathy in patients with multiple myeloma and Waldenström's macroglobulinemia (Davies-Jones and Sussman, 2001), but pathologically confirmed cases of neuropathy having this basis would appear to be rare, with malignant infiltration by lymphoma or leukemia being most often reported (Posner, 1995, p. 194). Ince et al. (1987) reported a patient with demyelinating peripheral neuropathy and an IgM paraprotein who had diffuse infiltration of the peripheral nerves by B-cell lymphoma. Malignant infiltration of the leptomeninges might cause a polyradiculopathy in which the clinical presentation might resemble peripheral neuropathy; neurophysiological studies are helpful in determining the site of nerve involvement.

### Neuropathy by Chance Association

Because idiopathic peripheral neuropathy, which is usually axonal in type, is not uncommon in older patients (perhaps related to aging or ischemic changes involving the peripheral nerves) (Notermans et al., 1993), and because MGUS is seen with increasing frequency with rising age, it is likely that some of the patients with paraproteinemia have a coincidental neuropathy (Latov, 1995; Notermans, 1996).

# Neurological Conditions That May Rarely Be Associated with Plasma Cell Dyscrasias

## Myopathy

Because reports of muscle disease in patients with paraproteinemias are infrequent, a chance association may be implied (Kissling and Michot, 1984). However, several distinct syndromes have been described in patients with either myeloma or MGUS in which a causative relation seems certain.

## Amyloid Myopathy

Weakness caused by amyloid deposition in skeletal muscles has been reported in a small number of patients with plasma cell dyscrasias (Jennekens and Wokke, 1987). The clinical presentation involves weakness and aching of the muscles, which might show pseudohypertrophy, a wooden consistency, and even palpable masses. Macroglossia might lead to difficulty in closing the mouth, and the voice might become hoarse. Weakness is generally proximal in distribution, and some patients with progressive weakness also develop atrophy of the muscles. There might be associated cardiac involvement. Muscle biopsy shows deposition of amyloid on the surface of muscle fibers but not within them. It has been suggested that this extracellular deposition of amyloid interferes with the normal propagation of the muscle action potential (Ringel and Claman, 1982). Alternatively, amyloid vasculopathy might cause ischemic myopathy (Bruni et al., 1977). Treatment of the plasma cell dyscrasia has little effect on the progression of the muscle disease (Jennekens and Wokke, 1987).

## Polymyositis

Jowitt et al. (1991) reported a patient with proximal weakness, which they attributed to polymyositis, evolving against a background of multiple myeloma with an IgGλ paraprotein. Although the muscle biopsy showed no evidence of active inflammation and there was evidence of vascular amyloid, they suggested that the muscle disorder may be a paraneoplastic myopathy. This hypothesis was developed by Al-Lozi et al. (1995), who demonstrated the deposition of IgMκ on the surface of muscle fibers taken from a patient with Waldenström's macroglobulinemia and an IgMκ paraprotein, who had a progressive proximal myopathy. They suggested that although there was no inflammatory infiltrate in the muscle, an autoimmune cause for the myopathy was likely.

## Inclusion Body Myositis

Inclusion body myositis is an acquired myopathic condition, usually seen in patients over 50 years of age with a male:female ratio of 3:1. Weakness is usually as marked distally as proximally; indeed, distal weakness might be more marked, leading to confusion with peripheral neuropathy and motor neurone disease. The cranial nerves are usually spared. Progression is usually slow and the creative kinase might be normal. Light microscopy shows typical inclusion bodies which, on electron microscopy, contain filamentous masses of amyloid material (Mendel et al., 1991). Dalakas et al. (1997) reported monoclonal gammopathy in 16 (23%)

of 70 patients with sporadic inclusion body myositis: IgG 13, IgM 2, and IgA 1. The IgG of these patients was seen to immunostain the myonuclei and various muscle proteins. It was uncertain whether the recognition of nuclear antigen by the monoclonal immunoglobulin was playing a pathogenic role in inclusion body myositis, but the findings support the view that this muscle disease might have an autoimmune basis.

## Neuromyotonia

Neuromyotonia (Isaac syndrome, the syndrome of continuous muscle fiber activity or undulant myokymia) is an uncommon neurologic condition in which spontaneous continuous muscle fiber contraction, which is usually visible as undulant myokymia, is associated with cramp (commonly triggered by voluntary contraction of the affected muscle), slowness of relaxation (pseudomyotonia), and excessive sweating. The electromyographic findings involve duplex, triplex, or multiplex single motor unit discharges with a high intraburst frequency. In addition, fibrillation and fasciculation are often seen. The discharges continue during sleep. Neuromyotonic discharges might arise from the anterior horn cell or from any site along the peripheral nerve to its termination. The condition might be autoimmune with antibodies directed against voltage-gated potassium channels (Shillito et al., 1995). Plasma exchange has led to dramatic clinical improvement and a reduction in the frequency of neuromyoclonic discharges. Zifko et al. (1994) reported a patient with cramp, fasciculation, myokymia seen in the limb muscles, and delayed relaxation of grip in association with the typical neurophysiological findings of neuromyotonia in association with multiple myeloma, a monoclonal IgM band, and Bence Jones proteinuria. Muscle cramps were relieved by treatment with carbamazepine.

## Optic Neuritis

In 1939 Langdon reported "retrobulbar neuritis" in a patient with multiple myeloma who also had other cranial nerve palsies, and Gudas (1971) described a patient with myelomatous infiltration of the optic nerve. Cox et al. (1988) reported a patient with multiple myeloma and an IgA paraproteinemia who developed progressive visual failure with bilateral central scotomata, which responded dramatically to treatment with prednisolone and melphalan. Because there was no evidence of compressive optic neuropathy, the authors favored an immunologically determined optic neuropathy rather than one caused by ischemia complicating amyloid infiltration of the vasa nervorum of the optic nerves, or direct infiltration of the optic nerves by myeloma or amyloid.

# Neurologic Consequences of Metabolic Complications of Myeloma

## Uremia

Deteriorating renal function is frequently encountered in patients with myeloma, and uremia is a common cause of death. Bence Jones proteinuria and hypercalcemia cause renal injury; acute renal failure might be precipitated by intravenous pyelograms. Declining renal function is often manifest by neurologic symptoms; uremic encephalopathy and neuropathy, the neurologic manifestations of uremia, have been reviewed by Raskin (2001).

## Uremic Encephalopathy

Impairment of cerebral function in patients with renal failure relates not only to the severity of uremia, but also its rate of onset, acute renal failure being less well tolerated than chronic uremia. Apathy, drowsiness, and poor concentration are followed by impairment of perception, hallucinosis, confusion, and eventually coma. Patients describe easy fatigue and generalized weakness. Dysarthria, tremulousness, and ataxia might be associated with hypertonicity, hyperreflexia, clonus, and extensor plantar responses. Pathologic reflexes such as pouting and the grasp reflex might be elicited. Truncal rigidity might be sufficiently marked to suggest meningism. In conscious patients, asterixis (negative myoclonus) can usually be elicited; this movement disorder (a nonspecific manifestation of metabolic encephalopathy) is best demonstrated by asking the patients to extend their arms with the hands dorsiflexed. The "flap" involves sudden downward movement of the fingers, which is then corrected. It is thought that these movements reflect a failure to sustain the original posture against gravity; hence, the term negative myoclonus (Shahani and Young, 1976). Asterixis might also be seen in the facial muscles by observing the patient's failure to maintain retraction of the corners of the mouth when showing the teeth. Asterixis can be demonstrated in stuporous or comatosed patients by flexing the knees when the patient is lying supine and allowing the legs to abduct; irregular jerking movements with alternating abduction and adduction develop (Noda et al., 1985). Seizures are a frequent manifestation of uremic encephalopathy, particularly in acute renal failure. Patients might also develop the syndrome of multifocal myoclonus in which brief, shock-like contractions of muscles occur irregularly involving the face, trunk, and limbs. Such movements might be difficult to distinguish from epileptic seizures, but the frequent, brief, irregular, nonstereotyped movements suggest myoclonus. Asterixis and myoclonus might interfere with voluntary movements in a manner that suggests either ataxia or chorea. The EEG in patients with uremic encephalopathy shows loss of normal rhythms, an excess of slow waves ($\theta$ and $\delta$ frequencies) and, in some cases, triphasic waves. In addition, epileptiform discharges might be seen, even in patients who have not experienced seizures. Asterixis and myoclonus generally have no EEG correlate.

## Uremic Neuropathy

Peripheral nerve dysfunction develops in over 50% of patients with chronic renal failure; a nonspecific mixed distal motor and sensory neuropathy usually begins in the legs and subsequently involves the upper limbs. Sensory symptoms are often predominant at the outset, with burning and painful dysesthesia affecting the feet. Restlessness of the legs is commonly reported; patients describe a need to move the legs in the context of unpleasant sensations of itching, tingling, crawling, or burning. Patients might become unable to sit for any length of time, and the condition, which is often worse when patients retire to bed, might interfere with sleep. Cramps might be prominent, sometimes as a manifestation of neuropathy, but also reflecting the metabolic abnormalities that occur in uremia. Some patients develop autonomic symptoms with postural hypotension and impotence (Campese et al., 1982). Progression of the neuropathy in some patients leads to marked loss of muscle bulk, severe weakness, and ataxia of gait. Neurophysiological studies show generalized slowing of motor and sensory conduction, which involves the proximal and distal segments of the limb nerves (Nielsen, 1973). Uremic neuropathy is usually seen as primarily axonal in type with secondary segmental demyelination (Dyck et al., 1971), although some authors have described predominantly demyelinating neuropathy (Said et al., 1983). Thus, in patients with myeloma and renal failure, it might be difficult to know whether neuropathy is uremic in origin or associated with paraproteinemia.

## Hypercalcemia

Myeloma is the hematologic malignancy most often associated with an elevated serum calcium (20% to 30% of patients become hypercalcemic). Osteoclastic osteolysis, caused by the local elaboration of an osteoclastic-activating factor by myeloma cells, is thought to be responsible. Hypercalcemia adversely affects neuromuscular transmission leading to fatigue and muscle weakness. Headache, lethargy, and decline in cognitive performance give way to confusion and eventually coma (usually only seen with very high calcium levels in excess of 14 mg/dL). Convulsions rarely occur.

# Neurology of Waldenström's Macroglobulinemia

Waldenström's macroglobulinemia is characterized by proliferation of lymphoplasmocytic cells, which secrete IgM paraprotein; malignant B cells might be present in the bone marrow, lymph nodes, and spleen. Neurologic symptoms are predominantly a consequence of the physicochemical properties of IgM paraprotein, which predisposes to hyperviscosity, cryoprecipitation, and hemorrhage, together with the immunologic effects of the paraprotein. Unlike myeloma, neurologic symptoms from direct bone involvement are rare; so too are hypercalcemia, renal failure, and amyloidosis.

Presentation often involves nonspecific symptoms of a neurologic nature, such as fatigue, weakness, headache, and visual disturbance. A hyperviscosity syndrome develops in at least one-fourth of patients and, in conjunction with hemorrhagic diathesis, patients might experience transient ischemic attacks, ischemic strokes, diffuse encephalopathy, spinal cord infarction, subarachnoid hemorrhage, cerebral hemorrhage, and spinal cord hemorrhage. The encephalopathy might present with headache, impaired cognitive performance leading to stupor and coma. Seizures are not infrequent. There is visual impairment associated with the retinopathy of hyperviscosity, and deafness might have this basis. Twenty-five percent of the patients with Waldenström's macroglobulinemia reported by Logothetis et al. (1960) developed neurologic manifestations.

Although neuropathy can occur as a feature of the hyperviscosity syndrome, it is rare; peripheral neuropathies, which frequently evolve in patients with Waldenström's macroglobulinemia, are more likely to relate to the binding of monoclonal IgM to peripheral nerves (as already discussed in the context of IgM MGUS). Dellagi et al. (1983) demonstrated that 40% of patients with Waldenström's macroglobulinemia and peripheral neuropathy had IgM antibody activity directed against the myelin sheath. Peripheral nerve dysfunction might occur as a consequence of direct infiltration of the peripheral nerves by malignant B cells, the development of amyloidosis, vasculitis, and neural hemorrhage. Symmetric mixed motor and sensory neuropathy is most frequently encountered, but multifocal mononeuropathy can also occur (Massey et al., 1978); the combination of multiple cranial and peripheral nerve lesions can sometimes evolve (Fraser et al., 1976). Individual cranial nerve involvement can occur; an isolated fourth nerve palsy was reported by

Moulis and Mamus (1989), and a complete unilateral ophthalmoplegia has also been described (Lossos et al., 1990). Paraneoplastic levodopa-resistant parkinsonism has been described (Rudnick et al., 1998). Plasmapheresis relieves the symptoms related to the hyperviscosity syndrome promptly, and improvement in the various neuropathies has been reported to follow treatment with cytotoxic drugs such as chlorambucil (Fraser et al., 1976; Lossos et al., 1990; Moulis and Mamus, 1989).

## REFERENCES

Abarbanel, J. M., Frisher, S., and Osimani, A. (1986). Primary amyloidosis with peripheral neuropathy and signs of motor neuron disease. *Neurology, 36*, 1125–1127.

Abitbol, J. J., Botte, M. J., Garfin, S. R., and Akeson, W. H. (1989). The treatment of multiple myeloma of the cervical spine with a halo vest. *Journal of Spinal Disorders, 2*, 263–267.

Adams, D., Kuntzer, T., Steck A. J., et al. (1993). Motor conduction block and high titres of anti-GM1 ganglioside antibodies: pathological evidence of a motor neuropathy in a patient with lower motor neuron syndrome. *Journal of Neurology, Neurosurgery and Psychiatry, 56*, 982–987.

Adams, D., and Said. G. (1998). Ultrastructural characterisation of the M-protein in nerve biopsy of patients with POEMS syndrome. *Journal of Neurology, Neurosurgery and Psychiatry, 64*, 809–812.

Adams, R. D., and Plank, C. R. (1973). Case records of the Massachusetts General Hospital. Case 3. *New England Journal of Medicine, 288*, 150–156.

Albers, J. W., and Kelly, J. J., Jr. (1989). Acquired inflammatory demyelinating polyneuropathies: clinical and electrodiagnostic features. *Muscle and Nerve, 12*, 435–451.

Alexanian, R., and Dimopoulos, M. (1994). The treatment of multiple myeloma. *New England Journal of Medicine, 330*, 484–489.

Al-Lozi, M. T., Pestronk, A., Yee, W. C., and Flaris, N. (1995). Myopathy and paraproteinaemia with serum IgM binding to a high molecular weight muscle fibre surface protein. *Annals of Neurology, 37*, 41–46.

Antoine, J. C., Steck, A., and Michel, D. (1993). Neuropathie peripherique mortelle a predominance mortice associee a une IgM monoclonale antiMAG. *Revue Neurologique, 149*, 496–499.

Arai, M., Yoshino, H., Kusano, Y., et al. (1992). Ataxic polyneuropathy and antiPr2 IgM-kappa M-proteinaemia. *Journal of Neurology, 239*, 147–151.

Auld, A. W., and Bueman, A. (1966). Metastatic spinal epidural tumours. An analysis of 50 cases. *Archives of Neurology, 15*, 100–108.

Azulay, J. P., Blin, O., Pouget, J., et al. (1994). Intravenous immunoglobulin treatment in patients with motor neuron syndromes associated with anti-GM1 antibodies: a double blind placebo controlled study. *Neurology, 44*, 429–432.

Bain, P. G., Britton, T. C., Jenkins, I. H., et al. (1996). Tremor associated with benign IgM paraproteinaemic neuropathy. *Brain, 119*, 789–799.

Barbieri, S., Nobile-Orazio, E., Baldini, L., et al. (1987). Visual evoked potentials in patients with neuropathy and macroglobulinaemia. *Annals of Neurology, 2*, 663–666.

Bardwick, P. A., Zvaifler, N. J., Gill, G. N., et al. (1980). Plasma cell dyscrasia with polyneuropathy, organomegaly, endocrinopathy, M protein, and skin changes: the POEMS syndrome. Report of two cases and a review of the literature. *Medicine (Baltimore), 59*, 311–322.

Barrier, J. H., Le Noan, H., Mussini, J. M., and Brisseau, J. M. (1989). Stabilisation of a severe case of POEMS syndrome after tamoxifen administration. *Journal of Neurology, Neurosurgery and Psychiatry, 52*, 286.

Benito-Leon, J., Lopez-Rios, F., Rodriguez-Martin, F. J., et al. (1998). Rapidly deteriorating polyneuropathy with osteosclerotic myeloma responsive to intravenous immunoglobulin and radiotherapy. *Journal of Neurological Sciences, 158*, 113–117.

Benson, W. J., Scarffe, J. H., Todd, I. D. H., et al. (1979). Spinal cord compression in myeloma. *British Medical Journal, i*, 1541–1544.

Berenson, J. R., Lichtenstein, A., Porter, L., et al. (1996). Efficacy of pamidronate in reducing skeletal events in patients with advanced multiple myeloma. *New England Journal of Medicine, 334*, 488–493.

Bergsagel, D. E., and Rider, W. D. (1985). Plasma cell neoplasms. In V. T. Devita, Jr., S. Hellman, and S. A. Rosenberg (Eds.), *Cancer. Principles and Practice of Oncology* (pp. 1776–1777). Philadelphia: Lippincott.

Bing, J., Fog, M., and Neel, A. V. (1937). Report of a third case of hyperglobulinaemia with affection of the central nervous system on a toxi-infectious basis. *Acta Medica Scandinavica, 91*, 409–427.

Bing, J., and Neel, A. V. (1936). Two cases of hyperglobulinaemia with affection of the central nervous system on a toxi-infectious basis. *Acta Medica Scandinavica, 88*, 492–506.

Bollensen, E., Schipper, H. I., and Steck, A. J. (1989). Motor neuropathy with activity of monoclonal IgM antibody to GDIa ganglioside. *Journal of Neurology, 236*, 353–355.

Brenner, B., Carter, A., Tatarsky, I., et al. (1982). Incidence prognostic significance and therapeutic modalities of CNS involvement in multiple myeloma. *Acta Haematologica, 68*, 77–83.

Brice, J., and McKissock, W. S. (1965). Surgical treatment of malignant extradural spinal tumours. *British Medical Journal, i*, 1339–1342.

Brouet, J. C., Clauvel, J. P., Danon, F., et al. (1974). Biologic and clinical significance of cryoglobulins. A report of 86 cases. *American Journal of Medicine, 57*, 775–788.

Brouet, J. C., Marriette, X., Chevalier, A., and Hauttecoure, B. (1992). Determination of the affinity of monoclonal human IgM for myelin associated glycoprotein and sulfated glucuronic paragloboside. *Journal of Neuroimmunology, 36*, 209–215.

Bruni, J., Bilbao, J. M., and Pritzker, K. P. H. (1977). Myopathy associated with amyloid angiopathy. *Canadian Journal of Neurological Sciences, 44*, 77–80.

Buskard, N. A., Galton, D. A. G., Goldman, J. R., et al. (1977). Plasma exchange in the longterm management of Waldenström's macroglobulinaemia. *Canadian Medical Association Journal, 117*, 135–137.

Byrne, T. N. (1992). Spinal cord compression from epidural metastases. *New England Journal of Medicine, 327*, 614–619.

Campese, Y. M., Procci, W. R., Levitan, D., et al. (1982). Autonomic nervous system dysfunction and impotence in uraemia. *American Journal of Nephrology, 2*, 140–143.

Capra, J. D., and Kunkel, H. G. (1970). Aggregation of $\gamma$G3 proteins. Relevance to the hyperviscosity syndrome. *Journal of Clinical Investigation, 49*, 610–621.

Cavaletti, G., Petruccioli, M. G., Crespi, V., et al. (1990). A clinico-pathological and follow-up study of 10 cases of essential type II cryoglobulinaemic neuropathy. *Journal of Neurology, Neurosurgery and Psychiatry, 53*, 886–889.

Chad, D., Pariser, K., Bradley, W. G., et al. (1982). The pathogenesis of cryoglobulinaemic neuropathy. *Neurology, 32*, 725–729.

Chandy, K. G., Stockley, R. A., Leonard, R. C. F., et al. (1981). Relationship between serum viscosity and intravascular IgA polymer concentration in IgA myeloma. *Clinical and Experimental Immunology, 46*, 653–661.

Chaudhry, V., Corse, A. M., Cornblath, D. R., et al. (1993). Multifocal motor neuropathy: response to human immune globulin. *Annals of Neurology, 33*, 237–242.

Christopherson, W. M., and Millar, A. J. (1950). A re-evaluation of solitary plasma cell myeloma of bone. *Cancer, 3*, 240–252.

Clarke, E. (1954). Cranial and intracranial myeloma. *Brain, 77*, 61–81.

Clarke, E. (1956). Spinal cord involvement in multiple myelomatosis. *Brain, 79*, 332–348.

Clemmensen, I., Jensen, B. A., Holund, B., et al. (1986). Circulating monoclonal IgM lambda cryoglobulinaemia with collagen type I affinity in vasculitis. *Clinical and Experimental Immunology, 64*, 587–596.

Cohen, D. M., Svien, H. J., and Dahlin, D. C. (1964). Long term survival of patients with myeloma of the vertebral column. *Journal of the American Medical Association, 187*, 914–917.

Comenzo, R. L., Vosburgh, E., Simms, R. W., et al. (1996). Dose intensive melphalan with blood stem cell support for the treatment of AL amyloidosis: one-year follow-up in five patients. *Blood, 88*, 2801–2806.

Connolly, A. M., Pestronk, A., Mehta, S., et al. (1997). Serum IgM monoclonal auto antibody binding to the 301–314 amino acid epitope of $\beta$tubulin: clinical association with slowly progressive demyelinating polyneuropathy. *Neurology, 48*, 243–248.

Cook, D., Dalakas, M., Galdi, A., et al. (1990). High dose intravenous immunoglobulin in the treatment of demyelinating neuropathy associated with monoclonal gammopathy. *Neurology, 40*, 212–214.

Cox, J. G., Steiger, M. J., and Pearce, J. M. S. (1988). Optic neuropathy and multiple myeloma. *British Journal of Hospital Medicine, 39*, 448.

Cream, J. J., Herne, J. E. C., Hughes, R. A. C., and Mackenzie, I. C. K. (1974). Mixed or immune complex cryoglobulinaemia and neuropathy. *Journal of Neurology, Neurosurgery and Psychiatry, 37*, 82–87.

Crow, R. S. (1956). Peripheral neuritis in myelomatosis. *British Medical Journal, 2*, 802–804.

Currie, S., and Henson, R. A. (1971). Neurological syndromes in the reticuloses. *Brain, 94*, 307–320.

Dabby, R., Weimer, L. H., Hays, A. P., et al. (2000). Antisulfatide antibodies in neuropathy. Clinical and electrophysiologic correlates. *Neurology, 54*, 1448–1452.

Dahlstrom, V., and Lindstrom, F. D. (1979). Paraplegia in myelomatosis: a study of 20 cases. *Acta Medica Scandinavica, 205*, 173–178.

Dalakas, M. C., Ilia, I., Gallardo, E., and Juarez, C. (1997). Inclusion body myositis and paraproteinaemia: incidence and immuno-pathologic correlations. *Annals of Neurology, 41*, 100–104.

Daune, G. C., Farrer, R. G., Dalakas, M. C., and Quarles, R. H. (1992). Sensory neuropathy associated with immunoglobulin M to GDIb ganglioside. *Annals of Neurology, 31*, 683–685.

Davies-Jones, G. A. B., and Esiri, M. M. (1971). Neuropathy due to amyloid in myelomatosis. *British Medical Journal, 2*, 444.

Davies-Jones, G. A. B., and Sussman, J. D. (2001). Neurological manifestations of haematological disorders. In M. J. Aminoff (Ed.), *Neurology and General Medicine*, 3rd ed (pp. 201–231). Philadelphia: Churchill Livingstone.

Dayan, A. D., and Lewis, P. D. (1966). Demyelinating neuropathy in macroglobulinaemia. *Neurology, 16*, 1141–1144.

Dellagi, K., Brouet, J. C., Perreau, J., and Paulin, D. (1982). Human monoclonal IgM with auto-antibody activity against intermediate filaments. *Proceedings of the National Academy of Science U S A, 79*, 446–450.

Dellagi, K., Dupouey, P., Brouet, J. C., et al. (1983). Waldenström's macroglobulinaemia and peripheral neuropathy. A clinical and immunologic study of 25 patients. *Blood, 62*, 280–285.

Diego Mirales, G., O'Fallon, J. R., and Talley, N. J. (1992). Plasma cell dyscrasia with polyneuropathy. *New England Journal of Medicine, 327*, 1919–1923.

Donofrio, P. D., Albers, J. W., Greenberg, H. S., and Mitchell, B. S. (1984). Peripheral neuropathy in osteosclerotic myeloma. Clinical and electrophysiological improvement with chemotherapy. *Muscle and Nerve, 7,* 137–141.

Drew, M. J. (2002). Plasmapheresis in the dysproteinemias. *Therapeutic Apheresis, 6,* 45–52.

Driedger, H., and Pruzanski, W. (1988). Plasma cell neoplasia with peripheral polyneuropathy. *Medicine (Baltimore), 59,* 301–310.

Dyck, P. J., Johnson, W. J., Lambert, E. H., and O'Brien, P. C. (1971). Segmental demyelination secondary to axonal degeneration in uraemic neuropathy. *Mayo Clinic Proceedings, 46,* 400–431.

Dyck, P. J., and Lambert, E. H. (1969). Dissociated sensation in amyloidosis: compound action potential, quantitative histologic and teased-fiber, and electron microscopic studies of sural nerve biopsies. *Archives of Neurology, 20,* 490–507.

Dyck, P. J., Low, P. A., Windebank, A. J., et al. (1991). Plasma exchange in polyneuropathy associated with monoclonal gammopathy of undetermined significance. *New England Journal of Medicine, 325,* 1482–1486.

Ellie, E., Vital, A., Steck, A., et al. (1996). Neuropathy associated with 'benign' antimyelin associated glycoprotein IgM gammopathy: clinical, immunological, neurophysiological, pathological findings and response to treatment in 33 cases. *Journal of Neurology, 243,* 34–43.

Enevoldson, T. P., and Harding, A. E. (1992). Improvement in the POEMS syndrome after administration of tamoxifen. *Journal of Neurology, Neurosurgery and Psychiatry, 55,* 71–72.

Eurelings, M., Moons, K. G. M., Notermans, N. C., et al. (2001). Neuropathy and IgM M-proteins. Prognostic value of antibodies to MAG SGPG and sulfatide. *Neurology, 56,* 228–233.

Feldman, E. L., Bromberg, M. B., Albers, J. W., and Pestronk, A. (1991). Immunosuppressive treatment in multifocal motor neuropathy. *Annals of Neurology, 30,* 397–401.

Findlay, G. F. G. (1984). Adverse effects of the management of malignant spinal cord compression. *Journal of Neurology, Neurosurgery and Psychiatry, 47,* 761–768.

Fraser, D. M., Parker, A. C., Amer, S., and Campbell, I. W. (1976). Mononeuritis multiplex in a patient with macroglobulinaemia. *Journal of Neurology, Neurosurgery and Psychiatry, 39,* 711–715.

Freddo, L., Sherman, W. H., and Latov, N. (1986b). Glycosaminoglycan antigens in peripheral nerve studies with antibodies from a patient with neuropathy and monoclonal gammopathy. *Journal of Neuroimmunology, 12,* 57–64.

Freddo, L., Yu, R. K., Latov, N., et al. (1986a). Gangliosides, GMI and GDlb are antigens for IgM M-protein in a patient with motor neurone disease. *Neurology, 36,* 454–458.

Freel, R. J., Maldonado, J. E., and Gleich, G. J. (1972). Hyperviscosity syndrome associated with immunoglobulin A myeloma. *American Journal of Medical Science, 264,* 117–122.

French, J. D. (1947). Plasmacytoma of the hypothalamus. *Journal of Neuropathology and Experimental Neurology, 6,* 265–270.

Gemignani, F., Pavesi, G., Fiocchi, A., et al. (1992). Peripheral neuropathy in essential mixed cryoglobulinaemia. *Journal of Neurology, Neurosurgery and Psychiatry, 55,* 116–120.

Gherardi, R. K., Chouaib, S., Malapert, D., et al. (1994). Early weight loss and high serum tumour necrosis factor alpha levels in polyneuropathy, organomegaly, endocrinopathy, M-protein, skin changes syndrome. *Annals of Neurology, 35,* 501–505.

Gilbert, R. W., Kim, J. H., and Posner, J. B. (1978). Epidural compression from metastatic tumour: diagnosis and treatment. *Annals of Neurology, 3,* 40–51.

Gillmore, J. D., Davies, J., Iqbal, A., et al. (1998). Allogenic bone marrow transplantation for systemic AL amyloidosis. *British Journal of Haematology, 100,* 226–228.

Glenner, G. G. (1980). Amyloid deposits and amyloidosis: the beta fibrilloses. *New England Journal of Medicine, 302,* 1283–1292, 1333–1343.

Gorson, K. C., Allam, G., and Ropper, A. H. (1997). Chronic inflammatory demyelinating polyneuropathy: clinical features and response to treatment in 67 consecutive patients with and without a monoclonal gammopathy. *Neurology, 48,* 321–328.

Gosselin, S., Kyle, R. A., and Dyck, P. J. (1991). Neuropathies associated with monoclonal gammopathies of undetermined significance. *Annals of Neurology, 30,* 54–61.

Gudas, P. P., Jr. (1971). Optic nerve myeloma. *American Journal of Ophthalmology, 71,* 1085–1089.

Haas, D. C., and Tatum, A. H. (1988). Plasmapheresis alleviates neuropathy accompanying IgM antimyelin-associated glycoprotein paraproteinaemia. *Annals of Neurology, 23,* 394–396.

Hansotia, P., Gani, K., and Friedenberg, W. (1983). Cerebrospinal fluid monoclonal gammopathy in multiple myeloma and Waldenström's macroglobulinaemia. *Neurology, 33,* 1411–1415.

Harbs, H., Arfmann, M., Frick, E., et al. (1985). Reactivity of sera and isolated monoclonal IgM from patients with Waldenström's macroglobulinaemia with peripheral nerve myelin. *Journal of Neurology, 232,* 43–48.

Harrington, K. D. (1984). Anterior cord decompression and spinal stabilization for patients with metastatic lesions of the spine. *Journal of Neurosurgery, 61,* 107–117.

Hayes, A. P., Latov, N., Takatsu, M., and Sherman, W. H. (1987). Experimental demyelination of nerve induced by serum of patients with neuropathy and an antiMAG IgM M-protein. *Neurology, 37,* 242–256.

Heisner, S., and Schwartzman J. J. (1952). Variations in the roentgen appearance of the skeletal system in myeloma. *Radiology, 58,* 178–191.

Henson, R. A., and Urich, H. (1982). *Cancer and the Nervous System. The Neurological Manifestations of Systemic Malignant Disease.* Oxford: Blackwell Scientific Publications.

Henze, T., and Krieger, G. (1995). Combined high-dose 7S-IgG and dexamethasone is effective in severe polyneuropathy of the POEMS syndrome. *Journal of Neurology, 242,* 482–483.

Hockaday, J. M., and Whitty, C. W. M. (1967). Patterns of referred pain in the normal subject. *Brain, 90,* 481–496.

Husain, M. M., Metzer, W. S., and Biner E. F. (1987). Multiple intraparenchymal brain plasmacytomas with spontaneous intratumoral haemorrhage. *Neurosurgery, 20,* 619–623.

Huang, C. C., and Chu, C. C. (1996). Poor response to intravenous immunoglobulin therapy in patients with Castleman's disease and the POEMS syndrome. *Journal of Neurology, 243,* 726–727.

Ilyas, A. A., Quarles, R. H., Dalakas, M. C., et al. (1985). Monoclonal IgM in a patient with paraproteinaemic polyneuropathy binds to gangliosides containing disialosyl groups. *Annals of Neurology, 18,* 655–659.

Ince, P. G., Shaw, P. J., Fawcett, P. R. W., and Bates, D. (1987). Demyelinating neuropathy due to primary IgM kappa B-cell lymphoma of peripheral nerves. *Neurology, 37,* 1231–1235.

Jaccard, A., Royer, B., Bordessoule, D., Brouet, J. C., and Fermand, J. P. (2002). High-dose therapy and autologous blood stem cell transplantation in POEMS syndrome. *Blood, 99,* 3057–3059.

Jacobs, J. M., and Scadding, J. W. (1990). Morphological changes in IgM paraproteinaemic neuropathy. *Acta Neuropathologica Berlin, 80,* 77–84.

Jamieson, D. R. S., Teasdale, E., and Willison, H. J. (1996). False localising signs in the spinal cord. *British Medical Journal, 312,* 243–244.

Jennekens, F. G. I., and Wokke, J. H. J. (1987). Proximal weakness of the extremities as main feature of amyloid myopathy. *Journal of Neurology, Neurosurgery and Psychiatry, 50,* 1353–1358.

Johnson, R. A. (1993). The management of acute spinal cord compression. *Journal of Neurology, Neurosurgery and Psychiatry, 56,* 1046–1054.

Jowitt, S. N., Liu Yin, J. A., and Schady, W. (1991). Polymyositis in association with multiple myeloma. *British Journal of Hospital Medicine, 45,* 234–235.

Kaji, R., Shibasaki, H., and Kimura, J. (1992). Multifocal demyelinating motor neuropathy: cranial nerve involvement and immunoglobulin therapy. *Neurology, 42*, 506–509.

Kaku, D. A., England, J. D., and Sumner, A. J. (1994). Distal accentiation of conduction slowing in polyneuropathy associated with antibodies to myelin-associated glycoprotein and sulphated glucuronyl paragloboside. *Brain, 117*, 941–947.

Kelly, J. J., Jr. (1990). The electrodiagnostic findings in polyneuropathies associated with IgM monoclonal gammopathies. *Muscle and Nerve, 13*, 1113–1117.

Kelly, J. J., Kyle, R. A., Miles, J. M., et al. (1981). The spectrum of peripheral neuropathy in myeloma. *Neurology, 31*, 24–31.

Kelly, J. J., Jr., Kyle, R. A., Miles, J. M., and Dyck, P. J. (1983). Osteosclerotic myeloma and peripheral neuropathy. *Neurology, 33*, 202–210.

Kernohan, J. W., and Woltman, H. W. (1942). Amyloid neuritis. *Archives of Neurology, 47*, 132–140.

Kissling, D., and Michot, F. (1984). Multiple myeloma occurring in association with a pre-existing neuromuscular disease (progressive muscular dystrophy). *Acta Haematologica, 72*, 94–104.

Konishi, T., Saida, K., Ohnishi, A., and Nishitani, H. (1982). Perineuritis in mononeuritis multiplex with cryoglobulinaemia. *Muscle and Nerve, 5*, 173–177.

Kopp, W. L., Beirne, G. J., and Byrnes, R. O. (1967). Hyperviscosity syndrome in multiple myeloma. *American Journal of Medicine, 43*, 141–146.

Kornberg, A. J., and Pestronk, A. (1995). Chronic motor neuropathies and lower motor neurone syndromes. *Bailliere's Clinical Neurology, 4*, 427–441.

Krumholz, A., Weiss, H. D., Jiji, V. H., et al. (1982). Solitary intracranial plasmacytoma: two patients with extended follow-up. *Annals of Neurology, 11*, 529–532.

Kuwabara, S., Hattori, T., Shimoe, Y., and Kamitsukasa, I. (1997). Long-term melphalan–prednisolone chemotherapy for POEMS syndrome. *Journal of Neurology, Neurosurgery and Psychiatry, 63*, 385–387.

Kyle, R. A., and Dyck, P. J. (1993). Amyloidosis and neuropathy. In P. J. Dyck, P. K. Thomas, and J. W. Griffin (Eds.), *Peripheral Neuropathy*, vol 2 (pp. 1294–1309). Philadelphia: WB Saunders.

Kyle, R. A., Eilers, S. G., Linscheid, R. L., and Gaffey, T. A. (1989). Amyloid localised to tenosynovium at carpal tunnel release. Natural history of 124 cases. *American Journal of Clinical Pathology, 91*, 393–397.

Kyle, R. A., and Garton, J. P. (1987). The spectrum of IgM monoclonal gammopathy in 430 cases. *Mayo Clinic Proceedings, 62*, 719–731.

Kyle, R. A., and Gertz, M. A. (1995), Primary systemic amyloidosis: clinical and laboratory features in 474 cases. *Seminars in Haematology, 32*, 45–59.

Kyle, R. A., Therneau, T. M., Rajkumar, S. V., et al. (2002). A long-term study of prognosis in monoclonal gammopathy of undetermined significance. *New England Journal of Medicine, 346*, 564–569.

Latov, N. (1995). Pathogenesis and therapy of neuropathies associated with monoclonal gammopathies. *Annals of Neurology, 37*(Suppl 1), 32–42.

Latov, N., Hays, A. P., Donofrio, P. D., et al. (1988b). Monoclonal IgM with unique specificity to gangliosides GMI and GDlb and to lacto N tetraose, associated with human motor neuron disease. *Neurology, 38*, 763–768.

Latov, N., Hays, A. P., and Sherman, W. H. (1988a). Peripheral neuropathy and antiMAG antibodies. *CRC Critical Reviews in Neurobiology, 3*, 301–332.

Latov, N, and Sherman, W. H. (1999). Therapy of neuropathy associated with antiMAG IgM monoclonal gammopathy with Rituxan. *Neurology, 52* (Suppl 2), A551.

Latov, N., and Steck, A. J. (1995). Neuropathies associated with anti-glycoconjugate antibodies and IgM monoclonal gammopathies.

In A. K. Asbury, and P. K. Thomas (Eds.), *Peripheral Nerve Disorders*, vol 2 (pp. 153–174). Oxford: Butterworth-Heinemann.

Leger, J. M., Oksenhendler, E., Bussel, A., et al. (1993). Treatment by chlorambucil with/without plasma exchange of polyneuropathy associated with monoclonal IgM. Prospective randomised controlled study in 44 patients. *Neurology, 43A*, 215–216.

Leger, J. M., Younes-Chennoufi, A. B., Chassande, B., et al. (1994). Human immunoglobulin treatment of multifocal motor neuropathy and polyneuropathy associated with monoclonal gammopathy. *Journal of Neurology, Neurosurgery and Psychiatry, 57*(Suppl), 46–49.

Levine, T. D., and Pestronk, A. (1999). IgM antibody related polyneuropathies: B-cell depletion chemotherapy using rituximab. *Neurology, 52*, 1701–1704.

Li, K., Kyle, R. A., and Dyck, P. J. (1992). Immunohistochemical characterisation of amyloid proteins in sural nerves and clinical associations in amyloid neuropathy. *American Journal of Pathology, 141*, 217–226.

Linke, R. P., Nathrath, W. B. J., and Eulitz, M. (1986). Classification of amyloid syndromes from tissue sections using antibodies against various amyloid fibril proteins: report of 142 cases. In G. G. Glenner, E. R. Osserman, and E. P. Benditt (Eds.), *Amyloidosis* (p. 599). New York: Plenum Press.

Logothetis, J., Silverstein, P., and Coe, J. (1960). Neurologic aspects of Waldenström's macroglobulinaemia. *Archives of Neurology, 5*, 564–573.

Lopate, G., Parks, B. J., Goldstein, M., et al. (1997). Polyneuropathies associated with high titre antisulphatide antibodies: characteristics of patients with and without serum monoclonal proteins. *Journal of Neurology, Neurosurgery and Psychiatry, 62*, 581–585.

Lossos, A., Averbuch-Heller, L., Reches, A., and Abramsky, O. (1990). Complete unilateral ophthalmoplegia as a presenting manifestation of Waldenström's macroglobulinaemia. *Neurology, 40*, 1801–1802.

Magnus-Levy, A. (1931). Bence Jones Eiweiss and Amyloid. *Zeitschrift fuer Klinische Medizin, 116*, 510–531.

Mancardi, G. L., and Mandybur, T. I. (1983). Solitary intracranial plasmacytoma. *Cancer, 51*, 2226–2233.

Mariette, X., Brouet, J.-C., Chevret, S., et al. (2000). A randomised double blind trial versus placebo does not confirm the benefit of α interferon in polyneuropathy associated with monoclonal IgM. *Journal of Neurology, Neurosurgery and Psychiatry, 69*, 279–280.

Mariette, X., Chastang, C., Clavelou, P., et al. (1997). A randomised clinical trial comparing interferon α and intravenous immunoglobulin in polyneuropathy associated with monoclonal IgM. *Journal of Neurology, Neurosurgery and Psychiatry, 63*, 28–34.

Massey, E. W., Pleet, A. B., and Brannon, W. L. (1978). Waldenström's macroglobulinaemia and mononeuritis multiplex. *Annals of Internal Medicine, 88*, 360–361.

Mathias, C. J. (1995). Autonomic neuropathy: aspects of diagnosis and management. In A. K. Asbury, and P. K. Thomas (Eds.), *Peripheral Nerve Disorders*, vol 2 (pp. 95–117). Oxford: Butterworth-Heinemann.

McKissock, W., Bloom, W. H., and Chynn, K. Y. (1961). Spinal cord compression caused by plasma-cell tumours. *Journal of Neurosurgery, 18*, 68–73.

McLain, R. F., and Weinstein, J. N. (1989). Solitary plasmacytomas of the spine: a review of 84 cases. *Journal of Spinal Disorders, 2*, 69–74.

Mendel, J. R., Sahenk, Z., Gales, T., and Paul, L. (1991). Amyloid filaments in inclusion body myositis. *Archives of Neurology, 48*, 1229–1234.

Miescher, G. C., and Steck, A. J. (1996). Paraproteinaemic neuropathies. *Bailliere's Clinical Neurology, 5*, 219–232.

Miralles, G. D., O'Fallon, J. R., and Talley, N. J. (1992). Plasma cell dyscrasia with polyneuropathy. The spectrum of POEMS syndrome. *New England Journal of Medicine, 327*, 1919–1923.

Miyatani, N., Baba, H., Sato, S., et al. (1987). Antibody to sialosyllac-tosaminyl-paragloboside in a patient with IgM paraproteinaemia and polyradiculoneuropathy. *Journal of Neuroimmunology, 14,* 189–196.

Monaco, S., Bonetti, B., Ferrari, S., et al. (1990). Complement mediated demyelination in patients with IgM monoclonal gammopathy and polyneuropathy. *New England Journal of Medicine, 322,* 649–652.

Moreau, P., Leblond, V., Bourquelot P., et al. (1998). Prognostic factors for survival and response after high dose therapy and autologous stem cell transplantation in systemic AL amyloidosis: a report on 21 patients. *British Journal of Haematology, 101,* 766–769.

Moulis, H., and Mamus, S. W. (1989). Isolated trochlear nerve palsy in a patient with Waldenström's macroglobulinaemia complete recovery with combination therapy. *Neurology, 39,* 1399.

Mueller, J., Hotson, J. R., and Langston, J. W. (1983). Hyperviscosity induced dementia. *Neurology, 33,* 101–103.

Mygland, A., and Monstad, P. (2003). Chronic acquired demyelinating symmetric polyneuropathy classified by pattern of weakness. *Archives of Neurology, 60,* 260–264.

Nakanishi, T., Sobue, I., Toyokura, Y., et al. (1984). The Crow-Fukase syndrome: a study of 102 cases in Japan. *Neurology, 34,* 712–720.

Nemni, R., Corbo, M., Fazio, R., et al. (1988). Cryoglobulinaemic neuropathy. A clinical, morphological, and immunocytochemical study of 8 cases. *Brain, 111,* 541–552.

Nemni, R., Fazio, R., Quattrini, A., et al. (1993). Antibodies to sulfatide and to chondroitin sulfate C in patients with chronic sensory neuropathy. *Journal of Neuroimmunology, 43,* 79–86.

Nielsen, V. K. (1973). The peripheral nerve function in chronic renal failure VI. The relationship between sensory and motor nerve conduction and kidney function, azotemia, age, sex, and clinical neuropathy. *Acta Medica Scandinavica, 194,* 455–462.

Nobile-Orazio, E., Baldini, L., Barbieri, S., et al. (1988). Treatment of patients with neuropathy and antiMAG IgM M-proteins. *Annals of Neurology, 24,* 93–97.

Nobile-Orazio, E., and Carpo, M. (2001). Neuropathy and monoclonal gammopathy. *Current Opinion in Neurology, 14,* 615–620.

Nobile-Orazio, E., Francomano, E., Daverio, R., et al. (1989). Antimyelin associated glycoprotein IgM antibody titres in neuropathy associated with macroglobulinaemia. *Annals of Neurology, 26,* 543–550.

Nobile-Orazio, E., Manfredini, E., Carpo, M., et al. (1994). Frequency and clinical correlates of anti-neural IgM antibodies in neuropathy associated with IgM monoclonal gammopathy. *Annals of Neurology, 36,* 416–424.

Nobile-Orazio, E., Marmiroli, P., Baldini, L., et al. (1987). Peripheral neuropathy in macroglobulinaemia: incidence and antigen specificity of M-proteins. *Neurology, 37,* 1506–1514.

Nobile-Orazio, E., Meucci, N., Baldini, L., et al. (2000). Long term prognosis of neuropathy associated with antiMAG IgM M-proteins and its relationship to immune therapies. *Brain, 123,* 710–717.

Nobile-Orazio, E., Meucci, N., Barbieri, S., et al. (1993). High dose intravenous immunoglobulin therapy in multifocal motor neuropathy. *Neurology, 43,* 537–544.

Noda, S., Ito, H., Umezaki, H., and Minato, S. (1985). Hip flexion—abduction to elicit asterixis in unresponsive patients. *Annals of Neurology, 18,* 96–97.

Notermans, N. C. (1996). Monoclonal gammopathy and neuropathy. *Current Opinion in Neurology, 9,* 334–337.

Notermans, N. C., Wokke, J. H. J., Franssen, H., et al. (1993). Chronic idiopathic polyneuropathy presenting in middle or old age: a clinical and electrophysiological study of 75 patients. *Journal of Neurology, Neurosurgery and Psychiatry, 56,* 1066–1071.

Notermans, N. C., Wokke, J. H. J., van den Berg, L. H., et al. (1996). Chronic idiopathic axonal polyneuropathy: comparison of patients with and without monoclonal gammopathy. *Brain, 119,* 421–427.

Obi, T., Kusunoki, S., Takatsu, M., et al. (1992). IgM M-protein in a patient with sensory dominant neuropathy binds preferentially to polysiayogangliosides. *Acta Neuroglica Scandinavica, 86,* 215–218.

Oda, K., Egawa, H., Okuhara, T., et al. (1991). Meningeal involvement in Bence Jones multiple myeloma. *Cancer, 67,* 1900–1902.

Oksenhendler, E., Chevret, S., Leger, J.-M., et al. (1995). Plasma exchange and chlorambucil in polyneuropathy associated with monoclonal IgM gammopathy. *Journal of Neurology, Neurosurgery and Psychiatry, 59,* 243–247.

Ono, K., Ito, M., Hotchi, M., et al. (1985). Polyclonal plasma cell proliferation with systemic capillary hemangiomatosis, endocrine disturbance, and peripheral neuropathy. *Acta Pathologica, Japan, 35,* 251–267.

Osserman, E. F., Takutsuki, K., and Talal, N. (1964). The pathogenesis of 'amyloidosis': studies on the role of abnormal gamma globulins and gamma globulin fragments of the Bence Jones (L-polypeptide) type in the pathogenesis of 'primary' and 'secondary' amyloidosis,' and the 'amyloidosis' associated with plasma cell myeloma. *Seminars in Hematology, 1,* 3–85.

Parker, D., and Malpas, J. S. (1979). Multiple myeloma. *Royal College of Physicians London Journal, 13,* 146–153.

Parry, G. J. G., and Clark, S. (1988). Multifocal acquired demyelinating neuropathy masquerading as motor neuron disease. *Muscle and Nerve, 11,* 103–107.

Patterson, W. P., Caldwell, C. W., and Doll, D. C. (1990). Hyperviscosity syndromes and coagulopathies. *Seminars in Oncology, 17,* 210–216.

Pestronk, A., Chaudhry, V., Feldman, E. L., et al. (1990). Lower motor neurone syndromes defined by patterns of weakness, nerve conduction abnormalities, and high titres of antiglycolipid antibodies. *Annals of Neurology, 27,* 316–326.

Pestronk, A., Li, F., Griffin, J., et al. (1991). Polyneuropathy syndromes associated with serum antibodies to sulfatide and myelin-associated glycoprotein. *Neurology, 41,* 357–362.

Posner, J. B. (1987). Back pain and epidural spinal cord compression. *Medical Clinics of North America, 71,* 185–205.

Posner, J. B. (1995). The neurologic complications of cancer, series number 45 (pp. 853–860). *The Contemporary Neurological Series.* Philadelphia: FA Davis.

Preston, F. E., Cooke, K. B., Foster, M. E., et al. (1978). Myelomatosis and hyperviscosity syndrome. *British Journal of Haematology, 38,* 517–530.

Pruzanski, W., and Watt, J. G. (1972). Serum viscosity and hyperviscosity syndrome in IgG multiple myeloma: report on ten patients and a review of the literature. *Annals of Internal Medicine, 77,* 853–860.

Puig, L., Moreno, A., Domingo, P., et al. (1985). Cutaneous angiomas in POEMS syndrome. *Journal of the American Academy of Dermatology, 12,* 961–964.

Quattrini, A., Corbo, M., Dhaliwal, S. K., et al. (1992). Antisulfatide antibodies in neurological disease: binding to rat dorsal root ganglia neurons. *Journal of the Neurological Sciences, 112,* 152–159.

Quattrini, A., Nemni, R., Fazio, R., et al. (1991). Axonal neuropathy in a patient with monoclonal IgM kappa reactive with Schmidt-Lanterman incisures. *Journal of Neuroimmunology, 33,* 73–79.

Quattrini, A., Nemni, R., Sferrazza, B., et al. (1998). Amyloid neuropathy simulating lower motor neurone disease. *Neurology, 51,* 600–602.

Rajkumar, S. V., Gertz, M. A., Kyle, R. A., et al. (1998). Prognosis of patients with primary systemic amyloidosis who present with dominant neuropathy. *American Journal of Medicine, 104,* 232–237.

Raskin, N. H. (2001). Neurological complications of renal failure. In M. J. Aminoff (Ed.), *Neurology and General Medicine,* 3rd ed (pp. 293–306). Philadelphia: Churchill Livingstone.

Resnick, D., Greenway, G. D., Bardwick, P. A., et al. (1981). Plasma-cell dyscrasia with polyneuropathy, organomegaly, endocrinopathy, M-protein, and skin changes: the POEMS syndrome: distinctive radiographic abnormalities. *Radiology, 140*, 17–22.

Ringel, S. P., and Claman, H. N. (1982). Amyloid associated muscle pseudohypertrophy. *Archives of Neurology, 39*, 413–417.

Ropper, A. H., and Gorson, K. C. (1998). Neuropathies associated with paraproteinaemia. *New England Journal of Medicine, 338*, 1601–1607.

Rudnicki, S. A., Harik, S. I., and Dhodapkar, M. (1998). Nervous system dysfunction in Waldenström macroglobulinemia: response to treatment. *Neurology, 51*, 1210–1213.

Russell, D. S., and Rubinstein, L. J. (1989). Pathology of tumours of the nervous system, 5th ed (pp. 618–619). London: Edward Arnold.

Said, G., Boudier, L., Selva, J., et al. (1983). Different patterns of uraemic polyneuropathy: clinicopathological study. *Neurology, 33*, 567–574.

Saperstein, D. S., Katz, J. S., Amato, A. A., and Barohn, R. J. (2001). Clinical spectrum of chronic acquired demyelinating polyneuropathies. *Muscle and Nerve, 24*, 311–324.

Scheinker, I. (1938). Myelom und Nervensystem: uber eine bisher nicht beschriebene mit eigentumlichen Hautveranderugen einhergehende Polyneuritis bei einem plasmazellularen. Myelom des Sternums. *Deutsche Zeitschrift fuer Nervenheilkunde, 147*, 247–273.

Schulman, P., Sun, T., Sharer, L., et al. (1980). Meningeal involvement in IgD myeloma with cerebrospinal fluid paraprotein analysis. *Cancer, 46*, 152–155.

Shahani, B. T., and Young, R. R. (1976). Asterixis—a disorder of the neurological mechanisms underlying sustained muscle contraction. In M. Shahani (Ed.), *The Motor System: Neurophysiology and Muscle Mechanisms* (pp. 301–316). New York: Elsevier.

Sherman, W. H., Latov, N., Hays, A. P., et al. (1983). Monoclonal IgMk antibody precipitating with chondroitin sulfate C from patients with axonal polyneuropathy and epidermolysis. *Neurology, 33*, 192–201.

Sherman, W. H., Latov, N., Lange, D., et al. (1994). Fludarabine for IgM antibody-mediated neuropathies. *Annals of Neurology, 36*, 326–327.

Sherman, W. H., Olarte, M. R., McKiernan, G., et al. (1984). Plasma exchange treatment of peripheral neuropathy associated with plasma cell dyscrasia. *Journal of Neurology, Neurosurgery and Psychiatry, 47*, 813–819.

Shillito, P., Molenaar, P. C., Vincent, A., et al. (1995). Acquired neuromyotonia: evidence for autoantibodies directed against K+ channels of peripheral nerves. *Annals of Neurology, 38*, 714–722.

Shimpo, S., Nishitani, H., Tsunematsu, T., et al. (1968). Solitary plasmacytoma with polyneuritis and endocrine disturbances. *Nippon Rinsho, 26*, 2444–2456.

Shy, M. E., Heiman-Paterson, T., Parry, G. J., et al. (1990). Lower motor neurone disease in a patient with antibodies against Gal (β1–3) GalNAc in gangliosides GMI and GDlb: improvement following immunotherapy. *Neurology, 40*, 842–844.

Siegal, T., and Siegal, T. (1989). Current considerations in the management of neoplastic spinal cord compression. *Spine, 14*, 223–228.

Silberstein, L. E., Dugan, D., and Berkman, E. M. (1985). Therapeutic trial of plasma exchange in osteosclerotic myeloma associated with the POEMS syndrome. *Journal of Clinical Apheresis, 2*, 253–257.

Silverstein, A., and Doniger, D. E. (1963). Neurologic complications of myelomatosis. *Archives of Neurology, 9*, 534–544.

Simmons, Z. (1999). Paraproteinaemia and neuropathy. *Current Opinion in Neurology, 12*, 589–595.

Simmons, Z., Albers, J. W., Bromberg, M. B., and Feldman, E. L. (1995). Long term follow up of patients with chronic inflammatory demyelinating polyradiculoneuropathy, with and without monoclonal gammopathy. *Brain, 118*, 359–368.

Simmons, Z., Albers, J. W., Bromberg, M. B., and Feldman, E. L. (1993a). Presentation and initial clinical course in patients with chronic inflammatory demyelinating polyradiculoneuropathy. Comparison of patients without and with monoclonal gammopathy. *Neurology, 43*, 2202–2209.

Simmons, Z., Blaivas, M., Aguilera, A. J., et al. (1993b). Low diagnostic yield of sural nerve biopsy in patients with peripheral neuropathy and primary amyloidosis. *Journal of Neurological Sciences, 120*, 60–63.

Sindic, C. J., Boucquey, D., Bisteau, M., et al. (1989). Monoclonal IgM gammopathy with antimyelin associated glycoprotein (MAG) activity and polyneuropathy: a study of three cases. *Acta Neurologlica Belgica, 89*, 331–345.

Sinoff, C. L., and Blumsohn, A. (1989). Spinal cord compression in myelomatosis: response to chemotherapy alone. *European Journal of Cancer and Clinical Oncology, 25*, 197–200.

Smith, E., Kochwa, S., and Wasserman, L. R. (1965). Cold aggregation of IgG globulin in vivo 1. The hyperviscosity syndrome in multiple myeloma. *American Journal of Medicine, 39*, 35–48.

Sod, L. M., and Wiener, L. M. (1959). Intradural extramedullary plasmacytoma: case report. *Journal of Neurosurgery, 16*, 107–109.

Sohier, W. D., and Richardson, E. P. (1971). Case reports of the Massachusetts General Hospital, case 32. *New England Journal of Medicine, 285*, 394–401.

Somer, T. (1987). Rheology of paraproteinemias and the hyperviscosity syndrome. *Balliere's Clinical Haematology, 1*, 695–723.

Sommer, C., and Schroder, J. M. (1989). Amyloid neuropathy: immunocytochemical localization of intra- and extracellular immunoglobulin light chains. *Acta Neuropathologlica, 79*, 190–199.

Spaar, F. W. (1980). Paraproteinaemias and multiple myeloma. In V. Bryn (Ed.), *Handbook of Clinical Neurology*, vol 39 (pp. 131–179). Amsterdam: Elsevier North Holland Biomedical Press.

Spiers, A. S. D., Halpern, R., Ross, S. C., et al. (1980). Meningeal *myelomatous. Archives of Internal Medicine, 140*, 256–259.

Steck, A. J. (1998). Neurological manifestations of malignant and non-malignant dysglobulinaemias. *Journal of Neurology, 245*, 634–639.

Stewart, P. M., McIntyre, M. A., and Edwards, C. R. W. (1989). The endocrinopathy of POEMS syndrome. *Scottish Medical Journal, 34*, 520–522.

Suarez, G. A., and Kelly, J. J., Jr. (1993). Polyneuropathy associated with monoclonal gammopathy of undetermined significance. Further evidence that IgM MGUS neuropathies are different from IgG MGUS. *Neurology, 43*, 1304–1308.

Svien, H. J., Price, R. D., and Bayrd, E. D. (1953). Neurosurgical treatment of compression of the spinal cord caused by myeloma. *Journal of the American Medical Association, 153*, 784–786.

Takatsuki, K., and Sanada, I. (1983). Plasma cell dyscrasia with polyneuropathy and endocrine disorder: clinical and laboratory features of 109 reported cases. *Japanese Journal of Clinical Oncology, 13*, 543–555.

Tatum, A. H. (1993). Experimental paraprotein neuropathy: demyelination by passive transfer of human IgM antiMAG. *Annals of Neurology, 33*, 502–506.

Thomas, P. K., and King, R. H. M. (1974). Peripheral nerve changes in amyloid neuropathy. *Brain, 97*, 395–406.

Thomas, P. K., Landon, D. N., and King, R. H. M. (1997). Disease of the peripheral nerves—amyloid neuropathy. In D. I. Graham, and P. L. Lantos (Eds.), *Greenfield's Neuropathology*, 6th ed, vol 2 (pp. 425–428). London: Arnold.

Traynor, A. E., Gertz, M. A., and Kyle, R. A. (1991). Cranial neuropathy associated with primary amyloidosis. *Annals of Neurology, 29*, 451–454.

Truong, L. D., Kim, H. S., and Estrada, R. (1982). Meningeal myeloma. *American Journal of Clinical Pathology, 78*, 532–535.

van den Berg, L. H., Kinsella, L. J., Corbo, M., et al. (1992). Antibodies to MAG and SGPG in neuropathy. *Annals of Neurology, 32*, 251.

van den Berg, L. H., Lankamp, C. L. A. M., de Jager, A. E. J., et al. (1993). Antisulfatide antibodies in peripheral neuropathy. *Journal of Neurology, Neurosurgery and Psychiatry, 56*, 1164–1168.

Veith, R. G., and Odom, G. L. (1965). Extradural spinal metastases and their neurosurgical treatment. *Journal of Neurosurgery, 23*, 501–508.

Verghese, J. P., Bradley, W. G., Nemni, R., and McAdam, K. P. W. J. (1983). Amyloid neuropathy in multiple myeloma and other plasma cell dyscrasias: a hypothesis of the pathogenesis of amyloid neuropathies. *Journal of the Neurological Sciences, 59*, 237–246.

Viard, J.-P., Lesavre, P., Boitard, C., et al. (1988). POEMS syndrome presenting as systemic sclerosis: clinical and pathologic study of a case with microangiopathic glomerular lesions. *American Journal of Medicine, 84*, 524–528.

Vital, A., Lagueny, A., Julien, J., et al. (2000). Chronic inflammatory demyelinating polyneuropathy associated with dysglobulinaemia: a peripheral nerve biopsy study in 18 cases. *Acta Neuropathologica, 100*, 63–68.

Vital, A., Vital, C., Julian, J., et al. (1989). Polyneuropathy associated with IgM monoclonal gammopathy. Immunological and pathological study in 31 patients. *Acta Neuropathologica Berlin, 79*, 160–167.

Waldenström, J. G. (1944). Incipient myelomatosis or 'essential hyperglobulinaemia with fibrinogenopaenia—a new syndrome?' *Acta Medica Scandinavica, 117*, 216–247.

Watanabe, O., Maruyama, I., Arimura, K., et al. (1998). Overproduction of vascular endothelial growth factor/vascular permeability factor is causative in Crow-Fukase (POEMS) syndrome. *Muscle and Nerve, 21*, 1390–1397.

Waterston, J. A., Brown, M. M., Ingram, D. A., and Swash, M. (1992). Cyclosporin A therapy in paraprotein-associated neuropathy. *Muscle and Nerve, 15*, 445–448.

Weber, H. (1867). Mollities ossium, doubtful whether carcinomatous or syphilitic. *Transactions of the Pathological Society of London, 18*, 206–209.

Weissman, D. E. (1988). Glucocorticoid treatment for brain metastases and epidural spinal cord compression: a review. *Journal of Clinical Oncology, 6*, 543–551.

Willison, H. J., O'Leary, C. P., Veitch, J., et al. (2001). The clinical and laboratory features of chronic sensory ataxic neuropathy with antidisialosyl IgM antibodies. *Brain, 124*, 1968–1977.

Willison, H. J., Trapp, B. D., Bacher, J. D., et al. (1988). Demyelination induced by intraneural injection of human antimyelin associated glycoprotein antibodies. *Muscle and Nerve, 11*, 1169–1176.

Wilson, H. C., Lunn, M. P. T., Schey, S., Hughes, R. A. C. (1999). Successful treatment of IgM paraproteinaemic neuropathy with fludarabine. *Journal of Neurology, Neurosurgery and Psychiatry, 66*, 575–580.

Woo E., Yu, Y. L., Ng, M., et al. (1986). Spinal cord compression in multiple myeloma: who gets it? *Australian and New Zealand Journal of Medicine, 16*, 671–675.

Woodruff, R. K., and Ireton, H. J. C. (1982). Multiple cranial nerve palsies as the presenting feature of meningeal myelomatosis. *Cancer, 49*, 1710–1712.

Woodruff, R. K., Whittle, J. H., and Malpas, J. S. (1979). Solitary plasmacytoma 1. Extra medullary soft tissue plasmacytoma. *Cancer, 43*, 2340–2343.

Wuhrmann, F. (1956). Uber das coma paraproteinaemicum bei myelomen und makroglobulinamien. *Schwiezerische Medizinische Wochenschrift, 86*, 623–625.

Yee, W. C., Hahn, A. F., Hearn, S. A., and Rupar, A. R. (1989). Neuropathy in IgM para proteinaemia: immunoreactivity to neural proteins and chondroitin sulfate. *Acta Neuropathologica, 78*, 57–64.

Young, R. F., Post, E. M., and King, G. A. (1980). Treatment of spinal epidural metastases: randomized prospective comparison of laminectomy and radiotherapy. *Journal of Neurosurgery, 53*, 741–748.

Yucki, N., Miyatani, N., Sato, S., et al. (1992). Acute relapsing sensory neuropathy associated with IgM antibody against B series gangliosides containing a GalNAc$\beta$1-4 (Gal3-2$\alpha$ Neu Ac 8-2$\alpha$ Neu Ac) $\beta$1-configuration. *Neurology, 42*, 686–689.

Zifko, U., Drlicek, M., Machacek, E., et al. (1994). Syndrome of continuous muscle fibre activity and plasmacytoma with IgM paraproteinaemia. *Neurology, 44*, 560–561.

# CHAPTER 18

## Myeloma: Patient and Caregiver Perspectives

MICHAEL S. KATZ
KARIN ISGUR BERGSAGEL
DANIEL E. BERGSAGEL

Myeloma presents difficult challenges for everyone it touches: patients, their families, friends, physicians, and other health care professionals. During the course of the disease, the failure of any of the above-named to understand the point of view of another can lead to strains in their relationships that can be unpleasant and, at times, harmful. Our purpose in writing this chapter is to provide explanations of certain interpersonal aspects of the disease, advice about where to look for more information, and explore coping mechanisms for patients and caregivers. We also describe various types of physician behaviors that patients with myeloma might encounter, so that they will have a better idea about what to expect. For physicians, we classify patient and caregiver emotional states. It is hoped that this will help them to better recognize patient needs and influence their design of the best treatment and support strategy for meeting these needs.

The authors' backgrounds provide 3 points of view about myeloma. One of the authors (M.S.K.) had a solitary plasmacytoma of the iliac crest discovered in 1990. He was treated successfully with surgical resection and radiation therapy. Subsequently, he progressed to multiple myeloma, which has been treated with multiple courses of radiation, a number of different steroids, chemotherapy, and, most recently, thalidomide. MSK consulted many knowledgeable specialists about his diagnosis and learned a great deal about the disease. He also became an executive board member and Vice President of the International Myeloma Foundation

(IMF) and established their Web site. Attendance at many IMF patient and family seminars and leading 2 in-person and 2 Internet-based support groups has introduced him to a large number of patients with myeloma, improved his knowledge about the disease, and allowed him to elicit survey responses from over 350 patients with myeloma. We present the result of this sampling of patient and caregiver opinions later in this chapter. M.S.K. has also served as co-chair of the Eastern Cooperative Oncology Group Patient Representatives Committee, chair of the National Cancer Institute Director's Consumer Liaison Group, and as a Patient Consultant for the Food and Drug Administration. K.I.B.'s husband, at age 48, was diagnosed with smoldering multiple myeloma in 1995 following a routine physical. He progressed to active myeloma by late 1996. His treatments included various chemotherapy protocols, including participation in clinical trials, autologous PBSCT, and radiation. Over the course of his illness he experienced most of the usual complications of myeloma: infections, plasmacytomas, kyphosis, pathologic fractures, lytic lesions, hypercalcemia, and anemia. He died at home, under hospice care, in 2001. K.I.B. was his caregiver. She became, and remains, an active member of the online myeloma community, bringing her into daily contact with over 1200 myeloma patients and caregivers. D.E.B. is a hematologist/oncologist with extensive experience in the management of patients with myeloma at the University of Texas Cancer Center in Houston (1955–1964) and at the Ontario Cancer Institute/Princess Margaret Hospital in Toronto (1965–1995).

We consider the following 6 topics:

1. Understanding the formidable challenge presented by myeloma
2. Special challenges for caregivers
3. Recognizing and dealing with patient and caregiver emotional states
4. The role of information in meeting the myeloma challenge
5. Different reactions physicians can elicit from patients and caregivers
6. Recognizing and managing positive and negative "fit factors" in physician and patient/caregiver interactions

## Understanding the Formidable Challenge Presented by Myeloma

If a patient has acute appendicitis, the choices are generally clear. Untreated, it can be fatal. However, with surgery and antibiotics, the prospects for a full recovery are excellent. An ordeal might lie ahead, but there is light at the end of the tunnel; there is a cure.

With multiple myeloma, the situation is more difficult. The disease is life threatening—fatal. There is no known cure. The medical profession has many approaches to help patients with myeloma live better and longer. As a result, people with myeloma can sometimes live for decades. Yet, there remains much controversy about how to treat the disease. The course of treatment is very much dependent on the specifics of the patient's physical, emotional, and family situation. Why is this?

- Because there is no known cure, treatments need to be viewed in terms of how long they are able to control the disease or relieve symptoms and how they affect the patient's quality of life.

- For some treatments, there is not enough clinical experience with patients to know what to expect. Furthermore, no 2 patients are alike so that predicting results for any treatment is a matter of probabilities; there are no guarantees.

- Virtually all of the treatments have potentially serious side effects; some treatments can lead to complications that might prove to be fatal. Patients, families, and physicians might have different perspectives about what constitutes acceptable risk. They also have different views about what is an acceptable outcome of treatment.

As a result, patients with a diagnosis of myeloma face difficult choices. Because there is typically no one right course of treatment, it is common to have conflicting medical opinions (International Myeloma Foundation, 2002).

Physicians play an important part in helping patients and their families make treatment decisions. However, anyone meeting large numbers of patients soon learns that each patient's role in treatment decisions and the criteria they apply tend to be quite different. A British study of 165 patients with Hodgkin's disease concluded, "Patients do not necessarily share doctors' priorities in decision-making or place the same emphasis on different types of morbidity" (Turner and Maher, 1996). The impact of treatment programs on quality of life and the patient's sense of well being is a very individual equation. For example, alopecia can have a more devastating impact on some patients' sense of well being than peripheral neuropathy or nausea. Treatment programs that require inpatient procedures can be anathema to people with active professional careers or young children. Many patients are looking for programs that allow them to self-administer much of the treatment (e.g., tablets or subcutaneous injections) or receive home care. Other patients prefer to have things totally taken care of in a clinical setting. When practical, physicians should endeavor to be sensitive to these differences to achieve the best outcome and to strengthen the patient/physician relationship.

Physicians face difficult issues in recommending diagnostic and treatment options for which the results generally cannot be assured. They face formidable choices in deciding what to communicate and how to convey it. The physician is often in the position of having to persuade the patient to pursue what can be frightening treatment options. Barring a crisis (e.g., spinal cord compression, hypercalcemia, kidney failure, hyperviscosity), the recommendation often lacks an ironclad rationale for immediate action.

It is important for patients and their families to understand which treatment decisions are critical and which can wait. When the situation permits, many would like the time to get more than one opinion before beginning a treatment program.

Treatment recommendations typically include multiple components, each with different objectives. Often, certain elements of the treatment program are more urgent than others and require quicker decisions. Others aim more at long-term management of the disease, allowing more time to decide (Table 18-1).

Beyond some tried and true stabilizing and palliative treatments, there are very few absolutes in myeloma treatment. Remission-inducing treatments, typically chemotherapy regimens, cannot guarantee results. Physicians have information on success rates and can use different factors (e.g., prognostic indicators such as chromosome 13 deletion, disease phenotype, beta 2 microglobulin) to help choose the programs that have the best probability of success. The same also can be said for peripheral stem cell auto and allo/mini-allotransplants, which aim at a cure. Thus, all parties face major challenges in dealing with the disease. Understanding the different perspectives that foster communications and trust can be key to achieving the best outcome.

Dr. Robert A. Kyle of the Mayo Clinic observed, "All patients with multiple myeloma need substantial and continuing emotional support. The approach must be positive and emphasize the potential benefits of therapy. It is reassuring to know that some patients survive for ten years or more. It is vital that the physician caring for patients with multiple myeloma has the interest and capacity to deal with an incurable disease over a span of years with assurance, sympathy, and resourcefulness."

# Special Challenges for Caregivers

As health care delivery evolves, more patients are cared for outside of the hospital setting by family members or friends acting as caregivers. The physician needs to be sensitive to the patient/caregiver relationship and to the role of the caregiver in patient care, because caregivers have a profound effect on quality of life and outcomes. It is important that the caregiver's personal needs are met so they can continue to care for the patient.

## TABLE 18-1
### Treatment Decision Timing

| | Objective | Examples | Time to Decide |
|---|---|---|---|
| Stabilizing | Countering the life-threatening disruptions to body chemistry and the immune system that can occur with myeloma | Drugs to reduce hypercalcemia might include bisphosphonates or chemotherapy<br>Hemodialysis when kidney function fails<br>Radiation to prevent spinal cord compression<br>Plasmapheresis to thin the blood and avoid stroke | Hours to days |
| Palliative | Relieving discomfort and increasing the patient's ability to function normally and enjoy life | Radiation to stop bone destruction and relieve pain<br>Erythropoietin to treat anemia<br>Orthopedic surgery to repair/strengthen bone | Days to months |
| Remission-inducing | Lessening the severity of the symptoms, slowing or temporarily arresting the course of the disease | Chemotherapy, steroids, immunomodulatory, or other drugs to kill malignant cells throughout the body<br>Radiation to kill malignant cells at a tumor site | Weeks to months |
| Cure | Permanent remission (although never achieved and confirmed, it remains the objective of experimental treatments) | Peripheral stem cell transplants as a means of delivering high-dose chemotherapy | Weeks to months |

Caregivers generally undertake 4 main functions. They might be primarily or partially responsible for the following:

1. Physical care, including monitoring health status, reporting symptoms, and administering medications or other forms of treatment

2. Information seeking and decision making

3. Providing emotional support

4. Acting as the main channel of communication between the patient and the health care team

Most family caregivers must assume additional responsibilities that the patient can no longer undertake. Care giving is usually added to an already full life, and balancing the needs of the patient against other roles and duties is a frequent concern of caregivers (Blanchard et al., 1997).

The role of the caregiver is intrinsically complex, as is the stress experienced, but it can be divided into physical and emotional components. Myeloma is a debilitating disease, and the care of the patient can be very taxing. Physically, the caregiver confronts fatigue and increased morbidity (Nijbooer et al., 1998). A subgroup of caregivers, who are characterized by having high caregiving demands, experiencing chronic stress associated with caregiving, and being physiologically compromised, has been shown to be at risk for negative health outcomes (Schultz and Beach, 1999).

Because the incidence of myeloma increases with age, many caregivers will themselves be elderly and have their own health problems. The Caregiver Health Effects Study (Schultz and Beach, 1999) observed a 63% increased mortality rate among older spousal caregivers who were experiencing mental or emotional strain and concluded "Caregivers who report strain are more likely to die than non-caregiver controls." Decreasing that associated strain on the caregiver is a very important intervention.

Emotionally, the caregiver confronts grief, anger, guilt, and the challenges of learning and assuming new roles. These challenges are all complicated by the impossibly high standards that most caregivers set for themselves. Many caregivers feel they must selflessly give themselves over to caregiving, ignoring their own needs.

Grief is a natural reaction to loss, and the myeloma caregiver experiences losses on multiple fronts. Caregivers typically grieve for the loss of the healthy person who has now been replaced by a patient, as well as loss of the lifestyle they led before being thrust into the role of caregiver. Work, health, finances, interests, family, and social life might all suffer in the wake of myeloma.

Anger is a common response and might be directed against the disease itself (known as "the beast" to many patients and caregivers). The perceived cause of the myeloma and the shortcomings of the medical establishment are also frequent choices. This anger might also be channeled constructively, into advocacy or fundraising efforts on behalf of the myeloma community. Hardest of all for caregivers to acknowledge or deal with is anger directed at the patient. Part of the "selfless caregiver" role that many adopt is an assumption that it is unacceptable to have any negative feelings toward the patient or to resent having to assume caregiving responsibilities.

Caregivers also experience a sort of "survivor's guilt" for not being the one with myeloma (Calhoun, 1998). "Why not me?" is an unanswerable paradox. This sense of guilt ("I don't deserve my good health.") is often responsible for the unreasonable expectations that many caregivers have for themselves and for their accompanying self-denial. The superhuman standards that perfectionist caregivers set for themselves would be impossible for anyone to meet; when they violate them, there is further guilt.

Rare indeed is the myeloma caregiver who is prepared to assume this challenging role. Most learn on the job, by trial and error. Spouses are frequently caregivers, and it is important to note that life-threatening illness can often cause severe marital stress (Glantz et al., 2001; Taylor-Brown et al., 2000) Husbands of terminally ill patients appear to be at increased risk for depression and find it more difficult to adjust to the rigors of caregiving than do the wives of ill husbands (Siegel et al., 1996).

This appears to be the result of less social support in men's networks than in women's. Patient and caregiver support groups are invaluable for helping both new and experienced caregivers to master the sometimes very steep learning curve of myeloma caretaking. Special attention should be paid to the support needs of male caregivers.

The following 4 characteristic types of patient/caregiver relationships in the management of myeloma are commonly observed:

1. Patient driven

2. Caregiver driven

3. Shared responsibility

4. "Team" caregiving

These categories can be somewhat fluid, depending on the stage of illness. Which model a particular patient and caregiver adopt will largely depend on their previous relationship style as well as the severity of the myeloma, and the consequent limitations on the patient's abilities. It will also depend on the individual skills and knowledge that each brings to the situation.

In the "patient-driven" model, the patient takes the initiative in managing his own care in cooperation with his physician. By contrast, in the "caregiver-driven" model, the caretaker takes primary responsibility for researching and making treatment decisions. The "shared responsibility" model has patient and caregiver sharing in decision making. In "team caregiving," more than one caregiver is involved, and caregivers and patient might play more defined roles. For example, one caregiver might specialize in researching treatment options and staying abreast of current developments whereas another provides emotional support or assistance with physical care.

Tensions arise when patient and caregiver have different perceptions of the situation. One or the other might feel overwhelmed by the bleak outlook that accompanies myeloma. Alternatively, one of them might be in denial about the severity of the illness. Stress can also arise when patient and caregiver have different goals. The patient's overriding concern might be for quality of life, whereas the caregiver might seek a "cure" at any cost; or the patient might want to pursue a promising but risky treatment whereas the caregiver would prefer a safer and more conservative course.

In most respects, the challenges confronting the myeloma caregiver parallel those facing the patient. Receiving the diagnosis of an obscure and incurable cancer, especially one with a complex pathophysiology and no single correct course of treatment, is overwhelming to both patient and caregiver. Just as physicians have become more aware of the emotional needs of patients, so they are now appreciating the needs of caregivers and have begun advocating "care for the carer." Harrison et al. observed that relatives of newly diagnosed cancer patients had 4 times more concerns than patients, concluding that "relatives of newly diagnosed cancer patients report high levels of concerns and psychological distress, and deserve greater attention than they currently receive" (Harrison et al., 1995).

# Recognizing and Dealing with Patient and Caregiver Emotional States

Patients and caregivers dealing with a diagnosis of myeloma are confronted with a terrifying reality. It can be a wrenching confrontation with mortality. Very often, patients will present with debilitating physical symptoms. Attendees at a November 2002 IMF Patient/Family Seminar reported that 65% had bone pain and 44% had pathologic fractures at diagnosis (see Table 18-2a).

At the same time, they might be dealing with a myriad of financial and emotional issues. Attendees at that same seminar were asked to rank their concerns at diagnosis (see Table 18-2b). Not surprisingly, they were most concerned about survival, as well as the impact on their family and lifestyle. Thus, diagnosis presents

---

**TABLE 18-2**

### Dealing with the Diagnosis

**a. Bone Problems at Diagnosis**

|  | Yes | No |
|---|---|---|
| Bone pain | 65% | 35% |
| Pathologic fractures | 44% | 56% |

**b. Patient/Caregiver Concerns at Diagnosis**

| Concern | Score |
|---|---|
| Survival | 9.1 |
| Family | 6.4 |
| Lifestyle | 6.2 |
| Pain | 3.8 |
| Job | 1.0 |
| Other | 0.5 |

**c. Patient/Caregiver Decisions at Diagnosis**

| Symptom at Diagnosis | Percent Reporting |
|---|---|
| Begin treatment | 58 |
| Seek a second opinion | 33 |
| Watch and wait | 9 |

Source: International Myeloma Foundation 2002 Seattle Seminar Attendee Survey (100 respondents).

---

the patient and caregiver(s) with formidable emotional turmoil.

Generally, the newly diagnosed patient is not in an ideal circumstance to make the very important decisions required. Seminar attendees confirmed that a substantial percentage of patients/caregivers (42%) do not make a treatment decision at time of diagnosis (see Table 18-2c). Beyond this, the patient's state of mind can attenuate the stress attendant with treatment and can also exact a physical toll.

Given these factors, attending to the psyche of the patient and caregiver is an important component of care and treatment. To help in this dimension, one should start by understanding these emotional issues and use this understanding to tailor the approach. Patients and caregivers should also be attentive to their state of mind, recognizing that certain behavior, while understandable given the situation, might cloud their judgment and potentially make an already bad situation worse.

After meeting large numbers of patients and caregivers, it is clear that there is no one right approach to dealing with the myeloma challenge. For the physician who is trying to help support and care for the patient, it is important to understand the emotional state and priorities of the patient and caregivers. This same understanding can help patients and families think about how to make decisions. More importantly,

## TABLE 18-3
## Patient and Caregiver Behavioral Factors

| | | | | |
|---|---|---|---|---|
| **Disease status** | Abnormal blood or urine proteins, normal marrow but otherwise asymptomatic | Disease previously active, now in remission | Active plasmacytoma(s) or diffuse disease, responsive to treatment | Disease active and not responsive to treatment (refractory) |
| **State of awareness about myeloma and the diagnosis** | No diagnosis suggesting cancer or myeloma | Diagnosed with myeloma symptoms, not aware condition is cancer | Diagnosed, aware that myeloma is a form of cancer | Diagnosed, very knowledgeable about the disease and its treatment |
| **Treatment history** | No prior treatment | Previously treated | Currently being treated | Refusing treatment |
| **Attitudes toward survival vs. quality of life** | Will not accept cancer therapies other than palliative (pain-relieving) measures | Want to minimize discomfort and disruption, will do what's absolutely necessary | Will pursue aggressive treatments with moderate costs/risks | Feel necessity to pursue potential cure(s), whatever the costs/risks |
| **Emotional posture** | Frightened, prone to despair | Concerned, aggressive | Accepting | Withdrawn |
| **Personal outlook** | Seriously depressed | Somewhat depressed | Calm | Upbeat |
| **Expectations of physician** | Does not want to deal with physicians | Wants strong recommendation about what to do next | Wants physician to present alternatives and explain pros and cons of each | Wants physician to present alternatives for discussion/debate |

Note: This table is a survey instrument used to gather patient/caregiver perceptions on each attribute (row). Common combinations of attribute perceptions observed are discussed below.

recognizing negative emotional states that can compromise support or treatment programs is an important first step in managing them.

Table 18-3 is proposed as a framework for thinking about patient and caregiver attitudes and behaviors. It undertakes to differentiate patient and caregiver attitudes and behaviors based not only on the disease status, but also taking into account attitudes and emotional states.

These factors provide some insight into the emotional state of the patient and caregivers and might prove helpful in categorizing and understanding their behavior. Questionnaires were distributed at patient/family seminars conducted by the IMF through the IMF's Web site and were included with information packages mailed to patients calling the IMF for help. Two hundred fifty responses were received over a 2-month period. The distribution of responses is shown in Table 18-4.

## TABLE 18-4
## Patient Caregiver Behaviors Survey Results (250 Respondents)

| | | | | |
|---|---|---|---|---|
| Disease status | No symptoms (10%) | Remission (34%) | Active (42%) | Refractory (14%) |
| Myeloma awareness | No Diagnosis (0%) | Not aware MM is cancer (2%) | Cancer (38%) | Knowledgeable (60%) |
| Treatment | No prior (10%) | Previous (20%) | Current (70%) | Refusing (0%) |
| Attitude toward treatment | Palliative (3%) | Minimize (22%) | Moderate (44%) | Cure (31%) |
| Emotional posture | Frightened (15%) | Concerned (38%) | Accepting (44%) | Withdrawn (3%) |
| Personal outlook | Seriously depressed (3%) | Somewhat depressed (31%) | Calm (36%) | Upbeat (30%) |
| Expectations of physician | Does not want to see (3%) | Recommendations (18%) | Alternatives (62%) | Debate (17%) |

This population is certainly not a random sample. All of the respondents had reached out for information as they had either contacted the IMF and/or attended an IMF seminar. Most had progressed beyond MGUS (monoclonal gammopathy of undetermined significance) and are currently being treated. They are aware that they are dealing with cancer and most characterize themselves as quite knowledgeable about the particulars of myeloma. The reality of the disease had taken an emotional toll, although 44% characterize themselves as "accepting." Most notably, 79% of this group want to hear about and/or debate alternative treatment options as opposed to receiving singular recommendations.

It is unclear what proportion of the patient/caregiver population is represented by the proactive individual who seeks both information and active involvement in the decision-making process. It has been observed that those who fall into this category were likely more stressed at diagnosis and more likely to have sought and received multiple opinions from multiple physicians/hospitals (Manfredi et al., 1993). For these individuals, the quest for information and an effort to exert control is an important element of their coping strategy and provides emotional benefits that border on being therapeutic. Most certainly, their level of aggression and desire to understand more of the pathology and the "why's" places higher demands on those involved in their treatment. Support organizations, patient networks, the Web, and printed material can play a helpful role in meeting these needs. However, "verbal communication, especially from the physician, is still the most popular choice for receiving information at treatment" (Hinds et al., 1995).

In a study of patients with prostate cancer, the majority (58%) preferred a passive decision-making role and had a correspondingly diminished appetite for information (Davison et al., 1995). Particularly with older patients and those with slowly progressing or early-stage disease, there are instances in which myeloma is managed as if it were a chronic disorder rather than a life-threatening malignancy. Such patients are typically treated with melphalan and prednisone and most recently, thalidomide, and might live for years without significant escalation of symptoms or dramatic disease progression, ultimately succumbing to unrelated age-related disorders.

Others who are less fortunate might have more aggressive disease but either cannot or will not face the reality of what is happening to them and/or mount a proactive struggle to fight the disease. There is a strong need to recognize and, at times, to actively manage a wide range of patient/caregiver behaviors. In fact, these attitudes and behaviors are every bit as diverse as myeloma itself, which presents and progresses in many different ways. Shown in Table 18-4 is a sampling of common patient/caregiver profiles, each represented by a catch phrase and a mapping to the framework shown previously.

Many patients with myeloma who are confronting myeloma take an aggressive, action-oriented posture, which can be characterized by the phrase "I'm going to beat this thing" (Table 18-5). In general, this is a constructive, positive attitude. These patients are likely to be good partners in treatment. They tend to be voracious in seeking information and diligent in pursuing the necessary diagnostic and treatment procedures. One cautionary note here is that this outlook can lead to forays into alternative and fringe treatments, risking serious impact on quality of life and deferral/avoidance of important, necessary treatment.

These patients are often unwilling to resign themselves to treatment programs whose results are all too predictable. They are eager to participate in clinical trials, although they frequently resist randomization (leaving the selection of alternative treatment options in a trial to chance). This is because they want to make sure that they receive the newest, most aggressive alternative. Many clinical trials, particularly in relapsed/refractory settings, address this concern by including crossover arms for nonresponders. Peripheral stem cell transplantation, although not proven to be curative, holds out the "hope" of a cure. To this group of patients, that hope can be as important as any immediate reduction in tumor mass or palliative effects. The therapeutic benefits of hope cannot be understated. Yet, there is a fine line to be drawn when weighing how far to go, particularly when considering highly aggressive options such as multiple transplants and/or allogeneic procedures (using marrow or stem cells from a related or unrelated donor vs. from the patient). Clearly, in all cases, the patient needs to be apprised of the risks and the extent of data on likely outcomes.

**TABLE 18-5**

### "I'm Going to Beat This Thing"

| Disease Status | Myeloma Awareness | Treatment History | Survival vs. Quality of Life | Emotional Posture | Personal Outlook | Expectations of Physician |
|---|---|---|---|---|---|---|
| Active | Knowledgeable | No prior treatment | Potential cure at any cost/risk | Concerned, aggressive | Somewhat depressed | Discussion, debate |

### TABLE 18-6
### "I'll Do What I Have To"

| Disease Status | Myeloma Awareness | Treatment History | Survival vs. Quality of Life | Emotional Posture | Personal Outlook | Expectations of Physician |
|---|---|---|---|---|---|---|
| Previously active | Knowledgeable | Previously treated | Minimize disruption | Accepting | Calm | Discussion, debate |

However, recognizing the overriding desire to "beat this thing," the physician needs to be very explicit and overcommunicate if the message is to be heard.

Many patients, particularly older patients, those with less aggressive disease, and those who have been through at least one treatment/remission/relapse cycle, tend to be relatively stoic about their disease. They have largely abandoned the idea that cure is possible and seek a careful balance between prolonged survival and quality of life. They will typically be quite rational partners in treatment, for they say, "I'll do what I have to" (Table 18-6). Although they are aggressive in seeking information and debating treatment options, they will generally be responsive to well-reasoned recommendations. By the same token, they tend to have an extensive knowledge base and a good understanding of the issues. Therefore, they can react quite badly to recommendations that are not grounded in sound logic.

Discussion of a full range of options, from conservative to experimental, is eminently reasonable with these patients. In the end, they will likely prefer to personally choose their treatment option. Physicians best serve the bulk of these patients by stepping them through a process to have them choose an appropriate treatment course rather than by being highly directive or by making strong recommendations. When the physician has strong feelings about the proper course that is at odds with the patient, gentle persuasion will likely work better than overt confrontation. Many patients run from an unpleasant recommendation, convincing themselves that it was the doctor, rather than the recommendation, that caused them to take flight.

Understandably, many are overwhelmed by the initial myeloma diagnosis or relapse and have extreme difficulty making the decisions necessary to proceed with treatment. Typically, these people are saying or thinking, "I cannot believe this is happening to me"

(Table 18-7). They will typically have active disease in need of treatment and are painfully aware of what myeloma is and the typical course of the disease. Serious depression and fear/despair go hand and hand with this state of mind. Most in this state of mind seek strong recommendations about what to do next. However, they tend to be biased toward minimalist treatment strategies. They would like to get out of the medical system quickly. Although the expectation might be unrealistic, they would like to get things back to normal as soon as possible. Extensive debate over numerous aggressive treatment options or clinical trials can be highly upsetting for these individuals, particularly when the results cannot be assured. Patients in this state tend to be looking for short-term physical and emotional relief above all else. Barring a clear clinical imperative (e.g., poor prognostic factors, dangerous symptoms, or a known cure), it is hard to argue in good conscience that they should not receive what they seek.

Such patients are likely candidates for traditional melphalan and prednisone therapy and should, at minimum, have that option explained to them. For the past few years, thalidomide with or without steroids has been helpful in treating relapsed/refractory patients and, most recently, for newly diagnosed patients and patients in first relapse. Clinical trials of new agents, such as Velcade (also known as PS-341, MLN-341), iMids (immunomodulatory thalidomide analogs such as Revimid), and controlled trials of thalidomide/dexamethasone are increasingly popular options for relapsed/refractory patients and some newly diagnosed patients. These regimens have proven to be well tolerated when the doses are kept in the low to moderate range. Other palliative/prophylactic measures, such as bisphosphonates (e.g., pamidronate/Aredia or zoledronic acid/Zometa, which help to minimize bone pain/fractures) are also eminently reasonable in these cases.

### TABLE 18-7
### "I Can't Believe This Is Happening to Me"

| Disease Status | Myeloma Awareness | Treatment History | Survival vs. Quality of Life | Emotional Posture | Personal Outlook | Expectations of Physician |
|---|---|---|---|---|---|---|
| Active | Aware | Untreated or previously treated | Minimize disruption | Frightened, prone to despair | Seriously depressed | Strong recommendation |

**TABLE 18-8**

**"I'm at the End of My Rope"**

| Disease Status | Myeloma Awareness | Treatment History | Survival vs. Quality of Life | Emotional Posture | Personal Outlook | Expectations of Physician |
|---|---|---|---|---|---|---|
| Refractory | Knowledgeable | Refusing treatment | Will consider palliative only | Withdrawn | Seriously depressed | Does not want to deal with them |

Therapies that are difficult to administer and/or have more severe side effects, such as VAD (Vincristine, Adriamycin, Dexamethasone) or other combination chemotherapy regimens, are not likely to be well tolerated (emotionally), regardless of the patient's health and performance status. More radical approaches, such as myeloablative high-dose therapies (i.e., bone marrow or stem cell transplantation) are likely to fly totally in the face of the patient's wishes. It would seem reasonable that these should only be pressed strongly when there is a clear rationale supported by prognostic factors and clinical research (i.e., there is reason to believe that the patient can only achieve remission through the more aggressive treatment).

If these patients are given palliative treatment and subsequently respond to conventional therapy, their outlook can change significantly, opening the door to a wider range of consolidation and/or salvage treatment options. Unfortunately, this approach might preclude future use of certain protocols that exclude previously treated patients or patients who have been treated with alkylating agents (e.g., melphalan). For example, extensive treatment with melphalan can damage the bone marrow or stem cells, making autologous transplant procedures difficult or impossible.

There comes a point in the bout with almost any terminal illness when the patient and caregivers are justifiably frustrated, frightened, and less tolerant of the discomfort and disruption of treatment programs. The phrase "I'm at the end of my rope" is often heard (Table 18-8).

They are often seriously depressed. These patients are likely to refuse treatment. They might also be resistant to diagnostic procedures or office visits. They will often reject critical care recommendations, such as dialysis, transfusions, or plasmapheresis.

The challenge here is to ensure that reasonable measures are taken to make the patient more comfortable and to manage potentially dangerous complications. At the same time, an effort should be made to get the patient back in the "I'll do what I have to" frame of mind.

Yet, assuming the patient and caregivers are lucid, the ultimate decision on how aggressively to treat and manage the disease must remain in their hands. Patient and caregiver attitudes are dynamic. These attitudes shift over time, most often in response to changes in the status of the disease or treatment experiences. Having put forward the patient attitudes framework and the common profiles encountered, we use these to describe common setbacks in patient and caregiver attitudes and suggest objectives for counselling and support.

Figure 18-1 shows common setbacks encountered. At diagnosis, patients and caregivers will typically present in states 1, 2, or 3. After presenting with positive

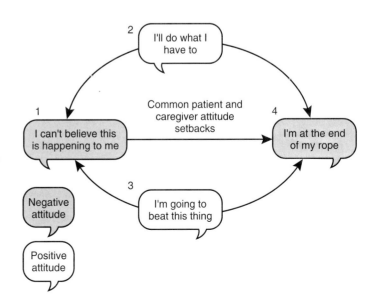

**Figure 18-1** *Common patient and caregiver attitude setbacks.*

attitudes (2 and 3), there can be setbacks that cause regression to negative attitudes (1 and 4). Regression to no. 4 will typically be triggered by a failed or particularly onerous treatment. Regression to no. 1 occurs most often as either a delayed reaction to the news or a delayed reaction as the weight of additional negative information or experience takes its toll. These negative attitude states are particularly dangerous to the patient because they can block the formation of an effective therapeutic partnership and stall treatment programs. These attitude states are just as dangerous when they afflict the patient's caregivers as when they affect the patient.

When the patient is in a negative state and the caregivers are still positive, the caregivers can be a powerful ally in helping bring the patient back to a positive state. When the caregivers are negative, the physician will have to be self-reliant or draw on other support services (e.g., social services, other patients, cancer support groups, and so on). Objectives for support/counselling should be decided up front and can be viewed using the same framework.

Patients and caregivers in state no. 1 are distraught, which often prevents them from focusing and dealing with the problems at hand. In attempting to help them to a positive state, one can aspire to either no. 2 or 3. Patients in state 4 are generally best helped toward no. 2 (Figure 18-2).

The most serious emotional setback confronting patient and caregivers is loss of hope. The negative states most often represent a loss of hope. "Cancer is a life-threatening disease that creates an uncertain and foreboding future, yet it is because of this future that hope can be accommodated." In a study of oncology patients receiving both conventional and complementary treatments (e.g., relaxation, visualization, diets, herbalism), patient satisfaction with "complementary treatments" was high, even when an anticancer effect was not perceived or achieved. These patients reported psychologic benefits in renewed hope and optimism (Poncar, 1994).

As myeloma runs its course, patients and their families are called on to make agonizing decisions and deal with often-onerous procedures and treatments. Paying close attention to behaviors, tailoring the approach to those behaviors, and actively managing those behaviors can make a world of difference for all concerned.

## The Role of Information in Meeting the Myeloma Challenge

Information can be a powerful tool to strengthen the patient/caregiver/physician partnership. It can also serve to help people in negative emotional states get into more positive frames of mind. Yet, there is some controversy surrounding the notion that patients and families should be better informed.

In some countries, doctors routinely do not disclose diagnoses of incurable cancer to their patients. The notion is that the knowledge would only cause the patient further distress that, heaped on top of the physical symptoms, could be devastating. Given that there is little that the patient can do to change the course of the disease or the ultimate outcome, why burden them? These patients are often treated with chemotherapy agents associated with significant morbidity without receiving any indication of their true condition. This approach is clearly extreme.

Yet, there are many physicians who have very mixed feelings about explaining too much about myeloma to

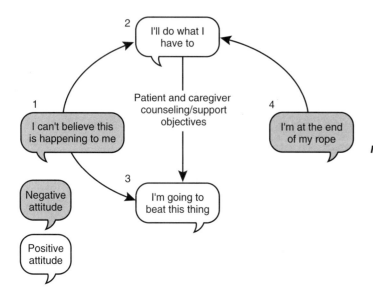

*Figure 18-2* Patient and caregiver counseling support objectives.

patients. In part, this seems to stem from the generally bleak prognosis and lack of a cure. Also, a factor is that many patients are elderly with other health issues who might have few treatment options. This sentiment likely flies in the face of patient and caregiver preferences. A recent report from Reuters (1996) stated that "Cancer patients want to know as much as possible about their disease and do not appreciate being 'spared' the truth." The same report suggested that "although sometimes relatives ask to keep a cancer patient in the dark about his or her illness while keeping the caregivers quietly informed, patients did not appreciate efforts by their families to keep bad news from them."

Dismissing for a moment the ethical and moral questions surrounding such practices, it is the authors' opinion that the vast majority of patients with myeloma and their families fare better when they are well-informed and proactive partners in treatment decisions. The patients and families participating in the IMF survey described previously are all actively engaged in learning more about the disease and its treatment. They know the seriousness of their situation, yet do not appear to have high instances of the negative emotional states that can impede support and treatment programs. They have met or talked to other patients with myeloma and found that these dialogues have helped them learn more about what to expect and about the patient's perspective on treatment. Physicians should encourage their patients to understand more about myeloma and engage in networking programs such as in-person or Internet-based support groups. Patients and caregivers should recognize that these efforts will help them understand their options and make better decisions about their treatment. In many instances, emotional or physical issues will dictate that these efforts be undertaken by the patient, a spouse, or relative of the patient. The important thing is that someone on the patient's team outside the clinical setting begins to build this knowledge and experience.

Patient and caregiver education about myeloma typically begins under less-than-ideal circumstances in consultation with the physician who makes the diagnosis. The shock of the diagnosis will confound all but the most articulate and persistent of physicians in their attempt to communicate more than the basics and the requisite immediate next steps. The physician will justifiably focus on immediate critical care needs. At this stage, the physician will attempt to communicate the basic facts to avoid overwhelming the patient and caregivers. It is important, however, to start the process of patient and caregiver outreach by providing information on where to go for support and information. Printed materials, such as the IMF Patient Handbook, can be very helpful, because they can be reviewed at a later time outside the clinical setting.

There is an unprecedented amount of information available to patients and caregivers about all aspects of myeloma and its treatment. With the emergence of the Internet and the establishment of targeted support organizations such as the International Myeloma Foundation (IMF; http://www.myeloma.org in the United States, http://www.myeloma.org.uk in the United Kingdom) and the Multiple Myeloma Research Foundation (MMRF; http://multiplemyeloma.org), patients and caregivers have many avenues they can pursue to educate themselves about myeloma.

With so much available, it is important to have an idea of where to start and to be able to put the information retrieved in perspective. Consequently, it is important for the patient and caregivers to have a strong relationship and good access to one or more hematologist/oncologists. In the end, physicians need to help patients and their families make treatment decisions. Physicians also need to administer treatments. It is clearly to the patient's and caregiver's advantage to have the physician as an active partner in the education and decision-making process. Most physicians will welcome patient and caregiver efforts in this area and will also value the involvement of another qualified physician. Establishing these partnerships is perhaps the most important element in the patient's and caregiver's battle against myeloma.

The International Myeloma Foundation offers a variety of information and services for patients with myeloma, their families, and the medical community. A telephone call to their hotline (800-452-CURE from the United States and Canada, 0800 980 3332 in the United Kingdom, 818-487-7455 elsewhere) offers the opportunity to talk to a knowledgeable person about myeloma and potential next steps. IMF's Web site (http://www.myeloma.org) offers a broad array of educational programs and information resources, including an international directory of in-person myeloma support groups (http://supportgroups.myeloma.org) as well as online support groups for myeloma and amyloidosis (http://listserv.myeloma.org). The MMRF offers educational programs and support and can be reached through their Web site (http://multiple myeloma.org) or by phone (203-972-1250). The British Association of Cancer United Patients (BACUP) is based in the United Kingdom and can be reached by telephone at (44) 171 696-9003 or by fax at (44) 171 696-9002. Leads on other support resources can often be obtained from the physician or cancer treatment center.

Moving from health care professionals and support organizations to print and electronic research implies a significant time commitment. More importantly, it requires that one build the vocabulary necessary to understand the materials one is likely to find. Also important to remember is that the literature is filled with potentially upsetting statistics about morbidity, survival, and mortality. Furthermore, there is no peer review and no professional standards for much of the information available on the Internet and elsewhere. As such, although there is much valuable material available, there is also a lot of misinformation. CancerGuide, an Internet resource developed by a cancer patient (Dunn, 2002), offers practical information about researching cancer, providing a balanced view of the pros and cons of taking this next step (Table 18-9).

The Internet is by far the most powerful channel readily available to the patient and caregiver community for conducting their own research about myeloma. Access to the Internet generally requires a personal computer, a cable, DSL, or analog modem, and an Internet service provider. For those using computers at corporate or institutional sites, there is increasingly a dedicated connection to the Internet through the local area network (LAN), which obviates the need for a modem. Internet access can include a variety of services such as electronic mail, access to the World Wide Web (WWW), File Transfer Protocol (FTP), Newsgroups, and Telnet. Each of these services requires software, typically provided by the Internet service provider or network manager. Information on Internet service providers should be available through local computer dealers.

A good place to start an Internet research effort is at the IMF and MMRF Web sites (http://myeloma.org and http://mutiplemyeloma.org). Other critical resources include the University of Pennsylvania Cancer Center's Oncolink site (http://www.oncolink.org) and the National Cancer Institute's myeloma resources (http://myeloma.cancer.gov). This site offers a broad sampling of literature on all types of cancer as well as general information useful to all patients with cancer. It also offers extensive information about other online resources. There are a number of quality commercial sites that offer valuable information. These sites often require registration and have commercial advertising and for-profit products and services. Among these sites are Medscape (http://www.medscape.com/hematology-oncologyhome) and CancerSource.com (http://www.cancersource.com/zones/cancer.cfm?DiseaseID=20).

Yahoo (http://yahoo.com), Google (http://google.com), and other commercial search engines are excellent tools to locate resources on the Internet. They provide extensive databases of Internet resources that can be searched using keywords or through hierarchical menus. The sites also offer links to many other databases and search facilities and are currently provided at no charge to the user (they are supported by commercial advertising revenues).

Already mentioned previously was CancerGuide (http://cancerguide.org), which was developed by a patient. The material includes an extensive discussion of the mechanics of electronic and print research. It also provides a patient's perspective on how to think about the research process and how to deal with the information one finds.

The US Government offers much information through a number of facilities. This includes basic information about the disease for physicians and laypersons as well as information about clinical trials and government research grants. Already mentioned previously was the National Cancer Institute's myeloma page (http://myeloma.cancer.gov.) The NCI also has online access to its Cancer Information Service (http://cis.nci.nih.gov/) and a publications locator and ordering service (https://cissecure.nci.nih.gov/ncipubs).

Medline is an extensive electronic database developed by the US National Library of Medicine. It covers major medical journals that include a wealth of information on the latest research about myeloma. Medline allows users to search using keywords (e.g., myeloma, plasmacytoma, melphalan, vincristine) to identify articles that might contain relevant information. Using Medline requires some trial and error, because keywords often turn up an overabundance of references, not all of which might be relevant. Furthermore, there can be numerous terms that refer to the same thing (e.g., myeloma vs. plasma cell neoplasm, lytic lesion vs. plasmacytoma), so searching one word might not yield all of the relevant references. Formerly available only through specialized software and hardware on a fee-per-use basis, it is now readily available to patients and their families in a number of forms. The National Library of Medicine's National Center for Biotechnology Information (NCBI) offers public access to the Medline database of medical and scientific journals through its PubMed service (http://www.ncbi.nlm.nih.gov/pubmed.) Medline can also be accessed on CD-ROM at many public libraries and medical libraries at no charge. It is also available at no charge through a variety of Internet-based services (the "free" services typically derive their revenue from commercial advertising). To gain access to those services, one should use the "Yahoo" World Wide Web search engine

========= **TABLE 18-9** =========

### Patient Information About Cancer

| Pros | Cons |
| --- | --- |
| It could save your life | It can be difficult and intimidating |
| It is empowering | You might make the wrong |
| You can make a more | decision (so be sure to work |
| informed decision | closely with your physician) |
| | You will have to confront the |
| | statistics |
| | There might not be any better |
| | treatment |

(http://www.yahoo.com) and search the word "Medline" to get a current list of service providers. Medline references generally include a citation or an abstract (summary) of journal articles. One must generally go to a medical library to retrieve the original article.

Much information is also available on the Web about clinical trials, which offer patients access to new agents and new treatment approaches under carefully controlled conditions. There are a number of useful Web-based resources to help patients and caregivers access basic information about clinical trials as well as tools to find clinical trials that might be appropriate for them (see Table 18-10a).

A new tool, called the Multiple Myeloma Profiler, developed by Nexcura, provides a decision support tool for patients with myeloma. By asking a series of detailed questions, it helps organize their information and determine the issues they should be discussing with their physicians. The tool can be accessed at http://nexcura.myeloma.org.

Besides the World Wide Web, electronic mail (e-mail) provides another valuable avenue of communications. E-mail can be used for personal communications with other patients. There are also electronic communities that are accessible through e-mail called Internet mailing lists. One joins an Internet mailing list by sending an e-mail message to the computer functioning as a "listserv." Once subscribed to a mailing list, all messages sent to the list will be routed to your personal mailbox. Messages you send to the list will be routed

to all subscribers, providing a very powerful forum for conducting discussion among people with similar interests. A number of mailing lists of potential interest to patients with myeloma are shown in Table 18-10b.

Mailing lists also offer a vehicle for meeting others with similar perspectives. Whereas those forums offer an opportunity for public discussions, participants can exchange e-mail addresses to communicate on a one-on-one basis through standard e-mail. One should approach these groups recognizing that virtually anyone can post messages and many messages are posted using pseudonyms. Although this open-door policy gives the medium vitality, it also allows for posting of questionable material, including exotic "cures" and commercial solicitations (i.e., the cyberspace equivalent of "junk mail"). Some of the mailing lists are moderated, which introduces some level of screening. However, in most cases, there are few controls on what is posted. Caution is advised.

The decision to learn more about myeloma is an important step in dealing with the disease. It requires a lot of hard work but does not require "re-inventing the wheel." There are a lot of patients and caregivers one can meet through the IMF and MMRF, in-person support groups, and online media to share valuable insights and favorite sources. The overall effect is generally to empower the patient and caregivers and provide them with useful information as well as emotional support that will strengthen the partnership with their physician.

---

**TABLE 18-10**

## Other Internet Resources

### a. Information About Clinical Trials

| Resource | World Wide Web Address |
| --- | --- |
| IMF clinical trials page | http://trials.myeloma.org |
| MMRF clinical trials page | http://multiplemyeloma.org/Trials-Grants.html |
| NCI literature about clinical trials | http://ncitrials.myeloma.org |
| NCI CancerTrials site | http://www.nci.nih.gov/clinical_trials |
| Coalition of National Cancer Cooperative groups | http://www.cancertrialshelp.org |
| EmergingMed Clinical Trials service | http://myeloma.org/emergingmed.html |
| CenterWatch Clinical Trials monitor | http://www.centerwatch.com/patient/studies/cat212.html |

### b. Mailing Lists of Potential Interest to Myeloma Patients

| List Name | E-Mail Address | To subscribe, send message with blank subject, filling in the text field as follows: |
| --- | --- | --- |
| MYELOMA (Multiple Myeloma) | LISTSERV@listserv.acor.org | Subscribe myeloma Your_Name |
| AMYLOID (Amyloidosis) | LISTSERV@listserv.acor.org | Subscribe amyloid Your_Name |
| Midwest Myeloma Exchange (Multiple Myeloma) | http://www.webspawner.com/users/myelomaexhange/ | Enter your email address in the space provided |
| BMT-Talk (Bone Marrow Transplant) | LISTSERV@listserv.acor.org | Subscribe BMT-TALK Your_Name |

## TABLE 18-11

### Patient/Caregiver Perceptions About Physicians

| Expertise about myeloma | General practitioner | Hematologist–oncologist, familiar with myeloma | Very knowledgeable about myeloma | Leading myeloma expert |
|---|---|---|---|---|
| Ability/willingness to explain medical issues | Professorial, sometimes too technical | Communicates essential concepts well | Communicates well but hard to get enough time to talk | Condescending, not anxious to discuss medical concepts |
| Demeanor | Caring | Caring but hurried | All business | Cold |
| Candor | Inspires trust | Provides a reasonable amount of information | Does not share as much information as desired | Does not provide a balanced perspective |
| Sensitivity | "Sugar coats" information, afraid to upset patients and family | Understands patient and family issues and improves state of mind | Makes an effort to understand patient and family issues | Focused solely on next treatment or diagnostic procedure |
| Objectivity | Presents too wide a range of options, bordering on bewildering | Provides a balanced view of a reasonable set of options | Discussed pros and cons of somewhat limited set of alternatives | Seems predisposed toward certain treatments |
| Medical facility and staff support | Well-managed, pleasant environment | Well managed, effort made to be accommodating | Somewhat disorganized, difficult to deal with | Disorganized, often exasperating |

Note: This table is a survey instrument used to gather patient/caregiver perceptions on each attribute (row). Common combinations of attribute perceptions observed are discussed below.

# Different Reactions Physicians Can Elicit from Patients and Caregivers

Physicians are just as diverse as patients and caregivers. It is reasonable to assume that different physicians are more likely to build strong relationships with certain types of patients and caregivers. Physicians can gain from more self-awareness about the responses they evoke from patients and caregivers. Patients and caregivers can benefit from awareness about physician behavior and how they can influence their very important relationship with the physician. To this end, we developed a framework to help understand patient/caregiver perceptions about physicians (Table 18-11).

The same IMF survey referenced previously was used to gather information about patients' perceptions of their physicians and treatment facilities. The results, based on the same 250 respondents, are shown in Table 18-12.

## TABLE 18-12

### Physician Perception Survey Results

| Physician expertise | GP (3%) | Hematology–oncology (50%) | Very knowledgeable (25%) | Leading expert (22%) |
|---|---|---|---|---|
| Explanations | Professorial (7%) | Communicates well (59%) | Pressed for Time (21%) | Condescending (13%) |
| Demeanor | Caring (61%) | Hurried (21%) | All business (14%) | Cold (4%) |
| Candor | Inspires trust (44%) | Reasonable information (29%) | Not enough information (22%) | Not balanced perspective (5%) |
| Sensitivity | Sugar coats (15%) | Understands issues (38%) | Tries to understand (44%) | Next procedure (3%) |
| Objectivity | Too many options (3%) | Resonable options (31%) | Limited options (36%) | Seems predisposed (30%) |
| Facility | Accommodating (3%) | Makes an effort (18%) | Somewhat difficult (62%) | Exasperating (17%) |

## TABLE 18-13

### "My Doctor Is Wonderful"

| Expertise about myeloma | Ability/willingness to explain medical issues | Demeanor | Candor | Sensitivity | Objectivity | Medical facility and staff support |
|---|---|---|---|---|---|---|
| Very knowledgeable or expert | Communicates essential concepts well | Caring | Inspires trust | Understands issues, improves state of mind | Balanced view of reasonable set of options | Well-managed, pleasant environment |

Again, the study group represents those who have decided that they need to be proactive and have some predictable patterns based on that decision. Virtually all (97%) see a hematologist/oncologist rather than a general practitioner. A full 80% rated their physicians good communicators, although 21% felt that time pressures did get in the way of information exchange. No one complained of being presented too many treatment options. Because these represent a population more likely to be seen at specialized facilities used to dealing with patients with cancer, it is encouraging to note that less than 20% are unhappy with their treatment facilities.

Like with the patient behavioral factors morphology, it can be used to represent typical physician perception profiles characterized by "catch phrases" and mapped to the framework. The first profile is characterized by the phrase "My doctor is wonderful" (Table 18-13).

There are few physicians who, treating patients with an incurable disease within the constraints imposed by today's health care infrastructure, can inspire this type of reaction. Those who are able to pull this off are very knowledgeable about the disease, treatment strategies, and research. They are able to project a relaxed, caring, competent persona while taking the patient and caregivers through serious and often complex decisions, diagnostic procedures, and treatment programs. These physicians are also highly adept at listening to patients and understanding how they and their families feel about the various issues they face. As such, they are able to sense the need to adapt their style and tailor their recommendations to achieve not only the optimal medical result, but also the best emotional outcome.

For many patients and caregivers, the medical experience and relationship with the physician is very positive. However, patient loads, administrative and operational lapses introduce tensions that stress the relationship with the physician (Table 18-14). The lament "My doctor tries very hard but is so busy" reflects a persona projected by physicians who genuinely care about their patients. Yet, the patients and caregivers feel the tyranny of the clock. They have to probe a little harder to get more detailed explanations. They feel that they should be discussing more details about more options. They are a bit frustrated with their treatment facility, be it a bout with too much paperwork, a long wait, or insurance hassles.

Unfortunately, given the level of stress associated with the disease and its attendant diagnostic and treatment procedures, most patients and caregivers will wind up with this perspective rather than joining those in the "My doctor is wonderful" camp. Add to these factors the frustration inherent in the lack of a proven cure or clearly advantaged treatment strategy and it really does seem like achieving this perception should be regarded as a victory.

Things do not always go that well. Some patients and caregivers will say "I don't trust my doctor" (Table 18-15). In some instances, this can be totally an artefact of the patient's situation: despair at news of disease progression or consternation about conflicting advice from other medical professional and

## TABLE 18-14

### "My Doctor Tries Very Hard But Is So Busy"

| Expertise about myeloma | Ability/willingness to explain medical issues | Demeanor | Candor | Sensitivity | Objectivity | Medical facility and staff support |
|---|---|---|---|---|---|---|
| Hematology–oncology knowledgeable or expert | Communicates well, hard to get enough time | Caring but hurried, all business | Reasonable or not enough information | Tries to understand issues | Pros and cons, limited set of options | Somewhat disorganized, difficult |

## TABLE 18-15
### "I Don't Trust My Doctor"

| Expertise about myeloma | Ability/willingness to explain medical issues | Demeanor | Candor | Sensitivity | Objectivity | Medical facility and staff support |
|---|---|---|---|---|---|---|
| Hematology–Oncology Knowledgeable or Expert | Condescending, not anxious to discuss medical concepts | Caring but hurried, all business | Not enough information or not a balanced perspective | Focused on next treatment or procedure | Seems predisposed toward certain treatments | Disorganized, often exasperating |

laypersons. In other cases, it can be the result of operational mishaps (e.g., a lab accident) or careless behavior by support personnel. However, this reaction can also be triggered by physician behavior. It could be lack of patience on the part of the physician. Strong recommendations without full discussion of alternatives and pros and cons can also trigger this reaction. If the patient or caregiver has reached this level of anxiety, it needs to be dealt with quickly if the relationship is to be salvaged.

Those at the top of their profession are always in high demand (Table 18-16). This exacerbates time pressures and tends to make it more difficult to devote the time necessary to fully answer patient and caregiver questions and tend to the human and interpersonal aspects of the relationship. Beyond this, more intermediaries tend to be introduced into the process to provide the needed leverage for the specialist (e.g., residents, more junior colleagues, nursing staff), further reducing the "personal touch." The research orientation of leading experts at major centers can also give the impression that patients are being too aggressively courted for participation in specific clinical trials. The individual feels that "my doctor is brilliant, but ..."; the overall experience loses much of the personal interchange that many look for when they seek medical help.

Except for the breakdown of trust, the tensions in the relationship with the physician seem to be the natural result of what are reasonable trade-offs. However, this would suggest that additional emphasis on demeanor, communications, and responsiveness to patient/caregiver preferences for participation in decision making could provide real benefit.

# Recognizing and Managing Positive and Negative "Fit Factors" in Physician and Patient/Caregiver Interactions

Patients and caregivers approach the medical experience from different perspectives. Physicians can project diverse impressions based on their focus and the facilities in which they practice. Given this, it is possible to anticipate certain patients and caregivers will be likely to have difficulties with certain physicians.

Table 18-17 shows patient/caregiver behaviors arrayed against perceptions of physicians with an

## TABLE 18-16
### "My Doctor Is Brilliant, But ..."

| Expertise about myeloma | Ability/willingness to explain medical issues | Demeanor | Candor | Sensitivity | Objectivity | Medical facility and staff support |
|---|---|---|---|---|---|---|
| Leading myeloma expert | Condescending, not anxious to discuss medical concepts | Cold | Does not provide a balanced perspective | Focused on next treatment or procedure | Seems predisposed toward certain treatments | Well managed, effort made to be accommodating |

## TABLE 18-17

### Patient/Caregiver–Physician Fit

| | "My doctor is wonderful" | "My doctor tries very hard but is so busy" | "My doctor is brilliant, but …" | "I don't trust my doctor" |
|---|---|---|---|---|
| "I'm going to beat this thing" | ● | ● | ● | ○ |
| "I'll do what I have to" | ● | ◑ | ◑ | ○ |
| "I can't believe this is happening to me" | ● | ◑ | ○ | ○ |
| "I'm at the end of my rope" | ● | ○ | ○ | ○ |

Legend: ● Strong Fit   ◑ Good Fit   ○ Poor Fit

assessment of likely fit/degree of comfort with the relationship.

No patient is likely to build a good working relationship with a physician who, for whatever reason, evokes the "I do not trust my doctor" response. Both parties need to recognize that this is happening and either fix it or sever the relationship as soon as possible.

The "I'm going to beat this thing" individual is determined and aggressive enough to hold their own in the face of any physician they feel they can trust. They are demanding and can prove a handful, particularly for the "pressed-for-time" physicians. They will typically build the strongest relationships with the physicians who provide what they perceive to be the most attractive treatment options.

Individuals who are "at the end of their rope" need lots of emotional support. They will not likely have a comfortable relationship with any physician who is not consistently evoking the "my doctor is wonderful" response.

Those who will "do what they have to" can get into trouble with physicians who evoke the "my doctor is brilliant, but …" response. These folks tend to have extensive fact bases and shy away from more aggressive and experimental approaches. They have consciously decided that they are working to manage quality and length of life as opposed to going for the cure. If the physician recognizes this and is responsive to it, things can proceed without a hitch.

Individuals who are clearly overwhelmed ("I can't believe this is happening to me") are likely to frustrate the "brilliant, but …" physician. They often shut out reality. Dealing with the unthinkable, they do not always listen to messages about their personal situation and treatment options. Treatment strategies they are willing to agree to are typically less aggressive than what is likely to be on the table with leading clinicians who have active research programs. It would seem that these individuals are best served by physicians who are comfortable with a conservative, largely patient-directed decision-making process and can devote the time and energy to working on the emotional issues to ensure the best result.

# Summary and Conclusions

People who have myeloma and the people who care for them are routinely dealing with serious medical and emotional issues. Modest investments of time and attention to the interpersonal dynamics and patient/caregiver education can significantly strengthen the therapeutic partnership. Perhaps just as important, it can dramatically reduce stress levels for all concerned. Although issues of emotional fit cannot always be considered in matching patients and families to physicians, recognizing likely areas of friction can help minimize their impact. It is our hope that the frameworks provided in this chapter would prove useful for both physicians and their patients as they strive to meet the myeloma challenge.

## REFERENCES

Blanchard, C. G., Albrecht, T. L., and Ruckdeschel, J. C. (1997). The crisis of cancer: psychological effect on family caregivers. *Oncology, 11*, 189–194.

Calhoun, R. D. (1998). What long-term survivors don't talk about. *Head's Up*. Brain Tumor Society. < http://www.tbts.org/longtermsurvivors.htm >

Davison, B. J., Degner, L. F., and Morgan, T. R. (1995). Information and decision-making preferences of men with prostate cancer. *Oncology Nursing Forum, 22*, 1401–1408.

Dunn, S. (2002). *CancerGuide*, < http://cancerguide.org >

Glantz, M. J., Cole, B. F., Mills, L., Cross, N., Edwards, K., Recht, L., Cobb, J., and Chamberlain, M. (2001). High incidence of marital disruptions in women but not men with primary brain tumors. American Society of Clinical Oncology 2001, abstract 227 < http://www.asco.org/asco/ascoMainConstructor/1,1003,_12-002324-00_29-00A-00_18-002001-00_19-00227,00.asp >

Harrison, J., Haddad, P., and Maguire, P. (1995). The impact of cancer on key relatives: a comparison of relative and patient concerns. *European Journal of Cancer, 31A*, 1731–1732.

Hinds, C., Streater, A., and Mood, D. (1995). Functions and preferred methods of receiving information related to radiotherapy. *Perceptions of Patients With Cancer*, p. 18. International Myeloma Foundation. (2002). *Patient Handbook*. Obtainable from: 4400 Coldwater Canyon, Ste. 200, Studio City, California 91406 < http:// www.myeloma.org > , e-mail: TheIMF@myeloma.org

Manfredi, C., Czaja, R., Price, R., Buis, M., and Janiszewski, R. (1993). Cancer patients' search for information. *Monographs of the National Cancer Institute, 14*, 93–104.

Nijbooer, C., Tempelaar, R., Sanderman, R., Triemstra, M., Spruijt, R. J., van den Bos, G. A. (1998). Cancer and caregiving: the impact on the caregiver's health. *PsychoOncology, 7*, 3–13.

Poncar, P. J. (1994). Inspiring hope in the oncology patient. *Journal of Psychosocial Nursing and Mental Health Services, 32*, 33–38.

Reuters. (1996). Sept. 20, 1996, London.

Schultz, R., and Beach, S. R. (1999). Caregiving as a risk factor for mortality. *Journal of the American Medical Society, 282*, 2215–2219.

Siegel, K., Karus, D. G., Raveis, V. H., Christ, G. H., and Mesagno, F. P. (1996). Depressive distress among the spouses of terminally ill cancer patients. *Cancer Practice, 4*, 25–30.

Taylor-Brown, J., Kilpatrick, M., Maunsell, E., and Dorval, M. (2000). Partner abandonment of women with breast cancer. Myth or reality? *Cancer Practice, 8*, 160–164.

Turner, S., and Maher, E. J. (1996). What are the information priorities for cancer patients involved in treatment decisions? An experienced surrogate study in Hodgkin's disease. *British Journal of Cancer, 73*, 222–227.

# PART IV

**Other Disorders Associated with Paraproteinemia**

# CHAPTER 19

# Monoclonal Gammopathies of Undetermined Significance

ROBERT A. KYLE
JOAN BLADÉ
S. VINCENT RAJKUMAR

## Introduction

Monoclonal gammopathies are disorders characterized by the proliferation of a single clone of plasma cells producing a homogeneous (monoclonal) protein (M component, M-protein, paraprotein). A current classification of monoclonal gammopathies is provided in Table 19-1. Although multiple myeloma (MM) constitutes the prototype of monoclonal gammopathies, the most common plasma cell disorder is the so-called benign monoclonal gammopathy (BMG) or monoclonal gammopathy of undetermined significance (MGUS). In fact, in a large institution such as Mayo Clinic, almost 60% of patients with a monoclonal gammopathy actually have MGUS (Fig. 19-1). Current definitions for the common monoclonal gammopathies are provided in Table 19-2. The nomenclature and structure of immunoglobulins as well as the pathophysiology of monoclonal gammopathies are discussed in Chapter 1.

### TABLE 19-1

## Classification of Monoclonal Gammopathies

I. Monoclonal gammopathy of undetermined significance
   A. Benign (IgG, IgA, IgD, IgM, and, rarely, free light chains)
   B. Associated with neoplasms of cell types not known to produce M-proteins
   C. Biclonal gammopathies
   D. Idiopathic Bence Jones proteinuria
II. Malignant monoclonal gammopathies
   A. Multiple myeloma (IgG, IgA, IgD, IgE, and free κ or λ light chains)
      1. Overt (symptomatic) multiple myeloma
      2. Smoldering (asymptomatic) multiple myeloma
      3. Plasma cell leukemia
      4. Nonsecretory myeloma
      5. IgD myeloma
      6. POEMS: polyneuropathy, organomegaly, endocrinopathy, M-protein, skin changes (osteosclerotic myeloma)
   B. Plasmacytoma
      1. Solitary plasmacytoma of bone
      2. Extramedullary plasmacytoma
   C. Malignant lymphoproliferative disorders
      1. Waldenström's macroglobulinemia (primary macroglobulinemia)
      2. Malignant lymphoma
      3. Chronic lymphocytic leukemia or lymphoproliferative disorders
   D. Heavy-chain diseases
      1. λ Heavy-chain disease
      2. α Heavy-chain disease
      3. μ Heavy-chain disease
   E. Amyloidosis
      1. Primary amyloidosis
      2. With multiple myeloma (secondary, localized, and familial amyloidosis have no M-protein)

M-protein, monoclonal protein.

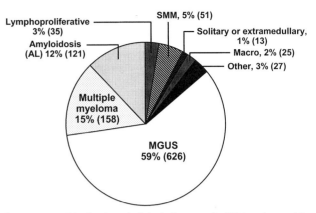

**Figure 19-1** *Distribution of clinical diagnoses in 1056 patients with a serum monoclonal protein detected at Mayo Clinic in 2002. AL, primary amyloidosis; Macro, macroglobulinemia; MGUS, monoclonal gammopathy of undetermined significance; SMM, smoldering multiple myeloma. (From Kyle, R. A., and Rajkumar, S. V. [2003 in press]. Monoclonal gammopathies of undetermined significance: a review.* Immunological Reviews. *By permission of the publisher.)*

immunoglobulins produces a broad-based peak or a broad band and is usually limited to the γ region. It is important to differentiate between an M-protein and a polyclonal increase, because the former is associated with a malignant or potentially malignant disorder, whereas the latter is associated with a reactive or

### TABLE 19-2

## Mayo Clinic Criteria for Diagnosis of MGUS, SMM, and MM

| | |
|---|---|
| MGUS: | Serum monoclonal protein <3 g/dL and bone marrow plasma cells <10% and absence of anemia, renal failure, hypercalcemia, and lytic bone lesions |
| SMM: | Serum monoclonal protein ≥3 g/dL or bone marrow plasma cells ≥10% and absence of anemia, renal failure, hypercalcemia, and lytic bone lesions |
| MM: | Presence of a serum or urine monoclonal protein, bone marrow plasmacytosis and anemia, renal failure, hypercalcemia, or lytic bone lesions; patients with primary systemic amyloidosis and ≥30% bone marrow plasma cells are considered to have both multiple myeloma and amyloidosis |

MGUS, monoclonal gammopathy of undetermined significance; MM, multiple myeloma (symptomatic); SMM, smoldering (asymptomatic) multiple myeloma.
Modified from Rajkumar, S. V., Dispenzieri, A., Fonseca, R., Lacy, M. Q., Geyer, S., Lust, J. A., Kyle, R. A., Greipp, P. R., Gertz, M. A., and Witzig, T. E. (2000). Thalidomide for previously untreated indolent or smoldering multiple myeloma. *Leukemia, 15,* 1274–1276. By permission of Nature Publishing Group.

# Recognition of Monoclonal Proteins

To detect the possible presence of an M-protein in the serum, a rapid and sensitive method is required. Agarose gel electrophoresis is more sensitive than cellulose acetate and is the preferred method of detection (Aguzzi et al., 1992; Howerton et al., 1986; Keren et al., 1999). Immunofixation with agarose gel (Roberts, 1986) should be used to confirm the presence of an M-protein and to distinguish the immunoglobulin class and its light-chain type (Kyle et al., 2002a).

An M-protein is usually seen as a narrow peak (like a church spire) in the γ, β, or β–γ region in the densitometer tracing, or as a dense, discrete band on the agarose gel. In contrast, an excess of polyclonal inflammatory process, especially chronic liver disease. In a group of 148 patients with a polyclonal gamma globulin level of 3.0 g/dL or more, liver disease was the most common association (61%), followed by connective tissue diseases (22%), chronic infections (6%), hematologic disorders (5%), and nonhematologic malignancies (3%) (Dispenzieri et al., 2001a). In approximately 8% of sera with an M-protein, there is an additional M-protein of a different immunoglobulin class (biclonal gammopathy) (Fig. 19-2).

The presence of an M-protein is indicative of MGUS, MM, primary amyloidosis (AL), Waldenström's macroglobulinemia (WM), or other lymphoproliferative disease. It is important to note that an M-protein can be present even if the total protein concentration, globulin levels, and quantitative immunoglobulin values are all within normal limits. A small M-protein may be hidden in the normal γ or β areas and could be overlooked. In addition, the presence of a monoclonal light chain (Bence Jones proteinemia) is rarely seen in the tracing, especially in patients with normal renal function. Immunofixation should be performed when a peak or a band is observed in the electrophoretic pattern or when a monoclonal gammopathy is suspected (Keren et al., 1999; Kyle et al., 2002a). Immunofixation is useful in the search for a small M-protein in AL, solitary plasmacytoma, or extramedullary plasmacytoma or after successful treatment of MM or WM (Kyle, 1994, 1999). Quantification of immunoglobulins is more useful than immunofixation for the detection of hypogammaglobulinemia. Quantification can be performed by radial immunodiffusion, but it is not recommended. Nephelometry is preferred because this technique is less subject to spurious abnormalities. However, levels of IgM obtained by nephelometry may

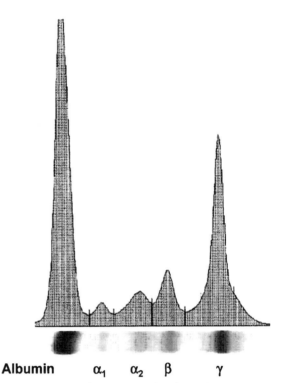

**Figure 19-3** *Pattern of serum monoclonal protein. (Top) Densitometer after electrophoresis on agarose gel showing tall, narrow-based peak of γ mobility. (Bottom) Electrophoresis of serum on agarose gel. Anode at left. Dense, localized band in γ area.*

**Albumin  α₁  α₂  β  γ**

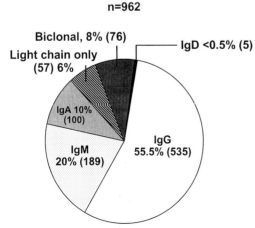

**n=962**

Biclonal, 8% (76)

Light chain only (57) 6%

IgD <0.5% (5)

IgA 10% (100)

IgM 20% (189)

IgG 55.5% (535)

**Figure 19-2** *Distribution of types of serum monoclonal proteins in 962 patients at Mayo Clinic in 2002. (From Kyle, R. A., and Rajkumar, S. V. [2003 in press]. Monoclonal gammopathies of undetermined significance: a review.* Immunological Reviews. *By permission of the publisher.)*

be 1000 to 2000 mg/dL higher than those expected on the basis of the serum protein electrophoresis tracing (Riches et al., 1991).

Dipstick tests used in many laboratories to screen for urinary proteins are often insensitive to Bence Jones protein. Consequently, sulfosalicylic acid or Exton's reagent is better for light-chain detection. Also, screening tests for Bence Jones proteinuria that use peculiar thermal properties are not recommended because of various shortcomings. Immunofixation of an adequately concentrated 24-hour urine specimen reliably detects Bence Jones protein. An M-protein appears as a dense, localized band on the agarose gel or as a tall, narrow, homogeneous peak in the densitometer tracing; its amount can be calculated on the basis of the size of the spike and the amount of total protein in the 24-hour urine specimen. It is not uncommon to have a negative reaction for protein, or even no obvious spike on electrophoresis, and to have a monoclonal light chain on immunofixation of a concentrated urine specimen. In MGUS, the M-protein is seen as a modest narrow peak or spike on the densitometer tracing or as a discrete band on the agarose gel (Fig. 19-3) in the γ or β regions, and it usually is a casual finding. Bence Jones proteinuria is generally absent or present in only small amounts.

# Monoclonal Gammopathy of Undetermined Significance (MGUS)

## Concept

The term "monoclonal gammopathy of undetermined significance" (MGUS) indicates the presence of an M-protein in persons with no evidence of MM, AL, WM, or other related disorders. Persons with MGUS have a serum M component less than 3 g/dL, none or a small amount of M-protein in the urine, less than 10% plasma cells in the bone marrow, and absence of lytic bone lesions, anemia, hypercalcemia, or impairment of renal function. The M-protein is an unexpected finding in the laboratory evaluation of an unrelated disorder, when investigating an increased erythrocyte sedimentation rate, or in a general health examination. When first described by Waldenström under the term "essential hypergammaglobulinemia" in 1952, this disorder was considered benign and, therefore, often called "benign monoclonal gammopathy" (Waldenström, 1961). Other terms for this condition have been idiopathic, asymptomatic, cryptogenic, or lanthanic monoclonal gammopathy, among others (Kyle, 1978). However, it is now well established that a proportion of cases will evolve to a symptomatic monoclonal gammopathy, and for this reason the term "MGUS" seems more appropriate (Kyle, 1978, 1984).

## Incidence

A monoclonal gammopathy was found in 64 (0.9%) of 6995 subjects older than 25 years in a mass health control study in Sweden (Axelsson et al., 1966). Similarly, an M-protein was detected in 0.7% of 102,000 sera samples from a general hospital in Italy (Malacrida et al., 1987) and in 1.2% of 73,630 hospitalized patients in the United States (Vladutiu, 1987). Also, in a population in Finistère, France, the frequency of serum M components was 1.1% among 30,279 adults (Saleun et al., 1982). The frequency of monoclonal gammopathies clearly increases with age. Thus, the frequency of M components is 1% in persons older than 50 years and approximately 3% in those older than 70 years (Axelsson et al., 1966; Fine et al., 1972; Kyle et al., 1972; Saleun et al., 1982). In subjects older than 80 years, the frequency of serum M components, as assessed by standard acetate cellulose electrophoresis, ranges from 4.1% to 5.2% (Axelsson et al., 1966; Fine et al., 1972; Kyle et al., 1972; Saleun et al., 1982). In a study in which high-resolution agarose gel electrophoresis and immunofixation were used, the frequency of M components in 111 residents of a retirement community who were 62 to 95 years old was 10%

(Crawford et al., 1987). In that series, M-proteins were present in 6% of subjects younger than 80 years but in 14% of those older than 90 years. In a study of persons in North Carolina, Cohen et al. (1998) reported MGUS in 3.6% in 816 persons 70 years or older. In contrast, the presence of an M-protein is rare in persons younger than 50 years. In this regard, in the studies by Axelsson et al. (1966) and Saleun et al. (1982), the frequency of M components in normal subjects younger than 50 years was only 0.15% (5 of 3321) and 0.2% (26 of 12,032), respectively. It is also of note that in the 2 series mentioned, no cases with M components were observed among 495 and 2747 individuals, respectively, younger than 30 years. In 2 studies (Schechter et al., 1990; Singh et al., 1990), the frequency of M components in the black population was higher than in whites. In the study by Cohen et al. (1998), an M-protein was found in 8.4% of 916 black patients and in 3.6% of whites. In contrast, only 2.7% of elderly Japanese patients had a monoclonal gammopathy (Bowden et al., 1993). Recently, Kurihara et al. (2000) found an M-protein in 71 (3.5%) of 2007 inpatients and outpatients in a Japanese University Hospital. When the 13 patients with myeloma and macroglobulinemia were excluded, MGUS was found in 2.9%, which is greater than previously reported.

More sensitive methods detect a higher incidence of M components. Thus, the frequency of a serum homogeneous band on high-resolution agarose gel electrophoresis in a healthy population aged 22 to 65 years was 5% (30 of 600), whereas in the same series cellulose acetate electrophoresis showed an M component in only 2 persons (0.33%) (Papadopoulos et al., 1982). In an unselected inpatient and outpatient population from a provincial hospital in northern Italy, M components were found on high-resolution serum electrophoresis in 7.8% of individuals older than 55 years (Aguzzi et al., 1992). In that study, almost 80% of M components were lower than 0.5 g/dL. Also, the frequency of monoclonal gammopathies determined by immunoisoelectric focusing in a population older than 45 years was 11% (22 of 200), 5 times more than that found by conventional serum electrophoresis (Sinclair et al., 1986a).

Considering the prevalence of MGUS, and that affected patients are usually seen by physicians in different fields of clinical practice, it is of particular importance to know whether the disorder will remain stable and benign or, on the contrary, will progress to a symptomatic monoclonal gammopathy requiring chemotherapy.

The cause of MGUS is unknown. In a population-based case-control study (565 subjects with MM and 2104 control subjects), the risk of MM was 3.7-fold higher for subjects who reported a first-degree relative with MM. The risk of hematolymphoproliferative

**TABLE 19-3**

Course of 241 Mayo Clinic Patients with Monoclonal Gammopathy
of Undetermined Significance

| | | Patients at Followup (24–38 y) | |
| | | No. | Percentage |
| Group | Description | | |
| --- | --- | --- | --- |
| 1 | No substantial increase of serum or urine monoclonal protein (benign) | 25 | 10 |
| 2 | Monoclonal protein ≥3.0 g/dL but no myeloma or related disease | 26 | 11 |
| 3 | Died of unrelated causes | 127 | 53 |
| 4 | Development of myeloma, macroglobulinemia, amyloidosis, or related disease | 63 | 26 |
| | Total | 241 | 100 |

Modified from Kyle, R. A. (1993) "Benign" monoclonal gammopathy: after 20 to 35 years of followup. *Mayo Clinic Proceedings, 68,* 26–36. By permission of Mayo Foundation.

cancers was also increased (1.7-fold) (Brown et al., 1999).

# Evolution of Monoclonal Gammopathy of Undetermined Significance

## Mayo Clinic Studies

At Mayo Clinic, a series of 241 individuals with MGUS has been followed for 24 to 38 years and periodically updated (Kyle, 1978, 1984, 1993). This series is composed of 140 males and 101 females; their median age at diagnosis was 64 years. Abnormal features on physical examination, such as hepatomegaly or splenomegaly and laboratory abnormalities such as anemia, thrombocytopenia, renal insufficiency, hypoalbuminemia, or hypercalcemia, were the result of unrelated disorders. The initial amount of M-protein ranged from 0.3 to 3.2 g/dL (median, 1.7 g/dL); the heavy-chain type was IgG in 73%, IgA in 11%, IgM in 14%, and biclonal in 2% of the patients. The type of light chain was κ in 62% and λ in 38%. Five patients had biclonal gammopathy. Fifteen patients had Bence Jones proteinuria, but the amount of urinary light chain was higher than 1 g/24 hours in only 3 patients. Twenty-eight percent had a reduction in the uninvolved immunoglobulin level. The median value of bone marrow plasma cells in the 109 patients in whom bone marrow aspiration was performed at diagnosis of MGUS was 3% (range, 1%–10%). One-fourth of the patients had no other abnormal findings at diagnosis of the monoclonal gammopathy.

After 24 to 38 years of followup, the 241 patients can be classified into four groups (Table 19-3 and Fig. 19-4). The number of patients in whom the M

component remained stable and who were classified as "benign" has decreased to 25 (10%) (group 1); however, they are still at risk for development of malignant transformation. The M component disappeared in 2 patients (IgGκ, IgAκ). Group 2 is composed of 26 patients in whom the serum M component increased to 3 g/dL or more, but they did not require chemotherapy for MM, WM, or AL. In this group, the pattern of increase was gradual in most patients, and only 3 patients had a sudden increase without malignant transformation. Slightly more than half of the patients (group 3) died of unrelated diseases without development of a malignant plasma cell or lymphoproliferative disorder, the most frequent causes of death being cardiac and cerebrovascular disorders. In approximately one-fourth of the patients (63 of the

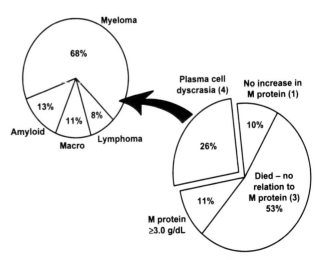

*Figure 19-4*  Evolution of monoclonal gammopathies in 241 patients at Mayo Clinic, 1956–1970. Macro, macroglobulinemia; M-protein, monoclonal protein.

## TABLE 19-4

### Development of Myeloma or Related Diseases in 63 Mayo Clinic Patients with Monoclonal Gammopathy of Undetermined Significance

| Disease | Patients | | Interval to Diagnosis (y)* | |
|---|---|---|---|---|
| | No. | % | Median | Range |
| Multiple myeloma | 43 | 68 | 10 | 2–29 |
| Macroglobulinemia | 7 | 11 | 8.5 | 4–20 |
| Amyloidosis | 8 | 13 | 9 | 6–19 |
| Lymphoproliferative disorder | 5 | 8 | 10.5 | 6–22 |
| Total | 63 | 100 | | |

*Actuarial rate was 16% at 10 years and 33% at 20 years.

241, 26%), malignant transformation developed during the median followup of 24 to 38 years (group 4): MM (43 cases), AL (8 cases), macroglobulinemia (7 cases), and other malignant lymphoproliferative disorders (5 cases) (Table 19-4). The actuarial rate of malignant transformation in the overall series was 16% at 10 years, 33% at 20 years, and 40% at 25 years (Fig. 19-5) (Kyle, 1993). The actuarial risk for development of a malignant gammopathy among 202 patients with IgG MGUS type was 14% at 10 years and 29% at 20 years, whereas the actuarial risk among 34 patients with IgM MGUS was 23% and 52% at 10 and 20 years, respectively. The risk of malignant transformation was not significantly different depending on the type of M-protein (IgG, IgA, or IgM).

In a long-term follow-up study of 430 subjects with an IgM serum M-protein, also conducted at Mayo Clinic (Kyle and Garton, 1987), 242 (56%) were considered to have IgM-type MGUS. At a median followup of 7 years (1714 patient-years), 40 (17%) of the 242 patients had a lymphoid malignancy: macroglobulinemia (22 patients), malignant lymphoproliferative disease (9), lymphoma (6), primary amyloidosis (2), and chronic lymphocytic leukemia (1). The median duration from the recognition of the M component to development of the malignant disorders ranged from 4 to 9 years (Kyle and Garton, 1987).

In an effort to confirm the findings of the original Mayo Clinic study, long-term followup was obtained in a group of patients with MGUS from southeastern Minnesota. MGUS was identified in 1384 patients who resided in the 11 counties of southeastern Minnesota. MGUS was diagnosed at Mayo Clinic between January 1, 1960, and December 31, 1994 (Kyle et al., 2002b). The study included 753 males (54%) and 631 females (46%). The median age at the time of diagnosis was 72 years, whereas it was 64 years in the original study of 241 patients. Only 2% were younger than 40 years, and 59% were 70 years or older. The M-protein value ranged from unmeasurable to 3.0 g/dL (median, 1.2 g/dL) (Fig. 19-6). On the basis of the heavy-chain type, 70% of the M-proteins were IgG, 12% IgA, and 15% IgM. Biclonal gammopathy was found in 45 patients (3%). The light chain was κ in 61% and λ in 39%. Uninvolved (normal or background) immunoglobulin was reduced in 38% of 840 patients in whom immunoglobulin was quantitated. Electrophoresis, immunoelectrophoresis, and immunofixation of urine were performed in 418 patients. Twenty-one percent had a monoclonal κ light chain and 10% had λ at the time of recognition of MGUS; 69% had negative results. Only 17% of the patients had a urinary M-protein value more than 150 mg/24 hours (Fig. 19-7).

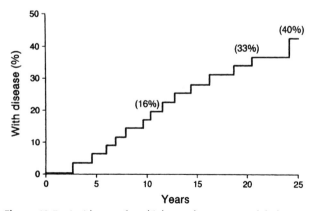

**Figure 19-5** *Incidence of multiple myeloma, macroglobulinemia, amyloidosis, or lymphoproliferative disease after recognition of monoclonal protein. (From Kyle, R. A. (1995). Monoclonal gammopathy of undetermined significance [MGUS]. Baillières Clinica Haematology, 8, 761–781. By permission of Baillière Tindall.)*

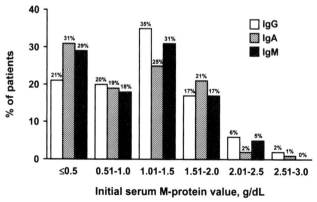

**Figure 19-6** *Initial serum monoclonal protein (M-protein) values in 1384 residents of southeastern Minnesota in whom monoclonal gammopathy of undetermined significance was diagnosed from 1960–1994.*

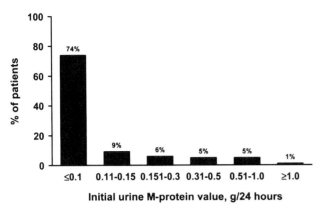

**Figure 19-7** *Initial urine monoclonal protein (M-protein) values in 1384 residents of southeastern Minnesota in whom monoclonal gammopathy of undetermined significance was diagnosed from 1960–1994. (From Kyle, R. A., and Rajkumar, S. V. [2003 in press]. Monoclonal gammopathies of undetermined significance: a review.* Immunological Reviews. *By permission of the publisher.)*

One hundred sixty patients (12%) had a bone marrow examination performed at the time of detection of the M-protein. The median percentage of bone marrow plasma cells was 3% (range, 0%–10%). The initial hemoglobin values ranged from 5.7 g/dL to 18.9 g/dL. The hemoglobin value was less than 10.0 g/dL in 7% and 12 g/dL or less in 23%. The anemia was the result of causes other than the plasma cell proliferative

process in each case. Only 3% of patients had a platelet value less than $100 \times 10^9$/L. The serum creatinine value was more than 2 mg/dL in 6% of the patients; this was attributed to unrelated causes such as diabetes, hypertension, and glomerulonephritis.

The 1384 patients were followed for a total of 11,009 person/years (median, 15.4 y; range, 0–35 y) (Table 19-5). Nine hundred sixty-three patients (70%) have died. During followup, MM, AL, lymphoma with an IgM serum M-protein, macroglobulinemia, plasmacytoma, or chronic lymphocytic leukemia developed in 115 patients (8%) (Table 19-6). Cumulative probability

## TABLE 19-5
### Follow-Up Data for 1384 Patients with Monoclonal Gammopathy of Undetermined Significance*

| Followup | |
| --- | --- |
| Person/years | 11,009 |
| Range (y) | 0–35 |
| Median (y) | 15.4 |
| Deaths | |
| No. | 963 |
| Percent | 70 |

*Mayo Clinic patients who were residents of southeastern Minnesota, diagnosis from 1960–1994.

## TABLE 19-6
### Risk of Progression Among 1384 Patients with Monoclonal Gammopathy of Undetermined Significance*

| Type of Progression | Patients (no.) Observed | Patients (no.) Expected[†] | Relative Risk (95% CI) |
| --- | --- | --- | --- |
| Multiple myeloma | 75 | 3.0 | 25.0 (20–32) |
| Lymphoma | 19[‡] | 7.8 | 2.4 (2–4) |
| Primary amyloidosis | 10 | 1.2 | 8.4 (4–16) |
| Macroglobulinemia | 7 | 0.2 | 46.0 (19–95) |
| Chronic lymphocytic leukemia | 3[§] | 3.5 | 0.9 (0.2–3) |
| Plasmacytoma | 1 | 0.1 | 8.5 (0.2–47) |
| Total | 115 | 15.8 | 7.3 (6–9) |

CI, confidence interval.

*Mayo Clinic patients who were residents of southeastern Minnesota, diagnosis from 1960–1994.

[†]Expected numbers of cases were derived from the age- and sex-matched white population of the Surveillance, Epidemiology, and End Results (SEER) Program (2001) in Iowa, except for primary amyloidosis, for which data are from Kyle et al. (1992).

[‡]All 19 patients had serum IgM monoclonal protein. If the 30 patients with IgM, IgA, or IgG monoclonal protein and lymphoma were included, the relative risk would be 3.9 (95% CI, 2.6–5.5).

[§]All 3 patients had serum IgM monoclonal protein. If all 6 patients with IgM, IgA, or IgG monoclonal protein and chronic lymphocytic leukemia were included, the relative risk would be 1.7 (95% CI, 0.6–3.7).

From Kyle, R. A., Therneau, T. M., Rajkumar, S. V., Offord, J. R., Larson, D. R., Plevak, M. F., and Melton, L. J. III (2002b). A long-term study of prognosis in monoclonal gammopathy of undetermined significance. *New England Journal of Medicine,* 346, 564–569. Copyright © 2002 Massachusetts Medical Society. All rights reserved.

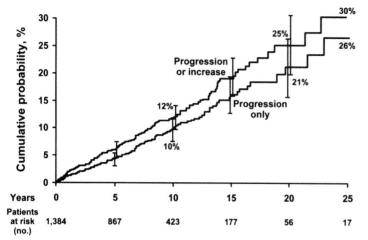

**Figure 19-8** *Probability of progression among 1384 residents of southeastern Minnesota in whom monoclonal gammopathy of undetermined significance (MGUS) was diagnosed from 1960–1994. The top curve shows the probability of progression to a plasma cell cancer (115 patients) or of an increase in the monoclonal protein concentration to more than 3 g/dL or the proportion of plasma cells in bone marrow to more than 10% (32 patients). The bottom curve shows only the probability of progression of MGUS to multiple myeloma, IgM lymphoma, primary amyloidosis, macroglobulinemia, chronic lymphocytic leukemia, or plasmacytoma (115 patients). The bars show 95% confidence intervals.*

of progression to one of these disorders was 10% at 10 years, 21% at 20 years, and 26% at 25 years (Fig. 19-8). The risk of progression was approximately 1% per year; in fact, patients were at risk of progression even after 25 years or more of stable MGUS. In addition, 32 patients had an M-protein value increase to more than 3 g/dL or a bone marrow increase to more than 10% but symptomatic MM or macroglobulinemia did not develop. Because patients who died are not included in Figure 19-8, the curves reflect the probability that a patient who has not died of other causes will experience plasma cell progression at each point in the followup; it therefore represents the natural history of the disease. Cumulative probability of progression to MM or a related disorder and an increase in the M-protein value to more than 3 g/dL or more than 10% bone marrow plasma cells was 12% at 10 years, 25% at 20 years, and 30% at 25 years (Fig. 19-8). At 10 years, the rate of progression to a plasma cell disorder was 6% and the rate of death from nonplasma cell disorders (such as cardiovascular and cerebrovascular diseases

and nonplasma cell cancers) was 53% (Fig. 19-9). At 25 years, the rate for progression to a plasma cell disorder was 11% and the rate of death from nonplasma cell diseases was 76%. These findings are not unexpected because the median age at diagnosis was 72 years. These findings confirm the results of the initial Mayo Clinic study (Fig. 19-10).

The number of patients with progression to a plasma cell disorder (115 patients) was 7.3 times the number expected on the basis of the incidence rates for those conditions in the general population (Table 19-6). The risk for development of MM was increased 25-fold, macroglobulinemia 46-fold, and AL 8.4-fold. The risk for development of lymphoma was only modestly increased at 2.4-fold, but this risk is underestimated because only lymphomas associated with an IgM counted in the observed number, whereas the incidence

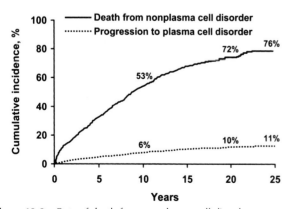

**Figure 19-9** *Rate of death from nonplasma cell disorders compared with progression to plasma cell disorders in 1384 residents of southeastern Minnesota in whom monoclonal gammopathy of undetermined significance was diagnosed from 1960–1994.*

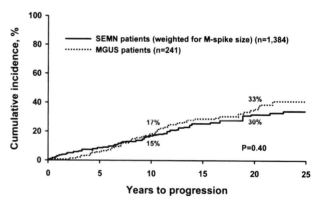

**Figure 19-10** *Progression to plasma cell disorders in the initial Mayo Clinic study of 241 patients with monoclonal gammopathy of undetermined significance (MGUS) and 1384 residents of southeastern Minnesota (SEMN) with MGUS diagnosed from 1960–1994. (From Kyle, R. A., and Rajkumar, S. V. [In press]. Monoclonal gammopathies of undetermined significance and smoldering multiple myeloma. In M. A. Gertz and P. R. Greipp (Eds). Handbook of Multiple Myeloma and Related Cell Disorders. By permission of Mayo Foundation for Medical Education and Research.)*

rates for lymphoma associated with IgG, IgA, and IgM were used to calculate the expected number. The risk for development of chronic lymphocytic leukemia was only slightly increased when all 6 cases were included.

MM developed in 65% of the 115 patients who had progressed to a plasma cell disorder. Three of the patients with myeloma also had AL, and 4 patients with MM had an initial plasmacytoma. MM was diagnosed more than 10 years after detection of the M-protein in 24 patients (32%). MM developed in 5 patients (7%) after 20 years of followup. The 75 patients with MM had the same characteristics as the 1027 patients with newly diagnosed MM referred to Mayo Clinic from 1985 to 1998, except that the southeastern Minnesota patients were older (median, 76 vs. 66 y) and were less likely to be male (46% vs. 60%) (Table 19-7). The pattern of increase in the level of the M-proteins is shown in Table 19-8. Degree of anemia, renal insufficiency, number of bone marrow plasma cells, size of the serum M-protein, occurrence of urine light chains, and reduction of uninvolved immunoglobulins were not different in the 2 groups; lytic lesions (66% vs. 46%) and hypercalcemia (13% vs. 7%) were more common in the referred patients. Light-chain myeloma was also more common in the referral group (16% vs. 0.3%), as expected, because all

## TABLE 19-8

### Pattern of Increase in Level of Monoclonal Protein Among Patients of Southeastern Minnesota with MGUS and Progression to Multiple Myeloma or Macroglobulinemia

| | Patients (no.) | |
| --- | --- | --- |
| **Pattern** | **Multiple Myeloma** | **Macro-Globulinemia** |
| Stable with sudden increase | 19 | 2 |
| Stable with gradual increase | 9 | 0 |
| Gradual increase | 9 | 3 |
| Sudden increase | 11 | 0 |
| Stable | 10 | 0 |
| Indeterminate | 17 | 2 |
| Total | 75 | 7 |

MGUS, monoclonal gammopathy of undetermined significance.

From Kyle, R. A., Therneau, T. M., Rajkumar, S. V., Offord, J. R., Larson, D. R., Plevak, M. F., and Melton, L. J. III (2002b). A long-term study of prognosis in monoclonal gammopathy of undetermined significance. *New England Journal of Medicine, 346,* 546–569. Copyright © 2002 Massachusets Medical Society. All rights reserved.

patients in the southeastern Minnesota group had a preceding serum M-protein and patients with an idiopathic Bence Jones protein were excluded. The median duration of survival of the patients with MM was shorter in the southeastern Minnesota group (16 vs. 33 mo). This difference is explained, at least partially, by their older age at diagnosis (median, 76 vs. 66 y).

The mode of development of MM among the patients with MGUS was variable (Fig. 19-11). The M-protein value increased within 2 years of the recognition of MGUS in 11 patients, was stable for more than 2 years and then increased within 2 years in 19 patients, increased gradually after having been stable for at least 2 years in 9 patients, and gradually increased during followup until symptomatic MM was diagnosed in 9 patients. In 10 patients the serum M-protein value remained essentially stable; the diagnosis of MM was unequivocal in these 10 patients because of an increase in bone marrow plasma cells, development of lytic lesions, or occurrence of anemia, renal insufficiency, or increased level of urine M-protein. Seventeen patients had an insufficient number of M-protein measurements to determine the pattern of increase. In macroglobulinemia, the M-protein value gradually increased in 3 patients and was stable and then suddenly increased in 2; data were insufficient in 2 patients (Table 19-8).

The M-protein disappeared during followup in 66 patients (5%). Only 17 of the 66 patients had a value more than 0.5 g/dL on diagnosis. The M-protein

## TABLE 19-7

### Characteristics of Patients with Multiple Myeloma

| | Patient Group | |
| --- | --- | --- |
| **Characteristic** | **SE Minnesota** (*n = 75*)* | **Referral** (*n = 1027*)† |
| Median age (y) | 76 | 66 |
| Male (%) | 47 | 59 |
| Hemoglobin < 12 g/dL (%) | 72 | 69 |
| Calcium > 11 mg/dL (%) | 7 | 13 |
| Creatinine ≥ 2 mg/dL (%) | 14 | 19 |
| Lytic lesions (%) | 46 | 66 |
| BMPC < 10% (%) | 6 | 4 |
| Median BMPC (%) | 40 | 50 |
| Median serum M protein (g/dL) | 3.2 | 3.2 |
| Urine M-protein present (%) | 81 | 78 |

BMPC, bone marrow plasma cells.

*Mayo Clinic patients who were residents of southeastern Minnesota.

†Patients with newly diagnosed multiple myeloma referred to Mayo Clinic from 1985–1998.

From Kyle, R. A., and Rajkumar, S. V. [in press]. Monoclonal gammopathies of undetermined significance and smoldering multiple myeloma. In M. A. Gertz and P. R. Greipp (Eds). *Handbook of Multiple Myeloma and Related Cell Disorders.* Berlin: Springer-Verlag. By permission of Mayo Foundation for Medical Education and Research.

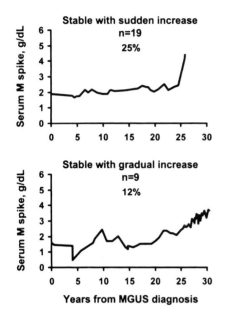

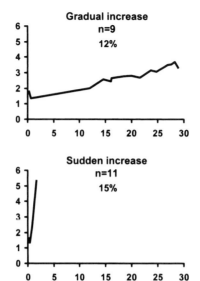

**Figure 19-11**  *Mode of development of multiple myeloma among 75 residents of southeastern Minnesota with monoclonal gammopathy of undetermined significance (MGUS) diagnosed from 1960–1994. M, monoclonal protein.*

disappeared in 39 patients in whom MM or lymphoma developed and required therapy or who had treatment for disorders such as idiopathic thrombocytopenic purpura or vasculitis unrelated to the monoclonal gammopathy. In 27 patients (2%), the M-protein disappeared without an apparent cause. Only 6 of these 27 patients (0.4% of all patients) had a discrete spike (median, 1.2 g/dL) on the densitometer tracing. These findings indicate that disappearance of the M-protein in MGUS is rare.

### Followup in Other Series

In the 20 years of followup in Axelsson's series (1986), 7 (11%) of the 64 patients who had an M-protein found in a screening health survey of 6995 individuals in 1964 had progression from their BMG. However, in that study, 3 patients with an increase in the M-protein value and a fourth patient with a large serum IgAκ protein and then light-chain proteinuria (evolving myeloma) were still alive without requiring chemotherapy at the time of the report. Fine et al. (1979), in a series of 20 patients with asymptomatic monoclonal gammopathy followed for 3 to 14 years, reported 4 patients with malignant evolution (MM in 2, WM in 2). In the series by Carter and Tatarsky (1980), 4 (6.2%) of 64 patients evolved from MGUS to MM after a long period of stability (range, 46–84 mo). A long-term followup in an Italian series of 313 subjects with MGUS has been reported (Paladini et al., 1989). In 14% of 213 patients followed for 5 to 8 years and in 18% of 100 patients with a followup of 8 to 13 years, malignant transformation developed. The average period from the first recognition of the M-protein until

the development of a serious disease was 63 months (range, 27–138 mo). In another series composed of 113 patients with MGUS, 10 evolved to a malignant plasma cell dyscrasia (MM in 8, AL in 2) after a median followup of 3 years (range, 1–17 y) (Manthorne et al., 1989). In that series, 16 additional patients also had a significant increase (more than 50%) in the initial M-component value. Belisle et al. (1990), in a series of 152 patients with BMG, found 19 patients with malignant evolution (MM in 15, AL in 3, and WM in 1) after a followup from 1 to 19 years. These authors stated that the risk of malignancy is apparent after 2 years.

In another series of 213 patients considered to have MGUS and who had a median followup of 38 months (range, 18–228 mo), 10 patients (4.6%) evolved to a malignant monoclonal gammopathy (MM in 8, WM in 1, and AL in 1) after a median period of 60 months (range, 11–124 mo) (Giraldo et al., 1991). In that series, the actuarial risk was 4.5% at 5 years, 15% at 10 years, and 26% at 15 years. Another series from Spain composed of 128 patients with MGUS followed for a median of 56 months (range, 12–156 mo) was reported (Bladé et al., 1992). Thirteen patients (10.2%) had malignant transformation: MM (10), AL (2), and WM (1). The actuarial probability of developing a malignant disease at 5 and 10 years was 8.5% and 19.2%, respectively. The median interval from recognition of the monoclonal gammopathy to the diagnosis of malignant transformation was 41.6 months (range, 12–155 mo).

In one study with a short followup (Ucci et al., 1993), 8 (3.3%) of 243 patients with MGUS progressed to MM with a median time from diagnosis to disease progression of 16 months (range, 6–18 mo). Van de Poel et al. (1995) reported that 22 (6.6%) of 334 patients with MGUS developed a malignant transformation after a median followup of 8.4 years. The median interval from recognition of the monoclonal gammopathy to the diagnosis of a malignant lymphoproliferative disease was 64 months (range, 7–143 mo). In the study by Isaksson et al. (1996), 15 (26%) of 57 patients developed a malignant plasma cell dyscrasia after a median followup of 8.4 years. Finally, in a recent report on 335 patients with MGUS, the frequency of progression after a median followup of 70 months was 6.8% (Baldini et al., 1996).

In a series of 263 cases of MGUS, the actuarial probability of development of malignancy was 31% at 20 years (Pasqualetti et al., 1997). Eleven (0.5%) of 2192 persons older than 21 years in a New Zealand town had an M-protein (Carrell et al., 1971). A hematologic malignancy developed in 7 of the 11 patients (MM in 4, macroglobulinemia in 2, and lymphoma in 1) after a 31-year followup of the 2192 persons. In a series of 1324 cases of MGUS in North Jutland County, Denmark, the standardized mortality ratio was 2.1. Malignant transformation was the cause of death in 97 patients (4.9 expected) (Gregersen et al., 2001a). In a series of 1229 patients with MGUS, the Danish Cancer Registry contained 64 new cases of malignancy (5.0 expected, relative risk 12.9). The risk for development of MM was 34.3-fold, WM 63.8-fold, and non-Hodgkin's lymphoma 5.9-fold. The relative risk of chronic lymphocytic leukemia was not significantly increased (Gregersen et al., 2000). In another series, MM developed in 10 of 88 patients with MGUS during a median followup of 6.75 years. The actuarial risk of progression was 9% at 5 years and 48% at 20 years (Van de Donk et al., 2001). Gregersen et al. (2001b) also reported that the relative risk of progression of IgA compared with IgG was 1.8. They also reported that the risk was higher with an increased concentration of immunoglobulin. High concentration of the immunoglobulin M component, female sex, and IgA type were all risk factors for progression. In 51 (10%) of 504 patients with MGUS from Iceland, a paraprotein malignancy developed after a median followup of 6 years. There was no association between monoclonal gammopathy and the subsequent development of non-hematologic malignancies (Ögmundsdóttir et al., 2002). In a group of 1104 patients with MGUS, more than 5% bone marrow plasmacytosis, presence of Bence Jones proteinuria, polyclonal immunoglobulin reduction, and high erythrocyte sedimentation rate were independent factors influencing MGUS transformation (Cesana et al., 2002). In summary, all studies confirm that the risk of progression from MGUS to MM or related disorders is approximately 1% per year. They also demonstrate that the risk does not disappear even after long-term followup.

## Pathophysiology of Malignant Transformation in MGUS

The sequence of events that are responsible for malignant transformation of MGUS to myeloma or related plasma cell proliferative disorder is still poorly understood. Clearly, alterations occur in both the myeloma cell and the bone marrow microenvironment during this transformation, but the specific pathogenetic role of these alterations remains unclear.

### Genetic Changes in MGUS and Myeloma

Cytogenetic changes are common in both myeloma and MGUS. The role of these changes in the initiation of the MGUS clone and progression to myeloma is being studied. Most studies indicate that when a chromosome abnormality is detected in MM and MGUS, it occurs in the majority of clonal plasma cells (Avet-Loiseau et al., 2000; Fonseca et al., 2001, 2002a).

### IgH Translocations

By fluorescence in situ hybridization (FISH) studies, 60% of patients with myeloma have IgH (14q32) translocations (Avet-Loiseau et al., 1998; Nishida et al., 1997). Furthermore, almost all myeloma cell lines have such translocations. Interestingly, studies indicate that these translocations are not unique to myeloma but also are present in the MGUS stage. In one series, 46% of patients with MGUS had IgH translocations, t(11;14)(q13;q32) being the most common (Avet-Loiseau et al., 1999a). More recently, Fonseca et al. (2002a) used a novel cytoplasmic immunoglobulin FISH technique (cIg-FISH) to study chromosome changes in individual plasma cells in MGUS. They found that 27 (46%) of 59 patients with MGUS had IgH translocations. This included t(11;14) (q13;q32) in 15 (25%) of 59 patients, t(4;14)(p16.3;q32) in 9%, and t(14;16)(q32;q23) in 5%.

IgH translocations are thought to be secondary to errors at the time of isotype class switching (Bergsagel et al., 1996, 1997; Chesi et al., 1996, 1997, 1998; Hallek et al., 1998). Specific partner chromosome loci are involved, including 4p16.3, 11q13, and 16q23 (Bergsagel et al., 1996, 1997; Chesi et al., 1996, 1997, 1998; Hallek et al., 1998). These translocations lead to dysregulation of putative oncogenes such as cyclin D1/myeov (11q13), c-maf (16q23), FGFR3/MMSET (4p16.3), and MUM-1 (6p25) (Chesi et al., 1996, 1997, 1998; Iida et al., 1997). For example, Fonseca et al. (2002a) recently confirmed the upregulation of FGFR3 by the t(4;14)(p16.3;q32) in MGUS.

The role of IgH translocations is still unclear. In myeloma, the presence of t(11;14)(q13;q32), as detected by FISH, appears to have specific biologic features and confers better survival (Fonseca et al., 2002b). Given that IgH translocations occur in both MGUS and myeloma, their primary role probably lies in initiation of the clone rather than progression of MGUS to myeloma.

## Deletions of Chromosome 13

Deletions of chromosome 13 have substantial adverse prognostic value in myeloma. However, even these cytogenetic abnormalities may start at the MGUS stage of the disease (Avet-Loiseau et al., 1999b; Konigsberg et al., 2000a). Although deletions of chromosome 13 confer an adverse effect once myeloma develops, it is unclear whether the rate of progression from MGUS to myeloma is accelerated because the frequency of deletion 13 is not very different between MGUS and MM (Avet-Loiseau et al., 1999b; Fonseca et al., 1997; Konigsberg et al., 2000a, 2000b). In fact, in a recent study using the cIg-FISH technique, deletion 13 was found in the clonal plasma cells in 50% of patients with MGUS. Bernasconi et al. (2002) reported that all 5 of 18 patients with MGUS who had a deletion of 13q had progression to MM within 6 to 12 months. They postulated that the deletion of 13q provided a growth advantage.

## Other Abnormalities

Several other cytogenetic abnormalities have been described, but little is known about their role in the pathogenesis or progression of MGUS. Aneuploidy does seem to be present in some patients with MGUS. Zandecki et al. (1995) detected trisomy in at least one of chromosomes 3, 7, 9, and 11 in 12% to 72% of bone marrow plasma cells in 12 of 14 patients with hyperdiploidy who had MGUS. Limited information is available about other abnormalities in MGUS such as p53.

## Angiogenesis in MGUS

In physiology, angiogenesis refers to the formation of new blood vessels, and it occurs during embryonal growth and in the female genital system during the menstrual cycle (Folkman, 1971, 1995; Rajkumar and Witzig, 2000). Pathologically, angiogenesis occurs during wound healing and is important for the proliferation and metastasis of most malignant neoplasms. In the absence of angiogenesis, tumors are unable to grow beyond 1 to 2 mm in size. Increased angiogenesis is an adverse prognostic factor in several tumors (Weidner et al., 1991; Weidner and Folkman, 1996). Recent evidence indicates that bone marrow angiogenesis is markedly increased in myeloma and has prognostic value in the disease (Rajkumar et al., 2000;

Vacca et al., 1994). Just like in solid tumors, angiogenesis may play a role in the transformation from premalignant stage (MGUS) to active myeloma. Increased angiogenesis probably is mediated by overexpression of angiogenic cytokines, such as vascular endothelial growth factor and basic fibroblast growth factor, in MGUS and MM.

Vacca et al. (1994) showed in a small study that bone marrow angiogenesis is increased in MM compared with MGUS. Recently, we studied bone marrow angiogenesis in 400 patients with various plasma cell disorders, including MGUS (76 patients), smoldering (indolent, early-stage) MM (112 patients), newly diagnosed, active MM (99 patients), relapsed (advanced) MM (26 patients), and AL (87 patients) (Rajkumar et al., 2002b). Forty-two normal control samples of bone marrow were studied for comparison. Bone marrow angiogenesis was studied in a blinded manner with immunohistochemical staining for CD34 to identify microvessels. The median (range) microvessel density was 1.3 (0–11) in the controls, 1.7 (0–10) in AL, 3 (0–23) in MGUS, 4 (1–30) in smoldering multiple myeloma, 11 (1–48) in MM, and 20 (6–47) in relapsed multiple myeloma ($p < 0.001$). This study showed that bone marrow angiogenesis progressively increases along the spectrum of plasma cell disorders from the more benign MGUS stage to advanced myeloma, indicating that angiogenesis might be related to disease progression (Rajkumar et al., 2002b). However, because of the low rate of transformation of MGUS to myeloma, estimated to be approximately 1% per year, we were unable to determine whether increased angiogenesis in MGUS led to increased risk of progression to myeloma.

Recently, Vacca et al. (1999) showed the angiogenic ability of myeloma cells in an *in vitro* chorioallantoic membrane angiogenesis assay. In this model, angiogenesis was found in 76% of purified myeloma samples and 20% of MGUS samples, further suggesting that increased angiogenesis is more a feature of myeloma than MGUS. However, more work needs to be done to determine whether angiogenesis is important in the progression from MGUS to MM. We think a serial follow-up study is needed of patients with MGUS over time to determine whether increased angiogenesis occurs right before progression to myeloma.

## Cytokines and Myeloma Bone Disease

The single most important clinical feature that differentiates myeloma from MGUS is the development of myeloma bone disease. Lytic bone lesions, osteopenia, hypercalcemia, and pathologic fractures in myeloma are a result of abnormal osteoclast activity induced by the neoplastic plasma cells (Callander and Roodman, 2001; Roodman, 2001; Yaccoby et al., 2002).

Osteoclasts are activated by stimulation of the transmembrane receptor RANK (receptor activator of nuclear factor κB), which belongs to the tumor necrosis factor receptor superfamily. Roodman hypothesized that the development of bone lesions in myeloma is the result of overexpression and interplay of various cytokines, most importantly RANKL (receptor activator of nuclear factor κB ligand) and MIP-1α (macrophage inflammatory protein-1α) (Roodman, 2002). The overproduction of RANKL by marrow stromal cells and possibly myeloma cells induces osteoclastogenesis (Roux et al., 2002). RANKL activity is modulated by a decoy receptor, osteoprotegerin (OPG), and thus stimulation of RANK is controlled by the ratio of RANKL to OPG (Croucher et al., 2001). Myeloma bone disease can thus occur as a result of excess RANKL and lower levels of OPG. Overproduction of interleukin-1β (IL-1β) and tumor necrosis factor-α by myeloma cells increases the RANKL/OPG ratio, thereby inducing osteoclast activation. MIP-1α is expressed by myeloma cells and is another candidate osteoclastogenic factor in myeloma (Abe et al., 2002; Han et al., 2001). MIP-1α probably directly affects osteoclast formation and enhances the activity of RANKL.

Lust and Donovan (1998) hypothesized that IL-1β plays an important role in the transformation from MGUS to myeloma and the development of myeloma bone disease. IL-1β is secreted by myeloma cells and induces osteoclast formation (Lacy et al., 1999; Lust and Donovan, 1999). Studies with an IL-β receptor antagonist in patients with high-risk MGUS are ongoing at Mayo Clinic.

Other cytokines such as tumor necrosis factor-α and IL-6 also have been implicated (Roodman, 2002). IL-6 is an important growth factor for myeloma cells. Increased levels of IL-6 have been found in patients with progressive myeloma in contrast to those with MGUS. IL-6 is another potent osteoclast-stimulating factor and thus may play a dual role in myeloma. Ely and Knowles (2002) reported that expression of CD56 was associated with the presence of lytic lesions. In summary, the progression of MGUS to MM may involve dysregulation of various cytokines in the myeloma cells and stromal cells, leading to osteoclast activation and lytic bone lesions.

### Helicobacter pylori

Malik et al. (2002) reported that 39 (66%) of 59 patients with MGUS also had a *Helicobacter pylori* infection. In 11 of these 39 patients, eradication of *H. pylori* led to normalization of the serum protein electrophoretic pattern and resolution of the gammopathy.

In one report of a patient with an IgM κ MGUS in whom a mucosa-associated lymphoid tissue lymphoma subsequently developed, the lymphoma disappeared

after successful treatment of the *H. pylori* infection. However, the MGUS persisted (Tursi and Modeo, 2002). Alternatively, serologic testing for *H. pylori* revealed that 30% of 93 patients with MGUS who were residents of Olmsted County had positive results, as did 32% of 98 control subjects from Olmsted County. In addition, 51 (33%) of 154 Mayo Clinic patients with MGUS were positive for *H. pylori*, and 365 (33%) of 1103 patients without MGUS also were positive for *H. pylori*. Thus, controversy exists concerning the role, if any, of *H. pylori* infection in MGUS (Rajkumar et al., 2002a).

### Predictors of Malignant Transformation in MGUS

No findings at diagnosis of MGUS can distinguish a patient whose condition will remain stable from one in whom a malignant condition will develop. Certain factors have been found useful for predicting the likelihood of progression from MGUS to MM. Although the diagnostic criteria for MGUS differ among studies, certain important findings emerge.

### Type of M-Protein

In Kyle's series (1993), patients with IgM-type MGUS had a higher probability of malignant evolution than those with IgG or IgA type, but the differences were not statistically significant. In a study by Bladé et al. (1992), patients with IgA-type MGUS had a greater probability for development of MM than the remainder. However, it should be pointed out that in their series only 21 subjects had an IgA M-protein. More recently, in the large series of 1384 Mayo Clinic patients, those with an IgM or an IgA M-protein had an increased risk of progression compared with patients who had an IgG M-protein ($p = 0.001$) (Fig. 19-12).

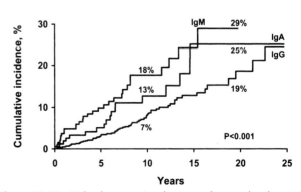

**Figure 19-12** *Risk of progression by type of monoclonal protein in 1384 residents of southeastern Minnesota with monoclonal gammopathy of undetermined significance diagnosed from 1960–1994 on the basis of immunoglobulin type.*

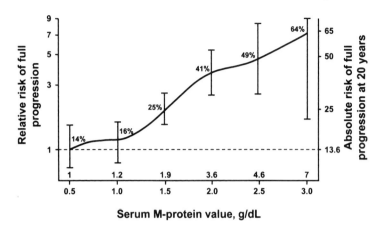

***Figure 19-13*** *Actuarial risk of full progression at 20 years by serum monoclonal protein (M-protein) value at diagnosis in 1384 residents of southeastern Minnesota with monoclonal gammopathy of undetermined significance diagnosed from 1960–1994.*

### Size of M-Protein

In the recent Mayo Clinic study of 1384 patients, the initial concentration of the serum M-protein was the most important risk factor for progression to a plasma cell disorder. The relative risk of progression was directly related to the concentration of M-protein in the serum at the time of diagnosis of MGUS. The risk of progression to MM or a related disorder 10 years after diagnosis of MGUS was 6% for an initial M-protein value of 0.5 g/dL or less, 7% for 1.0 g/dL, 11% for 1.5 g/dL, 20% for 2.0 g/dL, 24% for 2.5 g/dL, and 34% for 3.0 g/dL. Corresponding rates for progression at 20 years were 14%, 16%, 25%, 41%, 49%, and 64% (Fig. 19-13). The risk of progression with a serum M-protein value of 1.5 g/dL was almost twofold greater than the risk of progression with an M-protein value of 0.5 g/dL, and the risk of progression with 2.5 g/dL was 4.6 times that with a value of 0.5 g/dL (Fig. 19-14).

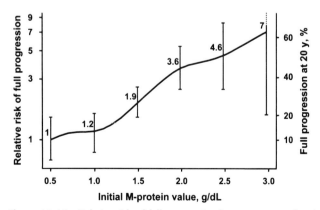

***Figure 19-14*** *Relative risk of full progression by serum monoclonal protein (M-protein) value at diagnosis in 1384 residents of southeastern Minnesota with monoclonal gammopathy of undetermined significance diagnosed from 1960–1994.*

### Bone Marrow Plasma Cells

In another study, Baldini et al. (1996) described 386 patients with nonmalignant monoclonal gammopathy. Most of the patients (335) had typical MGUS, whereas the remaining 51 patients fulfilled all the diagnostic criteria of MGUS except that their percentage of bone marrow plasma cells was 10% to 30%. The authors defined this latter group as having monoclonal gammopathy of borderline significance. The frequency of malignant transformation was 6.8% (median followup, 70 mo) in the MGUS group and 37% (median followup, 53 mo) in the group with monoclonal gammopathy of borderline significance. In a multivariate analysis, the variables that significantly correlated with evolution to MM in IgG cases were percentage of bone marrow plasma cells, reduction in polyclonal immunoglobulins, age, presence of light-chain proteinuria, and serum M-protein level. It is of interest that Baldini et al. (1996) identified a subset of patients with MGUS of IgG type with a low probability of progression to MM who exhibited no reduction in polyclonal immunoglobulins, no light-chain proteinuria, bone marrow plasma cell value less than 5%, and IgG value of 1.5 g/dL or less. This study by Baldini et al. indicated that the extent of bone marrow involvement may be an important predictor of progression to myeloma. Cesana et al. (2002) confirmed this in a large series of 1104 patients with MGUS. Patients with bone marrow plasma cell involvement of 6% to 9% had an increased risk of transformation.

Millá et al. (2001) reported that the presence of nucleoli was the most important feature in differentiating MM from MGUS. The percentage of plasma cells, cytoplasmic contour irregularities, and an anisocytosis also predicted a diagnosis of MM in multivariate analysis. Using these criteria they correctly identified 36 of 41 MGUS cases and all 21 cases of MM.

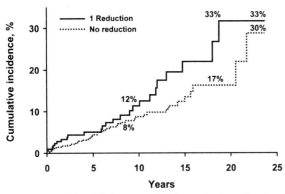

*Figure 19-15* Risk of full progression by reduction of uninvolved immunoglobulins in 1384 residents of southeastern Minnesota with monoclonal gammopathy of undetermined significance diagnosed from 1960–1994. (From Kyle, R. A., and Rajkumar, S. V. [In press]. Monoclonal gammopathies of undetermined significance and smoldering multiple myeloma. In M. A. Gertz and P. R. Greipp (Eds). Handbook of Multiple Myeloma and Related Cell Disorders. By permission of Mayo Foundation for Medical Education and Research.)

## Other Indicators of Progression

The presence of a urine M-protein (κ or λ) or reduction of one or more uninvolved immunoglobulins (Fig. 19-15) were not risk factors for progression in the 1384 Mayo Clinic patients (Tables 19-9 and 19-10). However, Cesana et al. (2002) reported that the presence of Bence Jones proteinuria, reduction of uninvolved immunoglobulins, and high erythrocyte sedimentation rate were independent factors of progression of MGUS.

In the 263 patients with MGUS reported by Pasqualetti et al. (1997), multivariate regression analysis showed that only age was significantly associated with the risk for development of a malignant immunoproliferative disease.

Blood clonal B-cell excess has been reported to be an important prognostic factor for the malignant evolution

### TABLE 19-9
#### Rates of Full Progression by Urinary Light Chain Among 1384 Patients with Monoclonal Gammopathy of Undetermined Significance*

| Light Chain | Rate of Full Progression (%) | | | |
| | 10 y | 20 y | 25 y | p |
| --- | --- | --- | --- | --- |
| κ or λ | 12 | 28 | NA | 0.12 |
| Negative | 11 | 34 | 34 | |

NA, not available.
*Mayo Clinic patients who were residents of southeastern Minnesota, diagnosis from 1960–1994.

### TABLE 19-10
#### Rates of Full Progression by Reduction of Uninvolved Immunoglobulins Among 1384 Patients with Monoclonal Gammopathy of Undetermined Significance*

| Uninvolved Immunoglobulin Reduction (no.) | Rate of Full Progression (%) | | | |
| | 10 y | 20 y | 25 y | p |
| --- | --- | --- | --- | --- |
| 1 | 12 | 33 | 33 | 0.15 |
| 2 | 22 | 22 | 22 | 0.09 |
| 0 | 8 | 17 | 30 | |

*Mayo Clinic patients who were residents of southeastern Minnesota, diagnosis from 1960–1994.

of MGUS (Isaksson et al., 1996). Bataille et al. (1996) showed that an excess of bone resorption is an early sign of malignancy in patients with MGUS and that it is significantly associated with progressive disease.

In the subset of patients who evolve to MM, MGUS constitutes the pre-myeloma phase, and MM usually develops after a prolonged period of stability. For some unknown reason, the plasma cell clone evades the influence of regulatory mechanisms and MM develops. In fact, when malignant transformation occurs, the type of M component is always the same as it was in the MGUS state. Also, patients with MM who achieve an objective response to therapy and enter into a stable "plateau phase" have a quiescent state similar to that in patients with MGUS and smoldering MM. The crucial difference between MGUS and MM in "plateau phase" is that virtually all patients with MM will eventually relapse, whereas only 25% of patients with MGUS will develop MM. In several instances, the onset of MM in subjects with MGUS is not gradual (as would be expected in an initially nonmalignant and slowly proliferative condition) but abrupt, resembling the relapses generally seen in patients with MM after the "plateau phase." Another finding of particular interest is that 32 (58%) of 55 patients diagnosed with MM in Olmsted County, Minnesota, had a preceding plasma cell disorder (MGUS, smoldering MM, or plasmacytoma) before the diagnosis of MM (Kyle et al., 1994). This finding suggests that a considerable portion of patients with MM actually had a previous monoclonal gammopathy.

## Characteristics of MM after MGUS

In Mayo Clinic series (Kyle, 1993), the mode of development of MM after MGUS was variable. Eleven patients gradually evolved to symptomatic MM from 1 to 4 years (median, 3 y) after a period of 4 to 18 years (median, 8 y) in which the M component remained stable. In 7 patients, the M-protein remained stable for 2 to 25 years (median, 8 y) and then abruptly increased along with the development of symptomatic myeloma. In 14 patients, there were not enough longitudinal M-component measurements to determine the mode of presentation of MM. The other 7 patients had initially fluctuating but gradually increasing serum M-component values until MM finally developed after a median of 12 years. In the overall series, the median interval from the diagnosis of MGUS to the diagnosis of MM was 10 years, and in 7 patients MM developed 20 or more years after the recognition of the M-protein. The median duration of survival after the diagnosis of MM was 34 months. In the study by Carter and Tatarsky (1980), the evolution of MM occurred suddenly in 3 of 4 patients after a long period in a stable condition. Similarly, in the series by Bladé et al. (1992), the evolution from MGUS to MM occurred abruptly in 8 of the 10 patients, 4 of them presenting with hypercalcemia (Salgado et al., 1993). Although 5 of the patients had an objective response to chemotherapy, the median survival was only 18 months (Salgado et al., 1993).

In summary, in a proportion of patients, the transition from MGUS to MM is abrupt after a long period of stability, and the outcome of patients who have MM after MGUS does not seem to be different from that of patients in whom MM develops without recognition of a prior MGUS.

### Life Expectancy in Patients with MGUS

Because MGUS is initially a benign condition with a median age at diagnosis ranging from 60 to 65 years, it is important to know whether such a disorder shortens the patient's life expectancy. Studies addressing this issue are particularly justified in elderly patients, in whom mortality results from the effects of both the underlying condition and the age-associated diseases. In the series by Bladé et al. (1992), the expected survival of the control population was calculated from the age-specific and sex-specific death rates of the 1970, 1975, 1980, and 1986 Spanish life tables, and in each patient the life table closest to the year of diagnosis was selected. Although in their study no significant differences were observed between the survival of patients with MGUS and that of the control population, a careful examination of the latter part of the curves shows a trend toward a shorter survival for the MGUS population. In fact, the lack of statistical significance is probably the result of the still relatively small number of patients evolving to a malignant monoclonal gammopathy. Kyle (1993) reported that survival of the 241 patients with MGUS diagnosed before 1971 was significantly shorter than that of an age- and sex-adjusted 1980 U.S. population (median, 13.7 vs. 15.7 y).

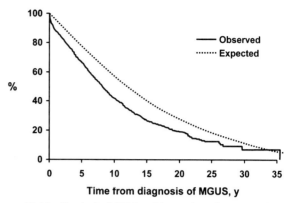

**Figure 19-16** *Survival of 1384 residents of southeastern Minnesota with monoclonal gammopathy of undetermined significance (MGUS) diagnosed from 1960–1994 compared with survival in a normal population (8.1 vs. 11.8 y, respectively) (p <0.001).*

However, it is of note that both curves run separately from the beginning when there is not a significant number of cases of malignant evolution, perhaps reflecting a naturally shorter expected survival in the MGUS population. In the study by van de Poel et al. (1995), the long-term survival of 334 patients with MGUS was slightly shorter than the expected survival of an age- and sex-adjusted population, but the difference was apparently not statistically significant. The median survival of the 1384 patients with MGUS from southeastern Minnesota was 8.1 years compared with 11.8 years (*p* < 0.001) expected for Minnesota residents of matched age and sex (Fig. 19-16).

## MGUS Variants

### IgD MGUS

Although the detection of an IgD M-protein in the serum is generally indicative of a malignant plasma cell proliferative disorder, at least one case of well-documented BMG of IgD type followed for more than 6 years has been reported (O'Connor et al., 1991). In this patient, the IgDλ M-protein value actually decreased during followup without any chemotherapy. Hobbs and Corbett (1969) described a patient who died of metastatic thyroid medullary carcinoma in whom a serum IgDλ protein was identified, but the bone marrow and radiologic examination for myeloma were negative. In that case, the IgD synthesis by the thyroid medullary carcinoma was reasonably excluded. A patient with IgDλ MGUS with axonal neuropathy has been reported (Hansen et al., 1989). However, in that case, the IgD level was only moderately increased and no follow-up information was given. At Mayo Clinic, one patient with IgD-type MGUS followed for more than 8 years with no malignant evolution also was recognized (Bladé and Kyle, 1994).

## Biclonal Gammopathies

Biclonal gammopathies are characterized by the production of 2 different M-proteins; they occur in at least 5% of patients with monoclonal gammopathies. The presence of 2 M-proteins may be the result of the proliferation of 2 different clones of plasma cells, each giving rise to an unrelated monoclonal immunoglobulin, or it could result from the production of 2 M-proteins by a single clone of plasma cells.

The characteristics of 57 patients with biclonal gammopathy were reviewed (Kyle et al., 1981): 65% had MGUS and the remainder had MM (16%) or a lymphoproliferative disorder (19%). The clinical features of biclonal gammopathies are similar to those of monoclonal gammopathies (Kyle et al., 1981). Serum protein electrophoresis showed only a single band on the cellulose acetate strip in many cases (31.6%), the second M-protein being unrecognized until immunoelectrophoresis or immunofixation was done.

Nilsson et al. (1986) reported that almost half of their 20 patients with biclonal gammopathy had biclonal gammopathy of undetermined significance. MM subsequently developed in 2 of them. In a series of 1135 patients with monoclonal gammopathy, 2.5% had biclonal gammopathy (Riddell et al., 1986). Sensorimotor peripheral neuropathy has been reported with biclonal gammopathy (Ilyas et al., 1988b). Sakashita et al. (1998) reported a patient with a single population of plasma cells producing an IgM and an IgG M-protein with the same λ light chain. The regulatory interactions between two monoclonal clones were emphasized by Pizzolato et al. (1998).

## Triclonal Gammopathies

Triclonal gammopathy was reported in a patient with plasma cell dyscrasia in whom acquired immunodeficiency syndrome subsequently developed (Ray et al., 1986; Ray and Schotters, 1986) and in a patient with non-Hodgkin's lymphoma (Berg et al., 1986). Murata et al. (1993) described a patient with triclonal gammopathy (IgMκ, IgGκ, and IgAκ) and a plasmacytoid lymphoma of the ileum and gastric wall. They thought that the 3 monoclonal proteins derived from a single clone of plasma cells that had undergone a "class switch." They noted that 11 of 15 patients with triclonal gammopathy described in the literature had a malignant lymphoma or lymphoproliferative disorder.

Grosbois et al. (1997) also described a patient with triclonal gammopathy (IgMκ, IgGκ, and IgAκ). In a review of the literature, they found that 16 patients with triclonal gammopathies were associated with a

malignant immunolymphoproliferative disorder, 5 appeared in nonhematologic diseases, and 3 were of undetermined significance. Saito et al. (1998) reported 2 patients with lymphoma with a triclonal gammopathy (IgMλ, IgGκ, and IgGλ; IgMλ, IgMκ, and IgGκ). They showed that the 3 immunoglobulins were synthesized at the same time in a single cell.

## Benign Bence Jones Proteinuria

The presence of light-chain proteinuria is frequently associated with malignant monoclonal gammopathy. However, patients excreting large amounts of Bence Jones protein who have a benign course have been well documented. Thus, 2 patients with a stable serum M component who also excreted 0.8 g or more of Bence Jones protein daily for almost 20 years without development of myeloma or amyloidosis had already been reported more than 3 decades ago (Kyle et al., 1973). Seven other patients without an M-protein in the serum and no evidence of a malignant plasma cell disorder at diagnosis who excreted more than 1 g per day of Bence Jones protein have been described (Kyle and Greipp, 1982). The plasma cell labeling index was low in all cases tested. During a follow-up period of 7 to 21 years, MM developed in 2 patients, evolving myeloma developed in 1 patient, and 2 patients died of unrelated causes. One patient developed AL; one patient has asymptomatic Bence Jones proteinuria at 25 years. Thus, although Bence Jones proteinuria of undetermined significance may remain stable for years, in most such patients MM or AL will ultimately develop. Consequently, these patients should be followed to ensure that treatment is started promptly if symptomatic disease develops.

# Differentiation of MGUS from MM

Asymptomatic patients with an M component of less that 3 g/dL, fewer than 10% bone marrow plasma cells, and absence of osteolytic lesions, anemia, hypercalcemia, or renal function impairment have MGUS. When these monoclonal gammopathies are first recognized, there are no clinical or biologic factors that can determine which patients will evolve to a symptomatic monoclonal gammopathy. Asymptomatic patients who have an M component of more than 3 g/dL or more than 10% bone marrow plasma cells fulfill the criteria for smoldering MM (Kyle and Greipp, 1980). They have no anemia, renal failure, hypercalcemia, lytic bone lesions, or other clinical manifestations related to the monoclonal gammopathy. Clinically and biologically these patients with smoldering MM are closer to having MGUS than overt MM. The recognition of these patients is extremely important because they should not be treated with chemotherapy until progression occurs.

In 75% to 80% of patients with MM, the levels of uninvolved (polyclonal) immunoglobulins are decreased (Bladé et al., 1984; Kyle, 1975). However, this criterion is not useful for differentiation because between 30% and 40% of patients with MGUS also have a decrease in the uninvolved immunoglobulins (Baldini et al., 1996; Bladé et al., 1992; Kyle, 1978; Lindström and Dahlström, 1978; Paladini et al., 1989).

Although the presence of Bence Jones proteinuria is suggestive of malignant gammopathy, it is not unusual to find small amounts of monoclonal light chains in the urine of patients with MGUS. Thus, 15 of the patients reported by Lindström and Dahlström (1978) also had Bence Jones proteinuria in the range of 50 to 500 mg/dL, and 39% of the patients in Mayo Clinic series had Bence Jones proteinuria (Kyle, 1978). In our MGUS cohort from southeastern Minnesota, 31% of the 418 tested patients had a monoclonal light chain in the urine. The value was more than 150 mg/24 hours in only 17%. However, the presence of a monoclonal light chain in the urine was not a risk factor for subsequent development of MM (Kyle et al., 2002b). In addition, some patients may excrete more than 1 g per day of Bence Jones protein and remain stable for many years (Kyle and Greipp, 1982).

Although in MM plasma cells tend to be more atypical, the authors have seen patients with a proportion of bone marrow plasma cells of more than 10% (smoldering myeloma), many of them with atypical features, who have remained stable for years or have never developed symptomatic myeloma. The plasma cell labeling index is the most useful measurement in differentiating MGUS or smoldering MM from overt MM (Greipp et al., 1987). A monoclonal antibody (BU-1) that reacts with 5-bromo-2-deoxyuridine detects cells synthesizing DNA. However, because the BU-1 antibody does not require denaturation, monoclonal plasma cells can be identified after staining with κ or λ antisera under immunofluorescence. There is a good correlation between the peripheral blood and the bone-marrow labeling index (Witzig et al., 1988). The labeling index study can be performed in 4 to 5 hours, and increased values strongly suggest that the patient has or will soon develop symptomatic disease. However, an increased labeling index is present in only a few patients with MGUS, whereas more than one-third of patients with overt MM have a normal value. Circulating Ki-67-positive lymphocytes may help to distinguish MGUS from MM (Miguel-Garcia et al., 1995).

The presence of circulating plasma cells in the peripheral blood is a good marker of active disease. Witzig et al. (1992) showed that monoclonal plasma cells can be detected in the peripheral blood of patients with active myeloma, even when they are not detectable in routine peripheral blood smears. A plasma cell concentration of $3 \times 10^6$/L or more in subjects with MGUS or smoldering MM indicates that the patient does not have a truly inactive disease and is at high risk of symptomatic myeloma within a few months (Witzig et al., 1994). A study by Billadeau et al. (1996) showed that clonal circulating cells are present in patients with MGUS, smoldering MM, and active myeloma. These authors analyzed blood mononuclear cells using 3 different methods to detect and quantify clonal cells: immunofluorescence microscopy; 3-color flow cytometry for CD38[+], CD45[−], and CD45[dim]; and the allele-specific oligonucleotide polymerase chain reaction. The polymerase chain reaction detected clonal cells in 13 of 16 patients with MGUS, and the immunofluorescence and flow cytometry techniques also detected clonal cells in 4 patients with MGUS. The finding of clonal cells in the peripheral blood of patients with MGUS demonstrates that the clone is present in the blood even at this early stage of monoclonal gammopathy. Because most of these patients will never develop a malignant disease, there must be additional factors that trigger the proliferation of these initially inactive clonal plasma cells.

Levels of $\beta_2$-microglobulin are not helpful in the differential diagnosis of MGUS and MM because there is a considerable overlap between the 2 entities (Garewal et al., 1984). The presence of J chains in malignant plasma cells, an increased level of plasma cell acid phosphatase, reduced numbers of CD4 cell subpopulation, increased numbers of monoclonal idiotype-bearing peripheral blood lymphocytes, and an increased number of immunoglobulin-secreting cells in peripheral blood are all characteristic of MM, but they are not reliable for differentiation because there is an overlap with MGUS (Kyle and Lust, 1991). In one study (Ong et al., 1996), serum neural cell adhesion molecule was shown to be useful in the differentiation of MM and nonmyelomatous monoclonal gammopathies.

Lytic bone lesions in the skeletal survey strongly suggest the diagnosis of MM. However, if a patient presents with constitutional symptoms (unusual in MM) and osteolytic lesions with fewer than 10% bone marrow plasma cells and a modest M component, the most probable diagnosis is metastatic carcinoma with an unrelated MGUS. Bataille et al. (1992) reported that increased bone resorption, assessed on quantitative bone biopsy, is almost a constant feature in patients with active myeloma, irrespective of the presence or absence of lytic bone lesions on the conventional radiographic examination. Interestingly, the degree of bone resorption was as pronounced in patients with smoldering or early myeloma as in those with overt MM (Bataille et al., 1991). In one study, Bataille et al. (1996) demonstrated that a quantifiable excess of bone resorption also can be found in patients with MGUS and that it is an early sign of malignant evolution. Interestingly, the excess of bone resorption may be detected several years before the features of MM develop.

A clear relationship between serum levels of IL-6 and different status of monoclonal gammopathies has been reported (Bataille et al., 1989; Solary et al., 1992). Thus, in the series by Bataille et al. (1989), only 1 of the 35 patients with MGUS or smoldering MM had a serum IL-6 level of more than 5 U/mL. However, 35 (41%) of 85 patients with newly diagnosed myeloma also had normal serum levels of IL-6. An increased IL-6 level probably reflects an advanced and aggressive disease already resistant to chemotherapy (Zhang et al., 1992). However, in 2 studies (DuVillard et al., 1995; Filella et al., 1996), serum IL-6 levels were increased in 15% and 14% of patients with MGUS, respectively. Patients with long-lasting MGUS and no associated infectious or inflammatory diseases who have high serum levels of IL-6 have been observed (Bladé J, unpublished data, December 2002). Therefore, the serum IL-6 level does not discriminate between MGUS and MM in patients with newly identified monoclonal gammopathies. The multidrug-resistant phenotype (MDR-1) expression together with the absence of the natural killer cell antigen (CD56) was reported to be useful for separating MGUS from smoldering MM (Sonneveld et al., 1993). However, other authors found a strong CD56 expression in patients with MGUS (Leo et al., 1992; Mathew et al., 1995) and concluded that the expression of CD56 does not help to distinguish MGUS from MM.

Conventional cytogenetic studies are not useful in the differentiation of MGUS from MM because abnormal karyotypes are rare in MGUS because of the small number of plasma cells and the low proliferative rate.

Ocqueteau et al. (1998) found a population of polyclonal plasma cells with CD38 expression and low forward light scatter. The plasma cells expressed CD19 but were negative for CD56. The monoclonal plasma cell population showed a lower CD38 expression and a higher forward light scatter population and expressed CD56 but not CD19. Ninety-eight percent of patients with MGUS had less than 3% normal polyclonal plasma cells, whereas only 1.5% of patients with MM had the same findings.

Bellaiche et al. (1997) reported that magnetic resonance imaging was normal in all 24 patients with MGUS but abnormalities were found in 86% of 44 patients with MM. Thus, magnetic resonance imaging may be useful for differentiating MGUS from MM.

Abnormal bone metabolism, manifested by increased levels of the C-terminal telopeptide of type I collagen, osteocalcin, and serum bone-specific alkaline phosphatase, may be present in patients with MM, but these abnormalities are not reliable for distinguishing MM from MGUS (Vejlgaard et al., 1997). Mathiot et al. (1996) reported that low soluble CD16 in MGUS was associated with a high likelihood of evolution to MM. In their study, low levels of soluble type III Fc gamma receptor (sCD16) discriminated myeloma from a control population.

Xu et al. (2001) reported that 21 of 27 patients with MM and 1 of 5 with MGUS had increased telomerase activity. Activation of telomerase may play a role in the transformation from MGUS to MM. In another study, the percentage of granular lymphocytes in the bone marrow was increased in 27% of patients with MGUS and in 15% of patients with MM. Natural killer cells (CD57$^+$CD16$^+$) were higher in MGUS than in MM (Sawanobori et al., 1997).

The frequency of methylation of p15$^{(INK4b)}$ and p16$^{(INK4a)}$ was similar in MGUS and MM, suggesting that methylation is an early event and is not associated with progression of MGUS to MM. Methylation of p15$^{(INK4b)}$ and p16$^{(INK4a)}$ may contribute to immortalization of plasma cells rather than malignant transformation (Guillerm et al., 2001).

IL-1β is produced by plasma cells in virtually all cases of MM but is undetectable in most patients with MGUS. IL-1β has strong osteoclast-activating factor activity that increases the expression of adhesion molecules and induces paracrine IL-6 production. Lytic lesions might result from stimulation of osteoclasts through the production of IL-1β as well as paracrine IL-6 secretion. IL-6 also stimulates osteoclasts through the production of IL-1β (Lacy et al., 1999; Lust and Donovan, 1998).

Vacca et al. (1994) reported that bone marrow angiogenesis was increased in MM but not in MGUS. Studies done at Mayo Clinic confirm this finding, although this test will have limited value in differentiating MGUS from MM because angiogenesis is not increased in approximately one-third of patients with MM (Rajkumar et al., 2000). Using the chick embryo chorioallantoic model, bone marrow samples were angiogenic in 76% of patients with myeloma and in only 20% of patients with MGUS (Vacca et al., 1999). Ellis et al. (2001) postulated that CD30$^+$ T cells may contribute to chronic activation of B cells through the production of IL-6.

In summary, the diagnosis of MGUS usually does not offer doubts, the M component being an unexpected finding in the course of an unrelated process or in a routine medical examination. However, at that time, no single factor can differentiate patients with BMG from those in whom a malignant plasma cell disorder will develop subsequently. The serum and urinary M-proteins must be periodically measured and a clinical evaluation conducted to determine whether MM, AL, WM, or another lymphoproliferative disorder has developed. If the patient has no features of MM or AL and the serum M-protein value is less than 1.5 g/dL, serum protein electrophoresis should be repeated at annual intervals. Bone marrow examination and skeletal radiographs usually are not necessary. If the asymptomatic patient has an M-protein level of 1.5 to 2.0 g/dL, a 24-hour urine specimen should be collected for electrophoresis and immunofixation. The serum protein electrophoretic pattern should be determined again in 3 to 6 months, and if the results are stable, the test should be repeated in 6 months and then annually (sooner if any symptoms occur).

If the IgG or the IgA serum M-protein level is more than 2.0 g/dL, a metastatic bone survey, including views of the humeri and femurs, and a bone marrow aspiration and biopsy should be done. The plasma cell labeling index test, cytogenetic studies, and a search for circulating plasma cells in the peripheral blood should be done if such tests are available. $\beta_2$-microglobulin and C-reactive protein levels also should be determined. If the patient has an IgM protein, aspiration and biopsy of the bone marrow and computed tomography of the abdomen are useful for recognizing macroglobulinemia or a related lymphoproliferative disorder. If results of these tests are satisfactory, serum protein electrophoresis should be repeated in 3 months, and if the results are stable the tests should be repeated at 6- to 12-month intervals. Patients should contact their physicians if there is any change in their clinical condition.

# Association of Monoclonal Gammopathies with Other Diseases

Monoclonal gammopathy is frequently a single abnormality, but it is sometimes associated with other diseases, as expected in an elderly population. The association of 2 diseases depends on the frequency with which each occurs independently. Thus, appropriate epidemiologic and statistical studies, especially valid control populations, should be used in evaluating these associations. Among the multitude of associations that have been reported, the following are the best established.

## Lymphoproliferative Disorders

Azar et al. (1957) reported that 13 patients with malignant lymphoma and chronic lymphocytic leukemia had a serum M-protein. In 1960, Kyle et al. described 6 patients with lymphoma and a serum or urinary M component in the electrophoretic pattern. In another series, an M-protein, predominantly of the IgM type, was found in 10 patients with different chronic lymphoproliferative disorders (Kim et al., 1973). In a large series of 1150 patients with lymphoma or chronic lymphocytic leukemia, an M-protein was found in 49 patients: IgM in 29, IgG in 15, and not typed in 5 (Alexanian, 1975). Among the 292 patients with a nodular histopathologic pattern, 4 had an M-protein (IgG in 3, not typed in 1). Similarly, only 1 of 218 patients with Hodgkin's disease had an IgG M-protein. In contrast, 44 of the 640 subjects with diffuse non-Hodgkin's lymphoma or chronic lymphocytic leukemia had a serum M component (IgM in 29, 4.5%; IgG in 11, 1.7%; and not typed in 4, 0.6%). None of the 510 patients with nodular lymphoma or Hodgkin's disease had an IgM peak, whereas 29 of the 640 patients with a diffuse histopathologic pattern had such a peak. Clinical response to therapy was associated with a reduction in the M-component size to a median of 20% of the pretreatment value (Alexanian, 1975). Ng et al. (1992) confirmed the infrequency of M-proteins in patients with Hodgkin's disease.

Using high-resolution agarose gel electrophoresis followed by immunofixation, Magrath et al. (1983) found an IgM M-protein in 12 of 21 patients with undifferentiated lymphomas of Burkitt and non-Burkitt type in advanced stage (C or D). Cellulose acetate electrophoresis failed to show any of these bands. Interestingly, these proteins disappeared after therapy and reappeared at relapse. Steinberg et al. (1988) reported that 2% of patients with angioimmunoblastic lymphadenopathy had monoclonal gammopathy. Others also have reported the presence of M-proteins in patients with angioimmunoblastic lymphadenopathy (Offit et al., 1986; Schauer et al., 1981). A polyclonal increase in immunoglobulins is much more common than monoclonal gammopathy in angioimmunoblastic lymphadenopathy. Castleman's disease (angiofollicular lymph node hyperplasia) may be associated with a monoclonal gammopathy (Hineman et al., 1982). Sjögren's syndrome has been reported with an IgA monoclonal gammopathy (Sugai et al., 1980). In 2 patients with Sjögren's syndrome and an M-protein, a malignant lymphoma subsequently developed (Humphrey et al., 1982). Ben-Chetrit et al. (1982) reported the presence of monoclonal gammopathy in a patient with Kaposi's sarcoma. Several cases of Kaposi's sarcoma and monoclonal gammopathy have been described (Strumia and Roveggio, 1994).

A serum M component is also present in approximately 5% of patients with chronic lymphocytic leukemia. In a series of 100 patients with this disorder and associated monoclonal gammopathy, the type of serum M component was IgG (51 cases), IgM (38 cases), light chains only (10 cases), and IgA (one case) (Noel and Kyle, 1987). No clinical differences were found depending on whether the patients had an IgG or an IgM M-protein. With the use of immunoisoelectric focusing, an M-protein, predominantly of the IgM type, was found in 34 (61%) of 56 patients with chronic lymphocytic leukemia (Sinclair et al., 1986b). In a series of 70 patients with hairy cell leukemia, 5 had paraproteinemia (Jansen et al., 1983). The coexistence of hairy cell leukemia and MM also has been described (Catovesky et al., 1981). A monoclonal gammopathy of the IgGκ type was found in 3 of 26 patients with adult T-cell leukemia (Matsuzaki et al., 1985). Cutaneous T-cell lymphomas also have been associated with monoclonal gammopathies. Thus, several patients with Sézary's syndrome and mycosis fungoides with associated monoclonal gammopathy have been described (Kövary et al., 1981; Venencie et al., 1984a, 1984b). B-cell acute lymphoblastic leukemia with hairy cell features was reported in a patient with monoclonal κ light chain in the serum and urine (Yetgin et al., 2000).

A series of 430 patients with serum IgM monoclonal gammopathy seen at Mayo Clinic between 1956 and 1978 was reviewed (Kyle and Garton, 1987). The categorization of these patients is shown in Table 19-11. Patients with MGUS had a serum M-protein value less than 3 g/dL and no symptoms or abnormal physical or laboratory findings resulting from the monoclonal gammopathy; they required no initial chemotherapy. Patients with WM had an IgM peak of 3 g/dL or more, together with an increase in lymphocytes or plasmacytoid lymphocytes in the bone marrow. Patients with malignant lymphoproliferative disease could not be assigned to any of the categories listed in Table 19-11 and were characterized by an IgM protein value less than 3 g/dL and bone marrow infiltration by lymphocytes and lymphoplasmacytoid cells; they required therapy because of constitutional symptoms or anemia. As previously mentioned, more than half of the patients had MGUS, and 17% of them subsequently

evolved to a malignant lymphoproliferative process requiring chemotherapy after a median followup of 4 years. The duration of survival of the subset of patients in whom WM developed after IgM MGUS was identical to that in patients with de novo WM.

## Other Hematologic Disorders

Monoclonal gammopathy was found in 6 (13.3%) of 45 patients with refractory anemia with or without excess of blasts (Economopoulus et al., 1985). Polyclonal hypergammaglobulinemia and serum M components have been observed in chronic myelomonocytic leukemia (Barnard et al., 1979; Ribera et al., 1987; Solal-Celigny et al., 1984). Chronic neutrophilic leukemia is a rare disorder characterized by persistent leukocytosis consisting of mature neutrophils, high leukocyte alkaline phosphatase value, and bone marrow granulocytic hyperplasia. In one-third of the patients, it is associated with paraproteinemia or myeloma (Rovira et al., 1990); this high frequency suggests that the association is not merely coincidental. Although the presentation of monoclonal gammopathy and chronic neutrophilic leukemia is usually simultaneous, one case of this disorder preceding the development of MM for 7 years was reported (Rovira et al., 1990). Interestingly, in this patient, the leukocyte counts became normal when myeloma developed. Dührsen et al. (1988) reported a concomitant plasma cell dyscrasia in 3 of 46 patients with idiopathic myelofibrosis, but no instances of monoclonal gammopathy in chronic granulocytic leukemia, polycythemia vera, and unclassifiable myeloproliferative disorders. These authors, reviewing 3 more series, found that the frequency of M components was 8.5% (16 of 188) among patients with idiopathic myelofibrosis.

Chronic myelocytic leukemia (Philadelphia chromosome-positive) and a monoclonal gammopathy were reported in 8 patients. Another case report described a patient with chronic myelocytic leukemia (Ph1+) who had subsequent development of a monocytic blast transformation associated with an IgGλ protein (Buonanno et al., 1986). Although chronic myelocytic leukemia and an M-protein have been reported, it is not known whether an association exists. Nagata et al. (2000) reported a patient with acute myelomonocytic leukemia and IgGκ monoclonal gammopathy. Acute promyelocytic leukemia was reported with an IgGκ M-protein in the serum (Atkins et al., 1989). Pasqualetti and Casale (1997) reported a patient with an IgGκ (2.0 g/dL) M-protein in whom plasma leukemia developed 5 months later. Data are not adequate to determine whether there is an increased incidence of M-protein in patients with leukemia. Three clonal disorders consisting of MGUS, paroxysmal nocturnal hemoglobinuria, and myelodysplastic syndrome that transformed into an acute

---

### TABLE 19-11

## Classification of IgM Monoclonal Gammopathies Among 430 Patients

| Classification | Patients | |
|---|---|---|
| | No. | Percent |
| Monoclonal gammopathy of undetermined significance | 242 | 56 |
| Waldenström's macroglobulinemia | 71 | 17 |
| Lymphoma | 28 | 7 |
| Chronic lymphocytic leukemia | 21 | 5 |
| Primary amyloidosis | 6 | 1 |
| Lymphoproliferative disease | 62 | 14 |
| Total | 430 | 100 |

myeloid leukemia have been reported (Watanabe et al., 2001).

Polyclonal hypergammaglobulinemia and oligoclonal and monoclonal gammopathies have been found in patients with Gaucher's disease (Marie et al., 1982; Marti et al., 1988; Pratt et al., 1968; Schoenfeld et al., 1990). The coexistence of Gaucher's disease and MM also has been reported in several instances (Garfinkel et al., 1982). The IgGκ protein decreased after splenectomy in one patient with Gaucher's disease, a change suggesting a direct relationship (Airó et al., 1993).

Cases of acquired von Willebrand's disease resulting from monoclonal gammopathy have been described (Castaman et al., 1989; Mannucci et al., 1984; Mant et al., 1973). In several cases, a specific interaction between the M component and the antigenic portion of the factor VIII molecule has been demonstrated (Bovill et al., 1986; Mohri et al., 1987). Lamboley et al. (2002) reported 7 new patients with MGUS and acquired von Willebrand's syndrome. An antibody inhibiting von Willebrand's factor was detected in all 7 patients. They noted that intravenous gamma globulin had a longer-lasting effect than did infusion of von Willebrand's factor concentrate. Federici et al. (1998) found that intravenous gamma globulin improved the laboratory abnormalities of bleeding in 8 patients with an IgG M-protein, whereas it was ineffective in 2 patients with an IgMκ M-protein. Severe bleeding may occur from binding of an M-protein by thrombin (Colwell et al., 1997).

Patients with monoclonal gammopathy and lupus anticoagulant activity have been described (Bellotti et al., 1989). An increased incidence of antiphospholipid antibodies has been reported in patients with MGUS (Stern et al., 1994). A patient with hydralazine-induced lupus erythematosus was reported with a transient IgMκ M-protein (Freestone and Ramsay, 1982).

Monoclonal gammopathies have been reported with pernicious anemia (Selroos and von Knorring, 1973). Three of 20 patients in a family with congenital dyserythropoietic anemia type III had an IgGκ M-protein (1 had MM) (Sandström et al., 1994). Six patients with pure red cell aplasia and an M-protein have been reported (Resegotti et al., 1978). Red cell aplasia might be caused by a block in the maturation of the erythroid burst-forming unit, which could be related to the M-protein (Balducci et al., 1984).

## Neurologic Disorders

Isobe and Osserman (1971) reported that 5.4% of 239 patients with MGUS had an associated peripheral neuropathy or myopathy. Conversely, Kelly et al. (1981) found 28 cases (10%) of monoclonal gammopathy in a series of 279 patients with a clinical picture of sensorimotor peripheral neuropathy of unknown cause: MGUS

(16 cases), AL (7 cases), MM (3 cases), WM (1 case), and γ heavy-chain disease (1 case). The type of M component was IgG in 15 cases, IgA in 3, IgM in 4, light chain only in 5, and γ heavy-chain type in 1. In that study, the monoclonal gammopathy was 3 times more common in polyneuropathy of unknown cause than it was in 358 patients with a polyneuropathy resulting from a known cause such as diabetes or alcoholism. In another report, 8 of 19 patients with MGUS had a clinical neuropathy (Vrethem et al., 1993). In an unselected series of patients with MGUS, neuropathy was noted in 2 (6%) of 34 patients with IgG, 2 (14%) of 14 with IgA, and 8 (31%) of 26 with IgM. The neuropathy was subclinical in 6 patients (Nobile-Orazio et al., 1992).

Baldini et al. (1994) reported that 14 of 31 patients with an IgM MGUS had peripheral neuropathy. There is no question that an association exists between MGUS and peripheral neuropathy. The incidence is variable and depends on patient selection bias, the vigor with which the presence of an M-protein is sought, and whether the diagnosis of peripheral neuropathy is made on electrophysiological grounds or clinical features. The association of neuropathies and monoclonal gammopathies has been the subject of excellent reviews (Kissel and Mendell, 1996; Latov, 1995; Ropper and Gorson, 1998).

In one-half of the patients with IgM gammopathy and polyneuropathy, IgM binds to the myelin-associated glycoprotein (MAG) (Hafler et al., 1986; Kelly et al., 1988). IgM M-proteins with anti-MAG activity react with P$_o$, the major glycoprotein of the peripheral myelin (Bollensen et al., 1988). The MAG-reactive polyneuropathies are characterized by a slowly progressive, mainly sensory neuropathy, beginning in the distal extremities and slowly extending proximally over a period of months to years. Motor involvement is less prominent than sensory. Cranial nerves and autonomic functions are characteristically spared. The clinical and electrodiagnostic features are similar to those of chronic inflammatory demyelinating polyneuropathy.

Patients with sensorimotor peripheral neuropathy might have an IgM protein binding to chondroitin sulfate (Freddo et al., 1986; Sherman et al., 1983; Yee et al., 1989), specific gangliosides (Ilyas et al., 1988a; Kusunoki et al., 1989), or glycolipids (Fredman, 1998; Ilyas et al., 1985; Kusunoki et al., 1987). Almost 80% of monoclonal IgM from patients with peripheral neuropathy reacts with some component of the peripheral nerve myelin (Brouet et al., 1990). An extensive review of antibodies associated with peripheral neuropathy has been published (Quarles and Weiss, 1999).

In a series of 40 patients with polyneuropathy associated with an IgM gammopathy, all but 1 had symmetric polyneuropathy. It was predominantly sensory in 13 patients and purely sensory in 17. Demyelination was noted in 83%. Anti-MAG antibodies were found in 65% and were associated only with demyelinating neuropathies (Chassande et al., 1998). In another series of 52 symptomatic patients with IgM monoclonal gammopathies, symptomatic neuropathy occurred in 3 of 4 patients with a high anti-MAG titer and in only 3 of 21 patients with a low anti-MAG titer (Meucci et al., 1999). In a comparison of 19 patients with IgM MGUS and 15 with IgG MGUS (Simovic et al., 1998), distal latencies of the median and ulnar motor nerves were prolonged in IgM MGUS. MAG antibodies failed to distinguish a subgroup of patients with IgM MGUS neuropathy.

The relationship of IgG and IgA M-proteins to peripheral neuropathy is less well documented than IgM-associated neuropathies (Kelly et al., 1987). Read et al. (1978) described 3 patients with an IgG M-protein and peripheral neuropathy. Bleasel et al. (1993) described 5 patients with peripheral neuropathy and IgG MGUS. IgA monoclonal gammopathy also has been reported in several patients with peripheral neuropathy (Bailey et al., 1986; Dhib-Jalbut and Liwnicz, 1986; Simmons et al., 1993a).

The relationship between chronic inflammatory demyelinating polyradiculoneuropathy (CIDP) and CIDP with MGUS is unclear. In a comparison of 77 patients with CIDP and 26 patients with CIDP and MGUS, patients in the latter group had a more indolent course, more frequent sensory loss, and less severe weakness. The outcome in the 2 groups was similar (Simmons et al., 1993b). In a comparison of 45 patients with CIDP and 15 with MGUS-associated neuropathy, the MGUS group had greater imbalance (ataxia), vibration loss in the hands, absent median and ulnar sensory potentials, and less severe muscular weakness (Gorson et al., 1997). In another report, patients with CIDP were more likely to have a relapsing course, whereas those with MGUS had a progressive clinical course. The MGUS group had less severe functional impairment and a lesser degree of weakness and sensory changes than did those with CIDP (Simmons et al., 1995). Alternatively, Maisonobe et al. (1996) found no significant clinical or electrophysiological difference between patients who had CIDP and an M-protein compared with patients who had CIDP. In short, CIDP might occur in any age, motor symptoms tend to predominate over sensory symptoms, there is a greater tendency for the course to be relapsing, and M-proteins are not found.

Hays et al. (1987) produced demyelination of the feline sciatic nerve by the intraneural injection of sera from patients who had IgM reactivity with MAG and an associated neuropathy. Demyelination was greater than that induced by sera from 6 patients with IgM monoclonal gammopathies who were unreactive to MAG (Steck et al., 1987). Demyelination characteristic of the human syndrome was found after injection of monoclonal IgM from patients with IgM peripheral neuropathy and anti-MAG. The report of a brother and sister with IgM monoclonal gammopathy and a demyelinating peripheral neuropathy raises the possibility of a genetic predisposition (Jønsson et al., 1988).

Although the overall results of the treatment of patients with peripheral neuropathy and monoclonal gammopathy have been disappointing, the results achieved in some patients are encouraging. Smith et al. (1987) reported that 9 of 13 patients with peripheral neuropathy and an IgM or IgG M-protein obtained clinical improvement, and 7 had electrophysiological improvement with plasmapheresis and chemotherapy. Hass and Tatum (1988) described a patient with peripheral neuropathy who had anti-MAG IgM protein and was successfully treated with plasmapheresis for more than 1 year. The patient's signs and symptoms correlated with variations in the serum IgM level. High-dose intravenously administered gamma globulin may benefit some patients with CIDP (Faed et al., 1989) and should be tried in patients with sensorimotor peripheral neuropathy and monoclonal gammopathy.

At Mayo Clinic, 39 patients with peripheral neuropathy and MGUS of the IgG, IgA, or IgM type were randomized to plasmapheresis or sham plasmapheresis in a double-blind trial (Dyck et al., 1991). In that study, plasma exchange significantly prevented worsening or ameliorated the neuropathy. Patients with IgG or IgA gammopathy had a better response to plasma exchange than those with IgM gammopathy. Plasma exchange produced benefit in 8 of 13 patients with monoclonal gammopathy and peripheral neuropathy (Mazzi et al., 1999).

Chlorambucil can be given to patients who do not respond to plasmapheresis when the M-protein is of the IgM type, or melphalan and prednisone can be used for IgG and IgA gammopathies. In a randomized study, 44 patients with an IgM M-protein and peripheral neuropathy received either chlorambucil orally or chlorambucil plus 15 courses of plasma exchange during the first 4 months of therapy. No difference was noted in the 2 treatment groups, which suggested that plasma exchange added no benefit to chlorambucil therapy (Oksenhendler et al., 1995). Notermans et al. (1996) reported that cyclophosphamide and prednisone produced benefit in 8 of 16 patients with monoclonal gammopathy and sensorimotor peripheral neuropathy.

Sherman et al. (1994) reported that fludarabine, a purine analogue, produced benefit in 7 of 10 patients with an IgM M-protein and neuropathy. In another report, 3 of 4 patients with an IgM M-protein and peripheral neuropathy had clinical and neurophysiological benefit from fludarabine (Wilson et al., 1999). Rituximab (Rituxan), a monoclonal antibody directed against CD20, produced benefit in all 5 patients with an

IgM M-protein and neuropathy (Levine and Pestronk, 1999). A randomized study comparing intravenous immunoglobulin and placebo followed by a crossover study revealed increased strength in 2 patients and improved sensorineuropathy in 1 other. Thus, fewer than 20% of patients obtained benefit (Dalakas et al., 1996).

Other neurologic disorders such as amyotrophic lateral sclerosis and progressive muscular atrophy have been reported with monoclonal gammopathies, but the association may be merely coincidental (Kyle and Lust, 1991). Of 120 patients with motor neuron disease, 11 (9%) had an associated M-protein: 10 had amyotrophic lateral sclerosis and 1 had progressive spinal muscular atrophy (Younger et al., 1990). Desai and Swash (1999) reported a patient with primary lateral sclerosis and IgM monoclonal gammopathy. Nemaline (rod) myopathy has been reported with an IgGκ monoclonal gammopathy (Deconinck et al., 2000).

Ataxia–telangiectasia, characterized by cerebellar ataxia, oculocutaneous telangiectasia, and both B- and T-lymphocyte deficiency, has been reported with monoclonal gammopathy (McDonald et al., 1998). Sadighi Akha et al. (1999) reported that 7 of 86 patients with ataxia–telangiectasia had gammopathy (monoclonal 3, biclonal 3, and triclonal 1).

## Osteosclerotic Myeloma (POEMS Syndrome)

POEMS syndrome is characterized by polyneuropathy, organomegaly, endocrinopathy, M-protein, and skin changes (Bardwick et al., 1980; Dispenzieri et al., in press; Driedger and Pruzanski, 1979; Kelly et al., 1983; Kyle and Dyck, 1993; Takatsuki and Sanada, 1983). The typical clinical features are chronic inflammatory demyelinating polyneuropathy, more motor than sensory, and sclerotic skeletal lesions. Cranial nerves are not involved except for the presence of papilledema, and autonomic functions are intact. Hepatomegaly is noted in one-half of the patients, and splenomegaly and lymphadenopathy may occur. Hyperpigmentation, hypertrichosis, angiomatous lesions on the trunk, gynecomastia, and testicular atrophy might be present. IgA is common, and most patients have a λ light chain. The M-component value (usually of the λ type) is almost always less than 3 g/dL, and the bone marrow aspirate usually contains less than 5% plasma cells. In contrast to MM (Kyle et al., 2003), the hemoglobin level is normal or increased, thrombocytosis is common, and hypercalcemia and renal insufficiency rarely occur. Biopsy of an osteosclerotic lesion is generally necessary to confirm the diagnosis. Patients with POEMS syndrome have higher levels of IL-1β, tumor necrosis factor-α, IL-6 (Gherardi et al., 1996), and vascular endothelial growth factor (Watanabe et al., 1998).

Single or multiple osteosclerotic lesions in a limited area should be treated with radiation in tumoricidal dosages of 40 to 50 cGy. Improvement occurs in more than one-half of patients, but it may be slow and require 2 to 3 years for maximum benefit. If the patient has widespread osteosclerotic lesions, systemic therapy is necessary. Five of 6 patients treated with melphalan and prednisone improved (Kuwabara et al., 1997). Autologous stem cell transplantation followed by high-dose melphalan therapy appears promising for younger patients with widespread osteosclerotic lesions (Dispenzieri et al., 2001b; Jaccard et al., 2002). Corticosteroids and plasma exchange generally have been of little benefit. Prognosis is better than in patients with typical MM.

## Dermatologic Diseases

Lichen myxedematosus (papular mucinosis, scleromyxedema), which is an uncommon disease characterized by dermal papules, macules, and plaques infiltrating the skin, is frequently associated with a cathodal IgGλ protein (James et al., 1967), although cases of an IgGκ M component also have been described (Danby et al., 1976). Skin biopsy shows a deposition of acid mucopolysaccharides. Scleredema (scleredema adultorum of Buschke) is another rare dermatologic disorder characterized by skin induration, which also has been found associated with monoclonal gammopathies (McFadden et al., 1987; Ohta et al., 1987). Hyperpigmentation and hyperlipoproteinemia also have been noted in scleredema associated with an IgG monoclonal gammopathy (McFadden et al., 1987).

Pyoderma gangrenosum is an unusual ulcerative disease of the skin that has been associated with several diseases (Powell et al., 1983b). The association of pyoderma gangrenosum and monoclonal gammopathy also is well established. Of 67 patients with pyoderma gangrenosum seen at Mayo Clinic over 12 years, 8 (11.9%) had monoclonal gammopathy (Powell et al., 1983b). In 7 of these 8 patients, the dermatologic process preceded the detection of the monoclonal gammopathy; 7 patients had an IgA M-protein. The high preponderance of IgA monoclonal gammopathy in this disease also has been reported by others (Holt et al., 1980; Sluis, 1966). Pyoderma gangrenosum may involve the oropharyngeal area (Setterfield et al., 2001). Rapidly progressive renal failure also has been noted in a patient with pyoderma gangrenosum (Akatsuka et al., 1997). In one series, necrobiotic xanthogranuloma was associated with IgG monoclonal gammopathy in 16 (73%) of 22 cases (Finan and Winkelmann, 1986; Mehregan and Winkelmann, 1992; Nestle et al., 1999). Discoid lupus erythematosus also has been reported to be associated with monoclonal gammopathies (Powell et al., 1983a). Monoclonal gammopathy has been found in patients with diffuse plane xanthomatosis (Bérard et al., 1986; Jones et al., 1979; Stockman et al., 2002) and in patients with psoriasis (Humbert et al., 1987). Schnitzler's syndrome, characterized by chronic urticaria and IgM monoclonal gammopathy, has been reported in 36 cases in the literature (Puddu et al., 1997). Subcorneal pustular dermatosis has been found with monoclonal gammopathy (Ryatt et al., 1981). In a report of 10 patients with subcorneal pustular dermatosis, an IgA M-protein was found in 3 and an IgG M-protein in 1 of the 7 patients in whom electrophoresis was performed (Lutz et al., 1998). Erythema elevatum diutinum has been reported with monoclonal gammopathy (Chowdhury et al., 2002; Dowd and Munro, 1983; Kavanagh et al., 1993). A comprehensive review of monoclonal gammopathies and skin disorders has been published (Daoud et al., 1999). The association between monoclonal gammopathies and cutaneous lymphomas has been discussed.

## Monoclonal Gammopathies and Immunosuppression

M-proteins have been found in association with acquired immunodeficiency syndrome (AIDS). In one small series, more than one-half of the patients with AIDS or lymphadenopathy syndrome had an M-protein in their sera (Heriot et al., 1985). In another series, 4 of 65 homosexual men with antibodies against human immunodeficiency virus (HIV) had a monoclonal gammopathy (Crapper et al., 1987). In a more recent series, 11 of 341 asymptomatic HIV-positive patients had a serum M-protein (Lefrère et al., 1993). In that study, after a median followup of 50 months (range, 19–69 m), the M-protein disappeared in 7 patients and persisted in the remaining 4. Finally, the presence of an M-protein in patients with asymptomatic HIV infection does not seem to influence the patient's outcome (Lefrère et al., 1993).

Hammarström and Smith (1987) reported the appearance of transient monoclonal gammopathies in 18 (43%) of 42 patients who underwent bone marrow transplantation. More recently, transient oligoclonal and monoclonal gammopathies were found in 31 (51.6%) of 60 patients who received an allogeneic (57 patients) or syngeneic (3 patients) bone marrow transplant. The monoclonal gammopathy appeared an average of 3 months after transplantation (range, 27–336 days) and persisted for approximately 6 months (range, 27–652 days) (Mitus et al., 1989). No association with patient age, sex, diagnosis, and type of prophylaxis for graft-versus-host disease was found. However, the development of graft-versus-host disease correlated strongly with the appearance of M-proteins. In both series, the most frequent immunoglobulin type was IgG (Hammarström and Smith, 1987; Mitus et al., 1989).

Gerritsen et al. (1993) reported that M-proteins appeared as early as 6 weeks after bone marrow transplantation in children. In another series (Zent et al., 1998) abnormal protein bands developed in 10% of 550 patients receiving an autologous stem cell transplant for MM. Forty-eight additional patients had oligoclonal bands and 23 had an isotope switch. It was thought that the isotope switch was the result of recovery of immunoglobulin production rather than recurrence of myeloma (Zent et al., 1998). Allogeneic bone marrow transplantation was associated with an M-protein in 12 of 47 patients. Eleven of the 12 patients had had a cytomegalovirus infection (Hebart et al., 1996).

Monoclonal gammopathies have been reported after liver transplantation. Twenty-eight percent of 201 patients had an M-protein after liver transplantation. Five of 7 in whom a posttransplantation lymphoproliferative disorder developed had an M-protein, whereas only 27% of 194 patients without posttransplantation lymphoproliferative syndrome had an M-protein (Badley et al., 1996). Pageaux et al. (1998) found M-proteins in 26 of 86 liver transplant recipients. In a series of 88 patients receiving a liver transplant, there was no difference in the incidence of M-proteins between those receiving cyclosporin A and those receiving FK506 (tacrolimus immunosuppression) (Pham et al., 1998). M-proteins have been reported in recipients of heart transplants, but they were small, transient, and of little clinical importance (Myara et al., 1991). Caforio et al. (2001) found a monoclonal protein in 25% of 308 patients undergoing heart transplantation. The incidence increased with older age. Frequent rejection episodes and immunosuppression played a role. The importance of posttransplantation MGUS is not completely known. Rostaing et al. (1994) found that the M-protein value increased after transplantation in 3 of 5 patients with MGUS. Smoldering myeloma developed in 2 of the 3 patients. In a patient in whom an IgGκ M-protein was recognized after kidney transplantation, AL developed 10 years later. More data are needed on posttransplantation monoclonal gammopathies (Dysseleer et al., 1999).

Monoclonal gammopathy was detected in 18 (12.7%) of 141 patients in whom renal transplantation was performed, the gammopathy being transient in 7 of them (Renoult et al., 1988). In another series (Radl et al., 1985), 70 (30%) of 232 patients who were receiving immunosuppressive therapy after renal transplantation were found to have monoclonal gammopathy. This incidence was 10 times greater than in a control group of 30 patients with chronic renal insufficiency in a dialysis program. Also in that series, the frequency of monoclonal gammopathy was age-related. In 74% of the 23 patients in whom a longitudinal study was available, the monoclonal gammopathy was transient.

These facts suggest that the immunosuppression leads to a temporary immunodeficiency state very similar to that observed with aging of the immune system (Radl et al., 1985). In 2 other series, an M component was found after renal transplantation in 3.6% (4 of 110) (Pollock et al., 1989) and 12.2% (26 of 213) (Stanko et al., 1989) of patients. In a study of 80 pediatric patients who had kidney transplantations, 57% of those with a cytomegalovirus infection had an M-protein, whereas only 8% without a cytomegalovirus infection had monoclonal gammopathy (Ginevri et al., 1998). An M-protein was found in 30% of 182 patients who had renal transplantation. The M-protein was thought to be a reflection of the T-cell immune defect (Ducloux et al., 1999).

## Monoclonal Gammopathies with Antibody Activity

An extensive overview on monoclonal gammopathies with antibody activity was published by Merlini et al. (1986). In patients with MGUS, MM, or macroglobulinemia, the M-protein has shown specificity against red blood cell polysaccharide membrane, acid polysaccharides such as those present on bacterial cells or animal tissues, dextran, antistreptolysin O, antistaphylolysin, antinuclear antibody, riboflavin, von Willebrand factor, thyroglobulin, insulin, single- and double-stranded DNA, apolipoprotein, thyroxine, cephalin, lactate dehydrogenase, anti-HIV, platelet glycoprotein IIIa, transferrin, seroalbumin, $\alpha_2$-macroglobulin, cardiolipin, chondroitin sulfate, group A streptococci, rubeola, cytomegalovirus, and antibiotics (Kyle and Lust, 1991; Merlini et al., 1986).

In a series of 612 patients with monoclonal gammopathy, 36 (5.9%) had a serum M component with antibody activity (Dighiero et al., 1983): 32 had antibodies against actin, and 4 against tubulin, myosin, thyroglobulin, and double-stranded DNA (one case each). Of the 31 patients for whom the clinical data were available, the presence of antibody activity had no clinical consequences. Twenty-six patients had a malignant plasma cell or lymphoproliferative disorder and 5 had MGUS. Eight of 70 monoclonal IgG gammopathies showed significant anti-DNA activity (Williams et al., 1997).

Farhangi and Osserman (1976) reported a patient with MM and xanthodermaxanthotrichia (unusually bright yellow coloration of the skin and hair) caused by an IgGλ M-protein with antiriboflavin antibody activity. Interestingly, the xanthoderma and xanthotrichia disappeared when the IgG level was reduced from 9.8 g/dL to less than 2 g/dL with melphalan therapy (Farhangi and Osserman, 1976). Another case with similar clinical and laboratory features also was recognized (Merlini et al., 1990).

The binding of calcium by M-protein may cause an increase in the total serum calcium level without pathologic consequences because the ionized calcium is normal (Merlini et al., 1984). This possibility should be considered to avoid treating patients for hypercalcemia (Annesly et al., 1982; Merlini et al., 1984). Pseudohypercalcemia was found because the IgM M-protein caused interference in the Aresenazo III dye binding method in 2 patients (Rhys et al., 1997). Copper-binding M-protein was recognized in 2 patients with MM (Baker and Hultquist, 1978), and hypercupremia was found in a patient with a benign IgGλ monoclonal gammopathy (Martin et al., 1983). A 10-fold increase in the serum copper level resulting from binding to a monoclonal IgGκ gammopathy produced deposition of copper on Descemet's membrane and the lens capsule (Probst et al., 1996). Pettersson et al. (1987) described a patient with an IgGκ protein that bound phosphate, which caused a false increase in the serum phosphorus level. Another cause of spurious hyperphosphatemia in monoclonal gammopathies, especially in IgG myeloma, is the interference of the M component with the phosphate chromogenic assay (Sonnenblick et al., 1986).

## Other Reported Associations

Several other diseases have been reported as having an association with MGUS. Because MGUS is common in the general population, whether these relationships are mere coincidence is unclear. We are currently pursuing a large population-based study to answer this question.

The association of monoclonal gammopathy and hyperparathyroidism has been reported (Dexter et al., 1972; Schnur et al., 1977). In 911 patients with hyperparathyroidism who were 50 years or older, immunoelectrophoresis demonstrated an M-protein in 9 patients (1%) (Mundis and Kyle, 1982). In another report, 4 of 386 patients with primary hyperparathyroidism had MGUS (Rao et al., 1991). In a recent report, 20 of 101 patients with hyperparathyroidism but only 2 of 127 control subjects had an M-protein (Arnulf et al., 2002). Thus, there is controversy concerning the association of hyperparathyroidism and MGUS.

Rheumatoid arthritis (Goldberg et al., 1969; Zawadzki and Benedek, 1969) and inflammatory seronegative polyarthritis (Hurst et al., 1987) have been reported to be associated with monoclonal gammopathies. MGUS was reported in 4 of 120 patients with systemic lupus erythematosus (Porcel et al., 1992). An M-protein was found in 1.3% of 555 cases of ankylosing spondylitis, but this incidence is similar to that expected in a normal population (Renier et al., 1992). Four patients with an IgGκ protein and polymyositis have been reported (Kiprov and Miller,

1984; Telerman-Toppet et al., 1982). In 3 of these patients, examination of muscle biopsy specimens with immunofluorescence disclosed linear deposits of IgGκ along the sarcolemmal basement membrane (Kiprov and Miller, 1984). Approximately 12 patients with an M-protein and polymyalgia rheumatica have been reported (Ilfeld et al., 1985; Kalra and Delamere, 1987). However, because monoclonal gammopathies and polymyalgia rheumatica occur typically in an older population, the causal relationship is doubtful.

Three patients with polymyositis and an IgGκ M-protein have been described (Kiprov and Miller, 1984). Dalakas et al. (1997) found an M-protein in 16 (23%) of 70 patients with inclusion body myositis. IgG accounted for 81% of the M-proteins. The association of scleroderma with an IgGκ M-protein and the subsequent development of MM have been reported (Nakanishi et al., 1989).

A patient with myelodysplasia and relapsing polychondritis who had a small IgMκ M-protein has been described (Banerjee et al., 2001). Fervenza et al. (1999) described a patient with recurrent Goodpasture's syndrome and an IgAκ M-protein.

Several cases of myasthenia gravis with a serum M component have been described (Soppi et al., 1985). In addition, one case of acute, rapidly fatal rhabdomyolysis associated with κ light-chain myeloma has been reported (Fernández-Solá et al., 1987). In that case, both the κ light-chain deposition in the sarcolemma, demonstrated by immunofluorescence, and the sarcolemmal damage, observed at the ultrastructural examination, suggested a pathogenetic mechanism between the κ light chain and rhabdomyolysis.

Angioneurotic edema caused by an acquired deficiency of C1-esterase inhibitor has been associated with monoclonal gammopathies. In the review by Gelfand et al. (1979), 5 of 15 patients had a serum IgM M-protein. Pascual et al. (1987) reported 2 patients with acquired C1-esterase inhibitor deficiency with recurrent episodes of panniculitis and hepatitis and an IgGκ M-protein. In another report, 12 of 19 patients with acquired angioedema type II had an MGUS (IgG in 4, IgA in 4, and IgM in 4). Two of the 12 patients had a lymphoma, and the remainder had MGUS. All but one patient had an M-protein of the same heavy-chain and light-chain isotype as the acquired antibody inhibitor. A patient with acquired inhibitor of the first component of complement (C1-INH) deficiency and an IgAκ M-protein that inactivated C1-INH also has been described (van Spronsen et al., 1998).

In a review of the literature, all 21 patients with capillary leak syndrome had a serum M-protein (IgGκ in 12, IgGλ in 7, IgA in 1, IgG in 1) (Droder et al., 1992).

Chronic liver disease is generally associated with polyclonal hypergammaglobulinemia, probably related to a persistent antigenic stimulation of the reticuloendothelial system (Feizi, 1968; Slavin et al., 1974; Zawadzki and Edwards, 1970). However, both chronic hepatitis and cirrhosis occasionally have been associated with monoclonal gammopathies (Slavin et al., 1974; Zawadzki and Edwards, 1970). Heer et al. (1984) found an M-protein in 11 of 31 patients with chronic active hepatitis who had either an M-protein spike or hypergammaglobulinemia on the serum electrophoretic pattern. In the same study, serum immunoelectrophoresis was performed in 50 randomly selected patients with chronic active hepatitis and no evidence of an M-protein spike on serum electrophoresis. In 13 (26%) of them, a monoclonal component was detected, the type of M-protein usually being IgG or IgM. M-proteins and MM also have been reported in patients with primary biliary cirrhosis (Bladé et al., 1981; Hendrick et al., 1986).

There is an association of hepatitis C virus (HCV) and monoclonal gammopathies. Sixty-nine percent of 94 patients with mixed cryoglobulinemia were HCV-positive, but only 14% of 107 without cryoglobulinemia were positive (Mussini et al., 1995). In another series, HCV infection was found in 16% of 102 patients with MM, macroglobulinemia, or MGUS, but only 5% of control subjects were HCV-positive (Mangia et al., 1996). An M-protein was found in 11% of 239 HCV-positive patients but in only 1% of 98 HCV-negative patients. Both HCV-positive and HCV-negative patients had chronic liver disease (Andreone et al., 1998). An increased prevalence of monoclonal gammopathy in association with carcinoma of the colon has been reported several times. However, in 2 large studies the prevalence of monoclonal gammopathies was no greater than that expected in a similar population (Migliorie and Alexanian, 1968; Talerman and Haije, 1973).

Many other conditions have been reported in patients with MGUS, such as Schönlein-Henoch purpura, bacterial endocarditis, Hashimoto's thyroiditis, septic arthritis, purpura fulminans, idiopathic pulmonary fibrosis, pulmonary alveolar proteinosis, idiopathic pulmonary hemosiderosis, sarcoidosis, thymoma, hereditary spherocytosis, and hyperlipidemia. However, the relationship of monoclonal gammopathy to these diseases is not clear and might well be fortuitous.

Active glomerular lesions consisting of epithelial crescents and a rapidly progressive glomerulonephritis have been reported with monoclonal gammopathy (Meyrier et al., 1984). The association of proliferative glomerulonephritis with monoclonal gammopathy has been recognized in 25 cases (Kebler et al., 1985), but the causal relationship is unknown.

We are not aware of any well-documented instances in which surgical removal of a nonhematologic tumor resulted in the disappearance of an M-protein. Chen and Carroll (1980) reported one case in which an IgG M-protein in the serum and urine disappeared 2 years after surgical removal of a carcinoma of the colon. However, the M-protein in the serum and urine was first recognized 2 months after operation, indicating that the tumor did not produce the M-protein.

The association of MGUS and silicone breast implants is controversial. Karlson et al. (2001) reported MGUS in 5 of 288 women with silicone breast implants and in 4 of 288 women without implants. Two patients with IgG MGUS had corneal crystal deposition (Hutchinson et al., 1998). The risk of bacteremia may be increased in MGUS. Gregersen et al. (1998) reported 40 episodes of bacteremia in 5500 person-years of followup compared with 18 episodes in the control population. They concluded that the overall risk is small and does not affect management of MGUS.

# Acknowledgments

This work was supported in part by Spanish grants from Fondo de Investigaciones Sanitarias de la Seguridad Social FISss 92/5462 and FISss 96/0397 and CA 62242 from the National Institutes of Health.

## REFERENCES

Abe, M., Hiura, K., Wilde, J., Moriyama, K., Hashimoto, T., Ozaki, S., Wakatsuki, S., Kosaka, M., Kido, S., Inoue, D., and Matsumoto, T. (2002). Role for macrophage inflammatory protein (MIP)-1alpha and MIP-1beta in the development of osteolytic lesions in multiple myeloma. *Blood, 100*, 2195–2202.

Aguzzi, F., Bergami, M. R., Gasparro, C., Bellotti, V., and Merlini, G. (1992). Occurrence of monoclonal components in general practice: clinical implications. *European Journal of Haematology, 48*, 192–195.

Airó, R., Gabusi, G., and Guindani, M. (1993). Gaucher's disease associated with monoclonal gammopathy of undetermined significance: a case report. *Haematologica, 78*, 129–131.

Akatsuka, T., Kawata, T., Hashimoto, S., Nakamura, S., and Koike, T. (1997). Rapidly progressive renal failure occurring in the course of pyoderma gangrenosum and IgA (lambda) monoclonal gammopathy. *Internal Medicine, 36*, 40–43.

Alexanian, R. (1975). Monoclonal gammopathy in lymphoma. *Archives of Internal Medicine, 135*, 62–66.

Andreone, P., Zignego, A. L., Cursaro, C., Gramenzi, A., Gherlinzoni, F., Fiorino, S., Giannini, C., Boni, P., Sabattini, E., Pileri, S., Tura, S., and Bernardi, M. (1998). Prevalence of monoclonal gammopathies in patients with hepatitis C virus infection. *Annals of Internal Medicine, 129*, 294–298.

Annesly, T. M., Burritt, M. F., and Kyle, R. A. (1982). Artifactual hypercalcemia in multiple myeloma. *Mayo Clinic Proceedings, 57*, 572–575.

Arnulf, B., Bengoufa, D., Sarfati, E., Toubert, M. E., Meignin, V., Brouet, J. C., and Fermand, J. P. (2002). Prevalence of monoclonal gammopathy in patients with primary hyperparathyroidism: a prospective study. *Archives of Internal Medicine, 162*, 464–467.

Atkins, H., Drouin, J., Izaguirre, C. A., and Sengar, D. S. (1989). Acute promyelocytic leukemia associated with a paraprotein that reacts with leukemic cells. *Cancer, 63*, 1750–1751.

Avet-Loiseau, H., Daviet, A., Sauner, S., and Bataille, R. (2000). Chromosome 13 abnormalities in multiple myeloma are mostly monosomy 13. *British Journal of Haematology, 111*, 1116–1117.

Avet-Loiseau, H., Facon, T., Daviet, A., Godon, C., Rapp, M. J., Harousseau, J. L., Grosbois, B., and Bataille, R. (1999a). 14q32 translocations and monosomy 13 observed in monoclonal gammopathy of undetermined significance delineate a multistep process for the oncogenesis of multiple myeloma: Intergroupe Francophone du Myelome. *Cancer Research, 59*, 4546–4550.

Avet-Loiseau, H., Li, J. Y., Facon, T., Brigaudeau, C., Morineau, N., Maloisel, F., Rapp, M. J., Talmant, P., Trimoreau, F., Jaccard, A., Harousseau, F. L., and Bataille, R. (1998). High incidence of translocations t(11;14)(q13;q32) and t(4;14)(p16;q32) in patients with plasma cell malignancies. *Cancer Research, 58*, 5640–5645.

Avet-Loiseau, H., Li, J. Y., Morineau, N., Facon, T., Brigaudeau, C., Harousseau, J. L., Grosbois, B., and Bataille, R. (1999b). Monosomy 13 is associated with the transition of monoclonal gammopathy of undetermined significance to multiple myeloma: Intergroupe Francophone du Myelome. *Blood, 94*, 2583–2589.

Axelsson, U. (1986). A 20-year follow-up study of 64 subjects with M-components. *Acta Medica Scandinavica, 219*, 519–522.

Axelsson, U., Bachmann, R., and Hällen, J. (1966). Frequency of pathological proteins (M-components) in 6995 sera from an adult population. *Acta Medica Scandinavica, 179*, 235–247.

Azar, H. A., Hill, W. T., and Osserman, E. F. (1957). Malignant lymphoma and lymphocytic leukemia associated with myeloma-type serum proteins. *American Journal of Medicine, 23*, 239–249.

Badley, A. D., Portela, D. F., Patel, R., Kyle, R. A., Habermann, T. M., Strickler, J. G., Ilstrup, D. M., Wiesner, R. H., de Groen, P., Walker, R. C., and Paya, C. V. (1996). Development of monoclonal gammopathy precedes the development of Epstein-Barr virus-induced posttransplant lymphoproliferative disorder. *Liver Transplant and Surgery: Official Publication of the American Association for the Study of Liver Diseases and the International Liver Transplantation Society, 2*, 375–382.

Bailey, R. O., Ritaccio, A. L., Bishop, M. B., and Wu, A. Y. (1986). Benign monoclonal IgAκ gammopathy associated with polyneuropathy and dysautonomia. *Acta Neurolgica Scandinavica, 73*, 574–580.

Baker, B. L., and Hultquist, D. E. (1978). A copper-binding immunoglobulin from a myeloma patient: purification, identification, and physical characteristics. *Journal of Biological Chemistry, 253*, 1195–1200.

Baldini, L., Guffanti, A., Cesana, B. M., Colombi, M., Chiorboli, O., Damilano, I., and Maiolo, A. T. (1996). Role of different hematologic variables in defining the risk of malignant transformation in monoclonal gammopathy. *Blood, 87*, 912–918.

Baldini, L., Nobile-Orazio, E., Guffanti, A., Barbieri, S., Carpo, M., Cro, L., Cesana, B., Damilano, I., and Maiolo, A. T. (1994). Peripheral neuropathy in IgM monoclonal gammopathy and Waldenström's macroglobulinemia: a frequent complication in elderly males with low MAG-reactive serum monoclonal component. *American Journal of Hematology, 45*, 25–31.

Balducci, L., Hardy, C., Dreiling, B., Tavassoli, M., and Steinberg, M. H. (1984). Pure red blood cell aplasia associated with paraproteinemia: in vitro studies of erythropoiesis. *Haematologia, 17*, 353–357.

Banerjee, S. S., Morris, D. P., Rothera, M. P., and Routledge, R. C. (2001). Relapsing polychondritis associated with monoclonal gammopathy in a patient with myelodysplastic syndrome. *Journal of Laryngology and Otology, 115*, 482–484.

Bardwick, P. A., Zvaifler, N. J., Gill, G. N., Newman, D., Greenway, G. D., and Resnick, D. L. (1980). Plasma cell dyscrasia with polyneuropathy, organomegaly, endocrinopathy, M protein, and skin changes: the POEMS syndrome. Report on two cases and a review of the literature. *Medicine (Baltimore), 59*, 311–322.

Barnard, D. L., Burns, G. F., Gordon, J., Cawley, J. C., Barker, C. R., Hayhoe, F. G. J., and Smith, J. L. (1979). Chronic myelomonocytic leukemia with paraproteinemia but no detectable plasmacytosis: a detailed cytological and immunological study. *Cancer, 44*, 927–936.

Bataille, R., Chappard, D., and Basle, M. F. (1996). Quantifiable excess of bone resorption in monoclonal gammopathy is an early symptom of malignancy: a prospective study of 87 bone biopsies. *Blood, 87*, 4762–4769.

Bataille, R., Chappard, D., and Klein, B. (1992). Mechanisms of bone lesions in multiple myeloma. *Hematology/Oncology Clinics of North America, 6*, 285–295.

Bataille, R., Chappard, D., Marcelli, C., Dessauw, P., Baldet, P., Sany, J., and Alexandre, C. (1991). Recruitment of new osteoblasts and osteoclasts is the earliest critical event in the pathogenesis of human multiple myeloma. *Journal of Clinical Investigation, 88*, 62–66.

Bataille, R., Jourdan, M., Zhang, X.-G., and Klein, B. (1989). Serum levels of interleukin 6, a potent myeloma cell growth factor, as a reflection of disease severity in plasma cell dyscrasias. *Journal of Clinical Investigation, 84*, 2008–2011.

Belisle, L. M., Case, D. C., Jr., and Neveux, L. (1990). Quantitation of risk of malignant transformation in patients with 'benign' monoclonal gammopathy (BMG) [Abstract]. *Blood, 76*(Suppl 1), 342a.

Bellaiche, L., Laredo, J. D., Liote, F., Koeger, A. C., Hamze, B., Ziza, J. M., Pertuiset, E., Bardin, T., and Tubiana, J. M. (1997). Magnetic resonance appearance of monoclonal gammopathies of unknown significance and multiple myeloma: the GRI Study Group. *Spine, 22*, 2551–2557.

Bellotti, V., Gamba, G., Merlini, G., Montani, N., Bucciarelli, E., Stoppini, M., and Ascari, E. (1989). Study of three patients with monoclonal gammopathies and 'lupus-like' anticoagulants. *British Journal of Haematology, 73*, 221–227.

Ben-Chetrit, E., Ben-Amitai, D., and Levo, Y. (1982). The association between Kaposi's sarcoma and dysgammaglobulinemia. *Cancer, 49*, 1649–1651.

Bérard, M., Antonucci, M., and Beaumont, J.-L. (1986). Cytotoxic effect of serum on fibroblasts in one case of normolipidemic plane xanthoma and myeloma IgGλ. *Atherosclerosis, 62*, 111–115.

Berg, A. R., Weisenburger, D. D., Linder, J., and Armitage, J. O. (1986). Lymphoplasmacytic lymphoma: report of a case with three monoclonal proteins derived from a single neoplastic clone. *Cancer, 57*, 1794–1797.

Bergsagel, P. L., Chesi, M., Nardini, E., Brents, L. A., Kirby, S. L., and Kuehl, W. M. (1996). Promiscuous translocations into immunoglobulin heavy chain switch regions in multiple myeloma. *Proceedings of the National Academy of Sciences of the United States of America, 93*, 13931–13936.

Bergsagel, P. L., Nardini, E., Brents, L., Chesi, M., and Kuehl, W. M. (1997). IgH translocations in multiple myeloma: a nearly universal event that rarely involves c-myc. *Current Topics in Microbiology and Immunology, 224*, 283–287.

Bernasconi, P., Cavigliano, P. M., Boni, M., Astori, C., Calatroni, S., Giardini, I., Rocca, B., Caresana, M., Crosetto, N., Lazzarino, M., and Bernasconi, C. (2002). Long-term followup with conventional cytogenetics and band 13q14 interphase/metaphase in situ hybridization monitoring in monoclonal gammopathies of undetermined significance. *British Journal of Haematology, 118*, 545–549.

Billadeau, D., Van Ness, B., Kimlinger, T., Kyle, R. A., Therneau, T. M., Greipp, P. R., and Witzig, T. E. (1996). Clonal circulating cells are common in plasma cell proliferative disorders: a comparison of monoclonal gammopathy of undetermined significance, smoldering multiple myeloma, and active myeloma. *Blood, 88*, 289–296.

Bladé, J., and Kyle, R. A. (1994). IgD monoclonal gammopathy with long-term followup. *British Journal of Haematology, 88*, 395–396.

Bladé, J., Lopez-Guillermo, A., Gozman, C., Cervantes, F., Salgado, C., Aguilar, J.-L., Vives-Corrons, J.-L., and Montserrat, E. (1992). Malignant transformation and life expectancy in monoclonal gammopathy of undetermined significance. *British Journal of Haematology, 81*, 391–394.

Bladé, J., Montserrat, E., Bruguera, M., Aranalde, J., Grañena, A., Cervantes, F., and Rozman, C. (1981). Multiple myeloma in primary biliary cirrhosis. *Scandinavian Journal of Haematology, 26*, 14–18.

Bladé, J., Rozman, C., Montserrat, E., Grañena, A., Brugués, R., Cervantes, F., et al. (1984). Mieloma múltiple: descripción de una serie de 170 casos. *Medicina Clinica (Barcelona), 82*, 287–294.

Bleasel, A. F., Hawke, S. H., Pollard, J. D., McLeod, J. G. (1993). IgG monoclonal paraproteinaemia and peripheral neuropathy. *Journal of Neurology, Neurosurgery, and Psychiatry, 56*, 52–57.

Bollensen, E., Steck, A. J., and Schachner, M. (1988). Reactivity with the peripheral myelin glycoprotein P$_0$ in serum from patients with monoclonal IgM gammopathy and polyneuropathy. *Neurology, 38*, 1266–1270.

Bovill, E. G., Ershler, W. B., Golden, E. A., Tindle, B. H., and Edson, J. R. (1986). A human myeloma-produced monoclonal protein directed against the active subpopulations of von Willebrand factor. *American Journal of Clinical Pathology, 85*, 115–123.

Bowden, M., Crawford, J., Cohen, H. J., and Noyama, O. (1993). A comparative study of monoclonal gammopathies and immunoglobulin levels in Japanese and United States elderly. *Journal of the American Geriatric Society, 41*, 11–14.

Brouet, J. C., Danon, F., Mihaesco, E., Bussel, A., and Oksenhendler, E. (1990). Peripheral polyneuropathies associated with monoclonal IgM: antibody activity of monoclonal IgM and therapeutic implications. *Nouvelle Revue Française d' Hematologie, 32*, 307–310.

Brown, L. M., Linet, M. S., Greenberg, R. S., Silverman, D. T., Hayes, R. B., Swanson, G. M., Schwartz, A. G., Schoenberg, J. B., Pottern, L. M., and Fraumeni, J. F., Jr. (1999). Multiple myeloma and family history of cancer among blacks and whites in the U.S. *Cancer, 85*, 2385–2390.

Buonanno, G., Pandolfi, F., Valente, A., Napolitano, M., Cafaro, A., and Gonnella, F. (1986). Monocytic blast cell crisis and IgG-lambda monoclonal gammopathy in a Ph1$^+$ chronic myelogenous leukemia: report of a case. *Haematologica, 71*, 489–492.

Caforio, A. L., Gambino, A., Belloni Fortina, A., Piaserico, S., Scarpa, E., Feltrin, G., Tona, F., Pompei, E., Tonin, E., Amadori, G., Thiene, G., Dalla Volta, S., Peserico, A., and Casarotto, D. (2001). Monoclonal gammopathy in heart transplantation: risk factor analysis and relevance of immunosuppressive load. *Transplantation Proceedings, 33*, 1583–1584.

Callander, N. S., and Roodman, G. D. (2001). Myeloma bone disease. *Seminars in Hematology, 38*, 276–285.

Carrell, R. W., Colls, B. M., and Murray, J. T. (1971). The significance of monoclonal gammopathy in a normal population. *Australian and New Zealand Journal of Medicine, 1*, 398–401.

Carter, A., and Tatarsky, I. (1980). The physiopathological significance of benign monoclonal gammopathy: a study of 64 cases. *British Journal of Haematology, 46*, 565–574.

Castaman, G., Rodeghiero, F., Di Bona, E., and Ruggeri, M. (1989). Clinical effectiveness of desmopressin in a case of acquired von Willebrand's syndrome associated with benign monoclonal gammopathy. *Blut, 58*, 211–213.

Catovesky, D., Costello, C., Leukopoulos, D., Fessas, P. R., Foxley, J. M., Traub, N. E., Mills, M. J., and O'Brien, M. (1981). Hairy cell leukemia and myelomatosis: chance association or clinical manifestations of the same B-cell disease spectrum. *Blood, 57*, 758–763.

Cesana, C., Klersy, C., Barbarano, L., Nosari, A. M., Crugnola, M., Pungolino, E., Gargantini, L., Granata, S., Valentini, M., and Morra, E. (2002). Prognostic factors for malignant transformation in monoclonal gammopathy of undetermined significance and smoldering multiple myeloma. *Journal of Clinical Oncology, 20*, 1625–1634.

Chassande, B., Leger, J. M., Younes-Chennoufi, A. B., Bengoufa, D., Maisonobe, T., Bouche, P., and Baumann, N. (1998). Peripheral neuropathy associated with IgM monoclonal gammopathy: correlations between M-protein antibody activity and clinical/electrophysiological features in 40 cases. *Muscle & Nerve, 21,* 55–62.

Chen, H. P., and Carroll, J. A. (1980). Monoclonal gammopathy in carcinoma of the colon. *American Journal of Clinical Pathology, 73,* 607–610.

Chesi, M., Bergsagel, P. L., Brents, L. A., Smith, C. M., Gerhard, D. S., and Kuehl, W. M. (1996). Dysregulation of cyclin D1 by translocation into an IgH gamma switch region in two multiple myeloma cell lines. *Blood, 88,* 674–681.

Chesi, M., Bergsagel, P. L., Shonukan, O. O., Martelli, M. L., Brents, L. A., Chen, T., Schrock, E., Ried, T., and Kuehl, W. M. (1998). Frequent dysregulation of the c-maf proto-oncogene at 16q23 by translocation to an Ig locus in multiple myeloma. *Blood, 91,* 4457–4463.

Chesi, M., Nardini, E., Brents, L. A., Schrock, E., Ried, T., Kuehl, W. M., and Bergsagel, P. L. (1997). Frequent translocation t(4;14)(p16.3;q32.3) in multiple myeloma is associated with increased expression and activating mutations of fibroblast growth factor receptor 3. *Nature Genetics, 16,* 260–264.

Chowdhury, M. M., Inaloz, H. S., Motley, R. J., and Knight, A. G. (2002). Erythema elevatum diutinum and IgA paraproteinaemia: 'a preclinical iceberg.' *International Journal of Dermatology, 41,* 368–370.

Cohen, H. F., Crawford, J., Rao, M. K., Pieper, C. F., and Currie, M. S. (1998). Racial differences in the prevalence of monoclonal gammopathy in a community-based sample of the elderly. *American Journal of Medicine, 104,* 439–444.

Colwell, N. S., Tollefsen, D. M., and Blinder, M. A. (1997). Identification of a monoclonal thrombin inhibitor associated with multiple myeloma and a severe bleeding disorder. *British Journal of Haematology, 97,* 219–226.

Crapper, R. M., Deam, D. R., and Mackay, I. R. (1987). Paraproteinemias in homosexual men with HIV infection: lack of association with abnormal clinical or immunologic findings. *American Journal of Clinical Pathology, 88,* 348–351.

Crawford, J., Eye, M. K., and Cohen, H. J. (1987). Evaluation of monoclonal gammopathies in the 'well' elderly. *American Journal of Medicine, 82,* 39–45.

Croucher, P. I., Shipman, C. M., Lippitt, J., Perry, M., Asosingh, K., Hijzen, A., Brabbs, A. C., van Beek, E. J., Holen, I., Skerry, T. M., Dunstan, C. R., Russell, G. R., Van Camp, B., and Vanderkerken, K. (2001). Osteoprotegerin inhibits the development of osteolytic bone disease in multiple myeloma. *Blood, 98,* 3534–3540.

Dalakas, M. C., Illa, I., Gallardo, E., and Juarez, C. (1997). Inclusion body myositis and paraproteinemia: incidence and immunopathologic correlations. *Annals of Neurology, 41,* 100–104.

Dalakas, M. C., Quarles, R. H., Farrer, R. G., Dambrosia, J., Soueidan, S., Stein, D. P., Cupler, E., Sekul, E. A., and Otero, C. (1996). A controlled study of intravenous immunoglobulin in demyelinating neuropathy with IgM gammopathy. *Annals of Neurology, 40,* 792–795.

Danby, F. W., Danby, C. W. E., and Pruzanski, W. (1976). Papular mucinosis with IgG (κ) M component. *Canadian Medical Association Journal, 114,* 920–922.

Daoud, M. S., Lust, J. A., Kyle, R. A., and Pittelkow, M. R. (1999). Monoclonal gammopathies and associated skin disorders. *Journal of the American Academy of Dermatology, 40,* 507–535.

Deconinck, N., Laterre, E. C., and Van den Bergh, P. Y. (2000). Adult-onset nemaline myopathy and monoclonal gammopathy: a case report. *Acta Neurologica Belgica, 100,* 34–40.

Desai, J., and Swash, M. (1999). IgM paraproteinemia in a patient with primary lateral sclerosis. *Neuromuscular Disorders: NMD, 9,* 38–40.

Dexter, R. N., Mullinax, F., Estep, H. L., and Williams, R. C., Jr. (1972). Monoclonal IgG gammopathy and hyperparathyroidism. *Annals of Internal Medicine, 77,* 759–764.

Dhib-Jalbut, S., and Liwnicz, B. H. (1986). Binding of serum IgA of multiple myeloma to normal peripheral nerve. *Acta Neurologica Scandinavica, 73,* 381–387.

Dighiero, G., Guilbert, B., Fermand, J.-P., Lymberi, P., Danon, F., and Avramea, S. (1983). Thirty-six human monoclonal immuno-globulins with antibody activity against cytoskeleton proteins, thyroglobulin, and native DNA: immunologic studies and clinical correlations. *Blood, 62,* 264–270.

Dispenzieri, A., Gertz, M. A., Therneau, T. M., and Kyle, R. A. (2001a). Retrospective cohort study of 148 patients with polyclonal gammopathy. *Mayo Clinic Proceedings, 76,* 476–487.

Dispenzieri, A., Kyle, R. A., Lacy, M. Q., et al. (2002). POEMS syndrome: definitions and long-term outcome. *Blood, 101,* 2496–2506.

Dispenzieri, A., Lacy, M. Q., Litzow, M. R., Tefferi, A., Inwards, D. J., Micallef, I. N., Gastineau, D. A., Ansell, S., Rajkumar, S. V., Fonseca, R., Witzig, T. E., Lust, J. A., Kyle, R. A., Greipp, P. R., and Gertz, M. A. (2001b). Peripheral blood stem cell transplant (PBSCT) in patients with POEMS syndrome [Abstract]. *Blood, 98,* 391b.

Dowd, P. M., and Munro, D. D. (1983). Erythema elevatum diutinum. *Journal of the Royal Society of Medicine, 76,* 310–313.

Driedger, H., and Pruzanski, W. (1979). Plasma cell neoplasia with osteosclerotic lesions: a study of five cases and a review of the literature. *Archives of Internal Medicine, 139,* 892–896.

Droder, R. M., Kyle, R. A., and Greipp, P. R. (1992). Control of systemic capillary leak syndrome with aminophylline and terbutaline. *American Journal of Medicine, 92,* 523–526.

Ducloux, D., Carron, P., Racadot, E., Rebibou, J. M., Bresson-Vautrin, C., Hillier, Y. S., and Chalopin, J. M. (1999). T-cell immune defect and B-cell activation in renal transplant recipients with monoclonal gammopathies. *Transplantation International: Official Journal of the European Society for Organ Transplantation, 12,* 250–253.

Dührsen, U., Uppenkamp, M., Meusers, P., König, E., and Brittinger, G. (1988). Frequent association of idiopathic myelofibrosis with plasma cell dyscrasias. *Blut, 56,* 97–102.

DuVillard, L., Guiguet, M., Casasnovas, R. O., Caillot, D., Monnier-Zeller, V., Bernard, A., Guy, H., and Solary, E. (1995). Diagnostic value of serum IL-6 level in monoclonal gammopathies. *British Journal of Haematology, 89,* 243–249.

Dyck, P. J., Low, P. A., Windebank, A. J., Jaradeh, S. S., Gosselin, S., Bourque, P., Smith, B. E., Krantz, K. M., Karnes, J. L., Evans, B. A., Pineda, A. A., O'Brien, P. C., and Kyle, R. A. (1991). Plasma exchange in polyneuropathy associated with monoclonal gammopathy of undetermined significance. *New England Journal of Medicine, 325,* 1482–1486.

Dysseleer, A., Michaux, L., Cosyns, J. P., Goffin, E., Hermans, C., and Pirson, Y. (1999). Benign monoclonal gammopathy turning to AL amyloidosis after kidney transplantation. *American Journal of Kidney Diseases: The Official Journal of the National Kidney Foundation, 34,* 166–169.

Economopoulos, T., Economidou, J., Giannopoulos, G., Terzoglou, C., Papageorgiou, E., Dervenoulas, J., Arseni, P., Hadjioannou, J., and Raptis, S. (1985). Immune abnormalities in myelodysplastic syndromes. *Journal of Clinical Pathology, 38,* 908–911.

Ellis, T. M., Le, P. T., DeVries, G., Stubbs, E., Fisher, M., and Bhoopalam, N. (2001). Alterations in CD30+ T cells in monoclonal gammopathy of undetermined significance. *Clinical Immunity, 98,* 301–307.

Ely, S. A., and Knowles, D. M. (2002). Expression of CD56/neural cell adhesion molecule correlates with the presence of lytic bone lesions in multiple myeloma and distinguishes myeloma from monoclonal gammopathy of undetermined significance and lymphomas with plasmacytoid differentiation. *American Journal of Pathology, 160,* 1293–1299.

Faed, J. M., Day, B., Pollock, M., Taylor, P. K., Nukada, H., and Hammond-Tooke, G. D. (1989). High-dose intravenous human immunoglobulin in chronic inflammatory demyelinating polyneuropathy. *Neurology, 39*, 422–425.

Farhangi, M., and Osserman, E. F. (1976). Myeloma with xanthoderma due to an IgG λ monoclonal anti-flavin antibody. *New England Journal of Medicine, 294*, 177–183.

Federici, A. B., Stabile, F., Castaman, G., Canciani, M. T., and Mannucci, P. M. (1998). Treatment of acquired von Willebrand syndrome in patients with monoclonal gammopathy of uncertain significance: comparison of three different therapeutic approaches. *Blood, 92*, 2707–2711.

Feizi, T. (1968). Immunoglobulins in chronic liver disease. *Gut, 9*, 193–198.

Fernández-Solá, J., Cases, A., Monforte, R., Pedro-Botet, J. C., Estruch, R., Grau, J. M., and Urbano-Márquez, A. (1987). A possible pathogenic mechanism for rhabdomyolysis associated with multiple myeloma. *Acta Haematologica, 77*, 231–233.

Fervenza, F. C., Terreros, D., Boutaud, A., Hudson, B. G., Williams, R. A., Jr., Donadio, J. V., Jr., and Schwab, T. R. (1999). Recurrent Goodpasture's disease due to a monoclonal IgA-kappa circulating antibody. *American Journal of Kidney Diseases: The Official Journal of the National Kidney Foundation, 34*, 549–555.

Filella, X., Bladé, J., López Guillermo, A., Molina, R., Rozman, C., and Ballesta, A. M. (1996). Cytokines (IL-6, TNF-α, IL-1α) and soluble interleukin-2 receptor as serum tumor markers in multiple myeloma. *Cancer Detection and Prevention, 20*, 52–56.

Finan, M. C., and Winkelmann, R. K. (1986). Necrobiotic xanthogranuloma with paraproteinemia: a review of 22 cases. *Medicine (Baltimore), 65*, 376–388.

Fine, J. M., Lambin, P., and Leroux, P. (1972). Frequency of monoclonal gammopathy ('M-components') in 13 400 sera from blood donors. *Vox Sanguinis, 23*, 336–343.

Fine, J. M., Lambin, P., and Muller, J. Y. (1979). The evolution of asymptomatic monoclonal gammopathies: a followup of 20 cases over periods of 3–14 years. *Acta Medica Scandinavica, 205*, 339–341.

Folkman, J. (1971). Tumor angiogenesis: therapeutic implications. *New England Journal of Medicine, 285*, 1182–1186.

Folkman, J. (1995). Seminars in Medicine of the Beth Israel Hospital, Boston: clinical applications of research on angiogenesis. *New England Journal of Medicine, 333*, 1757–1763.

Fonseca, R., Ahmann, G. J., Juneau, A. L., Jalal, S. M., Dewald, G. W., Larson, D. R., Therneau, T. M., Gertz, M. A., and Greipp, P. R. (1997). Cytogenetic abnormalities in systemic amyloidosis: a comparison of conventional cytogenetic analysis to fluorescent in-situ hybridization with simultaneous cytoplasmic immunoglobulin staining [Abstract]. *Blood, 90*(Suppl 1), 350a.

Fonseca, R., Bailey, R. J., Ahmann, G. J., Rajkumar, S. V., Hoyer, J. D., Lust, J. A., Kyle, R. A., Gertz, M. A., Greipp, P. R., and Dewald, G. W. (2002a). Genomic abnormalities in monoclonal gammopathy of undetermined significance. *Blood, 100*, 1417–1424.

Fonseca, R., Blood, E. A., Oken, M. M., Kyle, R. A., Dewald, G. W., Bailey, R. J., Van Wier, S. A., Henderson, K. J., Hoyer, J. D., Harrington, D., Kay, N. E., Van Ness, B., and Greipp, P. R. (2002b). Myeloma and the t(11;14)(q13;q32): evidence for a biologically defined unique subset of patients. *Blood, 99*, 3735–3741.

Fonseca, R., Oken, M. M., and Greipp, P. R. (2001). The t(4;14)(p16.3;q32) is strongly associated with chromosome 13 abnormalities in both multiple myeloma and monoclonal gammopathy of undetermined significance. *Blood, 98*, 1271–1272.

Freddo, L., Sherman, W. H., and Latov, N. (1986). Glycosaminoglycan antigens in peripheral nerve: studies with antibodies from a patient with neuropathy and monoclonal gammopathy. *Journal of Neuroimmunology, 12*, 57–64.

Fredman, P. (1998). The role of antiglycolipid antibodies in neurological disorders. *Annals of the New York Academy of Sciences, 845*, 341–352.

Freestone, S., and Ramsay, L. E. (1982). Transient monoclonal gammopathy in hydralazine-induced lupus erythematosus. *British Medical Journal (Clinical Research Edition), 285*, 1536–1537.

Garewal, H., Durie, B. G. M., Kyle, R. A., Finley, P., Bower, B., and Serokman, R. (1984). Serum beta₂-microglobulin in the initial staging and subsequent monitoring of monoclonal plasma cell disorders. *Journal of Clinical Oncology, 2*, 51–57.

Garfinkel, D., Sidi, Y., Ben-Bassat, M., Solomon, F., Hazaz, B., and Pinkhas, J. (1982). Coexistence of Gaucher's disease and multiple myeloma. *Archives of Internal Medicine, 142*, 2229–2230.

Gelfand, J. A., Boss, G. R., Conley, C. L., Reinhart, R., and Frank, M. M. (1979). Acquired C1 esterase inhibitor deficiency and angioedema: a review. *Medicine (Baltimore), 58*, 321–328.

Gerritsen, E. J., van Tol, M. J., Lankester, A. C., van der Weijden-Ragas, C. P., Jol-van der Zijde, C. M., Oudeman-Gruber, N. J., Radl, J., and Vossen, J. M. (1993). Immunoglobulin levels and monoclonal gammopathies in children after bone marrow transplantation. *Blood, 82*, 3493–3502.

Gherardi, R. K., Belec, L., Soubrier, M., Malapert, D., Zuber, M., Viard, J. P., Intrator, L., Degos, J. D., and Authier, F. J. (1996). Overproduction of proinflammatory cytokines imbalanced by their antagonists in POEMS syndrome. *Blood, 87*, 1458–1465.

Giraldo, M. P., Rubio-Félix, D., Perella, M., Gracia, J. A., Bergua, J. M., and Giralt, M. (1991). Gammapatías monoclonales de significado indeterminado: aspectos clínicos, biológicos y evolutivos de 397 casos. *Sangre (Barcelona), 36*, 377–382.

Ginevri, F., Nocera, A., Bonato, L., Losurdo, G., Rossi, G., Mangraviti, S., Fontana, I., Rabagliati, A. M., Basile, G., Barocci, S., Valente, U., and Gusmano, R. (1998). Cytomegalovirus infection is a trigger for monoclonal immunoglobulins in paediatric kidney transplant recipients. *Transplantation Proceedings, 30*, 2079–2082.

Goldberg, G. J., Paraskevas, F., and Israels, L. G. (1969). The association of rheumatoid arthritis with plasma cell and lymphocytic neoplasms. *Arthritis and Rheumatism, 12*, 569–579.

Gorson, K. C., Allam, G., and Ropper, A. H. (1997). Chronic inflammatory demyelinating polyneuropathy: clinical features and response to treatment in 67 consecutive patients with and without a monoclonal gammopathy. *Neurology, 48*, 321–328.

Gregersen, H., Ibsen, J. S., Mellemkjær, L., Dahlerup, J. F., Olsen, J. H., and Sørensen, H. T. (2001a). Mortality and causes of death in patients with monoclonal gammopathy of undetermined significance. *British Journal of Haematology, 112*, 353–357.

Gregersen, H., Madsen, K. M., Sørensen, H. T., Schønheyder, H. C., Ibsen, J. S., and Dahlerup, J. F. (1998). The risk of bacteremia in patients with monoclonal gammopathy of undetermined significance. *European Journal of Haematology, 61*, 140–144.

Gregersen, H., Mellemkjær, L., Ibsen, J. S., Dahlerup, J. F., Thomassen, L., and Sørensen, H. T. (2001b). The impact of M-component type and immunoglobulin concentration on the risk of malignant transformation in patients with monoclonal gammopathy of undetermined significance. *Haematologica, 86*, 1172–1179.

Gregersen, H., Mellemkjær, L., Salling Ibsen, J., Sørensen, H. T., Olsen, J. H., Pedersen, J. O., and Dahlerup, J. F. (2000). Cancer risk in patients with monoclonal gammopathy of undetermined significance. *American Journal of Haematology, 63*, 1–6.

Greipp, P. R., Witzig, T. E., Gonchoroff, N. J., Habermann, T. M., Katzmann, J. A., O'Fallon, W. M., and Kyle, R. A. (1987). Immunofluorescence labeling indices in myeloma and related monoclonal gammopathies. *Mayo Clinic Proceedings, 62*, 969–977.

Grosbois, B., Jego, P., de Rosa, H., Ruelland, A., Lancien, G., Gallou, G., and Leblay, R. (1997). Triclonal gammopathy and malignant immunoproliferative syndrome [French]. *Revue de Medecine Interne, 18*, 470–473.

Guillerm, G., Gyan, E., Wolowiec, D., Facon, T., Avet-Loiseau, H., Kuliczkowski, K., Bauters, F., Fenaux, P., and Quesnel, B. (2001). p16(INK4a) and p15(INK4b) gene methylations in plasma cells from monoclonal gammopathy of undetermined significance. *Blood, 98*, 244–246.

Hafler, D. A., Johnson, D., Kelly, J. J., Jr., Panitch, H., Kyle, R., and Weiner, H. L. (1986). Monoclonal gammopathy and neuropathy: myelin-associated glycoprotein reactivity and clinical characteristics. *Neurology, 36*, 75–78.

Hallek, M., Bergsagel, P. L., and Anderson, K. C. (1998). Multiple myeloma: increasing evidence for a multistep transformation process. *Blood, 91*, 3–21.

Hammarström, L., and Smith, C. I. E. (1987). Frequent occurrence of monoclonal gammopathies with an imbalanced light-chain ratio following bone marrow transplantation. *Transplantation, 43*, 447–449.

Han, J. H., Choi, S. J., Kurihara, N., Koide, M., Oba, Y., and Roodman, G. D. (2001). Macrophage inflammatory protein-1alpha is an osteoclastogenic factor in myeloma that is independent of receptor activator of nuclear factor kappaB ligand. *Blood, 97*, 3349–3353.

Hansen, P. R., Jønssonn, V., Schroder, H. D., Jensen, T. S., and Wiik, A. (1989). IgD-λ monoclonal gammopathy and axonal neuropathy [Letter]. *Journal of Internal Medicine, 225*, 289–290.

Hass, D. C., and Tatum, A. H. (1988). Plasmapheresis alleviates neuropathy accompanying IgM anti-myelin-associated glycoprotein paraproteinemia. *Annals of Neurology, 23*, 394–396.

Hays, A. P., Latov, N., Takatsu, M., and Sherman, W. H. (1987). Experimental demyelination of nerve induced by serum of patients with neuropathy and an anti-MAG IgM M-protein. *Neurology, 37*, 242–256.

Hebart, H., Einsele, H., Klein, R., Fischer, I., Buhler, S., Dietz, K., Jahn, G., Berg, P. A., Kanz, L., and Muller, C. A. (1996). CMV infection after allogeneic bone marrow transplantation is associated with the occurrence of various autoantibodies and monoclonal gammopathies. *British Journal of Haematology, 95*, 138–144.

Heer, M., Joller-Jemelka, H., Fontana, A., See-Feld, U., Schmid, M., and Ammann, R. (1984). Monoclonal gammopathy in chronic active hepatitis. *Liver, 4*, 255–263.

Hendrick, A. M., Mitchison, H. C., Bird, A. G., and James, O. F. W. (1986). Paraproteins in primary biliary cirrhosis. *Quarterly Journal of Medicine, 60*, 681–684.

Heriot, K., Hallquist, A. E., and Tomar, R. H. (1985). Paraproteinemia in patients with acquired immunodeficiency syndrome (AIDS) or lymphadenopathy syndrome (LAS). *Clinical Chemistry, 31*, 1224–1226.

Hineman, V. L., Phyliky, R. L., and Banks, P. M. (1982). Angiofollicular lymph node hyperplasia and peripheral neuropathy: association with monoclonal gammopathy. *Mayo Clinic Proceedings, 57*, 379–382.

Hobbs, J. R., and Corbett, A. A. (1969). Younger age of presentation and extraosseous tumour in IgD myelomatosis. *British Medical Journal, 1*, 412–414.

Holt, P. J. A., Davies, M. G., Saunders, K. C., and Nuki, G. (1980). Pyoderma gangrenosum: clinical and laboratory findings in 15 patients with special reference to polyarthritis. *Medicine, 59*, 114–133.

Howerton, D. A., Check, I. J., and Hunter, R. L. (1986). Densitometric quantitation of high resolution agarose gel protein electrophoresis. *American Journal of Clinical Pathology, 85*, 213–218.

Humbert, P., Blanc, D., Laurent, R., and Agache, P. (1987). Monoclonal IgG gammopathy in a case of pustular psoriasis. A ten-year follow-up [Letter]. *Blut, 54*, 61–62.

Humphrey, D. M., Cortez, E. A., and Spiva, D. A. (1982). Immunohistologic studies of cytoplasmic immunoglobulins in rheumatic diseases including two patients with monoclonal patterns and subsequent lymphoma. *Cancer, 49*, 2049–2069.

Hurst, N. P., Smith, W., and Henderson, D. R. (1987). IgG (kappa) paraproteinaemia and arthritis. *British Journal of Rheumatology, 26*, 142–146.

Hutchinson, K., Dal Pra, M., and Apel, A. (1998). Immunoglobulin G crystalline keratopathy associated with monoclonal gammopathy. *Australian and New Zealand Journal of Ophthalmology, 26*, 177–179.

Iida, S., Rao, P. H., Butler, M., Corradini, P., Boccadoro, M., Klein, B., Chaganti, R. S., and Dalla-Favera, R. (1997). Deregulation of MUM1/IRF4 by chromosomal translocation in multiple myeloma. *Nature Genetics, 17*, 226–230.

Ilfeld, D., Bazilay, J., Vana, D., Ben-Bassat, M., Joshua, H., and Pick, I. (1985). IgG monoclonal gammopathy in four patients with polymyalgia rheumatica [Letter]. *Annals of Rheumatic Disease, 44*, 501.

Ilyas, A. A., Li, S. C., Chou, D. K., Li, Y. T., Jungalwala, F. B., Dalakas, M. C., and Quarles, R. H. (1988a). Gangliosides GM2, IV4GalNAcGM1b, and IV4GalNAcGC1a as antigens for monoclonal immunoglobulin M in neuropathy associated with gammopathy. *Journal of Biological Chemistry, 263*, 4369–4373.

Ilyas, A. A., Quarles, R. H., Dalakas, M. C., and Brady, R. O. (1985). Polyneuropathy with monoclonal gammopathy: glycolipids are frequently antigens for IgM paraproteins. *Proceedings of the National Academy of Sciences of the United States of America, 82*, 6697–6700.

Ilyas, A. A., Willison, H. J., Dalakas, M. C., Whitaker, J. N., and Quarles, R. H. (1988b). Identification and characterization of gangliosides reacting with IgM paraproteins in three patients with neuropathy associated with biclonal gammopathy. *Journal of Neurochemistry, 51*, 851–858.

Isaksson, E., Bjorkholm, M., Holm, G., Johansson, B., Nilsson, B., Mellstedt, H., and Österborg, A. (1996). Blood clonal B-cell excess in patients with monoclonal gammopathy of undetermined significance (MGUS): association with malignant transformation. *British Journal of Haematology, 92*, 71–76.

Isobe, T., and Osserman, E. F. (1971). Pathologic conditions associated with plasma cell dyscrasias: a study of 806 cases. *Annals of the New York Academy of Sciences, 190*, 507–517.

Jaccard, A., Royer, B., Bordessoule, D., Brouet, J. C., and Fermand, J. P. (2002). High-dose therapy and autologous blood stem cell transplantation in POEMS syndrome. *Blood, 99*, 3057–3059.

James, K., Fudenberg, H., Epstein, W. L., and Shuster, J. (1967). Studies on a unique diagnostic serum globulin in papular mucinosis (lichen myxedematosus). *Clinical and Experimental Immunology, 2*, 153–166.

Jansen, J., Bolhuis, R. L. H., van Nieuwkoop, J. A., Schuit, H. R., and Kroese, W. (1983). Paraproteinaemia plus osteolytic lesions in typical hairy-cell leukaemia. *British Journal of Haematology, 54*, 531–541.

Jones, R. R., Baughan, A. S. J., Cream, J. J., Levantine, A., and Whicher, J. T. (1979). Complement abnormalities in diffuse plane xanthomatosis with paraproteinaemia. *British Journal of Dermatology, 101*, 711–716.

Jønsson, V., Schroder, H. D., Staehelin Jensen, T., Nolsoe, C., Stigsby, B., Trojaborg, W., Svejgaard, A., and Hippe, E. (1988). Autoimmunity related to IgM monoclonal gammopathy of undetermined significance: peripheral neuropathy and connective tissue sensibilization caused by IgM M-proteins. *Acta Medica Scandinavica, 223*, 255–261.

Kalra, L., and Delamere, J. P. (1987). Lymphoreticular malignancy and monoclonal gammopathy presenting as polymyalgia rheumatica. *British Journal of Rheumatology, 26*, 458–459.

Karlson, E. W., Tanasijevic, M., Hankinson, S. E., Liang, M. H., Colditz, G. A., Speizer, F. E., and Schur, P. H. (2001). Monoclonal gammopathy of undetermined significance and exposure to breast implants. *Archives of Internal Medicine, 161*, 864–867.

Kavanagh, G. M., Colaco, C. B., Bradfield, J. W., and Archer, C. B. (1993). Erythema elevatum diutinum associated with Wegener's granulomatosis and IgA paraproteinemia. *Journal of the American Academy of Dermatology, 28*, 846–849.

Kebler, R., Kithier, K., McDonald, F. D., and Cadnapaphornchai, P. (1985). Rapidly progressive glomerulonephritis and monoclonal gammopathy. *American Journal of Medicine, 78*, 133–138.

Kelly, J. J., Adelman, L. S., Berkman, E., and Bhan, I. (1988). Polyneuropathies associated with IgM monoclonal gammopathies. *Archives of Neurology, 45*, 1355–1359.

Kelly, J. J., Jr., Kyle, R. A., and Latov, N. (1987). *Polyneuropathies Associated With Plasma Cell Dyscrasias.* Boston: Martinus Nijhoff Publishing.

Kelly, J. J., Jr., Kyle, R. A., Miles, J. M., and Dyck, P. J. (1983). Osteosclerotic myeloma and peripheral neuropathy. *Neurology, 33*, 202–210.

Kelly, J. J., Jr., Kyle, R. A., O'Brien, P. C., and Dyck, P. J. (1981). Prevalence of monoclonal protein in peripheral neuropathy. *Neurology, 31*, 1480–1483.

Keren, D. F., Alexanian, R., Goeken, J. A., Gorevic, P. D., Kyle, R. A., and Tomar, R. H. (1999). Guidelines for clinical and laboratory evaluation of patients with monoclonal gammopathies. *Archives of Pathology and Laboratory Medicine, 123*, 106–107.

Kim, H., Heller, P., and Rappaport, H. (1973). Monoclonal gammopathies associated with lymphoproliferative disorders: a morphologic study. *American Journal of Clinical Pathology, 59*, 282–294.

Kiprov, D. D., and Miller, R. G. (1984). Polymyositis associated with monoclonal gammopathy. *Lancet, 2*, 1183–1186.

Kissel, J. T., and Mendell, J. R. (1996). Neuropathies associated with monoclonal gammopathies. *Neuromuscular Disorders, 6*, 3–18.

Konigsberg, R., Ackermann, J., Kaufmann, H., Zojer, N., Urbauer, E., Kromer, E., Jager, U., Gisslinger, H., Schreiber, S., Heinz, R., Ludwig, H., Huber, H., and Drach, J. (2000a). Deletions of chromosome 13q in monoclonal gammopathy of undetermined significance. *Leukemia, 14*, 1975–1979.

Konigsberg, R., Zojer, N., Ackermann, J., Kromer, E., Kittler, H., Fritz, E., Kaufmann, H., Nosslinger, T., Riedl, L., Gisslinger, H., Jager, U., Simonitsch, I., Heinz, R., Ludwig, H., Huber, H., and Drach, J. (2000b). Predictive role of interphase cytogenetics for survival of patients with multiple myeloma. *Journal of Clinical Oncology, 18*, 804–812.

Kövary, P. M., Suter, L., Macher, E., Niedorf, H., Grundmann, E., Lukitsch, O., Herzberg, J., Intorp, H., Schürmeyer, E., Kamanabroo, D., and Losse, H. (1981). Monoclonal gammopathies in Sézary syndrome: a report of four new cases and a review of the literature. *Cancer, 48*, 788–792.

Kurihara, Y., Shiba, K., Fukumura, Y., Kobayashi, I., and Kamei, S. (2000). Occurrence of serum M-protein species in Japanese patients older than 50 years based on relative mobility in cellulose acetate membrane electrophoresis. *Journal of Clinical Laboratory Analysis, 14*, 64–69.

Kusunoki, S., Kohriyama, T., Pachner, A. R., Latov, N., and Yu, R. K. (1987). Neuropathy and IgM paraproteinemia: differential binding of IgM M-proteins to peripheral nerve glycolipids. *Neurology, 37*, 1795–1797.

Kusunoki, S., Shimizu, T., Matsumura, K., Maemura, K., and Mannen, T. (1989). Motor dominant neuropathy and IgM paraproteinemia: the IgM M-protein binds to specific gangliosides. *Journal of Neuroimmunology, 21*, 177–181.

Kuwabara, S., Hattori, T., Shimoe, Y., and Kamitsukasa, I. (1997). Long-term melphalan-prednisolone chemotherapy for POEMS syndrome. *Journal of Neurology, Neurosurgery, and Psychiatry, 63*, 385–387.

Kyle, R. A. (1975). Multiple myeloma: review of 869 cases. *Mayo Clinic Proceedings, 50*, 29–40.

Kyle, R. A. (1978). Monoclonal gammopathy of undetermined significance: natural history in 241 cases. *American Journal of Medicine, 64*, 814–826.

Kyle, R. A. (1984). 'Benign' monoclonal gammopathy: a misnomer? *Journal of the American Medical Association, 251*, 1849–1854.

Kyle, R. A. (1993). 'Benign' monoclonal gammopathy: after 20 to 35 years of followup. *Mayo Clinic Proceedings, 68*, 26–36.

Kyle, R. A. (1994). The monoclonal gammopathies. *Clinical Chemistry, 40*, 2154–2161.

Kyle, R. A. (1999). Sequence of testing for monoclonal gammopathies. *Archives of Pathology and Laboratory Medicine, 123*, 114–118.

Kyle, R. A., Bayrd, E. D., McKenzie, B. F., and Heck, F. J. (1960). Diagnostic criteria for electrophoretic patterns of serum and urinary proteins in multiple myeloma: study of one hundred and sixty-five multiple myeloma patients and of seventy-seven non-myeloma patients with similar electrophoretic patterns. *Journal of the American Medical Association, 174*, 245–251.

Kyle, R. A., Beard, C. M., O'Fallon, W. M., and Kurland, L. T. (1994). Incidence of multiple myeloma in Olmsted County, Minnesota: 1978 through 1990, with a review of the trend since 1945. *Journal of Clinical Oncology, 12*, 1577–1583.

Kyle, R. A., and Dyck, P. J. (1993). Osteosclerotic myeloma (POEMS syndrome). In P. J. Dyck, P. K. Thomas, J. W. Griffin, P. A. Low, and J. F. Poduslo (Eds.), *Peripheral Neuropathy*, ed 3 (pp. 1288–1293). Philadelphia: WB Saunders Co.

Kyle, R. A., Finkelstein, S., Elveback, L. R., and Kurland, L. T. (1972). Incidence of monoclonal proteins in a Minnesota community with a cluster of multiple myeloma. *Blood, 40*, 719–724.

Kyle, R. A., and Garton, J. P. (1987). The spectrum of IgM monoclonal gammopathy in 430 cases. *Mayo Clinic Proceedings, 62*, 719–731.

Kyle, R. A., Gertz, M. A., Witzig, T. E., Lust, J. A., Lacy, M. Q., Dispenzieri, A., Fonseca, R., Rajkumar, S. V., Offord, J. R., Larson, D. R., Plevak, M. E., Therneau, T. M., and Greipp, P. R. (2003). Review of 1,027 patients with newly diagnosed multiple myeloma. *Mayo Clinic Proceedings, 78*, 21–33.

Kyle, R. A., and Greipp, P. R. (1980). Smoldering multiple myeloma. *New England Journal of Medicine, 302*, 1347–1349.

Kyle, R. A., and Greipp, P. R. (1982). 'Idiopathic' Bence Jones proteinuria: long-term followup in seven patients. *New England Journal of Medicine, 306*, 564–567.

Kyle, R. A., Katzmann, J. A., Lust, J. A., and Dispenzieri, A. (2002a). Immunochemical characterization of immunoglobulins. In N. R. Rose, R. G. Hamilton, and B. Detrick (Eds.), *Manual of Clinical Laboratory Immunology*, ed 6 (pp. 71–91). Washington, DC: ASM Press.

Kyle, R. A., and Lust, J. A. (1991). Monoclonal gammopathies of undetermined significance. In P. H. Wiernik, G. P. Cannelos, R. A. Kyle, and C. A. Schiffer (Eds.), *Neoplastic Diseases of the Blood*, ed 2 (pp. 571–594). New York: Churchill Livingstone.

Kyle, R. A., Maldonado, J. E., and Bayrd, E. D. (1973). Idiopathic Bence Jones proteinuria: a distinct entity? *American Journal of Medicine, 55*, 222–226.

Kyle, R. A., Robinson, R. A., and Katzmann, J. A. (1981). The clinical aspects of biclonal gammopathies: review of 57 cases. *American Journal of Medicine, 71*, 999–1009.

Kyle, R. A., Therneau, T. M., Rajkumar, S. V., Offord, J. R., Larson, D. R., Plevak, M. F., and Melton, L. J. III. (2002b). A long-term study of prognosis in monoclonal gammopathy of undetermined significance. *New England Journal of Medicine, 346*, 564–569.

Lacy, M. Q., Donovan, K. A., Heimbach, J. K., Ahmann, G. J., and Lust, J. A. (1999). Comparison of interleukin-1 beta expression by in situ hybridization in monoclonal gammopathy of undetermined significance and multiple myeloma. *Blood, 93*, 300–305.

Lamboley, V., Zabraniecki, L., Sie, P., Pourrat, J., and Fournie, B. (2002). Myeloma and monoclonal gammopathy of uncertain significance associated with acquired von Willebrand's syndrome: seven new cases with a literature review. *Joint, Bone, Spine: Revue du Rheumatisme, 69*, 62–67.

Latov, N. (1995). Pathogenesis and therapy of neuropathies associated with monoclonal gammopathies. *Annals of Neurology, 37*(Suppl 1), S32–S42.

Lefrère, J.-J., Debbia, M., and Lambin, P. (1993). Prospective follow-up of monoclonal gammopathies in HIV-infected individuals. *British Journal of Haematology, 84,* 151–155.

Leo, R., Boeker, M., Peest, D., Hein, R., Bartl, R., Gessner, J. E., Selbach, J., Wacker, G., and Deicher, H. (1992). Multiparameter analyses of normal and malignant human plasma cells: CD38++, CD56+, CD54+, cIg+ is the common phenotype of myeloma cells. *Annals of Hematology, 64,* 132–139.

Levine, T. D., and Pestronk, A. (1999). IgM antibody-related polyneuropathies: B-cell depletion chemotherapy using Rituximab. *Neurology, 52,* 1701–1704.

Lindström, F. D., and Dahlström, U. (1978). Multiple myeloma or benign monoclonal gammopathy? A study of differential diagnostic criteria in 44 cases. *Clinical Immunology and Immunopathology, 10,* 168–174.

Lust, J. A., and Donovan, K. A. (1998). Biology of the transition of monoclonal gammopathy of undetermined significance (MGUS) to multiple myeloma. *Cancer Control: Journal of the Moffitt Cancer Center, 5,* 209–217.

Lust, J. A., and Donovan, K. A. (1999). The role of interleukin-1 beta in the pathogenesis of multiple myeloma. *Hematology/Oncology Clinics of North America, 13,* 1117–1125.

Lutz, M. E., Daoud, M. S., McEvoy, M. T., and Gibson, L. E. (1998). Subcorneal pustular dermatosis: a clinical study of ten patients. *Cutis: Cutaneous Medicine for the Practitioner, 61,* 203–208.

Magrath, I., Benjamin, D., and Papadopoulos, N. (1983). Serum monoclonal immunoglobulin bands in undifferentiated lymphomas of Burkitt's and non-Burkitt's types. *Blood, 61,* 726–731.

Maisonobe, T., Chassande, B., Verin, M., Jouni, M., Leger, J. M., and Bouche, P. (1996). Chronic dysimmune demyelinating polyneuropathy: a clinical and electrophysiological study of 93 patients. *Journal of Neurology, Neurosurgery, and Psychiatry, 61,* 36–42.

Malacrida, V., De Francesco, D., Banfi, G., Porta, F. A., and Riches, P. G. (1987). Laboratory investigation of monoclonal gammopathy during 10 years of screening in a general hospital. *Journal of Clinical Pathology, 40,* 793–797.

Malik, A. A., Ganti, A. K., Potti, A., Levitt, R., and Hanley, J. F. (2002). Role of *Helicobacter pylori* infection in the incidence and clinical course of monoclonal gammopathy of undetermined significance. *American Journal of Gastroenterology, 97,* 1371–1374.

Mangia, A., Clemente, R., Musto, P., Cascavilla, I., La Floresta, P., Sanpaolo, G., Gentile, R., Viglotti, M. L., Facciousso, D., Carotenuto, M., Rizzetto, M., and Andriulli, A. (1996). Hepatitis C virus infection and monoclonal gammopathies not associated with cryoglobulinemia. *Leukemia, 10,* 1209–1213.

Mannucci, P. M., Lombardi, R., Bader, R., Horellou, M. H., Finazzi, G., Besana, C., Conard, J., and Samama, M. (1984). Studies of the pathophysiology of acquired von Willebrand's disease in seven patients with lymphoproliferative disorders or benign monoclonal gammopathies. *Blood, 64,* 614–621.

Mant, M. J., Hirsh, J., Gauldie, J., Bienenstock, J., Pines, G. F., and Luke, K. H. (1973). von Willebrand's syndrome presenting as an acquired bleeding disorder in association with a monoclonal gammopathy. *Blood, 42,* 429–436.

Manthorne, L. A., Dudley, R. W., Case, D. C., Jr., Turgeon, W. P., and Ritchie, R. F. (1989). A longitudinal study of monoclonal gammopathy of undetermined significance (MGUS) [Abstract]. *Clinical Research, 36,* 414A.

Marie, J. P., Tulliez, M., Tricottet-Paczinski, V., Reynes, M., and Diebold, J. (1982). Gaucher's disease with monoclonal gammopathy: significance of splenic plasmacytosis. *Scandinavian Journal of Haematology, 28,* 54–58.

Marti, G. E., Ryan, E. T., Papadopoulos, N. M., Filling-Katz, M., Barton, N., Fleischer, T. A., Rick, M., and Gralnick, H. R. (1988). Polyclonal B-cell lymphocytosis and hypergammaglobulinemia in patients with Gaucher disease. *American Journal of Hematology, 29,* 189–194.

Martin, N. F., Kincaid, M. C., Stark, W. J., Petty, B. G., Surer, J. L., Hirst, L. W., and Green, W. R. (1983). Ocular copper deposition associated with pulmonary carcinoma, IgG monoclonal gammopathy, and hypercupremia: a clinicopathologic correlation. *Ophthalmology, 90,* 110–116.

Mathew, P., Ahmann, G. J., Witzig, T. E., Roche, P. C., Kyle, R. A., and Greipp, P. R. (1995). Clinicopathological correlates of CD56 expression in multiple myeloma: a unique entity? *British Journal of Haematology, 90,* 459–461.

Mathiot, C., Mary, J. Y., Tartour, E., Facon, T., Monconduit, M., Grosbois, B., Pollet, J. P., Michaux, J. L., Euller Ziegler, L., Sautes, C., Bataille, R., and Fridman, W. H. (1996). Soluble CD16 (sCD16), a marker of malignancy in individuals with monoclonal gammopathy of undetermined significance (MGUS). *British Journal of Haematology, 95,* 660–665.

Matsuzaki, H., Yamaguchi, K., Kagimoto, T., Nakai, R., Takatsuki, K., and Oyama, W. (1985). Monoclonal gammopathies in adult T-cell leukemia. *Cancer, 56,* 1380–1383.

Mazzi, G., Raineri, A., Zucco, M., Passadore, P., Pomes, A., and Orazi, B. M. (1999). Plasma-exchange in chronic peripheral neurological disorders. *International Journal of Artificial Organs, 22,* 40–46.

McDonald, P. S., Cora-Bramble, D., and De Palma, L. (1998). Monoclonal gammopathy of the immunoglobulin A class in a two-year-old girl with ataxia–telangiectasia. *Pediatric Developmental Pathology: The Official Journal of the Society for Pediatric Pathology and the Paediatric Pathology Society, 1,* 319–321.

McFadden, N., Ree, K., Søyland, E., and Larsen, T. E. (1987). Scleroedema adultorum associated with a monoclonal gammopathy and generalized hyperpigmentation. *Archives of Dermatology, 123,* 629–632.

Mehregan, D. A., and Winkelmann, R. K. (1992). Necrobiotic xanthogranuloma. *Archives of Dermatology, 128,* 94–100.

Merlini, G., Bruening, R., Kyle, R. A., and Osserman, E. F. (1990). The second riboflavin-binding myeloma IgGλ[DOT]. I. Biochemical and functional characterization. *Molecular Immunology, 27,* 385–394.

Merlini, G., Farhangi, M., and Osserman, E. F. (1986). Monoclonal immunoglobulins with antibody activity in myeloma, macroglobulinemia and related plasma cell dyscrasias. *Seminars in Oncology, 13,* 350–365.

Merlini, G., Fitzpatrick, L. A., Siris, E. S., Bilezikian, J. P., Birken, S., Beychok, S., and Osserman, E. F. (1984). A human myeloma immunoglobulin G binding four moles of calcium associated with asymptomatic hypercalcemia. *Journal of Clinical Oncology, 4,* 185–196.

Meucci, N., Baldini, L., Cappellari, A., Di Troia, A., Allaria, S., Scarlato, G., and Nobile-Orazio, E. (1999). Antimyelin-associated glycoprotein antibodies predict the development of neuropathy in asymptomatic patients with IgM monoclonal gammopathy. *Annals of Neurology, 46,* 119–122.

Meyrier, A., Simon, P., Mignon, F., Striker, L., and Ramee, M. P. (1984). Rapidly progressive (crescentic) glomerulonephritis and monoclonal gammopathies. *Nephron, 38,* 156–162.

Migliore, P. J., and Alexanian, R. (1968). Monoclonal gammopathy in human neoplasia. *Cancer, 21,* 1127–1131.

Miguel-Garcia, A., Matutes, E., Tarin, F., Garcia-Talavera, J., Miguel-Sosa, A., Carbonell, F., and Catovsky, D. (1995). Circulating Ki67 positive lymphocytes in multiple myeloma and benign monoclonal gammopathy. *Journal of Clinical Pathology, 48,* 835–839.

Millá, F., Oriol, A., Aguilar, J., Aventin, A., Ayats, R., Alonso, E., Domingo, A., Feliu, E., Florensa, L., López, A., Perez-Vila, E., Rozman, M., Sanchez, C., Vallespi, T., and Woessner, S. (2001). Usefulness and reproducibility of cytomorphologic evaluations to differentiate myeloma from monoclonal gammopathies of unknown significance. *American Journal of Clinical Pathology, 115,* 127–135.

Mitus, A. J., Stein, R., Rappaport, J. M., Antin, J. H., Weinstein, H. J., Alper, C. A., and Smith, B. R. (1989). Monoclonal and oligoclonal gammopathy after bone marrow transplantation. *Blood, 74,* 2764–2768.

Mohri, H., Noguchi, T., Kodama, F., Itoh, A., and Ohkubo, T. (1987). Acquired von Willebrand disease due to inhibitor of human myeloma protein specific for von Willebrand factor. *American Journal of Clinical Pathology, 87,* 663–668.

Mundis, R. J., and Kyle, R. A. (1982). Primary hyperparathyroidism and monoclonal gammopathy of undetermined significance. *American Journal of Clinical Pathology, 77,* 619–621.

Murata, T., Fujita, H., Harano, H., Hukawa, M., Kanamori, H., Matsuzaki, M., Mohri, H., Kudoh, J., Shimizu, N., and Okubo, T. (1993). Triclonal gammopathy (IgAκ, IgGκ, and IgMκ) in a patient with plasmacytoid lymphoma derived from a monoclonal origin. *American Journal of Hematology, 42,* 212–216.

Mussini, C., Ghini, M., Mascia, M. T., Zanni, G., Lattuada, I., Giovanardi, P., Bonacorsi, G., and Artusi, T. (1995). HCV and monoclonal gammopathies. *Clinical and Experimental Rheumatology, 13*(Suppl 13), S45–S49.

Myara, I., Quenum, G., Storogenko, M., Tenenhaus, D., Guillemain, R., and Moatti, N. (1991). Monoclonal and oligoclonal gammopathies in heart-transplant recipients. *Clinical Chemistry, 37,* 1334–1337.

Nagata, T., Mugishima, H., Yoden, A., Yoshikawa, K., Oguni, T., Yamashiro, K., Yamamori, S., and Harada, K. (2000). A case of monoclonal gammopathy associated with acute myelomonocytic leukemia with eosinophilia suggested to be the result of lineage infidelity. *American Journal of Hematology, 65,* 66–71.

Nakanishi, H., Takehara, K., Soma, Y., and Ishibashi, Y. (1989). Atypical scleroderma associated with multiple myeloma. *Dermatologica, 178,* 176–178.

Nestle, F. O., Hofbauer, G., and Burg, G. (1999). Necrobiotic xanthogranuloma with monoclonal gammopathy of the IgG lambda type. *Dermatology, 198,* 434–435.

Ng, J. P., Jones, E. L., Pati, A., Strevens, M. J., and Guha, T. (1992). Hodgkin's disease and paraproteinaemia: a case report and review of the literature. *Clinical and Laboratory Haematology, 14,* 257–261.

Nilsson, T., Norberg, B., Rudolphi, O., and Jacobsson, L. (1986). Double gammopathies: incidence and clinical course of 20 patients. *Scandinavian Journal of Haematology, 36,* 103–106.

Nishida, K., Tamura, A., Nakazawa, N., Ueda, Y., Abe, T., Matsuda, F., Kashima, K., and Taniwaki, M. (1997). The Ig heavy chain gene is frequently involved in chromosomal translocations in multiple myeloma and plasma cell leukemia as detected by in situ hybridization. *Blood, 90,* 526–534.

Nobile-Orazio, E., Barbieri, S., Baldini, L., Marmiroli, P., Carpo, M., Premoselli, S., Manfredini, E., and Scarlato, G. (1992). Peripheral neuropathy in monoclonal gammopathy of undetermined significance: prevalence and immunopathogenetic studies. *Acta Neurologica Scandinavica, 85,* 383–390.

Noel, P., and Kyle, R. A. (1987). Monoclonal proteins in chronic lymphocytic leukemia. *American Journal of Clinical Pathology, 87,* 385–388.

Notermans, N. C., Lokhorst, H. M., Franssen, H., Van der Graaf, Y., Teunissen, L. L., Jennekens, F. G., Van den Berg, L. H., and Wokke, J. H. (1996). Intermittent cyclophosphamide and prednisone treatment of polyneuropathy associated with monoclonal gammopathy of undetermined significance. *Neurology, 47,* 1227–1233.

O'Connor, M. L., Rice, D. T., Buss, D. H., and Muss, H. B. (1991). Immunoglobulin D benign monoclonal gammopathy: a case report. *Cancer, 68,* 611–616.

Ocqueteau, M., Orfao, A., Almeida, J., Bladé, J., Gonzalez, M., Garcia-Sanz, R., Lopez-Berges, C., Moro, M. J., Hernandez, J., Escribano, L., Caballero, D., Rozman, M., and San Miguel, J. F. (1998). Immunophenotypic characterization of plasma cells from monoclonal gammopathy of undetermined significance patients: implications for the differential diagnosis between MGUS and multiple myeloma. *American Journal of Pathology, 152,* 1655–1665.

Offit, K., Macris, N. T., and Finkbeiner, J. A. (1986). Monoclonal hypergammaglobulinemia without malignant transformation in angioimmunoblastic lymphadenopathy with dysproteinemia. *American Journal of Medicine, 80,* 292–294.

Ögmundsdóttir, H. M., Haraldsdóttir, V., Jóhannesson, G. M., Ólafsdóttir, G., Bjarnadóttir, K., Sigvaldason, H., and Tulinius, H. (2002). Monoclonal gammopathy in Iceland: a population-based registry and follow-up. *British Journal of Haematology, 118,* 166–173.

Ohta, A., Uitto, J., Oikarinen, A. I., Palatsi, R., Mitrane, M., Bancila, E. A., Seibold, J. R., and Kim, H. C. (1987). Paraproteinemia in patients with scleredema: clinical findings and serum effects on skin fibroblasts in vitro. *Journal of the American Academy of Dermatology, 16,* 96–107.

Oksenhendler, E., Chevret, S., Leger, J. M., Louboutin, J. P., Bussel, A., and Brouet, J. C. (1995). Plasma exchange and chlorambucil in polyneuropathy associated with monoclonal IgM gammopathy: IgM-associated Polyneuropathy Study Group. *Journal of Neurology, Neurosurgery, and Psychiatry, 59,* 243–247.

Ong, F., Kaiser, U., Seelen, P. J., Hermans, J., Wijermans, P. W., de Kieviet, W., Jaques, G., and Kluin-Nelemans, J. C. (1996). Serum neural cell adhesion molecule differentiates multiple myeloma from paraproteinemias due to other causes. *Blood, 87,* 712–716.

Pageaux, G. P., Bonnardet, A., Picot, M. C., Perrigault, P. F., Coste, V., Navarro, F., Fabre, J. M., Domergue, J., Descomps, B., Blanc, P., Michel, H., and Larrey, D. (1998). Prevalence of monoclonal immunoglobulins after liver transplantation: relationship with posttransplant lymphoproliferative disorders. *Transplantation, 65,* 397–400.

Paladini, G., Fogher, M., Mazzanti, G., Parma, A., Fabiani, M. G., Sala, P. G., et al. (1989). Gammapatia monoclonale idiopatica: Studio a lungo termine di 313 casi. *Recenti Progressi in Medicina, 80,* 123–132.

Papadopoulos, N. M., Elin, R. J., and Wilson, D. M. (1982). Incidence of γ-globulin banding in a healthy population by high-resolution electrophoresis. *Clinical Chemistry, 28,* 707–708.

Pascual, M., Widmann, J.-J., and Schifferli, J. A. (1987). Recurrent febrile panniculitis and hepatitis in two patients with acquired complement deficiency and paraproteinemia. *American Journal of Medicine, 83,* 959–962.

Pasqualetti, P., and Casale, R. (1997). Monoclonal gammopathy of undetermined significance evolving directly in primary plasma cell leukemia. *Biomedical Pharmacotherapy, 51,* 284–285.

Pasqualetti, P., Festuccia, V., Collacciani, A., and Casale, R. (1997). The natural history of monoclonal gammopathy of undetermined significance: a 5- to 20-year followup of 263 cases. *Acta Haematologica, 97,* 174–179.

Pettersson, T., Hortling, L., Teppo, A. M., Tötterman, J., and Fyhrquist, F. (1987). Phosphate binding by a myeloma protein. *Acta Medica Scandinavica, 222,* 89–91.

Pham, H., Lemoine, A., Salvucci, M., Azoulay, D., Frenoy, N., Samuel, D., Reynes, M., Bismuth, H., and Debuire, B. (1998). Occurrence of gammopathies and lymphoproliferative disorders in liver transplant recipients randomized to tacrolimus (FK506)- or cyclosporine-based immunosuppression. *Liver Transplantation Surgery: Official Publication of the American Association for the Study of Liver Diseases and the International Liver Transplantation Society, 4,* 146–151.

Pizzolato, M., Bragantini, G., Bresciani, P., Pavlovsky, S., Chuba, J., Vidal, R., Rostagno, A., and Ghiso, J. (1998). IgG1-kappa biclonal gammopathy associated with multiple myeloma suggests a regulatory mechanism. *British Journal of Haematology, 102,* 503–508.

Pollock, C. A., Mahony, J. F., Ibels, L. S., Caterson, R. J., Waugh, D. A., Wells, J. V., and Sheil, A. G. R. (1989). Immunoglobulin abnormalities in renal transplant recipients. *Transplantation, 47,* 952–956.

Porcel, J. M., Ordi, J., Tolosa, C., Selva, A., Castro-Salomo, A., and Vilardell, M. (1992). Monoclonal gammopathy in systemic lupus erythematosus. *Lupus, 1,* 263–264.

Powell, F. C., Greipp, P. R., and Su, W. P. D. (1983a). Discoid lupus erythematosus and monoclonal gammopathy. *Br J Dermatol, 109,* 355–360.

Powell, F. C., Schroeter, A. L., Su, W. P. D., and Perry, H. O. (1983b). Pyoderma gangrenosum and monoclonal gammopathy. *Arch Dermatol, 119,* 468–472.

Pratt, P. W., Estren, S., and Kochwa, S. (1968). Immunoglobulin abnormalities in Gaucher's disease: report of 16 cases. *Blood, 31,* 633–640.

Probst, L. E., Hoffman, E., Cherian, M. G., Yang, J., Feagan, B., Adams, P., and Nichols, B. (1996). Ocular copper deposition associated with benign monoclonal gammopathy and hypercupremia. *Cornea, 15,* 94–98.

Puddu, P., Cianchini, G., Girardelli, C. R., Colonna, L., Gatti, S., and de Pita, O. (1997). Schnitzler's syndrome: report of a new case and a review of the literature. *Clinical and Experimental Rheumatology, 15,* 91–95.

Quarles, R. H., and Weiss, M. D. (1999). Autoantibodies associated with peripheral neuropathy. *Muscle & Nerve, 22,* 800–822.

Radl, J., Valentijn, R. M., Haaijman, J. J., and Paul, L. C. (1985). Monoclonal gammopathies in patients undergoing immunosuppressive treatment after renal transplantation. *Clinical Immunology and Immunopathology, 37,* 98–102.

Rajkumar, S. V., Kyle, R. A., Plevak, M. F., Murray, J. A., and Therneau, T. M. (2002a). *Helicobacter pylori* infection and monoclonal gammopathy of undetermined significance. *British Journal of Haematology, 119,* 706–708.

Rajkumar, S. V., Leong, T., Roche, P. C., Fonseca, R., Dispenzieri, A., Lacy, M. Q., Lust, J. A., Witzig, T. E., Kyle, R. A., Gertz, M. A., and Greipp, P. R. (2000). Prognostic value of bone marrow angiogenesis in multiple myeloma. *Clinical Cancer Research: An Official Journal of the American Association for Cancer Research, 6,* 3111–3116.

Rajkumar, S. V., Mesa, R. A., Fonseca, R., Schroeder, G., Plevak, M. F., Dispenzieri, A., Lacy, M. Q., Lust, J. A., Witzig, T. E., Gertz, M. A., Kyle, R. A., Russell, S. J., and Greipp, P. R. (2002b). Bone marrow angiogenesis in 400 patients with monoclonal gammopathy of undetermined significance, multiple myeloma, and primary amyloidosis. *Clinical Cancer Research, 8,* 2210–2216.

Rajkumar, S. V., and Witzig, T. E. (2000). A review of angiogenesis and antiangiogenic therapy with thalidomide in multiple myeloma. *Cancer Treatment Review, 26,* 351–362.

Rao, D. S., Antonelli, R., Kane, K. R., Kuhn, J. E., and Hetnal, C. (1991). Primary hyperparathyroidism and monoclonal gammopathy. *Henry Ford Hospital Medical Journal, 39,* 41–44.

Ray, R. A., and Schotters, S. B. (1986). Triclonal gammopathy in a patient with AIDS. *Clinical Chemistry, 32,* 2000.

Ray, R. A., Schotters, S. B., Jacobs, A., and Rodgerson, D. O. (1986). Triclonal gammopathy in a patient with plasma cell dyscrasia. *Clinical Chemistry, 32,* 205–206.

Read, D. J., Vanhegan, R. I., and Matthews, W. B. (1978). Peripheral neuropathy and benign IgG paraproteinaemia. *Journal of Neurology, Neurosurgery, and Psychiatry, 41,* 215–219.

Renier, G., Renier, J. C., Gardembas-Pain, M., Chevailler, A., Boasson, M., and Herez, D. (1992). Ankylosing spondylitis and monoclonal gammopathies. *Annals of Rheumatic Disease, 51,* 951–954.

Renoult, E., Bertrand, F., and Kessler, M. (1988). Monoclonal gammopathies in HBsAg-positive patients with renal transplants [Letter]. *New England Journal of Medicine, 318,* 1205.

Resegotti, L., Dolci, C., Palestro, G., and Peschle, C. (1978). Paraproteinemic variety of pure red cell aplasia: immunological studies in 1 patient. *Acta Haematologica, 60,* 227–232.

Rhys, J., Oleesky, D., Issa, B., Scanlon, M. F., Williams, C. P., Harrison, C. B., and Child, D. F. (1997). Pseudohypercalcaemia in two patients with IgM paraproteinaemia. *Annals of Clinical Biology, 34,* 694–696.

Ribera, J.-M., Cervantes, F., and Rozman, C. (1987). A multivariate analysis of prognostic factors in chronic myelomonocytic leukaemia according to the FAB criteria. *British Journal of Haematology, 65,* 307–311.

Riches, P. G., Sheldon, J., Smith, A. M., and Hobbs, J. R. (1991). Overestimation of monoclonal immunoglobulin by immunochemical methods. *Annals of Clinical Biochemistry, 28,* 253–259.

Riddell, S., Traczyk, Z., Paraskevas, F., and Israels, L. G. (1986). The double gammopathies: clinical and immunological studies. *Medicine (Baltimore), 65,* 135–142.

Roberts, R. T. (1986). Usefulness of immunofixation electrophoresis in the clinical laboratory. *Clinical Laboratory Medicine, 6,* 601–605.

Roodman, G. D. (2001). Biology of osteoclast activation in cancer. *Journal of Clinical Oncology, 19,* 3562–3571.

Roodman, G. D. (2002). Multiple myeloma: biology of myeloma bone disease. In V. C. Broudy, J. L. Abkowitz, and J. M. Vose (Eds.), *Hematology 2002: American Society of Hematology Education Program Book* (pp. 227–232). Washington, DC: American Society of Hematology.

Ropper, A. H., and Gorson, K. C. (1998). Neuropathies associated with paraproteinemia. *New England Journal of Medicine, 338,* 1601–1607.

Rostaing, L., Modesto, A., Abbal, M., and Durand, D. (1994). Long-term followup of monoclonal gammopathy of undetermined significance in transplant patients. *American Journal of Nephrology, 14,* 187–191.

Roux, S., Meignin, V., Quillard, J., Meduri, G., Guiochon-Mantel, A., Fermand, J. P., Milgrom, E., and Mariette, X. (2002). RANK (receptor activator of nuclear factor-kappaB) and RANKL expression in multiple myeloma. *British Journal of Haematology, 117,* 86–92.

Rovira, M., Cervantes, F., Nomdedeu, B., and Rozman, C. (1990). Chronic neutrophilic leukaemia preceding for seven years the development of multiple myeloma. *Acta Haematologica, 83,* 94–95.

Ryatt, K. S., Dodman, B. A., and Cotterill, J. A. (1981). Subcorneal pustular dermatosis and IgA gammopathy. *Acta Dermato-Venereolgica, 61,* 560–562.

Sadighi Akha, A. A., Humphrey, R. L., Winkelstein, J. A., Loeb, D. M., and Lederman, H. M. (1999). Oligo-/monoclonal gammopathy and hypergammaglobulinemia in ataxia–telangiectasia: a study of 90 patients. *Medicine (Baltimore), 78,* 370–381.

Saito, N., Hirai, K., Torimoto, Y., Taya, N., Kohgo, Y., Takemori, N., Tokuyasu, Y., and Miyokawa, N. (1998). Plural immunoglobulin synthesis in a single cell: an ultrastructural study of two cases with three M-proteins. *Ultrastructural Pathology, 22,* 421–429.

Sakashita, C., Saito, T., Kurosu, T., Yoshinaga, H., Kumagai, T., Yamamoto, K., Miki, T., Koyama, T., Miura, O., Nemoto, T., Asakawa, H., and Hirosawa, S. (1998). Two M-components in a single cell lineage in a patient with a dual isotype secretory B-cell tumour. *British Journal of Haematology, 102,* 791–794.

Saleun, J. P., Vicariot, M., Deroff, P., and Morin, J. F. (1982). Monoclonal gammopathies in the adult population of Finistère, France. *Journal of Clinical Pathology, 35,* 63–68.

Salgado, C., Bladé, J., López-Guillermo, A., Cervantes, F., Montserrat, E., and Rozman, C. (1993). Mieloma múltiple tras gammapatía monoclonal de significado incierto. Estudio de 10 casos. *Sangre, 38,* 371–374.

Sandström, H., Wahlin, A., Eriksson, M., Bergstrom, I., and Wickramasinghe, S. N. (1994). Intravascular haemolysis and increased prevalence of myeloma and monoclonal gammopathy in congenital dyserythropoietic anaemia, type III. *European Journal of Haematology, 52,* 42–46.

Sawanobori, M., Suzuki, K., Nakagawa, Y., Inoue, Y., Utsuyama, M., and Hirokawa, K. (1997). Natural killer cell frequency and serum cytokine levels in monoclonal gammopathies: correlation of bone marrow granular lymphocytes to prognosis. *Acta Haematologica, 98*, 150–154.

Schauer, P. K., Straus, D. J., Bagley, C. M., Jr., Rudolph, R. H., McCracken, J. D., Huff, J., Glucksburg, H., Bauermeister, D. E., and Clarkson, B. D. (1981). Angioimmunoblastic lymphadenopathy: clinical spectrum of disease. *Cancer, 48*, 2493–2498.

Schechter, G. P., Shoff, N., Chan, C., and Hawley, H. P. (1990). The frequency of monoclonal gammopathy of unknown significance (MGUS) in black and Caucasian veterans in a hospital population [Abstract]. *Blood, 76*(Suppl 1), 371a.

Schnur, M. J., Appel, G. B., and Bilezikian, J. P. (1977). Primary hyperparathyroidism and benign monoclonal gammopathy. *Archives of Internal Medicine, 137*, 1201–1203.

Schoenfeld, Y., Berliner, S., Pinkhas, J., and Beutler, E. (1990). The association of Gaucher's disease and dysproteinemias. *Acta Haematologica, 64*, 241–243.

Selroos, O., and von Knorring, J. (1973). Immunoglobulins in pernicious anaemia: including a report on a patient with pernicious anaemia, IgA deficiency and an M component of kappa-type IgG. *Acta Medica Scandinavica, 194*, 571–574.

Setterfield, J. F., Shirlaw, P. J., Challacombe, S. J., and Black, M. M. (2001). Pyoderma gangrenosum associated with severe oropharyngeal involvement and IgA paraproteinaemia. *British Journal of Dermatology, 144*, 393–396.

Sherman, W. H., Latov, N., Hays, A. P., Takatsu, M., Nemni, R., Galassi, G., and Osserman, E. F. (1983). Monoclonal IgM kappa antibody precipitating with chondroitin sulfate C from patients with axonal polyneuropathy and epidermolysis. *Neurology, 33*, 192–201.

Sherman, W. H., Latov, N., Lange, D., Hays, R., and Younger, D. (1994). Fludarabine for IgM antibody-mediated neuropathies [Abstract]. *Annals of Neurology, 36*, 326–327.

Simmons, Z., Albers, J. W., Bromberg, M. B., and Feldman, E. L. (1993a). Presentation and initial clinical course in patients with chronic inflammatory demyelinating polyradiculoneuropathy: comparison of patients without and with monoclonal gammopathy. *Neurology, 43*, 2202–2209.

Simmons, Z., Albers, J. W., Bromberg, M. B., and Feldman, E. L. (1995). Long-term followup of patients with chronic inflammatory demyelinating polyradiculoneuropathy, without and with monoclonal gammopathy. *Brain, 118*, 359–368.

Simmons, Z., Bromberg, M. B., Feldman, E. L., and Blaivas, M. (1993b). Polyneuropathy associated with IgA monoclonal gammopathy of undetermined significance. *Muscle & Nerve, 16*, 77–83.

Simovic, D., Gorson, K. C., and Ropper, A. H. (1998). Comparison of IgM-MGUS and IgG-MGUS polyneuropathy. *Acta Neurologica Scandinavica, 97*, 194–200.

Sinclair, D., Dagg, J. H., Dewar, A. E., Mowat, A.McI., Parrott, D. M. V., Stockdill, G., and Stott, D. I. (1986a). The incidence, clonal origin, and secretory nature of serum paraproteins in chronic lymphocytic leukaemia. *British Journal of Haematology, 64*, 725–735.

Sinclair, D., Sheehan, T., Parrott, D. M. V., and Stott, D. I. (1986b). The incidence of monoclonal gammopathy in a population over 45 years old determined by isoelectric focusing. *British Journal of Haematology, 64*, 745–750.

Singh, J., Dudley, A. W., Jr., and Kulig, K. A. (1990). Increased incidence of monoclonal gammopathy of undetermined significance in blacks and its age-related differences with whites on the basis of a study of 397 men and one woman in a hospital setting. *Journal of Laboratory and Clinical Medicine, 116*, 785–789.

Slavin, S., Zlotnick, A., Levij, I. S., and Eliakim, M. (1974). Clinical implications of monoclonal gammopathy in chronic liver disease. *American Journal of Digestive Diseases, 19*, 223–234.

Sluis, I. V. D. (1966). Two cases of pyoderma (ecthyma) gangraenosum associated with the presence of an abnormal serumprotein ($\beta_2$ A-paraprotein): with a review of the literature. *Dermatologica, 132*, 409–424.

Smith, T., Sherman, W., Olarte, M. R., and Lovelace, R. E. (1987). Peripheral neuropathy associated with plasma cell dyscrasia: a clinical and electrophysiological follow-up study. *Acta Neurologica Scandinavica, 75*, 244–248.

Solal-Celigny, P., Desaint, B., Herrera, A., Chastang, C., Amar, M., Vroclans, M., Brousse, N., Mancilla, F., Renoux, M., Bernard, J.-F., and Boivin, P. (1984). Chronic myelomonocytic leukemia according to FAB classification: analysis of 35 cases. *Blood, 63*, 634–638.

Solary, E., Guignet, M., Zeller, V., Casasnovas, R.-O., Caillot, D., Chavanet, P., Guy, H., and Mack, G. (1992). Radioimmunoassay for the measurement of serum IL-6 and its correlation with tumour cell mass parameters in multiple myeloma. *American Journal of Hematology, 39*, 163–171.

Sonnenblick, M., Eylath, U., Brisk, R., Eldad, C., and Hershko, C. (1986). Paraprotein interference with colorimetry of phosphate in serum of some patients with multiple myeloma. *Clinical Chemistry, 32*, 1537–1539.

Sonneveld, P., Durie, B. G. M., Lokhorst, H. M., Frutiger, Y., Schoester, M., and Vela, E. E. (1993). Analysis of multidrug-resistance (MDR-1) glycoprotein and CD56 expression to separate monoclonal gammopathy from multiple myeloma. *British Journal of Haematology, 83*, 63–67.

Soppi, E., Eskola, J., Roytta, M., Veromaa, T., Panelius, M., and Lehtonen, A. (1985). Thymoma with immunodeficiency (Good's syndrome) associated with myasthenia gravis and benign IgG gammopathy. *Archives of Internal Medicine, 145*, 1704–1707.

Stanko, C. K., Jeffrey, J. R., and Rush, D. N. (1989). Monoclonal and multiclonal gammopathies after renal transplantation. *Transplantation Proceedings, 21*, 3330–3332.

Steck, A. J., Murray, N., Dellagi, K., Brouet, J. C., and Seligmann, M. (1987). Peripheral neuropathy associated with monoclonal IgM autoantibody. *Annals of Neurology, 22*, 764–767.

Steinberg, A. D., Seldin, M. F., Jaffe, E. S., Smith, H. R., Klinman, D. M., Krieg, A. M., and Cossman, J. (1988). NIH conference: angioimmunoblastic lymphadenopathy with dysproteinemia. *Ann Intern Med, 108*, 575–584.

Stern, J. J., Ng, R. H., Triplett, D. A., and McIntyre, J. A. (1994). Incidence of antiphospholipid antibodies in patients with monoclonal gammopathy of undetermined significance. *American Journal of Clinical Pathology, 101*, 471–474.

Stockman, A., Delanghe, J., Geerts, M.-L., and Naeyaert, J. M. (2002). Diffuse plane normolipaemic xanthomatosis in a patient with chronic lymphatic leukaemia and monoclonal gammopathy. *Dermatology, 204*, 351–354.

Strumia, R., and Roveggio, C. (1994). Kaposi's sarcoma and monoclonal gammopathy. *Dermatology, 188*, 76–77.

Sugai, S., Konda, S., Shoraski, Y., Murayama, T., and Nishikawa, T. (1980). Non-IgM monoclonal gammopathy in patients with Sjögren's syndrome. *American Journal of Medicine, 68*, 861–866.

*Surveillance, Epidemiology, and End Results (SEER) Program public-use data (1973–1998)*. Bethesda, MD: National Cancer Institute, Cancer Statistics Branch, April 2001.

Takatsuki, K., and Sanada, I. (1983). Plasma cell dyscrasia with polyneuropathy and endocrine disorder: clinical and laboratory features of 109 reported cases. *Japanese Journal of Clinical Oncology, 13*, 543–555.

Talerman, A., and Haije, W. G. (1973). The frequency of M-components in sera of patients with solid malignant neoplasms. *British Journal of Cancer, 27*, 276–282.

Telerman-Toppet, N., Wittek, M., Bacq, M., Dajez, P., Coërs, C., and Fassotte, A. (1982). Benign monoclonal gammopathy and relapsing polymyositis [Letter]. *Muscle & Nerve, 5*, 490–491.

Tursi, A., and Modeo, M. E. (2002). Monoclonal gammopathy of undetermined significance predisposing to *Helicobacter pylori*-related gastric mucosa-associated lymphoid tissue lymphoma. *Journal of Clinical Gastroenterology, 34*, 147–149.

Ucci, G., Riccardi, A., Luoni, R., and Ascari, E. (1993). Presenting features of monoclonal gammopathies: an analysis of 684 newly diagnosed cases. Cooperative Group for the Study and Treatment of Multiple Myeloma. *Journal of Internal Medicine, 234*, 165–173.

Vacca, A., Ribatti, D., Presta, M., Minischetti, M., Iurlaro, M., Ria, R., Albini, A., Bussolino, F., and Dammacco, F. (1999). Bone marrow neovascularization, plasma cell angiogenic potential, and matrix metalloproteinase-2 secretion parallel progression of human multiple myeloma. *Blood, 93*, 3064–3073.

Vacca, A., Ribatti, D., Roncali, L., Ranieri, G., Serio, G., Silvestris, F., and Dammacco, F. (1994). Bone marrow angiogenesis and progression in multiple myeloma. *British Journal of Haematology, 87*, 503–508.

Van De Donk, N., De Weerdt, O., Eurelings, M., Bloem, A., and Lokhorst, H. (2001). Malignant transformation of monoclonal gammopathy of undetermined significance: cumulative incidence and prognostic factors. *Leukemia and Lymphoma, 42*, 609–618.

van de Poel, M. H., Coebergh, J. W., and Hillen, H. F. (1995). Malignant transformation of monoclonal gammopathy of undetermined significance among out-patients of a community hospital in southeastern Netherlands. *British Journal of Haematology, 91*, 121–125.

van Spronsen, D. J., Hoorntje, S. J., Hannema, A. J., and Hack, C. E. (1998). Acquired angio-oedema caused by IgA paraprotein. *The Netherlands Journal of Medicine, 52*, 22–25.

Vejlgaard, T., Abildgaard, N., Jans, H., Nielsen, J. L., and Heickendorff, L. (1997). Abnormal bone turnover in monoclonal gammopathy of undetermined significance: analyses of type I collagen telopeptide, osteocalcin, bone-specific alkaline phosphatase and propeptides of type I and type III procollagens. *European Journal of Haematology, 58*, 104–108.

Venencie, P. Y., Winkelmann, R. K., Friedman, S. J., Kyle, R. A., and Puissant, A. (1984a). Monoclonal gammopathy and mycosis fungoides: report of four cases and review of the literature. *Journal of the American Academy of Dermatology, 11*, 576–579.

Venencie, P. Y., Winkelmann, R. K., Puissant, A., and Kyle, R. A. (1984b). Monoclonal gammopathy in Sézary syndrome: report of three cases and review of the literature. *Archives of Dermatology, 120*, 605–608.

Vladutiu, A. O. (1987). Prevalence of M-proteins in serum of hospitalized patients: physicians' response to finding M-proteins in serum protein electrophoresis. *Annals of Clinical Laboratory Sciences, 17*, 157–161.

Vrethem, M., Cruz, M., Wen-Sin, H., Malm, C., Holmgren, H., and Ernerudh, J. (1993). Clinical, neurophysiological and immunological evidence of polyneuropathy in patients with monoclonal gammopathies. *Journal of Neurological Sciences, 114*, 193–199.

Waldenström, J. (1961). Studies on conditions associated with disturbed gamma globulin formation (gammopathies). *Harvey Lectures, 56*, 211–231.

Watanabe, J., Kondo, H., Iwazaki, H., Hatake, K., and Horikoshi, N. (2001). An unusual association of monoclonal gammopathy, paroxysmal nocturnal haemoglobinuria and myelodysplastic syndrome transformed into acute myeloid leukaemia: coexistence of triple clonal disorders. *Leukemia and Lymphoma, 42*, 813–817.

Watanabe, O., Maruyama, I., Arimura, K., Kitajima, I., Arimura, H., Hanatani, M., Matsuo, K., Arisato, T., and Osame, M. (1998). Overproduction of vascular endothelial growth factor/vascular permeability factor is causative in Crow-Fukase (POEMS) syndrome. *Muscle & Nerve, 21*, 1390–1397.

Weidner, N., and Folkman, J. (1996). Tumoral vascularity as a prognostic factor in cancer. *Important Advances in Oncology*, 167–190.

Weidner, N., Semple, J. P., Welch, W. R., and Folkman, J. (1991). Tumor angiogenesis and metastasis: correlation in invasive breast carcinoma. *New England Journal of Medicine, 324*, 1–8.

Williams, R. C., Jr., Malone, C. C., Silvestris, F., and Nickerson, K. G. (1997). Benign monoclonal gammopathy with IgG anti-DNA, anti-Sm and anti-F(ab')2 activity. *Clinical and Experimental Rheumatology, 15*, 33–38.

Wilson, H. C., Lunn, M. P., Schey, S., and Hughes, R. A. (1999). Successful treatment of IgM paraproteinaemic neuropathy with fludarabine. *Journal of Neurology, Neurosurgery, and Psychiatry, 66*, 575–580.

Witzig, T. E., Gonchoroff, N. J., Katzmann, J. A., Therneau, T. M., Kyle, R. A., and Greipp, P. R. (1988). Peripheral blood B cell labeling indices are a measure of disease activity in patients with monoclonal gammopathies. *Journal of Clinical Oncology, 6*, 1041–1046.

Witzig, T. E., Kyle, R. A., and Greipp, P. R. (1992). Circulating peripheral blood plasma cells in multiple myeloma. *Current Topics in Microbiology and Immunology, 182*, 195–199.

Witzig, T. E., Kyle, R. A., O'Fallon, W. M., and Greipp, P. R. (1994). Detection of peripheral blood plasma cells as a predictor of disease course in patients with smouldering multiple myeloma. *British Journal of Haematology, 87*, 266–272.

Xu, D., Zheng, C., Bergenbrant, S., Holm, G., Bjorkholm, M., Yi, Q., and Gruber, A. (2001). Telomerase activity in plasma cell dyscrasias. *British Journal of Cancer, 84*, 621–625.

Yaccoby, S., Pearse, R. N., Johnson, C. L., Barlogie, B., Choi, Y., and Epstein, J. (2002). Myeloma interacts with the bone marrow microenvironment to induce osteoclastogenesis and is dependent on osteoclast activity. *British Journal of Haematology, 116*, 278–290.

Yee, W. C., Hahn, A. F., Hearn, S. A., and Rupar, A. R. (1989). Neuropathy in IgM lambda paraproteinemia: immunoreactivity to neural proteins and chondroitin sulfate. *Acta Neuropathologica, 78*, 57–64.

Yetgin, S., Olcay, L., Yel, L., Tuncer, M., Tezcan, I., Erdemli, E., Oner, A. F., and Behm, F. G. (2000). T-ALL with monoclonal gammopathy and hairy cell features. *American Journal of Hematology, 65*, 166–170.

Younger, D. S., Rowland, L. P., Latov, N., Sherman, W., Pesce, M., Lange, D. J., Trojaborg, W., Miller, J. R., Lovelace, R. E., Hays, A. P., and Kim, T. S. (1990). Motor neuron disease and amyotrophic lateral sclerosis: relation of high CSF protein content to paraproteinemia and clinical syndromes. *Neurology, 40*, 595–599.

Zandecki, M., Obein, V., Bernardi, F., Soenen, V., Flactif, M., Lai, J. L., François, M., and Facon, T. (1995). Monoclonal gammopathy of undetermined significance: chromosome changes are a common finding within bone marrow plasma cells. *British Journal of Haematology, 90*, 693–696.

Zawadzki, Z. A., and Benedek, T. G. (1969). Rheumatoid arthritis, dysproteinemic arthropathy, and paraproteinemia. *Arthritis and Rheumatism, 12*, 555–568.

Zawadzki, Z. A., and Edwards, G. A. (1970). Dysimmunoglobulinemia associated with hepatobiliary disorders. *American Journal of Medicine, 48*, 196–202.

Zent, C. S., Wilson, C. S., Tricot, G., Jagannath, S., Siegel, D., Desikan, K. R., Munshi, N., Bracy, D., Barlogie, B., and Butch, A. W. (1998). Oligoclonal protein bands and Ig isotype switching in multiple myeloma treated with high-dose therapy and hematopoietic cell transplantation. *Blood, 91*, 3518–3523.

Zhang, X. G., Bataille, R., Widjenes, J., and Klein, B. (1992). Interleukin-6 dependence of advanced malignant plasma cell dyscrasias. *Cancer, 69*, 1373–1376.

# CHAPTER 20

# Plasmacytoma

JAMES S. MALPAS
JAMIE D. CAVENAGH

## Introduction

The plasma cell dyscrasias (PCD) constitute a wide spectrum of disorders.

1. Monoclonal gammopathy of undetermined significance (MGUS).

2. Localized plasmacytoma
    a. Solitary plasmacytoma of bone
    b. Extramedullary plasmacytoma

3. Diffuse plasmacytoma
    a. Smoldering MM
    b. Indolent MM
    c. MM (overt)
    d. Plasma cell leukemia

Localized plasmacytomas are tumors of plasma cell origin composed of sheets of plasma cells of varying maturity, involving bone or soft tissue, which are histologically similar to MM. They develop either in bone (solitary plasmacytoma of bone [SPB]) or in the soft tissues (extramedullary plasmacytoma [EMP]). Both forms are rare disorders and account for less than 10% of all plasma cell neoplasms.

SPB might involve any bone but arises most commonly in the marrow-containing bones in the axial skeleton. EMP, in contrast, might occur in a variety of soft tissue sites but usually presents in the head and neck, arising in the upper air passages. SPB progresses to MM more frequently than EMP, which normally remains localized. SPB and EMP have clinicopathologic features that distinguish them from each other and from MM; these are discussed in detail in this chapter.

# Solitary Plasmacytoma of Bone (SPB)

SPB was first described in 1897 (Wiltshaw, 1976). The concept of a plasma cell tumor occurring as an isolated lesion of bone was first recognized in 1923 when Shaw reported a case of "solitary plasma cell myeloma" in a 29-year-old man who presented with a plasmacytoma of the right humerus.

## Clinical Features

SPB is an uncommon plasma cell tumor occurring in 3% to 5% of patients with plasma cell neoplasms (Conklin and Alexanian, 1975; Dimopoulous et al., 1992; Knowling et al., 1983; Tsang et al., 2001). The disease occurs predominantly in males (male:female ratio 2:1). It might affect any age group from childhood to old age, the median age being 55, approximately 10 years less than in patients with MM.

The most common mode of presentation is pain at the site of the skeletal lesion occurring in 70% to 80% (Frassica et al., 1989; Jackson and Scarffe, 1990; Knowling et al., 1983). Neurologic dysfunction in the form of nerve root compression or spinal cord compression is another common form of presentation occurring predominantly in patients with SPB in the vertebral column. Other forms of presentation are pathologic fractures, soft tissue extensions of SPB resulting in mass lesions, and more rare manifestations such as peripheral neuropathy with or without endocrine abnormalities, lymphadenopathy, and skin abnormalities.

In more than half the cases of skeletal SPB, the presentation is in the axial skeleton. The remaining presentations occur in the appendicular skeleton (Bataille and Sarny, 1981; Frassica et al., 1989; Tsang et al., 2001). In the vertebral column the thoracic vertebrae are the most commonly affected followed by the lumbar, sacral, and cervical vertebrae in that order. The sites of SPB based on pooled data from cases reported in the literature are shown in Tables 20-1 and 20-2.

## Diagnostic Criteria of SPB

The diagnostic criteria of SPB have not been well defined as yet. Various studies have applied different criteria in diagnosis, some authors including patients with multiple lesions (Corwin and Lindberg, 1979; Tong et al., 1980), whereas others have excluded patients whose disease progressed to MM within 2 or

### TABLE 20-1

Sites of Lesions in 343 Patients with SPB

| Axial Skeleton (n = 235, 68%) | | Appendicular Skeleton (n = 108, 32%) | |
|---|---|---|---|
| Skull | 31 | Shoulder girdle | 26 |
| Vertebral column | 160 | Pelvic girdle | 47 |
| Ribs | 38 | Extremities | 35 |
| Sternum | 6 | | |

Sources: Bataille and Sarny, 1981; Chak et al., 1987; Corwin and Lindberg, 1979; Dimopoulos et al., 1992; Frassica et al., 1989; Greenberg et al., 1987; Holland et al., 1992; Jackson and Scarffe, 1990; Knowling et al., 1983; Meis et al., 1987; Mendenhall et al., 1980; Meyr et al., 1990; Tong et al., 1980; Tsang et al., 2001; Woodruff et al., 1979a.

3 years (Christopherson and Miller, 1950; Meyer and Schultz, 1974; Tong et al., 1980). The interpretation of bone marrow has also been a subject of debate, some authors using a cut-off point of 10% infiltration with plasma cells (Corwin and Lindberg, 1979; Frassica et al., 1989; Mayr et al., 1990; Mendenhall et al., 1980; Tong et al., 1980; Wasserman, 1987) whereas others included only those patients with a normal bone marrow, that is, less than 5% plasma cells of normal cytology (Bush et al., 1981; Castro et al., 1973; Dimopoulos et al., 1992; Knowling et al., 1983; Meyer and Schultz, 1974; Woodruff et al., 1979a). Most series included patients with minor serum protein abnormalities (Chak et al., 1987; Frassica et al., 1989; Mayr et al., 1990; Mendenhall et al., 1980; Meyer and Schultz, 1974; Tong et al., 1980; Woodruff et al., 1979a), whereas some include them only if the abnormalities decrease with specific therapy (Corwin and Lindberg, 1979; Knowling et al., 1983).

Despite the reported differences, certain diagnostic criteria stand out as essential whereas others are retrospective or nonessential for the diagnosis of SPB.

They are subsequently summarized.

1. Essential diagnostic criteria for SPB
   a. Solitary bone lesion on skeletal survey

### TABLE 20-2

Sites of Spinal Lesions in 252 Patients with SPB (141 [56%] had spinal involvement)

| Site | No. of Total | Percentage |
|---|---|---|
| Thoracic vartebrae | 81/141 | 58 |
| Lumbar vertebrae | 33/141 | 23 |
| Sacrum | 17/141 | 12 |
| Cervical | 10/141 | 7 |

Note: This includes 19 cases of SPB of the spine only (Delauche-Cavallier et al., 1988), thirty-two cases from Holland et al., (1992), and 45 cases of Dimopoulos et al., (1992) were excluded because no exact site for the vertebral involvement was given.

b. Histologically proven plasmacytoma in a biopsy of the tumor

c. Bone marrow aspirate showing less than 5% of plasma cells

d. Absence of anemia, hypercalcemia, or impairment of renal function

e. Absence of monoclonal paraprotein or low concentration of monoclonal component using immunoelectrophoresis (IgG less than 35 g/L; IgA less than 20 g/L, Bence Jones protein excretion less than 1 g in 24 h).

2. Nonessential criteria (retrospective) of SPB

a. Disappearance of monoclonal component after surgery or radiation

b. Normal levels of immunoglobulins or low levels that return to normal after surgery or radiation

Most centers depend on a negative skeletal survey to exclude other bone lesions in patients with SPB. However, special techniques such as CT or MRI scanning have detected abnormalities in bones previously reported normal by conventional radiography (Dimopoulos et al., 1992).

MRI scanning has helped with the diagnosis of early systemic MM in cases referred with presumed SPB.

## Investigations

When a diagnosis of SPB is suspected, investigation should proceed as follows:

1. Normally recommended investigations

a. History and examination

b. Hematology: erythrocyte sedimentation rate, full blood count, bone marrow aspiration, and biopsy

c. Biochemistry: renal function tests, liver function tests, LDH, calcium, serum protein and urinary electrophoresis or immunoelectrophoresis, serum immunoglobulins

d. Radiology: plain radiograph of involved site, skeletal survey

2. Special investigations: CT and MRI, immunoperoxidase staining for mAb on biopsied tissue, immunostaining to detect light chain restriction on biopsied tissue

## Management of SPB

Definitive local radiotherapy is the mainstay of treatment for SPB, although optimal management might depend on other factors such as the site of the tumor and clinical presentation. In summary, treatment consists of the following: Local radiotherapy (RT) is the treatment of choice; the treatment field includes the tumor and a margin of normal tissues. The recommended dose is 4000 to 5000 cGy and duration of treatment is 3 to 5 weeks. For spinal lesions such as epidural

plasmacytoma and compressive myelopathy, a laminectomy might be needed to make the diagnosis. This is then followed by radiotherapy (RT). If neurologic dysfunction is minimal, dexamethasone followed by RT is the treatment of choice. Surgical excision of the tumor might also be achieved and other surgical procedures such as the insertion of Harrison's rods or internal fixation of fractures might be necessary.

An optimal dose of radiotherapy has not been established owing to the small number of cases seen in any individual center. The majority of studies recommend 4000 to 5000 cGy spread over 3 to 5 weeks (Bush et al., 1981; Frassica et al., 1989; Greenberg et al., 1987; Holland et al., 1992; Mayr et al., 1990; Mendenhall et al., 1980; Meyer and Schultz, 1974; Woodruff et al., 1979a), whereas some consider 3500 cGy sufficient for local control (Harwood et al., 1981; Knowling et al., 1983). Following adequate radiotherapy virtually all patients experience relief of pain, and local control is established in 87% to 100% of patients (Bataille and Sarny, 1981; Chak et al., 1987; Dimopoulos et al., 1992).

In 45 patients treated in a single center with RT doses varying from 3500 to 5000 cGy, there was no clear relationship between the dose of local radiotherapy and the onset of MM (Dimopoulos et al., 1992). Tsang et al. (2001), updating the Princess Margaret Hospital experience of plasmacytoma, reported a long-term followup of 46 patients treated with 3500 cGy for solitary plasmacytoma and showed that local control was related to tumor size. All tumors less than 5 cm in bulk in 34 patients were controlled by RT. They recommended that tumors greater than 5 cm in bulk should be treated with chemotherapy and radiotherapy to increase local control. Aviles et al. (1996), in a randomized trial in which melphalan and prednisolone were given after RT in one arm, showed that with a median followup of 8.9 years, 15 of 25 (54%) of patients on the RT-only arm of the study progressed to MM whereas only 3 of 25 (12%) in the combined therapy group did so. However, this study was criticized because of the sample size and the hazard of long-term effects from the use of melphalan. Bolek et al. (1996) found no advantage in giving chemotherapy; this area evidently needs further investigation.

Surgical intervention might include internal fixation of pathologic fractures, prophylactic fixation to prevent fractures, stabilization of the spinal lesions by the use of Harrington's rods (Harrington, 1981; Loftus et al., 1983), and decompression of spinal lesions. Compressive myelopathy caused by spinal epidural plasmacytoma might be treated by laminectomy followed by RT (Bacci et al., 1982; Loftus et al., 1983). Complete or almost-complete reversal of neurologic dysfunction might be observed in all cases of spinal cord compression (Delauche-Cavallier et al., 1988). Some authors advocate RT alone for SPB of the spine with minimal neurologic deficit (Cohen et al., 1964;

Gilbert et al., 1978; Kaplan and Bennett, 1968). Surgical excision only of lesions in easily accessible sites has been advocated (Durie and Salmon, 1975), but a combination of surgical excision followed by RT is probably the best approach.

### Prognostic Features

The local or distant recurrence of SPB is related to age at diagnosis. Higher relapse rates are seen in older patients; location of the primary is also important with peripheral lesions having a better prognosis than axial lesions (Bataille and Sarny, 1981); the disappearance of paraprotein after treatment is also associated with a better prognosis (Dimopolous et al., 1992; Dimopolous et al., 1999).

Initial absence of paraprotein is known to correlate with limited tumor mass and is reported to be associated with longer disease-free intervals (Delauche-Cavallier et al., 1988). Holland et al. (1992) have shown that the size of the lesion (median size, 7 cm), total serum protein levels (median, 7.55 mg/dL), and presence of a monoclonal spike on serum electrophoresis correlates with the development of MM. Despite all these factors, it still remains impossible to determine a patient's prognosis at diagnosis. Jackson and Scarffe (1990) found that only generalized osteoporosis and immunoparesis were adverse prognostic factors.

### Natural History

Long-term followup of patients with SPB indicates a disease-free survival rate of over 40% at 5 years (Dimopoulos et al., 1992; Mayr et al., 1990) and 15% to 30% at 10 years (Alexanian et al., 1980; Bataille and

Sarny, 1981; Frassica et al., 1989). The pattern of progression over a 10-year period is variable and includes the development of a new solitary lesion at another site in 15% of patients or local recurrence in 3% to 12%. In most cases (44% to 64%) eventual progression to MM occurs (Dimopoulos et al., 1992; Jackson and Scarffe, 1990; Mayr et al., 1990).

The overall prognosis of SPB is good with a median survival of over 10 years in most series. The clinical outcome of SPB in some major series is shown in Table 20-3.

## Extramedullary Plasmacytoma (EMP)

EMP is a rare soft tissue plasma cell tumor, which was first described by Schridde in 1905. These tumors are known to arise in a variety of anatomic sites, although approximately 90% arise in the head and neck region (Batsakis et al., 1964; Poole and Marchetta, 1968) and most of these arise in the upper respiratory air passages, including the paranasal sinuses (Castro et al., 1973; Knowling et al., 1983; Webb et al., 1962; Wiltshaw, 1976; Woodruff et al., 1979b). EMPs constitute less than 5% of all plasma cell tumors, are more responsive to therapy, and generally remain localized.

### Clinical Features

EMPs are reported to have a strong male preponderance, with a male:female ratio of at least 2:1 and in some series a ratio of 5:1 has been reported (Knowling et al., 1983). The median age at presentation is 60 years but the condition has been reported in childhood and

---

### TABLE 20-3
#### Clinical Outcome of Patients with SPB

| | Study | | | | | | | |
| Parameter | Alexanian (1981) | Bataille (1981) | Knowling (1983) | Chak (1987) | Frassica (1989) | Mayr (1990) | Jackson (1990) | Dimopoulos (1992) |
|---|---|---|---|---|---|---|---|---|
| Number of patients | 29 | 18 | 25 | 20 | 46 | 13 | 32 | 45 |
| Median age (y) | 52 | 51 | 50 | 58 | 56 | 61 | 62 | 53 |
| Spinal disease (%) | 40 | 60 | 40 | 55 | 54 | 76 | 72 | 33 |
| Myeloma protein (%) | 55 | 33 | 24 | 40 | 54 | 50 | 34 | 58 |
| Local recurrence (%) | 5 | 11 | N/A | 5 | 11 | 12 | 3 | 4 |
| Progression to myeloma | — | 44 | 52 | 55 | 54 | 53 | 69 | 46 |
| Median time to progression to myeloma (mo) | — | — | — | — | — | 36 | 46 | 36 |
| Disease-free survival at 10 years (%) | 30 | 15 | 16 | 23 | 25 | N/A | N/A | N/A |
| Median survival (y) | 12 | N/A | 7 | 11 | 8 | N/A | 10 | 13 |

SPB, Solitary plasmacytoma.

adolescence (Bertoni-Salateo et al., 1998). Clinical presentation varies according to site and organ involved, and EMPs are seldom diagnosed purely on their clinical features because diagnosis can only be made on histologic examination. The most common sites of primary tumors are the nose, paranasal sinuses, nasopharynx, and tonsil. Patients might be symptom-free or might have nasal discharge, epistaxes, nasal obstruction, sore throat, hoarseness, hemoptysis, or dyspnea (Fu and Perzin, 1978; Medini et al., 1980; Meis et al., 1987; Poole and Marchetta, 1968). Pain and tenderness over the maxillary sinus, if this is the primary site, has been reported by Fu and Perzin (1978). Examination of the air passages might reveal a smooth, fleshy, sessile, or pedunculated dark-red or grayish-red or gray tumor, confined to the submucosa, obstructing the lumen of the involved structure or it might be ulcerated on its surface. Less commonly involved sites in the head and neck region are the salivary glands, skin, cervical lymph nodes, orbit, larynx, and thyroid (Fishkin and Spiegelberg, 1976; Gorenstein et al., 1977; Hellwig, 1943; Johnson and Taylor, 1970; Macpherson et al., 1981; Pahor, 1977; Rodman and Font, 1972; Shimaoka et al., 1978; Webb et al., 1962). EMP of the thyroid presents with painless, nontender, nontoxic goiter and the diagnosis is only confirmed on histologic examination (Shimaoke et al., 1978).

Other relatively rare sites of origin include the gastrointestinal tract, liver, spleen, and pancreas and other organs such as the breast and testis (Deodhare et al., 1975; Douglass et al., 1971; Remigio and Klaum, 1971; Sharma and Shrivastav, 1961; Wiltshaw, 1976). De Chiara et al. (2001) reported on a breast plasmacytoma, reviewed the histologic features of previously reported cases, and emphasized the difficulties that might arise in diagnosing from frozen sections. EMP of the gastrointestinal tract commonly involves the small intestine, the stomach, and less commonly the large bowel; abdominal pain, gastrointestinal bleeding, and weight loss are the usual presenting features. Uceda-Montanes et al. (2000) and Honavar et al. (2001) reported an EMP of the orbit in one patient and of the choroid in another. Both occurrences are extremely rare but these patients survive at 4 and 9 years. Testicular plasmacytomas were reported by Suzuki et al. (2001) and Ramadan et al. (2000). In the latter report the patient had acquired AIDS, a condition that is leading to an increased frequency of plasmacytomas at an earlier age. The sites of EMP based on pooled data from the literature is shown in Table 20-4.

## Diagnostic Criteria

The diagnosis of EMP is based on the following criteria: solitary plasma cell tumor presenting in the head and neck (multiple tumors are included only

### TABLE 20-4

Sites of Lesions in 382 Patients with EMP

| Site | No. of Patients Affected |
|---|---|
| Upper air passages and perinasal sinuses (includes palate, tongue, tonsils, and epiglottis) | — 309 |
| Lower air passages and lungs | 16 |
| Lymph nodes and spleen | 22 |
| Gastrointestinal tract | 10 |
| Thyroid | 10 |
| Other | 3 |

Sources: Corwin and Lindberg, 1979; Greenberg et al., 1987; Knowling et al., 1983; Mayr et al., 1990; Meis et al., 1987; Mendenhall et al., 1980; Petrovich et al., 1977; Poole and Marchetta, 1968; Tsang et al., 2001; Wiltshaw, 1976; Woodruff et al., 1979b.

if they occur in other sites of primary involvement), histologic confirmation of EMP, normal bone marrow taken from a distant site, and a low concentration of paraprotein.

Histologic diagnosis is complicated by the difficulty of differentiating EMP from benign reactive plasmacytosis. The demonstration of intracellular polyclonal Ig using immunoperoxidase staining can help to exclude reactive plasmacytosis. Monoclonal cytoplasmic pattern of Ig is seen in both EMP and malignant lymphoma but is more easily detectable in EMP and invariably positive (Kapadia et al., 1982). Hotz et al. (1999), in reviewing 24 patients with morphologically diagnosed EMP treated in a single center, found that using immunophenotyping only 14 satisfied the criteria of true monoclonal plasmacytomas.

## Investigations

Investigations might be carried out like for SPB, but in view of the frequency of nasopharyngeal presentations, all surgically removed polyps should be sent for histologic examination.

## Management

Surgery was at first the only form of treatment available for EMP. RT is now the preferred form of therapy because EMPs are highly radiosensitive. The majority of small mucosal EMPs can be controlled with 3000 to 4000 cGy (Corwin and Lindberg, 1979; Knowling et al., 1983; Mayr et al., 1990; Poole and Marchetta, 1968; Wasserman, 1987; Wiltshaw, 1976; Woodruff et al., 1979b). Mayr et al. (1990) reported seeing no recurrences when using 4000 cGy in 20 fractions. The recommended dose is therefore 4000 to 5000 cGy over

4 to 5 weeks, higher doses only being used in extensive involvement or if the tumor appears more resistant. Some centers also prophylactically irradiate local lymph nodes because there is a 25% risk of local recurrence at these sites.

## Natural History

Local tumor control, defined as permanent eradication of the tumor from the treated area with resolution of the soft tissue mass or stabilization of the lytic area on radiologic examination, is achieved in over 50% of patients treated with RT. Regional failures, that is, patients developing lymph node metastases, vary from 8% to 15% (Knowling et al., 1983; Mayr et al., 1990; Tong et al., 1980). Progression to MM is reported as occurring in from 0% to 40% (Chak et al., 1987; Corwin and Lindberg, 1979; Knowling et al., 1983; Mayr et al., 1990; Mendenhall et al., 1980; Tong et al., 1980; Woodruff et al., 1979b). Metastasis to bone with single osteolytic lesions is also reported, these lesions differing from those seen in MM both in distribution and radiologic appearance (Wiltshaw, 1976). Soft tissue spread has also occurred to other sites such as skin and subcutaneous tissue. Very rarely, EMP may spread to organs such as the liver, spleen, lungs, gastrointestinal tract, and genitourinary tract.

The median survival of patients with EMP varies from 4 to 10 years; the prognosis for nasopharyngeal EMP that has responded well to treatment is usually very good.

## Prognostic Factors

Localized EMPs of the upper air passages have a better prognosis than large tumors arising outside the head and neck. Destruction of underlying bone has been reported by some as being an adverse prognostic factor (Batsakis et al., 1964; Hellwig, 1943; Rainer, 1970; Webb et al., 1962). However, in a later study, this was not considered a significant factor (Corwin and Lindberg, 1979). Lymph node involvement is not considered an adverse prognostic feature.

## Other Rare Presentations

Peripheral neuropathy in solitary plasmacytoma is rare with one small series reported by Read and Warlow (1978). Patients with solitary plasmacytoma usually present with peripheral neuropathy in contrast to patients with MM. It occurs in a younger age group than MM; predominantly in males; is progressive, symmetric, atrophic, areflexic, and sensorimotor in type; and occurs in the arms and legs. Occasionally pure sensory or motor neuropathy occurs and even facial paresis has been reported (Dreidger and

Pruzanski, 1980). Axonal degeneration and demyelinization is seen histologically (Morley and Schwieger, 1967; Victor et al., 1958). Treatment with RT or excision (Mankodi et al., 1999) might cure the neuropathy or at least halt its progress.

## POEMS Syndrome

POEMS syndrome is seen in patients with solitary plasmacytoma and is discussed fully in Chapter 19.

# Relationship Between SPB, EMP, and Multiple Myeloma (MM)

SPB, EMP, and MM are identifiable as separate entities by their distinct clinical features and natural histories, as outlined earlier. However, in a certain percentage of cases they might be linked, in that some patients with MM can develop secondary EMP or even osseous plasmacytoma; similarly, some patients with SPB or EMP eventually develop disseminated myeloma. Rarely, a patient with SPB might develop EMP at a later stage and finally progress to MM (Ganjoo et al., 1993). Preliminary studies of ploidy in SPB and EMP (Guida et al., 1994) have shown an almost complete aneuploid cell population in SPB (80%) compared with only 2% aneuploidy in a patient with EMP. The number of cells in S phase was 16% and 1%, respectively, suggesting that SPB is a more aggressive form of plasma cell malignancy. These features will need confirmation. Multiple intraosseous plasmacytomas without generalized myelomatosis, although rare, have also been observed. These patients eventually develop MM after decades of normal health.

## REFERENCES

Alexanian, R. (1980). Localized and indolent myeloma. *Blood, 56*, 521–525.

Aviles, A., Huerta-Guzman, J., and Delgado, S. (1996). Improved outlook in solitary bone plasmacytoma with combined therapy. *Haematology Oncology, 14*, 111-117.

Bacci, G., Savini, R., Calderoni, P., Gnudi, S., Mintutillo, A., et al. (1982). Solitary plasmacytoma of the vertebral column. A report of 15 cases. *Tumori, 68*, 271–275.

Bataille, R., and Sarny, J. (1981). Solitary myeloma: clinical and prognostic features of a review of 114 cases. Cancer, 48, 845–851.

Batsakis, J. G., Fried, G. T., Goldman, R. T., and Karlsberg, R. C. (1964). Upper respiratory tract plasmacytoma. *Archives of Otolaryngology, 79*, 613–618.

Bertoni-Salateo, R., De Camargo, B., Soares, F., Chozniac, F., and Penna, V. (1998). Solitary plasmacytoma of bone in an adolescent. *Journal of Pediatric Hemotology Oncology, 20*, 574-576.

Bolek, T. W., Marcus, R. B., and Mendenhall, N. P. (1996). Solitary plasmacytoma of bone and soft tissues. *International Journal of Radiation Oncology, Biology, Physics, 36*, 329–333.

Bush, S. E., Goffinet, D. R., and Bagshaw, M. A. (1981). Extramedullary plasmacytoma of the head and neck. *Radiology*, *104*, 801–805.

Castro, E. B., Lewis, J. S., and Strong, E. W. (1973). Plasmacytoma of paranasal sinuses and nasal cavity. *Archives of Otolaryngology*, *97*, 326–329.

Chak, L. Y., Cox, R. S., Bostwick, D. G., and Hoppe, R. T. (1987). Solitary plasmacytoma of bone: treatment, progression and survival. *Journal of Clinical Oncology*, *5*, 1811–1815.

Christopherson, W. M., and Miller, A. J. (1950). A re-evaluation of solitary plasma-cell myeloma of bone. *Cancer*, *3*, 240–252.

Cohen, D. M., Svien, H. J., and Dublin, D. C. (1964). Long-term survival of patients with myeloma of the vertebral column. *Journal of the American Medical Association*, *187*, 914–917.

Conklin, R., and Alexanian, R. (1975). Clinical classification of plasma cell myeloma. *Archives of Internal Medicine*, *135*, 139–143.

Corwin, J., and Lindberg, R. D. (1979). Solitary plasmacytoma of bone vs. extramedullary plasmacytoma and their relationship to multiple myeloma. *Cancer*, *43*, 1007–1013.

De Chiara, A., Losito, S., Terracciano, L. D., Giacomo, R., Iccarino, G., et al. (2001). Primary plasmacytoma of the breast. *Archives of Pathology and Laboratory Medicine*, *125*, 1078–1080.

Delauche-Cavallier, M. C., Laredo, J. D., Wybier, M., Bard, M., Mazabrand, A., Darne, J. L. L., et al. (1988). Solitary plasmacytoma of the spine. Long-term clinical course. *Cancer*, *61*, 1707–1714.

Deodhare, S. G., Pujari, B. D., Apte, P. G., and Gujar, A. G. (1975). Plasmacytomas of gastro-intestinal tract. *Journal of Postgraduate Medicine*, *21*, 145–150.

Dimopoulos, M. A., Goldstein, J., Fuller, L., Delasalle, K., and Alexanian, R. (1992). Curability of solitary bone plasmacytoma. *Journal of Clinical Oncology*, *10*, 587–590.

Dimopoulos, M. A., Kiamouris, C., and Moulopoulos, L. A. (1999). Solitary plasmacytoma of bone and extramedullary plasmacytoma. *Haematology and Oncology Clinics of North America*, *13*, 1249–1257.

Douglass, H. O., Sika, J. V., and Le Veen, H. H. (1971). Plasmacytoma: a not so rare tumour of the small intestine. *Cancer*, *28*, 456–460.

Driedger, H., and Pruzanski, W. (1980). Plasma cell neoplasia with peripheral polyneuropathy. A study of five cases and a review of the literature. *Medicine*, *59*, 301–310.

Durie, B. G. M., and Salmon, S. E. (1975). A clinical staging system for multiple myeloma: correlation of measured myeloma cell mass with presenting clinical features, response to treatment and survival. *Cancer*, *36*, 842–854.

Fishkin, B. G., and Spiegelberg, H. I. (1976). Cervical lymph node metastasis as the first manifestation of localised extramedullary plasmacytoma. *Cancer*, *38*, 1641–1644.

Frassica, D. A., Frassica, F. J., Schray, M. F., Sino, F. H., and Kyle, R. A. (1989). Solitary plasmacytoma of bone: Mayo Clinic experience. *International Journal of Radiation Oncology, Biology and Physics*, *16*, 43–48.

Fu, Y. S., and Perzin, K. H. (1978). Nonepithelial tumours of the nasal cavity, paranasal sinuses and nasopharynx: a clinicopathologic study. IX. Plasmacytomas. *Cancer*, *42*, 2399–2406.

Ganjoo, R. K., Malpas, J. S., and Plowman, P. N. (1993). Solitary plasmacytoma of bone – a rare disorder with an unusual evolution. *Postgraduate Medical Journal*, *69*, 153–154.

Gilbert, R. W., Kim, J.-H., and Posner, J. B. (1978). Epidural spinal cord compression from metastatic tumour. Diagnosis and treatment. *Annals of Neurology*, *3*, 40–51.

Gorenstein, A., Neal, H. B., Devine, K. D., and Weiland, L. H. (1977). Solitary extramedullary plasmacytoma of the larynx. *Archives of Otolaryngology*, *103*, 159–161.

Greenberg, P., Parker, R. G., Fu, Y. S., and Abemayor, E. (1987). The treatment of solitary plasmacytoma of bone and extramedullary plasmacytoma. *American Journal of Clinical Oncology (CCT)*, *10*, 199–204.

Guida, M., Cassamassima, A., Abbate, I., Paradiso, A., Zito, A., Marzullo, F., et al. (1994). Solitary plasmacytosis of bone and extramedullary plasmacytoma—two different nosobiological entities? *Tumori*, *80*, 370–377.

Harrington, K. D. (1981). The use of methylmethacrylate for vertebral body replacement and anterior stabilisation of pathological fracture—dislocation of the spine due to metastatic malignant disease. *Journal of Bone and Joint Surgery [Am]*, *63*, 36–46.

Harwood, A. R., Knowling, M. A., and Bergsagel, D. E. (1981). Radiotherapy of extramedullary plasmacytoma of the head and neck. *Clinical Radiology*, *32*, 31–36.

Hellwig, C. A. (1943). Extramedullary plasma-cell tumours as observed in various locations. *Archives of Pathology*, *36*, 95.

Holland, J., Trenkner, D. A., Wasserman, T. H., and Fineberg, B. (1992). Plasmacytoma: treatment results and conversion to myeloma. *Cancer*, *69*, 1513–1517.

Honavar, S. G., Shields, J. A., Shields, C. L., Demirci, H., and Ehya, H. (2001). Extramedullary plasmacytoma confined to the choroids. *American Journal of Ophthalmology*, *131*, 277–278.

Hotz, M.-A., Bosq, J., Schawb, G., and Munck, J.-N. (1999). Extramedullary solitary plasmacytoma of the head and neck, a clinicopathological study. *Annals of Otology, Rhinology and Laryngology*, *108*, 495–500.

Jackson, A., and Scarffe, J. H. (1990). Prognostic significance of osteopenia and immunoparesis at presentation in patients with solitary myeloma of bone. European Journal of *Cancer*, *26*, 363–371.

Johnson, W. H., and Taylor, B. G. (1970). Solitary extramedullary plasmacytoma of the skin. A review of the world literature and the report of an additional case. *Cancer*, *26*, 65–68.

Kapadia, S. B., Desai, U., and Cheng, V. S. (1982). Extramedullary plasmacytoma of the head and neck. A clinicopathologic study of 20 cases. *Medicine*, *61*, 317–329.

Kaplan, G. A., and Bennett, J. (1968). Solitary myeloma of the lumbar spine successfully treated with radiation. *Radiology*, *91*, 10–18.

Knowling, M. A., Harwood, A. R., and Bergsagel, D. E. (1983). Comparison of extramedullary plasmacytomas with solitary and multiple plasma cell tumours of bone. Journal of Clinical *Oncology*, *1*, 255–262.

Loftus, C. M., Michelson, C. B., Rapoport, F., and Antunes, J. L. (1983). Management of plasmacytomas of the spine. *Neurosurgery*, *13*, 30–36.

Macpherson, T. A., Dekker, A., and Kapadia, S. B. (1981). Thyroid-gland plasma cell neoplasm (plasmacytoma). *Archives of Pathology and Laboratory Medicine*, *105*, 570–572.

Mayr, N. A., Wen, B. C., Hussey, D. H., Burns, C. P., Staples, J. J., et al. (1990). The role of radiation therapy in the treatment of solitary plasmacytomas. *Radiotherapy and Oncology*, *17*, 293–303.

Mankodi, A. K., Rao, C. V., and Katrak, S. M. (1999). Solitary plasmacytoma presenting as peripheral neuropathy, a case report. *Neurology India*, *47*, 234–237.

Medini, E., Ras, Y., and Levitt, S. H. (1980). Solitary extramedullary plasmacytoma of the upper respiratory and digestive tracts. *Cancer*, *45*, 2893–2896.

Meis, J. N., Butler, J. J., Osborne, B. M., and Ordonez, N. G. (1987). Solitary plasmacytomas of bone and extramedullary plasmacytomas. A clinicopathologic and immunohistochemical study. *Cancer*, *59*, 1475–1485.

Mendenhall, C. M., Thar, T. L., and Million, R. R. (1980). Solitary plasmacytoma of bone and soft tissue. *International Journal of Radiation Oncology, Biology and Physics*, *6*, 1497–1501.

Meyer, J. E., and Schultz, M. D. (1974). 'Solitary' myeloma of bone. A review of 12 cases. *Cancer*, *34*, 438–440.

Morley, J. B., and Schwieger, A. C. (1967). The relation between chronic polyneuropathy and osteosclerotic myeloma. *Journal of Neurology, Neurosurgery and Psychiatry, 30*, 432–442.

Pahor, A. L. (1977). Extramedullary plasmacytoma of the head and neck, parotid and sub-mandibular salivary glands. *Journal of Laryngology and Otology, 91*, 241–258.

Petrovich, Z., Fishkin, B., Hittle, R. E., Acquarelli, M., and Barton, R. (1977). Extramedullary plasmacytoma of the upper respiratory passages. *International Journal of Radiation Oncology, Biology and Physics, 2*, 723–730.

Poole, A. G., and Marchetta, F. C. (1968). Extramedullary plasmacytoma of the head and neck. *Cancer, 22*, 14–21.

Rainer, E. H. (1970). Extramedullary plasmacytoma of upper respiratory tract. *Journal of Laryngology and Otology, 84*, 909–919.

Ramadan, A., Naab, T., Frederick, W., and Green, W. (2000). Testicular plasmacytoma in a patient with the acquired immunodeficiency syndrome. *Tumour, 86*, 480–482.

Read, D., and Warlow, C. (1978). Peripheral neuropathy and solitary plasmacytoma. *Journal of Neurology, Neurosurgery and Psychiatry, 41*, 177–184.

Remigio, P. A., and Klaum, A. (1971). Extramedullary plasmacytoma of stomach. *Cancer, 27*, 562–568.

Rodman, H. I., and Font, R. L. (1972). Orbital involvement in multiple myeloma. Review of the literature and report of three cases. *Archives of Ophthalmology, 87*, 30–35.

Schridde, H. (1905). Weitere untersuchungen uber die koernelungen der pharmazellen. *Zentralblatte fur Allgemeine Pathologie und Pathologische Anatomie, 16*, 433–435.

Sharma, K. D., and Shrivastav, J. D. (1961). Extramedullary plasmacytoma of gastrointestinal tract. A case report of plasmoma of the rectum and a review of the literature. *Archives of Pathology, 71*, 229–233.

Shaw, A. F. B. (1923). A case of plasma cell myeloma. *Journal of Pathology and Bacteriology, 26*, 125–126.

Shimaoka, K., Gailani, S., Tsukada, Y., and Barcos, M. (1978). Plasma cell neoplasm involving the thyroid. *Cancer, 41*, 1140–1146.

Suzuki, K., Shioji, Y., Morita, T., and Tokue, A. (2001). Primary testicular plasmacytoma with hydrocele of the testis. *International Journal of Urology, 8*, 139–140.

Tong, D., Griffin, T. W., Laramore, G. E., Kurtz, J. M., Russell, A. H., et al. (1980). Solitary plasmacytoma of bone and soft tissues. *Radiology, 135*, 195–198.

Tsang, R. W., Gospodarowicz, M. K., Pintilie, M., Bezjak, A., Wells, W., et al. (2001). Solitary plasmacytoma treated with radiotherapy, impact of tumour size on outcome. *International Journal of Radiation Oncology, Biology, Physics, 50*, 113–120.

Uceda-Montanes, A., Blanco, G., Saornil, M. A., Gonzalez, C., Sarasia, et al. (2000). Extramedullary plasmacytoma of the orbit. *Acta Opthalmologica Scandinavica, 78*, 601–603.

Victor, M., Banker, B. Q., and Adams, R. D. (1958). The neuropathy of multiple myeloma. *Journal of Neurology, Neurosurgery and Psychiatry, 21*, 73–88.

Wasserman, T. H. (1987). Diagnosis and management of plasmacytomas. *Oncology, 1*, 37–41.

Webb, H. E., Harrison, E. G., Masson, J. K., and Remine, W. H. (1962). Solitary extramedullary myeloma (plasmacytoma) of the upper part of the respiratory tract and aroplaryer. *Cancer, 15*, 1142–1155.

Wiltshaw, E. (1976). The natural history of extramedullary plasmacytoma and its relation to solitary myeloma of bone and myelomatosis. *Medicine, 55*, 217–237.

Woodruff, R. K., Malpas, J. S., and White, F. E. (1979a). Solitary plasmacytoma. II. Solitary plasmacytoma of bone. *Cancer, 43*, 2344–2347.

Woodruff, R. K., Whittle, J. M., and Malpas, J. S. (1979b). Solitary plasmacytoma. I. Extramedullary soft tissue plasmacytoma. *Cancer, 43*, 2340–2343.

# CHAPTER 21

# Amyloidosis

## PHILIP N. HAWKINS

## Introduction

Amyloidosis is a disorder of protein folding in which normally soluble proteins are deposited as abnormal, insoluble fibrils that progressively disrupt tissue structure and cause disease (Dobson et al., 2001). Some 20 different unrelated proteins can form amyloid *in vivo*, and clinical amyloidosis is classified according to the fibril protein type (Tables 21-1 and 21-2). In systemic amyloidosis, deposits might occur in all tissues except within the brain, and are present to some extent in blood vessels throughout the body. Systemic amyloidosis is potentially fatal, although its prognosis has been improved by hemodialysis, kidney, liver and heart transplantation, and by increasingly effective treatment of the various conditions that underlie amyloid deposition. There are also various localized forms of amyloidosis in which the deposits are confined to specific foci or to a particular organ or tissue. These might be clinically silent or trivial, or they might be associated with serious disease such as hemorrhage in local respiratory or urogenital tract AL amyloid. In addition, there are important diseases associated with local amyloid deposition in which the pathogenetic role of the amyloid is still unclear, for example, Alzheimer's disease, the prion disorders, and type II diabetes mellitus. Although these conditions are not discussed here, it should be noted that therapeutic strategies aimed at inhibiting amyloid fibrillogenesis and/or promoting regression of amyloid deposits in systemic amyloidosis might also be applicable to localized amyloidosis and vice versa.

In addition to the fibrils, amyloid deposits always contain the normal plasma protein serum amyloid P component (SAP), because it undergoes specific calcium-dependent binding to amyloid fibrils (Pepys et al., 1997). SAP contributes to

## TABLE 21-1
### Acquired Amyloidosis Syndromes

| Clinical Syndrome | Fibril Protein |
| --- | --- |
| Systemic AL amyloidosis, associated with immunocyte dyscrasia, myeloma, monoclonal gammopathy, occult dyscrasia | AL fibrils derived from monoclonal immunoglobulin light chains |
| Local nodular AL amyloidosis (skin, respiratory tract, urogenital tract, etc) associated with focal immunocyte dyscrasia | AL fibrils derived from monoclonal immunoglobulin light chains |
| Reactive systemic AA amyloidosis, associated with chronic active diseases | AA fibrils derived from serum amyloid A protein (SAA) |
| Senile systemic amyloidosis | Transthyretin (TTR) derived from plasma TTR |
| Focal senile amyloidosis | |
|     Atria of the heart | Atrial natriuretic peptide |
|     Brain | $\beta$-protein |
|     Joints | Not known |
|     Seminal vesicles | Seminal vesicle exocrine protein |
|     Prostate | $\beta_2$-microglobulin |
| Nonfamilial Alzheimer's disease, Down syndrome | $\beta$-protein derived from $\beta$-amyloid protein precursor (AAP) |
| Sporadic cerebral amyloid angiopathy | $\beta$-protein derived from $\beta$-amyloid precursor protein (AAP) |
| Sporadic Creutzfeldt-Jakob disease, kuru (transmissible spongiform encephalopathies, prion diseases) | Prion protein (PrP) derived from prion protein precursor |
| Type II diabetes mellitus | Islet amyloid polypeptide (IAPP), amylin, derived from its precursor protein |
| Endocrine amyloidosis, associated with APUDomas | Peptide hormones or fragments thereof (e.g., precalcitonin in medullary carcinoma of thyroid) |
| Hemodialysis-associated amyloidosis; localized to osteoarticular tissues or systemic | $\beta_2$-microglobulin derived from high plasma levels |
| Primarily localized cutaneous amyloid (macular, popular) | ? Keratin-derived |
| Ocular amyloid (cornea, conjunctiva) | Includes monoclonal immunoglobulin light chains |
| Orbital amyloids | AH fibrils derived from immunoglobulin heavy chain in one case, monoclonal immunoglobulin light chains in others |

List not exhaustive

amyloidogenesis (Botto et al., 1997), and radio-labeled SAP is a specific, quantitative, and highly informative tracer for scintigraphic imaging of systemic amyloid deposits (Hawkins et al., 1990a). The treatment of amyloidosis comprises measures to support impaired organ function, including dialysis and transplantation, along with vigorous efforts to control underlying conditions responsible for production of fibril precursors (Gillmore et al., 1997). Serial SAP scintigraphy has demonstrated that reduction of the supply of amyloid fibril precursor proteins leads to regression of amyloid deposits and clinical benefit in many cases.

## Pathogenesis of Amyloidosis

Amyloidogenesis involves substantial refolding of the native structures of the various amyloid precursor proteins enabling them to autoaggregate in a highly ordered manner to form fibrils with a characteristic $\beta$-sheet structure (Booth et al., 1997; Sunde et al.,

1997). Amyloid deposition occurs *in vivo* under several conditions. First, when a normal protein is present for a sufficient time at an abnormally high concentration, for example, serum amyloid A protein (SAA) and $\beta_2$-microglobulin ($\beta_2$M) during chronic inflammation and renal failure, respectively. Second, in the presence of an ordinary concentration of a normal but inherently weak amyloidogenic protein over a very prolonged period, such as in the case of transthyretin in senile cardiac amyloidosis. Third, when there is an acquired or inherited variant protein with abnormal amyloidogenic structure, such as some monoclonal immunoglobulin light chains or variants of transthyretin, lysozyme, apolipoprotein AI, fibrinogen A $\alpha$-chain, and so on.

### Amyloid Fibrils

Regardless of their very diverse protein subunits, amyloid fibrils of all different types are remarkably similar: straight, rigid, nonbranching, of indeterminate length and 10 to 15 nm in diameter. They are insoluble

## TABLE 21-2
### Hereditary Amyloidosis Syndromes

| Clinical Syndrome | Fibril Protein |
|---|---|
| Predominant peripheral nerve involvement, familial amyloid polyneuropathy (FAP), autosomal-dominant | Transthyretin (TTR) genetic variants (most commonly Met30, but over 80 others described) |
| Predominant peripheral nerve involvement, familial amyloid polyneuropathy (FAP), autosomal-dominant | Apolipoprotein AI (apoAI) N-terminal fragment of genetic variant Arg26 |
| Predominant cranial nerve involvement with lattice corneal dystrophy, autosomal-dominant | Gelsolin, fragment of genetic variant Asn187 or Tyr187 |
| Nonneuropathic, prominent visceral involvement, autosomal-dominant | ApoAI, N-terminal fragment of genetic variants Arg26, Arg50, Argo60, and so on |
| Nonneuropathic, prominent visceral involvement, autosomal-dominant | Lysozyme genetic variant Thr56, Arg64, His67 |
| Nonneuropathic, prominent visceral involvement, autosomal-dominant | Fibrinogen α-chain, fragment of genetic variants, Leu554 or Val526 |
| Nonneuropathic, prominent visceral involvement, autosomal-dominant | ApoAII novel extension associated with loss of stop codon at residue 78 |
| Predominant cardiac involvement, no clinical neuropathy, autosomal-dominant | TTR genetic variants Thr45, Ala60, Ser84, Met111, Ile122, and so on |
| Hereditary cerebral haemorrhage with amyloidosis (cerebral amyloid angiopathy), autosomal-dominant | |
|     Icelandic type (major asymptomatic systemic amyloid also present) | Cystatin C, fragment of genetic variant Glu68 |
|     Dutch type | β-protein derived from genetic variant APP Gln693 |
| Familial Alzheimer's disease | β-protein derived from genetic variant APP Ile717, Phe717 or Gly717 |
| Familial dementia–probable Alzheimer's disease | β-protein derived from genetic variant APP Asn670, Leu671 |
| Familial Creutzfeldt-Jakob disease, Gerstmann-Sträussler-Scheinker syndrome (hereditary spongiform encephalopathies, prion diseases) | Prion protein (PrP) derived from genetic variants of PrP precursor protein 51-91 insert, Leu102, Val117, Asn178, Lys200 |
| Familial mediterranean fever, prominent renal involvement, autosomal-recessive | AA derived from SAA |
| Muckle-Well's syndrome, nephropathy, deafness, urticaria, limb pain, other inherited chronic inflammatory disease | AA derived from SAA |

in physiological solutions (although curiously soluble in distilled water), relatively resistant to proteolysis, and bind Congo red dye in an ordered manner producing pathognomonic green birefringence when viewed under cross-polarized light. Electron microscopy reveals that each fibril consists of 2 or more protofilaments, the precise number varying with the fibril type. The x-ray diffraction patterns of the different *ex vivo* amyloid fibrils, and of synthetic fibrils formed *in vitro*, that have been studied demonstrate the presence of a common core structure within the filaments in which the subunit proteins are arranged in a stack of twisted antiparallel β-pleated sheets lying with their long axes perpendicular to the fibril long axis. Recent observations show that many different proteins, including molecules totally unrelated to amyloidosis *in vivo*, can be refolded after denaturation *in vitro* to form typical, stable, Congophilic cross β fibrils. Although it is not clear why only the 20 or so known amyloidogenic proteins adopt

the amyloid fold and persist as fibrils *in vivo*, a major unifying theme currently emerging is that in all cases studied the precursors are relatively unstable. Even under physiological or other conditions they may encounter *in vivo*, they populate partly unfolded states, involving loss of tertiary or higher order structure, which readily aggregate with retention of β-sheet secondary structure into protofilaments and fibrils. Once the process has started, seeding may also play an important facilitating role so that amyloid deposition may progress exponentially as expansion of the amyloid template "captures" further precursor molecules.

## Glycosaminoglycans

Amyloidotic organs contain more glycosaminoglycans than normal tissues, some of which is a tightly bound, integral part of the amyloid fibrils. These fibril-associated glycosaminoglycans are heparan sulphate and dermatan sulphate in all forms of amyloid that have been investigated. Fibrils isolated by water extraction and separated from other tissue components contain 1% to 2% by weight of glycosaminoglycan, none of which is covalently associated with the fibril protein. Interestingly, studies in systemic AA and AL amyloidosis have shown marked restriction in the heterogeneity of the glycosaminoglycan chains, suggesting that particular subclasses of heparan and dermatan sulphates are involved. Immunohistochemical studies demonstrate the presence of proteoglycan core proteins in all amyloid deposits, and that these are closely related to fibrils at the ultrastructural level. However, in isolated fibril preparations much of the glycosaminoglycan material is free carbohydrate chains, and it is not yet clear whether this represents aberrant glycosaminoglycan metabolism related to amyloidosis or just an artefact.

The significance of glycosaminoglycans in amyloid remains unclear, but their universal presence, intimate relationship with the fibrils, and restricted heterogeneity all suggest that they might be important. Glycosaminoglycans are known to participate in the organization of some normal structural proteins into fibrils, and they might have comparable fibrillogenic effects on certain amyloid fibril precursor proteins. Polysulphonated drug molecules, which act as low-molecular-weight glycosaminoglycan analogues, have lately begun to be tested for amyloid-inhibiting properties in clinical trials.

## Serum Amyloid P Component

All amyloid deposits in all species contain the non-fibrillar glycoprotein amyloid P component (AP) (Pepys et al., 1997). Amyloid P component is identical to and derived from the normal circulating plasma protein, serum amyloid P component (SAP), a member of the pentraxin protein family, which includes C-reactive protein (CRP). Human SAP is secreted only by hepatocytes and is a trace constituent of plasma present at a steady concentration of approximately 20 to 30 mg/L. Within the amyloid deposits it is by far the most abundant protein apart from the fibrils themselves.

SAP consists of 5 identical noncovalently associated subunits, each with a molecular mass of 25,462 Da, which are noncovalently associated in a pentameric disc-like ring. SAP is a calcium-dependent ligand-binding protein, the best defined specificity of which is for the 4,6-cyclic pyruvate acetal of $\beta$–D-galactose, but it also binds avidly and specifically to DNA, to chromatin, to glycosaminoglycans, particularly heparan and dermatan sulphates, and to all known types of amyloid fibrils. This latter interaction is responsible for the unique, specific accumulation of SAP in amyloid deposits. In addition to being a plasma protein, SAP is also a normal constituent of certain extracellular matrix structures.

It is covalently associated with collagen and/or other matrix components in the *lamina rara interna* of the human glomerular basement membrane and is present on the microfibrillar mantle of elastin fibers throughout the body.

The SAP molecule is highly resistant to proteolysis and, although not itself a proteinase inhibitor, its binding to amyloid fibrils *in vitro* protects them against proteolysis. Once bound to amyloid fibrils *in vivo*, SAP persists for very prolonged periods and is not catabolized at all, in contrast to its rapid clearance from the plasma, half-life of 24 hours, and prompt catabolism in the liver (Hawkins et al., 1990b). These observations suggest that SAP might contribute to persistence of amyloid deposits *in vivo*, and indeed SAP knockout mice show retarded and reduced development of experimentally induced AA amyloidosis, confirming that SAP is significantly involved in pathogenesis of amyloidosis.

## Other Proteins in Amyloid

A number of plasma proteins, other than the fibril proteins themselves and SAP, have been detected immunohistochemically in some amyloid deposits. These include $\alpha_1$-antichymotrypsin, some complement components, apolipoprotein E, and various extracellular matrix or basement membrane proteins. None of these match the universality, quantitative or selective importance of SAP, and their role, if any, in pathogenesis of amyloid deposition or its effects is not known.

## Mechanisms by Which Amyloid Causes Disease

The mechanisms by which amyloid deposits damage tissues and compromise organ function are incompletely understood. Massive deposits, which might amount to kilograms, are structurally disruptive and incompatible with normal function, as are strategically located small deposits, for example, in the glomeruli or nerves. However, the relationship between quantity of amyloid and organ dysfunction differs greatly between individuals, and there is a strong impression that the rate of new amyloid deposition is at least as important a determinant of progressive organ failure as the amyloid load itself. *In vitro* studies have suggested that isolated amyloid fibrils, and in particular newly formed fibrils, are toxic and might induce death of cultured cells both by necrosis and apoptosis.

Major unanswered questions concern the tissue distribution and time of appearance of amyloid deposits as well as their variable clinical consequences. Although many features of the various forms of amyloidosis overlap, the clinical phenotype associated with a particular fibril type can also be enormously variable, even between families with identical amyloidogenic mutations and even within single kindreds. There are clearly major genetic and environmental factors that influence amyloidogenesis *in vivo* other than simply the presence of an adequate supply of an amyloidogenic protein.

# Acquired Systemic Amyloidosis

Acquired systemic amyloidosis is the cause of death in more than 1 in 1500 of the British population, and is probably much underdiagnosed in the elderly population in which it probably occurs most frequently. Systemic AL amyloidosis is the most serious and commonly diagnosed form, and presently outnumbers referrals of AA amyloidosis to the UK National Amyloidosis Centre by a factor of approximately 8:1. Although less serious, dialysis-related $\beta_2$-microglobulin amyloidosis affects approximately one million patients receiving long-term renal replacement therapy worldwide and causes much suffering. Senile systemic amyloidosis, which predominantly involves the heart, often known as senile cardiac amyloidosis, occurs in approximately one-fourth of individuals over the age of 80 years, a sector of the population that is ever rising.

## Reactive Systemic Amyloidosis, AA Amyloidosis

AA amyloidosis is a complication of chronic infections and inflammatory diseases, and indeed any condition that stimulates overproduction of the acute phase protein, serum amyloid A protein (SAA). The amyloid fibrils are composed of AA protein, an *N*-terminal fragment of SAA, and AA amyloidosis has a lifetime incidence of approximately 1% to 5% among patients with rheumatoid arthritis, juvenile idiopathic arthritis, and Crohn's disease. Most patients present with nephropathy, and although liver and gastrointestinal involvement might occur at a late stage, the heart and nerves are rarely affected clinically.

### AA Fibril Protein

The AA protein is a single nonglycosylated polypeptide chain usually of mass approximately 8000 Da and containing 76 residues corresponding to the *N*-terminal portion of the 104 residue SAA protein. Smaller and larger AA fragments, even whole molecules, have also been reported in AA fibrils. SAA is an apolipoprotein of high-density lipoprotein particles and is the polymorphic product of a set of genes located on the short arm of chromosome 11. SAA is highly conserved in evolution and is a major acute-phase reactant. Most of the SAA in plasma is produced by hepatocytes in which the synthesis is under transcriptional regulation by cytokines, especially interleukin 1 (IL-1), interleukin 6 (IL-6), and tumour necrosis factor. After secretion, SAA rapidly associates with high-density lipoproteins from which it displaces apolipoprotein AI. The circulating concentration can rise from normal levels of up to 3 mg/L to over 1500 mg/L within 24 to 48 hours of an acute stimulus and can remain persistently high with ongoing chronic inflammation.

Amyloid AA protein is derived from circulating SAA by proteolytic cleavage, but it is not known whether this occurs before, during, or after aggregation of monomers in the process of AA fibril formation. Persistent overproduction of SAA causing sustained high circulating levels is a necessary prerequisite for deposition of AA amyloid, but it is not known why only some individuals in this state get amyloid. In mice, only 1 of the 3 major isoforms of murine SAA is the precursor of AA in amyloid fibrils. Human SAA isoforms are more complex but homozygosity for particular types seems to favor amyloidogenesis, although there might also be ethnic differences.

The functions of SAA are not known, but might include modulating effects on reverse cholesterol transport and on lipid functions in the microenvironment of inflammatory foci. Regardless of its physiological role, the behavior of SAA as an exquisitely sensitive acute-phase protein with an enormous dynamic range that makes it an extremely valuable empiric clinical marker. It can be used to objectively monitor the extent and activity of infective, inflammatory, necrotic, and some neoplastic diseases. Monitoring of SAA is vital in the management of all patients with AA amyloid because control of the primary inflammatory process sufficient to reduce SAA production is essential if amyloidosis is to be halted or enabled to regress. Automated immunoassay systems for SAA are available standardized on a World Health Organization International Reference Standard (Wilkins et al., 1994).

### Associated Conditions

AA amyloidosis occurs in association with chronic inflammatory disorders, chronic local or systemic microbial infections, and occasionally neoplasms. In Western Europe and the United States the most frequent predisposing conditions are idiopathic rheumatic diseases. The lifetime incidence of AA amyloidosis in patients with rheumatoid arthritis and juvenile idiopathic arthritis in Europe is 1% to 5%, although for reasons that are not clear, the incidence appears to be lower in the United States and might generally be decreasing. Amyloidosis is exceptionally rare in systemic lupus erythematosus and related connective tissue diseases, and in ulcerative colitis because only a modest acute-phase response occurs in these conditions. Tuberculosis and leprosy are important causes of AA amyloidosis in some parts of the world. Chronic osteomyelitis, bronchiectasis, chronically infected burns and decubitus ulcers, and the chronic pyelonephritis of paraplegia are other well-recognized associations. Hodgkin's disease and renal carcinoma, which often cause a major acute-phase response, are the malignancies most commonly associated with systemic AA amyloid. Approximately 5% to 10% of patients with AA amyloidosis do not have an overt chronic inflammatory disease, and these patients are prone to be diagnosed to have AL amyloidosis in error. The most common underlying pathology in such cases in our series has been Castleman's disease tumors of the solitary plasma cell type located in either the mediastinum or gut mesentery (Lachmann et al., 2002b).

## Clinical Features

AA amyloid involves the viscera but might be widely distributed without causing clinical symptoms. More than 90% of patients present with nonselective proteinuria resulting from glomerular deposition, and nephrotic syndrome might develop before progression to end-stage renal failure. Hematuria, isolated tubular defects, nephrogenic diabetes insipidus, and diffuse renal calcification occur rarely. Kidney size is usually normal, but might be enlarged, or, in advanced cases, reduced. End-stage chronic renal failure is the cause of death in 40% to 60% of cases, but acute renal failure might be precipitated by hypotension and/or salt and water depletion after surgery, excessive use of diuretics, or intercurrent infection, and might be associated with renal vein thrombosis. The second most common presentation is with organ enlargement, such as hepatosplenomegaly or occasionally thyroid goiter, with or without overt renal abnormality, but in any case amyloid deposits are almost always widespread at the time of presentation. Clinically significant involvement of the heart is rare, as is liver failure, but gastrointestinal dysfunction, including bleeding, is common in advanced disease.

AA amyloidosis can become clinically evident just 1 year along the course of the associated inflammatory disorder, but the incidence increases with time, and the median duration before diagnosis of amyloid is approximately 10 years. The prognosis is closely related to the degree of renal dysfunction and the effectiveness of treatment for the underlying inflammatory condition. In the presence of persistent, uncontrolled inflammation, 50% of patients with AA amyloid die within 10 years of the amyloid being diagnosed, but if the acute-phase response can be consistently suppressed, proteinuria can be resolved, renal function might be retained, and the prognosis is much better (see under "Treatment" subsequently in this chapter) (Gillmore et al., 2001). Availability of chronic hemodialysis and

transplantation prevents early death from uremia per se, but amyloid deposition in extrarenal tissues is responsible for a less favorable prognosis than in other causes of end-stage renal failure.

## Amyloidosis Associated with Immunocyte Dyscrasia, AL Amyloidosis

AL amyloidosis is a complication of monoclonal gammopathies, which in most cases are very subtle. AL fibrils are derived from monoclonal light chains and have a unique structure in each patient, probably accounting for the extremely heterogeneous clinical features of this disease. Any organ other than the brain might be affected, commonly including the heart, and the prognosis is poor.

## AL Fibril Proteins

AL proteins are derived from the *N*-terminal region of monoclonal immunoglobulin light chains and consist of the whole or part of the variable ($V_L$) domain. Intact light chains might rarely be found, and the molecular weight therefore varies between approximately 8000 and 30,000 Da. The light chain of the monoclonal paraprotein is either identical to, or clearly the precursor of, AL fibrils isolated from the amyloid deposits.

AL is more commonly derived from $\lambda$ chains than from $\kappa$ chains, despite the fact that $\kappa$ chains predominate among both normal immunoglobulins and the paraprotein products of immunocyte dyscrasias. A new $\lambda$ chain subgroup, $\lambda_{VI}$, was identified first as an AL protein in 2 cases of immunocyte dyscrasia-associated amyloidosis before it had been recognized in any other form, and it has subsequently been observed in many more cases of AL amyloidosis. Furthermore, there is increasing evidence from sequence analyses of Bence Jones proteins of both $\kappa$ and $\lambda$ type from patients with AL amyloidosis, and of AL proteins themselves, that these polypeptides contain unique amino acid replacements or insertions compared with non-amyloid monoclonal light chains. In some cases these changes involve replacement of hydrophilic framework residues by hydrophobic residues, changes likely to promote aggregation and insolubilization, and in others the monoclonal light chains from amyloid patients have been demonstrated directly to have decreased solubility and a greater propensity for precipitation than control non-amyloid proteins (Wetzel, 1997). The inherent "amyloidogenicity" of particular monoclonal light chains has been elegantly confirmed in an *in vivo* model in which isolated Bence Jones proteins are injected into mice (Solomon et al., 1992). Animals receiving light chains from AL amyloid patients developed typical amyloid deposits composed of the human protein, whereas animals receiving light chains from myeloma patients without amyloid did not. Recently developed ultra-high sensitivity assays have shown that free monoclonal immunoglobulin light chains can be identified in the serum of almost all patients with systemic AL amyloidosis in contrast to most patients with monoclonal gammopathies of undetermined significance, suggesting that the presence of light chains in free form is another factor that influences their amyloidogenicity.

## Associated Conditions

Almost any dyscrasia of cells of the B lymphocyte lineage, including multiple myeloma, malignant lymphomas, and macroglobulinemia, might be complicated by immunoglobulin light chain (AL) amyloidosis, but well over 80% of cases are associated with low-grade and otherwise "benign" monoclonal gammopathy. Histologic studies suggest that amyloid deposition occurs in up to 15% of cases of myeloma, but often in small and clinically insignificant amounts, and it probably occurs in less than 5% of patients with "benign" monoclonal gammopathy. In some cases deposition of AL amyloid might be the only evidence of the dyscrasia. A monoclonal paraprotein or free light chains can be detected in serum or urine by conventional electrophoresis and immunofixation in only approximately 80% to 90% of patients with AL amyloid (Kyle and Greipp, 1983), but highly sensitive bone marrow immunophenotyping techniques and high sensitivity light chain assays (see subsequent paragraphs in this chapter) can confirm a monoclonal gammopathy in most remaining cases. Subnormal levels of some or all serum immunoglobulins or increased numbers of marrow plasma cells might provide less direct clues to the underlying etiology. Until recently it has been the practice to diagnose apparently "primary" cases of amyloidosis with no previous predisposing inflammatory condition or family history of amyloidosis as AL type by exclusion. However, it has lately been recognized that autosomal-dominant hereditary amyloidosis, particularly that caused by variant forms of fibrinogen A α-chain and transthyretin, might be poorly penetrant and have a late onset, so that there may be no family history. The coincident occurrence of a monoclonal gammopathy might then be gravely misleading, and it is essential to exclude all known amyloidogenic mutations (see subsequent paragraphs in this chapter) when immunohistochemical or biochemical identification of the amyloid fibril protein has not given positive results.

## Clinical Features

AL amyloid occurs equally in men and women, usually over the age of 50 but as early as the third decade. It has a lifetime incidence, and is the cause of death of between 0.5 to 1 per thousand individuals in the United Kingdom. The clinical manifestations are protean, because virtually any tissue other than the brain may be directly involved (Kyle and Gertz, 1995). Uremia, heart failure, or other effects of the amyloid usually cause death within 1 to 2 years of diagnosis unless the underlying B cell clone is suppressed.

The heart is affected pathologically in up to 90% of AL patients, in 30% of whom restrictive cardiomyopathy is the presenting feature and in up to one-half of whom it is fatal. Other cardiac presentations include arrhythmias and angina. Renal AL amyloid has the same manifestations as renal AA amyloid but the prognosis is worse. Gut involvement may cause motility disturbances (often secondary to autonomic neuropathy), malabsorption, perforation, hemorrhage, or obstruction. Macroglossia occurs rarely but is almost pathognomonic. Hyposplenism sometimes occurs in both AA and AL amyloidosis. Painful sensory polyneuropathy with early loss of pain and temperature sensation followed later by motor deficits is seen in 10% to 20% of cases and carpal tunnel syndrome in 20%. Autonomic neuropathy leading to orthostatic hypotension, impotence, and gastrointestinal disturbances might occur alone or together with the peripheral neuropathy and has a very poor prognosis. Skin involvement takes the form of papules, nodules, and plaques usually on the face and upper trunk, and involvement of dermal blood vessels results in purpura occurring either spontaneously or after minimal trauma and is quite common. Articular amyloid is rare but the symptoms may mimic an inflammatory polyarthritis. Infiltration of the glenohumeral joint and surrounding soft tissues occasionally produces the characteristic "shoulder pad" sign. A rare but serious manifestation of AL amyloid is an acquired bleeding diathesis that might be associated with deficiency of factor X, and sometimes also factor IX, or with increased fibrinolysis. It does not occur in AA amyloidosis, although in both AL and AA disease there might be serious bleeding in the absence of any identifiable factor deficiency.

## Localized AL Amyloidosis

Localized foci of AL amyloid can occur anywhere in the body, the most common sites being the skin, upper airways and respiratory tract, and the urogenital tract. They may be associated with a local plasmacytoma or B cell lymphoma producing a monoclonal immunoglobulin, but much more often the clonal cell population, which must be present to produce the amyloidogenic protein, is very inconspicuous. Amyloid deposits in the eye cause local problems in the cornea or conjunctiva. Orbital amyloid presents as mass lesions that can disrupt eye movement and the structure of the orbit; the fibril protein in one such case was identified as an immunoglobulin heavy chain fragment (Tan et al., 1994). The clinical problems caused by these space-occupying amyloidomas may be helped by surgical resection, but this is not always possible.

In primary, localized, cutaneous amyloidosis, which presents in adult life as macular or papular lesions, the fibrils might be derived from keratin. Hereditary cutaneous amyloid lesions are rare, of unknown fibril type, and sometimes associated with other non-amyloid, multisystem disorders.

## Dialysis-Related Amyloidosis (DRA), $\beta_2$-Microglobulin Amyloidosis

### Fibril Protein and Associated Conditions

The amyloid fibril precursor protein is $\beta_2$-microglobulin, which is the invariant chain of the MHC class I molecule, and is expressed by all nucleated cells. It is synthesized at an average rate of 150 to 200 mg per day and in normal circumstances is freely filtered at the glomerulus and then reabsorbed and catabolized by the proximal tubular cells. Decreasing renal function causes a proportionate rise in levels. $\beta_2$-microglobulin amyloidosis was first described in 1980 and occurs in patients who have been on dialysis for several years or very occasionally those with longstanding severe chronic renal impairment. DRA is better recognized in the hemodialysis population but also occurs in patients on CAPD. Relatively few patients have yet been maintained on peritoneal dialysis for the 5 to 10 years required to develop symptomatic $\beta_2$-microglobulin amyloid, but histologic studies of early subclinical deposits suggests that the incidence of DRA is similar among patients receiving the 2 modalities of dialysis. Indeed, $\beta_2$-microglobulin amyloid deposits are present in 20% to 30% of patients within 3 years of beginning dialysis for end-stage renal failure.

### Clinical Features

$\beta_2$-microglobulin amyloidosis is preferentially deposited in articular and periarticular structures, and its manifestations are largely confined to the locomotor system. Carpal tunnel syndrome is usually the first clinical manifestation of $\beta_2$-microglobulin amyloidosis. Some individuals develop symptoms within 3 to 5 years and by 20 years the prevalence is almost 100% (Drüeke, 1998). Older patients appear to be more susceptible to the disease and tend to exhibit symptoms more rapidly. Amyloid arthropathy tends to occur a little later but eventually affects the most patients on dialysis. The arthralgia of $\beta_2$-microglobulin amyloidosis affects the shoulders, knees, wrists, and small joints of the hand and is associated with joint swelling,

chronic tenosynovitis and, occasionally, hemarthroses. Spondyloarthropathies are also well recognized, as is cervical cord compression. $\beta_2$-microglobulin amyloid deposition within the periarticular bone produces typical appearances of subchondral erosions and cysts, which can contribute to pathologic fractures, particularly of the femoral neck, cervical vertebrae, and scaphoid. Although $\beta_2$-microglobulin amyloidosis is a systemic form of amyloid, manifestation outside the musculoskeletal system are rare, but there have been reports of $\beta_2$-microglobulin amyloidosis causing congestive cardiac failure, gastrointestinal bleeding, perforation or pseudo-obstruction, and macroglossia.

### Senile (ATTR) Amyloidosis

Senile (ATTR) amyloidosis is a disease that occurs in up to 25% of the very elderly who have deposits of transthyretin (TTR) amyloid involving the heart and blood vessel walls, smooth and striated muscle, fat tissue, renal papillae, and alveolar walls. In contrast to most other forms of systemic amyloidosis, including hereditary transthyretin amyloid caused by point mutations in the transthyretin gene, the spleen and renal glomeruli are rarely affected. The brain is not involved. Deposits in the heart can be substantial and may cause significant impairment of cardiac function and be fatal, but clinical cardiac involvement is extremely rare before 65 years of age. The transthyretin involved is probably usually of the normal wild-type, but transthyretin variants have been described and analysis of the TTR gene is advisable in all patients who are found to have amyloid of TTR type.

### Endocrine Amyloidosis

Many endocrine tumors that produce peptide hormones have amyloid deposits in their stroma. These are probably composed of the hormone peptides and in the case of medullary carcinoma of the thyroid the fibril subunits are derived from procalcitonin. In insulinomas the amyloid fibril protein is a novel peptide first identified in that site and subsequently shown to be the fibril protein in the amyloid of the islets of Langerhans in type II diabetes. This peptide is called islet amyloid polypeptide (IAPP), and also amylin, and shows appreciable homology with calcitonin gene-related peptide. IAPP-amyloid is an almost universal feature of the pancreatic islets in type II diabetes and becomes more extensive with increasing duration and severity of the disease. Although it is not clear whether the amyloid itself is initially responsible for the metabolic defect in this form of diabetes, it seems likely that progressive amyloid deposition leading to islet destruction subsequently does contribute to its course.

# Hereditary Systemic Amyloidosis

Hereditary systemic amyloidosis is caused by deposition of genetically variant proteins as amyloid fibrils, and is associated with mutations in the genes for transthyretin, cystatin C, gelsolin, apolipoprotein AI, apolipoprotein AII, lysozyme and fibrinogen A α-chain. These diseases are all inherited in an autosomal-dominant pattern with variable penetrance and present clinically at various times from the teens to old age, although usually in adult life. By far the most common hereditary amyloidosis is caused by transthyretin variants and usually presents as familial amyloid polyneuropathy with peripheral and autonomic neuropathy, often with prominent cardiac involvement. Cystatin C amyloidosis presents as cerebral amyloid angiopathy with recurrent cerebral hemorrhage and clinically silent systemic deposits and has been reported only in Icelandic families. Gelsolin amyloidosis presents with cranial neuropathy but is also extremely rare. Apolipoprotein AI, apolipoprotein AII, lysozyme and fibrinogen α-chain amyloidosis almost always present as nonneuropathic systemic amyloidosis that can affect any or all the major viscera, with renal involvement typically being prominent. These latter conditions are readily misdiagnosed as acquired AL amyloidosis and are less rare than previously thought (Lachmann et al., 2002a).

## Familial Amyloidotic Polyneuropathy

Familial amyloidotic polyneuropathy (FAP) is caused by point mutations in the gene for the plasma protein transthyretin (TTR) and is an autosomal-dominant syndrome with variable penetrance. Symptoms typically present between the third and seventh decades (Benson and Uemichi, 1996). The disease is characterized by progressive and disabling peripheral and autonomic neuropathy and varying degrees of visceral amyloid involvement. Severe cardiac amyloidosis is common. Deposits within the vitreous of the eye occur in a proportion of cases and are very characteristic, but renal, thyroid, spleen, and adrenal deposits are usually asymptomatic. There are well-recognized foci in Portugal, Japan, and Sweden, but FAP has been reported in most ethnic groups throughout the world. There is considerable phenotypic variation in the age of onset, rate of progression, involvement of different systems, and disease penetrance generally, although within families the pattern may be quite consistent. More than 80 variant

forms of TTR are associated with FAP, the most frequent of which is the substitution of methionine for valine at residue 30. TTR alanine 60 is the most frequent cause of FAP in the British population, and usually presents after age 50 years, often with predominant cardiac amyloidosis.

## Familial Amyloid Polyneuropathy with Predominant Cranial Neuropathy

Originally described in Finland but now reported in other ethnic groups, this is a very rare autosomal-dominant form of hereditary amyloidosis that presents in adult life with cranial neuropathy, lattice corneal dystrophy, and a mild distal peripheral neuropathy. There may be skin, renal, and cardiac manifestations but these are usually covert and life expectancy approaches normal. The mutant gene responsible encodes a variant form of gelsolin, which is an actin-modulating protein. The functional role of circulating gelsolin is unknown but may be related to clearance of actin filaments released by apoptotic cells. There is no specific treatment for this disorder, which is progressively disfiguring and very distressing during its late stages.

## Hereditary Nonneuropathic Systemic Amyloidosis

Ostertag first described the syndrome of hereditary systemic amyloidosis in a German family in 1932. He reported 2 families with autosomal-dominantly inherited renal amyloidosis without neuropathy. This disorder is now known to be caused by mutations in the genes for lysozyme, apolipoprotein AI, and fibrinogen A α-chain (Benson et al., 1993). A family with this phenotype has also been reported with mutation in the gene for apolipoprotein AII in which loss of a stop codon results in a 21-residue extension at the C-terminus of the protein.

### Lysozyme Amyloidosis

Hereditary nonneuropathic systemic amyloidosis has been described in association with 3 lysozyme variants (Booth et al., 1997): the substitution of histidine for aspartic acid at position 67, threonine for isoleucine at position 56, and arginine for tryptophan at position 64. Most patients present in middle age with proteinuria, very slowly progressive renal impairment, and sometimes hepatosplenomegaly with or without purpuric rashes. Virtually all patients have substantial gastrointestinal amyloid deposits, and although these are often asymptomatic, they are important because gastrointestinal hemorrhage or perforation is a frequent cause of death.

### Apolipoprotein AI Amyloidosis

Apolipoprotein AI is a major constituent of high-density lipoprotein. Eleven amyloidogenic variants are known, 8 of which are single amino acid substitutions, 2 are deletions, and 1 a deletion/insertion. Depending on the mutation, patients can present with massive abdominal visceral amyloid involvement, predominant cardiomyopathy, or an FAP-like syndrome. Several of the variants in the *C*-terminal region are also associated with hoarseness resulting from laryngeal amyloid deposits. The majority of patients eventually develop renal failure, but despite extensive hepatic amyloid deposition, liver function usually remains well preserved. Normal wild-type apolipoprotein AI amyloid is itself weakly amyloidogenic, and is the precursor of small amyloid deposits that occur quite frequently in aortic atherosclerotic plaques.

### Fibrinogen A α-Chain Amyloidosis

Fibrinogen A α-chain was first isolated from amyloid fibrils in 1993. Four amyloidogenic mutations have been described in 8 unrelated kindreds. These include 2-frame shifting deletion mutations and a leucine for arginine substitution at codon 554. However, much of the most common mutation results in the substitution of valine for glutamic acid at position 526 (Uemichi et al., 1994). We have lately shown that this mutation is unexpectedly frequent in the northern European population, and that, overall, it has quite low penetrance. Indeed, most patients with this form of hereditary amyloidosis do not give a family history of similar disease. Five percent of patients referred to the UK National Amyloidosis Centre with a diagnosis of acquired AL amyloidosis have been shown on further investigation to have hereditary fibrinogen A α-chain valine 526 amyloidosis (Lachmann et al., 2002a). Most patients present in middle age with proteinuria or hypertension and over the following 4 to 10 years progress to end-stage renal failure. Amyloid deposition is seen in the kidneys, spleen, and sometimes the liver but is usually asymptomatic in the latter 2 sites. The majority of patients have an excellent outcome on dialysis, and the limited experience with renal transplantation is extremely encouraging.

## Diagnosis of Amyloidosis

The diagnosis of amyloidosis usually requires histologic confirmation (Hawkins, 1994a). The pathognomonic tinctorial property of amyloidotic tissue is apple green/red birefringence when stained with Congo red dye and viewed under intense cross-polarized light. Immunohistochemical staining of amyloid-containing tissue sections is the most accessible method for characterizing the amyloid fibril protein type. However, histology cannot provide information about the overall whole body load or distribution of amyloid deposits, and does not permit monitoring of the natural history of amyloidosis or its response to treatment. To overcome these problems, we developed radio-labeled human SAP as a specific, non-invasive, quantitative *in vivo* tracer for amyloid deposits and have used it as a routine tool in our clinical practice for 10 years (Hawkins et al., 1988, 1990a). We have performed over 3000 studies, and scintigraphy and metabolic turnover studies with labeled SAP have contributed greatly to the diagnosis, monitoring, and evaluation of response to treatment in all types of systemic amyloidosis.

### Clinical Diagnosis of Amyloid

Amyloid might be an unexpected finding on histologic study of virtually any surgical specimen. On the other hand, certain clinical features by themselves might alert the physician to the diagnosis, especially when other conditions known to be associated with amyloidosis are present. For example, proteinuria in a patient with a chronic inflammatory disorder or a monoclonal gammopathy may be the result of AA or AL amyloidosis, respectively. However, with the occasional exception of hepatic or splenic enlargement, patients with AA amyloid rarely have other suggestive clinical signs. By contrast, in AL amyloidosis certain features (Gertz and Kyle, 1989), including cutaneous purpura around the eyes and macroglossia, are highly characteristic. Carpal tunnel syndrome, peripheral and autonomic neuropathy, and/or restrictive cardiomyopathy should also strongly suggest AL amyloidosis in patients with clonal B cell dyscrasias. Hereditary amyloid syndromes are less rare than previously thought, and although these syndromes are caused by point mutations in the genes for various proteins and transmitted in an autosomal-dominant manner, penetrance may be incomplete and a family history is often absent. In a study of 350 patients attending the UK National Amyloidosis Centre who had been thought to have acquired AL type, an alternative diagnosis of hereditary amyloid was demonstrated in 10% of cases after the introduction of routine DNA analysis (Lachmann et al., 2002a). The hereditary amyloid in most of these patients with apparent sporadic amyloidosis was of variant TTR and fibrinogen A α-chain type. All patients receiving long-term dialysis for end-stage renal failure are at risk of developing β₂M amyloidosis (Gejyo et al., 1985; Gorevic et al., 1985). A high index of suspicion for amyloid should therefore be maintained in subjects with any of these predisposing clinical or genetic disorders.

## Histochemical Diagnosis of Amyloid

### Biopsy

The diagnosis of amyloid is usually made after a biopsy of the kidneys, liver, heart, bowel, peripheral nerve, lymph node, skin, thyroid, or bone marrow. When amyloidosis is suspected clinically, biopsy of subcutaneous fat or the rectum is less invasive. Amyloid is present in these sites in 50% to 80% of cases of systemic AA or AL. Alternatively, clinically affected tissue may be biopsied directly, which has a higher yield but a greater risk of hemorrhage and other complications.

### Congo Red and Other Histochemical Stains

Many cotton dyes, fluorochromes, and metachromatic stains have been used, but Congo red staining, and its resultant green birefringence when viewed with high-intensity polarized light, is the pathognomonic histochemical test for amyloidosis. The stain is unstable and must be freshly prepared every 2 months or less. Thick sections of 5 to 10 µm and inclusion in every staining run of a positive control tissue containing modest amounts of amyloid are critical.

### Immunohistochemistry

Although many amyloid fibril proteins can be identified immunohistochemically, the demonstration of amyloidogenic proteins in tissues does not, on its own, establish the presence or type of amyloid. Congo red staining and green birefringence are always required and immunostaining might then enable the amyloid fibril protein to be classified. Antibodies to serum amyloid A protein are commercially available and virtually always stain AA deposits, as is the case with antibodies to $\beta_2$-microglobulin in hemodialysis-associated amyloid. In AL amyloid the deposits are stainable with antibodies to $\kappa$ or $\lambda$ immunoglobulin light chains in only approximately one-half of all cases, probably because the light-chain fragment in the fibrils is chiefly the *N*-terminal variable domain, which is unique for each monoclonal protein. Immunohistochemical staining of transthyretin and other hereditary amyloid fibril proteins may require pretreatment of sections with formic acid, alkaline guanidine, or deglycosylation, and, even then, may not give definitive results in some cases.

## Electron Microscopy

Amyloid fibrils cannot always be convincingly identified ultrastructurally, and a diagnosis of amyloidosis made through electron microscopy alone should be regarded with caution because other fibrillar deposition diseases occur.

## Problems of Histologic Diagnosis

The tissue sample must be adequate (for example, the inclusion of submucosal vessels in a rectal biopsy specimen), and failure to find amyloid does not exclude the diagnosis. The unavoidable sampling problem means that biopsy cannot reveal the extent or distribution of amyloid. Experience with Congo red staining is required if clinically important false-negative and false-positive results are to be avoided. Immunohistochemical staining requires positive and negative controls, including demonstration of specificity of staining by absorption of positive antisera with isolated pure antigens.

## Nonhistologic Investigations

Two-dimensional echocardiography showing small, concentrically hypertrophied ventricles, generally impaired contraction, dilated atria, homogeneously echogenic valves, and increased echodensity of ventricular walls is virtually diagnostic of cardiac amyloidosis. However, clinically significant restrictive diastolic impairment might be difficult to detect even by comprehensive Doppler and other functional studies. Imaging after injection of isotope-labeled calcium-seeking tracers has poor sensitivity and specificity and is of no routine clinical value.

In cases of known or suspected hereditary amyloidosis the gene defect must be characterized. If amyloidotic tissue is available, the fibril protein might be known and the corresponding gene can then be studied, but if no tissue containing amyloid is available, screening of the genes for known amyloidogenic proteins must be undertaken.

Biochemical and immunochemical screening tests for the presence in the plasma of amyloidogenic variant protein products of mutant genes also exist, but molecular genetic analysis of DNA is the most direct approach. However, it remains essential to corroborate DNA findings by confirming one way or another that the respective protein is indeed the main constituent of the amyloid.

## Detection of Serum Free Light Chains in AL Amyloidosis Using High-Sensitivity Nephelometry

A high-sensitivity latex-enhanced serum immunoassay has lately been developed that can quantify circulating free immunoglobulin light chains with remarkable precision (Bradwell et al., 2001). The assay uses antibodies directed against free light-chain epitopes that are hidden in whole intact immunoglobulin molecules and has a sensitivity of < 5 mg/L. This compares with typical detection limits of 150 to 500 mg/L by immunofixation and 500 to 2000 mg/L by electrophoresis. Monoclonal free light chains are identified as values for kappa or lambda that exceed the respective reference ranges and that produce an abnormal kappa to lambda ratio. This assay has numerous applications in multiple myeloma and can also identify monoclonal free light chains in the serum of virtually all patients with systemic AL amyloidosis. In a series of 262 patients undergoing assessment at the UK National Amyloidosis Centre, a monoclonal immunoglobulin could not be detected at presentation by electrophoresis or immunofixation in either serum or urine in 55 (21%) cases. In another 67 patients (26%) monoclonal light chains could only be detected qualitatively by immunofixation of serum or urine. By contrast, monoclonal-free immunoglobulin light chains were quantified in the serum using the high-sensitivity latex-enhanced immunoassay in 98% of these patients. This assay also has a major application in monitoring the response to chemotherapy of the clonal disease in patients with AL amyloidosis enabling such treatment to be given on a much more rational basis than has previously been possible.

## Radiolabeled Serum Amyloid P Component Scintigraphy and Natural History of Amyloid

The universal presence in amyloid deposits of AP, derived from circulating SAP, is the basis for use of radioisotope-labeled SAP as a diagnostic tracer in amyloidosis (Hawkins et al., 1988, 1990a). No localization or retention of labeled SAP occurs in healthy subjects or in patients with diseases other than amyloidosis. Radio-iodinated SAP has a short half-life (24 h) in the plasma and is rapidly catabolized with complete excretion of the iodinated breakdown products in the urine. However, in patients with systemic or localized extracerebral amyloidosis, the tracer rapidly and specifically localizes to the deposits, in proportion to the quantity of amyloid present, and persists there without breakdown or modification (Fig. 21-1). For clinical purposes, highly purified SAP is isolated from the plasma of single accredited donors and is oxidatively iodinated with the pure gamma emitter [123]iodine. The dose of radioactivity administered (less than 4 mSv) is well within accepted safety limits. In addition to the images, the uptake of tracer into various organs can be precisely and repeatedly quantified (Hawkins, 2002; Hawkins et al., 1990b, 1993a).

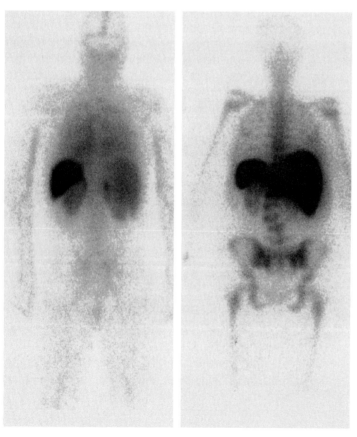

**A**

**B**

*Figure 21-1* Whole-body [123]I-SAP scintigraphy: **(A)** posterior view of a patient with familial Mediterranean fever complicated by AA amyloidosis. There is uptake of tracer in the spleen, kidneys, and adrenal glands, and some tracer remaining in the blood pool reflecting a relatively small whole body amyloid load; **(B)** posterior views of a patient with AL amyloidosis associated with a subtle monoclonal gammopathy. The tracer has localized within extensive amyloid deposits in the liver, spleen, kidneys, and bones. There is no blood pool or bladder signal because nearly all of the tracer has been taken up into very substantial amyloid deposits. The bone marrow uptake is pathognomonic for AL amyloidosis.

Important observations regarding amyloid, which have been made for the first time *in vivo*, include the following: the different distribution of amyloid in different forms of the disease; amyloid in anatomic sites not available for biopsy (adrenals, spleen); major systemic deposits in forms of amyloid previously thought to be organ-limited; a poor correlation between the quantity of amyloid present in a given organ and the level of organ dysfunction; a nonhomogeneous distribution of amyloid within individual organs; and evidence for rapid progression and regression of amyloid deposits with different rates in different organs. The impression that amyloid deposition is irreversible and inexorably progressive is misleading and largely reflects the persistent nature of the acquired or hereditary conditions that underlie it. Many case reports have described improvement in organ function, suggesting regression of amyloid, when underlying conditions have been controlled, and serial SAP scintigraphy has systematically shown regression of amyloid under these circumstances. This has been observed when supply of amyloid fibril precursor proteins has been reduced in AA amyloidosis by vigorous control of rheumatic inflammation (Hawkins et al., 1993b), in AL amyloidosis with clonal suppression by cytotoxic drugs (Gillmore et al., 1999c), in hemodialysis-associated amyloidosis after renal transplantation (Tan et al., 1996), and in hereditary transthyretin (Rydh et al., 1998) and fibrinogen A α-chain amyloidosis after liver transplantation (Gillmore et al., 2000). It is now clear that amyloid deposits exist generally in a state of dynamic turnover with encouraging implications for patient management.

Labeled SAP studies thus make a valuable contribution to the diagnosis and management of patients with systemic amyloidosis and are now performed routinely at the NHS National Amyloidosis Centre at the Royal Free Hospital, London.

## Management of Amyloidosis

In the absence of any treatment that specifically causes regression of amyloid deposits, the aim of therapy is to reduce the supply of amyloid fibril precursor proteins in the hope that progression of the disease will be slowed down or halted. However, few clinical trials have been performed and the approach to treatment remains somewhat empiric. Relatively radical approaches may be justified when the prognosis is otherwise poor (Table 21-3) and significant clinical benefits can be obtained, including the preservation and restoration of vital organ function as well as improved survival. Speculation that amyloid deposits might regress under these circumstances has now been systematically confirmed using SAP scintigraphy in AA (Gillmore et al., 2001), AL (Hawkins, 1994b), $\beta_2$M (Tan et al., 1996), and variant TTR (Rydh et al., 1998) amyloidosis. However, it is important to appreciate that clinically significant regression of amyloid might not be evident for months or years after the supply of the fibril precursor has been reduced.

Supportive therapy remains a critical component of management, with the potential for delaying target organ failure, maintaining quality of life, and prolonging survival while therapy directed against the underlying metabolic defect can be instituted. Replacement of vital organ function, notably with renal dialysis, might be necessary and cardiac (Dubrey et al., 2001; Hall and Hawkins, 1994; Hosenpud et al., 1991) and other transplant (Pasternack et al., 1986) procedures have a role in selected cases. Rigorous control of hypertension

=== TABLE 21-3 ===

## Reducing the Supply of Fibril Precursors in Systemic Amyloidosis

| Disease | Aim of Treatment | Example of Treatment |
|---|---|---|
| AA amyloid | Suppress acute phase response | Anti-inflammatory and immunosuppressive therapy in rheumatoid arthritis, Still's disease (e.g., anti-TNF and chlorambucil); colchicine for familial mediterranean fever, even if clinical episodes not fully suppressed; surgery for osteomyelitis, and rare cytokine-producing tumors |
| AL amyloid | Suppress production of monoclonal immunoglobulin light chains | Chemotherapy directed at monoclonal gammopathy |
| Hereditary amyloidosis | Eliminate source of genetically variant protein | Orthotopic liver transplantation for variant transthyretin-associated familial amyloid polyneuropathy |
| Hemodialysis amyloidosis | Reduce plasma concentration of $\beta_2$M | Renal transplantation |

is vital in renal amyloidosis. Surgical resection of amyloidotic tissue is occasionally beneficial but, in general, a conservative approach to surgery, anesthesia, and other invasive procedures is best. Should any such procedure be undertaken, meticulous attention to blood pressure and fluid balance is essential, especially in patients with renal and/or cardiac involvement. Amyloidotic tissues might heal poorly and are liable to hemorrhage. Diuretics and vasoactive drugs should be used cautiously in cardiac amyloidosis because they can reduce cardiac output substantially. Dysrhythmias may respond to conventional pharmacologic therapy or pacing.

Prevention of amyloidosis is sometimes possible. Deposition of AA amyloid can be almost completely inhibited in familial Mediterranean fever (FMF) by the long-term prophylactic use of colchicine (Goldfinger, 1972; Livneh et al., 1992; Zemer et al., 1986) and dialysis-related amyloidosis is avoided by early renal transplantation. Mutant genes associated with hereditary forms of amyloidosis can now be identified *in utero*, giving the option of elective termination, and orthotopic hepatic transplantation is potentially curative in established cases associated with variant forms of TTR (Holmgren et al., 1993).

## Reactive Systemic (AA) Amyloid

Chronic idiopathic inflammatory diseases are the most common causes of AA amyloidosis in the Western world. Median survival is approximately 5 to 10 years in untreated patients. The few systematic treatment studies that have been performed have been in rheumatoid arthritis (RA) and juvenile rheumatoid arthritis (JRA). The aim of therapy is to suppress the underlying disease process and hence reduce acute-phase synthesis of serum amyloid A protein (SAA), from which AA amyloid fibrils are derived.

### Anti-inflammatory Treatment

The effect of treating chronic inflammatory rheumatic disease on the course of AA amyloidosis has been reported by several groups (Ahlmen et al., 1987; Berglund et al., 1987, 1993; David, 1991; Falck et al., 1979; Schnitzer and Ansell, 1977). In these studies, response to treatment was defined in terms of organ function and survival. Histologic information has rarely been sought, although regression of AA amyloid has lately been documented using prospective SAP scintigraphy (Gillmore et al., 2001).

Seminal observations regarding the management of AA amyloidosis were made in a study of 51 patients with JRA who were treated with chlorambucil (Schnitzer and Ansell, 1977). Proteinuria was present in each case at diagnosis but in only 36% after 3 years

or more continuous administration of the drug. Survival was 100% at 5 years, and after 15 years (David, 1991) 68% of the patients were still alive. In contrast, no patient survived among a nonrandomized control group that did not receive chlorambucil.

In 1980 a Finnish group reported remission from nephrotic syndrome in 5 of 7 patients with AA amyloidosis complicating RA after treatment with cyclophosphamide and low-dose prednisolone (Falck et al., 1979). Repeat renal biopsy performed in one of these patients after 2 years of therapy suggested regression of amyloid. Renal function was preserved in all responders and cumulative survival of the treatment group after 5 years was far superior to 53 untreated control subjects. The treatment group was, however, very small and was intentionally highly selected for patients with normal renal function and blood pressure at the outset.

The only randomized, prospective treatment trial so far reported in AA amyloidosis compared cytotoxic therapy in 11 patients with RA with 11 untreated control subjects (Ahlmen et al., 1987). End-stage renal disease developed after 54 months in 2 patients treated with a podophyllotoxin derivative, chlorambucil, cyclophosphamide, or azathioprine, in contrast to 7 patients after 46 months who received no such treatment ($p < 0.04$). The glomerular filtration rate declined initially in both groups but leveled off among treated patients. Proteinuria was not reported. These investigators subsequently reported that plasma SAA levels were reduced substantially in the patients who had received cytotoxics.

Another study has also suggested major improvements in renal survival and mortality of patients with inflammatory rheumatic diseases treated with alkylating agents (Berglund et al., 1993). Sixteen consecutive patients with AA amyloidosis complicating RA, JRA, and ankylosing spondylitis were followed up for 10 to 21 years during which time courses of chlorambucil or cyclophosphamide were administered repeatedly when there was evidence of deteriorating renal function in association with active inflammatory disease. The median duration of each course of treatment was 13 months (range, 4–45 mo). Two patients were lost to followup and acute renal failure occurred in another 2 cases, thought to be related to renal vein thrombosis and infection, respectively. Renal function was preserved among all of the remainder after 10 years (75% of total). Alkylating drug therapy was well tolerated and associated with reduction of C-reactive protein (CRP), and therefore presumably SAA as well, to virtually normal levels in 15 of 17 courses of the drug. Proteinuria was much reduced in most cases at 10 years compared with baseline, although estimation of glomerular filtration showed a median deterioration of 35% among the 10 long-term survivors. Histologic evidence for regression of amyloid was not sought.

Although there were no control subjects in this study, the clinical outcome and survival of these patients were much superior to that expected without treatment. The importance of managing hypertension, intercurrent infections, surgery and general anesthesia with meticulous care was emphasized.

In a long-term study performed in our center (Gillmore et al., 2001), amyloidotic organ function and survival were studied prospectively for 12 to 117 months in 80 patients with systemic AA amyloidosis in whom serum SAA concentration was measured monthly and the visceral amyloid deposits were evaluated annually by serum amyloid P component scintigraphy. The causative underlying inflammatory diseases were treated as vigorously as possible. Amyloid deposits regressed in 25 of 42 patients whose median SAA values were sustained within the reference range ( <10 mg/L) and amyloidotic organ function stabilized or improved in 39 of these cases. Outcome varied substantially between patients whose median SAA concentration exceeded 10 mg/L, but amyloid load increased and organ function deteriorated in most patients whose SAA remained above 50 mg/L. The survival at 10 years estimated by Kaplan-Meier analysis was 90% in patients whose median SAA was under 10 mg/L and 40% among those whose median SAA exceeded this value ($p < 0.0009$). More than half of the patients with AA amyloidosis complicating inflammatory arthritis in this study had responded extremely well to oral chlorambucil treatment. The protocol for treatment with oral chlorambucil used in our center comprises a starting dose of 2 mg per day, increased by 2-mg increments every 6 to 8 weeks up to a dose of 6 to 8 mg per day, until plasma SAA concentration has fallen substantially or borderline total leukopenia occurs. A response might take up to 6 months, and slow progressive reduction in dose is advised after 1 year in patients who have responded. Chlorambucil is not licensed for this indication in the United Kingdom; it causes permanent infertility in males and premature menopause in women. It is potentially teratogenic and carcinogenic, although these risks are relatively small even after long-term treatment. The new generation of tumor necrosis factor (TNF)-blocking biologic agents represent a more recently available alternative treatment for AA amyloidosis complicating inflammatory arthritis, which can be extremely effective in suppressing acute-phase SAA production in these patients. We presently think there are strong grounds for a therapeutic trial of anti-TNF before resorting to alkylating cytotoxic drugs for this indication.

Many patients with AA amyloidosis now have a prolonged life expectancy, and although the amyloid deposits frequently regress after successful treatment, follow-up SAP scintigraphy has shown that substantial deposits remain present in some such patients for decades, long after the function of amyloidotic organs

has recovered. It is important to recognize that such patients remain at increased risk of acute renal failure under intercurrent stresses, including dehydration, surgery, or pregnancy. They also might reaccumulate damaging quantities of amyloid extremely rapidly should they develop a further acute-phase response, probably because their amyloid deposits serve as a template for ongoing amyloid deposition as soon as a supply of SAA is available in the plasma.

### Colchicine

FMF is a unique example of an inflammatory disease, which is frequently complicated by AA amyloid and for which a specific and effective treatment exists (Goldfinger, 1972; Livneh et al., 1992, 1994; Zemer et al., 1986). Colchicine taken continuously on a prophylactic basis prevents the symptoms of FMF completely in 65% of patients and partially in 30% but, interestingly, appears to prevent the development of amyloidosis in almost all cases, including the 5% of patients who continue to have frequent clinical attacks. Even after the appearance of amyloid, colchicine has beneficial effects, and remission of proteinuria and nephrotic syndrome are well documented among patients with preserved renal function. Doses of at least 1.5 mg per day are often required. The drug also prevents graft amyloidosis in FMF patients who have received a renal transplant (Livneh et al., 1992). Colchicine appears to be remarkably safe, the agent having been given in the long term to children (Zemer et al., 1991) and pregnant women without adverse effects. Although one-third of FMF patients do not respond fully to the drug in terms of clinical episodes, there is no evidence that colchicine inhibits amyloidosis by any means other than through suppressing the cumulative acute-phase production of SAA, much of which might occur when these patients are asymptomatic.

Some case reports suggest colchicine might also be beneficial in the treatment of AA amyloidosis secondary to other conditions, but this approach has not been investigated systematically. However, these observations, along with the fact that colchicine can suppress the acute-phase response in experimental animals, do suggest that there are grounds for further study of the value of this drug in AA amyloidosis generally. There is no evidence that colchicine is of benefit in other forms of amyloidosis.

### Surgery

Occasionally, the stimulus for the acute-phase response is localized to a single anatomic site. Successful surgical excision can lead to the dramatic resolution of clinical symptoms and biochemical abnormalities and be followed by substantial regression of amyloid deposits. This has occurred after tumor resection in renal carcinoma, hepatic adenomas, and Castleman's disease (Lachmann et al., 2002b), bowel resection in ulcerative colitis and Crohn's disease, and amputations of affected limbs in chronic osteomyelitis that has failed to respond to antibiotics.

## Monoclonal Immunoglobulin (AL) Amyloidosis

AL amyloid is a progressive systemic disease with a prognosis far worse than the AA type. In the extensive Mayo Clinic experience (Kyle and Gertz, 1995) comprising over 400 cases of AL amyloidosis, median survival was only 12 to 15 months. Some 50% of deaths are cardiac and in cases in which heart failure is evident at presentation, median survival is only approximately 6 months (Kyle and Greipp, 1978). The aim of treatment is to suppress the underlying plasma cell/B-cell clone and, therefore, production of the AL amyloid fibril precursor protein. There are, however, many difficulties. Chemotherapy regimes are based on those used in multiple myeloma, whereas the plasma cell dyscrasias in most patients with AL amyloidosis are low grade and might be less chemosensitive. The diagnosis can be difficult and many patients have advanced multisystem disease at presentation. It is often impossible to monitor response to treatment because the monoclonal protein cannot be measured by conventional assays. Finally, the prognosis is often too short for any cytotoxic regime to lead to clinical benefit.

### Melphalan and Prednisolone

After the immunoglobulin nature of AL amyloid was established, case reports appeared in the literature claiming beneficial responses to cytotoxic therapy, but only the efficacy of melphalan and prednisolone has been studied systematically in controlled clinical trials. A definitive study performed by the Mayo Clinic group comprised a prospective, randomized trial of 219 patients with AL in whom 3 treatment regimes comprising melphalan and prednisolone, melphalan and prednisolone, plus colchicine and colchicine alone were compared (Kyle et al., 1997). Colchicine was effectively a placebo in this study, and median survival was 17 months, 16 months, and 8.5 months for the 3 groups, respectively. Similar results had previously been obtained by the Boston group who found that in a prospective series of 100 AL patients, those randomized to colchicine alone survived for a median of 10.5 months and those who received melphalan and prednisolone plus colchicine had a median survival of 14.8 months ($p = 0.032$) (Skinner et al., 1994).

Alkylating cytotoxic therapy with low-dose oral melphalan and prednisolone thus appears to be of significant, albeit rather limited, benefit in AL amyloidosis, whereas colchicine is almost certainly of no value. In an attempt to identify which patients with AL were likely to derive the greatest benefit from therapy with melphalan and prednisolone, the Mayo Clinic investigators reported long-term followup of 153 patients who received this regime for a planned 24 to 36 months (Gertz et al., 1991). The very stringent criteria used to define a treatment response are worthy of close scrutiny; patients with nephrotic syndrome were required to show a 50% reduction in proteinuria without any increase in serum creatinine level or a complete return to a normal creatinine level if it had been increased before treatment; patients with hepatic involvement had to have complete return to normal such that the liver was no longer palpable along with normalization of the serum alkaline phosphatase level; and patients with cardiomyopathy had to have total resolution of congestive heart failure. In addition, the complete disappearance of any monoclonal protein present in the serum or urine had to be demonstrated. A total of 27 patients (18%) responded. Among patients with nephrotic syndrome, a normal serum creatinine, and no evidence of cardiac amyloidosis, the response rate was 39% (12 of 31). Five of 34 patients with amyloid cardiomyopathy responded, 2 of whom were alive 10 years after diagnosis. None of 18 patients with peripheral neuropathy showed evidence of disease regression. The median time to achieve a response was 11.7 months and the median survival of the 27 responders was an impressive 89.4 months. Twenty-one patients were alive at 5 years and 8 survived for at least 90 months. Among the 126 patients who did not "respond," but whose disease might of course have been partially ameliorated by treatment, median survival was 14.7 months and 7% survived for 5 years. Unfortunately, melphalan and prednisolone therapy is not without toxicity and one-fourth of the responders died of acute leukemia or myelodysplasia.

There is substantial variation in the gastric absorption of melphalan, which might in addition be affected adversely by amyloid involvement of the gut, so that adequate absorption and delivery of the drug should be confirmed by escalating the dose of melphalan given in 6 weekly cycles until midcycle leukopenia or thrombocytopenia occurs. In renal failure, the dose of melphalan must be reduced and, given the idiosyncratic absorption of the drug, safer alternatives such as weekly doses of oral cyclophosphamide are often used instead. Myeloma studies have offered little evidence that the addition of prednisolone confers any clear advantage over the use of melphalan alone, and it is probably reasonable to omit the drug in patients in whom corticosteroids are considered undesirable.

Although dose-intensive chemotherapy regimens (see subsequent paragraphs) have not been tested as rigorously as low-dose oral melphalan and prednisolone, the evidence that they might be substantially more efficacious is quite compelling, and nowadays low-dose oral therapy tends to be used as first-line treatment mainly in elderly patients.

## Vincristine, Doxorubicin (Adriamycin), and Dexamethasone (VAD) and Similar Regimens

The VAD infusional regimen is an established induction regimen in myeloma. It is associated with a high response rate of 60% to 80%, a complete response rate of 10% to 25%, and a rapid reduction in tumor burden (Alexanian et al., 1990; Samson et al., 1989). It therefore has theoretical advantages in treating AL amyloidosis when a rapid response is desirable. In addition, it does not deplete stem cell reserve, keeping open the option for subsequent peripheral blood stem cell transplantation (PBSCT). Potential problems with the use of VAD in AL amyloidosis are cardiotoxicity of Adriamycin and, probably more importantly in practice, exacerbation of peripheral and autonomic neuropathy by vincristine. High-dose dexamethasone can cause severe fluid retention in patients with renal or cardiac amyloidosis and can lead to bone fractures and vertebral collapse in those with bone involvement. Amyloid cardiomyopathy has not been reported to have been exacerbated by Adriamycin, but caution is recommended.

There have been anecdotal reports of good responses to VAD in AL amyloidosis although the regimen has not been assessed in a randomized, controlled trial. The most substantial experience of this approach has been obtained in 98 patients with AL amyloidosis who were evaluated and followed up at the UK National Amyloidosis Centre. These patients received a median of 4 cycles of standard-dose VAD or C-VAMP as first-line therapy. Their median age was 55.5 years (range, 29–77 y); 36% had echocardiographic features of cardiac involvement and 10% were dialysis-dependent. Patients with symptomatic heart failure, autonomic neuropathy, or severe peripheral neuropathy were excluded. The treatment-related mortality as defined by death during chemotherapy or within 100 days of completing treatment was 7%. The underlying clonal plasma cell dyscrasia responded in 53 patients (representing 63% of 84 evaluable patients), as defined by a fall in the amyloidogenic class of serum-free light-chain concentration by more than 50%. In more than 50% of these responders, SAP scintigraphy demonstrated subsequent regression of amyloid deposits. The function of organs predominantly affected by amyloid improved in one-half of all patients. There was subsequent progression of the

plasma cell dyscrasia in 11 of the 53 responding patients after a median of 20 months (range, 7–54 mo), associated in 6 cases with reaccumulation of amyloid. After a median followup of 21 months, the projected overall median survival was 50 months.

## Intermediate-Dose Intravenous Melphalan (IDM)

The variable absorption of melphalan from the gastrointestinal tract led Schey et al. (1998) to investigate the use of intravenous intermediate-dose melphalan (25 mg/m$^2$) and oral dexamethasone in patients with untreated multiple myeloma. Their results showed that this treatment could be delivered safely on an outpatient basis in patients up to the age of 78 years; 82% of patients achieved an objective response and 30% a complete hematologic and clinical remission. Median overall survival for their study group was 37 months. This regimen has been used as first-line therapy in 33 patients with AL amyloidosis who have been evaluated and followed up at the National Amyloidosis Centre. These patients were selected for IDM on the basis that they were not fit enough to receive VAD-based treatment, either because of age, poor performance status, severe amyloid cardiomyopathy, or neuropathy. Their median age was 64 years (range, 47–77 y); 51% had echocardiographic features of cardiac involvement and 15% were dialysis-dependent. Treatment-related mortality as defined by death during chemotherapy or within 100 days of completing treatment was 18%, and at median followup of 8 months 20 of 33 (61%) patients were alive. The underlying clonal plasma cell dyscrasia responded completely or partially in 55% of evaluable patients, in more than 70% of whom SAP scintigraphy demonstrated subsequent regression of existing amyloid deposits.

It might be prudent to harvest stem cells from patients in whom IDM is considered, who may subsequently benefit from PBSCT because the IDM regimen might deplete stem cell reserve.

## Autologous Peripheral Blood Stem Cell Transplantation (PBSCT)

Use of high-dose melphalan therapy and PBSCT in patients with AL amyloidosis was first reported in 1996, and a series of 25 patients was reported shortly afterward (Comenzo et al., 1998). Since then, encouraging results have been reported in several series of patients in various centers (Gertz et al., 2000a; Gillmore et al., 1999a; Moreau et al., 1998; Sanchorawala et al., 2001). However, the efficacy of PBSCT in AL amyloidosis has yet not been investigated in any controlled comparative study, and procedure-related mortality has been consistently and substantially higher among patients with amyloid than those with multiple myeloma. The 100-day mortality rate in 2 experienced single-center US studies has been approximately 14% (Gertz et al., 2002; Sanchorawala et al., 2001) and in 2 multicenter European studies 39% (Gillmore et al., 1999a; Moreau et al., 1998). This reflects compromised function of multiple organ systems by amyloid and, therefore, refinement of patient selection and improvement of peritransplantation clinical management are priorities.

HDT and PBSCT can result in reversal of the clinical manifestations of AL amyloidosis in up to approximately 60% of patients who survive the procedure. This is associated with regression of AL deposits on SAP scanning (Fig. 21-2), reduction or elimination of the causative clonal plasma cell disorder, and improved performance status and quality of life for patients.

Transplant-related mortality of PBSCT is associated with the number of organ systems involved with amyloid, based on standard clinical evaluations of the kidneys, heart, liver/gastrointestinal system, and peripheral/autonomic nervous system. Of 43 patients transplanted in 2 single-center studies (Comenzo et al., 1998; Gertz et al., 2000b), patients with ≤2 organ systems involved had significantly superior 100-day survival (81%, 25 of 31) compared with those who had >2 organ systems involved (33%, 4 of 12; $p$ <0.01,

Fisher's exact test). Similar conclusions have been reported in multicenter studies (Gillmore et al., 1999a; Moreau et al., 1998). The causes of death included cardiac arrhythmias, intractable hypotension, multiorgan failure, and gastrointestinal bleeding. Patients with poor renal function and those who are already dialysis-dependent fare very badly (Gertz et al., 2002).

There is also a significant risk, including death, associated with stem cell mobilization in patients with AL amyloidosis, even when G-CSF is used alone (Gertz et al., 2000b). Complications have included sudden onset of pulmonary edema, and/or an unexplained syndrome of progressive hypoxia and hypotension, which might occur in patients without cardiac amyloid. It is therefore recommended that patients receive twice-daily dosing of G-CSF, and collections might need to be interrupted because of worsening hypoxia or edema. Measures that can reduce morbidity and mortality during the PBSCT procedure itself include avoidance of substantial prehydration, administering the melphalan in 2 divided doses, using a dose of >5 × 10⁶ CD34+ cells/kg, and avoiding G-CSF support (Comenzo and Gertz, 2002).

The high TRM associated with PBPCT is a major concern. Moreover, although outcome is apparently better than that reported for standard-dose treatment, this might substantially reflect patient selection. Dispenzieri et al. (2001) examined data from patients

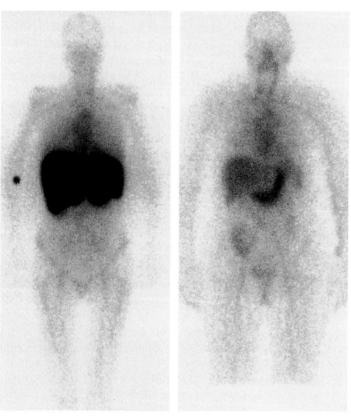

**A**     **B**

*Figure 21-2* Serial anterior whole-body ¹²³I-SAP scintigraphs in a woman with AL amyloidosis presenting in 1998 **(A)** with hepatomegaly. Initially there was massive uptake in the spleen and liver, obscuring any renal signal. She underwent high-dose chemotherapy and the follow-up scan in 2002 **(B)** shows that the deposits have regressed substantially. Chemotherapy was complicated by end-stage renal failure, but she subsequently received a renal transplant producing a normal faint blood-pool outline in the right iliac fossa on the follow-up scan. The stomach signal in this scan is artefactual as a result of a small quantity of free iodine that sometimes accumulates in this site.

with AL amyloid treated at the Mayo Clinic from 1983 to 1997 and identified 229 patients who would now have been eligible for PBPCT based on age less than 70 years and well-preserved cardiac, renal, and hepatic function. At a median followup of 52 months, their median survival was 42 months and 5- and 10-year survival rates were 36% and 15%, respectively.

The role of PBPCT therefore remains unclear, and because of its special problems in AL amyloidosis, it is recommended that such patients be treated in units with expertise of this particular disease. It seems reasonable to restrict PBSCT to younger patients with 1 or 2 involved organs who have not had previous amyloid-related gastrointestinal bleeding and who do not have severe cardiomyopathy, advanced renal failure, or are dialysis-dependent. Our own practice is to rarely recommend PBSCT as first-line therapy, but to consider its role in patients who have not responded adequately to VAD and/or IDM.

### Allogeneic BMT

The first successful allogeneic BMT for AL amyloidosis was reported in 1998 (Gillmore et al., 1998), and 3 years post-BMT was associated with complete clinical recovery. This supports the hypothesis that like in myeloma, a small proportion of patients might derive significant clinical benefit from the procedure but at present it remains experimental and is likely to be associated with extremely high treatment-related mortality in this setting. There is currently no data on the use of reduced-intensity conditioning in AL amyloid.

### Other Regimes

The effect of interferon-$\alpha$2b was evaluated in an open trial at the Mayo Clinic in 15 patients with AL amyloidosis who had failed traditional cytotoxic therapy (Gertz and Kyle, 1993). None of the patients showed any objective evidence of improvement, and the authors concluded that interferon did not appear to have a place in the treatment of AL amyloidosis.

An anthracycline derivative 4'-iodo-4'-deoxydoxorubicin (I-DOX) has been shown to bind avidly to amyloid fibrils *in vitro* and inhibits amyloid fibril formation under experimental conditions (Merlini et al., 1995), but early promising results in 8 patients with AL amyloidosis (Gianni et al., 1995) have not yet been extended in further studies. I-DOX is cytotoxic and cardiotoxic.

### Thalidomide

Several groups are presently evaluating the role of thalidomide in AL amyloidosis, and early impressions are that clonal plasma cell disease responses occur in a similar proportion of patients like in those with multiple myeloma. Adverse effects of thalidomide, including somnolence, constipation, development of neuropathy, and risk of venous and arterial thrombosis, limit its use in patients with AL amyloidosis.

### Supportive Treatment and Organ Transplantation

Supportive care has an important role in the management of AL amyloidosis. Most renal units in the United Kingdom readily accept patients in end-stage renal failure into their dialysis programs (discussed further later in this chapter), and this substantially prolongs survival, especially if there is no echocardiographic evidence of cardiac amyloid (Brown and Doherty, 1993; Gertz et al., 1992; Martinez-Vea et al., 1990; Moroni et al., 1992). Renal transplantation, which has also been used in AL amyloidosis, is discussed elsewhere. When AL amyloidosis is limited to the heart, death usually occurs suddenly or as a result of progressive heart failure. Cardiac transplantation has been performed in a small number of these patients (Dubrey et al., 2001; Hosenpud et al., 1991), although the procedure remains controversial because of the scarcity of donor hearts, the high transplant-related mortality (as a result of extracardiac amyloid), and the likelihood of amyloid deposition in the graft. Chemotherapy used in association with cardiac and other organ transplantation is required to prevent recurrence of amyloid or its progression in other organ systems.

Systemic AL amyloidosis involving the spleen is occasionally accompanied by acquired deficiency of clotting factors IX and/or X, which may lead to catastrophic hemorrhage (Griepp et al., 1981). Splenectomy can be an effective way of correcting the clotting defect, although there are case reports of resolution of the coagulopathy following chemotherapy with melphalan and steroids (Camoriano et al., 1987).

## Overview of Chemotherapy for AL Amyloidosis

The objective of chemotherapy in AL amyloidosis is to suppress production of disease-causing amyloidogenic monoclonal immunoglobulin light chains as quickly and safely as possible, but the relative efficacies of different chemotherapy regimens have not been determined. Recent experience at the National Amyloidosis Centre suggests that treatment strategies in individual patients are presently best guided by their early effect on quantitative measurements of circulating free immunoglobulin light chains (Bradwell et al., 2001). Indeed, reduction in the concentration of the amyloidogenic class of free immunoglobulin light chain by just 50% is associated with substantial survival benefit regardless of the type of chemotherapy used.

More intensive suppression of the underlying clonal disease is unnecessary in some patients, and efforts to minimize toxicity from chemotherapy should be paramount. Clinical improvement following chemotherapy in AL amyloidosis is always delayed for months or even years after adequate suppression of the underlying clonal disease, and amyloidotic organ function might deteriorate in some patients even when the clonal disease has responded completely to chemotherapy.

## $\beta_2$-Microglobulin Amyloidosis

The disabling arthralgia of $\beta_2$-microglobulin amyloidosis might respond partially to nonsteroidal antiinflammatory drugs or corticosteroids, but the only really effective treatment for this condition is renal transplantation (Drüeke, 1998). Serum levels of $\beta_2$-microglobulin fall rapidly after transplantation, and this is usually accompanied by a very rapid and substantial improvement in symptoms. Although prospective SAP scintigraphy has shown that $\beta_2$-microglobulin amyloid deposits can gradually regress, the resolution of symptoms within days or weeks of renal transplantation implicates other factors. These might include the antiinflammatory properties of immunosuppression after transplantation and some effect of discontinuation of the dialysis procedure itself. In contrast to the symptoms, radiologic bone cysts heal very slowly indeed and unsurprisingly amyloid can be demonstrated histologically many years after renal transplantation. Within a few years of renal transplantation, arthralgic symptoms might reappear very rapidly if the graft is lost, providing further evidence that dialysis is required for the clinical expression of disease associated with $\beta_2$-microglobulin amyloid deposits. Possible explanations of this phenomenon are that newly deposited $\beta_2$-microglobulin amyloid is more damaging than old, or that the cytokine-modulating effects of dialysis are involved. Certainly, $\beta_2$-microglobulin amyloid deposits are unusual in that they are often associated with a degree of inflammation and macrophage infiltration.

The risks of developing symptomatic $\beta_2$-microglobulin amyloidosis might be increased in patients dialyzed using less "biocompatible" cuprophane membranes, and the use of more permeable membrane systems that remove $\beta_2$-microglobulin more efficiently might be relatively protective (Miyata et al., 1998).

Drug treatment of established disease includes nonsteroidal anti-inflammatory analgesics, systemic and intra-articular corticosteroid therapy, but none of these is especially effective and long-term steroid therapy is particularly undesirable in this population of patients. Surgery might be required to relieve carpal tunnel compression, stabilize the cervical spine, or to treat bone fractures.

## Hereditary Amyloidosis

Hepatic transplantation is effective in familial amyloid polyneuropathy associated with transthyretin gene mutations because the variant amyloidogenic protein is produced mainly in the liver (Holmgren et al., 1993). Successful liver transplantation has now been reported in hundreds of patients with this condition and although the peripheral neuropathy usually only stabilizes, autonomic function can improve and the associated visceral amyloid deposits have been shown to regress in most cases. Important questions remain about the timing of the procedure but, so far, early intervention seems advisable. Disappointingly, there is evidence that wild-type TTR, an inherently but weakly amyloidogenic protein, might in some cases continue to be deposited after liver transplantation on an existing "template" of amyloid in the heart and in the vitreous (Stangou et al., 1998).

Fibrinogen is also synthesized only in the liver, and hepatic transplantation therefore has a potential role in the management of hereditary fibrinogen A α-chain amyloidosis. Successful, and most likely curative, liver transplants have been performed in a small number of these patients who have had unusually severe and early-onset disease. However, renal support, including renal transplantation, offers most patients with hereditary fibrinogen A α-chain amyloidosis an excellent quality of life and a relatively normal life expectancy.

The most common forms of hereditary apolipoprotein AI amyloidosis present with slowly progressive renal disease, which is probably managed optimally by renal transplantation. Although this does not alter the supply of the amyloidogenic precursor protein, which is produced in the liver and small intestine, renal and other solid organ grafts are rarely damaged by "recurrent" amyloid deposition in the medium- to long-term.

Hereditary lysozyme amyloidosis usually runs an exceptionally slow course, and patients with renal failure merit strong consideration for renal transplantation (Gillmore et al., 1999b).

# Supportive Measures

Supportive therapy remains critical in systemic amyloidosis, with the potential for delaying target organ failure, maintaining quality of life, and prolonging survival while the underlying process can be treated. Rigorous control of hypertension is vital in renal amyloidosis. Surgical resection of amyloidotic tissue is occasionally beneficial but, in general, a conservative approach to surgery, anesthesia, and other invasive procedures is advisable. Should any such procedure be undertaken, meticulous attention to blood pressure and fluid balance is essential. Amyloidotic tissues might heal poorly and are liable to bleed. Diuretics and vasoactive drugs should be used cautiously in cardiac amyloidosis because they can reduce cardiac output substantially. Dysrhythmias might respond to conventional pharmacologic therapy or pacing. Replacement of vital organ function, notably dialysis, might be necessary and cardiac, renal, and liver transplant procedures have a role in selected cases.

### Role of Renal Replacement Therapy

Renal failure is a major cause of death in systemic amyloidosis, and the introduction of hemodialysis and CAPD has improved the prognosis considerably (Cantaluppi, 1988; Gertz et al., 1992; Martinez-Vea et al., 1990; Moroni et al., 1992). Amyloidosis now accounts for 1% to 2% of all patients with end-stage renal failure who are accepted into European dialysis programs.

There is little information on the proportion of patients with systemic amyloidosis who require renal replacement therapy. However, among a series of 211 patients seen at the Mayo Clinic between 1969 and 1982, 37 required dialysis (Gertz et al., 1992). The median time between diagnosis and need for dialysis was 14 months and median survival from the start of dialysis was 8 months. No patient who had a normal serum creatinine and proteinuria < 2 g per day at diagnosis required dialysis.

Survival of patients with AL amyloid requiring dialysis compares favorably with those not requiring dialysis, and the overall survival on dialysis in amyloidosis is comparable to that of patients with other systemic diseases, including diabetes. Cardiovascular and circulatory complications associated with amyloidosis are the main causes of death among dialysis patients, both with AA and AL types. Cardiac amyloid, even if subclinical, is the most important predictor of poor survival in patients with AL amyloidosis undergoing dialysis whereas a history of rapid deterioration of renal function, short disease duration, older age, and evidence for significant amyloid involvement in other organ systems predicts poor survival in both AA and AL types (Gertz et al., 1992; Martinez-Vea et al., 1990; Moroni et al., 1992).

CAPD has inherent advantages over hemodialysis, which could be of particular significance in amyloidosis, especially in patients with cardiac involvement. It is not associated with the circulatory stress of intermittent hemodialysis, hemoglobin levels are better preserved and vascular access is not required, but so far there have been no prospective, comparative studies. Little information is available regarding the rate of bacterial infection among CAPD patients undergoing chemotherapy and, although some such patients have done well (Korzets et al., 1990), temporary conversion to hemodialysis is worth considering.

Systemic extrarenal amyloid deposition is likely to progress during dialysis unless the underlying cause of amyloidosis is treated successfully or undergoes spontaneous remission. Amyloid involvement of other organ systems, notably the gut (Lovat et al., 1997), adrenal glands (Danby et al., 1990), heart, and autonomic nerves, might be responsible for many nonspecific features ranging from nausea to circulatory failure and might go undetected for prolonged periods in the setting of uremia and hemodialysis. Gut and very occasionally cardiac amyloid deposits can progress sufficiently to become of major clinical significance even in AA amyloidosis (Ylinen et al., 1992). Eventually, most patients die of progressive systemic amyloidosis rather than complications of dialysis, indicating that attempts to halt the progression of amyloid must not be abandoned even when end-stage renal failure has occurred.

### Renal Transplantation

Renal transplantation is effective in both AA and AL amyloidosis. Five-year patient and graft survival at 65% and 62%, respectively (Hartmann et al., 1992) compare favorably with survival in other groups of patients, including those with nonsystemic causes of renal failure. Survival is similar in AL and AA patients and is significantly higher in patients under 45 years (Hartmann et al., 1992; Shmueli et al., 1992).

There is a high, early posttransplant mortality as a result of infection in amyloid patients (Hartmann et al., 1992; Isoniemi et al., 1989; Kilicturgay et al., 1992; Pasternack et al., 1986), pneumonia and septicemia being especially frequent during the first 3 months. In contrast, outcome after 1 year is much improved. Mortality is markedly reduced and the incidence of rejection episodes and overall survival was better than that of non-amyloid patients in one study comprising 45 individuals (Pasternack et al., 1986). Recurrence of amyloid in the transplanted organ might occur, but this rarely causes graft failure, even after 15 years of follow-up (Hartmann et al., 1992). Measures to limit this and to retard the progression of extrarenal amyloidosis should be instituted whenever possible.

## New Approaches

Improved understanding of the protein-folding mechanisms underlying amyloid fibrillogenesis, and recognition that relative instability of the precursor molecules is a key factor in amyloidogenesis, have identified novel therapeutic possibilities. These include investigation of small molecules, peptides, and glycosaminoglycan analogues that bind to and stabilize fibril precursors, or interfere with refolding and/or aggregation into the cross-β core structure common to amyloid fibrils. Some of these agents have already been shown to be effective in experimental murine AA amyloidosis. Our own efforts to develop specific therapy are focused on the avid binding of SAP to amyloid fibrils, which significantly contributes to pathogenesis of amyloidosis (Botto et al., 1997). The removal of SAP from amyloid deposits might facilitate their clearance, and we have identified a pharmacologic compound that inhibits the SAP-fibril interaction and which is presently being evaluated in clinical trials at the Royal Free Hospital (Pepys et al., 2002).

## Acknowledgments

This work was supported in part by grants from the Medical Research Council (UK) and The Wellcome Trust, and by NHS Research and Development Funds.

## REFERENCES

Ahlmen, M., Ahlmen, J., Svalander, C., et al. (1987). Cytotoxic drug treatment of reactive amyloidosis in rheumatoid arthritis with special reference to renal insufficiency. *Clinical Rheumatology, 6*, 27–38.

Alexanian, R., Barlogie, B., and Tucker, S. (1990). VAD-based regimens as primary treatment for multiple myeloma. *American Journal of Hematology, 33*, 86–89.

Benson, M. D., Liepnieks, J., Uemichi, T., et al. (1993). Hereditary renal amyloidosis associated with a mutant fibrinogen α-chain. *Nature Genetics, 3*, 252–255.

Benson, M. D., and Uemichi, T. (1996). Transthyretin amyloidosis. *Amyloid: International Journal of Experimental Clinical Investigation, 3*, 44–56.

Berglund, K., Keller, C., and Thysell, H. (1987). Alkylating cytostatic treatment in renal amyloidosis secondary to rheumatic disease. *Annals of the Rheumatic Diseases, 46*, 757–762.

Berglund, K., Thysell, H., and Keller, C. (1993). Results, principles and pitfalls in the management of renal AA-amyloidosis; a 10–21-year followup of 16 patients with rheumatic disease treated with alkylating cytostatics. *Journal of Rheumatology, 20*, 2051–2057.

Booth, D. R., Sunde, M., Bellotti, V., et al. (1997). Instability, unfolding and aggregation of human lysozyme variants underlying amyloid fibrillogenesis. *Nature, 385*, 787–793.

Botto, M., Hawkins, P. N., Bickerstaff, M. C. M., et al. (1997). Amyloid deposition is delayed in mice with targeted deletion of the serum amyloid P component gene. *Nature Medicine, 3*, 855–859.

Bradwell, A. R., Carr-Smith, H. D., Mead, G. P., et al. (2001). Highly sensitive, automated immunoassay for immunoglobulin free light chains in serum and urine. *Clinical Chemistry, 47*, 673–680.

Brown, J. H., and Doherty, C. C. (1993). Renal replacement therapy in multiple myeloma and systemic amyloidosis. *Postgraduate Medical Journal, 69*, 672–678.

Camoriano, J. K., Greipp, P. R., Bayer, G. K., et al. (1987). Resolution of acquired factor X deficiency and amyloidosis with melphalan and prednisone therapy. *New England Journal of Medicine, 316*, 1133–1135.

Cantaluppi, A. (1988). CAPD and systemic diseases. *Clinical Nephrology, 30* (Suppl 1), S8–12.

Comenzo, R. L., and Gertz, M. A. (2002). Autologous stem cell transplantation for primary systemic amyloidosis. *Blood, 99*, 4276–4282.

Comenzo, R. L., Vosburgh, E., Falk, R. H., et al. (1998). Dose-intensive melphalan with blood stem-cell support for the treatment of AL (amyloid light-chain) amyloidosis: survival and responses in 25 patients. *Blood, 91*, 3662–3670.

Danby, P., Harris, K. P. G., Williams, B., et al. (1990). Adrenal dysfunction in patients with renal amyloid. *Quarterly Journal of Medicine, 76*, 915 922.

David, J. (1991). Amyloidosis in juvenile chronic arthritis. *Clinical and Experimental Rheumatology, 9*, 73–78.

Dispenzieri, A., Lacy, M. Q., Kyle, R. A., et al. (2001). Eligibility for hematopoietic stem-cell transplantation for primary systemic amyloidosis is a favorable prognostic factor for survival. *J Clinical Oncology, 19*, 3350–3356.

Dobson, C. M., Ellis, R. J., and Fersht, A. R. (Eds.). (2001). Protein misfolding and disease. *Philosophical Transaction of the Royal Society of London: Series B: Biological Sciences, 356*, 127–227.

Drüeke, T. B. (1998). Dialysis-related amyloidosis. *Nephrology, Dialysis, Transplantation, 13*, 58–64.

Dubrey, S. W., Burke, M. M., Khaghani, A., et al. (2001). Long-term results of heart transplantation in patients with amyloid heart disease. *Heart, 85*, 202–207.

Falck, H. M., Törnroth, T., Skrifvars, B., et al. (1979). Resolution of renal amyloidosis secondary to rheumatoid arthritis. *Acta Med Scand, 205*, 651–656.

Gejyo, F., Yamada, T., Odani, S., et al. (1985). A new form of amyloid protein associated with chronic hemodialysis was identified as β$_2$-microglobulin. *Biochemical and Biophysical Research Communities, 129*, 701–706.

Gertz, M. A., and Kyle, R. A. (1989). Primary systemic amyloidosis—a diagnostic primer. *Mayo Clinic Proceedings, 64*, 1505–1519.

Gertz, M. A., and Kyle, R. A. (1993). Phase II trial of recombinant interferon alfa-2 in the treatment of primary systemic amyloidosis. *American Journal of Hematology, 44*, 125–128.

Gertz, M. A., Kyle, R. A., and Greipp, P. R. (1991). Response rates and survival in primary systemic amyloidosis. *Blood, 77*, 257–262.

Gertz, M. A., Kyle, R. A., and O'Fallon, W. M. (1992). Dialysis support of patients with primary systemic amyloidosis. A study of 211 patients. *Archives of Internal Medicine, 152*, 2245–2250.

Gertz, M. A., Lacy, M. Q., and Dispenzieri, A. (2000a). Myeloablative chemotherapy with stem cell rescue for the treatment of primary systemic amyloidosis: a status report. *Bone Marrow Transplant, 25*, 465–470.

Gertz, M. A., Lacy, M. Q., Dispenzieri, A., et al. (2002). Stem cell transplantation for the management of primary systemic amyloidosis. *American Journal of Medicine, 113*, 549–555.

Gertz, M. A., Lacy, M. Q., Gastineau, D. A., et al. (2000b). Blood stem cell transplantation as therapy for primary systemic amyloidosis (AL). *Bone Marrow Transplant, 26*, 963–969.

Gianni, L., Bellotti, V., Gianni, A. M., et al. (1995). New drug therapy of amyloidoses: resorption of AL-type deposits with 4'-iodo-4'-deoxydoxorubicin. *Blood, 86*, 855–861.

Gillmore, J. D., Apperley, J. F., Pepys, M. B., et al. (1999a). High dose chemotherapy for systemic AL amyloidosis. *Kidney International, 55*, 2103.

Gillmore, J. D., Booth, D. R., Madhoo, S., et al. (1999b). Hereditary renal amyloidosis associated with variant lysozyme in a large English family. *Nephrology, Dialysis, Transplantation, 14*, 2639–2644.

Gillmore, J. D., Booth, D. R., Rela, M., et al. (2000). Curative hepatorenal transplantation in systemic amyloidosis caused by the

Glu526Val fibrinogen α-chain variant in an English family. *Quarterly Journal of Medicine, 93*, 269–275.

Gillmore, J. D., Davies, J., Iqbal, A., et al. (1998). Allogeneic bone marrow transplantation for systemic AL amyloidosis. *British Journal of Haematology, 100*, 226–228.

Gillmore, J. D., Hawkins, P. N., and Pepys, M. B. (1997). Amyloidosis: a review of recent diagnostic and therapeutic developments. *British Journal of Haematology, 99*, 245–256.

Gillmore, J. D., Lovat, L. B., Persey, M. R., et al. (2001). Amyloid load and clinical outcome in AA amyloidosis in relation to circulating concentration of serum amyloid A protein. *Lancet, 358*, 24–29.

Gillmore, J. D., Persey, M. R., Lovat, L. B., et al. (1999c). Serum amyloid P component scintigraphy in AL amyloidosis. In: R. A. Kyle, and M. A. Gertz (Eds.), *Amyloid and Amyloidosis 1998* (p. 148), Pearl River, NY: Parthenon Publishing.

Goldfinger, W. E. (1972). Colchicine for familial Mediterranean fever. *New England Journal of Medicine, 287*, 1302.

Gorevic, P. D., Casey, T. T., Stone, W. J., et al. (1985). Beta-2 microglobulin is an amyloidogenic protein in man. *Journal of Clinical Investigations, 76*, 2425–2429.

Griepp, P. R., Kyle, R. A., and Bowie, E. J. W. (1981). Factor X deficiency in amyloidosis: a critical review. *American Journal of Hematology, 11*, 443–450.

Hall, R., and Hawkins, P. N. (1994). Cardiac transplantation for AL amyloidosis: a personal account. *British Medical Journal, 309*, 1135–1137.

Hartmann, A., Holdaas, H., Fauchald, P., et al. (1992). Fifteen years' experience with renal transplantation in systemic amyloidosis. *Transplant International, 5*, 15–18.

Hawkins, P. N. (1994a). Diagnosis and monitoring of amyloidosis. In G. Husby (Ed.), *Baillière's Clinical Rheumatology: Reactive Amyloidosis and the Acute Phase Response*, vol 8 (p. 635–659). London: Baillière Tindall.

Hawkins, P. N. (1994b). Studies with radiolabelled serum amyloid P component provide evidence for turnover and regression of amyloid deposits *in vivo*. *Clinical Science, 87*, 289–295.

Hawkins, P. N. (2002). Serum amyloid P component scintigraphy for diagnosis and monitoring amyloidosis. *Current Opinion in Nephrology and Hypertension, 11*, 649–655.

Hawkins, P. N., Lavender, J. P., and Pepys, M. B. (1990a). Evaluation of systemic amyloidosis by scintigraphy with [123]I-labeled serum amyloid P component. *New England Journal of Medicine, 323*, 508–513.

Hawkins, P. N., Myers, M. J., Lavender, J. P., et al. (1988). Diagnostic radionuclide imaging of amyloid: biological targeting by circulating human serum amyloid P component. *Lancet, i*, 1413–1418.

Hawkins, P. N., Richardson, S., MacSweeney, J. E., et al. (1993a). Scintigraphic quantification and serial monitoring of human visceral amyloid deposits provide evidence for turnover and regression. *Quarterly Journal of Medicine, 86*, 365–374.

Hawkins, P. N., Richardson, S., Vigushin, D. M., et al. (1993b). Serum amyloid P component scintigraphy and turnover studies for diagnosis and quantitative monitoring of AA amyloidosis in juvenile rheumatoid arthritis. *Arthritis and Rheumatism, 36*, 842–851.

Hawkins, P. N., Wootton, R., and Pepys, M. B. (1990b). Metabolic studies of radioiodinated serum amyloid P component in normal subjects and patients with systemic amyloidosis. *Journal of Clinical Investigation, 86*, 1862–1869.

Holmgren, G., Ericzon, B.-G., Groth, C.-G., et al. (1993). Clinical improvement and amyloid regression after liver transplantation in hereditary transthyretin amyloidosis. *Lancet, 341*, 1113–1116.

Hosenpud, J. D., DeMarco, T., Frazier, O. H., et al. (1991). Progression of systemic disease and reduced long-term survival in patients with cardiac amyloidosis undergoing heart transplantation. *Circulation, 84*, 338–343.

Isoniemi, H., Eklund, B., Hockerstedt, K., et al. (1989). Renal transplantation in amyloidosis. *Transplantation Proceedings, 21*, 2039–2040.

Kilicturgay, S., Tokyay, R., Arslan, G., et al. (1992). The results of transplantation of patients with amyloid nephropathy. *Transplantation Proceedings, 24*, 1788–1789.

Korzets, A., Tam, F., Russell, G., et al. (1990). The role of continuous ambulatory peritoneal dialysis in end-stage renal failure due to multiple myeloma. *American Journal of Kidney Diseases, 16*, 216–223.

Kyle, R. A., and Gertz, M. A. (1995). Primary systemic amyloidosis: clinical and laboratory features in 474 cases. *Seminars in Hematology, 32*, 45–59.

Kyle, R. A., Gertz, M. A., Greipp, P. R., et al. (1997). A trial of three regimens for primary amyloidosis: colchicine alone, melphalan and prednisone, and melphalan, prednisone, and colchicine. *New England Journal of Medicine, 336*, 1202–1207.

Kyle, R. A., and Greipp, R. R. (1978). Primary systemic amyloidosis: comparison of melphalan and prednisone versus placebo. *Blood, 52*, 818–827.

Kyle, R. A., and Greipp, P. R. (1983). Amyloidosis (AL): clinical and laboratory features in 229 cases. *Mayo Clinic Proceedings, 58*, 665–683.

Lachmann, H. J., Booth, D. R., Booth, S. E., et al. (2002a). Misdiagnosis of hereditary amyloidosis as AL (primary) amyloidosis. *New England Journal of Medicine, 346*, 1786–1791.

Lachmann, H. J., Gilbertson, J. A., Gillmore, J. D., et al. (2002b). Unicentric Castleman's disease complicated by systemic AA amyloidosis: a curable disease. *Quarterly Journal of Medicine, 95*, 211–218.

Livneh, A., Zemer, D., Langevitz, P., et al. (1994). Colchicine treatment of AA amyloidosis of familial Mediterranean fever. An analysis of factors affecting outcome. *Arthritis and Rheumatism, 37*, 1804–1811.

Livneh, A., Zemer, D., Siegal, B., et al. (1992). Colchicine prevents kidney transplant amyloidosis in familial Mediterranean fever. *Nephron, 60*, 418–422.

Lovat, L. B., Pepys, M. B., and Hawkins, P. N. (1997). Amyloid and the gut. *Digestive Diseases, 15*, 155–171.

Martinez-Vea, A., Garcia, C., Carreras, M., et al. (1990). End-stage renal disease in systemic amyloidosis: clinical course and outcome on dialysis. *American Journal of Nephrology, 10*, 283–289.

Merlini, G., Ascari, E., Amboldi, N., et al. (1995). Interaction of the anthracycline 4′-iodo-4′-deoxydoxorubicin with amyloid fibrils: inhibition of amyloidogenesis. *Proceedings of the National Academy of the Sciences of the United States of America, 92*, 2959–2963.

Miyata, T., Jadoul, M., Kurokawa, K., et al. (1998). Beta-2 microglobulin in renal disease. *Journal of the American Society of Nephrology, 9*, 1723–1735.

Moreau, P., Leblond, V., Bourquelot, P., et al. (1998). Prognostic factors for survival and response after high-dose therapy and autologous stem cell transplantation in systemic AL amyloidosis: a report on 21 patients. *British Journal of Haematology, 101*, 766–769.

Moroni, G., Banfi, G., Montoli, A., et al. (1992). Chronic dialysis in patients with systemic amyloidosis: the experience in Northern Italy. *Clinical Nephrology, 38*, 81–85.

Pasternack, A., Ahonen, J., and Kuhlback, B. (1986). Renal transplantation in 45 patients with amyloidosis. *Transplantation, 42*, 598–601.

Pepys, M. B., Booth, D. R., Hutchinson, W. L., et al. (1997). Amyloid P component. A critical review. *Amyloid: International Journal of Experimental Clinical Investigation, 4*, 274–295.

Pepys, M. B., Herbert, J., Hutchinson, W. L., et al. (2002). Targeted pharmacological depletion of serum amyloid P component for treatment of human amyloidosis. *Nature, 417*, 254–259.

Rydh, A., Suhr, O., Hietala, S.-O., et al. (1998). Serum amyloid P component scintigraphy in familial amyloid polyneuropathy: regression of visceral amyloid following liver transplantation. *European Journal of Nuclear Medicine, 25*, 709–713.

Samson, D., Gaminara, E., Newland, A., et al. (1989). Infusion of vincristine and doxorubicin with oral dexamethasone as first-line therapy for multiple myeloma. *Lancet, ii*, 882–885.

Sanchorawala, V., Wright, D. G., Seldin, D. C., et al. (2001). An overview of the use of high-dose melphalan with autologous stem cell transplantation for the treatment of AL amyloidosis. *Bone Marrow Transplant, 28*, 637–642.

Schey, S. A., Kazmi, M., Ireland, R., et al. (1998). The use of intravenous intermediate dose melphalan and dexamethasone as induction treatment in the management of *de novo* multiple myeloma. *European Journal of Haematology, 61*, 306–310.

Schnitzer, T. J., and Ansell, B. M. (1977). Amyloidosis in juvenile chronic polyarthritis. *Arthritis and Rheumatism, 20*, 245–252.

Shmueli, D., Lustig, S., Nakache, R., et al. (1992). Renal transplantation in patients with amyloidosis due to familial Mediterranean fever. *Transplantation Proceedings, 24*, 1783–1784.

Skinner, M., Anderson, J., Wang, M., et al. (1994). Treatment of patients with primary amyloidosis. In R. Kisilevsky, M. D. Benson, B. Frangione, et al. (Eds.), *Amyloid and Amyloidosis 1993* (p. 232–234). Pearl River, NY: Parthenon Publishing.

Solomon, A., Weiss, D. T., and Pepys, M. B. (1992). Induction in mice of human light chain-associated amyloidosis. *American Journal of Pathology, 140*, 629–637.

Stangou, A. J., Hawkins, P. N., Heaton, N. D., et al. (1998). Progressive cardiac amyloidosis following liver transplantation for familial amyloid polyneuropathy: implications for amyloid fibrillogenesis. *Transplantation, 66*, 229–233.

Sunde, M., Serpell, L. C., Bartlam, M., et al. (1997). Common core structure of amyloid fibrils by synchrotron x-ray diffraction. *Journal of Molecular Biology, 273*, 729–739.

Tan, S. Y., Irish, A., Winearls, C. G., et al. (1996). Long-term effect of renal transplantation on dialysis-related amyloid deposits and symptomatology. *Kidney International, 50*, 282–289.

Tan, S. Y., Murdoch, I. E., Sullivan, T. J., et al. (1994). Primary localized orbital amyloidosis composed of the immunoglobulin γ heavy chain CH3 domain. *Clin Sci, 87*, 487–491.

Uemichi, T., Liepnieks, J. J., and Benson, M. D. (1994). Hereditary renal amyloidosis with a novel variant fibrinogen. *Journal of Clinical Investigation, 93*, 731–736.

Wetzel, R. (1997). Domain stability in immunoglobulin light chain deposition disorders. *Advances in Protein Chemistry, 50*, 183–242.

Wilkins, J., Gallimore, J. R., Tennent, G. A., et al. (1994). Rapid automated enzyme immunoassay of serum amyloid A. *Clinical Chemistry, 40*, 1284–1290.

Ylinen, K., Gronhagen-Riska, C., Honkanen, E., et al. (1992). Outcome of patients with secondary amyloidosis in dialysis treatment. *Nephrology, Dialysis, and Transplantation, 7*, 908–912.

Zemer, D., Livneh, A., Danon, Y. L., et al. (1991). Long-term colchicine treatment in children with familial Mediterranean fever. *Arthritis and Rheumatism, 34*, 973–977.

Zemer, D., Pras, M., Sohar, E., et al. (1986). Colchicine in the prevention and treatment of amyloidosis of familial Mediterranean fever. *New England Journal of Medicine, 314*, 1001–1005.

# CHAPTER 22

---

# Heavy Chain Disease

### DIETLIND L. WAHNER-ROEDLER
### ROBERT A. KYLE

## Introduction

The heavy chain diseases (HCD) represent a proliferative process of lymphoplasma cells involving B cells and are characterized by the production of incomplete heavy chains devoid of light chains. They have been described for the 3 main immunoglobulin (Ig) classes. The most frequent is α-HCD; μ-HCD is rare. The incidence of γ-HCD is intermediate.

## γ Heavy Chain Disease

γ-HCD is a serologically determined entity. Since the first report by Franklin et al. (1964), approximately 120 patients with γ-HCD have been described in the literature.

### Clinical Features

γ-HCD has been recognized throughout the world and has been noted in black and Asian as well as in white patients. The median age at diagnosis is approximately 60 years. However, the disease can occur in children or very young adults (Bender et al., 1978; Bloch et al., 1973; Dammacco et al., 1976; Pruzanski et al., 1979; Rabin and Moon, 1973; Woods et al., 1970). Although γ-HCD has been reported to occur equally in men and women (Fermand et al., 1989; Wester et al., 1982), there was a clear predominance of women in a recently reported series, which included 15 women and 8 men (Wahner-Roedler et al., 2003).

In contrast to the uniformity of findings associated with α-HCD, γ-HCD has a great variety of clinical and pathologic features. In general, γ-HCD can be placed into 3 broad categories on the basis of the underlying pathologic process and its distribution: disseminated lymphoproliferative disease, localized proliferative disease, and no proliferative disease.

## Disseminated Lymphoproliferative Disease

Disseminated lymphoproliferative disease is present in most patients at the time of diagnosis of γ-HCD and has been reported in 57% to 66% of patients in various series (Fermand et al., 1989; Wahner-Roedler et al., 2003; Wester et al., 1982). The lymphoid proliferation may be associated with an autoimmune disorder, as observed in 23% of patients with γ-HCD and disseminated lymphoproliferative disease (Wahner-Roedler et al., 2003). Lymphadenopathy and constitutional symptoms are the usual features in these patients. On physical examination at the time of diagnosis of γ-HCD, lymphadenopathy was present in 62%, splenomegaly in 38%, and hepatomegaly in 8% of 13 patients who had an underlying disseminated lymphoproliferative disorder (Wahner-Roedler et al., 2003). In reviewing the literature, Fermand et al. (1989) reported lymphadenopathy in 56%, splenomegaly in 52%, and hepatomegaly in 37% of 81 patients with a diagnosis of γ-HCD. Lymphadenopathy obstructing the vena cava has been noted (Bloch et al., 1973; Gallart et al., 1978). Edema of the uvula and palate has occasionally been observed, presumably because of lymphatic obstruction resulting from involvement of the Waldeyer ring of lymph nodes. Spontaneous rupture of the spleen has occurred (Fermand et al., 1989). A free γ heavy chain was observed in serum and urine after high-dose chemotherapy and autologous peripheral blood stem cell transplantation in a patient with IgG-κ multiple myeloma. The isolated heavy chain was detected 2 months after transplantation, persisted for an additional 2 months, and was eventually replaced by an intact IgG-κ monoclonal protein (Butch et al., 2001).

## Localized Proliferative Disease

The lymphoproliferative process is localized in approximately 25% of patients with γ-HCD. Localized disease may be extramedullary or may involve only the bone marrow (Fermand et al., 1989; Wahner-Roedler et al., 2003).

Various extrahematopoietic lesions have been described and might be a presenting symptom. Skin lesions in general have been reported to be the most frequent extrahematopoietic manifestation of γ-HCD (Lassoued et al., 1990), and several patients showed cutaneous or subcutaneous involvement featured by an extranodal mass (Fermand et al., 1989; Kyle et al., 1981a; Osserman and Takatsuki, 1964; Wahner-Roedler et al., 2003) or skin nodules (Case records of the Massachusetts General Hospital, 1970; Dickson et al., 1989; Gallart et al., 1978; Kanoh et al., 1988; Kanoh and Nakasato, 1987; Kyle et al., 1981a; Lassoued et al., 1990; O'Conor et al., 1985; Rabin and Moon, 1973; Roda et al., 1985a). Several authors described patients presenting with extramedullary plasmacytoma of the thyroid (Kyle et al., 1981a; Matsubayashi et al., 1985; Ottó et al., 1986; Rouesse et al., 1972; Westin et al., 1972) or parotid or submandibular swelling (Faguet et al., 1977; Franklin et al., 1964; Kyle et al., 1981a; Wahner-Roedler et al., 2003). A patient with dysphagia and hoarseness from an oropharyngeal mass consisting of plasma cells was reported (Blum et al., 1985). A 12-year-old Turkish girl presented with malabsorption and marked infiltration of the intestine with lymphoplasmacytoid cells (similar to α-HCD) (Bender et al., 1978), and a 63-year-old woman with γ-HCD associated with mucosa-associated lymphoid tissue lymphoma of the duodenum has been reported in the Japanese literature (Ieko et al., 1998). In several other cases, the initial symptoms were caused by a gastric lymphoid tumor (Papae et al., 1978; Roda et al., 1985b; Virella et al., 1977).

Of the patients in whom the disease was localized to the bone marrow only, one presented with an infection resulting from absolute neutropenia and one had lymphoproliferative disease with plasmacytoid differentiation revealed by bone marrow examination after a γ heavy chain was coincidentally detected in the serum (Wahner-Roedler et al., 2003).

## No Apparent Proliferative Disease

No proliferative disease is apparent in 9% to 17% of patients with γ-HCD. In most of these patients, an underlying autoimmune disorder has been reported. Autoimmune diseases documented in patients with γ-HCD with or without associated lymphoproliferative disease include rheumatoid arthritis in approximately 12 patients (Chernokhvostova et al., 1991; Creyssel et al., 1977; Dickson et al., 1989; Fermand et al., 1989; Gaucher et al., 1977; Husby, 2000; Husby et al., 1998; Ibuka et al., 1974; Jacqueline et al., 1978; Kretschmer et al., 1974; Loyau et al., 1975; Ockhuizen et al., 1983; Stühlinger et al., 1987; Wahner-Roedler et al., 2003; Zawadzki et al., 1969), systemic lupus erythematosus

(Jones et al., 1974), discoid lupus (Westin et al., 1972), vasculitis with or without associated rheumatoid arthritis (Fermand et al., 1989; Kretschmer et al., 1974; Stühlinger et al., 1987), livedoid vasculitis (Cooper et al., 1991; Wahner-Roedler et al., 2003), Sjögren syndrome (Castelino et al., 1994; Wager et al., 1969; Wahner-Roedler et al., 2003), and Coombs'-positive hemolytic anemia (Lyons et al., 1975; Wahner-Roedler et al., 2003). Neurologic manifestations such as peripheral neuropathy (Ellman and Bloch, 1968; Fermand et al., 1989; Leloup et al., 1989), myasthenia gravis (Fermand et al., 1989; Westin et al., 1972), and Guillain-Barré syndrome (Kyle et al., 1981a) were reported in several patients with γ-HCD. Herpes zoster involved the eye of one patient (Chury et al., 1971) and was generalized in another (Baker et al., 1977). Solid tumors diagnosed in patients with γ-HCD included prostate cancer (Ellman and Bloch, 1968; Kyle et al., 1981a), uterine sarcoma (Fermand et al., 1989; Loyau et al., 1975), gastric carcinoma (Fermand et al., 1989), and pancreatic cancer (Adlersberg et al., 1978); these tumors were probably fortuitous. There have been several patients with γ-HCD with features of benign monoclonal gammopathy or monoclonal gammopathy of undetermined significance (Albutt et al., 1981; Galanti et al., 1995; Lenders et al., 1984; Wahner-Roedler et al., 2003; Westin et al., 1972). In many patients with γ-HCD the diagnosis of a lymphoproliferative or autoimmune disease preceded the diagnosis of γ-HCD by a few weeks to many years. In 22 patients, the median time interval between the diagnosis of an underlying disease (lymphoproliferative, autoimmune, or both) and the diagnosis of γ-HCD was 71 months (range, 0–540 mo) (Wahner-Roedler et al., 2003).

## Protein Findings

The serum protein electrophoretic pattern might not suggest monoclonal gammopathy. Indeed, in 12 of 28 cases (40%) reported by Fermand et al. (1989), the abnormal component was not detectable by electrophoresis. In a more recent series, a monoclonal peak, albeit small and apparently inconsequential, was detected on serum protein electrophoresis in 19 of 22 patients (86%) (Wahner-Roedler et al., 2003). When a localized band was detected, it was most commonly in the $\beta_1$ or $\beta_2$ region. The median monoclonal peak at diagnosis in the 19 patients was 1.59 g/dL (range, 0.40–3.91 g/dL), and monoclonal peaks of more than 2 g/dL were found in 5 patients (Wahner-Roedler et al., 2003). Analysis of the distribution of the IgG subclasses in γ-HCD shows a lower than expected incidence of IgG2 HCD protein. The most common subclass is IgG1, which occurs in 65% of cases. IgG3 has been identified in 27%, IgG4 in 5%, and IgG2 in 3% of patients

(Fermand et al., 1989), whereas the normal distribution of IgG subclasses is IgG1, 64% to 70%; IgG2, 23% to 28%; IgG3, 4% to 7%; and IgG4, 3% to 4% (Schur, 1972). A hybrid γ-HCD protein with features of IgG3 and IgG1 has been reported (Arnaud et al., 1981). IgA and IgM are usually reduced in γ–HCD.

The amount of γ-HCD protein present in the urine ranges from nondetectable to 20 g per 24 hours and is less than 1 g per 24 hours in most instances. A median of 0.23 g/24 hours (range, 0.02–4.12 g/24 hours) was observed in 19 patients in the urine at the time of diagnosis (Wahner-Roedler et al., 2003). The electrophoretic mobility of the monoclonal protein in the urine is the same as in the serum with only rare exceptions (Bloch et al., 1973).

With high-resolution electrophoresis and immunofixation, relatively homogeneous fragments of γ chains unaccompanied by light chains may be found during examination of urine. Such fragments should not be confused with the γ-HCD protein (Charles and Valdes, 1994). Differentiation from the γ-HCD protein can be accomplished by gel diffusion analysis. However, from a practical point of view, such studies are not required because the γ-HCD protein is always present in the serum and migrates into the β-γ region, whereas the free fragments of γ chain described by Charles and Valdes (1994) are found only in the urine and migrate in the $\alpha_2$ region. These fragments are of no known clinical importance.

The response to the Bence Jones heat test is, in general, negative. Five patients with γ-HCD and Bence Jones proteinuria have been described (Chernokhvostova et al., 1991; Hauke et al., 1992; Marcenò et al., 1984; Wahner-Roedler et al., 2003).

## Structural Protein Abnormalities

Structural studies have shown that most γ-HCD proteins are dimers of deleted heavy chains devoid of light chains. The molecular weight of the monomeric γ chain ranges from 27,000 to 49,000. The length of the γ chain varies from case to case but usually is one-half to three-fourths the length of its normal counterpart (Seligmann et al., 1979). All γ-HCD proteins show deletion of the $C_H1$ domain. Often, the deletions are internal, with a portion of the V sequence present at the amino terminus, ruling out postsynthetic degradation. The resumption of the normal sequence occurs precisely at the beginning of a domain. On the basis of their structure, the γ-HCD proteins can be placed into several groups (Fig. 22-1).

Most γ-HCD proteins in the first group contain a fragment of the V region. Usually they have a normal V region amino terminus followed by an internal deletion of the V and the entire $C_H1$ domain. In all HCD

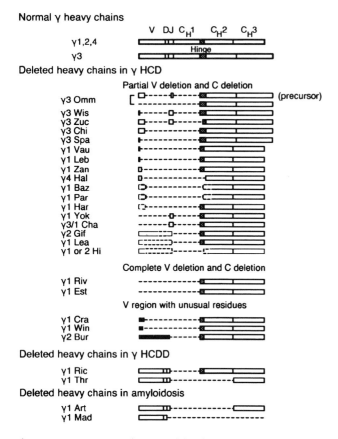

**Figure 22-1** *Structure of various deleted γ heavy chains in γ heavy chain disease (γ-HCD), γ heavy chain deposition disease (γ-HCDD), and amyloidosis compared with that of normal chains. Hatched bars correspond to hinge regions, closed bars indicate unusual sequences, dotted bars indicate regions potentially present but not sequenced, and dotted lines indicate deletions. V, variable region; D, diversity; J, joining; $C_H$, constant region. Omm (Adlersberg et al., 1978; Alexander et al., 1982, 1988), Wis (Frangione et al., 1980; Franklin et al., 1979b), Zuc (Wolfenstein-Todel et al., 1976), Chi (Frangione, 1976), Spa (Frangione and Franklin, 1979), Vau and Leb (Franklin et al., 1979a), Zan (Franklin et al., 1979b), Hal (Frangione et al., 1973), Baz (Smith et al., 1978), Par (Calvanico et al., 1972), Har (Frangione et al., 1978), Yok (Nabeshima and Ikenaka, 1976), Cha (Arnaud et al., 1981), Gif (Cooper et al., 1972), Lea (Frangione et al., 1978), Hi (Terry and Ohms, 1970), Riv (Guglielmi et al., 1988), Est (Biewenga et al., 1980), Cra (Frangione et al., 1978; Franklin and Frangione, 1971), Win (Hauke et al., 1992), Bur (Prelli and Frangione, 1992), Ric (Khamlichi et al., 1995), Thr (Khamlichi et al., 1995), Art (Eulitz et al., 1990), and Mad (Solomon et al., 1994). (Modified from Cogné, M., Preud'homme, J. L., and Guglielmi, P. [1989]. Immunoglobulin gene alterations in human heavy chain disease. Research in Immunology, 140, 487–502; Cogné et al. [1992]. By permission of The American Society of Hematology and Elsevier Science Publishers.)*

proteins with an internal V region deletion, the residues corresponding to the VDJ junction are missing. Some of these proteins contain a portion of this region and feature 2 noncontiguous deletions (γ3 Omm, γ3 Wis, γ3 Zuc). γ3 Omm has been shown to undergo postsynthetic degradation to yield an $NH_2$ terminal deleted protein.

The second group consists of γ-HCD proteins that lack the entire V and $C_{H1}$ domains, with the sequence starting within the hinge region (γ$^1$ Riv, γ$^1$ Est).

The third group is characterized by an unusual amino acid sequence preceding the deletion. An abnormal sequence of 10 residues has been found in protein γ$^1$ Cra and in 7 residues in γ$^1$ Win. The complete sequence of γ$^2$-HCD Bur has been reported. This mutant is composed of a complete V region, hinge, $C_{H2}$, and $C_{H3}$ domains.

γ-HCD cells usually do not secrete light chains. There are, however, a few cases in which light chains or light-chain fragments were documented. In γ-HCD patient Win, λ Bence Jones protein was found in the serum and urine (Hauke et al., 1991, 1992). In another patient, IgG-κ and IgM-λ were detected in the serum, and κ and λ Bence Jones proteins were detected in the urine (Chernokhvostova et al., 1991). In 3 additional patients, light chains were detected in the urine during the course of γ-HCD, κ in 2 and λ in 3 patients (Marcenò et al., 1984; Wahner-Roedler et al., 2003). In 1 of 9 patients with γ-HCD, nonsecreted monotypic light chains were found by direct immunofluorescence in the cytoplasm and at the surface of blood and bone marrow cells (Preud'homme et al., 1979). Small amounts of a truncated κ chain were documented in a cytoplasmic extract by internal labeling when HCD protein Riv was studied (Cogné et al., 1988, 1992).

In most cases of HCD, the association of several distinct gene alterations is responsible for both the complex structural abnormalities found among these proteins and the usual absence of light-chain synthesis. The alterations found in 2 γ heavy-chain genes (γ-HCD protein Omm and γ-HCD protein Riv) and in one light-chain gene (κ Riv) include somatic mutations, deletions, and insertions in rearranged V genes. HCD protein γ3 Omm was found to be the product of 2 deletions, a splice correction and postsynthetic $NH_2$ terminal proteolysis (Alexander et al., 1988). Sequencing of the γ1 Riv gene revealed that it had undergone $V_H$-$J_H$ and H chain class switch recombinations. However, normal RNA splice sites had been eliminated by a DNA insertion/deletion ($V_H$ acceptor site), mutations ($J_H$ donor site), or a large deletion ($C_{H1}$ region). These DNA alterations resulted in aberrant mRNA processing in which the leader region was spliced directly to the hinge region, accounting for the HCD protein (Guglielmi et al., 1988) (Fig. 22-2).

Similar to genes encoding HCD proteins, the κ chain gene of patient Riv showed deletions, insertions, and a very high rate (25%) of somatic mutations in the VJ region. Mutations of spliced sites bounding the $V_κ J_κ$ region resulted in exon skipping and splicing of the leader peptide exon onto the $C_κ$ exon. A short mRNA was present and coded for a $C_κ$ fragment devoid of the V domain (Cogné et al., 1988).

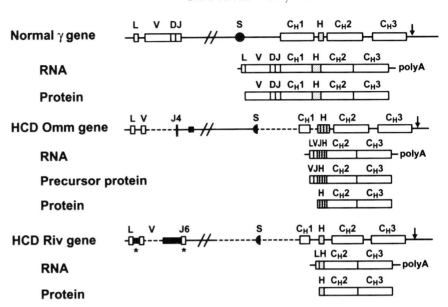

**Figure 22-2** *Structure of γ heavy chain disease (HCD) gene, RNA transcript, and protein compared with their normal rearranged counterpart. S, switch region; V, variable region; L, leader; H, hinge; CH, constant region; D, diversity; J, joining. Asterisks indicate altered splice site; solid bars represent insertions in coding (large bar) or noncoding (small bar) regions; dashed lines indicate deletion. (From Fermand, J. P., and Brouet, J. C. [1999]. Heavy-chain diseases.* Hematological Oncology Clinic of North America, *13, 1281–1294. By permission of WB Saunders Company.)*

The rearranged λ light-chain gene in Omm HCD cell lines was shown to have a mutation in the splice donor site at the 3′ end of the leader J exon, resulting in direct splicing of the 3′ end of the leader to the acceptor site of the constant region. The cells contained mRNA consisting of the leader-coding region joined directly to the constant region. The V-region exon was skipped and the shortened mRNA translated into a truncated protein containing no V-region amino acids. It was further noted that Omm cells produced an excess of heavy- to light-chain mRNA as well as protein. The excess was found to be independent of the structural gene abnormality and was thought to be the result of a low level of light-chain transcription, suggesting that Omm cells either lack a transcription factor or have a functional repressor of light-chain transcription (Teng et al., 2000).

## Hematologic Abnormalities

Anemia is frequent. It is usually normochromic, normocytic, and moderate, except in cases with autoimmune hemolytic anemia. The median hemoglobin for 22 patients at time of diagnosis of γ-HCD was 11.2 g/dL (range, 8.4–14.3 g/dL). In 8 of these patients, the hemoglobin was less than 10 g/dL (Wahner-Roedler et al., 2003). Coombs' positive autoimmune hemolytic anemia has been reported in several cases (Chernokhvostova et al., 1991; Kuroyanagi et al., 1979; Kyle et al., 1981a; Lyons et al., 1975; Rabin and Moon, 1973; Shirakura et al., 1976; Wahner-Roedler et al., 2003) and was sometimes associated with idiopathic thrombocytopenic purpura (Evans syndrome) (Kyle et al., 1981a; Rabin and Moon, 1973; Wahner-Roedler et al., 2003). The leukocyte count and differential are usually normal, but leukopenia and leukocytosis might

be present. Lymphocytosis with or without atypical lymphocytes may occur, and occasionally a patient presents with chronic lymphocytic leukemia (Wahner-Roedler et al., 2003). In some cases, rare circulating plasma cells have been noted. Plasma cell leukemia was reported in 2 patients (Keller et al., 1970; Woods et al., 1970). Eosinophilia might occur. Thrombocytopenia caused by an autoimmune process, hypersplenism, or, less frequently, bone marrow failure has been reported (Fermand et al., 1989).

Bone marrow aspirates and biopsies might reveal an increase of plasma cells, lymphocytes, or plasmacytoid lymphocytes similar to the bone marrow findings in Waldenström macroglobulinemia. These lymphocytoid plasma cells express pan-B cell markers and cytoplasmic γ heavy chain without light chain, and they are negative for CD5 and CD10 (Jaffe et al., 2001). The typical bone marrow features of multiple myeloma (Ruiz-Arguelles et al., 1984; Solling and Askjaer, 1973) or chronic lymphocytic leukemia (Fermand et al., 1989; Kyle et al., 1981a; Wahner-Roedler et al., 2003) are rarely observed. Marrow changes consistent with a myeloproliferative disorder were noted in a few patients (Ellis et al., 1992; Pontet et al., 1988; Wahner-Roedler et al., 2003; Wester et al., 1982). The presence of mast cells has been mentioned (Van Bergeijk et al., 1980). In many instances, the bone marrow aspirate and biopsy specimens are normal, which was the case in 15 of 22 patients with γ-HCD who underwent a bone marrow examination in one series; the bone marrow of the other 7 patients revealed involvement by a lymphoplasma cell proliferative disorder with a median involvement of 30% (range, 9%–70%). In 2 patients, the marrow involvement was estimated to be 50% or greater (Wahner-Roedler et al., 2003). Other series reported bone marrow involvement in 58% to 63% of cases (Fermand et al., 1989).

## Other Features

The bones usually appear normal radiographically, although a case with osteolytic lesions simulating advanced multiple myeloma has been described (Kanoh et al., 1988; Kanoh and Nakasato, 1987). Only 3 other cases with skeletal involvement have been reported (Fermand et al., 1989; Prévot et al., 1977; Ruiz-Arguelles et al., 1984). Hypercalcemia was noted in 5 cases (Bloch et al., 1973; Case records of the Massachusetts General Hospital, 1970; Eisner and Mitnick, 1986; Kanoh and Nakasato, 1987; Kyle et al., 1981a; Wahner-Roedler et al., 2003), without apparent skeletal involvement in 3. Renal insufficiency is uncommon but may occur in association with hypercalcemia. Lymphoid infiltration involving the kidneys (Kyle et al., 1981a; Shirakura et al., 1976), adrenals (Ogawa et al., 1978; Osserman and Takatsuki, 1964), lungs (Kyle et al., 1981a; O'Conor et al., 1985), and central nervous system (Kretschmer et al., 1974) has been detected mainly at postmortem examinations.

## Lymph Node Pathology

There is no consistent morphologic pattern corresponding to serologically defined γ-HCD. Non-Hodgkin lymphoma was diagnosed in 18 (38%) of 47 patients in whom lymph nodes were examined (Wester et al., 1982). Lymphoplasmacytic proliferation, with or without atypia, was present in 36% of cases. Hyperplastic nodes and plasmacytoma each made up 11% of the total. There was 1 case of Hodgkin disease and 1 case of probable Hodgkin disease (Wester et al., 1982). Five additional cases of γ-HCD associated with Hodgkin disease have been reported (Cozzolino et al., 1982; Di Benedetto et al., 1989; Hudnall et al., 2001; Roda et al., 1985a; Wahner-Roedler et al., 2003). In 2 cases, the subtype was nodular sclerosing (Cozzolino et al., 1982; Roda et al., 1985a); in 1, mixed cellularity (Di Benedetto et al., 1989); in 1, nodular lymphocytic predominance (Hudnall et al., 2001); and in another, lymphocytic depletion (Wahner-Roedler et al., 2003).

## Cytogenetic Abnormalities

Cytogenetic abnormalities were reported in 7 of 15 patients; 4 of these had aneuploidy (Fermand et al., 1989; Kyle et al., 1981a; Loyau et al., 1975; Roda et al., 1985a), and 3 others had trisomy 7 (O'Conor et al., 1985), trisomy 21 (Pruzanski et al., 1979), or multiple chromosome abnormalities (Fermand et al., 1989). Three of these patients (Fermand et al., 1989; Loyau et al., 1975) had previously received chemotherapy, which might have caused some of the abnormalities. No cytogenetic abnormalities were found in 8 other patients (Delmas-Marsalet et al., 1971; Faguet et al., 1977; Fermand et al., 1989; Franklin et al., 1964; Gaucher et al., 1977; Zawadzki et al., 1969). N-ras oncogene activation was demonstrated in 1 patient with γ-HCD (patient Omm) (Moskovits et al., 1992).

## Diagnosis

γ-HCD can present with diverse clinical features. The diagnosis is established by immunofixation or immunoelectrophoresis of the serum and a concentrated urine specimen using specific antisera. A modified immunoselection technique for the diagnosis of heavy chain disease has been described (Sun et al., 1994). Two-dimensional electrophoresis and immunoblotting have also been used for the recognition of γ-HCD (Blangarin et al., 1984; Mitchell et al., 1990). Tissot et al. (1998) showed that the combination of serum protein agarose electrophoresis and 2-dimensional electrophoresis can be used to further characterize abnormal protein bands detected by immunofixation. We think γ-HCD is underdiagnosed and urge that immunofixation of serum and urine be performed in all cases of atypical lymphoplasma cell proliferative diseases.

## Clinical Course

The clinical course of γ-HCD may range from an asymptomatic, benign, or transient process to a rapidly progressive neoplasm leading to death within a few weeks. Patients with features of benign monoclonal gammopathy or monoclonal gammopathy of undetermined significance have remained clinically well for 2 to 7 years of followup after a persistent γ heavy chain was documented (Albutt et al., 1981; Galanti et al., 1995; Lenders et al., 1984; Wahner-Roedler et al., 2003; Westin et al., 1972). Disappearance of the γ-HCD protein has also been reported. In 1 patient, the γ heavy chain protein was detected during a recurrent febrile illness but disappeared after cholecystectomy (Biewenga and van Loghem, 1979; Van Bergeijk et al., 1980). In another patient, the monoclonal γ heavy chain disappeared from the serum 8 months after irradiation for a thyroid mass and cervical lymphadenopathy; in that case biopsy specimens had shown an invasive plasmacytic proliferation (Rouesse et al., 1972). In 3 other patients with rheumatoid arthritis, the γ-HCD protein disappeared (Fermand et al., 1989; Gaucher et al., 1977; Ockhuizen et al., 1983). One of these patients was followed for more than 10 years; at last followup, despite slowly progressive rheumatoid arthritis, the γ-HCD protein had not reappeared and overt lymphoid proliferation had not developed (Fermand et al., 1989).

When an underlying lymphoid malignancy exists, knowledge of the histopathologic pattern is essential for determination of prognosis. The presence of the γ-HCD protein by itself does not seem to influence the course of the underlying disorder (Fermand et al., 1989).

## Treatment

γ-HCD represents a heterogeneous condition that does not fit the designation of a disease process and, as suggested by Roda et al. (1985a), should rather be named "monoclonal γ heavy chain" or "Franklin's protein associated with…" Therefore, the course of therapy depends on the underlying clinicopathologic features rather than on the presence of the abnormal protein. If the abnormal protein is an accidental finding in an asymptomatic patient, no therapy is indicated. Any associated autoimmune disease should be treated with standard therapy regardless of the presence of a γ-HCD protein.

In symptomatic patients with a low-grade lymphoplasmacytic malignancy, a trial of chlorambucil may be beneficial. Melphalan and prednisone can be used if the proliferation is predominantly plasmacytic. For patients with symptomatic γ-HCD and evidence of a progressive lymphoplasma cell proliferative process or non-Hodgkin lymphoma, cyclophosphamide, vincristine, and prednisone should be tried. If there is no response to this regimen, doxorubicin should be added.

Agrawal et al. (1994) reported a patient who had complete remission with disappearance of the heavy chain after 6 courses of fludarabine. Successful treatment of γ-HCD with low-dose etoposide was reported in a Japanese patient whose disease was unresponsive to combination chemotherapy (Ishikawa et al., 1997). In one patient in whom a lymph node biopsy specimen revealed follicles containing CD20-positive B lymphocytes, rituximab was used with good response after a temporary response to fludarabine, mitoxantrone, and dexamethasone (Wahner-Roedler et al., 2003). Apparent complete response, including disappearance of the monoclonal component from serum and urine, has been induced by chemotherapy (Agrawal et al., 1994; Fermand et al., 1989), irradiation (Fermand et al., 1989; Rouesse et al., 1972), or surgical removal of a localized process (Matsubayashi et al., 1985; Ottó et al., 1986). In some instances, however, the γ-HCD protein does not vary in parallel with the associated process, and relapse can occur without the reappearance of the pathologic protein (Fermand et al., 1989; Orth et al., 1994).

In a series of 23 patients reported by Wahner-Roedler et al. (2003), 16 patients were treated for an underlying lymphoplasma cell proliferative disorder or an associated autoimmune disorder, in 5 patients treatment was thought to be unnecessary, and 2 patients

were thought to be too sick for treatment. Of the 16 patients treated, 6 had a complete clinical response; the γ heavy chain disappeared in 2 patients and persisted in 2, and no serologic followup was available for 2 patients. Ten patients had persisting clinical disease; the γ heavy chain disappeared in 3 of these patients and persisted in 6, and no serologic followup was available for 1. Of the 7 patients who were not treated, 2 died, 1 within 1 month and 1 within 5 months. Two patients had no evidence of clinical disease at last followup, although γ heavy chain persisted in urine or serum. The other 3 patients had no change in clinical or serologic status. The median length of followup for the 23 patients from time of diagnosis of γ-HCD was 2.75 years (range, 0.08–21.75 y). At the time of last followup, 15 patients had died. The cause of death was known in 12 patients and was not related to the underlying disease in 7 of these. The median survival of the 23 patients was 7.4 years (range, 1 mo to more than 21 y).

## Monoclonal Immunoglobulin and γ Heavy Chain Disease

Biclonal gammopathy has been reported in approximately 1% to 3% of all patients with serum monoclonal components (Creyssel et al., 1976; Kyle et al., 1981b; Pick et al., 1979). In contrast, the association between γ-HCD and other monoclonal gammopathies occurs at a much higher rate. In a literature review of 56 patients with γ-HCD, 9 patients (16%) had biclonal gammopathy with an intact monoclonal immunoglobulin in the serum and a monoclonal γ heavy chain in the serum or urine (Kyle et al., 1981a). In a series of 23 patients with γ-HCD, 7% were found to have IgM-λ intact monoclonal immunoglobulin (Wahner-Roedler et al., 2003). In a review by Presti (1990), the average age of 13 patients with γ-HCD and an associated monoclonal gammopathy was 56 years, and men predominated 2:1.

The associated monoclonal immunoglobulin has been of the IgM type (Creyssel et al., 1977; Feremans et al., 1979; Fermand et al., 1989; Keller et al., 1970; Ockhuizen et al., 1984; Presti et al., 1990; Roda et al., 1985b; Virella et al., 1977; Wahner-Roedler et al., 2003; Wang et al., 1978) or IgG type (Adlersberg et al., 1978; Fine et al., 1968; Guardia et al., 1976; Kretschmer et al., 1974; Isobe and Osserman, 1974; Lebreton et al., 1967, 1982). No association between γ-HCD and monoclonal IgA has yet been described, although the IgG–IgA association was the most frequent in several series of biclonal gammopathies (Kyle et al., 1981b; van Camp et al., 1978). A higher frequency of λ than κ chain expression was seen (Presti et al., 1990). One patient described by Lebreton et al. (1982) was unique in that the serum contained 2 deleted γ chains of different subclasses (IgG1 and IgG2).

All reported cases except one (Kretschmer et al., 1974) have been associated with a lymphoplasma proliferative process. The median duration of survival in patients with biclonal disease has been reported to be 22 months (Presti et al., 1990). The reason for the relative tendency of γ-HCD to coexist with other unrelated paraproteins remains unclear, although different mechanisms have been proposed (van Camp et al., 1978).

## γ Heavy Chain Deposition Disease

Monoclonal immunoglobulin deposition disease is a well-recognized, pathologically defined entity. Continuous linear deposits of κ or λ immunoglobulin light chains are the immunohistologic hallmark of light chain deposition disease (LCDD). Some cases of monoclonal immunoglobulin deposition disease have deposits of both light and heavy chains (LHCDD) (Buxbaum et al., 1990). In 1992, Tubbs et al. described 2 patients for whom they proposed the term "pseudo-γ-HCDD." Both patients presented with acute renal failure. Results of renal biopsy demonstrated nodular intercapillary glomerulopathy and continuous electron-dense granular deposits associated with a linear pattern of IgG4 heavy-chain deposition in vascular, tubular, and glomerular basement membranes. Light-chain deposits were absent in one patient and very faint and limited to the glomerular basement membrane in the other. The authors thought these immunohistologic findings were best explained by a change in the 3-dimensional conformational structure of the protein after entrapment and binding to the basement membrane, rendering the light chain antigenic sites inaccessible to antibody reagent and thereby undetectable. Therefore, they proposed the designation "pseudo-γ heavy-chain deposition disease." In view of subsequent reports describing kidney deposits containing short heavy chains but no detectable light chains, the cases reported by Tubbs et al. (1992) are now considered examples of γ heavy-chain deposition disease (γ-HCDD) (Aucouturier et al., 1993; Katz et al., 1994). Since then, not more than two dozen documented cases of γ-HCDD have been reported in the literature (Lesavre et al., 2001). They have included the full subgroup spectrum of γ1 (7 patients) (Khamlichi et al., 1995; Lin et al., 2001; Mougenot et al., 1983; Moulin et al., 1999; Yasuda et al., 1995), γ2 (1 patient) (Herzenberg et al., 2000), γ3 (5 patients) (Herzenberg et al., 1996; Husby, 2000; Husby et al., 1998; Kambham et al., 1999; Lin et al., 2001; Rott et al., 1998), and γ4 (5 patients) (Aucouturier et al., 1993; Katz et al., 1994; Lin et al., 2001; Tubbs et al., 1992). In several other cases, the subtypes were not determined (Bridoux et al., 2001; Chiara et al., 2000; Imai, 2001; Lin et al., 2001; Polski et al., 1999; Strom et al., 1994).

In all cases of γ-HCDD in which the constant domains have been studied, the common feature is $C_{H^1}$ deletion (patient Ric, Fig. 22-1) (Khamlichi et al., 1995). In addition to the $C_{H^1}$ deletion, absence of the hinge and $C_{H^2}$ domain have been reported in another patient (patient Thr, Fig. 22-1) (Khamlichi et al., 1995). The γ3 heavy chain from a patient with articular γ-HCDD was documented to start at the normal γ3 hinge region (Danevad et al., 2000), similar to the findings for HCD protein γ3 Omm. The most common clinical findings in γ-HCDD are nephrotic syndrome, hypertension, microhematuria, renal failure, and, in some cases, hypocomplementemia. A positive hepatitis C virus (HCV) antibody test with HCV undetectable by polymerase chain reaction has been reported in some patients with γ-HCDD (Lin et al., 2001). Renal insufficiency is usually present at the time of diagnosis. Besides important renal involvement, there may be heavy-chain deposits in other organs such as skin and skeletal muscle, as described by Rott et al. (1998) in 1 patient, and in synovial tissue, as described by Husby et al. (1998, 2000) in a patient with seronegative rheumatoid arthritis. The characteristic lesion on renal biopsy is nodular sclerosing glomerulopathy, sometimes with crescents. Immunofluorescence and electron microscopy show heavy-chain deposition in the mesangium and basement membranes of glomeruli, tubules, and blood vessels. Except for the composition of the deposits detected by immunofluorescence, the renal biopsy findings are otherwise indistinguishable from those of LCDD and LHCDD. In contrast to LCDD, in γ-HCDD, nodular glomerulosclerosis is a constant feature, hypertension and microhematuria are more frequent, and the hematologic disorder is generally mild. In most cases of γ-HCDD, a monoclonal protein can be documented in the serum, urine, or bone marrow biopsy specimen, although its demonstration might require special studies. Often, the monoclonal proteins are detected in only minute quantities in serum or urine, probably in large part because the heavy chains have avid tissue-binding properties.

There is no consensus on treatment of γ-HCDD, and in most cases the renal outcome is poor (Kambham et al., 1999). For γ-HCDD associated with myeloma, which has been reported in 4 patients (Aucouturier et al., 1993; Kambham et al., 1999; Moulin et al., 1999), Moulin et al. suggested that conventional chemotherapy should be used in patients older than 60 years but that intensive therapy with blood stem-cell autografting should be considered in younger patients. Treatment of nonmyeloma patients should be modulated according to clinical presentation. Five patients with γ-HCDD without associated multiple myeloma reported by Lin et al. (2001) received melphalan and prednisone (1 patient), pulse dexamethasone (1 patient), prednisone plus chlorambucil (1 patient), or no treatment (2 patients). Follow-up data showed that 2 patients had stable serum creatinine (over 5 mo each) and 3 had either end-stage renal disease or a requirement for immediate dialysis. One patient received a renal transplant from a living related donor and was doing well 8 months posttransplantation without recurrence of proteinuria. In a patient reported by Herzenberg et al. (2000), a renal transplant resulted in recurrent γ-HCDD in the transplant.

### Heavy Chain-Associated Amyloidosis

Two heavy chain-associated amyloid proteins have been described. Protein γ1 Art (Eulitz et al., 1990) lacks the $C_{H^1}$, hinge, and $C_{H^2}$ domains. Amyloid protein Mad has a virtually intact $V_H$ region plus a D segment but lacks the $J_H$ segment and the entire $C_H$ region (Fig. 22-1) (Solomon et al., 1994). These reports are compatible with the hypothesis that constant domain deletion in heavy chains might be responsible for free heavy chain secretion, whereas variable-domain conformational singularities rather than gross structural alterations might promote either HCDD or heavy chain-associated amyloidosis (Khamlichi et al., 1995; Preud'homme et al., 1994a, 1994b).

# α-Heavy Chain Disease

Since the first description by Seligmann et al. in 1968, more than 400 cases of α-HCD have been described in the literature (Seligmann, 1993). The disease is defined as a lymphoid proliferation involving the IgA secretory system and producing a homogeneous population of Ig molecules consisting of incomplete α chains devoid of light chains. The initial, benign-appearing, antibiotic-responsive immunoproliferative lesions often evolve to fatal, highly malignant lymphoma. α-HCD might be considered as a model showing the complex interactions of the environment with genetic factors and the complex infection-immunity-cancer interrelationships originating from the same proliferating clone.

### Epidemiology and Etiology

Most reported cases of α-HCD have originated from the Mediterranean area or the Middle East. However, the disease is not restricted to a specific ethnic group. Numerous cases have been reported in inhabitants of Eastern Europe, the Indian subcontinent, the Far East, Central, North, and South America, and sub-Saharan Africa. In developed countries, α-HCD often occurs among immigrants from developing countries and underprivileged native populations (Arista-Nasr et al., 1994). The incidence is slightly greater in men than in women and is highest in the third decade of life. Nevertheless, α-HCD has been reported in children (Altuntas and Ensari, 2000; Bowie and Hill, 1988; Faux et al., 1973; Joller et al., 1984; Savilahti et al., 1980; Stoop et al., 1971) and in the seventh decade of life (Geraci et al., 1985). A common denominator of these patients is poor socioeconomic status and hygiene resulting in repeated acute infectious diarrhea and chronic parasitic infestation. Geophagia since early infancy was almost always found in subjects at risk in Tunisia (Rambaud et al., 1990).

The cause of α-HCD is unknown. Current clinical, histologic, molecular, and immunologic data indicate that the evolutionary cause of α-HCD is a complex, multistep process. The peculiar epidemiologic features suggest strongly that environmental factors operating from early infancy could play a major role in the pathogenesis of the disease. No specific microorganism has been found (Harzic et al., 1985). Bacterial lipopolysaccharides, dietary lectins (Rambaud and Matuchansky, 1973; Ramot and Rechavi, 1992; Seligmann and Rambaud, 1978), enterotoxins of *Vibrio* cholera (Al-Saleem, 1978), oncogenic viruses (Arista-Nasr et al., 1993; Seligmann and Rambaud, 1978), and asbestosis (Rouhier et al., 1982) have been suspected of providing antigenic stimulation triggering the histoimmunopathologic changes. Although the Epstein-Barr virus, which has been associated with B cell lymphoproliferative disorders, was documented to play no role in the induction of B cell proliferation in immunoproliferative small intestine disease (IPSID) in 8 patients (Baddoura et al., 1994), ultrastructural studies of a lymph node of a patient with α-HCD described by Arista-Nasr et al. (1993) revealed viruses that resembled the Epstein-Barr virus.

A report of spontaneous remission of α-HCD after departure from an endemic area (Sala et al., 1983) and a decline in the incidence rate of IPSID-associated primary small intestine lymphoma among Jews born in Israel compared with Jewish immigrants with a relatively low socioeconomic standard from North Africa and Asia (Selzer et al., 1979) support the influence of environmental factors. The postulated environmental antigenic stimulation might be associated with an underlying immunodeficiency. An increase of circulating B lymphocytes, a decrease of T lymphocytes, and a decrease in cellular immunity have been found in patients and first-degree relatives of patients with α-HCD (Al-Mondhiry, 1986; Alsabti, 1978; Alsabti et al., 1979; Kharazmi et al., 1978). A genetic element is suggested by the finding that patients with α-HCD have a greater association of the HLA-AW19 and HLA-B12 antigen than normal blood donors or patients with malabsorption (Nikbin et al., 1979). However, familial α-HCD has not been recognized.

## Clinical Features

α-HCD most commonly manifests in the "digestive form." Diarrhea, steatorrhea, weight loss, abdominal pain, and vomiting are the most common presenting symptoms (Rambaud and Seligmann, 1976). Chronic small bowel obstruction or abdominal surgical emergencies may sometimes reveal the disease (Comelli and Paris, 1990), and abdominal masses may be present. However, these "tumoral" signs are more often observed in the late stages of α-HCD (Rambaud et al., 1978). Ascites, tetany, or edema might be present; clubbing of the fingers and retardation of physical growth and secondary sexual characteristics might occur (Tabbane et al., 1976). Hepatosplenomegaly and peripheral lymphadenopathy are uncommon findings (Al-Bahrani et al., 1978).

α-HCD may be confined to the respiratory tract, but this "respiratory form" is rare. Stoop et al. (1971) described an 8-year-old girl with pulmonary infiltrates, hilar adenopathy, skull lesions, and a pharyngeal tumor. Another patient presented with dyspnea and had diffuse interstitial pulmonary fibrosis, pleural effusion, and mediastinal nodes (Florin-Christensen et al., 1974). A 3-year-old boy who had recurrent respiratory infections was found to have hypogammaglobulinemia and an α-heavy chain fragment (Faux et al., 1973).

Three cases of "lymphoma form" α-HCD have been described in Japan (Itoh et al., 1991; Furuta et al., 1982, as cited in Takahashi et al., 1988; Takahashi et al., 1988; Tezuka et al., 1986). A striking clinical feature in 2 of these cases was long-standing and recurring skin eruptions that developed 2 years before the occurrence of lymph node swelling. The third patient had a history of rheumatoid arthritis and had marked cervical and inguinal lymphadenopathy. α-Heavy chain was identified in serum and urine. The site of α-chain synthesis was the cytoplasm of infiltrating malignant cells in the lymph nodes. The gastrointestinal and the respiratory tract were not involved in these patients. α-HCD has been reported in a patient with goiter from a plasmacytoma of the thyroid (Tracy et al., 1984b) and in a patient with amyloidosis (Sakka et al., 1986). Lymphomatous infiltration of duodenum, jejunum, nasopharynx, and bone marrow was described in a Mauritanian man with α-HCD (Lucidarme et al., 1993).

## Protein Findings

The characteristic sharp spike of a monoclonal gammopathy is not detected on serum protein electrophoresis in α-HCD. In approximately half of cases, an abnormal broad band is seen in the $α_2$- or β-globulin region. This broad band is probably the result of the propensity of α-heavy chains to form polymers (Seligmann, 1975). In the other half of cases, serum protein electrophoresis shows no evidence of an abnormal protein. In most patients, the α-HCD protein can be found in the serum, but its concentration is often low (Seligmann and Rambaud, 1978). The concentration of α-HCD protein in the urine is low, and Bence Jones proteinuria has never been found. In most patients studied, when the α-HCD protein was documented in the serum it was also found in the jejunal fluid (Rambaud et al., 1990; Rambaud and Halphen, 1989). Interestingly, however, in 2 cases the α-HCD protein was found in the intestinal or gastric lumen but was undetectable in the serum and urine despite the use of the most sensitive techniques (Coulbois et al., 1986; Rambaud et al., 1983). Whether α-HCD protein in the jejunal fluid is or is not linked to the secretory component has been disputed (Brandtzaeg and Savilahti, 1978; Doe et al., 1972; Hibi et al., 1982; Joller et al., 1984; Savilahti et al., 1980; Seligmann et al., 1969). A possible mechanism explaining such a link was described by Lucidarme et al. (1993).

## Structural Protein Abnormalities

In all cases studied so far, the α-HCD protein belonged to the $α_1$ subclass. Most α-HCD proteins consist of multiple polymers. The monomeric unit has a molecular weight ranging from 29,000 to 34,000, and its length varies from one-half to three-fourths that of a normal α chain. The shortening results from an internal deletion involving most of the $V_H$ and first constant domains.

Sequence data are available for several α-HCD proteins: Def (Wolfenstein-Todel et al., 1974), Ait (Wolfenstein-Todel et al., 1975), Mal (Tsapis et al., 1989), and Yao (Bentaboulet et al., 1989). In all instances, the normal sequence of the $α_1$ chain constant region resumes at the hinge (Fig. 22-3). Studies by Wolfenstein-Todel et al. (1974, 1975) indicate that synthesis of protein Def and protein Ait as internally deleted α chains is followed by postsynthetic amino terminal proteolysis. α-HCD proteins Mal and Yao are devoid of $V_H$ and $C_{H1}$ domains. In a study of the nucleotide sequence of mRNA Mal (Tsapis et al., 1989) and Yao (Bentaboulet et al., 1989) and the nucleotide sequence of α mRNA for 6 other cases of α-HCD (Ben, Arf, Mec, Lte, Har, Ayo) (Fakhfakh et al., 1992), all 8 mRNAs lacked the $V_H$ and $C_{H1}$ sequences (Fig. 22-4). They contained inframe inserts of unknown origin between the leader peptide and the normal $C_{H2}$ and $C_{H3}$ coding sequences. These inserts had variable lengths and were unrelated; thus, it is unlikely that they originated from an infectious agent.

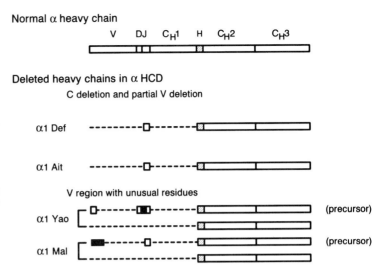

**Figure 22-3** *Structure of α heavy chain disease (HCD) proteins compared with that of normal chain. Hatched bars correspond to hinge regions, closed bars indicate unusual sequences, and dotted lines indicate deletions. V, variable region; D, diversity; J, joining; C_H, constant region; H, hinge region. α1 Def (Wolfenstein-Todel et al., 1974), α1 Ait (Wolfenstein-Todel et al., 1975), α1 Yao (Bentaboulet et al., 1989), and α1 Mal (Tsapis et al., 1989). (Modified from Cogné, M., Preud'homme, J. L., and Guglielmi, P. [1989]. Immunoglobulin gene alterations in human heavy chain disease. Research in Immunology, 140, 487–502; Cogné et al. [1992]. By permission of The American Society of Hematology and Elsevier Science Publishers.)*

The presence of inserted sequences of unknown origin appears to be a common feature of an α-HCD productive mRNA. Because the amino acid sequence of α-HCD proteins begins with the C_H2 domain, the amino terminal sequence encoded by these inserts most probably is cleaved intracellularly before secretion. Two molecular species of α-HCD protein Ben have been described: one starting at the beginning of the hinge region and another shorter one missing the 2 first amino acids of the hinge region. Intracellular cleavage or limited postsecretion proteolysis might explain these findings (Fakhfakh et al., 1993).

Molecular biologic studies also indicate that genomic abnormalities such as multiple deletion/insertion processes, mutations, or duplications that are focused in the V_H – J_H and C_H1 regions are at least partly responsible for the production of α-HCD proteins (Goossens et al., 1998; Klein et al., 1998). These proteins are monoclonal even in the early stage of the disease (Fakhfakh et al., 1991). By studying a murine cell line model of α-HCD, Chou and Morrison (1993) showed that the failure of light-chain synthesis resulted from a disruption in the normal splicing pattern caused by the insertion of a 358-nucleotide non-Ig sequence into the intron separating the leader exon from Vκ.

## Hematologic and Metabolic Abnormalities

Anemia is usually mild or moderate and of variable type, with low iron, folate, or vitamin B_{12} serum levels. The serum albumin level is nearly always low. Electrolyte imbalance, especially hypokalemia, is frequent. Hypocalcemia and hypomagnesemia are also common. The frequent high level of serum alkaline phosphatase

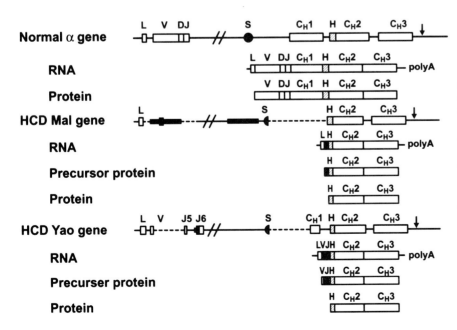

**Figure 22-4** *Structure of α heavy chain disease (HCD) productive gene, RNA transcript, and protein compared with their normal rearranged counterpart. S, switch region; V, variable region; L, leader; H, hinge; CH, constant region; D, diversity; J, joining. Solid bars represent insertions in coding (large bar) or noncoding (small bar) regions; dashed lines indicate deletion. (From Fermand, J. P., and Brouet, J. C. [1999]. Heavy-chain diseases. Hematological Oncology Clinic of North America, 13, 1281–1294. By permission of WB Saunders Company.)*

is usually explained by the increase in the intestinal isoenzyme fraction (Doe et al., 1972). Serum lipid levels are low even if steatorrhea is mild. The Schilling test with intrinsic factor yields low values in two-thirds of cases. The D-xylose test almost always shows abnormal results. Fecal fat (24-h values) ranged from 6 g to 15 g in 43% and was more than 15 g in 52% of patients studied (Rambaud and Seligmann, 1976).

## Radiographic Abnormalities

Radiographs of the small intestine show hypertrophic and pseudopolypoid mucosal folds in the duodenum and jejunum, sometimes associated with strictures or filling defects suggesting extrinsic compression by hypertrophic peripancreatic or mesenteric lymph nodes (Rambaud and Seligmann, 1976). Double-contrast studies are helpful in evaluating IPSID (Matsumoto et al., 1990).

## Endoscopic Abnormalities

α-HCD intestinal lesions nearly always affect the duodenum and the jejunum. Five primary endoscopic patterns have been defined, occurring alone or in various combinations. The infiltrated pattern is the most common and specific finding, followed by the nodular pattern. Other primary lesions (ulcerations, mosaic pattern, and mucosal fold thickening alone) are nonspecific (Halphen et al., 1986).

## Cytogenetic Abnormalities

Cytogenetic abnormalities have been found in the lymphoid cells of patients with α-HCD. Berger et al. (1986) reported abnormal karyotypes in 3 of 4 patients. In 2 instances, a rearrangement of 14q32 resulting from a t(9;14)(p11;q32) and a t(2;14)(p12;q32) translocation was observed. Cloning and sequencing of the der breakpoint of a chromosome translocation involving the 14q32 Ig locus revealed that the translocation originated from a local pairing of 2 chromosomes, 9 and 14 (Pellet et al., 1989, 1990). One case showed complex rearrangements, including t(5;9). An abnormal chromosome marker (D14q+) has been reported in the marrow of a patient with α-HCD (Gafter et al., 1980).

## Pathology

In its digestive form, α-HCD manifests as IPSID. This condition is a subtype of mucosa-associated lymphoid tissue lymphoma (Ben Rejeb et al., 1991; Isaacson, 1994; Isaacson et al., 1989; Isaacson and Spencer, 1987; Papadaki et al., 1995; Spencer and Isaacson, 1987). The pathologic features usually extend throughout the small bowel. Three histopathologic

stages have been described (Galian et al., 1977). In stage A, a mature plasmacytic or lymphoplasmacytic infiltration of the mucosal lamina propria is noted. Stage B is characterized by the presence of atypical plasmacytic or lymphoplasmacytic cells and more or less atypical immunoblast-like cells extending at least to the submucosa. Subtotal or total villous atrophy is present. Stage C corresponds to an immunoblastic lymphoma, either forming discrete ulcerated tumors or extensively infiltrating long segments involving the entire intestinal wall (Galian et al., 1977; Khojasteh et al., 1983a). Involvement of the liver, spleen, and peripheral lymph nodes is uncommon.

The histologic lesions may progress at any given site from stage A to stage B or from stage B to stage C. However, it should be kept in mind that different stages can be found at the same time in different organs or even at different sites of the same organ. This asynchronism must be kept in mind for staging.

In a few cases, intestinal lesions spare the duodenum and even the jejunum or are limited to a segment of the latter (Galian et al., 1983; Rambaud et al., 1990). Spread of the disease outside the enteromesenteric area is common, even when intestinal lesions are stage A. Often, gastric and colorectal mucosae, which belong to the IgA secretory system, are involved (Rambaud et al., 1983; Rhodes et al., 1980). α-HCD confined to the stomach (Coulbois et al., 1986; Guardia et al., 1980; Tungekar et al., 1987) or presenting as a colonic mass (Cho et al., 1982) has been reported.

The major lymphoma cell type in patients with α-HCD is immunoblastic lymphoma with various degrees of plasmacytoid differentiation (Rambaud et al., 1990). A patient with α-HCD associated with multiple polypoid lymphocytic lymphoma and leukemic manifestations without evidence of bone marrow involvement has been described. Cytogenetic analysis showed the same abnormal karyotypes of neoplastic clones in the intestinal tumor cells as in the circulating leukemic cells (Chang et al., 1992).

There has been some confusion in regard to the terminology of "Mediterranean" lymphoma. In 1976, the World Health Organization suggested the term *immunoproliferative small intestinal disease* (IPSID) (Alpha-chain disease, 1976). This term should be restricted to small intestine lesions whose pathologic features are identical to those of α-HCD at any of its histologic stages irrespective of the type of Ig synthesized by the proliferating cells (Fine and Stone, 1999; Isaacson, 1994; Papadaki et al., 1995). Because previously used methods to detect the protein were not very sensitive, data regarding the presence of the abnormal protein vary (Khojasteh and Haghighi, 1990). In the experience of Rambaud et al. (1990), among 19 consecutive patients with the epidemiologic, clinical, and pathologic features of IPSID, 16 had α-HCD protein in their serum and one had it in the jejunal fluid only. In one case, immunofluorescence study of the small bowel mucosa showed that most of the infiltrating cells were positive for α chains and negative for other heavy or light chains (nonsecretory) (Rambaud et al., 1983). The 19th patient showed a massive infiltration of the small intestine by polyclonal plasma cells (Colombel et al., 1988).

In a few patients with the typical clinical and pathologic features of α-HCD, another monoclonal Ig (γ-HCD protein) (Bender et al., 1978), a complete monoclonal IgA (Chantar et al., 1974; Marquez et al., 1993; Rodriguez Gomez et al., 1994; Tangun et al., 1975), or a polyclonal expression of IgA was found (Colombel et al., 1988; Pohl et al., 1991).

A few cases with the respiratory form of α-HCD have been reported. The pathologic changes in these cases are poorly documented. In a case of lymph node form or lymphoma form, lymph node biopsy showed diffuse plasmacytic lymphoma (Takahashi et al., 1988).

In a patient with a history of IPSID, histologic assessment of persistent ulcerated lesions on her gingiva revealed several features in common with the intestinal lesions of IPSID. There was no mention of the presence of an α-HCD protein (Bartold and Henning, 1990).

## Diagnosis

Because α-HCD in its intestinal form nearly always affects the duodenum and the jejunum, endoscopy has been advocated as the first diagnostic procedure in the investigation of patients clinically suspected of having α-HCD. Enteric presentation of γ-HCD (Bender et al., 1978), monoclonal IgA secretion with a complete molecule (Chantar et al., 1974; Marquez et al., 1993; Rodriguez Gomez et al., 1994; Tangun et al., 1975), variable immunodeficiency (Neudorf et al., 1983), and acquired immunodeficiency syndrome (Ullrich et al., 1989) with clinicopathologic features simulating IPSID must be excluded.

The diagnosis of α-HCD depends on the identification of free α-heavy chains. Several methods might be used to document α-HCD protein in biologic fluids (Doe et al., 1979). A modified immunoselection technique described by Sun et al. (1994) appears to be simple, convenient, and specific.

The quantity of abnormal α chains in the sera seems to be related to the nature (plasma cell type or immunoblastic type) of cells predominantly present in the intestinal mucosa or the mesenteric lymph nodes. α-HCD protein hyposecretion might be found early as well as during the terminal evolutionary stage of the disease (Rabhi et al., 1988, 1989b).

When α-HCD is suspected but the α-HCD protein cannot be documented in the serum or intestinal fluid, immunohistochemical or immunocytochemical studies

might be helpful. In these nonsecreting forms, synthesis of the α-HCD protein by proliferating cells has been demonstrated by immunochemical or immunocytochemical methods and by biosynthesis studies in vitro (Buxbaum and Preud'homme, 1972; Cogné and Preud'homme, 1990; Matuchansky et al., 1989; Rambaud et al., 1983; Seligmann et al., 1969; Sopeña et al., 1992; Tashiro et al., 1995; Zahner et al., 1994).

Once the diagnosis of α-HCD has been established, a staging laparotomy should be performed, because the histopathologic lesions are frequently asynchronic (Martin and Aldoori, 1994; Rambaud et al., 1990). Whether improved diagnostic tools such as computed tomography or magnetic resonance imaging will reduce the need for staging laparotomy remains to be seen.

## Course, Prognosis, and Treatment

The course of α-HCD is variable but generally progressive in the absence of therapy. Spontaneous clinical and immunologic remission of α-HCD in an Italian adult with the digestive form of the disease was reported after the patient's departure from Libya (Sala et al., 1983). The abnormal protein disappeared after total thyroidectomy in another patient with α-HCD who presented with a goiter from an extramedullary plasmacytoma (Tracy et al., 1984b).

Treatment depends on knowledge of the extension and histologic stage of the disease. Present therapeutic guidelines are as follows. Patients with stage A lesions limited to the bowel and to mesenteric lymph nodes should be treated initially with oral antibiotics (either metronidazole and ampicillin or tetracycline). Any documented parasite should be eradicated. Eradication of Helicobacter pylori has led to complete remission in 2 patients with α-HCD (Fischbach et al., 1997; Zamir et al., 1998), one of whom was unresponsive to prior combination chemotherapy (Fischbach et al., 1997). A minimum 6-month trial of tetracycline (1–2 g per day) is the prerequisite for establishing responsiveness. El Sagir (1995) recommends giving tetracycline for 2 years. Of interest is the finding of a persistently abnormal α chain mRNA, despite an apparently complete clinical, pathologic, and immunopathologic remission after tetracycline therapy in one patient. Consistent with this finding was the subsequent rapid recurrence of α-HCD with transformation to immunoblastic lymphoma (Matuchansky et al., 1989).

In patients with stage B or C disease, antiparasitic and antibiotic treatments are often useful in improving the malabsorption syndrome. Patients with stage B or C lesions, or stage A lesions without marked improvement after a 6-month course of antibiotic treatment, should be given chemotherapy. In a prospective, randomized study, a doxorubicin-based regimen (CHOP: cyclophosphamide, doxorubicin hydrochloride, vincristine, and prednisone) provided a higher response rate than a non-doxorubicin-containing protocol (C-MOPP: cyclophosphamide, vincristine, procarbazine, prednisone) or total abdominal radiation (Khojasteh et al., 1983b). Similar results were noted in a retrospective study by Salimi and Spinelli (1996). Encouraging results have been obtained in a treatment trial of cyclophosphamide, doxorubicin, teniposide, and prednisone with or without alternation with bleomycin, vinblastine, and doxorubicin (Ben-Ayed et al., 1989).

Chemotherapy with CEOP-IMVP-Dexa (cyclophosphamide, epidoxorubicin, vincristine, prednisolone, ifosfamide, VP-16, dexamethasone, methotrexate) resulted in a complete remission in a patient with α-HCD associated with a high-grade malignant non-Hodgkin lymphoma (Hubmann et al., 1995).

Immunotherapy with rituximab, an anti-CD20 monoclonal antibody, has been a major advance in the treatment of indolent non-Hodgkin lymphoma (McLaughlin et al., 1998). Because α-HCD is a disease of the B cells, it is likely that rituximab might be of benefit as a single agent or combined with chemotherapy in patients whose neoplastic cells express CD20. However, there have been no reports to date of rituximab use in patients with α-HCD.

When a focal or bulky transmural lymphomatous tumor is found during staging laparotomy, surgical resection of the bowel segment bearing the tumor may be used to debulk or prevent perforation or obstruction (Khojasteh and Haghighi, 1990; Tabbane et al., 1988). This approach, followed by combination chemotherapy, may induce complete remission (Rambaud et al., 1990). Because most patients are young, those with disseminated stage C disease showing a good response to conventional or salvage chemotherapy could be candidates for autologous bone marrow transplantation (Perrot et al., 1988).

It is difficult to evaluate the optimal treatment on the basis of the literature, partly because of the small number of cases in any one study, but mainly because of the poor long-term followup in most series. Because of the rarity of the disease, precise therapeutic protocols performed as multicenter studies are needed.

In a prospective study (Ben-Ayed et al., 1989), 20 of 21 Tunisian patients with α-HCD underwent laparotomy. Staging was done according to the histopathologic staging system of Galian et al. (1977). Six patients were classified as having stage A, 2 as stage B, and 13 as stage C. Survival of the total group was 90% at 2 years and 67% at 3 years. Akbulut et al. (1997) reported 5-year treatment results of 23 Turkish patients with IPSID, including 5 with the secretory type. Seven patients had stage A disease and were treated with tetracycline for a median of 7 months, whereas the remaining 16 patients (9 stage B, 7 stage C) received combination chemotherapy (cyclophosphamide, vincristine, procarbazine, and prednisolone [COPP]). The

median followup was 68 months. In patients with stage A disease, tetracycline yielded a complete response in 71% and a disease-free survival rate of 43%. Eleven of the 16 patients (69%) with stage B or C disease who received the COPP regimen achieved a complete response, and only 2 patients had a recurrence (disease-free survival rate of 56%). The 5-year overall survival rate for the entire group was 70%, and the 5-year disease-free survival rate for patients with a complete response was 75%. However, the median overall survival rate for 3 patients with immunoblastic lymphoma was only 7 months.

Price (1990) studied 13 patients who had IPSID associated with α-HCD. Of 3 patients with high-grade lymphoma at presentation, 1 died untreated at 2 months, and 2 were alive at 34 and 91 months. Of 10 patients with low-grade disease, 2 died, one at 76 months and the other after transformation to high-grade lymphoma at 73 months. The 8 other patients were alive at an average of 67 months after presentation. Abdominal irradiation was thought to be useful in several of these cases.

Shih et al. (1994) reported 6 patients who had α-HCD with lymphoma. All patients responded poorly to chemotherapy; the median duration of survival was 10.5 months. Malik et al. (1995) studied 12 patients with IPSID. Six presented with stage A disease. Four of the 6 responded to antibiotics or steroids. In 2 patients, stage A disease evolved into stage C, 1 patient was lost to followup, and 1 patient is alive with disease. Three patients presented with stage B disease. Two responded completely to chemotherapy; the third refused treatment and died after 16 months. Three patients with stage C disease at diagnosis received aggressive combination chemotherapy and remain in complete remission after a median followup of 2.2 years.

Preliminary results suggest that flow cytometric analysis of S-phase fraction may be useful as a prognostic indicator and in the clinical management of patients with IPSID (Demirer et al., 1995). Followup should include a periodic search for α-heavy chain protein, bowel radiography, and esophagogastroduodenojejunal endoscopy in which multilevel biopsy specimens are obtained and studied by immunohistochemical techniques. A second-look laparotomy may be necessary for accurate evaluation (Rambaud et al., 1990). Relapses, sometimes after a long disease-free interval, may occur after treatment at any stage of the disease.

Because antibiotic therapy in the early stage of intestinal α-HCD can result in full clinical remission, awareness of the incidence and increased efforts to detect the disease before the lymphomatous phase are of importance (De Franco et al., 1991; Fernandes et al., 1994; Nair et al., 1998; Pramoolsinsap et al., 1993; Smith et al., 1987). The development of abdominal lymphadenopathy and thickening of the small intestine wall can be monitored by sequential ultrasound examinations (Kaufmann et al., 1994). The disease may well be eradicated without any medical intervention by improving the socioeconomic status of the underprivileged population in underdeveloped countries.

## α-Heavy Chain Deposition Disease

Three patients with α-HCDD have been reported in the literature. Cheng et al. (1996) described a patient who presented with many of the clinicopathologic features common to patients with γ-HCDD, namely, hypertension, progressive renal failure, and nephrotic syndrome with a renal biopsy showing crescentic nodular glomerulosclerosis and refractile granular electron dense deposits in the glomerular and tubular basement membranes. The immune deposits stained for α Ig heavy chain only but not for γ and μ Ig heavy chains and light chains and not with anti-α 1 and anti-α 2 subclass-specific reagents. On the basis of these findings, the authors hypothesized that the abnormally short α Ig heavy chain may arise from a genetic mutation that deletes the genomic sequences that encode the $C_{H^1}$ and $C_{H^2}$ domains, similar to the findings in patients with γ-HCDD. Lin et al. (2001) described a patient with α-HCDD who met the criteria for multiple myeloma. The third case, reported by Chauveau et al. (2000), presented with renal and skin deposits of a $C_{H^1}$ deleted α-1 heavy chain.

# μ-Heavy Chain Disease

μ-HCD is rare. Since the first report in 1970 (Ballard et al., 1970; Forte et al., 1970), only 32 additional cases have been reported in the world literature (Bedu-Addo et al., 2000; Campbell and Juneja, 2000; Cogné et al., 1993; Iwasaki et al., 1997; Wahner-Roedler and Kyle, 1992; Witzens et al., 1998).

## Clinical Features

Most patients with μ-HCD are older than 40 years. The median age at the time of diagnosis in 27 patients with μ-HCD was 57.5 years (range, 15–80 y) (Wahner-Roedler and Kyle, 1992). Of the 33 reported patients, 18 were men; 26 were white, 4 were black (Bedu-Addeo et al., 2000; Bonhomme et al., 1974; Danon et al., 1975; O'Reilly et al., 1981), 2 were Asian (Fujii et al., 1982; Iwasaki et al., 1997), and 1 was of unknown ethnic origin (Campbell and Juneja, 2000). An associated lymphoplasma cell proliferative disorder (chronic lymphocytic leukemia, lymphoma, Waldenström disease, or myeloma) was noted at some time during the disease in 22 of 27 patients (Wahner-Roedler and Kyle, 1992). μ-HCD protein has also been described in one patient each with systemic lupus erythematosus (Leach et al., 1987), hepatic cirrhosis (Danon et al., 1975),

hepatosplenomegaly with ascites (O'Reilly et al., 1981), pulmonary infection (Biserte et al., 1973), splenomegaly with pancytopenia (Bonhomme et al., 1974), and myelodysplasia (Witzens et al., 1998). Although most patients with μ HCD have an associated lymphoproliferative disorder, μ-chain secretion is a rare feature of chronic lymphocytic leukemia. Bonhomme et al. (1974) were unable to detect any cases when they screened more than 150 patients with chronic lymphocytic leukemia for this abnormality.

Splenomegaly and hepatomegaly are common in μ-HCD and were noted in 21 of 22 and 15 of 21 patients, respectively. Peripheral lymphadenopathy is less frequent and was described in 10 of 25 patients (Wahner-Roedler and Kyle, 1992). In one patient, massive pelvic lymphadenopathy resulted in bilateral hydronephrosis (Campbell and Juneja, 2000).

## Protein Findings

A monoclonal spike on routine serum protein electrophoresis was found in less than half of a series of patients with μ-HCD (8 of 19) (Wahner-Roedler and Kyle, 1992). Three of 33 reported patients had a biclonal gammopathy: IgA κ and μ (Josephson et al., 1973), IgG and μ (Silva-Moreno et al., 1983), and IgG κ and μ (Leach et al., 1987). Hypogammaglobulinemia was noted in 10 of 22 patients. Hyperimmunoglobulinemia with a polyclonal immunoglobulin expansion in the γ-globulin fraction was described in one case (Witzens et al., 1998). Fourteen of 22 patients had Bence Jones proteinuria: 11 excreted a κ chain, 2 excreted a λ chain, and in 1 patient the type of light chain was not reported (Wahner-Roedler and Kyle, 1992). μ-HCD protein was found in the urine of only 2 patients (Bonhomme et al., 1974; O'Reilly et al., 1981).

Bence Jones proteinuria may lead to the occurrence of cast nephropathy. Preud'homme et al. (1997) described a patient with μ-HCD in whom renal failure developed after a 3-year followup. Kidney biopsy showed numerous tubular eosinophilic casts that stained for κ chain determinants by immunofluorescence. Hence, this report paradoxically puts μ-HCD in the list of immunoproliferative disorders with light chain-related visceral complications.

## Structural Protein Abnormalities

The molecular weight of the μ-HCD protein determined in 8 patients varied between 26,500 and 158,000 (Bakhshi et al., 1986a; Ballard et al., 1970; Bonhomme et al., 1974; Dammacco et al., 1974; Danon et al., 1975; Forte et al., 1969, 1970; Fujii et al., 1982; Pruzanski et al., 1978; Wetter et al., 1979). The higher molecular weights are thought to be the result of polymerization of the μ-chain fragments. The μ-heavy chain fragments from 6 patients were subjected to detailed chemical

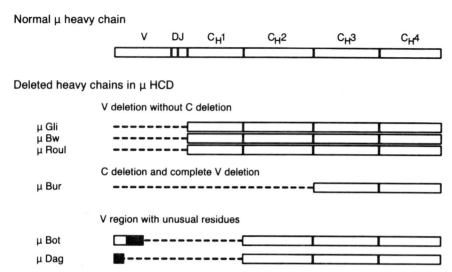

**Figure 22-5** *Structure of 6 μ heavy chain disease (HCD) proteins compared with that of normal μ chain. Closed bars indicate unusual sequences; dotted lines indicate deletions. V, variable region; D, diversity; J, joining; $C_H$, constant region. Gli (Franklin et al., 1976), Bw (Bakhshi et al., 1986b), Roul (Cogné et al., 1993), Bur (Lebreton et al., 1975), Bot (Mihaesco et al., 1980; Barnikol-Watanabe et al., 1984), and Dag (Mihaesco et al., 1990). (Modified from Cogné, M., Preud'homme, J. L., and Guglielmi, P. [1989]. Immunoglobulin gene alterations in human heavy chain disease. Research in Immunology, 140, 487–502; Cogné et al. [1992]. By permission of The American Society of Hematology and Elsevier Science Publishers.)*

analysis (Bakhshi et al., 1986a; Barnikol-Watanabe et al., 1984; Cogné et al., 1993; Franklin et al., 1976; Lebreton et al., 1974, 1975; Mihaesco et al., 1980, 1990; Roussel et al., 1974). Figure 22-5 depicts the structure of these 6 μ-HCD proteins compared with that of the normal μ heavy chain. The $V_H$ domain is absent in all cases. The normal sequence begins with $C_{H^1}$ in 3 cases, $C_{H^2}$ in 2 cases, and $C_{H^3}$ in 1.

In proteins Bot (Barnikol-Watanabe et al., 1984; Mihaesco et al., 1980) and Dag (Mihaesco et al., 1990), the deleted chains start with an aberrant amino acid sequence (extra sequence) displaying no known homology with the protein sequences in the databases currently available. Figure 22-6 depicts the structure of a μ-HCD gene, RNA transcript, and protein compared with the normal rearranged counterpart.

The reasons for the failure to assemble a complete immunoglobulin are not understood. Bakhshi et al. (1986a, 1986b) suggested that a defect at the level of immunoglobulin gene structure or assembly is responsible for the synthesis of the truncated μ-HCD protein Bw by deleting coding information or formation of aberrant RNA.

Studies with transgenic mice by Corcos et al. (1995) suggest that amino terminal truncation of heavy chains could play a role in the genesis of HCD neoplasia; however, it is unlikely that this by itself would be sufficient to produce carcinogenesis.

## Hematologic Abnormalities

Anemia is frequent, but lymphocytosis and thrombocytopenia are rare. Bone marrow lymphocytosis and plasmacytosis are common findings. Plasmacytosis was noted in 18 of 20 cases; in 13 of these, vacuolated plasma cells were found (Wahner-Roedler and Kyle, 1992).

## Radiographic Abnormalities

Lytic bone lesions are rare and were described in 3 of 15 patients (Andreeva et al., 1976; Brouet et al., 1979; Chernokhvostova et al., 1977; Pruzanski et al., 1978), and osteoporosis was mentioned in 3 others (Ballard et al., 1970; Brouet et al., 1979; Dammacco et al., 1974; Forte et al., 1969, 1970).

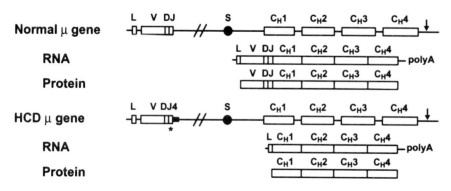

**Figure 22-6** *Structure of μ heavy chain disease (HCD) productive gene, RNA transcript, and protein compared with their normal rearranged counterpart. S, switch region; V, variable region; L, leader; CH, constant region; D, diversity; J, joining. Asterisk indicates altered splice site; solid small bar represents insertion in noncoding region. (From Fermand, J. P., and Brouet, J. C. [1999]. Heavy-chain diseases. Hematological Oncology Clinic of North America, 13, 1281–1294. By permission of WB Saunders Company.)*

## Diagnosis

The diagnosis of μ-HCD requires awareness on the part of the clinician. The finding of Bence Jones proteinuria in a patient with a lymphoproliferative disorder and vacuolated plasma cells in the bone marrow should prompt further investigation to exclude μ-HCD. Once μ-HCD is suspected, immunofixation or immunoelectrophoresis of both serum and urine should be performed. Sometimes these procedures yield ambiguous results; in this situation, 2-dimensional gel electrophoresis is a useful additional tool (Tracy et al., 1984a).

## Clinical Course

The median duration of survival from the time of diagnosis is 24 months (range, less than 1 mo to 11 y) (Wahner-Roedler and Kyle, 1992). In one patient (Wetter et al., 1979), the hematologic data became normal and the μ-heavy chain disappeared after 2 years without any specific treatment. μ-HCD can exist as benign monoclonal gammopathy for years before the development of a malignant lymphoproliferative disorder (Wahner-Roedler and Kyle, 1992).

## Treatment

There is no specific treatment for μ-HCD. Currently, the finding of a μ-HCD protein in the serum of an apparently normal patient should be considered to represent monoclonal gammopathy of undetermined significance, and the patient should be followed closely for the development of a symptomatic lymphoplasma cell proliferative disorder. Once this develops, chemotherapy is given. Initially, a combination of cyclophosphamide, vincristine, and prednisone is a reasonable choice. If there is no response, either doxorubicin or BCNU (carmustine) or both should be added. If the patient presents with a non-lymphoplasma cell proliferative clinical disease, this should be treated according to current standard therapy.

### Nonsecretory μ-Heavy Chain Disease

In 3 cases of nonsecretory μ-HCD, the presenting features were lymphadenopathy and splenomegaly in one (Gordon et al., 1981), osteoporosis and lytic lesions of the spine in one (Guglielmo et al., 1982), and fever and splenomegaly in one (Leglise et al., 1983). μ-Heavy chains were documented by immunofluorescence on the cell surface of proliferative lymphocytes in 1 patient and in bone marrow plasma cells of the 2 others.

### μ-Heavy Chain Deposition Disease

Liapis et al. (2000) described a 68-year-old Greek woman with hypertension, decreased renal clearance, and proteinuria. No abnormal protein was detected in

the patient's serum, and Bence Jones protein was not found in the urine. A renal biopsy performed to evaluate the cause of the proteinuria showed nodular glomerulosclerosis. Monotypic μ-heavy chain mesangial deposits without κ and λ chains were identified by immunofluorescence. No evaluation was done to determine whether the deposited μ-heavy chain was normal or deleted. Two years after the diagnosis, the patient had stable renal disease and had not required dialysis.

# δ-Heavy Chain Disease

One case of possible δ-HCD has been described (Vilpo et al., 1980). This patient presented with renal insufficiency and features of multiple myeloma. However, the possibility that the documented δ heavy chain represented a degradation product from an intact IgD monoclonal protein could not be ruled out. A marked susceptibility of δ chains to cleavage has been demonstrated (Goyert et al., 1977; Rabhi et al., 1989a).

## REFERENCES

Adlersberg, J. B., Grann, V., Zucker-Franklin, D., Frangione, B., and Franklin, E. C. (1978). An unusual case of a plasma cell neoplasm with an IgG3 lambda myeloma and a gamma 3 heavy chain disease protein. *Blood, 51,* 85–96.

Agrawal, S., Abboudi, Z., Matutes, E., and Catovsky, D. (1994). First report of fludarabine in gamma-heavy chain disease. *British Journal of Haematology, 88,* 653–655.

Akbulut, H., Soykan, I., Yakaryilmaz, F., Icii, F., Aksoy, F., Haznedaroglu, S., and Yildirim, S. (1997). Five-year results of the treatment of 23 patients with immunoproliferative small intestinal disease. A Turkish experience. *Cancer, 80,* 8–14.

Al-Bahrani, Z., Al-Saleem, T., Al-Mondhiry, H., Bakir, F., Yahia, H., Taha, I., and King, J. (1978). Alpha heavy chain disease (report of 18 cases from Iraq). *Gut, 19,* 627–631.

Albutt, E. C., Hawker, P. C., Hine, K. R., and Northam, B. E. (1981). Diagnosis of gamma heavy-chain disease. *Ann Clin Biochem, 18,* 207–210.

Alexander, A., Anicito, I., and Buxbaum, J. (1988). Gamma heavy chain disease in man. Genomic sequence reveals two noncontiguous deletions in a single gene. *Journal of Clinical Investigation, 82,* 1244–1252.

Alexander, A., Steinmetz, M., Barritault, D., Frangione, B., Franklin, E. C., Hood, L., and Buxbaum, J. N. (1982). Gamma heavy chain disease in man. cDNA sequence supports partial gene deletion model. *Proceedings of the National Academy of Sciences of the United States of America, 79,* 3260–3264.

Al-Mondhiry, H. (1986). Primary lymphomas of the small intestine. East-west contrast. *American Journal of Hematology, 22,* 89–105.

Alpha-chain disease and related small-intestinal lymphoma. A memorandum. (1976). *Bulletin of the World Health Organization, 54,* 615–624.

Alsabti, E. A. (1978). Paraproteinemia in normal family members of eight cases with primary intestinal lymphomas in Iraq. *Oncology, 35,* 68–72.

Alsabti, E. A., Safo, M. H., and Shaheen, A. (1979). Lymphocytes subpopulation in normal family members of patients with alpha-chain disease. *Journal of Surgical Oncology, 11,* 365–374.

Al-Saleem, T. I. (1978). Evidence of acquired immune deficiencies in Mediterranean lymphoma. A possible aetiological link. *Lancet, 2,* 709–712.

Altuntas, B., and Ensari, A. (2000). Alpha heavy chain disease in a child. *Pediatrics International, 42,* 306–309.

Andreeva, N. E., Antipova, L. G., Chernokhvostova, E. V., and Batalova, T. N. (1976). Disease of heavy chains mu (new forms of paraproteinemic hemoblastoses) [Russian]. *Terapevticheskii arkhiv, 48,* 10–15.

Arista-Nasr, J., Armando, G., and Hernandez-Pando, R. (1993). Immunoproliferative small intestinal disease. Report of a case with immunohistochemical and ultrastructural study [Spanish]. *Revista de investigacion clinica; organo del Hospital de Enfermedades de la Nutricion, 45,* 275–280.

Arista-Nasr, J., Gonzalez-Romo, M. A., Mantilla-Morales, A., Lazos-Ochoa, M., and Ortiz-Hidalgo, C. (1994). Immunoproliferative small intestinal disease in Mexico. Report of four cases and review of the literature. *Journal of Clinical Gastroenterology, 18,* 67–71.

Arnaud, P., Wang, A. C., Gianazza, E., Wang, I. Y., Lasne, Y., Creyssel, R., and Fudenberg, H. H. (1981). Gamma heavy chain disease protein CHA. Immunological and structural studies. *Molecular Immunology, 18,* 379–384.

Aucouturier, P., Khamlichi, A. A., Touchard, G., Justrabo, E., Cogné, M., Chauffert, B., Martin, F., and Preud'homme, J. L. (1993). Brief report. Heavy-chain deposition disease. *New England Journal of Medicine, 329,* 1389–1393.

Baddoura, F. K., Unger, E. R., Mufarrij, A., Nassar, V. H., and Zaki, S. R. (1994). Latent Epstein-Barr virus infection is an unlikely event in the pathogenesis of immunoproliferative small intestinal disease. *Cancer, 74,* 1699–1705.

Baker, A. S., Lankford, P., Krantz, S. B., and Buchanan, R. D. (1977). Gamma heavy chain disease—presenting as pancytopenia and splenomegaly. *Southern Medical Journal, 70,* 495–497.

Bakhshi, A., Guglielmi, P., Coligan, J. E., Gamza, F., Waldmann, T. A., and Korsmeyer, S. J. (1986a). A pre-translational defect in a case of human mu heavy chain disease. *Molecular Immunology, 23,* 725–732.

Bakhshi, A., Guglielmi, P., Siebenlist, U., Ravetch, J. V., Jensen, J. P., and Korsmeyer, S. J. (1986b). A DNA insertion/deletion necessitates an aberrant RNA splice accounting for a mu heavy chain disease protein. *Proceedings of the National Academy of Sciences of the United States of America, 83,* 2689–2693.

Ballard, H. S., Hamilton, L. M., Marcus, A. J., and Illes, C. H. (1970). A new variant of heavy-chain disease (mu-chain disease). *New England Journal of Medicine, 282,* 1060–1062.

Barnikol-Watanabe, S., Mihaesco, E., Mihaesco, C., Barnikol, H. U., and Hilschmann, N. (1984). The primary structure of mu-chain-disease protein BOT. Peculiar amino-acid sequence of the N-terminal 42 positions. *Hoppe-Seyler's Zeitschrift für Physiologische Chemie, 365,* 105–118.

Bartold, P. M., and Henning, F. R. (1990). Oral manifestation of immunoproliferative small intestinal disease. A case report. *Journal of Periodontology, 61,* 710–713.

Bedu-Addo, G., Sheldon, J., and Bates, I. (2000). Massive splenomegaly in tropical West Africa. *Postgraduate Medicine Journal, 76,* 107–109.

Ben Rejeb, A., Khediri, F., Souissi, H., Machghoul, S., Ben Othman, M., Gamoudi, A., Bahri, M., Chouikha, M., and Ben Ayed, F. (1991). Malt digestive system lymphomas and alpha heavy chain diseases. Histological and immunohistochemical study. Apropos of 3 cases [French]. *Archives d'anatomie et de cytologie pathologiques, 39,* 27–33.

Ben-Ayed, F., Halphen, M., Najjar, T., Boussene, H., Jaafoura, H., Bouguerra, A., Ben Salah, N., Mourali, N., Ayed, K., Ben Khalifa, H., Garoui, H., Gargouri, M., and Tufrali, G. (1989). Treatment of alpha chain disease. Results of a prospective study in 21 Tunisian

patients by the Tunisian-French Intestinal Lymphoma Study Group. *Cancer, 63,* 1251–1256.

Bender, S. W., Danon, F., Preud'homme, J. L., Posselt, H. G., Roettger, P., and Seligmann, M. (1978). Gamma heavy chain disease simulating alpha chain disease. *Gut, 19,* 1148–1152.

Bentaboulet, M., Mihaesco, E., Gendron, M. C., Brouet, J. C., and Tsapis, A. (1989). Genomic alterations in a case of alpha heavy chain disease leading to the generation of composite exons from the JH region. *European Journal of Immunology, 19,* 2093–2098.

Berger, R., Bernheim, A., Tsapis, A., Brouet, J. C., and Seligmann, M. (1986). Cytogenetic studies in four cases of alpha chain disease. *Cancer, Genetics, and Cytogenetics, 22,* 219–223.

Biewenga, J., Frangione, B., Franklin, E. C., and van Loghem, E. (1980). A γ1 heavy-chain disease protein (EST) lacking the entire VH and CH1 domains. *Scandinavian Journal of Immunology, 11,* 601–607.

Biewenga, J., and van Loghem, E. (1979). A new case of gamma-3 heavy chain disease. Biochemical and immunological investigations. *Vox Sanguinis, 36,* 193–198.

Biserte, G., Lebreton, J. P., Ropartz, C., Tijou, G., Mouty, B., Rodat, G., Maillet, J. Y., Letournou, A., Guimbretiere, J., Bray, B., and Doudart, D. (1973). A case of mu heavy chain disease [French]. *Nouvelle presse medicale, 2,* 1997.

Blangarin, P., Deviller, P., Kindbeiter, K., and Madjar, J. J. (1984). Gamma heavy chain disease studied by two-dimensional electrophoresis and immunoblotting techniques. *Clinical Chemistry, 30,* 2021–2025.

Bloch, K. J., Lee, L., Mills, J. A., and Haber, E. (1973). Gamma heavy chain disease—an expanding clinical and laboratory spectrum. *American Journal of Medicine, 55,* 61–70.

Blum, D. J., Doyle, J. A., Greipp, P. R., and McDonald, T. J. (1985). Gamma heavy-chain disease involving upper airway. *Otolaryngology—head and neck surgery, 93,* 677–679.

Bonhomme, J., Seligmann, M., Mihaesco, C., Clauvel, J. P., Danon, F., Brouet, J. C., Bouvry, P., Martine, J., and Clerc, M. (1974). Mu-chain disease in an African patient. *Blood, 43,* 485–492.

Bowie, M. D., and Hill, I. D. (1988). Alpha-chain disease in children. *Journal of Pediatrics, 112,* 46–49.

Brandtzaeg, P., and Savilahti, E. (1978). Further evidence for a role of secretory component (SC) and J chain in the glandular transport of IgA. *Advances in Experimental Medical and Biology, 107,* 219–226.

Bridoux, F., Goujon, J. M., Binaut, R., Fleury, D., Moulin, B., Bataille, P., Vanhille, P., Bauwens, M., Mougenot, B., Droz, D., Preud'homme, J. L., and Touchard, G. (2001). Randall-type monoclonal immunoglobulin deposition disease (MIDD). Clinico-pathological features and outcome [Abstract]. *Journal of the American Society of Nephrology, 12,* 94A.

Brouet, J. C., Seligmann, M., Danon, F., Belpomme, D., and Fine, J. M. (1979). Mu-chain disease. Report of two new cases. *Archives of Internal Medicine, 139,* 672–674.

Butch, A. W., Badros, A., Desikan, K. R., and Munchi, N. C. (2001). Expression of a free gamma heavy chain in serum following autologous stem cell transplantation for IgG kappa multiple myeloma. *Bone Marrow Transplantation, 27,* 663–666.

Buxbaum, J. N., Chuba, J. V., Hellman, G. C., Solomon, A., and Gallo, G. R. (1990). Monoclonal immunoglobulin deposition disease. Light chain and light and heavy chain deposition diseases and their relation to light chain amyloidosis. Clinical features, immunopathology, and molecular analysis. *Annals of Internal Medicine, 112,* 455–464.

Buxbaum, J. N., and Preud'homme, J. L. (1972). Alpha and gamma heavy chain diseases in man. Intracellular origin of the aberrant polypeptides. *Journal of Immunology, 109,* 1131–1137.

Calvanico, N., Rabin, B., Plaut, A., and Tomasi, T. B., Jr. (1972). Studies on a new gamma heavy chain disease protein [Abstract]. *Federation Proceedings, 31,* 771.

Campbell, J. K., and Juneja, S. K. (2000). Test and teach. Number one hundred and four. Mu heavy chain disease (mu-HCD). *Pathology, 32*, 202–203, 227.

Case records of the Massachusetts General Hospital. Weekly clinico-pathological exercises. Case 50. (1970). *New England Journal of Medicine, 283*, 1332–1339.

Castelino, D., Gray, F., D'Apice, A., Paspaliaris, B., Riglar, A., McLachlan, R., and Murphy, B. (1994). Primary Sjögren's syndrome and gamma heavy chain disease. *Pathology, 26*, 337–338.

Chang, C. S., Lin, S. F., Chen, T. P., Liu, H. W., Liu, T. C., Li, C. Y., Chao, M. C., and Wu, P. L. (1992). Leukemic manifestation in a case of alpha-chain disease with multiple polypoid intestinal lymphocytic lymphoma. *American Journal of Hematology, 41*, 209–214.

Chantar, C., Escartin, P., Plaza, A. G., Corugedo, A. F., Arenas, J. I., Sanz, E., Anaya, A., Bootello, A., and Segovia, J. M. (1974). Diffuse plasma cell infiltration of the small intestine with malabsorption associated to IgA monoclonal gammopathy. *Cancer, 34*, 1620–1630.

Charles, E. Z., and Valdes, A. J. (1994). Free fragments of gamma chain in the urine. A possible source of confusion with gamma heavy-chain disease. *American Journal of Clinical Pathology, 101*, 462–464.

Chauveau, D. L., Noel, H., Cogné, M., Aucouturier, P., Grunfeld, J. P., and Lesavre, P. (2000). Renal and skin deposits of a Ch1 deleted alpha-1 heavy chain [Abstract]. *Journal of the American Society of Nephrology, 11*, 543A.

Cheng, I. K., Ho, S. K., Chan, D. T., Ng, W. K., and Chan, K. W. (1996). Crescentic nodular glomerulosclerosis secondary to truncated immunoglobulin alpha heavy chain deposition. *American Journal of Kidney Diseases, 28*, 283–288.

Chernokhvostova, E. V., Batalova, T. N., Andreeva, N. E., and Antipova, L. G. (1977). Immunochemical study of serum in the diagnosis of mu-chain disease [Russian]. *Zhurnal Mikrobiologii Epidemiologii I Immunobiologii, 2*, 42–48.

Chernokhvostova, E. V., German, G. P., Varlamova, E., Andreeva, N. E., and Kotova, T. S. (1991). An unusual case of heavy gamma-chain disease with several monoclonal components. IgG kappa, IgM lambda, Bence Jones proteins kappa and lambda [Russian]. *Terapevticheskii Arkhiv, 63*, 80–85.

Chiara, M., Belardi, P., Dragonetti, A., Mazzucco, G., Calosso, L., Fortunato, M., Gioacchino, F., Sena, L. M., and Roccatello, D. (2000). Heavy chain deposition disease [Abstract]. *Nephrology Dialysis Transplantation, 15*(9), A51.

Cho, C., Linscheer, W. G., Bell, R., and Smith, R. (1982). Colonic lymphoma producing alpha-chain disease protein. *Gastroenterology, 83*, 121–126.

Chou, C. L., and Morrison, S. L. (1993). An insertion-deletion event in murine immunoglobulin kappa gene resembles mutations at heavy-chain disease loci. *Somatic Cell and Molecular Genetics, 19*, 131–139.

Chury, Z., Jansa, P., Jedlickova, J., Rosprimova, L., and Sabacky, J. (1971). A contribution to Franklin's disease. *Folia haematologica (Leipzig), 96*, 43–58.

Cogné, M., Aucouturier, P., Brizard, A., Dreyfus, B., Duarte, F., and Preud'homme, J. L. (1993). Complete variable region deletion in a mu heavy chain disease protein (ROUL). Correlation with light chain secretion. *Leukemia Research, 17*, 527–532.

Cogné, M., Bakhshi, A., Korsmeyer, S. J., and Guglielmi, P. (1988). Gene mutations and alternate RNA splicing result in truncated Ig L chains in human gamma H chain disease. *Journal of Immunology, 141*, 1738–1744.

Cogné, M., and Preud'homme, J. L. (1990). Gene deletions force non-secretory alpha-chain disease plasma cells to produce membrane-form alpha-chain only. *Journal of Immunology, 145*, 2455–2458.

Cogné, M., Silvain, C., Khamlichi, A. A., and Preud'homme, J. L. (1992). Structurally abnormal immunoglobulins in human immunoproliferative disorders. *Blood, 79*, 2181–2195.

Colombel, J. R., Rambaud, J. C., Vaerman, J. P., Galian, A., Delacroix, D. L., Nemeth, J., Duprey, F., Halphen, M., Godeau, P., and Dive, C. (1988). Massive plasma cell infiltration of the digestive tract. Secretory component as the rate-limiting factor of immunoglobulin secretion in external fluids. *Gastroenterology, 95*, 1106–1113.

Comelli, A. M., and Paris, B. (1990). Alpha heavy chain disease. A clinical study of 3 cases and review of the literature [Italian]. *Giornale di Clinica Medica, 71*, 339–341, 344–348.

Cooper, D. L., Bolognia, J. L., and Lin, J. T. (1991). Atrophie blanche in a patient with gamma-heavy-chain disease. *Archives of Dermatology, 127*, 272–273.

Cooper, S. M., Franklin, E. C., and Frangione, B. (1972). Molecular defect in a gamma-2 heavy chain. *Science, 176*, 187–189.

Corcos, D., Dunda, O., Butor, C., Cesbron, J. Y., Lores, P., Bucchini, D., and Jami, J. (1995). Pre-B-cell development in the absence of lambda 5 in transgenic mice expressing a heavy-chain disease protein. *Current Biology, 5*, 1140–1148.

Coulbois, J., Galian, P., Galian, A., Couteaux, B., Danon, F., and Rambaud, J. (1986). Gastric form of alpha chain disease. *Gut, 27*, 719–725.

Cozzolino, F., Vercelli, D., Castigli, E., Becucci, A., and Di Guglielmo, R. (1982). A new case of gamma-heavy chain disease. Clinical and immunochemical studies. *Scandinavian Journal of Haematology, 28*, 145–150.

Creyssel, R., Brizard, C. P., Gibaud, A., Cordier, J. F., and Gibaud, H. (1977). Maladie des chaines lourdes gamma d'apparition secondaire au cours de l'evolution d'une macroglobulinemie. *Lyon Medical, 237*, 215.

Creyssel, R., Gibaud, A., Arnaud, Ph., and Cordier, J. F. (1976). Gammopathies biclonales et oligoclonales. Problèmes posés par la coexistence chez le même sujet de plusieurs constituants immunoglobuliniques d'hétérogénéité restreinte. *Lyon Medical, 236*, 101–115.

Dammacco, F., Bonomo, L., and Franklin, E. C. (1974). A new case of mu heavy chain disease: clinical and immunochemical studies. *Blood, 43*, 713–719.

Dammacco, F., Rigoli, E., Ferrarese, M., and Bonomo, L. (1976). Gamma heavy chain disease in a young girl. *Haematologica, 61*, 278–290.

Danevad, M., Sletten, K., Gaarder, P. I., Mellbye, O. J., and Husby, G. (2000). The amino acid sequence of a monoclonal gamma 3-heavy chain from a patient with articular gamma-heavy chain deposition disease. *Scandinavian Journal of Immunology, 51*, 602–606.

Danon, F., Mihaesco, C., Bouvry, M., Clerc, M., and Seligmann, M. (1975). A new case of heavy mu-chain disease. *Scandinavian Journal of Haematology, 15*, 5–9.

De Franco, A., Brizi, M. G., Barbaro, B., Buffa, V., Vecchioli, A., and Marano, P. (1991). Primary lymphoma of the small intestine: clinico-radiological correlations [Italian]. *La Radiologica Medica, 81*, 459–463.

Delmas-Marsalet, Y., Voisin, D., Hennache, G., Bauters, F., and Goudemand, M. (1971). Clinical and biological study of heavy gamma chain disease. Apropos of a new case [French]. *Nouvelle Revue Francaise d Hematologie, 11*, 717–734.

Demirer, T., Uzunalimoglu, O., Anderson, T., Koethe, S. M., McFadden, P. W., Demirer, S., Uzunalimoglu, B., and Kucuk, O. (1995). Flow cytometric measurement of proliferation-associated nuclear antigen P105 and DNA content in immuno-proliferative small intestinal disease (IPSID). *Journal of Surgical Oncology, 58*, 25–30.

Di Benedetto, G., Cataldi, A., Verde, A., Gloghini, A., Nicolo, G., and Pistoia, V. (1989). Gamma heavy chain disease associated with Hodgkin's disease. Clinical, pathologic, and immunologic features of one case. *Cancer, 63*, 1804–1809.

Dickson, J. R., Harth, M., Bell, D. A., Komar, R., and Chodirker, W. B. (1989). Gamma heavy chain disease and rheumatoid arthritis. *Seminars in Arthritis and Rheumatism, 18*, 247–251.

Doe, W. F., Danon, F., and Seligmann, M. (1979). Immunodiagnosis of alpha chain disease. *Clinical and Experimental Immunology, 36,* 189–197.

Doe, W. F., Henry, K., Hobbs, J. R., Jones, F. A., Dent, C. E., and Booth, C. C. (1972). Five cases of alpha chain disease. *Gut, 13,* 947–957.

Eisner, S. B., and Mitnick, P. D. (1986). Hypercalcemia and reversible renal failure in heavy-chain disease. *Southern Medical Journal, 79,* 507–509.

Ellis, V. M., Cowley, D. M., Taylor, K. M., and Marlton, P. (1992). Gamma heavy chain disease developing in association with myelodysplastic syndrome. *British Journal of Haematology, 81,* 125–126.

Ellman, L. L., and Bloch, K. J. (1968). Heavy-chain disease. Report of a seventh case. *New England Journal of Medicine, 278,* 1195–1201.

el Saghir, N. S. (1995). Combination chemotherapy with tetracycline and aggressive supportive care for immunoproliferative small-intestinal disease lymphoma. *Journal of Clinical Oncology, 13,* 794–795.

Eulitz, M., Weiss, D. T., and Solomon, A. (1990). Immunoglobulin heavy-chain-associated amyloidosis. *Proceedings of the National Academy of Sciences of the United States of America, 87,* 6542–6546.

Faguet, G. B., Barton, B. P., Smith, L. L., and Garver, F. A. (1977). Gamma heavy chain disease. Clinical aspects and characterization of a deleted, noncovalently linked gamma 1 heavy chain dimer (BAZ). *Blood, 49,* 495–505.

Fakhfakh, F., Ayadi, H., Bouguerra, A., Fourati, R., Ben Ayed, F., Tsapis, A., and Dellagi, K. (1991). Rearrangement of immunoglobulin genes in alpha heavy chain disease. A criterion of monoclonality [French]. *Archives de l Institut Pasteur de Tunis, 68,* 251–259.

Fakhfakh, F., Dellagi, K., Ayadi, H., Bouguerra, A., Fourati, R., Ben Ayed, F., Brouet, J. C., and Tsapis, A. (1992). Alpha heavy chain disease alpha mRNA contain nucleotide sequences of unknown origins. *European Journal of Immunology, 22,* 3037–3040.

Fakhfakh, F., Mihaesco, E., Ayadi, H., Brouet, J. C., and Tsapis, A. (1993). Alpha heavy chain disease. Molecular analysis of a new case [French]. *Presse Medicale, 22,* 1047–1051.

Faux, J. A., Crain, J. D., Rosen, F. S., and Merler, E. (1973). An alpha heavy chain abnormality in a child with hypogammaglobulinemia. *Clinical Immunology and Immunopathology, 1,* 282–290.

Feremans, W., Caudron, M., and Bieva, C. (1979). A case of gamma 3 heavy chain disease with vacuolated plasma cells. A clinical, immunological, and ultrastructural study. *Journal of Clinical Pathology, 32,* 334–343.

Fermand, J. P., Brouet, J. C., Danon, F., and Seligmann, M. (1989). Gamma heavy chain 'disease.' Heterogeneity of the clinicopathologic features. Report of 16 cases and review of the literature. *Medicine (Baltimore), 68,* 321–335.

Fernandes, P. M., Capucho, R., Brandao, F., Ferreira, A., Macedo, F., Fonseca, E., Rodrigues Gomes, M., and Castro, I. (1994). Right atrial septic thrombus in a patient with alpha-heavy chain disease. *Arquivos de Medicina, 8,* 19–21.

Fine, J. M., Zakin, M. M., Faure, A., and Boffa, G. A. (1968). Myeloma with a serum gammaG paraprotein and urinary elimination of a fragment of gammaG devoid of light chains [French]. *Revue Francaise d Etudes Cliniques et Biologiques, 13,* 175–178.

Fine, K. D., and Stone, M. J. (1999). Alpha-heavy chain disease, Mediterranean lymphoma, and immunoproliferative small intestinal disease. A review of clinicopathological features, pathogenesis, and differential diagnosis. *American Journal of Gastroenterology, 94,* 1139–1152.

Fischbach, W., Tacke, W., Greiner, A., Konrad, H., and Muller, H. (1997). Regression of immunoproliferative small intestinal disease after eradication of *Helicobacter pylori. Lancet, 349,* 31–32.

Florin-Christensen, A., Doniach, D., and Newcomb, P. B. (1974). Alpha-chain disease with pulmonary manifestations. *British Medical Journal, 2,* 413–415.

Forte, F. A., Prelli, F., Yount, W. J., Jerry, L. M., Kochwa, S., Franklin, E. C., and Kunkel, H. G. (1970). Heavy chain disease of the μ (γM) type. Report of the first case. *Blood, 36,* 137–144.

Forte, F. A., Prelli, F., Yount, W., Kochwa, S., Franklin, E. C., and Kunkel, H. (1969). Heavy chain disease of the μ type: report of the first case [Abstract]. *Blood, 34,* 831.

Frangione, B. (1976). A new immunoglobulin variant. Gamma 3 heavy chain disease protein CHI. *Proceedings of the National Academy of Sciences of the United States of America, 73,* 1552–1555.

Frangione, B., Franklin, E. C., and Smithies, O. (1978). Unusual genes at the aminoterminus of human immunoglobulin variants. *Nature, 273,* 400–401.

Frangione, B., Lee, L., Haber, E., and Bloch, K. J. (1973). Protein Hal. Partial deletion of a "γ" immunoglobulin gene(s) and apparent reinitiation at an internal AUG codon. *Proceedings of the National Academy of Sciences of the United States of America, 70,* 1073–1077.

Frangione, B., Rosenwasser, E., Prelli, F., and Franklin, E. C. (1980). Primary structure of human gamma 3 immunoglobulin deletion mutant. Gamma 3 heavy-chain disease protein Wis. *Biochemistry, 19,* 4304–4308.

Franklin, E. C., and Frangione, B. (1971). The molecular defect in a protein (CRA) found in gamma-1 heavy chain disease, and its genetic implications. *Proceedings of the National Academy of Sciences of the United States of America, 68,* 187–191.

Franklin, E. C., Frangione, B., and Prelli, F. (1976). The defect in mu heavy chain disease protein GLI. *Journal of Immunology, 116,* 1194–1195.

Franklin, E. C., Kyle, R., Seligmann, M., and Frangione, B. (1979a). Correlation of protein structure and immunoglobulin gene organization in the light of two new deleted heavy chain disease proteins. *Molecular Immunology, 16,* 919–921.

Franklin, E. C., Lowenstein, J., Bigelow, B., and Meltzer, M. (1964). Heavy chain disease—a new disorder of serum γ-globulins. Report of the first case. *American Journal of Medicine, 37,* 332–350.

Franklin, E. C., Prelli, F., and Frangione, B. (1979b). Human heavy chain disease protein WIS. Implications for the organization of immunoglobulin genes. *Proceedings of the National Academy of Sciences of the United States of America, 76,* 452–456.

Fujii, H., Shimizu, T., Seki, S., Isemura, T., Yamamoto, K., Kanoh, T., and Ohno, Y. (1982). Combined features of mu-heavy chain disease and primary macroglobulinemia in a single patient. Clinical and immunological studies [Japanese]. *Nippon Ketsueki Gakkai Zasshi, 45,* 622–632.

Furuta, T., Ooba, Y., Hirai, R., and Tezuka, T. Cited by Takahashi, K., Naito, M., Matsuoka, Y., and Takatsuki, K. (1988). A new form of alpha-chain disease with generalized lymph node involvement. *Pathology, Research and Practice (Stuttgart), 183,* 717–723.

Gafter, U., Kessler, E., Shabtay, F., Shaked, P., and Djaldetti, M. (1980). Abnormal chromosomal marker (D14 q +) in a patient with alpha heavy chain disease. *Journal of Clinical Pathology, 33,* 136–144.

Galanti, L. M., Doyen, C., Vander Maelen, C., Dapare, N., Bosly, A., Puthier, F., and Vaerman, J. P. (1995). Biological diagnosis of a gamma-1-heavy chain disease in an asymptomatic patient. *European Journal of Haematology, 54,* 202–204.

Galian, A., Le Charpentier, Y., and Rambaud, J. C. (1983). La Maladie des Chaines Lourdes Alpha. In C. Nezelof (Ed.), *Nouvelles Acquisitions en Pathologie* (p. 73). Paris: Hermann.

Galian, A., Lecestre, M. J., Scotto, J., Bognel, C., Matuchansky, C., and Rambaud, J. C. (1977). Pathological study of alpha-chain disease, with special emphasis on evolution. *Cancer, 39,* 2081–2101.

Gallart, M. T., Canals, J., Canadell, E., Cortez, L., Moragas, A., and Schwartz, S. (1978). A new case of gamma-heavy chain disease. *Acta Haematologica, 59,* 262–276.

Gaucher, A., Bertrand, F., Brouet, J. C., Pourel, J., Netter, P., Faure, G., and Seligmann, M. (1977). Gamma heavy chain disease associated with rheumatoid arthritis. Spontaneous disappearance of the pathologic protein [French]. *Semaine des Hopitaux, 53*, 2117–2120.

Geraci, L., Merlini, G., Spadano, A., Di Matteo, S., Torlontano, G., and Ascari, E. (1985). Alpha heavy chain disease. Report of two cases. *Haematologica, 70*, 431–436.

Goossens, T., Klein, U., and Kuppers, R. (1998). Frequent occurrence of deletions and duplications during somatic hypermutation. Implications for oncogene translocations and heavy chain disease. *Proceedings of the National Academy of Sciences of the United States of America, 95*, 2463–2468.

Gordon, J., Hamblin, T. J., Smith, J. L., Stevenson, F. K., and Stevenson, G. T. (1981). A human B-cell lymphoma synthesizing and expressing surface mu-chain in the absence of detectable light chain. *Blood, 58*, 552–556.

Goyert, S. M., Hugli, T. E., and Spiegelberg, H. L. (1977). Sites of 'spontaneous' degradation of IgD. *Journal of Immunology, 118*, 2138–2144.

Guardia, J., Mirada, A., Moragas, A., Armengol, J. R., and Martinez-Vazquez, J. M. (1980). Alpha chain disease of the stomach. *Hepatogastroenterology, 27*, 238–239.

Guardia, J., Rubies-Prat, J., Gallart, M. T., Moragas, A., Martinez-Vazquez, J. M., Bacardi, R., and Vilaseca, J. (1976). The evolution of alpha heavy chain disease. *American Journal of Medicine, 60*, 596–602.

Guglielmi, P., Bakhshi, A., Cogné, M., Seligmann, M., and Korsmeyer, S. J. (1988). Multiple genomic defects result in an alternative RNA splice creating a human γ H chain disease protein. *Journal of Immunology, 141*, 1762–1768.

Guglielmo, P., Granata, P., Di Raimondo, F., Lombardo, T., Giustolisi, R., and Cacciola, E. (1982). 'μ' Heavy chain type 'non-excretory' myeloma. *Scandinavian Journal of Haematology, 29*, 36–40.

Halphen, M., Najjar, T., Jaafoura, H., Cammoun, M., and Tufrali, G. (1986). Diagnostic value of upper intestinal fiber endoscopy in primary small intestinal lymphoma. A prospective study by the Tunisian-French Intestinal Lymphoma Group. *Cancer, 58*, 2140–2145.

Harzic, M., Girard-Pipau, F., Halphen, M., Ferchal, F., Perol, Y., and Rambaud, J. C. (1985). Bacteriological, parasitological and virological study of the digestive flora in alpha-chain disease [French]. *Gastroenterologie Clinique et Biologique (Paris), 9*, 472–479.

Hauke, G., Krawinkel, U., Schiltz, E., Metz, B., Hollmann, A., and Peter, H. H. (1991). Gamma-1 heavy chain disease with the demonstration of Bence-Jones proteins [German]. *Immunitat und Infektion (Munchen), 19*, 89–90.

Hauke, G., Schiltz, E., Bross, K. J., Hollmann, A., Peter, H. H., and Krawinkel, U. (1992). Unusual sequence of immunoglobulin L-chain rearrangements in a gamma heavy chain disease patient. *Scandinavian Journal of Immunology, 36*, 463–468.

Herzenberg, A. M., Kiaii, M., and Magil, A. B. (2000). Heavy chain deposition disease. Recurrence in a renal transplant and report of IgG(2) subtype. *American Journal of Kidney Diseases, 35*, E25.

Herzenberg, A. M., Lien, J., and Magil, A. B. (1996). Monoclonal heavy chain (immunoglobulin G3) deposition disease. Report of a case. *American Journal of Kidney Diseases, 28*, 128–131.

Hibi, T., Asakura, H., Kobayashi, K., Munakata, Y., Kano, S., Tsuchiya, M., Teramoto, T., and Uematsu, Y. (1982). Alpha heavy chain disease lacking secretory alpha chain, with cobblestone appearance of the small intestine and duodenal ulcer demonstrated by endoscopy. *Gut, 23*, 422–427.

Hubmann, R., Kaiser, W., Radaszkiewicz, T., Fridrik, M., and Zazgornik, I. (1995). Malabsorption associated with a high-grade-malignant non-Hodgkin's lymphoma, alpha-heavy chain disease and immunoproliferative small intestinal disease. *Zeitschrift fur Gastroenterologie, 33*, 209–213.

Hudnall, S. D., Alperin, J. B., and Petersen, J. R. (2001). Composite nodular lymphocyte-predominance Hodgkin disease and gamma-heavy-chain disease. A case report and review of the literature. *Archives of Pathology and Laboratory Medicine, 125*, 803–807.

Husby, G. (2000). Is there a pathogenic link between gamma heavy chain disease and chronic arthritis? *Current Opinions in Rheumatology, 12*, 65–70.

Husby, G., Blichfeldt, P., Brinch, L., Brandtzaeg, P., Mellbye, O. J., Sletten, K., and Stenstad, T. (1998). Chronic arthritis and gamma heavy chain disease. Coincidence or pathogenic link? *Scandinavian Journal of Rheumatology, 27*, 257–264.

Ibuka, T., Shimoyama, M., Sakano, T., Sakai, Y., Kimura, K., Mukojimi, T., and Ooboshi, S. (1974). Gamma heavy chain disease. Report of a case. *Rinsho Ketsueki—Japanese Journal of Clinical Hematology, 15*, 671–672.

Ieko, M., Kohno, M., Ohmoto, A., Notoya, A., Fukazawa, Y., Yasukouchi, T., Sawada, K., and Koike, T. (1998). Gamma-heavy chain disease associated with MALT lymphoma of the duodenum [Japanese]. *Rinsho Ketsueki, 39*, 512–518.

Imai, H. (2001). Heavy chain deposition disease: report of a case and review of the literature [Japanese]. *Rinsho Byori—Japanese Journal of Clinical Pathology, 49*, 695–698.

Isaacson, P. G. (1994). Gastrointestinal lymphoma. *Human Pathology, 25*, 1020–1029.

Isaacson, P. G., Dogan, A., Price, S. K., and Spencer, J. (1989). Immunoproliferative small-intestinal disease. An immunohistochemical study. *American Journal of Surgical Pathology, 13*, 1023–1033.

Isaacson, P. G., and Spencer, J. (1987). Malignant lymphoma of mucosa-associated lymphoid tissue. *Histopathology, 11*, 445–462.

Ishikawa, K., Hira, M., Tsutsumi, H., Kumakawa, T., Mori, M., and Masami, M. (1997). Successful treatment of heavy-chain disease with etoposide [Japanese]. *Nippon Ronen Igakkai Zasshi, 34*, 221–225.

Isobe, T., and Osserman, E. F. (1974). Plasma cell dyscrasia associated with the production of incomplete (? deleted) IgGλ molecules, gamma heavy chains, and free lambda chains containing carbohydrate. Description of the first case. *Blood, 43*, 505–526.

Itoh, Y., Ohtaki, H., Ono, T., Mori, N., Kawaoi, A., and Kawai, T. (1991). A case of lymphoma-type alpha-chain disease. *Acta Haematologica, 86*, 107–110.

Iwasaki, T., Hamano, T., Kobayashi, K., and Kakishita, E. (1997). A case of mu-heavy chain disease. Combined features of mu-chain disease and macroglobulinemia. *International Journal of Hematology, 66*, 359–365.

Jacqueline, F., Renversez, J. C., Groslambert, P., and Fine, J. M. (1978). Gamma heavy chain disease during rheumatoid polyarthritis. A clinical and immunochemical study [French]. *Revue du Rhumatisme et des Maladies Osteo—Articulaires, 45*, 661–665.

Jaffe, E. S., Harris, N. L., Stein, H., and Vardiman, J. W. (Eds.). (2001). *Pathology and Genetics of Tumours of Haematopoietic and Lymphoid Tissues* (p 154). Lyon. IARC Press.

Joller, P. W., Joller-Jemelka, H. I., Shmerling, D. H., and Skvaril, F. (1984). Immunological and biochemical studies of an unusual alpha heavy chain protein in a 9-year-old boy. *Journal of Clinical Laboratory Immunology, 15*, 167–172.

Jones, W. G., Elvy, R. J., Pedersen, N. (1974). Heavy-chain disease in Australia [Letter]. *Lancet, 1*, 570.

Josephson, A. S., Nicastri, A., Price, E., and Biro, L. (1973). H chain fragment and monoclonal IgA in a lymphoproliferative disorder. *American Journal of Medicine, 54*, 127–135.

Kambham, N., Markowitz, G. S., Appel, G. B., Kleiner, M. J., Aucouturier, P., and D'Agati, V. D. (1999). Heavy chain deposition disease. The disease spectrum. *American Journal of Kidney Diseases, 33*, 954–962.

Kanoh, T., and Nakasato, H. (1987). Osteolytic gamma heavy chain disease. *European Journal of Haematology, 39,* 60–65.

Kanoh, T., Takigawa, M., and Niwa, Y. (1988). Cutaneous lesions in gamma heavy-chain disease. *Archives of Dermatology, 124,* 1538–1540.

Katz, A., Zent, R., and Bargman, J. M. (1994). IgG heavy-chain deposition disease. *Modern Pathology, 7,* 874–878.

Kaufmann, H. P., Schmitt, W., and Seib, H. J. (1994). Alpha-heavy chain disease—Mediterranean lymphoma [German]. *Leber, Magen, Darm, 24,* 32–35.

Keller, H., Spengler, G. A., Skvaril, F., Flury, W., Noseda, G., and Riva, G. (1970). Heavy chain disease. A case of IgG-heavy-chain-fragment and IgM-type K-paraproteinemia with plasma cell leukemia [German]. *Schweizerische Medizinische Wochenschrift. Journal Suisse de Medecine, 100,* 1012–1022.

Khamlichi, A. A., Aucouturier, P., Preud'homme, J. L., and Cogné, M. (1995). Structure of abnormal heavy chains in human heavy-chain-deposition disease. *European Journal of Biochemisrty, 229,* 54–60.

Kharazmi, A., Rezai, M. H., Abadi, P., Nasr, K., Haghighi, P., and Haghshenas, M. (1978). T and B lymphocytes in alpha-chain disease. *British Journal of Cancer, 37,* 48–54.

Khojasteh, A., and Haghighi, P. (1990). Immunoproliferative small intestinal disease: portrait of a potentially preventable cancer from the Third World. *American Journal of Medicine, 89,* 483–490.

Khojasteh, A., Haghshenass, M., and Haghighi, P. (1983a). Current concepts immunoproliferative small intestinal disease. A 'Third-World lesion.' *New England Journal of Medicine, 308,* 1401–1405.

Khojasteh, A., Saalabian, M. J., and Haghshenass, M. (1983b). Randomized comparison of abdominal irradiation (AI) vs CHOP vs C-MOPP for the treatment of immunoproliferative small intestinal disease (IPSID) associated lymphoma (AL) [Abstract]. *Proceedings of the Annual Meeting of the American Society of Clinical Oncologists, 2,* 207.

Klein, U., Goossens, T., Fischer, M., Kanzler, H., Braeuninger, A., Rajewsky, K., and Kuppers, R. (1998). Somatic hypermutation in normal and transformed human B cells. *Immunology Reviews, 162,* 261–280.

Kretschmer, R. R., Pizzuto, J., Gonzalez, J., and Lopez, M. (1974). Heavy chain disease, rheumatoid arthritis and cryoglobulinemia. *Clinical Immunology and Immunopathology, 2,* 195–215.

Kuroyanagi, T., Kura, K., Akamatsu, Y., and Arao, T. (1979). A case report of the immunodysplasia syndrome and heavy chain disease associated with subacute bacterial endocarditis. *Tohoku Journal of Experimental Medicine, 128,* 325–331.

Kyle, R. A., Greipp, P. R., and Banks, P. M. (1981a). The diverse picture of gamma heavy-chain disease. Report of seven cases and review of literature. *Mayo Clinic Proceedings, 56,* 439–451.

Kyle, R. A., Robinson, R. A., and Katzmann, J. A. (1981b). The clinical aspects of biclonal gammopathies. Review of 57 cases. *American Journal of Medicine, 71,* 999–1008.

Lassoued, K., Picard, C., Danon, F., Pocidalo, M., Grossin, M., Crickx, B., and Belaich, S. (1990). Cutaneous manifestations associated with gamma heavy chain disease. Report of an unusual case and review of literature. *Journal of the American Academy of Dermatology, 23,* 988–991.

Leach, I. H., Jenkins, J. S., Murray-Leslie, C. F., and Powell, R. J. (1987). Mu-heavy chain and monoclonal IgG K paraproteinaemia in systemic lupus erythematosus. *British Journal of Rheumatology, 26,* 460–462.

Lebreton, J. P., Fontaine, M., Rousseaux, J., Youinou, P., Hurez, D., Rivat-Peran, L., and Bernards, J. P. (1982). Deleted IgG1 and IgG2 H chains in a patient with an IgG subclass imbalance. *Clinical and Experimental Immunology, 47,* 206–216.

Lebreton, J. P., Rivat, C., Rivat, L., Guillemot, L., and Ropartz, C. (1967). An unrecognized immunoglobinopathy. Heavy chain disease [French]. *Presse Medicale, 75,* 2251–2254.

Lebreton, J. P., Ropartz, C., and Biserte, G. (1974). Partial study of a case of heavy mu chain disease [French]. *Lille Medica, 19,* 126–131.

Lebreton, J. P., Ropartz, C., Rousseaus, J., Roussel, P., Dautrevaus, M., and Biserte, G. (1975). Immunochemical and biochemical study of a human Fc mu-like fragment (mu-chain disease). *European Journal of Immunology, 5,* 179–184.

Leglise, M. C., Briere, J., Abgrall, J. F., and Hurez, D. (1983). Non-secretory myeloma of heavy mu-chain type [French]. *Nouvelle Revue Francaise d Hematologie, 25,* 103–106.

Leloup, E., Gallinari, C., Bouchon, J. P., and Benis, Y. (1989). Heavy gamma-chain diseases. A new case and review of the literature. *Annales de Médicine Interne (Paris), 140,* 274–278.

Lenders, J. W., Holdrinet, R. S., Nguyen, C. T., and De Waal, R. (1984). A case of gamma-heavy chain monoclonal gammopathy of undetermined significance. *Netherlands Journal of Medicine, 27,* 412–416.

Lesavre, P., Droz, D., Noël, L. H., Hummel, A., Aucouturier, P., Chauveau, D., and Grünfeld, J. P. (2001). Amylose AL et maladies par dépôts d'immunoglobulines monoclonales. *Revue de Médicine Interne, 22*(suppl 1), 16–17.

Liapis, H., Papadakis, I., and Nakopoulou, L. (2000). Nodular glomerulosclerosis secondary to mu heavy chain deposits. *Human Pathology, 31,* 122–125.

Lin, J., Markowitz, G. S., Valeri, A. M., Kambham, N., Sherman, W. H., Appel, G. B., and D'Agati, V. D. (2001). Renal monoclonal immunoglobulin deposition disease: the disease spectrum. *Journal of the American Society of Nephrology, 12,* 1482–1492.

Loyau, G., Barre, J. P., L'Hirondel, J. L., Maniece, M., and Preud'Homme, J. L. (1975). Gamma heavy chain disease. A new case [French]. *Nouvelle Presse Medicale, 4,* 957–959.

Lucidarme, D., Colombel, J. F., Brandtzaeg, P., Tulliez, M., Chaussade, S., Marteau, P., Dehennin, J. P., Vaerman, J. P., and Rambaud, J. C. (1993). Alpha-chain disease: analysis of alpha-chain protein and secretory component in jejunal fluid. *Gastroenterology, 104,* 278–285.

Lyons, R. M., Chaplin, H., Tillack, T. W., and Majerus, P. W. (1975). Gamma heavy chain disease. Rapid, sustained response to cyclophosphamide and prednisone. *Blood, 46,* 1–9.

Malik, I. A., Shamsi, Z., Shafquat, A., Aziz, Z., Shaikh, H., Jafri, W., Khan, M. A., and Khan, A. H. (1995). Clinicopathological features and management of immunoproliferative small intestinal disease and primary small intestinal lymphoma in Pakistan. *Medical Pediatric Oncology, 25,* 400–406.

Marcenò, R., Majolino, I., Cavallaro, A. M., and Caronia, F. (1984). An unusual case of plasma cell dyscrasia with gamma heavy chains in the serum and free kappa chains in the urine. *Haematologica, 69,* 715–720.

Marquez, J. L., Mota, R., Herrera, J. M., Narvaez, I., and Saenz de Santamaria, J. (1993). Immunoproliferative disease of the small intestine. Report of a case [Spanish]. *Revista Española de Enfermedades Digestivas, 83,* 381–383.

Martin, I. G., and Aldoori, M. I. (1994). Immunoproliferative small intestinal disease. Mediterranean lymphoma and alpha heavy chain disease. *British Journal of Surgery, 81,* 20–24.

Matsubayashi, S., Tamai, H., Suzuki, T., Matsuzuka, F., Miyauchi, A., Kobayashi, N., Fukata, S., Kuma, K., Yanaihara, N., and Nagataki, S. (1985). Extramedullary plasmacytoma of the thyroid gland producing gamma heavy chain. *Endocrinologia Japonica, 32,* 427–433.

Matsumoto, T., Iida, M., Matsui, T., Tanaka, H., and Fujishima, M. (1990). The value of double-contrast study of the small intestine in immunoproliferative small intestinal disease. *Gastrointestinal Radiology, 15,* 159–163.

Matuchansky, C., Cogné, M., Lemaire, M., Babin, P., Touhard, G., Chamaret, S., and Preud'homme, J. L. (1989). Nonsecretory alpha-chain disease with immunoproliferative small-intestinal disease. *New England Journal of Medicine, 320,* 1534–1539.

McLaughlin, P., Grillo-Lopez, A. J., Link, B. K., Levy, R., Czuczman, M. S., Williams, M. E., Heyman, M. R., Bence-Bruckler, I., White, C. A., Cabanillas, F., Jain, V., Ho, A. D., Lister, J., Wey, K., Shen, D., and Dallaire, B. K. (1998). Rituximab chimeric anti-CD20 monoclonal antibody therapy for relapsed indolent lymphoma. Half of patients respond to a four-dose treatment program. *Journal of Clinical Oncology, 16*, 2825–2833.

Mihaesco, C., Ferrara, P., Guillemot, J. C., Congy, N., Gendron, M. C., Roy, J. P., Sizaret, P. Y., and Mihaesco, E. (1990). A new extra sequence at the amino terminal of a mu heavy chain disease protein (DAG). *Mol Immunol, 27*, 771–776.

Mihaesco, E., Barnikol-Watanabe, S., Barnikol, H. U., Mihaesco, C., and Hilschmann, N. (1980). The primary structure of the constant part of mu-chain-disease protein BOT. *European Journal of Biochemistry, 111*, 275–286.

Mitchell, P. E., Ford, R. P., Coughtrie, M. W., Heppleston, A. D., and Fraser, C. G. (1990). A case of heavy chain disease. Diagnosis and monitoring using assays of immunoglobulin heavy and light chains. *Scottish Medical Journal, 35*, 18–19.

Moskovits, T., Jacobson, D. R., and Buxbaum, J. (1992). N-ras oncogene activation in a patient with gamma heavy chain disease. *American Journal of Hematology, 41*, 302–303.

Mougenot, B., Brouet, J. C., Ronco, P. M., Kourilsky, O., Dupouët, L., and Aucouturier, P. (1983). Kidney deposition of immunoglobulin truncated heavy chains [Abstract]. *Journal of the American Society of Nephrology, 4*, 684.

Moulin, B., Deret, S., Mariette, X., Kourilsky, O., Imai, H., Dupouët, L., Marcellin, L., Kolb, I., Aucouturier, P., Brouet, J. C., Ronco, P. M., and Mougenot, B. (1999). Nodular glomerulosclerosis with deposition of monoclonal immunoglobulin heavy chains lacking C(H)1. *Journal of the American Society of Nephrology, 10*, 519–528.

Nabeshima, Y., and Ikenaka, T. (1976). N- and C-terminal amino acid sequences of a gamma-heavy chain disease protein YOK. *Immunochemistry, 13*, 245–249.

Nair, S., Mathan, M., Ramakrishna, B. S., and Mathan, V. I. (1998). Immunoproliferative small intestinal disease in South India. A clinical and immunomorphological study. *Journal of Gastroenterology Hepatology, 13*, 1207–1211.

Neudorf, S., Snover, D., and Filipovich, A. (1983). Immunoproliferative small intestinal disease [Letter]. *New England Journal of Medicine, 309*, 1126.

Nikbin, B., Banisadre, M., Ala, F., and Mojtabai, A. (1979). HLA AW19, B12 in immunoproliferative small intestinal disease. *Gut, 20*, 226–228.

Ockhuizen, T., Jilderda, J. F., and Cazemier, T. (1984). Sequential development of Waldenström's macroglobulinemia and gamma-1-heavy chain disease in a single patient. Clinical, immunochemical, immunofluorescent and protein studies. *Acta Haematologica, 71*, 53–59.

Ockhuizen, T., Smit, J. W., and van Leeuwen, M. (1983). Rheumatoid arthritis associated with transient gamma 2-heavy chain disease. *Rheumatology International, 3*, 167–172.

O'Conor, G. T., Jr., Wyandt, H. E., Innes, D. J., Normansell, D. E., and Hess, C. E. (1985). Gamma heavy chain disease. Report of a case associated with trisomy of chromosome 7. *Cancer, Genetics, and Cytogenetics, 15*, 1–5.

Ogawa, K., Imai, M., Tanigawa, T., Tsuji, T., and Arima, T. (1978). Pathological studies on a long-term survived case of gamma heavy chain disease—a brief review of 30 reported cases and a proposal for histological typing. *Acta Pathologica Japonica, 28*, 759–778.

O'Reilly, D. S., Adjukiewicz, A., and Whicher, J. T. (1981). Biochemical findings in a case of mu-chain disease. *Clinical Chemistry, 27*, 331–333.

Orth, H. B., Hurwitz, N., Lohri, A., Weber, W., and Herrmann, R. (1994). Gamma-heavy chain production as an epiphenomenon in non-Hodgkin's lymphoma [German]. *Deutsche Medizinische Wochenschriff, 119*, 1235–1238.

Osserman, E. F., and Takatsuki, K. (1964). Clinical and immunochemical studies of four cases of heavy ($H^{\gamma 2}$) chain disease. *American Journal of Medicine, 37*, 351–373.

Ottó, S., Peter, I., Vegh, S., Juhos, E., and Besznyak, I. (1986). Gamma-chain heavy-chain disease with primary thyroid plasmacytoma. *Archives of Pathological Laboratory Medicine, 110*, 893–896.

Papadaki, Th., Afendaki, S., Economidou, I., Kosmas, C., Stamatopoulos, K., Vaslamatzis, M., Alexopoulos, C., Loukopoulos, D., and Anagnostou, D. (1995). Immunoproliferative small intestinal disease (IPSID) associated with alpha heavy-chain disease [Abstract]. *Proceedings of ASCO, 14*, 403.

Papae, R. J., Rosenstein, R. W., Richards, F., and Yesner, R. (1978). Gamma heavy chain disease seen initially as gastric neoplasm. *Archives of Internal Medicine, 138*, 1151–1153.

Pellet, P., Berger, R., Bernheim, A., Brouet, J. C., and Tsapis, A. (1989). Molecular analysis of a t(9;14)(p11;q32) translocation occurring in a case of human alpha heavy chain disease. *Oncogene, 4*, 653–657.

Pellet, P., Tsapis, A., and Brouet, J. C. (1990). Alpha heavy chain disease of patient MAL: structure of the non-functional rearranged alpha gene translocated on chromosome 9. *European Journal of Immunology, 20*, 2731–2735.

Perrot, S., Delchier, J.-C., Farcet, J.-P., Kuentz, M., Haioun, C., and Soulé, J.-C. (1988). Maladie des chaines lourdes α (MCL α) disseminee. Resultats preliminaires d'un traitement par chimiotherapie intensive et autogreffe de moelle [Abstract]. *Gastroenterology and Clinical Biology, 12*, A264.

Pick, A. I., Shoenfeld, Y., Frohlichmann, R., Weiss, H., Vana, D., and Schreibman, S. (1979). Plasma cell dyscrasia. Analysis of 423 patients. *Journal of the American Medical Association, 241*, 2275–2278.

Pohl, C., Eidt, S., Ziegenhagen, D., and Kruis, W. (1991). Immunoproliferative disease of the small intestine. A rare differential diagnosis of Crohn's disease [German]. *Deutsche Medizinische Wochenschriff, 116*, 1265–1269.

Polski, J. M., Galvin, N., and Salinas-Madrigal, L. (1999). Non-amyloid fibrils in heavy chain deposition disease. *Kidney International, 56*, 1601–1602.

Pontet, F., Gue, X., Dosquet, C., Caen, J., and Rousselet, F. (1988). Rapid evolution in the immunochemical findings of a gamma heavy chain disease. *Clinical Chemistry, 34*, 439–443.

Pramoolsinsap, C., Kurathong, S., Atichartakarn, V., and Nitiyanand, P. (1993). Immunoproliferative small intestinal disease (IPSID) in Thailand. *Southeast Asian Journal of Tropical Medicine and Public Health, 24*, 11–17.

Prelli, F., and Frangione, B. (1992). Franklin's disease. Ig gamma 2 H chain mutant BUR. *Journal of Immunology, 148*, 949–952.

Presti, B. C., Scioto, C. G., and Marsh, S. G. (1990). Lymphocytic lymphoma with associated gamma heavy chain and IgM-lambda paraproteins. An unusual biclonal gammopathy. *American Journal of Clinical Pathology, 93*, 137–141.

Preud'homme, J. L., Aucouturier, P., Touchard, G., Khamlichi, A. A., Rocca, A., Denoroy, L., and Cogné, M. (1994a). Monoclonal immunoglobulin deposition disease. A review of immunoglobulin chain alterations. *International Journal of Immunopharmacology, 16*, 425–431.

Preud'homme, J. L., Aucouturier, P., Touchard, G., Striker, L., Khamlichi, A. A., Rocca, A., Denoroy, L., and Cogné, M. (1994b). Monoclonal immunoglobulin deposition disease (Randall type). Relationship with structural abnormalities of immunoglobulin chains. *Kidney International, 46*, 965–972.

Preud'homme, J. L., Bauwens, M., Dumont, G., Goujon, J. M., Dreyfus, B., and Touchard, G. (1997). Cast nephropathy in mu heavy chain disease. *Clinical Nephrology, 48*, 118–121.

Preud'homme, J. L., Brouet, J. C., and Seligmann, M. (1979). Cellular immunoglobulins in human gamma- and alpha-heavy chain diseases. *Clinical and Experimental Immunology, 37*, 283–291.

Prévot, P., Loyau, G., Heron, J. P., Hirondel, J. L., Chaix, G., Laniece, M., Broulet, J. L., Danon, F., and Seligmann, M. (1977). Gamma heavy chain disease. A recent case with plasmocytic proliferation and cranial lacunae [French]. *Annales De Medecine Interne (Paris), 128*, 151–157.

Price, S. K. (1990). Immunoproliferative small intestinal disease. A study of 13 cases with alpha heavy-chain disease. *Histopathology, 17*, 7–17.

Pruzanski, W., Hasselback, R., Katz, A., and Parr, D. M. (1978). Multiple myeloma (light chain disease) with rheumatoid-like amyloid arthropathy and mu-heavy chain fragment in the serum. *American Journal of Medicine, 65*, 334–341.

Pruzanski, W., Parr, D. M., Prchal, J., and Chan, E. Y. (1979). Gamma 3-heavy-chain disease (gamma 3-HCD) in a young patient with Down syndrome. Study of peripheral blood lymphocytes and of susceptibility to infection. *Clinical Immunology and Immunopathology, 12*, 253–262.

Rabhi, H., Ghaffor, M., and Abbadi, M. C. (1989a). Spontaneous enzymatic cleavage of IgD myeloma protein giving a pattern of delta heavy chain disease. *Archives de l'Institut Pasteur d'Algerie, 57*, 135–140.

Rabhi, H., Ghaffor, M., Abbadi, M. C., Boucekkine, T., and Illoul, G. (1988). Abnormal protein hyposecretion in early and late course of alpha chain disease. *Archives de l'Institut Pasteur d'Algerie, 56*, 187–195.

Rabhi, H., Ghaffor, M., Benhalima-Bouali, M., and Abbadi, M. C. (1989b). Cells expressing intracytoplasmic immunoglobulins in secreting and hyposecreting cases of alpha chain disease. *Archives de l'Institut Pasteur d'Algerie, 57*, 125–134.

Rabin, B. S., and Moon, J. (1973). Clinical findings in a case of newly defined gamma heavy chain disease protein. *Clinical and Experimental Immunology, 14*, 563–568.

Rambaud, J. C., Galian, A., Danon, F. G., Preud'homme, J. L., Brandtzaeg, P., Wassef, M., Le Carrer, M., Mehaut, M. A., Voinchet, O. L., Perol, R. G., and Chapman, A. (1983). Alpha-chain disease without qualitative serum IgA abnormality. Report of two cases, including a "nonsecretory" form. *Cancer, 51*, 686–693.

Rambaud, J. C., Galian, A., Matuchansky, C., Danon, F., Preud'Homme, J. L., Brouet, J. C., and Seligmann, M. (1978). Natural history of alpha-chain disease and the so-called Mediterranean lymphoma. *Recent Results of Cancer Research, 64*, 271–276.

Rambaud, J. C., and Halphen, M. (1989). Immunoproliferative small intestinal disease (IPSID). Relationships with alpha-chain disease and "Mediterranean" lymphomas. *Gastroenterology International, 2*, 33–41.

Rambaud, J. C., Halphen, M., Galian, A., and Tsapis, A. (1990). Immunoproliferative small intestinal disease (IPSID). Relationships with alpha-chain disease and "Mediterranean" lymphomas. *Springer Seminars in Immunopathy, 12*, 239–250.

Rambaud, J. C., and Matuchansky, C. (1973). Alpha-chain disease. Pathogenesis and relation to Mediterranean lymphoma. *Lancet, 1*, 1430–1432.

Rambaud, J. C., and Seligmann, M. (1976). Alpha-chain disease. *Clinical Gastroenterology, 5*, 341–358.

Ramot, B., and Rechavi, G. (1992). Non-Hodgkin's lymphomas and paraproteinaemias. *Baillieres Clinical Haematology, 5*, 81–99.

Rhodes, J. M., Jewell, D. P., and Janossy, G. (1980). Alpha-chain disease diagnosed by rectal biopsy. *British Medical Journal, 280*, 1043–1044.

Roda, L., David, M. J., Biron, P., Souche, S., and Creyssel, R. (1985a). Gamma heavy chain disease DUB. Clinical, immunochemical and pathological studies. *Haematologica, 70*, 232–235.

Roda, L., David, M. J., Souche, S., Coiffier, B., and Creyssel, R. (1985b). Gamma 3 heavy chain disease and monoclonal IgMκ in a patient with a gastrointestinal lymphoma. *Haematologica, 70*, 115–119.

Rodriguez Gomez, S. J., Jaras Hernandez, M. J., Sanchez Molini, P., and Jimenez Alonso, I. (1994). Immunoproliferative disease of the small intestine, associated with IgA kappa monoclonal gammapathy with good clinical and histologic response to the treatment with tetracyclines [Spanish]. *Anales de Medicina Interna, 11*, 566–567.

Rott, T., Vizjak, A., Lindic, J., Hvala, A., Perkovic, T., and Cernelc, P. (1998). IgG heavy-chain deposition disease affecting kidney, skin, and skeletal muscle. *Nephrology Dialysis Transplantation, 13*, 1825–1828.

Rouesse, J., Gerard-Marchant, R., Chevalier, A., and Seligmann, M. (1972). Gamma heavy chain disease with thyroid involvement [French]. *Rev Eur Etud Clin Biol, 17*, 405–411.

Rouhier, D., Andre, C., Allard, C., Gillon, J., and Brette, R. (1982). Malignant alpha chain disease and exposure to asbestos. *Environmental Research, 27*, 222–225.

Roussel, P., Dautrevaux, M., and Rousseaux, J. (1974). Biochemical study of a case of heavy mu chain disease [French]. *Lille Medical, 19*, 131–133.

Ruiz-Arguelles, A., Valls-de-Ruiz, M., Dominguez-Barranco, A., Ruiz-Arguelles, G., and Ruiz-Reyes, G. (1984). 'Incomplete' pyroglobulin-gamma disease in a patient with osteosclerotic myeloma. *Scandinavian Journal of Haematology, 33*, 351–355.

Sakka, T., Meknini, B., Ayed, K., Ben Jilani, S., Ben Maiz, H., Ben Moussa, F., Ben Mami, N., and Derouiche, N. (1986). An unusual case of heavy alpha chain disease associated with amyloidosis [French]. *Tunisie Medicale, 64*, 161–164.

Sala, P., Tonutti, E., Mazzolini, S., Antonutto, G., and Bramezza, M. (1983). Alpha-heavy chain disease. Report of a case with spontaneous regression. *Scandinavian Journal of Haematology, 31*, 149–154.

Salimi, M., and Spinelli, J. J. (1996). Chemotherapy of Mediterranean abdominal lymphoma. Retrospective comparison of chemotherapy protocols in Iranian patients. *American Journal of Clinical Oncology, 19*, 18–22.

Savilahti, E., Brandtzaeg, P., and Kuitunen, P. (1980). Atypical intestinal alpha-chain disease evolving into selective immunoglobulin A deficiency in a Finnish boy. *Gastroenterology, 79*, 1303–1310.

Schur, P. H. (1972). Human gamma-g subclasses. *Progress in Clinical Immunology, 1*, 71–104.

Seligmann, M. (1975). Immunochemical, clinical, and pathological features of alpha-chain disease. *Archives of Internal Medicine, 135*, 78–82.

Seligmann, M. (1993). Heavy chain diseases [French]. *Rev Prat, 43*, 317–320.

Seligmann, M., Danon, F., Hurez, D., Mihaesco, E., and Preud'homme, J. L. (1968). Alpha-chain disease. A new immunoglobulin abnormality. *Science, 162*, 1396–1397.

Seligmann, M., Mihaesco, E., Hurez, D., Mihaesco, C., Preud'homme, J. L., and Rambaud, J. C. (1969). Immunochemical studies in four cases of alpha chain disease. *Journal of Clinical Investigation, 48*, 2374–2389.

Seligmann, M., Mihaesco, E., Preud'homme, J. L., Danon, F., and Brouet, J. C. (1979). Heavy chain diseases. Current findings and concepts. *Immunology Review, 48*, 145–167.

Seligmann, M., and Rambaud, J.-C. (1978). α-Chain disease. A possible model for the pathogenesis of human lymphomas. In J. J. Twomey, and R. A. Good (Eds.), *The Immunopathology of Lymphoreticular Neoplasms. Comprehensive Immunology*, vol 4 (p. 425). New York: Plenum Medical Book Co.

Selzer, G., Sacks, M., Sherman, G., and Naggan, L. (1979). Primary malignant lymphoma of the small intestine in Israel. Changing incidence with time. *Israeli Journal of Medical Science, 15*, 390–396.

Shih, L. Y., Liaw, S. J., Dunn, P., and Kuo, T. T. (1994). Primary small-intestinal lymphomas in Taiwan. Immunoproliferative small-intestinal disease and nonimmunoproliferative small-intestinal disease. *Journal of Clinical Oncology, 12*, 1375–1382.

Shirakura, T., Kobayashi, Y., Murai, Y., Inoue, T., and Imamura, Y. (1976). A case of gamma heavy chain disease associated with autoimmune haemolytic anaemia. Clinical, haematological, immunological and pathological details. *Scandinavian Journal of Haematology, 16,* 387–393.

Silva-Moreno, M., Ruiz-Arguelles, G. J., Lopez-Karpovitch, X., and Labardini-Mendez, J. (1983). Heavy chain disease. Report of four cases [Spanish]. *Sangre, 28,* 89–98.

Smith, L. L., Barton, B. P., Garver, F. A., Chang, L. S., McGuire, B., Faguet, G. B., and Lutcher, C. L. (1978). Physicochemical and immunochemical properties of gamma 1 heavy chain disease protein BAZ. *Immunochemistry, 15,* 323–329.

Smith, W. J., Price, S. K., and Isaacson, P. G. (1987). Immunoglobulin gene rearrangement in immunoproliferative small intestinal disease (IPSID). *Journal of Clinical Pathology, 40,* 1291–1297.

Solling, K., and Askjaer, S. A. (1973). Multiple myeloma with urinary excretion of heavy chain components of IgG and nodular glomerulosclerosis. *Acta Medica Scandinavica, 1–2,* 23–30.

Solomon, A., Weiss, D. T., and Murphy, C. (1994). Primary amyloidosis associated with a novel heavy-chain fragment (AH amyloidosis). *American Journal of Hematology, 45,* 171–176.

Sopeña, F., Lopez Zaborras, J., Nerin, J. M., Soria, J., Sousa, F. L., and Freile, E. (1992). Deficiency polyneuropathy secondary to immunoproliferative disease of the small intestine [Spanish]. *Revista Española de Enfermedades Digestivas, 82,* 423–426.

Spencer, J., and Isaacson, P. G. (1987). Immunology of gastrointestinal lymphoma. *Baillieres Clinical Gastroenterology, 1,* 605–621.

Stoop, J. W., Ballieux, R. E., Hijmans, W., and Zegers, B. J. (1971). Alpha-chain disease with involvement of the respiratory tract in a Dutch child. *Clinical and Experimental Immunology, 9,* 625–635.

Strom, E. H., Fogazzi, G. B., Banfi, G., Pozzi, C., and Mihatsch, M. J. (1994). Light chain deposition disease of the kidney. Morphological aspects in 24 patients. *Virchows Archiv-An International Journal of Pathology, 425,* 271–280.

Stühlinger, W., Berek, K., Lapin, A., Jaschke, E., and Pastner, D. (1987). Gamma 1 heavy chain disease with immune vasculitis and rheumatoid arthritis [German]. *Klinische Wochenschrift, 65,* 359–368.

Sun, T., Peng, S., and Narurkar, L. (1994). Modified immunoselection technique for definitive diagnosis of heavy-chain disease. *Clinical Chemistry, 40,* 664.

Tabbane, F., Mourali, N., Cammoun, M., and Najjar, T. (1988). Results of laparotomy in immunoproliferative small intestinal disease. *Cancer, 61,* 1699–1706.

Tabbane, S., Tabbane, F., Cammoun, M., and Mourali, N. (1976). Mediterranean lymphomas with alpha heavy chain monoclonal gammopathy. *Cancer, 38,* 1989–1996.

Takahashi, K., Naito, M., Matsuoka, Y., and Takatsuki, K. (1988). A new form of alpha-chain disease with generalized lymph node involvement. *Pathology Research and Practice, 183,* 717–723.

Tangun, Y., Saracbasi, Z., Inceman, S., Danon, F., and Seligmann, M. (1975). IgA myeloma globulin and Bence Jones proteinuria in diffuse plasmacytoma of small intestine [Letter]. *Annals of Internal Medicine, 83,* 673.

Tashiro, T., Sato, H., Takahashi, T., Genda, T., Sugitani, S., Yoshida, T., Funakoshi, K., Tukada, Y., Narisawa, R., Nomoto, M., Kamimura, T., Asakura, H., Ohta, T., and Watanabe, H. (1995). Non-secretory alpha chain disease involving stomach, small intestine and colon. *Internal Medicine, 34,* 255–260.

Teng, M. H., Rosen, S., Gorny, M. K., Alexander, A., and Buxbaum, J. (2000). Gamma heavy chain disease in man. Independent structural abnormalities and reduced transcription of a functionally rearranged lambda L-chain gene result in the absence of L-chains. *Blood Cells, Molecules and Diseases, 26,* 177–185.

Terry, W. D., and Ohms, J. (1970). Implications of heavy chain disease protein sequences for multiple gene theories of immuno-globulin synthesis. *Proceedings of the National Academy of Sciences of the United States of America, 66,* 558–563.

Tezuka, T., Hirai, R., Takahashi, M., Furuta, I., Ohba, Y., Tsubaki, K., and Horiuchi, A. (1986). Alpha-heavy-chain disease with erythematous skin lesions. *Archives of Dermatology, 122,* 1243–1244.

Tissot, J. D., Tridon, A., Ruivard, M., Layer, A., Henry, H., Philippe, P., and Schneider, P. (1998). Electrophoretic analyses in a case of monoclonal gamma chain disease. *Electrophoresis, 19,* 1771–1773.

Tracy, R. P., Kyle, R. A., and Leitch, J. M. (1984a). Alpha heavy-chain disease presenting as goiter. *American Journal of Clinical Pathology, 82,* 336–339.

Tracy, R. P., Kyle, R. A., and Young, D. S. (1984b). Two-dimensional gel electrophoresis as an aid in the analysis of monoclonal gammopathies. *Human Pathology, 15,* 122–129.

Tsapis, A., Bentaboulet, M., Pellet, P., Mihaesco, E., Thierry, D., Seligmann, M., and Brouet, J. C. (1989). The productive gene for alpha-H chain disease protein MAL is highly modified by insertion-deletion processes. *Journal of Immunology, 143,* 3821–3827.

Tubbs, R. R., Berkley, V., Valenzuela, R., McMahon, J. T., Gephardt, G. N., Fishleder, A. J., Nally, J. V., Pohl, M. A., Bukowski, R. M., and Lichtin, A. E. (1992). Pseudo-gamma heavy chain (IgG4 lambda) deposition disease. *Modern Pathology, 5,* 185–190.

Tungekar, M. F., Omar, Y. T., and Behbehani, K. (1987). Gastric alpha heavy chain disease. *Oncology, 44,* 360–366.

Ullrich, R., Zeitz, M., Heise, W., L'Age, M., Hoffken, G., and Riecken, E. O. (1989). Small intestinal structure and function in patients infected with human immunodeficiency virus (HIV). Evidence for HIV-induced enteropathy. *Annals of Internal Medicine, 111,* 15–21.

Van Bergeijk, L., Biewenga, J., and Langenhuijsen, M. M. (1980). Gamma heavy chain disease with an unusually benign course. *Clinical Laboratory Haematology, 2,* 83–88.

van Camp, B. G., Shuit, H. R., Hijmans, W., and Radl, J. (1978). The cellular basis of double paraproteinemia in man. *Clinical Immunology and Immunopathology, 9,* 111–119.

Vilpo, J. A., Irjala, K., Viljanen, M. K., Klemi, P., Kouvonen, I., and Ronnemaa, T. (1980). Delta-heavy chain disease. A study of a case. *Clinical Immunology and Immunopathology, 17,* 584–594.

Virella, G., Monteiro, J. M., Lopes-Virella, M. F., Ducla Soares, A., and Fudenberg, H. H. (1977). Asynchronous development of two monoclonal proteins (IgM lambda and delta 1 chains) in a patient with abdominal lymphoma. *Cancer, 39,* 2247–2253.

Wager, O., Rasanen, J. A., Lindeberg, L., and Makela, V. (1969). Two cases of IgG heavy-chain disease. *Acta Pathologica Microbiologica Scandinavica, 75,* 350–352.

Wahner-Roedler, D. L., and Kyle, R. A. (1992). Mu-heavy chain disease. Presentation as a benign monoclonal gammopathy. *American Journal of Hematology, 40,* 56–60.

Wahner-Roedler, D. L., Witzig, T. E., Loehrer, L. L., and Kyle, R. A. (2003) Gamma heavy chain disease. The Mayo Clinic experience. Review of 23 cases, *Medicine, 82,* 236–250.

Wang, A. C., Arnaud, P., Fudenberg, H. H., and Creyssel, R. (1978). Monoclonal IgM cryoglobulinemia associated with gamma-3 heavy chain disease. Immunochemical and biochemical studies. *European Journal of Immunology, 8,* 375–379.

Wester, S. M., Banks, P. M., and Li, C. Y. (1982). The histopathology of gamma heavy-chain disease. *American Journal of Clinical Pathology, 78,* 427–436.

Westin, J., Eyrich, R., Falsen, E., Lindholm, L., Lundin, P., Lonnroth, I., and Weinfeld, A. (1972). Gamma heavy chain disease. Reports of three patients. *Acta Medica Scandinavica, 192,* 281–292.

Wetter, O., Schmidt, C. G., Linder, K. H., and Leene, W. (1979). Heavy chain disease. Humoral and cellular findings in six patients with mu chain disease [author's translation; German]. *Journal of Cancer Research and Clinical Oncology, 94,* 207–223.

Witzens, M., Egerer, G., Stahl, D., Werle, E., Goldschmidt, H., and Haas, R. (1998). A case of mu heavy-chain disease associated with hyperglobulinemia, anemia, and a positive Coombs test. *Annals of Hematology, 77*, 231–234.

Wolfenstein-Todel, C., Frangione, B., Prelli, F., and Franklin, E. C. (1976). The amino acid sequence of "heavy chain disease" protein ZUC. Structure of the Fc fragment of immunoglobulin G3. *Biochemical and Biophysical Research Communications, 71*, 907–914.

Wolfenstein-Todel, C., Mihaesco, E., and Frangione, B. (1974). "Alpha chain disease" protein def. Internal deletion of a human immunoglobulin A1 heavy chain. *Proceedings of the National Academy of Sciences of the United States of America, 71*, 974–978.

Wolfenstein-Todel, C., Mihaesco, E., and Frangione, B. (1975). Variant of a human immunoglobulin. "Alpha chain disease" protein AIT. *Biochemical and Biophysical Research Communications, 65*, 47–53.

Woods, R., Glumenshein, G. R., and Terry, W. D. (1970). A new type of human gamma heavy chain disease protein. Immunochemical and physical characteristics. *Immunochemistry, 7*, 373–381.

Yasuda, T., Fujita, K., Imai, H., Morita, K., Nakamoto, Y., and Miura, A. B. (1995). Gamma-heavy chain deposition disease showing nodular glomerulosclerosis. *Clinical Nephrology, 44*, 394–399.

Zahner, J., Kirchner, T., Ott, G., and Schneider, W. (1994). Immunoproliferative small intestinal disease (IPSID). An unusual form of gastrointestinal lymphoma [German]. *Schweizerische Medizinische Wochenschrift. Journal Suisse de Medecine, 124*, 1227–1231.

Zamir, A., Parasher, G., Moukarzel, A. A., Guarini, L., Zeien, L., and Feldman, F. (1998). Immunoproliferative small intestinal disease in a 16-year-old boy presenting as severe malabsorption with excellent response to tetracycline treatment. *Journal of Clinical Gastroenterology, 27*, 85–89.

Zawadzki, Z. A., Benedek, T. G., Ein, D., and Easton, J. M. (1969). Rheumatoid arthritis terminating in heavy-chain disease. *Annals of Internal Medicine, 70*, 335–347.

# CHAPTER 23

# Waldenström's Macroglobulinemia

## ROBERT A. KYLE
## RAFAEL FONSECA

## Introduction

In 1944, Waldenström described 2 patients with oronasal bleeding, severe normocytic normochromic anemia, excessive erythrocyte sedimentation, lymphadenopathy, and low serum fibrinogen values. Both had an abnormally large amount of a homogeneous gamma globulin with a sedimentation coefficient of 19S to 20S, corresponding to a molecular weight of more than 1,000,000. Both had a high serum viscosity, and in one patient the serum gelled at low temperatures. (The description of a third patient does not permit a definite diagnosis of macroglobulinemia.) Subsequently, the serum globulin was identified as an immunoglobulin and was designated IgM. As an entity, macroglobulinemia bears similarities to multiple myeloma, lymphoma, and chronic lymphocytic leukemia (Ries, 1988). The basic abnormality in macroglobulinemia is the proliferation of cells with lymphocyte and plasma cell characteristics producing a large IgM monoclonal protein.

Macroglobulinemia is characterized by the proliferation of B lymphocytes that produce an IgM monoclonal protein. This broad definition includes persons with monoclonal gammopathy of undetermined significance (MGUS), chronic lymphocytic leukemia (CLL), lymphoma (LY), primary amyloidosis (AL), and Waldenström's macroglobulinemia (WM). We have previously defined WM as a malignant B cell proliferative disorder with an IgM monoclonal protein value of

3 g/dL or more. However, in a review of 430 patients with an IgM monoclonal gammopathy, we defined WM as an IgM monoclonal protein value of 3.0 g/dL or more and an increase in lymphocytes or plasmacytoid lymphocytes in the bone marrow; LY as lymphadenopathy or an extranodal lymphoid tumor and biopsy findings consistent with LY; CLL as more than 9000 lymphocytes/mm$^3$ in a peripheral blood specimen; AL as histologic proof of amyloid in a biopsy specimen; MGUS as an IgM monoclonal protein value of less than 3 g/dL, no constitutional symptoms, no hepatosplenomegaly or lymphadenopathy, no anemia, and no need for therapy; and malignant lymphoproliferative disease (LP), which would not be classified in the other categories (Kyle and Garton, 1987). Patients with LP had an IgM protein value of less than 3 g/dL, usually had bone marrow infiltration with lymphocytes or plasmacytoid lymphocytes, and required therapy because of anemia or constitutional symptoms. No difference in survival or other features, except the size of the monoclonal protein and hyperviscosity in WM, differentiated LP from WM. Consequently, no rationale exists for separation of these entities, and LP and WM can be combined in future prospective studies. The presence of a monoclonal protein does not alter the clinical picture or course of CLL, LY, or AL. WM has been reviewed (Dimopoulos and Alexanian, 1994).

## Etiology

The cause of macroglobulinemia is unknown, but this condition has been reported in several families. In one, 2 brothers had macroglobulinemia with a very similar clinical picture and protein abnormality; the serum from their mother also showed a narrow band on electrophoresis and increased IgM with immunoelectrophoresis (Massari et al., 1962). In another report, a patient with an IgM spike of 2.73 g/dL, and his father, with a globulin value of 7.6 g/dL, both had symptomatic macroglobulinemia (Gétaz and Staples, 1977). Blattner and associates (1980) described a father and 2 children with an IgM monoclonal protein and a lymphoproliferative process and a third child with WM. All had HLA haplotype A2, B8, and DRw3, as well as the B cell alloantigens Ia-172 and 350. WM has also been reported in monozygotic twins (Fine et al., 1986). Four brothers, all with an IgM monoclonal protein in the serum, had WM, MGUS, MGUS with peripheral neuropathy, or primary amyloidosis. The 4 brothers did not share a common HLA-A, -B, or -DR haplotype; a genetic linkage to the HLA complex could not be ascertained. Five of 12 relatives had increased serum immunoglobulin levels; 2 were IgM (Renier et al., 1989). In another family, 2 sisters had an IgM monoclonal protein and a symptomatic lymphoproliferative

process. Four siblings had an increased IgM concentration but no monoclonal component (Taleb et al., 1991). Two studies of relatives of other patients with WM revealed an increased frequency of IgM monoclonal proteins and quantitative abnormalities (Kalff and Hijmans, 1969; Seligmann et al., 1967). Thus, there is a genetic influence in some families.

Although radiation can cause acute leukemia, there is only one reported case of WM occurring after radiotherapy, which was given for ankylosing spondylitis (Epenetos et al., 1980). However, the long duration of 29 years between radiation and macroglobulinemia raises serious doubts about the relationship.

Occupational exposure may play a role in a few cases. Williamson et al. (1989) reported 3 patients with overt macroglobulinemia who had worked for more than 40 years in a family shoe repair business and had been exposed to leather, rubber adhesives, dyes, and paints. Another patient with an interstitial pulmonary infiltrate consisting of foamy histiocytes, lymphocytes, plasma cells, and mast cells had an IgM monoclonal protein value of 2.6 g/dL and bone marrow containing a lymphoplasmacytic infiltration. He had been exposed to a canary and its droppings. The patient's IgM monoclonal protein was purified and produced a precipitin line on Ouchterlony double immunodiffusion against canary droppings, a finding raising the possibility of a relationship between the patient's disease and his exposure to the canary (James et al., 1987).

In a case-control study of 65 cases of WM compared with 213 hospital control subjects, there were no differences in sociodemographic factors, prior medical conditions, medication use, cigarette smoking, alcohol consumption, specific occupational exposures, employment in any particular industry or occupation, or familial cancer history. Two relatives had MGUS. Almost 40% of family members had diverse immunologic abnormalities (Linet et al., 1993).

## Chromosome Abnormalities

Various chromosome abnormalities have been reported in WM, but no specific changes have been recognized. Carbone et al. (1992) noted clonal chromosome changes in 10 of 17 patients. In another series, 17 of 19 patients (89%) had clonal chromosome abnormalities. The chromosome number ranged from 40 to 50. It was impossible to identify the primary chromosome abnormalities because many patients were studied late in the course of their disease (Palka et al., 1987). An isochromosome (6p) was reported in most metaphases in 2 cases of macroglobulinemia (White et al., 1992). Sister chromatid exchange was reported in all 12 patients with WM in one study (Carbone et al., 1993). The frequency of sister chromatid exchange was significantly increased in phytohemagglutinin-stimulated cultures. Abnormal cytogenetic findings correlated with a poor prognosis in 37 cases (Mansoor et al., 2001).

Translocations of the IgH locus occasionally have been described in multiple myeloma, but they do not seem to play a predominant role in the pathogenesis of WM. A Burkitt's lymphoma-like translocation (t[8;14] [q24.1;q32]) has been reported (Chong et al., 1998). A t(9;14) p13 q32 has been reported in approximately half of patients with lymphoplasmacytic lymphoma without paraproteinemia. In our series of 74 patients with documented WM, we did not find any patients with t(9;14), t(11;18), or other translocations involving the immunoglobulin heavy-gene locus. The most common abnormality was deletion of 6q21, which was found in 42% of patients (Schop et al., 2002b). We have noted that patients with macroglobulinemia who have 17p13.1 (p53) deletions have a higher percentage of involvement of clonal cells in the bone marrow (Schop et al., 2002a). None of 11 patients with WM had detectable interleukin (IL)-1β expression, whereas 2 patients with IgM multiple myeloma expressed IL-1β mRNA at high levels (Donovan et al., 2002). The presence of a 14q+ marker and a complex karyotype was reported in one patient with a short survival (Cigudosa et al., 1994).

# Clinical Findings

## Incidence, Age, and Sex

An incidence rate of 0.61 per 100,000 in white men and 0.25 per 100,000 in white women has been reported (Herrinton and Weiss, 1993). In a study from the United States, the incidence of WM was 0.3 per 100,000 in white men and 0.17 per 100,000 in white women; approximately 1400 new cases occur in the United States each year (Groves et al., 1998). The incidence increased markedly with age, from 0.1 at less than 45 years to 36.3 per 100,000 at age 75 years or older for males. There was no change in rates over the 7-year study. The rates were higher in whites than blacks in contrast to multiple myeloma (Groves et al., 1998). However, 5 cases of macroglobulinemia have been reported in young black adults (Ahmed et al., 1999). WM and LP occur approximately one-sixth as often as multiple myeloma (MM) in our practice. The median age in our series of 71 patients was 63 years (range, 30–89 y) (Kyle and Garton, 1987). It rarely occurs before the age of 40 years, and approximately 60% of patients are male.

## Clinical Symptoms

The onset is usually insidious and characterized by weakness and fatigue. Bleeding in the oronasal area is not uncommon. Blurring or other impairment of vision may be a major symptom (Hanlon et al., 1958; Martin, 1968). In a series of 260 patients with macroglobulinemia, fatigue was present in 85%, bleeding in 60%, and neurologic symptoms in 17% (MacKenzie, 1996). Recurrent infections, dyspnea, congestive heart failure, loss of weight, and neurologic symptoms occur. In contrast to MM, bone pain is rare.

## Physical Findings

Pallor is a frequent finding. Hepatomegaly occurs in approximately one-fourth of patients at diagnosis, whereas splenomegaly and lymphadenopathy are slightly less frequent. Retinal lesions, including hemorrhages, exudates, and venous congestion with vascular segmentation ("sausage" formation), may be impressive (Fig. 23-1). These findings might also result from

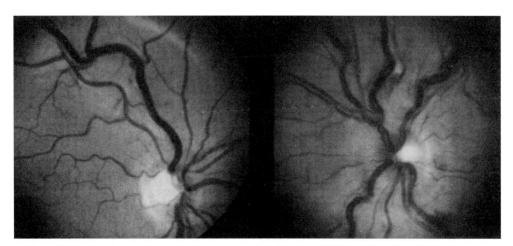

***Figure 23-1*** *Ocular fundi of patient with macroglobulinemia of Waldenström. (From Kyle, R. A., and Bayrd, E. D. (1976). The Monoclonal Gammopathies: Multiple Myeloma and Related Plasma-Cell Disorders [p. 200]. Springfield, IL: Charles C Thomas Publishers. With permission of the publisher.)*

hyperviscosity from other causes. Purpura and gross bleeding may also occur.

## Laboratory Findings

Anemia is found in most patients with symptomatic macroglobulinemia. The anemia is caused by inadequate red cell synthesis, decreased erythrocyte survival, and iron deficiency (Cline et al., 1963). Anemia (hemoglobin <10 g/dL) has been reported in 27% to 38% of patients (Facon et al., 1993; Garcia-Sanz et al., 2001). Increased viscosity may reduce erythropoietin production and contribute to the anemia of macroglobulinemia (Singh et al., 1993). Autoimmune hemolytic anemia may occur. Coombs'-positive hemolytic anemia was reported in 16% of 57 patients with WM (Jønsson et al., 1999). Increased plasma volume is a frequent finding (MacKenzie et al., 1970) and is responsible for spuriously low hemoglobin and hematocrit levels. Thus, the anemia is often more apparent than real. Rouleaux formation is striking, and the erythrocyte sedimentation is usually greatly increased. The leukocyte count is usually normal, but lymphocytosis or monocytosis is not uncommon. Thrombocytopenia may be present initially, but the platelet count is rarely less than $50,000/mm^3$. Serum cholesterol levels are frequently very low. Hyperuricemia may be present, but the serum creatinine value is almost always normal. Serum IL-6 levels have been reported as higher in patients with macroglobulinemia than in healthy control subjects. The value decreased with successful therapy (Hatzimichael et al., 2001).

## Serum and Urine Protein Abnormalities

The serum protein electrophoretic pattern is indistinguishable from that of MM, namely, a sharp, narrow spike or dense band almost always migrating in the γ area. In our series of 71 cases, the monoclonal protein value ranged from 3.0 to 7.9 g/dL (median, 4.3 g/dL) (Kyle and Garton, 1987). Seventy-five percent of the IgM proteins were κ. The IgM level is always increased. The value obtained by nephelometry may be 2000 or 3000 mg/dL more than that found in the serum protein electrophoretic spike. Consequently, one must measure the protein abnormality by the same technique during followup. The IgG level is reduced in approximately 60% of patients, and the IgA level is decreased in approximately 20% (Kyle and Garton, 1987). The reduction in uninvolved immunoglobulins is less striking than that in MM. The presence of an IgM monoclonal protein and its light-chain type must be determined by immunoelectrophoresis (Fig. 23-2) or immunofixation (Fig. 23-3). Macroglobulins may precipitate in the cold (cryoglobulins) or when heated (pyroglobulins) (Cagnoni et al., 1995).

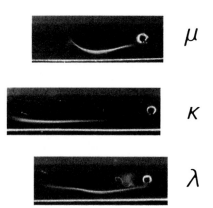

*Figure 23-2* Serum immunoelectrophoretic pattern. **Top:** Antiserum to IgM (μ) shows a thickened arc. **Middle:** Antiserum to κ chains shows a normal-appearing arc. **Bottom:** Antiserum to λ light chains shows bowing corresponding to IgM arc. Patient's serum contains IgM λ protein. (From Kyle, R. A., and Garton, J. P. [1986]. Laboratory monitoring of myeloma proteins. Seminars in Oncol, 13, 310–317. With permission of W. B. Saunders.)

Bence Jones proteinuria is found in 70% to 80% of patients with immunoelectrophoresis or immunofixation of an appropriately concentrated urine specimen (Krajny and Pruzanski, 1976; Kyle and Garton, 1987).

## Bone Marrow Examination

The bone marrow aspirate is often hypocellular; however, the biopsy specimen is usually hypercellular and extensively infiltrated with lymphoid or plasmacytoid cells. The presence of Dutcher bodies (intranuclear

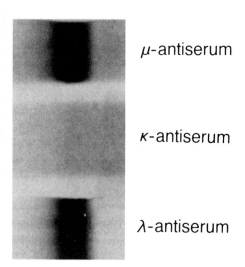

*Figure 23-3* Serum immunofixation. **Top:** Dense, localized band with IgM (μ) antiserum. **Middle:** No band with κ antiserum. **Bottom:** Dense band with λ antiserum corresponding to IgM band. Patient has IgM λ monoclonal protein. (From Kyle, R. A., and Garton, J. P. [1986]. Laboratory monitoring of myeloma proteins. Seminars in Oncology, 13, 310–317. With permission of W. B. Saunders.)

vacuoles) is common in macroglobulinemia (Dutcher and Fahey, 1959). These inclusion bodies consist of the IgM monoclonal protein (Boyd, 1980).

The cells in macroglobulinemia are B cells with a low proliferative rate. The B cells express CD19, CD20, and CD22 and only one type of light chain (κ in approximately 75% of cases) (Jensen et al., 1991). CD9, CD10 (common acute lymphocytic leukemia antigen), and CD11-B also may be expressed. CD5 is expressed in 5% to 15% (Remstein et al., personal communication, September 2002). In a series of 111 cases of WM, bone marrow infiltration by small lymphocytes showed a diffuse pattern in 58%, interstitial in 32%, nodular in 6%, and paratrabecular in 4%. Ninety percent of the lymphocytes were CD19+, CD20+, CD5−, CD10−, and CD23− (Owen et al., 2001a). The number of plasma cells is usually greater than normal. Mast cells may be increased and could help differentiate macroglobulinemia from myeloma or lymphoma. Rywlin et al. (1975) were unable to establish a correlation between IgM levels and other histologic features in the bone marrow, including the presence of Dutcher bodies or periodic acid-Schiff-positive intravascular or extravascular material.

The presence of small lymphocytes, normal mature plasma cells, and transitional lymphoplasmacytic cells characteristic of WM does not always indicate the presence of macroglobulinemia. These morphologic findings may also be associated with the production of IgG or IgA monoclonal proteins (Tursz et al., 1977).

Lytic bone lesions are uncommon but have been reported in up to 20% of patients with macroglobulinemia (Vermess et al., 1972). Bone marrow morphology was not helpful in differentiating patients with lytic lesions from those without (Leb et al., 1977). In our experience, fewer than 5% of patients with typical WM have lytic bone lesions (Kyle and Garton, 1987).

## Pulmonary Involvement

WM may be manifested by diffuse pulmonary infiltrates, isolated masses, or pleural effusion. In a review of 20 patients with macroglobinemia, 5 had pulmonary involvement with multiple asymmetric nodular infiltrates in both lungs (in 4 patients) and unilateral pleural effusion (in 1 patient). The chest radiograph was abnormal in most cases. The major symptoms were cough and dyspnea. Infiltration of the lung, pleura, or hilar lymph nodes by lymphocytes and plasmacytoid cells is often seen. The natural course is one of progression (Winterbauer et al., 1974). The pulmonary manifestations often respond to alkylating agents or irradiation and do not seem to affect prognosis adversely (Rausch and Herion, 1980). Pulmonary involvement also has been reported in 2 patients with a large IgM serum protein but no evidence of bone marrow involvement (Kyrtsonis et al., 2001a). Plasma cell interstitial pneumonia has also been reported with macroglobulinemia (Essig et al., 1974).

## Renal Involvement

Renal insufficiency is uncommon in macroglobulinemia. Deposits of IgM on the endothelial aspect of the basement membrane may become large enough to occlude the capillary lumen and resemble thrombi. Morphologic appearance and the composition of these deposits suggest a passive deposition of circulating IgM. Infiltration of lymphocytes or plasmacytoid cells identical to those found in the bone marrow is frequent. Tubular casts, which are common in MM, are never seen (Morel-Maroger et al., 1970). Nephrotic syndrome is rare in WM, but when present it is usually caused by amyloidosis. However, 5 cases of non-amyloid nephrotic syndrome have been reported (Hory et al., 1987; Tsuji et al., 1990). Hyponatremia from inappropriate antidiuresis has been recognized in macroglobulinemia (Braden et al., 1986). Acute renal failure may be precipitated by dehydration in macroglobulinemia (Argani and Kipkie, 1964). Macroglobulinemia may be associated with a perirenal tumor. Lorigan et al. (1988) reported a patient who had macroglobulinemia (IgM κ monoclonal proteins 7.2 g/dL) with massive bilateral perirenal masses that consisted of a well-differentiated lymphocytic lymphoma.

## Gastrointestinal Tract

Diarrhea and steatorrhea are uncommon features of macroglobulinemia (Bedine et al., 1973; Cabrera et al., 1964; Koivisto et al., 1989; Tait et al., 1993). In many cases with intestinal involvement, deposits of an amorphous hyaline-like material appeared in the small intestine. A patient with such abnormalities and severe malabsorption had extracellular amorphous material in the lamina propria and in the dilated mucosal lymphatics of the upper duodenum and jejunum. The material was periodic acid-Schiff-positive and did not stain for amyloid. Immunofluorescence studies showed strong, specific staining for IgM and λ light chains, confirming the presence of a monoclonal immunoglobulin. Moderate numbers of plasma cells, small lymphocytes, and eosinophils were present in the deeper layers of the lamina propria (Pruzanski et al., 1973).

In another case, hyaline deposits consisting of IgM were found in the villi of the small bowel. There was no lymphoplasmacytic infiltration. The patient had diarrhea, but evidence of malabsorption was not well documented (Case records of the Massachusetts General Hospital, 1990). Deposits of monoclonal IgM or the infiltration of lymphocytes and plasma cells may be responsible for diarrhea and steatorrhea (Brandt et al., 1981). A patient with WM presented with a malabsorption syndrome. Examination of the intestinal villi revealed lymphangiectasia with dilated lymphatics containing a homogeneous eosinophilic material, presumably IgM λ (Tait et al., 1993). Obstructive jaundice caused by bleeding into the biliary tract has been reported in 2 patients with macroglobulinemia (Elias et al., 1972). Portal hypertension may result from infiltration of the portal tracts with lymphocytoid cells (Brooks, 1976).

Computed tomography scans of the abdomen may show retroperitoneal and mesenteric lymph nodes and splenomegaly and can be useful in following the course of macroglobulinemia (Aspelin et al., 1989). Moulopoulos et al. (1993) reported large nodes in 10 (43%) of 23 patients with WM studied by computed tomography. The retrocrural, retroperitoneal, iliac, and inguinal nodes were most commonly involved.

## Neurologic Abnormalities

Approximately 25% of patients with WM have neurologic abnormalities, including peripheral neuropathy, Guillain-Barré-like syndrome, encephalopathy, and subarachnoid hemorrhage (Logothetis et al., 1960). Cranial nerve palsies, mononeuropathy, and mononeuritis multiplex may result from infiltration of nerves by tumor cells, hyperviscosity, or a bleeding diathesis (Kelly et al., 1987). Often the neuropathy is a distal, symmetric, and slowly progressive sensorimotor process. The lower extremities are usually more involved than the upper ones.

Biopsy of the sural nerve reveals myelin degeneration but no significant infiltration by lymphocytes or plasma cells in most cases (Darnley, 1962; Dayan and Lewis, 1966). However, cellular infiltration of the nerve may occur (Vital et al., 1982). The incidence of peripheral neuropathy is higher if one relies on electrophysiologic tests rather than clinical manifestations. Anti-myelin-associated glycoprotein (anti-MAG) activity by the monoclonal IgM protein is found in approximately one-half of patients with a sensorimotor peripheral neuropathy. The IgM protein may also react with chondroitin sulfate and various gangliosides (Kelly et al., 1987). Sural nerve biopsies reveal demyelination and IgM deposits on the myelin sheath in many instances (Nobile-Orazio et al., 1987); however, it is impossible to determine whether the presence of IgM in the biopsy specimen is a causative factor or whether it represents passive deposition of IgM in an already damaged nerve.

Amyloid deposition in the nerve may be responsible for sensorimotor peripheral neuropathy. Peripheral neuropathy may progress and produce Charcot's joint (Scott et al., 1973). The presence of peripheral neuropathy in an older person should always bring the possibility of macroglobulinemia to mind because it may precede and dominate other manifestations of the disease.

Neurologic symptoms normally associated with hyperviscosity such as headache, dizziness, vertigo, ataxia, and altered consciousness as well as diplopia, seizures, and coma have been referred to as the Bing-Neel syndrome. Whether the first 2 patients described by Bing and Neel (1936) had macroglobulinemia is doubtful, but another patient that the authors thought to have CLL most likely had macroglobulinemia (Bichel et al., 1950).

Multifocal leukoencephalopathy has been reported in macroglobulinemia (Lyon et al., 1971; Scheithauer et al., 1984). Progressive spinal muscular atrophy responding to chlorambucil was described in one patient (Peters and Clatanoff, 1968). Sudden deafness, first in one ear and then in the other, was noted in a case of macroglobulinemia (Ruben et al., 1969). Six patients have been reported with hearing loss as a presenting symptom of macroglobulinemia (Syms et al., 2001). WM should be considered in the differential diagnosis of sudden sensorineural hearing loss or vestibular symptoms of sudden onset (Ronis et al., 1966). Hyperviscosity is the probable cause of hearing loss in macroglobulinemia. It is characterized by sudden onset of the cochlear type, and patients may benefit from plasmapheresis or alkylating agents (Wells et al., 1977).

Infiltration of the meninges by plasmacytoid lymphocytes has been noted in WM (Torrey and Katakkar, 1984). Shimizu et al. (1993) described a patient with well-documented WM who had confusion without hyperviscosity. Magnetic resonance imaging showed an area of abnormal intensity in the left frontal lobe, which on histologic examination consisted of small lymphocytes, lymphoplasmacytic cells, and mature plasma cells. The cells stained with IgM and λ antisera. Radiation produced a reduction in the size of the left frontal lobe tumor. In a subsequent report of apparently the same patient, she was doing well 3 years after radiation therapy (Imai et al., 1995). 2-Chlorodeoxyadenosine (2-CdA) produced a complete response in one patient with meningeal involvement (Richards, 1995). In 4 patients with macroglobulinemia, lower limb sensorimotor neuropathy developed from leptomeningeal and nerve root lymphoplasmacytoid infiltration (Abad et al., 1999). The presence of mental nerve neuropathy with IgM deposition on the myelin sheath has been seen (Klokkevold et al., 1989).

## Other Organ Involvement

Involvement of the orbit producing proptosis and reduced motility of the eye from a retro-orbital tumor consisting of lymphoid and plasmacytic cells was reported in a patient with long-standing WM (Ettl et al., 1992). Dry eyes may occur and may respond to chlorambucil and prednisone for WM (Cordido et al., 1995).

In a patient with WM, congestive heart failure subsequently developed from massive infiltration of plasmacytoid cells containing cytoplasmic IgM involving the right atrium and obstructing the tricuspid valve (Brawn et al., 1988). Deposition of IgM κ in the myocardium produced atrial flutter and progressive heart failure in a patient with WM. The echocardiogram showed a restrictive pattern suggestive of amyloidosis, but only a homogeneous interstitial material staining with IgM κ was found (Yowell and Hammond, 1994).

## Bleeding Diathesis

A bleeding diathesis in macroglobulinemia is common. Perkins et al. (1970) reported bleeding in 5 of 14 patients and stressed prolongation of the bleeding time; abnormalities in platelet adhesiveness, prothrombin time, and thromboplastin generation; and decreased levels of factor VIII. Abnormalities of platelet function are most important. Abnormal bleeding times, platelet adhesiveness, or interference with the capacity to release platelet factor III may play a role (Rozenberg and Dintenfass, 1965). In one case, the IgM λ protein (5.4 g/dL) exhibited specific activity against factor VIII, thus producing a hemophilia-like condition (Castaldi and Penney, 1970). Hyperviscosity is an important factor in bleeding and probably exerts its effect from abnormalities of platelet function. Thrombocytopenia from marrow infiltration is a contributing factor in some instances. In one case of macroglobulinemia, the monoclonal IgM protein exhibited antiplatelet activity. The patient had significant thrombocytopenia and petechiae (Varticovski et al., 1987).

## Dermatologic Involvement

The presence of an IgM monoclonal protein and erythematous urticarial skin lesions (Schnitzler's syndrome) has been reported (Schnitzler et al., 1974). Many of the more than 20 reported patients have not fulfilled the complete criteria for WM. One patient with biclonal gammopathy (IgM κ, 3.1 g/dL; IgA λ) had pseudoxanthoma elasticum in addition to urticaria (Machet et al., 1992). Rarely, cold urticaria is the presenting symptom (Török et al., 1993).

Infiltration of the dermis with malignant lymphoplasmacytoid cells producing papulonodular and macular lesions analogous to lymphoma and leukemia cutis may be seen (Bergroth et al., 1981). An IgM monoclonal protein may be deposited in the skin and produce pruritic papules. In one case, the circulating IgM κ protein expressed anti-epidermal basement membrane zone antibody. The deposition of IgM was associated with infiltration of mononuclear T cells and eosinophils but no B cells were seen (Cobb et al., 1992). In another case of macroglobulinemia, erythematous papules of the skin consisted of deposits of the M protein, which histologically resembled amyloid deposition (Lowe et al., 1992). In another case of typical WM, a solitary nodule of the skin developed that was recognized as a granulocytic sarcoma; myeloid leukemia subsequently developed (Choi et al., 1989).

## Infection

The incidence of infection in macroglobulinemia is twice that in normal persons (Fahey et al., 1963). Antibody production may be a factor, as suggested in one study in which IgM antibody production was decreased when stimulated by sheep cell stroma. Brucellin, which is a more potent antigen, produced antibodies (Pitts and McDuffie, 1967). *Pneumocystis carinii* and cytomegalic inclusion disease have been found in macroglobulinemia (Font and Zimmerman, 1970). Antibody response to pneumococcal antigen in macroglobulinemia is similar to that in controls, in contrast to patients with MM (Jacobson et al., 1988).

## Association with Other Diseases

WM has been reported in association with various other diseases. However, caution must be used in linking macroglobulinemia with any other entity unless one has an adequate control population to exclude a fortuitous association.

Rheumatoid arthritis (Gothoni et al., 1965), xanthomatosis and hypercholesterolemia (Petersen, 1973), xanthoma disseminatum (Goodenberger et al., 1990), polycythemia vera (Franzén et al., 1966), discoid lupus erythematosus, and CLL (Abdou and Abdou, 1975) have been reported to be associated with macroglobulinemia. Chronic calcific pancreatitis has been noted but the relationship is unclear (Hertan and Pitchumoni, 1991). α₁-Antitrypsin deficiency has been reported in WM (Sebastián Domingo and Nuñez Olarte, 1988). Another patient's monoclonal IgM protein actually bound thyroxine, resulting in hypothyroidism (Trimarchi et al., 1982).

An increased incidence of nonlymphoid malignancies has been seen. In one series, 8 of 40 patients with macroglobulinemia had carcinoma. In addition, 3 patients had basal cell carcinomas (MacKenzie and Fudenberg, 1972). In contrast, Yamaguchi (1973) found only one carcinoma (gastric) in 35 autopsy cases of macroglobulinemia. It is impossible to know whether the incidence of carcinoma is increased in macroglobulinemia. Two cases of Hodgkin's disease have been reported with Waldenström's macroglobulinemia; in one the conditions occurred simultaneously, and in the other Hodgkin's disease developed 15 years later (Rosales et al., 2001). Acute monocytic leukemia (FAB M5b) was reported in a patient with untreated Waldenström's macroglobulinemia (Murashige et al., 2002).

Primary systemic amyloidosis has been reported with WM (Cohen et al., 1966; Lindemalm et al., 1988; Stevens and Whitehouse, 1976). Fifty patients were reported to have an IgM monoclonal protein and systemic amyloidosis (Gertz et al., 1993). Six patients had an M-component of more than 3 g/dL. The bone marrow was consistent with WM in 10 cases, a plasma cell proliferative disorder in 10, and a lymphoproliferative process in 11. In the 8 patients studied, the amyloid deposits consisted of a monoclonal immunoglobulin light chain (Gertz et al., 1993).

Lin et al. (2001) reported the second case of myasthenia gravis and Waldenström's macroglobulinemia. The relationship between the 2 entities is not clear. Another autoimmune disease, thrombocytopenic purpura, was reported in 4 of 105 cases of macroglobulinemia (Owen et al., 2001b).

## Hyperviscosity

Although hyperviscosity of serum has been noted since 1929 (Bannick and Greene), its significance was little appreciated by clinicians until the review by Fahey et al. in 1965. Bleeding is the most common symptom. Chronic nasal bleeding and oozing from the gums are characteristic, and postsurgical or gastrointestinal bleeding may also occur. Patients may report blurring or loss of vision. Neurologic symptoms include dizziness, headaches, vertigo, nystagmus, loss of hearing, ataxia, paresthesias, or diplopia. Congestive heart failure may also occur. Somnolence, stupor, coma, and cerebral hemorrhage develop in some cases. Retinal vein engorgement and flame-shaped hemorrhages are common. Papilledema may also be present.

Serum viscosity should be determined when the IgM serum M-spike is more than 4 g/dL or in any patient with oronasal bleeding, blurred vision, or neurologic symptoms suggestive of hyperviscosity. The Ostwald-100 viscometer is a satisfactory instrument for this purpose, but a Wells-Brookfield viscometer (Brookfield Engineering Laboratories, Stoughton, MA) is preferred because it is more accurate, requires less serum (1 mL), and can perform at different shear rates and at variable temperatures. In addition, determinations can be made more rapidly, especially if the viscosity of the serum is high.

Although most patients have symptoms when the relative viscosity is more than 4 centipoise (cP), the relationship between serum viscosity and clinical manifestations is imprecise. Symptoms are rarely attributable to hyperviscosity when the relative viscosity is less than 4 cP (normal, 1.8 cP or less). Most patients have symptoms when the viscosity reaches 6 to 7 cP, but the authors have seen a patient with a serum viscosity of 15 cP but no symptoms or findings of hyperviscosity.

The viscosity-protein concentration curve for monoclonal IgM is nonlinear. At low serum IgM concentrations, the addition of 1 to 2 g/dL produces only a small increase in the serum viscosity, but at higher levels (4–5 g/dL), an increment of 1 to 2 g/dL greatly increases the relative viscosity (Fahey et al., 1965). The specific viscosity level at which clinical symptoms occur is probably affected not only by the serum protein concentration, molecular characteristics of the protein, or aggregation of protein molecules, but also by a combination of other factors, including the presence of disease involving the microvasculature, hematocrit level, cardiac status, local pH, and ionic strength (Bloch and Maki, 1973).

In our experience, the serum viscosity was more than 4.0 cP in 15 (29.4%) of 51 patients with WM. Surprisingly, 5 patients had no symptoms related to hyperviscosity. Nine of 15 patients had bleeding; this was manifested by epistaxis in 7 patients. Three patients had bleeding from the gums, and blurred vision occurred in 3 patients. The size of the monoclonal protein ranged from 4.3 to 8.0 g/dL (median, 5.5 g/dL) in the 15 patients who had a serum viscosity of more than 4.0 cP (Kyle and Garton, 1987). Crawford et al. (1985) reported that 6 of 8 patients with a serum viscosity of more than 5 cP had symptoms. None of their patients had symptoms of hyperviscosity if the level was less than 3 cP.

# Diagnosis of Macroglobulinemia

WM must be differentiated from multiple myeloma, lymphoma, CLL, undifferentiated lymphoproliferative disorders, and MGUS of the IgM type.

The diagnosis of macroglobulinemia depends on the presence of signs and symptoms in association with the monoclonal proliferation of lymphocytes or plasmacytoid cells in the marrow and a serum monoclonal protein (Dimopoulos et al., 2000; Gertz et al., 2000). A physician must consider the entire clinical and laboratory presentation to differentiate MGUS of the IgM type from macroglobulinemia. The presence of a lymphoplasmacytic infiltrate of the bone marrow or an IgM monoclonal protein does not necessarily provide the diagnosis of macroglobulinemia because other B cell neoplasms also may have plasmacytic differentiation and associated IgM monoclonal proteins.

A combination of typical symptoms and physical findings, more than 3 g/dL of IgM monoclonal protein (some patients have a value <3 g/dL), and a lymphocyte-plasma cell infiltration of the bone marrow provides the diagnosis of WM. Major problems in the differential diagnosis center around the distinction among MM, CLL, lymphoma, undifferentiated lymphoproliferative disease, and MGUS of the IgM type. These conditions are closely related, and some patients have characteristics of more than one of these disorders.

The presence of an IgM monoclonal protein level of less than 3.0 g/dL; the absence of anemia, hepatosplenomegaly, or lymphadenopathy; mild lymphocytic infiltration of the bone marrow; and no constitutional symptoms are suggestive of MGUS of the IgM type. A long-term followup of 242 patients with MGUS of IgM type revealed that 40 (17%) had development of a serious disease (WM in 22, lymphoproliferative disease in 9, lymphoma in 6, amyloidosis in 2, and CLL in 1) during followup. The median duration from recognition of MGUS until the development of serious disease ranged from 4 to 9 years. An additional 19 patients had an increase in the serum M-spike during followup, but the diagnosis of macroglobulinemia or malignant lymphoproliferative disease could not yet be made (Kyle and Garton, 1987).

A total of 213 patients with IgM MGUS were identified in southeastern Minnesota from 1960 to 1994. The patients were followed for a total of 1567 person-years (median, 6.3 y; range, 0–20.6 y). Lymphoma developed in 17 patients (relative risk [RR], 14.8), WM in 6 (RR, 262), primary systemic amyloidosis in 3 (RR, 16.5), and CLL in 3 (RR, 5.7). The relative risk of progression was 16-fold higher in patients with IgM MGUS than in the white population of the Iowa Surveillance Epidemiology and End Results Program. The cumulative incidence of progression was 10% at 5 years, 18% at 10 years, and 24% at 15 years. Multivariate analysis revealed that the concentration of the serum monoclonal protein and the level of serum albumin at diagnosis were the major risk factors for progression to lymphoma or a related disorder. Age, sex, reduction of IgA or IgG immunoglobulins, presence or concentration of the urine monoclonal protein, and size of the liver were not prognostic features. The risk of progression to lymphoma or a related disorder at 10 years after diagnosis of MGUS was 14% for patients with an initial monoclonal protein value of 0.5 g/dL or less, 26% with 1.5 g/dL, 34% for 2.0 g/dL, and 41% with more than 2.5 g/dL. The risk of progression at 10 years with an initial monoclonal protein value of 1.5 g/dL was 1.8 times the risk of progression with an initial value of 0.5 g/dL or less, whereas the risk of progression with a monoclonal protein value of 2.5 g/dL or more was 3.1 times the risk of progression with an initial value of 0.5 g/dL or less. The rate of progression of MGUS of IgM type of lymphoma or related disorders averaged 1.5% per year throughout the period of observation (Kyle et al., 2002). A patient with MGUS must be followed because, in many patients with an apparently benign monoclonal gammopathy, WM or related disorders develop subsequently.

The author and coworkers have seen some patients with IgG or IgA MM who had many lymphocytoid cells in the bone marrow and no lytic bone lesions (Maldonado et al., 1966). Levine et al. (1980) described 6 patients with lymphocytic-plasmacytoid morphology and an IgG or IgA monoclonal protein. Mast cell infiltration was not conspicuous in contrast to WM. The author and coworkers classify such patients as having IgG or IgA myeloma. Alternatively, patients who had anemia, oronasal bleeding, blurred vision, and large amounts of IgM protein in the serum have been seen who also had lytic bone lesions and immature plasma cells in the bone marrow, which are characteristic of MM and are classified as IgM myeloma (Takahashi et al., 1986; Zarrabi et al., 1981). Recent information suggests that IgM myeloma frequently has IgH translocations, particularly (11;14) (q13;q32) (Avet-Loiseau, 2003), whereas WM does not have them (Schop et al., 2002a).

## Course and Prognosis

Cohen et al. (1966) reported a survival of 55 months (range, 23–152 mo) from the date of clinical onset of WM and a survival of 35 months from the date of diagnosis. In another series, the mean survival after diagnosis was 49.2 months in patients responding to chemotherapy and 24.1 months in the nonresponders (MacKenzie and Fudenberg, 1972). McCallister et al. (1967) reported a survival of 5.3 years from the onset of symptoms and 3.2 years from the time of diagnosis. The median survival of 74 patients with macroglobulinemia from Malmö, Sweden, was 7 years (Waldenström, 1980).

In our series of 71 patients, the median survival of patients with WM was 5 years (Kyle and Garton, 1987). Bartl et al. (1983) distinguished 3 types of macroglobulinemia based on bone marrow involvement: lymphoplasmacytoid (47%), lymphoplasmacytic (42%), and polymorphous (11%). The median survivals for the 3 groups were 74 months, 25 months, and 12 months, respectively.

In a series of 167 patients with WM from a single institution, the median survival was 60 months. Shorter survival was associated with age 60 years or older, male sex, presence of general symptoms, hemoglobin value less than 10 g/dL, leukocyte count less than $4 \times 10^9$/L, neutrophil count less than $1.7 \times 10^9$/L, and platelet count less than $150 \times 10^9$/L. Organomegaly, signs of hyperviscosity, renal failure, serum IgM level at diagnosis, blood lymphocytosis, and percentage of bone marrow lymphoid cells did not significantly influence survival. With use of the Cox multivariate regression analysis, male sex, neutrophil value less than $1.7 \times 10^9$/L, age older than 60 years, and hemoglobin concentration less than 10 g/dL were the most important adverse prognostic factors for survival (Facon et al., 1993). In a study of prognostic factors in clinically overt macroglobulinemia requiring therapy, multivariate analysis revealed that age (70 y), hemoglobin value (9 g/dL), and the presence or absence of weight loss or cryoglobulinemia were the most significant prognostic factors (Gobbi et al., 1994). In another group of 28 patients with WM, the $\beta_2$-microglobulin level was of no value in determining response to chemotherapy or survival. In addition, the $\beta_2$-microglobulin level was not helpful in differentiating WM from benign monoclonal gammopathy of the IgM type (Belisle and Case, 1991).

Patients with lymphoplasmacytoid features have a better prognosis than those with a polymorphous appearance, which is characterized by a wide spectrum of lymphoid cells ranging from lymphocytes, plasma cells, and plasmacytoid cells to immunoblasts, lymphoblasts, and centroblasts. Tumor cell mass correlates inversely with survival (Bartl et al., 1983).

In a study of patients with clinically overt macroglobulinemia requiring therapy, age older than 70 years, hemoglobin concentration less than 9.0 g/dL, and either weight loss or the presence of cryoglobulinemia were the most significant adverse prognostic factors (Gobbi et al., 1994). In a series of 232 French patients with macroglobulinemia, age 65 years or older, albumin value less than 4 g/dL, and the presence of one or more cytopenias were the major factors adversely affecting survival. The 5-year survival rate was 87% in patients at low risk (≤1 adverse factor), 62% in those at intermediate risk (2 adverse factors), and 25% in those at high risk (≥3 adverse factors) (Morel et al., 2000). In a series of 60 patients with macroglobulinemia, the major prognostic features were age 65 years or older, presence of lymphadenopathy, and bone marrow infiltration of 50% or more (Kyrtsonis et al., 2001b).

Macroglobulinemia may follow a typical course for several years and then develop into a rapidly progressive reticulum cell sarcoma (Wanebo and Clarkson, 1965) or lymphoblastic lymphosarcoma (Wood and Frenkel, 1967). Large cell lymphoma may occur during the course of WM (Case records of the Massachusetts General Hospital, 1991). In one case, IgM κ was detected on the surface of the lymphocytes in the macroglobulinemia, but the diffuse, large cell lymphoma exhibited IgM λ markers, indicating that 2 distinct clones had developed (Chubachi et al., 1991).

The development of immunoblastic sarcoma (Richter's syndrome) has been seen in WM (Leonhard et al., 1980). It may occur from 3 months to 16 years after the recognition of WM. Response to initial treatment plays no role. The most frequent features of Richter's syndrome are the deterioration in the patient's performance and the rapid development of lymphadenopathy. In many instances, the IgM level is reduced. The median survival is short (García et al., 1993). Immunoblastic transformation is not always fatal. Winter et al. (1995) reported a patient with WM who had a rapidly enlarging spleen. Splenectomy was performed and immunoblastic transformation was documented. The patient was given chlorambucil and 45 months later was doing well. The development of acute lymphoblastic leukemia has been noted in more than 12 cases of macroglobulinemia (Angelopoulos et al., 1989).

## Therapy

If symptoms of hyperviscosity are present, plasmapheresis will alleviate the symptoms quickly (Schwab and Fahey, 1960; Solomon and Fahey, 1963). Currently, plasmapheresis is best accomplished with a cell separator.

Specific therapy should be directed against the proliferating lymphocytes and plasma cells. Chlorambucil given continuously was reported as beneficial in 4 cases of macroglobulinemia more than 40 years ago (Bayrd, 1961). Forty-six patients with symptomatic macroglobulinemia were randomized to receive 0.1 mg/kg chlorambucil per day or 0.3 mg/kg chlorambucil per day orally for 7 days every 6 weeks. Criteria for response included a 50% or more reduction of the serum monoclonal protein, increase in hemoglobin level of 2 g/dL without transfusion, 50% or more decrease of urine monoclonal protein, or a reduction of 2 cm or more in the size of the liver, spleen, or lymph nodes. Continuous chlorambucil therapy produced an objective response in 79% of patients by either reduction of serum monoclonal protein or increase in hemoglobin, whereas 68% given chlorambucil intermittently had an objective response. The size of the liver decreased by 2 cm or more in 55% of patients, and the size of the spleen decreased 2 cm or more in 67%. Lymphadenopathy decreased in 71%. Acute leukemia or refractory anemia developed in 4 patients. The median duration of survival was 5.4 years, and there was no difference between the 2 regimens (Kyle et al., 2000). In a series of 180 patients with symptomatic macroglobulinemia, 80% received chlorambucil. A myelodysplastic syndrome developed in only 3 (Garcia-Sanz et al., 2001). Kyrtsonis et al. (2001b) reported a 92% response rate to intermittent oral chlorambucil therapy in 50 patients with macroglobulinemia. Thus, chlorambucil, in an initial dosage of 6 to 8 mg per day, is a useful agent. The dosage of chlorambucil must be altered depending on the leukocyte and platelet counts, which should be determined every

2 weeks. Treatment should be continued until the patient reaches a plateau state—resolution of constitutional symptoms and stabilization of the IgM protein level. The patient should then be followed without therapy and chlorambucil therapy can be reinstituted at the time of relapse. Responses have also been achieved with cyclophosphamide given orally for prolonged periods (Bouroncle et al., 1964).

Combinations of alkylating agents have also been reported as beneficial. Case et al. (1991) found that 27 of 33 patients with symptomatic WM treated with the M2 protocol (BCNU: cyclophosphamide, vincristine, melphalan, and prednisone) obtained some benefit. Survival ranged from 1 month to more than 120 months; 58% of patients were projected to be alive at 10 years. Ten patients were alive 10 years or more after beginning therapy. The patients were said to have only mild to moderate hematologic toxicity. Sepsis developed in only 2 patients. In another series of 31 evaluable patients, melphalan, cyclophosphamide, and prednisone for a total of 12 courses produced some response in 74%. Eight of the 31 evaluable patients (26%) had a complete response. The overall median event-free survival duration was 66 months (Petrucci et al., 1989).

The use of alkylating agents may be associated with the development of acute leukemia. Rosner and Grünwald (1980) described 10 patients with WM in whom acute leukemia developed 16 to 72 months after the diagnosis of macroglobulinemia. Acute myelogenous leukemia has also been reported (Majumdar and Slater, 1993); the patient had received 3 courses of chlorambucil. Cytogenetic studies were not done. Several other similar cases have been reported (Cardamone et al., 1974; Effron et al., 1978).

Fludarabine and cladribine, nucleoside analogues, have been evaluated in patients with macroglobulinemia. These agents produce responses, but there are no long-term data indicating that they are more effective than chlorambucil or other alkylating agents. Both are more inconvenient to administer and have more side effects than chlorambucil. Fludarabine produced responses in 10 of 28 patients who were given a dosage of 20 to 30 mg/m$^2$ intravenously per day for 5 days or 30 mg/m$^2$ intravenously per day for 3 days. Treatment was continued until maximal response was achieved. Only 2 patients were previously untreated. Eight of 26 patients (31%) who were resistant to prior therapy responded. The median duration of unmaintained remissions was 38 months (Dimopoulos et al., 1993). In a group of 78 patients with low-grade lymphoma, including patients with macroglobulinemia and lymphoplasmacytic lymphoma, fludarabine produced a complete response in 15% and a median duration of response of 2.5 years (Foran et al., 1999). The treatment-related mortality was 5%. The authors stated that

fludarabine was active but complete remission rates were low. Dhodapkar et al. (2001) reported a complete response in 2% and a partial response in 34% of 182 patients treated with 30 mg/m$^2$ fludarabine intravenously per day for 5 days every 4 weeks for 4 cycles. The estimated rates of 5-year overall survival were 62% for previously untreated patients and 32% for previously treated patients. $\beta_2$-microglobulin values of 3 mg/L or more and a serum monoclonal protein value less than 4 g/dL were associated with poorer survival. In 71 patients with macroglobulinemia that was previously treated, fludarabine produced an objective response in 30%. The median number of courses of fludarabine was 6. No patients had a complete response (Leblond et al., 1998). Ninety-two patients with primary resistant or relapsed macroglobulinemia after alkylating agent therapy were randomized to either 25 mg/m$^2$ fludarabine intravenously on days 1 through 5 or a combination of cyclophosphamide, doxorubicin (Adriamycin), and prednisone (CAP) every 4 weeks for 6 courses (Leblond et al., 2001). Partial responses were obtained in 30% of patients receiving fludarabine and 11% receiving CAP, but overall survival was not different. There was no difference in hematologic or infectious toxicities between the 2 arms, but patients receiving CAP had more mucositis and alopecia. In a separate analysis of the study, the quality-adjusted time without symptoms or toxicity was 5.9 months longer in the fludarabine group than in the CAP group (Levy et al., 2001).

Cladribine in a 2-hour infusion over 5 consecutive days every 4 weeks for 4 cycles produced one complete response and 8 partial responses in 10 patients with previously untreated macroglobulinemia (Fridrik et al., 1997). Cladribine given in 2-hour infusions to 9 patients with untreated macroglobulinemia and 13 with relapsed disease produced a complete response in 4.5% (1 patient) and a partial response in 36.4%. There was no significant difference in the response rate of the 2 groups (Hellmann et al., 1999). Autoimmune hemolytic anemia occurred in 4 patients a median of 40 months from cladribine administration. Only 1 of the 4 patients responded to corticosteroids (Tetreault and Saven, 2000). Complete responses were attained in 5% and partial responses in 50% of 20 patients with previously untreated or treated macroglobulinemia given cladribine by a bolus injection (0.12 mg/kg per day by 2-h intravenous infusion for 5 consecutive days at monthly intervals for 3 courses) (Liu et al., 1998). The overall response rates were similar in previously untreated and treated patients. Survival at a median followup of 1.7 years was 85%. The major toxicity was myelosuppression; 60% of patients had grade 3 or 4 neutropenia. Cladribine also may be given subcutaneously. Twenty-five patients with previously treated symptomatic macroglobulinemia received subcutaneous cladribine (total dose of 0.5 mg/kg per cycle over 5 days at ≥4-week intervals for a maximum of 6 cycles). The overall response rate, including disease stabilization, was 68% (Betticher et al., 1997). Cladribine has been given in combination with cyclophosphamide and prednisone for low-grade proliferative disorders. The overall response rate was 88%, and a complete response was achieved in 21% (Laurencet et al., 1999).

Cladribine was given to 26 patients with previously untreated, symptomatic WM. Two courses were given at a dosage of 0.1 mg/kg per day for a 7-day continuous infusion. Twenty-two (85%) responded, including 3 patients who had a complete response. Five patients had relapse during a median followup of 13 months, but all retreated patients again responded (Dimopoulos et al., 1994a). Twenty of 46 patients resistant to an alkylating agent and a glucocorticoid responded to 27-day courses of cladribine. The median duration of survival after treatment was 28 months. Only 22% of patients with refractory disease late in their course responded to cladribine (Dimopoulos et al., 1995). Three of 4 patients who had previously responded to fludarabine and were relapsing from unmaintained remission achieved a partial response with cladribine. However, only 1 of 10 patients with disease resistant to fludarabine responded to cladribine (Dimopoulos et al., 1994c). In another series, less impressive results were reported. Only 7 of 18 patients with WM (5 untreated and 13 previously treated) obtained a partial response (Delannoy et al., 1994). Paclitaxel produced no response in six patients with previously untreated WM (Dimopoulos et al., 1994b).

Rituximab (Rituxan), manufactured by IDEC Pharmaceuticals in San Diego, is an anti-CD20 monoclonal antibody that is directed against an antigenic determinant on the surface of lymphoid cells in macroglobulinemia. Byrd et al. (1999) reported a 50% reduction in monoclonal protein value in 3 of 7 patients with heavily pretreated macroglobulinemia. In another report, 8 of 30 patients with previously treated macroglobulinemia obtained a partial response with rituximab. No complete responses were found. The median time to treatment failure for the patients with a partial response was 8 months (Treon et al., 2001). In a recently reported study, 6 (40%) of 15 patients with previously untreated disease and 6 (50%) of 12 patients with pretreated disease responded to rituximab. The median time to progression was 16 months (Dimopoulos et al., 2002). The monoclonal protein level may initially increase shortly after the infusion of rituximab. In this case, the patient should be observed because the monoclonal protein level frequently decreases. Clinically meaningful responses to rituximab may occur several months after completion of therapy.

Thalidomide produced a partial response in 3 of 10 patients with previously untreated disease and 2 of 10 patients with pretreated macroglobulinemia. None of the patients who had treatment during refractory relapse or with disease duration of more than 2 years responded. Only low doses of thalidomide were tolerated because of adverse side effects (Dimopoulos et al., 2001).

Seven patients with macroglobulinemia (previously untreated in 4) received dexa-BEAM chemotherapy (dexamethasone, BCNU [carmustine], etoposide, cytarabine, and melphalan) and then myeloablative therapy consisting of total body irradiation 2 Gy twice a day for 3 days followed by cyclophosphamide. All patients responded, but immunofixation revealed a monoclonal protein in 5 patients. There was no sign of clinical or serologic progression at 3 to 30 months (Dreger et al., 1999). Six patients with previously treated macroglobulinemia were given 200 mg/m$^2$ melphalan or 140 mg/m$^2$ melphalan with added total body irradiation followed by infusion with peripheral blood stem cells. One patient had a complete response and the remainder had a partial response. Four patients were event-free at 52, 15, 12, and 2 months after transplantation. The authors advised that stem cells should be collected before extensive use of purine analogues because 2 patients with prior extensive fludarabine therapy required a second attempt at stem cell mobilization (Desikan et al., 1999). In another report, 3 of 4 patients with refractory macroglobulinemia obtained a partial response from autologous stem cell transplantation. One patient died of a cerebrovascular accident on day 30 (Anagnostopoulos et al., 2001).

Allogeneic transplantation from HLA-identical donors in 2 patients with aggressive macroglobulinemia resulted in an event-free survival of more than 3 and 9 years (Martino et al., 1999). In another report of 3 patients with refractory macroglobulinemia, an allogeneic transplant resulted in a partial response in one patient and no response in one patient; one patient died of graft-versus-host disease on day 39 (Anagnostopoulos et al., 2001).

Some benefit has also been found using $\alpha_2$-interferon. In one report, 2 of 5 patients previously treated with chemotherapy obtained some response (Quesada et al., 1988). De Rosa et al. (1989) reported 3 patients, 2 of whom had been previously treated with alkylating agents, who responded to $\alpha_2$-interferon. In another report of a patient previously treated with chlorambucil, cyclophosphamide, and plasma exchange, $\alpha_2$-interferon produced benefit (Bhavnani et al., 1990). In a group of 36 patients with WM, 12 had a major and 6 had a minor response to $\alpha_2$-interferon. In contrast, a study of 41 evaluable patients with IgM MGUS showed only 2 with a major response and 6 with a minor response (Rotoli et al., 1994).

The administration of prednisone (O'Reilly and MacKenzie, 1967) or dexamethasone (Jane and Salem,

1988) has produced a reduction in protein levels. Pentostatin (2'-deoxycoformycin) may provide benefit in macroglobulinemia (Riddell et al., 1986). Sequential hemibody radiation has also been used (Jacobs et al., 1992). Splenectomy produced a complete response in 2 patients who were refractory to chemotherapy. Both remained free of disease at 12 and 13 years after splenectomy (Humphrey and Conley, 1995). Another patient with refractory macroglobulinemia responded to splenectomy with a response duration of 6 years (Takemori et al., 1997).

# Acknowledgments

This work was supported in part by Research Grant CA 62242 from the National Institutes of Health.

## REFERENCES

Abad, S., Zagdanski, A. M., Brechignac, S., Thioliere, B., Brouet, J. C., and Mariette, X. (1999). Neurolymphomatosis in Waldenström's macroglobulinaemia. *British Journal of Haematology, 106,* 100–103.

Abdou, N. I., and Abdou, N. L. (1975). Idiotypic immunoglobulin (ID-IG) on monoclonal lymphocytes (Ly) of human multiple myeloma (MM): effects of therapy [Abstract]. *Clinical Research, 23,* 408A.

Ahmed, S., Shurafa, M. S., Bishop, C. R., and Varterasian, M. (1999). Waldenström's macroglobulinemia in young African-American adults. *American Journal of Hematology, 60,* 229–230.

Angelopoulos, N., Camerone, G., Guzzini, F., and Polli, N. (1989). A case of Waldenström macroglobulinemia terminating in acute lymphoblastic leukemia. *Haematologica, 74,* 309–312.

Anagnostopoulos, A., Dimopoulos, M. A., Aleman, A., Weber, D., Alexanian, R., Champlin, R., and Giralt, S. (2001). High-dose chemotherapy followed by stem cell transplantation in patients with resistant Waldenström's macroglobulinemia. *Bone Marrow Transplantation, 27,* 1027–1029.

Argani, I., and Kipkie, G. F. (1964). Macroglobulinemic nephropathy: acute renal failure in macroglobulinemia of Waldenström. *American Journal of Medicine, 36,* 151–157.

Aspelin, P., Adielsson, G., Dimitrov, N., Nyman, U., and Waldenström, J. (1989). Abdominal computed tomography in macroglobulinemia (Waldenström's disease): report of a case. *Acta Radiologica, 30,* 197–200.

Avet-Loiseau, H., Garand, R., Lode, L., Harousseau, J. L., and Bataille, R. (2003). Translocation t(11;14)(q13;q32) is the hallmark of IgM, IgE, and nonsecretory multiple myeloma variants. *Blood, 101,* 1570–1571.

Bannick, E. G., and Greene, C. H. (1929). Renal insufficiency associated with Bence-Jones proteinuria: report of thirteen cases with a note on the changes in the serum proteins. *Archives of Internal Medicine, 44,* 486–501.

Bartl, R., Frisch, B., Mahl, G., Burkhardt, R., Fateh-Moghadam, A., Pappenberger, R., Sommerfeld, W., and Hoffmann-Fezer, G. (1983). Bone marrow histology in Waldenström's macroglobulinaemia: clinical relevance of subtype recognition. *Scandinavian Journal of Haematology, 31,* 359–375.

Bayrd, E. D. (1961). Continuous chlorambucil therapy in primary macroglobulinemia of Waldenström: report of four cases. *Proceedings of the Staff Meetings of the Mayo Clinic, 36,* 135–147.

Bedine, M. S., Yardley, J. H., Elliott, H. L., Banwell, J. G., and Hendrix, T. R. (1973). Intestinal involvement in Waldenström's macroglobulinemia. *Gastroenterology, 65,* 308–315.

Belisle, L., and Case, D. C., Jr. (1991). β-2 microglobulin (β 2M) levels in Waldenström's macroglobulinemia and IgM "benign" gammopathy (BMG) [Abstract]. *Proceedings of the American Society of Clinical Oncology, 10,* 304.

Bergroth, V., Reitamo, S., Konttine, Y. T., and Wegelius, O. (1981). Skin lesions in Waldenström's macroglobulinaemia. *Acta Medica Scandinavica, 209,* 129–131.

Betticher, D. C., Hsu Schmitz, S. F., Ratschiller, D., von Rohr, A., Egger, T., Pugin, P., Stalder, M., Hess, U., Fey, M. F., and Cerny, T. (1997). Cladribine (2-CDA) given as subcutaneous bolus injections is active in pretreated Waldenström's macroglobulinaemia: Swiss Group for Clinical Cancer Research (SAKK) *British Journal of Haematology, 99,* 358–363.

Bhavnani, M., Marples, J., and Liu Yin, J. A. (1990). Treatment of Waldenström's macroglobulinaemia with α interferon. *Journal of Clinical Pathology, 43,* 437.

Bichel, J., Bing, J., and Harboe, N. (1950). Another case of hyperglobulinemia and affection of the central nervous system. *Acta Medica Scandinavica, 138,* 1–14.

Bing, J., and Neel, A. V. (1936). Two cases of hyperglobulinaemia with affection of the central nervous system on a toxic-infectious basis. *Acta Medica Scandinavica, 88,* 492–506.

Blattner, W. A., Garber, J. E., Mann, D. L., McKeen, E. A., Henson, R., McGuire, D. B., Fisher, W. B., Bauman, A. W., Goldin, L. R., and Fraumeni, J. F., Jr. (1980). Waldenström's macroglobulinemia and autoimmune disease in a family. *Annals of Internal Medicine, 93,* 830–832.

Bloch, K. J., and Maki, D. G. (1973). Hyperviscosity syndrome associated with immunoglobulin abnormalities. *Seminars in Hematology, 10,* 113–124.

Bouroncle, B. A., Datta, P., and Frajola, W. J. (1964). Waldenström's macroglobulinemia: report of three patients treated with cyclophosphamide. *Journal of the American Medical Association, 189,* 729–732.

Boyd, J. F. (1980). Immunohistochemical staining of the Dutcher-Fahey intranuclear inclusion body in a case of Waldenström's macroglobulinaemia. *Journal of Pathology, 132,* 81–91.

Braden, G. L., Mikolich, D. J., White, C. F., Germain, M. J., and Fitzgibbons, J. P. (1986). Syndrome of inappropriate antidiuresis in Waldenström's macroglobulinemia. *American Journal of Medicine, 80,* 1242–1244.

Brandt, J. L., Davidoff, A., Bernstein, L. H., Biempica, L., Rindfleisch, B., and Goldstein, M. L. (1981). Small-intestinal involvement in Waldenström macroglobulinemia: case report and review of the literature. *Digestive Diseases and Sciences, 26,* 174–180.

Brawn, L. A., Parsons, M. A., Allamby, P., Ramsay, L. E., and Preston, F. E. (1988). Massive cardiac disease in a patient with Waldenström macroglobulinaemia [Letter]. *Journal of Clinical Pathology, 41,* 475–478.

Brooks, A. P. (1976). Portal hypertension in Waldenström's macroglobulinaemia. *British Medical Journal, 1,* 689–690.

Byrd, J. C., White, C. A., Link, B., Lucas, M. S., Velasquez, W. S., Rosenberg, J., and Grillo-Lopez, A. J. (1999). Rituximab therapy in Waldenström's macroglobulinemia: preliminary evidence of clinical activity. *Annals of Oncology, 10,* 1525–1527.

Cabrera, A., de la Pava, S., and Pickren, J. W. (1964). Intestinal localization of Waldenström's disease. *Archives of Internal Medicine, 114,* 399–407.

Cagnoni, P. J., Lenzi, R., Wisch, N., Seremetis, S., and Rand, J. H. (1995). Spurious fibrinogen levels secondary to pyroglobulinemia in Waldenström's macroglobulinemia. *American Journal of Hematology, 48,* 126–127.

Carbone, P., Caradonna, F., Granata, G., and Barbata, G. (1993). Sister chromatid exchange in Waldenström's macroglobulinemia. *Cancer, Genetics, and Cytogenetics, 66,* 63–69.

Carbone, P., Caradonna, F., Granata, G., Marcenò, R., Cavallaro, A. M., and Barbata, G. (1992). Chromosomal abnormalities in

Waldenström's macroglobulinemia. *Cancer, Genetics, and Cytogenetics, 61*, 147–151.

Cardamone, J. M., Kimmerle, R. I., and Marshall, E. Y. (1974). Development of acute erythroleukemia in B-cell immunoproliferative disorders after prolonged therapy with alkylating drugs. *American Journal of Medicine, 57*, 836–842.

Case, D. C., Ervin, T. J., Boyd, M. A., and Redfield, D. L. (1991). Waldenström's macroglobulinemia: long-term results with the M-2 protocol. *Cancer Invest, 9*, 1–7.

Case records of the Massachusetts General Hospital. (1990). *New England Journal of Medicine, 322*, 183–192, case 3.

Case records of the Massachusetts General Hospital. (1991). *New England Journal of Medicine, 324*, 1267–1277, case 18.

Castaldi, P. A., and Penney, R. (1970). A macroglobulin with inhibitory activity against coagulation factor VIII. *Blood, 35*, 370–376.

Choi, H. S. H., Orentreich, D., Kornblee, L., and Muhlfelder, T. W. (1989). Granulocytic sarcoma presenting as a solitary nodule of skin in a patient with Waldenstrom's macroglobulinemia: an immunohistochemical and electron-microscopic study. *American Journal of Dermatopathology, 11*, 51–57.

Chong, Y. Y., Lau, L. C., Lui, W. O., Lim, P., Lim, E., Tan, P. H., Tan, P., and Ong, Y. Y. (1998). A case of t(8;14) with total and partial trisomy 3 in Waldenström macroglobulinemia. *Cancer, Genetics, and Cytogenetics, 103*, 65–67.

Chubachi, A., Ohtani, H., Sakuyama, M., Nimura, T., Mamiya, S., Saitoh, M., Watanuki, T., and Miura, A. B. (1991). Diffuse large-cell lymphoma occurring in a patient with Waldenström's macroglobulinemia: evidence for the two different clones in Richter's syndrome. *Cancer, 68*, 781–785.

Cigudosa, J. C., Calasanz, M. J., Pérez, C., Rifón, J., Cuesta, B., and Gullon, A. (1994). Complex karyotype including 14q+ marker in a case of Waldenström's macroglobulinemia. *Cancer, Genetics, and Cytogenetics, 73*, 169–170.

Cline, M. J., Solomon, A., Berlin, N. I., and Fehey, J. L. (1963). Anemia in macroglobulinemia. *American Journal of Medicine, 34*, 213–220.

Cobb, M. W., Domloge-Hultsch, N., Frame, J. N., and Yancey, K. B. (1992). Waldenström macroglobulinemia with an IgM-κ antiepidermal basement membrane zone antibody. *Archives of Dermatology, 128*, 372–376.

Cohen, R. J., Bohannon, R. A., and Wallerstein, R. O. (1966). Waldenström's macroglobulinemia: a study of ten cases. *American Journal of Medicine, 41*, 274–284.

Cordido, M., Fernández-Lago, C., Fernández-Vigo, J., and López-Nieto, C. (1995). Dry eye in Waldenström's macroglobulinemia: improvement after systemic chemotherapy. *Cornea, 14*, 210–211.

Crawford, J., Cox, E. B., and Cohen, H. J. (1985). Evaluation of hyperviscosity in monoclonal gammopathies. *American Journal of Medicine, 79*, 13–22.

Darnley, J. D. (1962). Polyneuropathy in Waldenström's macroglobulinemia: case report and discussion. *Neurology, 12*, 617–623.

Dayan, A. D., and Lewis, P. D. (1966). Demyelinating neuropathy in macroglobulinemia. *Neurology, 16*, 1141–1144.

Delannoy, A., Ferrant, A., Martiat, P., Bosly, A., Zenebergh, A., and Michaux, J. L. (1994). 2-Chlorodeoxyadenosine therapy in Waldenström's macroglobulinemia. *Nouvelle Revue Française d' Hematologie, 36*, 317–320.

De Rosa, G., De Renzo, A., Buffardi, S., and Rotoli, B. (1989). Treatment of Waldenström's macroglobulinemia with interferon. *Haematologica, 74*, 313–315.

Desikan, R., Dhodapkar, M., Siegel, D., Fassas, A., Singh, J., Singhal, S., Mehta, J., Vesole, D., Tricot, G., Jagannath, S., Anaissie, E., Barlogie, B., and Munshi, N. C. (1999). High-dose therapy with autologous haemopoietic stem cell support for Waldenström's macroglobulinaemia. *British Journal of Haematology, 105*, 993–996.

Dhodapkar, M. V., Jacobson, J. L., Gertz, M. A., Rivkin, S. E., Roodman, G. D., Tuscano, J. M., Shurafa, M., Kyle, R. A., Crowley, J. J., and Barlogie, B. (2001). Prognostic factors and response to fludarabine therapy in patients with Waldenström macroglobulinemia: results of United States Intergroup Trial (Southwest Oncology Group S9003). *Blood, 98*, 41–48.

Dimopoulos, M. A., and Alexanian, R. (1994). Waldenström's macroglobulinemia. *Blood, 83*, 1452–1459.

Dimopoulos, M. A., Kantarjian, H., Weber, D., O'Brien, S., Estey, E., Delasalle, K., Rose, E., Cabanillas, F., Keating, M., and Alexanian, R. (1994a). Primary therapy of Waldenström's macroglobulinemia with 2-chlorodeoxyadenosine. *Journal of Clinical Oncology, 12*, 2694–2698.

Dimopoulos, M. A., Luckett, R., and Alexanian, R. (1994b). Primary therapy of Waldenström's macroglobulinemia with paclitaxel [Letter]. *Journal of Clinical Oncology, 12*, 1998.

Dimopoulos, M. A., O'Brien, S., Kantarjian, H., Pierce, S., Delasalle, K., Barlogie, B., Alexanian, R., and Keating, M. J. (1993). Fludarabine therapy in Waldenström's macroglobulinemia. *American Journal of Medicine, 95*, 49–52.

Dimopoulos, M. A., Panayiotidis, P., Moulopoulos, L. A., Sfikakis, P., and Dalakas, M. (2000). Waldenström's macroglobulinemia: clinical features, complications, and management. *Journal of Clinical Oncology, 18*, 214–226.

Dimopoulos, M. A., Weber, D., Delasalle, K. B., Keating, M., and Alexanian, R. (1995). Treatment of Waldenström's macroglobulinemia resistant to standard therapy with 2-chlorodeoxyadenosine: identification of prognostic factors. *Annals of Oncology, 6*, 49–52.

Dimopoulos, M. A., Weber, D. M., Kantarjian, H., Keating, M., and Alexanian, R. (1994c). 2-Chlorodeoxyadenosine therapy of patients with Waldenström macroglobulinemia previously treated with fludarabine. *Annals of Oncology, 5*, 288–289.

Dimopoulos, M. A., Zervas, C., Zomas, A., Kiamouris, C., Viniou, N. A., Grigoraki, V., Karkantaris, C., Mitsouli, C., Gika, D., Christakis, J., and Anagnostopoulos, N. (2002). Treatment of Waldenström's macroglobulinemia with rituximab. *Journal of Clinical Oncology, 20*, 2327–2333.

Dimopoulos, M. A., Zomas, A., Viniou, N. A., Grigoraki, V., Galani, E., Matsouka, C., Economou, O., Anagnostopoulos, N., and Panayiotidis, P. (2001). Treatment of Waldenström's macroglobulinemia with thalidomide. *Journal of Clinical Oncology, 19*, 3596–3601.

Donovan, K. A., Lacy, M. Q., Gertz, M. A., and Lust, J. A. (2002). IL-1beta expression in IgM monoclonal gammopathy and its relationship to multiple myeloma. *Leukemia, 16*, 382–385.

Dreger, P., Glass, B., Kuse, R., Sonnen, R., von Neuhoff, N., Bolouri, H., Kneba, M., and Schmitz, N. (1999). Myeloablative radiochemotherapy followed by reinfusion of purged autologous stem cells for Waldenström's macroglobulinaemia. *British Journal of Haematology, 106*, 115–118.

Dutcher, T. F., and Fahey, J. L. (1959). The histopathology of macroglobulinemia of Waldenström. *Journal of the National Cancer Institute, 22*, 887–917.

Effron, M. K., Rosenbaum, J., and Greenberg, P. L. (1978). Remission of acute myelogenous leukemia complicating Waldenström macroglobulinemia. *Western Journal of Medicine, 129*, 337–339.

Elias, E. G., Holyoke, E. D., and Mittelman, A. (1972). Obstructive jaundice in macroglobulinemia. *Journal of Surgical Oncology, 4*, 380–384.

Epenetos, A. A., Rohatiner, A., Slevin, M., and Woothipoom, W. (1980). Ankylosing spondylitis and Waldenström's macroglobulinaemia: a case report. *Clinical Oncology, 6*, 83–84.

Essig, L. J., Timms, E. S., Hancock, D. E., and Sharp, G. C. (1974). Plasma cell interstitial pneumonia and macroglobulinemia: a response to corticosteroid and cyclophosphamide therapy. *American Journal of Medicine, 56*, 398–405.

Ettl, A. R., Birbamer, G. G., and Philipp, W. (1992). Orbital involvement in Waldenström's macroglobulinemia: ultrasound, computed tomography and magnetic resonance findings. *Ophthalmologica, 205*, 40–45.

Facon, T., Brouillard, M., Duhamel, A., Morel, P., Simon, M., Jouet, J. P., Bauters, F., and Fenaux, P. (1993). Prognostic factors in Waldenström's macroglobulinemia: a report of 167 cases. *Journal of Clinical Oncology, 11*, 1553–1558.

Fahey, J. L., Barth, W. F., and Solomon, A. (1965). Serum hyperviscosity syndrome. *Journal of the American Medical Association, 192*, 464–467.

Fahey, J. L., Scogins, R., Utz, J. P., and Szwed, C. F. (1963). Infection, antibody response and gamma globulin components in multiple myeloma and macroglobulinemia. *American Journal of Medicine, 35*, 698–707.

Fine, J. M., Muller, J. Y., Rochu, D., Marneux, M., Gorin, N. C., Fine, A., and Lambin, P. (1986). Waldenström's macroglobulinemia in monozygotic twins. *Acta Medica Scandinavica, 220*, 369–373.

Font, R. L., and Zimmerman, L. E. (1970). Macroglobulinemia complicated by *Pneumocystis* pneumonia and cytomegalic inclusion disease including postmortem examination of the eyes: report of a case. *Medical Annals of the District of Columbia, 39*, 428–432.

Foran, J. M., Rohatiner, A. Z., Coiffier, B., Barbui, T., Johnson, S. A., Hiddemann, W., Radford, J. A., Norton, A. J., Tollerfield, S. M., Wilson, M. P., and Lister, T. A. (1999). Multicenter phase II study of fludarabine phosphate for patients with newly diagnosed lymphoplasmacytoid lymphoma, Waldenström's macroglobulinemia, and mantle-cell lymphoma. *Journal of Clinical Oncology, 17*, 546–553.

Franzén, S., Johansson, B., and Kaigas, M. (1966). Primary polycythemia associated with multiple myeloma. *Acta Medica Scandinavica Supplement, 445*, 336–343.

Fridrik, M. A., Jager, G., Baldinger, C., Krieger, O., Chott, A., and Bettelheim, P. (1997). First-line treatment of Waldenström's disease with cladribine: Arbeitsgemeinschaft Medikamentose Tumortherapie. *Annals of Hematology, 74*, 7–10.

García, R., Hernández, J. M., Caballero, M. D., González, M., and San Miguel, J. F. (1993). Immunoblastic lymphoma and associated non-lymphoid malignancies following two cases of Waldenström's macroglobulinemia: a review of the literature [Letter]. *European Journal of Haematology, 50*, 299–301.

Garcia-Sanz, R., Montoto, S., Torrequebrada, A., de Coca, A. G., Petit, J., Sureda, A., Rodriguez-Garcia, J. A., Masso, P., Perez-Aliaga, A., Monteagudo, M. D., Navarro, I., Moreno, G., Toledo, C., Alonso, A., Besses, C., Besalduch, J., Jarque, I., Salama, P., Rivas, J. A., Navarro, B., Bladé, J., and Miguel, J. F. (2001). Waldenström macroglobulinaemia: presenting features and outcome in a series with 217 cases. *British Journal of Haematology, 115*, 575–582.

Gertz, M. A., Fonseca, R., and Rajkumar, S. V. (2000). Waldenström's macroglobulinemia. *Oncologist, 5*, 63–67.

Gertz, M. A., Kyle, R. A., and Noel, P. (1993). Primary systemic amyloidosis: a rare complication of immunoglobulin M monoclonal gammopathies and Waldenström's macroglobulinemia. *Journal of Clinical Oncology, 11*, 914–920.

Gétaz, E. P., and Staples, W. G. (1977). Familial Waldenström's macroglobulinaemia: a case report. *South African Medical Journal, 51*, 891–892.

Gobbi, P. G., Bettini, R., Montecucco, C., Cavanna, L., Morandi, S., Pieresca, C., Merlini, G., Bertoloni, D., Grignani, G., Pozzetti, U., Caporali, R., and Ascari, E. (1994). Study of prognosis in Waldenström's macroglobulinemia: a proposal for a simple binary classification with clinical and investigational utility. *Blood, 83*, 2939–2945.

Goodenberger, M. E., Piette, W. W., Macfarlane, D. E., and Argenyi, Z. B. (1990). Xanthoma disseminatum and Waldenström's macroglobulinemia. *Journal of the American Academy of Dermatology, 23*, 1015–1018.

Gothoni, G., Wasastjerna, C., and Jeglinsky, B. (1965). Macroglobulinaemia: primary (Waldenström) and symptomatic in rheumatoid arthritis. *Acta Medica Scandinavica, 177*, 263–273.

Groves, F. D., Travis, L. B., Devesa, S. S., Ries, L. A., and Fraumeni, J. F., Jr. (1998). Waldenström's macroglobulinemia: incidence patterns in the United States, 1988–1994. *Cancer, 82*, 1078–1081.

Hanlon, D. G., Bayrd, E. D., and Kearns, T. P. (1958). Macroglobulinemia: report of four cases. *Journal of the American Medical Association, 167*, 1817–1820.

Hatzimichael, E. C., Christou, L., Bai, M., Kolios, G., Kefala, L., and Bourantas, K. L. (2001). Serum levels of IL-6 and its soluble receptor (sIL-6R) in Waldenström's macroglobulinemia. *European Journal of Haematology, 66*, 1–6.

Hellmann, A., Lewandowski, K., Zaucha, J. M., Bieniaszewska, M., Halaburda, K., and Robak, T. (1999). Effect of a 2-hour infusion of 2-chlorodeoxyadenosine in the treatment of refractory or previously untreated Waldenström's macroglobulinemia. *European Journal of Haematology, 63*, 35–41.

Herrinton, L. J., and Weiss, N. S. (1993). Incidence of Waldenström's macroglobulinemia. *Blood, 82*, 3148–3150.

Hertan, H. I., and Pitchumoni, C. S. (1991). Chronic calcific pancreatitis in a patient with Waldenström's macroglobulinemia. *American Journal of Gastroenterology, 86*, 633–634.

Hory, B., Saunier, F., Wolff, R., Saint-Hillier, Y., Coulon, G., and Perol, C. (1987). Waldenström macroglobulinemia and nephrotic syndrome with minimal change lesion. *Nephron, 45*, 68–70.

Humphrey, J. S., and Conley, C. L. (1995). Durable complete remission of macroglobulinemia after splenectomy: a report of two cases and review of the literature. *American Journal of Hematology, 48*, 262–266.

Imai, F., Fujisawa, K., Kiya, N., Ninomiya, T., Ogura, Y., Mizoguchi, Y., Sano, H., and Kanno, T. (1995). Intracerebral infiltration by monoclonal plasmacytoid cells in Waldenström's macroglobulinemia: case report. *Neurologia Medico-Chirurgica (Tokyo), 35*, 575–579.

Jacobs, P., Wood, L., and Shuttleworth, M. (1992). Long-term response to sequential hemibody radiotherapy in Waldenström's macroglobulinemia [Letter]. *Journal of Clinical Apheresis, 7*, 219–220.

Jacobson, D. R., Ballard, H. S., and Schiffman, G. S. (1988). Antibody response to pneumococcal vaccination in patients with nodular small cleaved cell lymphoma and Waldenström's macroglobulinemia [Abstract]. *Blood, 72*(suppl 1), 244a.

James, J. M., Brouet, J. C., Orvoenfrija, E., Capron, F., Brechot, J., Danon, F., Diebold, J., Rochemaure, J., and Zittoun, R. (1987). Waldenström's macroglobulinaemia in a bird breeder: a case history with pulmonary involvement and antibody activity of the monoclonal IgM to canary's droppings. *Clinical and Experimental Immunology, 68*, 397–401.

Jane, S. M., and Salem, H. H. (1988). Treatment of resistant Waldenström's macroglobulinemia with high-dose glucocorticosteroids. *Australian and New Zealand Journal of Medicine, 18*, 77–78.

Jensen, G. S., Andrews, E. J., Mant, M. J., Vergidis, R., Ledbetter, J. A., and Pilarski, L. M. (1991). Transitions in CD45 isoform expression indicate continuous differentiation of a monoclonal CD5+ CD11b+ B lineage in Waldenström's macroglobulinemia. *American Journal of Hematology, 37*, 20–30.

Jønsson, V., Kierkegaard, A., Salling, S., Molander, S., Andersen, L. P., Christiansen, M., and Wiik, A. (1999). Autoimmunity in Waldenström's macroglobulinaemia. *Leukemia and Lymphoma, 34*, 373–379.

Kalff, M. W., and Hijmans, W. (1969). Immunoglobulin analysis in families of macroglobulinaemia patients. *Clinical and Experimental Immunology, 5*, 479–498.

Kelly, J. J., Jr., Kyle, R. A., and Latov, N. (1987). *Polyneuropathies Associated With Plasma Cell Dyscrasias* (pp. 51–72). Boston: Martinus Nijhoff.

Klokkevold, P. R., Miller, D. A., and Friedlander, A. H. (1989). Mental nerve neuropathy: a symptom of Waldenström's macroglobulinemia. *Oral Surg Oral Med Oral Pathol, 67,* 689–693.

Koivisto, P. V. I., Karhunen, P. J., Färkkilä, M. A., and Kahri, A. (1989). Endoscopic appearance of intestinal involvement in Waldenström's macroglobulinemia. *Endoscopy, 21,* 155–156.

Krajny, M., and Pruzanski, W. (1976). Waldenström's macroglobulinemia: review of 45 cases. *Can Med Assoc J, 114,* 899–905.

Kyle, R. A., and Garton, J. P. (1987). The spectrum of IgM monoclonal gammopathy in 430 cases. *Mayo Clinic Proceedings, 62,* 719–731.

Kyle, R. A., Greipp, P. R., Gertz, M. A., Witzig, T. E., Lust, J. A., Lacy, M. Q., and Therneau, T. M. (2000). Waldenström's macroglobulinaemia: a prospective study comparing daily with intermittent oral chlorambucil. *British Journal of Haematology, 108,* 737–742.

Kyle, R. A., Therneau, T. M., Rajkumar, S. V., Offord, J. R., Larson, D. R., Plevak, M. L., and Melton, L. J. III. (2002). Long-term followup of IgM monoclonal gammopathy of undetermined significance (MGUS) [Abstract]. *Blood, 100,* 104a.

Kyrtsonis, M. C., Angelopoulou, M. K., Kontopidou, F. N., Siakantaris, M. P., Dimopoulou, M. N., Mitropoulos, F., Kalovidouris, A., Vaiopoulos, G. A., and Pangalis, G. A. (2001a). Primary lung involvement in Waldenström's macroglobulinaemia: report of two cases and review of the literature. *Acta Haematologica, 105,* 92–96.

Kyrtsonis, M. C., Vassilakopoulos, T. P., Angelopoulou, M. K., Siakantaris, P., Kontopidou, F. N., Dimopoulou, M. N., Boussiotis, V., Gribabis, A., Konstantopoulos, K., Vaiopoulos, G. A., Fessas, P., Kittas, C., and Pangalis, G. A. (2001b). Waldenström's macroglobulinemia: clinical course and prognostic factors in 60 patients. Experience from a single hematology unit. *Annals of Hematology, 80,* 722–727.

Laurencet, F. M., Zulian, G. B., Guetty-Alberto, M., Iten, P. A., Betticher, D. C., and Alberto, P. (1999). Cladribine with cyclophosphamide and prednisone in the management of low-grade lymphoproliferative malignancies. *British Journal of Cancer, 79,* 1215–1219.

Leb, L., Grimes, E. T., Balough, K., and Merritt, J. A., Jr., (1977). Monoclonal macroglobulinemia with osteolytic lesions: a case report and review of the literature. *Cancer, 39,* 227–231.

Leblond, V., Ben-Othman, T., Deconinck, E., Taksin, A. L., Harousseau, J. L., Delgado, M. A., Delmer, A., Maloisel, F., Mariette, X., Morel, P., Clauvel, J. P., Duboisset, P., Entezam, S., Hermine, O., Merlet, M., Yakoub-Agha, I., Guibon, O., Caspard, H., and Fort, N. (1998). Activity of fludarabine in previously treated Waldenström's macroglobulinemia: a report of 71 cases. Groupe Cooperatif Macroglubulinemie. *Journal of Clinical Oncology, 16,* 2060–2064.

Leblond, V., Levy, V., Maloisel, F., Cazin, B., Fermand, J. P., Harousseau, J. L., Remenieras, L., Porcher, R., Gardembas, M., Marit, G., Deconinck, E., Desablens, B., Guilhot, F., Philippe, G., Stamatoullas, A., and Guibon, O. (2001). Multicenter, randomized comparative trial of fludarabine and combination of cyclophosphamide-doxorubicin-prednisone in 92 patients with Waldenström macroglobulinemia in first relapse or with primary refractory disease. *Blood, 98,* 2640–2644.

Leonhard, S. A., Muhleman, A. F., Hurtubise, P. E., and Martelo, O. J. (1980). Emergence of immunoblastic sarcoma in Waldenström's macroglobulinemia. *Cancer, 45,* 3102–3107.

Levine, A. M., Lichtenstein, A., Gresik, M. V., Taylor, C. R., Feinstein, D. I., and Lukes, R. J. (1980). Clinical and immunologic spectrum of plasmacytoid lymphocytic lymphoma without serum monoclonal IgM. *British Journal of Haematology, 46,* 225–233.

Levy, V., Porcher, R., Leblond, V., Fermand, J. P., Cazin, B., Maloisel, F., Harousseau, J. L., Remenieras, L., Guibon, O., and Chevret, S. (2001). Evaluating treatment strategies in advanced Waldenström macroglobulinemia: use of quality-adjusted survival analysis. *Leukemia, 15,* 1466–1470.

Lin, Y. T., Kuo, H. C., Chang, Y. T., and Chang, M. H. (2001). Myasthenia gravis and Waldenström's macroglobulinemia: a case report and review of the literature. *Acta Neurologica Scandinavica, 104,* 246–248.

Lindemalm, C., Biberfeld, P., Christensson, B., Eriksson, C., Haverling, M., Tornling, G., Unge, G., and Mellstedt, H. (1988). Bilateral pleural effusions due to amyloidosis in a case of Waldenström's macroglobulinemia. *Haematologica, 73,* 407–409.

Linet, M. S., Humphrey, R. L., Mehl, E. S., Morris Brown, L., Pottern, L. M., Bias, W. B., and McCaffrey, L. (1993). A case-control and family study of Waldenström's macroglobulinemia. *Leukemia, 7,* 1363–1369.

Liu, E. S., Burian, C., Miller, W. E., and Saven, A. (1998). Bolus administration of cladribine in the treatment of Waldenström macroglobulinaemia. *British Journal of Haematology, 103,* 690–695.

Logothetis, J., Silverstein, P., and Coe, J. (1960). Neurologic aspects of Waldenström's macroglobulinemia: report of a case. *Archives of Neurology, 3,* 564–573.

Lorigan, J. G., David, C. L., Shirkhoda, A., Eftekhari, F., and Alexanian, R. (1988). Macroglobulinaemic lymphoma presenting with perirenal masses. *British Journal of Radiology, 61,* 1077–1078.

Lowe, L., Fitzpatrick, J. E., Huff, J. C., Shanley, P. F., and Golitz, L. E. (1992). Cutaneous macroglobulinosis: a case report with unique ultrastructural findings. *Archives of Dermatology, 128,* 377–380.

Lyon, L. W., McCormick, W. F., and Schochet, S. S., Jr. (1971). Progressive multifocal leukoencephalopathy. *Archives of Internal Medicine, 128,* 420–426.

Machet, L., Vaillant, L., Machet, M. C., Esteve, E., de Muret, A., Khallouf, R., Arbeille, B., Muller, C., and Lorette, G. (1992). Schnitzler's syndrome (urticaria and macroglobulinemia) associated with pseudoxanthoma elasticum. *Acta Dermato-Venereologica (Stockholm), 72,* 22–24.

MacKenzie, M. R. (1996). Macroglobulinemia. In P. H. Wiernick, G. P. Canellos, and J. D. Dutcher (Eds.), *Neoplastic Diseases of the Blood*, ed 3 (p. 601). New York: Churchill Livingstone.

MacKenzie, M. R., Brown, E., Fudenberg, H. H., and Goodenday, L. (1970). Waldenström's macroglobulinemia: correlation between expanded plasma volume and increased serum viscosity. *Blood, 35,* 394–408.

MacKenzie, M. R., and Fudenberg, H. H. (1972). Macroglobulinemia: an analysis for forty patients. *Blood, 39,* 874–889.

Majumdar, G., and Slater, N. G. P. (1993). Waldenström's macroglobulinaemia terminating in acute myeloid leukaemia: report of a case and review of the literature. *Leukemia and Lymphoma, 9,* 513–516.

Maldonado, J. E., Kyle, R. A., Brown, A. L., Jr., and Bayrd, E. D. (1966). "Intermediate" cell types and mixed cell proliferation in multiple myeloma: electron microscopic observations. *Blood, 27,* 212–226.

Mansoor, A., Medeiros, L. J., Weber, D. M., Alexanian, R., Hayes, K., Jones, D., Lai, R., Glassman, A., and Bueso-Ramos, C. E. (2001). Cytogenetic findings in lymphoplasmacytic lymphoma/Waldenström macroglobulinemia: chromosomal abnormalities are associated with the polymorphous subtype and an aggressive clinical course. *American Journal of Clinical Pathology, 116,* 543–549.

Martin, N. H. (1968). Macroglobulinaemia. *Clinica Chemica Acta, 22,* 15–25.

Martino, R., Shah, A., Romero, P., Brunet, S., Sierra, J., Domingo-Albos, A., Fruchtman, S., and Isola, L. (1999). Allogeneic bone marrow transplantation for advanced Waldenström's macroglobulinemia. *Bone Marrow Transplantation, 23,* 747–749.

Massari, R., Fine, J. M., and Metais, R. (1962). Waldenström's macroglobulinemia observed in two brothers [Letter]. *Nature, 196,* 176–178.

McCallister, B. D., Bayrd, E. D., Harrison, E. G., Jr., and McGuckin, W. F. (1967). Primary macroglobulinemia: review with a report on thirty-one cases and notes on the value of continuous chlorambucil therapy. *American Journal of Medicine, 43,* 394–434.

Morel, P., Monconduit, M., Jacomy, D., Lenain, P., Grosbois, B., Bateli, C., Facon, T., Dervite, I., Bauters, F., Najman, A., de Gramont, A., and Wattel, E. (2000). Prognostic factors in Waldenström macroglobulinemia: a report on 232 patients with the description of a new scoring system and its validation on 253 other patients. *Blood, 96,* 852–858.

Morel-Maroger, L., Basch, A., Danon, F., Verroust, P., and Richet, G. (1970). Pathology of the kidney in Waldenström's macroglobulinemia: study of sixteen cases. *New England Journal of Medicine, 283,* 123–129.

Moulopoulos, L. A., Dimopoulos, M. A., Varma, D. G. K., Manning, J. T., Johnston, D. A., Leeds, N. E., and Libshitz, H. I. (1993). Waldenström macroglobulinemia: MR imaging of the spine and CT of the abdomen and pelvis. *Radiology, 188,* 669–673.

Murashige, N., Tabanda, R., and Zalusky, R. (2002). Occurrence of acute monocytic leukemia in a case of untreated Waldenström's macroglobulinemia. *American Journal of Hematology, 71,* 94–97.

Nobile-Orazio, E., Marmiroli, P., Baldini, L., Spagnol, G., Barbieri, S., Moggio, M., Polli, N., Polli, E., and Scarlato, G. (1987). Peripheral neuropathy in macroglobulinemia: incidence and antigen-specificity of M proteins. *Neurology, 37,* 1506–1514.

O'Reilly, R. A., and MacKenzie, M. R. (1967). Primary macrocryoglobulinemia: remission with adrenal corticosteroid therapy. *Archives of Internal Medicine, 120,* 234–238.

Owen, R. G., Barrans, S. L., Richards, S. J., O'Connor, S. J., Child, J. A., Parapia, L. A., Morgan, G. J., and Jack, A. S. (2001a). Waldenström macroglobulinemia: development of diagnostic criteria and identification of prognostic factors. *American Journal of Clinical Pathology, 116,* 420–428.

Owen, R. G., Lubenko, A., Savage, J., Parapia, L. A., Jack, A. S., and Morgan, G. J. (2001b). Autoimmune thrombocytopenia in Waldenström's macroglobulinemia. *American Journal of Hematology, 66,* 116–119.

Palka, G., Spadano, A., Geraci, L., Fioritoni, G., Dragani, A., Calabrese, G., Guanciali Franci, P., and Stuppia, L. (1987). Chromosome changes in 19 patients with Waldenström's macroglobulinemia. *Cancer, Genetics, and Cytogenetics, 29,* 261–269.

Perkins, H. A., MacKenzie, M. R., and Fudenberg, H. H. (1970). Hemostatic defects in dysproteinemias. *Blood, 35,* 694–707.

Peters, H. A., and Clatanoff, D. V. (1968). Spinal muscular atrophy secondary to macroglobulinemia: reversal of symptoms with chlorambucil therapy. *Neurology, 18,* 101–108.

Petersen, H. S. (1973). Waldenström's macroglobulinemia with xanthomatosis and hypercholesterolaemia: report of a case. *Acta Medica Scandinavica, 193,* 573–576.

Petrucci, M. T., Avvisati, G., Tribalto, M., Giovangrossi, P., and Mandelli, F. (1989). Waldenström's macroglobulinemia: results of a combined oral treatment in 34 newly diagnosed patients. *Journal of Internal Medicine, 226,* 443–447.

Pitts, N. C., and McDuffie, F. C. (1967). Defective synthesis of IgM antibodies in macroglobulinemia. *Blood, 30,* 767–771.

Pruzanski, W., Warren, R. E., Goldie, J. H., and Katz, A. (1973). Malabsorption syndrome with infiltration of the intestinal wall by extracellular monoclonal macroglobulin. *American Journal of Medicine, 54,* 811–818.

Quesada, J. R., Alexanian, R., Kurzrock, R., Barlogie, B., Saks, S., and Gutterman, J. U. (1988). Recombinant interferon gamma in hairy cell leukemia, multiple myeloma, and Waldenström's macroglobulinemia. *American Journal of Hematology, 29,* 1–4.

Rausch, P. G., and Herion, J. C. (1980). Pulmonary manifestations of Waldenström macroglobulinemia. *American Journal of Hematology, 9,* 201–209.

Renier, G., Ifrah, N., Chevailler, A., Saint-Andre, J. P., Boasson, M., and Herez, D. (1989). Four brothers with Waldenström's macroglobulinemia. *Cancer, 64,* 1554–1559.

Richards, A. I. (1995). Response of meningeal Waldenström's macroglobulinemia to 2-chlorodeoxyadenosine [Letter]. *Journal of Clinical Oncology, 13,* 2476.

Riddell, S., Johnston, J. B., Rayner, H. L., and Israels, L. G. (1986). Response of Waldenström's macroglobulinemia to pentostatin (2'-deoxycoformycin). *Cancer Treatment Reports, 70,* 546–548.

Ries, C. A. (1988). Waldenström's macroglobulinemia. *West Journal of Medicine, 148,* 320–323.

Ronis, M. L., Rojer, C. L., and Ronis, B. J. (1966). Otologic manifestations of Waldenström's macroglobulinemia. *Laryngoscope, 76,* 513–523.

Rosales, C. M., Lin, P., Mansoor, A., Bueso-Ramos, C., and Medeiros, L. J. (2001). Lymphoplasmacytic lymphoma/Waldenström macroglobulinemia associated with Hodgkin disease: a report of two cases. *American Journal of Clinical Pathology, 116,* 34–40.

Rosner, F., and Grünwald, H. W. (1980). Multiple myeloma and Waldenström's macroglobulinemia terminating in acute leukemia: review with emphasis on karyotypic and ultrastructural abnormalities. *New York State Journal of Medicine, 80,* 558–570.

Rotoli, B., De Renzo, A., Frigeri, F., Buffardi, S., Marcenò, R., Cavallaro, A. M., Ruggeri, P., Liso, V., Musto, P., Andriani, A., Callea, V., Pizzuti, M., Iannitto, E., Cimino, R., Molica, S., Citarrella, P., Musolino, C., Guarino, S., Lucarelli, G., Espinosa, A., and Del Vecchio, L. (1994). A phase II trial on alpha-interferon (α IFN) effect in patients with monoclonal IgM gammopathy. *Leukemia and Lymphoma, 13,* 463–469.

Rozenberg, M. C., and Dintenfass, L. (1965). Platelet aggregation in Waldenström's macroglobulinaemia. *Thrombosis et Diathesis Haemorrhagica, 14,* 202–208.

Ruben, R. J., Distenfeld, A., Berg, P., and Carr, R. (1969). Sudden sequential deafness as the presenting symptom of macroglobulinemia. *Journal of the American Medical Association, 209,* 1364–1365.

Rywlin, A. M., Civantos, F., Ortega, R. S., and Dominguez, C. J. (1975). Bone marrow histology in monoclonal macroglobulinemia. *American Journal of Clinical Pathology, 63,* 769–778.

Scheithauer, B. W., Rubinstein, L. J., and Herman, M. M. (1984). Leukoencephalopathy in Waldenström's macroglobulinemia: immunohistochemical and electron microscopic observations. *Journal of Neuropathology and Experimental Neurology, 43,* 408–425.

Schnitzler, L., Schubert, B., Boasson, M., Gardais, J., and Tourmen, A. (1974). Uritcaire chronique, lésions osseuses, macroglobulinémie IgM: maladie de Waldenström? *Bulletin de la Societé de Française de Dermatologie et de Syphiligraphie, 81,* 363.

Schop, R. F., Jalal, S. M., Van Wier, S. A., Ahmann, G. J., Bailey, R. J., Kyle, R. A., Greipp, P. R., Rajkumar, S. V., Gertz, M. A., Lust, J. A., Lacy, M. Q., Dispenzieri, A., Witzig, T. E., and Fonseca, R. (2002b). Deletions of 17p13.1 and 13q14 are uncommon in Waldenström macroglobulinemia clonal cells and mostly seen at the time of disease progression. *Cancer, Genetics, and Cytogenetics, 132,* 55–60.

Schop, R. F., Kuehl, W. M., Van Wier, S. A., Ahmann, G. J., Price-Troska, T., Bailey, R. J., Jalal, S. M., Qi, Y., Kyle, R. A., Greipp, P. R., and Fonseca, R. (2002a). Waldenström macroglobulinemia neoplastic cells lack immunoglobulin heavy chain locus translocations but have frequent 6q deletions. *Blood, 100,* 2996–3001.

Schwab, P. J., and Fahey, J. L. (1960). Treatment of Waldenström's macroglobulinemia by plasmapheresis. *New England Journal of Medicine, 263,* 574–579.

Scott, R. B., Elmore, S. M., Brackett, N. C., Jr., Harris, W. O., Jr., and Still, W. J. S. (1973). Neuropathic joint disease (Charcot joints) in Waldenström's macroglobulinemia with amyloidosis. *American Journal of Medicine, 54*, 535–538.

Sebastián Domingo, J. J., and Nuñez Olarte, J. M. (1988). Waldenström's macroglobulinaemia associated with alpha-antitrypsin deficiency [Letter]. *American Journal of Hematology, 29*, 122.

Seligmann, M., Danon, F., Mihaesco, C., and Fudenberg, H. H. (1967). Immunoglobulin abnormalities in families of patients with Waldenström's macroglobulinemia. *American Journal of Medicine, 43*, 66–83.

Shimizu, K., Fujisawa, K., Yamamoto, H., Mizoguchi, Y., and Hara, K. (1993). Importance of central nervous system involvement by neoplastic cells in a patient with Waldenström's macroglobulinemia developing neurologic abnormalities. *Acta Haematologica, 90*, 206–208.

Singh, A., Eckardt, K. U., Zimmermann, A., Gotz, K. H., Hamann, M., Ratcliffe, P. J., Kurtz, A., and Reinhart, W. H. (1993). Increased plasma viscosity as a reason for inappropriate erythropoietin formation. *Journal of Clinical Investigation, 91*, 251–256.

Solomon, A., and Fahey, J. L. (1963). Plasmapheresis therapy in macroglobulinemia. *Annals of Internal Medicine, 58*, 789–800.

Stevens, D. B., and Whitehouse, G. H. (1976). Waldenström's macroglobulinaemia with amyloidosis: lymphographic findings. *Lymphology, 9*, 142–144.

Syms, M. J., Arcila, M. E., and Holtel, M. R. (2001). Waldenström's macroglobulinemia and sensorineural hearing loss. *American Journal of Otolaryngology, 22*, 349–353.

Tait, R. C., Oogarah, P. K., Houghton, J. B., Farrand, S. E., and Haeneye, M. R. (1993). Waldenström's macroglobulinaemia secreting a paraprotein with lupus anticoagulant activity: possible association with gastrointestinal tract disease and malabsorption. *Clinical Pathology, 46*, 678–680.

Takahashi, K., Yamamura, F., and Motoyama, H. (1986). IgM myeloma: its distinction from Waldenström's macroglobulinemia. *Acta Pathologica Japonica, 36*, 1553–1563.

Takemori, N., Hirai, K., Onodera, R., Kimura, S., and Katagiri, M. (1997). Durable remission after splenectomy for Waldenström's macroglobulinemia with massive splenomegaly in leukemic phase. *Leukemia and Lymphoma, 26*, 387–393.

Taleb, N., Tohme, A., Abi Jirgiss, D., Kattan, J., and Salloum, E. (1991). Familial macroglobulinemia in a Lebanese family with two sisters presenting with Waldenström's disease. *Acta Oncology, 30*, 703–705.

Tetreault, S. A., and Saven, A. (2000). Delayed onset of autoimmune hemolytic anemia complicating cladribine therapy for Waldenström macroglobulinemia. *Leukemia and Lymphoma, 37*, 125–130.

Török, L., Borka, I., and Szabó, G. (1993). Waldenström's macroglobulinaemia presenting with cold urticaria and cold purpura. *Clinical and Experimental Dermatology, 18*, 277–279.

Torrey, J. J., and Katakkar, S. B. (1984). Treatable meningeal involvement in Waldenström's macroglobulinemia. *Annals of Internal Medicine, 101*, 345–347.

Treon, S. P., Agus, T. B., Link, B., Rodrigues, G., Molina, A., Lacy, M. Q., Fisher, D. C., Emmanouilides, C., Richards, A. I., Clark, B., Lucas, M. S., Schlossman, R., Schenkein, D., Lin, B., Kimby, E., Anderson, K. C., and Byrd, J. C. (2001). CD20-directed antibody-mediated immunotherapy induces responses and facilitates hematologic recovery in patients with Waldenström's macroglobulinemia. *Journal Immunotherapy, 24*, 272–279.

Trimarchi, F., Benvenga, S., Fenzie, G., Mariotti, S., and Consolo, F. (1982). Immunoglobulin binding of thyroid hormones in a case of Waldenström's macroglobulinemia. *Journal of Clinical Endocrinology and Metabolism, 54*, 1045–1050.

Tsuji, M., Ochiai, S., Taka, T., Hishitani, Y., Nagareda, T., and Mori, H. (1990). Nonamyloidotic nephrotic syndrome in Waldenström's macroglobulinemia. *Nephron, 54*, 176–178.

Tursz, T., Brouet, J. C., Flandrin, G., Danon, F., Clauvel, J. P., and Seligmann, M. (1977). Clinical and pathologic features of Waldenström's macroglobulinemia in seven patients with serum monoclonal IgG or IgA. *American Journal of Medicine, 63*, 499–502.

Varticovski, L., Pick, A. I., Schattner, A., and Schoenfeld, Y. (1987). Anti-platelet and anti-DNA IgM in Waldenström macroglobulinemia and ITP. *American Journal of Hematology, 24*, 351–355.

Vermess, M., Pearson, K. D., Einstein, A. B., and Fahey, J. L. (1972). Osseous manifestations of Waldenström's macroglobulinemia. *Radiology, 102*, 497–504.

Vital, C., Vallat, J. M., Deminiere, C., Loubet, A., and Leboutet, M. J. (1982). Peripheral nerve damage during multiple myeloma and Waldenström's macroglobulinemia: an ultrastructural and immunopathologic study. *Cancer, 50*, 1491–1497.

Waldenström, J. (1944). Incipient myelomatosis or "essential" hyperglobulinemia with fibrinogenopenia: a new syndrome? [Editorial] *Acta Medica Scandinavica, 216*, 433–434.

Waldenström, J. G. (1980). The prognosis of myeloma and macroglobulinemia. *Annals of Life Insurance and Medicine, 6*, 93–98.

Wanebo, H. J., and Clarkson, B. D. (1965). Essential macroglobulinemia: report of a case including immunofluorescent and electron microscopic studies. *Annals of Internal Medicine, 62*, 1025–1045.

Wells, M., Michaels, L., and Wells, D. G. (1977). Otolaryngological disturbances in Waldenström's macroglobulinaemia. *Clinical Otolaryngology, 2*, 327–338.

White, A. D., Clark, R. E., and Jacobs, A. (1992). Isochromosome (6p) in Waldenström's macroglobulinemia. *Cancer, Genetics, and Cytogenetics, 58*, 89–91.

Williamson, L. M., Greaves, M., Waters, J. R., and Harling, C. C. (1989). Waldenström's macroglobulinaemia: three cases in shoe repairers. *British Medical Journal, 298*, 498–499.

Winter, A. J., Obeid, D., and Jones, E. L. (1995). Long survival after splenic immunoblastic transformation of Waldenström's macroglobulinaemia. *British Journal of Haematology, 91*, 412–414.

Winterbauer, R. H., Riggins, R. C. K., Griesman, F. A., and Bauermeister, D. E. (1974). Pleuropulmonary manifestations of Waldenström's macroglobulinemia. *Chest, 66*, 368–375.

Wood, T. A., and Frenkel, E. P. (1967). An unusual case of macroglobulinemia. *Archives of Internal Medicine, 119*, 631–637.

Yamaguchi, K. (1973). Pathology of macroglobulinemia: a review of Japanese cases. *Acta Pathologica Japonica, 23*, 917–952.

Yowell, R. L., and Hammond, E. H. (1994). Cardiac paraprotein associated with Waldenström's macroglobulinemia: a case report. *Ultrastructural Pathology, 18*, 229–232.

Zarrabi, M. H., Stark, R. S., Kane, P., Dannaher, C. L., and Chandor, S. (1981). IgM myeloma, a distinct entity in the spectrum of B-cell neoplasia. *American Journal of Clinical Pathology, 75*, 110.

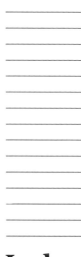

# Index

Note: Page numbers followed by the letter f refer to figures and those followed by the letter t refer to tables.

ISBN 0–7216–0006–9

9 780721 600062